Antifungal Therapy
Second Edition

Edited by

Mahmoud A. Ghannoum
John R. Perfect

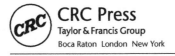

CRC Press
Taylor & Francis Group
Boca Raton London New York

CRC Press is an imprint of the
Taylor & Francis Group, an **informa** business

CRC Press
Taylor & Francis Group
6000 Broken Sound Parkway NW, Suite 300
Boca Raton, FL 33487-2742

First issued in paperback 2020

© 2019 by Taylor & Francis Group, LLC
CRC Press is an imprint of Taylor & Francis Group, an Informa business

No claim to original U.S. Government works

ISBN-13: 978-1-4987-6814-6 (hbk)
ISBN-13: 978-0-367-65594-5 (pbk)

Library of Congress Cataloging-in-Publication Data

Names: Ghannoum, Mahmoud A. (Mahmoud Afif), editor. | Perfect, John R., 1949- editor.
Title: Antifungal therapy / [edited by] Mahmoud Ghannoum, John R. Perfect.
Description: Second edition. | New York, NY : CRC Press, [2019] | Includes bibliographical references and index.
Identifiers: LCCN 2018033731| ISBN 9781498768146 (hardback : alk. paper) | ISBN 9780429402012 (ebook)
Subjects: | MESH: Mycoses--drug therapy | Antifungal Agents--therapeutic use
Classification: LCC RM410 | NLM WC 450 | DDC 615.7/92--dc23
LC record available at https://lccn.loc.gov/2018033731

Visit the Taylor & Francis Web site at
http://www.taylorandfrancis.com

and the CRC Press Web site at
http://www.crcpress.com

Contents

Preface

This book is designed to provide a comprehensive but insightful examination of antifungal therapy in the changing clinical milieu of modern medicine. It is an update from the original work almost a decade ago. It is clear that as medicine advances to treat and cure severe underlying diseases, the collateral consequences of this management can be immunosuppression and opportunistic fungal infections. Furthermore, there are a series of primary fungal infections, such as dermatophytosis and endemic mycoses, which continue to plague normal hosts. Additionally, the pandemic of HIV, which has impacted the entire world, laid in its immunosuppressive path the rise of invasive mycoses. It is clear that most clinicians who care for the seriously sick will be faced at times with the appearance of a fungal infection and a need to manage its disease. There are many aspects of invasive mycoses, including genetic susceptibility, risk factor predictions, diagnosis, epidemiology, and outcome of underlying diseases, that require a present and future knowledge base for medical practice. In this book, we have attempted to focus the presentation on the updated management aspects of fungal diseases. With the rising number of fungal infections worldwide and the development and clinical use of a variety of antifungal agents, it is quite clear that the statement: "Amphotericin B is the gold standard for the invasive mycoses" is no longer true. We have safer and effective alternative drugs to use. It is our mission in this book to provide clinicians with a foundation and insights into current antifungal management and the second edition has allowed us the ability to revisit the subjects as they have changed over the last decade. The book has repeated the original list of topics.

First, we approach some general antifungal agent issues, from the history of antifungal agents, fungal epidemiology, antifungal agent preclinical development to drug resistance. Second, we examine in depth the antifungal classes of drugs. Third, there is an attempt to provide clinical management issues and strategies around specific fungal infections that the clinician may face frequently or rarely, depending on the patient population in their practice. In these sections, there are insights provided into dosing, choice of drugs, concerns about complications, and outcomes, which are evidence-based but mixed with personal opinions and experiences. Fungal infections are treated "one patient at a time," and there is no "cookbook recipe" that fits all patients all the time. In fact, the underlying disease simply gets in the way too often or our evidence-based material is either weak or non-existent. Finally, we conclude with the management of several risk groups, or unique patient populations or infection sites, and their fungal infections. It is not an exhaustive list but provides illustrative exposure to these patients. It also lays the ground work/foundation for the principles of managing other risk groups which occur today or may occur tomorrow.

Fungal diseases have risen to prominence over the last 50 years. They have paralleled the technological advances in the care of serious medical diseases. Fungi, as eukaryotic organisms, play an interesting role in the human condition. They have been harnessed to help make our bread and beverages. In fact, we eat some of them and, during the traffic of life, we are constantly exposed to millions of them. During health, they are rarely a problem for us and after death they degrade us. Many of our critical exposures for health and fungi come between these stations of life. It is in this arena as a "human petri dish" that fungal disease raises its ugly consequences. It is the hope of these authors that this book reveals the tools, strategies, and insights to manage these irritating, costly, and life-threatening infections, and they have updated them to meet the rapidly changing clinical landscape. At times, it may seem the patient is defenseless against these marauders, but, in fact, present antifungal therapy is very good and applied early and correctly can make a difference in patient outcome. This success story is told in the following pages. In this second edition, we have made an effort to insightfully update the fast-moving field over the last decade, so all available tools and principles are recognized. Vulnerable patients continue to integrate into the fabric of modern medicine; thus, invasive fungal diseases consistently follow these patients. From the specialists to the generalists, we must "all be in" when it comes to successful management of fungal diseases.

Mahmoud A. Ghannoum
John R. Perfect

Editors

Mahmoud A. Ghannoum, PhD, MBA, FIDSA, FAAM joined Case Western Reserve University and University Hospitals Case Medical Center in 1996 from prior positions at the UCLA School of Medicine and Kuwait University. Dr. Ghannoum has spent his entire academic career studying medically important fungi encompassing different fungal pathogens including *Candida*, *Aspergillus*, and *Cryptococcus*, the major causes of fungal infections. He has published more than 350 peer-reviewed articles addressing various aspects of superficial and systemic fungal infections. More recently, he published the first study describing the oral mycobiome of healthy individuals. He has published extensively in the area of fungal pathogenesis with special focus on virulence factors including phospholipase B, germination, adhesion, and bio-film formation, both *in vitro* and *in vivo*. Dr. Ghannoum is a professor and director of the Center for Medical Mycology at Case Western Reserve University and University Hospitals Case Medical Center. This center of excellence, which he directs, is a multidisciplinary center that combines basic and translational research investigating fungi from the test tube to the bedside. He has performed several studies investigating the mechanisms underlying *Candida* pathogenesis. He is the recipient of the Freedom to Discover Award from Bristol-Myers Squibb and the Rhoda Benham Award from the Medical Mycological Society of the Americas. He served as a chairman of the Subcommittee on Antifungal Susceptibility Testing, Clinical Laboratory Standards Institute, and was selected as a "Most Interesting Person" by Cleveland Magazine in 2013. Dr. Ghannoum is an entrepreneur-scientist who has launched a number of companies focusing on the treatment of biofilm infections and microbial dysbiosis as it relates to gut health. He coined the term 'Mycobiome'.

John R. Perfect, MD, is James B. Duke Professor of Medicine at Duke University Medical Center, a faculty member of the Duke University Interdisciplinary Program in Genetics, and director of the Duke University Mycology Research Unit. He is chief of the Division of Infectious Diseases in the Department of Medicine at Duke Medical Center. Dr. Perfect is a diplomat of the American Board of Internal Medicine and American Board of Infectious Diseases. After receiving an undergraduate degree in biology from Wittenberg University, Dr. Perfect went on to receive a medical degree from the Medical College of Ohio at Toledo. He then completed an internship at the Riverside Methodist Hospital in Columbus, Ohio; a residency in internal medicine at the University of Michigan Medical Center in Ann Arbor; and a fellowship in infectious diseases at Duke University Medical Center. He is a fellow of the American Society for Microbiology and the Infectious Diseases Society of America. Dr. Perfect is also a fellow of the American Association for Advancement of Science and member of International Society for Human and Animal Mycology, and Immunocompromised Host Society (ISHAM). He is president of the Mycoses Study Group and Educational Research Consortium and president-elect of ISHAM. Dr. Perfect has served on numerous committees and advisory boards. He received the Rhoda Benham Award from Medical Mycology Society of the Americas and the Lucille Georg Award from ISHAM. Dr. Perfect's research interests focus on the understanding of fungal pathogenesis through the study of *Cryptococcus neoformans* as well as clinical studies on the epidemiology, diagnosis, and management of invasive mycoses.

Contributors

Barbara D. Alexander
Department of Medicine/Infectious Diseases
Duke University Medical Center
Durham, North Carolina

Ali Abdul Lattif Ali
Rudolph H. Raabe College of Pharmacy
Ohio Northern University
Ada, Ohio

J. Andrew Alspaugh
Department of Medicine
Duke University School of Medicine
and
Department of Molecular Genetics and
Microbiology
Duke University School of Medicine
Durham, North Carolina

Elizabeth S. Dodds Ashley
Division of Infectious Diseases and
International Health
Duke University
Durham, North Carolina

Jeffery J. Auletta
Hematology/Oncology/BMT & Infectious Diseases
Nationwide Children's Hospital
and
Clinical Pediatrics
The Ohio State University College of Medicine
The James Comprehensive Cancer Center
Columbus, Ohio

Daniel K. Benjamin, Jr.
Department of Pediatrics
Duke University Medical Center
and
Duke Clinical Research Institute
Durham, North Carolina

Jyotsna Chandra
Department of Dermatology
Center of Medical Mycology
University Hospitals Cleveland Medical Center
Case Western Reserve University
Cleveland, Ohio

Jasmine Chung
Division of Medicine/Infectious Diseases
Duke University Medical Center
Durham, North Carolina
and
Department of Infectious Diseases,
Singapore General Hospital, Singapore

Sylvia F. Costa
Department of Medicine/Infectious Diseases
Duke University Medical Center
Durham, North Carolina

Sharvari Dharmaiah
Center for Medical Mycology
University Hospitals Cleveland Medical Center
Case Western Reserve University
Cleveland, Ohio

Richard H. Drew
Duke University School of Medicine
Durham, North Carolina
and
Campbell University College of Pharmacy and Health
Sciences
Buies Creek, North Carolina

Najla El-Jurdi
Division of Hematology/Oncology
Department of Medicine
University Hospitals Cleveland Medical Center
Case Western Reserve University
Cleveland, Ohio

Frank Esper
Center for Pediatric Infectious Diseases
Cleveland Clinic Children's Hospital
Cleveland, Ohio

Mahmoud A. Ghannoum
Center for Medical Mycology
University Hospitals Cleveland Medical Center
Case Western Reserve University
Cleveland, Ohio

Rachel G. Greenberg
Department of Pediatrics
Duke University Medical Center
and
Duke Clinical Research Institute
Durham, North Carolina

Christopher L. Hager
Center for Medical Mycology
University Hospitals Cleveland Medical Center
Case Western Reserve University
Cleveland, Ohio

Kimberly E. Hanson
Department of Clinical Microbiology
ARUP Laboratories
and
Department of Infectious Diseases
University of Utah
Salt Lake City, Utah

Nour Hasan
Department of Pediatric Infectious Disease
University Hospitals Cleveland Medical Center
Cleveland, Ohio

Jeffery Hu
Case Western Reserve University School of Medicine
Cleveland, Ohio

Yoshifumi Imamura
Department of Molecular Microbiology and Immunology
Nagasaki University Graduate School of Biomedical Sciences
Nagasaki, Japan

Nancy Isham
Center for Medical Mycology
University Hospitals Cleveland Medical Center
Case Western Reserve University
Cleveland, Ohio

Vidya Jagadeesan
Clinical Microbiology
ARUP Laboratories
Salt Lake City, Utah

Melissa D. Johnson
Division of Infectious Diseases
Department of Medicine
Duke University Medical Center
Durham, North Carolina

Steven W. Johnson
Campbell University College of Pharmacy and Health Sciences
Buies Creek, North Carolina
and
Novant Health Forsyth Medical Center
Winston-Salem, North Carolina

Frederic Lamoth
Service of Infectious Diseases and Institute of Microbiology
Lausanne University Hospital
Lausanne, Switzerland

Emily L. Larkin
Center for Medical Mycology
Department of Dermatology
University Hospitals Case Medical Center
Case Western Reserve University
Cleveland, Ohio

Hillard M. Lazarus
Department of Medicine
Case Western Reserve University
Cleveland, Ohio

Tracy Lemonovich
Division of Infectious Diseases and HIV Medicine
University Hospitals Cleveland Medical Center
Case Western Reserve University
Cleveland, Ohio

Jessica C. Lloyd
Section of Female Pelvic Medicine and Reconstructive Surgery
Glickman Urology and Kidney Institute
Cleveland Clinic Lerner College of Medicine of Case Western Reserve University
Cleveland, Ohio

Lisa Long
Center for Medical Mycology
University Hospitals Cleveland Medical Center
Case Western Reserve University
Cleveland, Ohio

John Mohr
Medical Affairs Strategic Solutions, LLC
Acton, Massachusetts

Ahmad Mourad
Division of Infectious Diseases
Department of Medicine
Duke University Medical Center
Durham, North Carolina

Pranab K. Mukherjee
Department of Dermatology
Center of Medical Mycology
University Hospitals Cleveland Medical Center
Case Western Reserve University
Cleveland, Ohio

John R. Perfect
Division of Infectious Diseases
Department of Medicine
Duke University Medical Center
Durham, North Carolina

Melanie W. Pound
Campbell University College of Pharmacy and Health
Sciences
Buies Creek, North Carolina
and
New Hanover Regional Medical Center
Wilmington, North Carolina

Margaret Powers-Fletcher
Department of Pathology and Laboratory Medicine
College of Medicine
University of Cincinnati
Cincinnati, Ohio

Raymond R. Rackley
Surgery
Glickman Urology and Kidney Institute
Cleveland Clinic Lerner College of Medicine of Case
Western Reserve University
Cleveland, Ohio

Daniel R. Richardson
Division of Hematology/Oncology
Department of Internal Medicine
The University of North Carolina at Chapel Hill
Chapel Hill, North Carolina

Marcie L. Riches
Division of Hematology/Oncology
Department of Internal Medicine
The University of North Carolina at Chapel Hill
Chapel Hill, North Carolina

Iman Salem
Center for Medical Mycology
University Hospitals Cleveland Medical Center
Case Western Reserve University
Cleveland, Ohio

Rania A. Sherif
Center for Medical Mycology
University Hospitals Cleveland Medical Center
Case Western Reserve University
Cleveland, Ohio

William J. Steinbach
Department of Pediatrics
and
Department of Molecular Genetics & Microbiology
Duke University Medical Center
Durham, North Carolina

Kim Swindell
Martinsburg, Pennsylvania

Mary L. Townsend
Campbell University College of Pharmacy and Health
Sciences
Buies Creek, North Carolina
and
Durham Veterans Administration Health Care
System
Durham, North Carolina

Richard R. Watkins
Division of Infectious Diseases
Cleveland Clinic Akron General
Akron, Ohio
and
Northeast Ohio Medical University
Rootstown, Ohio

Aimee K. Zaas
Division of Infectious Diseases
Duke University Medical Center
Durham, North Carolina

History of antifungals

EMILY L. LARKIN, ALI ABDUL LATTIF ALI, AND KIM SWINDELL

INTRODUCTION

Over the past decades, the incidence and diversity of fungal infections has grown in association with an increasing number of immunocompromised patients. The human immunodeficiency virus (HIV) epidemic, technological improvements in the fields of solid organ transplantation medicine, stem cell transplantation, neonatology, coupled with the advent of new immunosuppressive drugs have collectively attributed to an increase in the incidence of systemic fungal infections, including those caused by *Candida*, *Aspergillus*, *Cryptococcus*, *Coccidioides*, *Pneumocystis*, and *Zygomycetes* species. More recently, other species have begun to rival *Candida albicans* as major causative agents of fungal disease. For example, fluconazole-resistant non-*albicans Candida* species, such as *C. glabrata*, are now more prevalent in some hospitals [1,2]. Likewise, molds, such as *Scedosporium*, *Fusarium*, *Rhizopus*, and *Mucor* species, are now increasingly responsible for superficial and systemic mycoses in humans [3,4].

Healthcare professionals must carefully consider the expanded role of medically important fungi in order to provide optimal treatment of fungal infections in immunocompromised patient populations. Coincidently, novel therapies that target host defenses, fungal biofilm physiology, and emerging resistances must be developed in order to keep pace with changes in the etiology and the resistance patterns of fungal pathogens.

EARLY TREATMENTS

Antifungal therapies evolved slowly during the early years of the past century. For example, from the beginning of the twentieth century until after World War II, potassium iodide was the standard treatment for cutaneous fungal infections, including actinomycosis, blastomycosis, sporotrichosis, and tinea [5]. First derived from sea algae, potassium iodide was considered to exert a direct antifungal effect, although the complete mechanism of action remains unclear [6–8]. Contemporarily, radiation was used to treat severe tinea capitis infections, often with significant complications, including skin cancer and brain tumors [9].

In the 1940s, Mayer et al. [10] demonstrated that sulfonamide drugs, such as sulfadiazine, exhibited both fungistatic and fungicidal activities against *Histoplasma capsulatum* [11]. This discovery led to the formation and the use of sulfonamide derivatives for the treatment of blastomycosis, nocardiosis, and cryptococcosis [12–14].

Griseofulvin, a compound derived from *Penicillium griseofulvum*, has been widely used to treat superficial fungal infections since its isolation in 1939 [15]. In 1958, Gentles [16] reported the successful treatment of ringworm in guinea pigs using oral griseofulvin.

These successful attempts to develop novel and effective antifungal drugs encouraged the further study and discovery of new agents.

ANTIFUNGALS FOR THE TREATMENT OF INVASIVE INFECTIONS

Polyenes

In 1946, polyene antifungals (Figure 1.1), which are effective against organisms with sterol-containing cell membranes (e.g., yeast, algae, and protozoa), were developed from the fermentation of *Streptomyces* [17,18]. These drugs disrupt the fungal cell membrane by binding to ergosterol, the main cell fungal membrane sterol moiety. As a result, holes form in the membrane allowing leakage of essential cytoplasmic materials, such as potassium, leading to cell death. From the 1950s until the advent of effective azole compounds in the 1960s, polyene antifungal agents were standard therapy for systemic fungal infections [19].

NYSTATIN

In 1949, while conducting research at the Division of Laboratories and Research of the New York State Department of Health, Elizabeth Lee Hazen and Rachel Fuller Brown discovered nystatin, a polyene derived from *Streptomyces noursei* [20–22]. In 1955, Sloane [23] reported topical nystatin to be particularly effective for treatment of noninvasive moniliasis (candidiasis), a frequent complication observed in children enrolled in early chemotherapeutic leukemia trials underway during this period [24].

Nystatin exhibited good activity against *Candida* and modest activity against *Aspergillus* species.

In aqueous solutions, nystatin forms aggregates that are toxic to mammalian cells both *in vitro* and *in vivo*. The insolubility and toxicity precluded its use as an intravenous therapy for systemic mycoses.

Subsequently, (Nyotran^OR), a more soluble liposomal nystatin formulation with reduced toxicity was developed [25]. The liposomal formulation consists of a freeze-dried, solid dispersion of nystatin mixed with a dispersing agent, such as a poloxamer or polysorbate [26,27]. The dispersing agent prevents aggregate formation in solution, increasing the drug's solubility and decreasing toxicity while maintaining efficacy [27,28]. Liposomal nystatin has good activity *in vitro* against a variety of *Candida* species, including some amphotericin B–resistant isolates [28].

Studies by Oakley et al. [29] showed that Nyotran^OR was more effective than liposomal amphotericin against *Aspergillus* species. Although the liposomal form of nystatin was less toxic than conventional nystatin, unacceptable infusion-related toxicity unfortunately caused a halt in the development of this drug [30–32].

AMPHOTERICIN B

Amphotericin B is a fungicidal polyene antibiotic and, like other members of the polyene class, is effective against organisms with sterol-containing cell membranes [19].

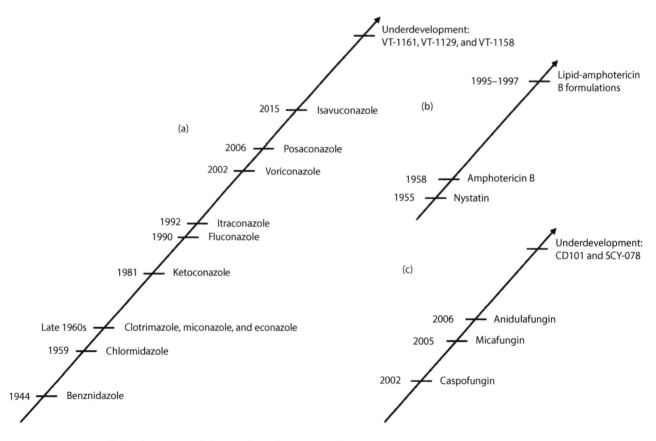

Figure 1.1 Historical development of the antifungal agents, including novel antifungals: **(a)** azoles, **(b)** polyenes, and **(c)** echinocandins (1,3-β-glucan synthase inhibitors).

Amphotericin B was extracted from *Streptomyces nodosus*, a filamentous bacterium, at the Squibb Institute for Medical Research in 1955 and subsequently served as the standard treatment for many invasive fungal infections [33].

Amphotericin B provided activity against invasive *Aspergillus* superior to that of previously available antifungal agents [33,34]. Amphotericin B continues to be effective for the treatment of fluconazole-resistant fungal infections [19,30]. Like other polyenes, amphotericin B exhibits dose-dependent toxicities including renal impairment and hypokalemia [19,30,34,35]. Renal toxicity associated with polyene antibiotics is believed to be mediated by the drug interaction with cholesterol within the mammalian cell membrane, resulting in pore formation, abnormal electrolyte flux, decrease in adenosine triphosphate (ATP), and eventually a loss of cell viability [19].

In the early 1980s, several research groups developed a new liposomal amphotericin B formulation. Graybill et al. [36] published the first extensive study investigating the treatment of murine cryptococcosis with liposome-associated amphotericin B. The tissues of Crytococcus-infected mice treated with the liposome-associated formulation were demonstrated to have lower tissue fungal burden than the tissues of similarly-infected mice treated with conventional amphotericin B. Liposome-associated amphotericin B demonstrated increased efficacy attributed to the ability to treat with higher doses (due to its lesser toxicity) than was possible with amphotericin B deoxycholate (conventional amphotericin B formulation) [36,37].

In the past decades, three novel liposomal formulations of amphotericin B have been approved for use in the United States: amphotericin B colloidal dispersion (ABCD; Amphocil^OR or Amphotec^OR), amphotericin B lipid complex (ABLC; Abelcet^OR), and small unilamellar vesicle liposomal formulation (L-AmB; Ambisome^OR).

The development of lipid-based amphotericin B formulations afforded significant advantages in treatment of systemic fungal infections, including decreased toxicity and improved tolerance [38–40].

Despite the introduction of newer antifungal agents for the treatment of systemic mycoses, amphotericin B remains the standard treatment for many severe, invasive fungal infections. However, because of toxicities associated with its intravenous use, along with the expanded availability of safer treatment options, it is frequently reserved for patients who have severe, life-threatening invasive fungal infections or who are unable to tolerate alternative antifungal agents.

Azole antifungals

Progress in the development of new antifungal agents lagged behind that of antibacterial antibiotics. The delay can be explained by two factors: (*i*) before the HIV/AIDS period, the occurrence of fungal infections was believed to be too low to warrant aggressive research by the pharmaceutical industry; and (*ii*) the apparent lack of a highly selective fungal target not present in other mammalian cells limited the number of potential pharmacologic mechanisms not associated with shared pathogen–host cell toxicity [19,41].

The discovery of the azole antifungal drugs (Figure 1.1) was seminal in the history of antifungal development. Until the discovery of azoles, amphotericin B was the only available agent to treat disseminated fungal infections including invasive aspergillosis—although not without concerns regarding nephrotoxicity and administration.

Azoles inhibit the synthesis of ergosterol, the major sterol in the fungal cell membrane, via inhibition of the cytochrome P450 enzyme, lanosterol demethylase [41,42]. This inhibition results in disruption of cell membrane integrity with eventual death.

EARLY AZOLES

In 1944, Woolley [43] described the antifungal activity of the first azole, benzimidazole. Descriptions of the antifungal properties of substituted benzimidazole were followed by the discovery of chlormidazole [44–46].

In the late 1960s, clotrimazole was developed in Germany by Bayer [17]. Miconazole and econazole were developed subsequently by Janssen Pharmaceutica, Antwerp, Belgium [46]. The early imidazoles, such as clotrimazole, miconazole, and tioconazole, showed good topical antifungal activity, but were of limited value for treating systemic infections.

SECOND GENERATION AZOLES

In 1981, the Food and Drug Administration (FDA) approved the systemic use of ketoconazole, an imidazole derivative synthesized and developed by Janssen Pharmaceutica, Antwerp, Belgium [45]. Ketoconazole was also available commercially as an anti-dandruff shampoo, branded (Nizoral^OR) by the same company. For almost a decade, ketoconazole was regarded as the standard oral agent for treatment of fungal infections, including chronic mucocutaneous candidiasis [47]. Mendes et al. [48] considered azole derivatives as the drugs of choice for the treatment of eumycetomas. The oral formulation of ketoconazole is now regarded as a treatment option only when all others fail [49]. There are serious hepatic issues that can develop with its use. In fact, it was taken off the market across Europe and in Australia in 2013 [50]. Its topical formulation is still in use because it does not share the same toxicity concerns as its oral counterpart.

In 1978, Pfizer developed fluconazole, a drug suitable for oral and intravenous treatment of superficial and systemic fungal infections [47,48,51]. Fluconazole was shown to have a good safety profile and was approved for the treatment of oropharyngeal, esophageal, vaginal, peritoneal, and genito-urinary candidal infections, disseminated candidiasis, and cryptococcal meningitis. Unlike ketoconazole, fluconazole is highly water soluble and can be administered parenterally. Recently, the utility of fluconazole has been limited by the emergence of resistant organisms, such as *C. krusei* and *C. glabrata*, against which fluconazole has poor activity [52,53].

In 1992, the FDA approved itraconazole, a broad spectrum triazole antifungal agent developed by Janssen Pharmaceutica (Sporanox[OR]). Itraconazole was shown to be less toxic than previous azoles, with a spectrum of activity broader than that of ketoconazole [52,53]. Consequently, itraconazole has replaced ketoconazole as the treatment of choice for invasive aspergillosis [52].

Although the discovery of fluconazole and itraconazole represented a major advancement in the management of systemic fungal infections, these triazole antifungal agents have some important limitations [54,55]. Fluconazole activity has a narrow spectrum, targeting mainly yeast (*Cryptococcus neoformans*, *C. albicans*) and dimorphic fungi, with no activity against molds [56,57]. In comparison, itraconazole has a broader spectrum that includes activity against *Aspergillus* species and some yeast strains that are intrinsically resistant to fluconazole, such as *C. krusei* and *C. glabrata* [56,57].

THIRD GENERATION AZOLES

Voriconazole, a derivative of fluconazole, is a synthetic third-generation triazole developed in the late 1980s by Pfizer Pharmaceuticals, Antwerp, Belgium [58,59] and approved by the FDA in May 2002. Voriconazole is more active than fluconazole and itraconazole against *Candida* species [60]. The activity of voriconazole against filamentous fungi, particularly *Aspergillus*, was found to be superior to that of amphotericin B [57,58]. Voriconazole is now considered the gold standard for the treatment of aspergillosis [61–63].

Posaconazole, a hydroxylated analogue of itraconazole, was developed by the Schering-Plough Research Institute and approved for use in 2006 [64]. Posaconazole is effective against opportunistic and endemic fungi, such as *Aspergillus* spp., *Zygomycetes*, and *Candida* species [64,65]. Posaconazole has been shown to be superior to amphotericin B, fluconazole, and itraconazole against most common fungal pathogens in *in vitro* and animal studies [66]. It is approved for prophylaxis of invasive fungal infections (aspergillosis and candidiasis) in immunocompromised patients and for the treatment of oropharyngeal candidiasis. Recently, a delayed-release formula was created that allows patients to be dosed once to twice daily in the hospital or at home [67].

Isavuconazole (Basilea Pharmaceutica, Antwerp, Belgium) and marketed by Astellas Pharma was approved by the FDA in 2015 for the treatment of invasive aspergillosis and invasive mucormycosis in adults [68]. It is a broad-spectrum antifungal affective against *Candida* species, *Aspergillus*, some *Zygomycetes*, *C. neoformans*, *Cryptococcus*, and several other molds, including Mucorales [69]. It has been shown to be as effective as voriconazole and is highly water soluble, unlike voriconazole and posaconazole. This allows for it to be administered without a cyclodextrin vehicle. Cyclodextrin vehicles are associated with nephrotoxicity and, since isavuconazole and its inactive, prodrug form isacuconazonium sulfate do not require this

vehicle, this antifungal is associated with lower toxicity in humans.

Azoles underdevelopment that show great promise are several compounds by Viamet Pharmaceuticals [70]. VT-1161, VT-1129, and VT-1598 are all azoles that have been molecularly altered to substantially reduce the interactions these azoles have with cytochrome P450 and to increase their half-lives [70,71]. Since azoles effects on cytochrome P450 is the main driving force behind drug-drug interactions of azoles, Viamet's compounds have markedly less drug-drug complications leading to their ability to be used in more circumstances than previously allowed [72]. VT-1161 was recently evaluated in phase II clinical trials for both vaginal candidiasis and onychomycosis, while VT-1129 and VT-1598 are still undergoing *in vitro* and *in vivo* testing [73].

Echinocandin antifungals

The advent of echinocandins (Figure 1.1), was heralded by the development and approval of caspofungin acetate (Cancidas; Merck & Co., Inc.) for the treatment of candidiasis in 2002 [66]. The echinocandins are a group of large, semisynthetic, cyclic lipopeptides discovered in the 1970s. Large molecular weight may explain their poor absorption through the digestive tract. Therefore, all three commercially available echinocandin compounds—caspofungin acetate, micafungin, and anidulafungin—are used only intravenously [74,75]. Echinocandins inhibit synthesis of 1,3-ß-D-glucan, an essential component of the fungal cell wall [76]. The synthesis of caspofungin acetate based on pneumocandin B0 requires chemical modification at two sites of the peptide core, reduction of a primary amide to an amine, and condensation of the hemiaminal moiety with ethylenediamine [76].

Caspofungin acetate (Cancidas[OR]) is fungicidal against yeasts and dimorphic fungi such as *C. albicans*, including triazole-resistant isolates, and fungistatic against *Aspergillus* species [77]. *Aspergillus fumigatus* is unable to sustain polarized growth in the presence of multiple doses of caspofungin, leading to significant fungal cell death in tissues [74,78]. Isham and Ghannoum [79] concluded that voriconazole demonstrated greater *in vitro* inhibitory activity than caspofungin against the non-*albicans* isolates.

Micafungin (Mycamine[OR], Astellas Pharma, Japan) and anidulafungin (Eraxis[OR], Pfizer, Inc., New York) were approved for use in 2006. Micafungin was first isolated from the culture broth of *Coleophoma empedri* [80]. It is a novel water-soluble lipopeptide derived by semisynthetic modification of FR901379, a naturally occurring cyclic hexapeptide with a fatty acryl side chain and is similar in structure to echinocandins and pneumocandins [80,81]. Micafungin is useful in the treatment of infections due to azole-resistant *Candida* [82].

Anidulafungin is a derivative of a naturally occurring candin, echinocandin B, produced by *Aspergillus nidulans* or *A. rugulosis* [83]. Cilofungin was the first semisynthetic derivative of echinocandin B to be evaluated in clinical trials; however, the trials were discontinued due to associated nephrotoxicity. Further structure modification of cilofungin led to the synthesis of anidulafungin [83].

The newest echinocandin underdevelopment is CD101 (Cidara Therapeutics), which is more stable and, thus, has a longer half-life than the previous echinocandins [84]. This stability also leads to the ability for CD101 to be used topically [85]. This allows for its use in skin and vaginal infections as well as systemic infections. Like the other echinocandins, there is no oral formulation. It is in clinical trials for vaginal and invasive candidiasis [85,86].

New antifungals underdevelopment

SCY-078 (Scynexis, Inc., New Jersey), another 1,3-β-glucan synthase inhibitor that continues to be evaluated in clinical trials, unlike echinocandins, is an orally bioavailable triterpene with a spectrum of activity similar to echinocandins [87,88]. SCY-078 has been demonstrated to have similar in vitro efficacy as echinocandins with regard to several species of Candida and Aspergillus including those that are resistant [88].

There are also a couple novel antifungals with unique mechanisms of action: APX001 (previously E1210; Amplyx Pharmaceuticals Inc., San Diego, CA) and F901318 (F2G Ltd., Manchester, UK). APX001 inhibits Gwp1p, an enzyme involved in the glycosylphophtidylinositol-anchoring pathway, which causes the cell wall to weaken [89]. While humans contain a homolog to Gwp1p, APX001 does not inhibit the mammalian version and, therefore, this drug has demonstrated low toxicity in in vivo models [89,90]. APX001 has demonstrated effectiveness against both yeast and molds, including Candida, Aspergillus, and Fusarium [91–94]. APX001 has begun undergoing clinical trials to further evaluate its safety, pharmacokinetics and tolerability.

F901318 impedes pyrimidine biosynthesis by inhibiting the fungal enzyme dihydroorotate dehydrogenase [95]. This new antifungal is ineffective against Candida species but is highly active against molds such as Aspergillus, Scedosporium, and Lomentospora, including azole-resistant types [95–97]. Like APX001, humans have their own version of dihydroorotate dehydrogenase, which is not inhibited by F901318, indicating that it will have a low toxicity that has been demonstrated in in vivo models [95]. Clinical trials to evaluate its tolerability and safety have been undertaken.

The development of the new antifungals that belong to triazole and echinocandin classes as well as novel antifungals will provide clinicians new alternatives for the treatment of invasive and resistant systemic fungal infections.

TOPICAL ANTIFUNGALS

Superficial fungal infections, such as cutaneous and mucosal candidiasis, dermatophytoses, and tinea versicolor are among the most frequently encountered infections worldwide [98,99]. These infections are commonly caused by Candida, Trichophyton, Microsporum, and Malassezia species and most often involve the skin, nails, buccal or vaginal mucosa, or eyes [98]. Historically, compounds such as gentian violet and Balsam of Peru were used for topical antifungal therapy. However, in the past decades, fungistatic azole drugs with imidazole- and triazole-containing compounds (e.g., miconazole and itraconazole, respectively) have been the mainstay of topical antifungal therapy [100,101]. The advent of fungicidal allylamines (e.g., terbinafine) has improved treatment outcomes, as cure rates are higher with fungicidal drugs. Other new agents such as topical echinocandins (caspofungin), ciclopirox, efinaconazole, and tavaborole offer additional options for the treatment of superficial fungal infections [102–104].

FUTURE AGENTS

Powerful historical precedents support the use of antibody-based therapies to treat infectious diseases [105,106]. However, although still in the early stages of development, newer approaches to the treatment of fungal infections will likely include the consideration of the host immune system and the interplay of drugs and host immunomodulators [107,108].

Immunomodulator therapies can be categorized as either pathogen specific or pathogen nonspecific [107]. Pathogen-specific immunomodulators include antibody reagents and vaccines, whereas cytokines, antimicrobial peptides, and probiotics are considered pathogen nonspecific immunomodulators [109]. Studies have shown immune sera to be protective in animal models of systemic candidiasis [107,109–115].

The immunodominant fungal antigen heat shock protein 90 (HPS90), expressed on the cell surfaces of yeasts and certain malignant cells, has been investigated as a potential target for antibody therapy [116,117]. Mycograb^OR (NeuTec Pharma, Antwerp, Belgium), a human recombinant monoclonal antibody against HSP90, was shown to have synergistic activity with amphotericin B, fluconazole, and caspofungin in vitro against a broad spectrum of Candida species [118–120]. Mycograb^OR consists of an antigen-binding variable domain of heavy and light chains linked together to create a recombinant protein that can be expressed in Escherichia coli. This drug demonstrated activity in clinical trials and looked like it would be an excellent addition to the antifungal armamentarium [119,121]. Unfortunately, the Committee for Medicinal Products for Human Use released an opinion against the use of the product in combination [120]. The main reason for this negative opinion was because the protein could fold incorrectly and aggregate [120]. Alterations to the protein have been made to fix this issue; however, the new molecule, Mycgrab C28Y, does not increase survival rates compared to amphotericin B alone.

Other new antifungal agents under study include naturally derived molecules with antifungal properties, such as the antifungal proteins secreted by fungus, bacteria, or derived from plants such as Clitoria ternatea [122–125].

Antifungal proteins interfere with the physiological properties of fungus leading to fungal cell death [122–125].

The history of antifungal agents continues to evolve, and no doubt will produce novel agents that, it is hoped, will target the organism as well as the host immunity.

REFERENCES

1. Li L, Redding S, Dongari-Bagtzoglou A. *Candida glabrata*, an emerging oral opportunistic pathogen. *J Dent Res* 2007;86(3):204–215.
2. Bille J, Marchetti O, Calandra T. Changing face of health-care associated fungal infections. *Curr Opin Infect Dis* 2005;8:314–319.
3. Castagnola E, Cesaro S, Giacchino M, et al. Fungal infections in children with cancer: A prospective, multicenter surveillance study. *Pediatr Infect Dis J* 2006;25:634–639.
4. Bethge WA, Schmalzing M, Stuhler G, et al. Mucormycoses in patients with hematologic malignancies: An emerging fungal infection. *Haematologica* 2005;90:ECR22.
5. Richardson MD, Warnock DW (Eds.). *Fungal Infection: Diagnosis and Management*, 3rd ed. Malden, MA: Blackwell Publishing, 1993.
6. Frankenberg BE, Litvineko AN. Treatment of cervicofacial actinomycosis with massive doses of potassium iodide. *Stomatologiia (Mosk)* 1952;6(4):26–30.
7. Dostrovsky A, Rauitschek F, Paz ZE, et al. The treatment of tinea capitis with oral potassium iodide. *J Invest Dermatol* 1960;34:347–349.
8. Urabe H, Nagashima T. Mechanism of antifungal action of potassium iodide on sporotrichosis. *Dermatol Int* 1969;8:36–39.
9. Shore RE, Moseson M, Xue X, et al. Skin cancer after X-ray treatment for scalp ringworm. *Radiat Res* 2002;157:410–418.
10. Mayer RL, Eisman PC, Geftic S, et al. Sulfonamides and experimental histoplasmosis. *Antibiot Chemother* 1956;6:215–225.
11. Mahgoub ES. Treatment of actinomycetoma with sulphamethoxazole plus trimethoprim. *Am J Trop Med Hyg* 1972;21(3):332–335.
12. Lamb JH. Combined therapy in histoplasmosis and coccidioidomycosis; methyltestosterone and meth-dia-mer-sulfonamides. *AMA Arch Derm Syphilol* 1954;70:695–712.
13. Webster BH. Pulmonary nocardiosis; a review with a report of seven cases. *Am Rev Tuber Pulmonary Dis* 1956;73:485–500.
14. Weed LA, Andersen HA, Good CA, et al. Nocardiosis; clinical, bacteriologic and pathological aspects. *New Engl J Med* 1955;253:1137–1143.
15. Oxford AE, Raistrick H, Simonart P. Studies in the biochemistry of micro-organisms: Griseofulvin, C(17)H(17)O(6)Cl, a metabolic product of penicillium griseo-fulvum dierckx. *Biochem J* 1939;33(2):240–248.
16. Gentles JC. Experimental ringworm in guinea pigs: Oral treatment with griseofulvin. *Nature* 1958;182(4633):476–477.
17. Whiffen AJ, Bohonos N, Emerson RL. The production of an antifungal antibiotic by *streptomyces griseus*. *J Bacteriol* 1946;52(5):610–611.
18. Steffen C, Dupree MT. The introduction of griseofulvin. *Skin Med* 2004;3(2):105–106.
19. Ghannoum MA, Rice LB. Antifungal agents: Mode of action, mechanisms of resistance, and correlation of these mechanisms with bacteria resistance. *Clin Microbiol Rev* 1999;12(4):501–517.
20. Fromtling RA. Overview of medically important antifungal azole derivatives. *Clin Microbiol Rev* 1988;1:187–219.
21. Brown R, Hazen EL. Present knowledge of nystatin, an antifungal antibiotic. *Trans N Y Acad Sci* 1957;19(5):447–456.
22. Brown R, Hazen EL. Nystatin. *Ann NY Acad Sci* 1960;89:258–266.
23. Sloane MB. A new antifungal antibiotic, mycostatin (nystatin), for the treatment of moniliasis: A preliminary report. *J Invest Dermatol* 1955;24(6):569–571.
24. Mehta RT, Hopfer RL, Gunner LA, et al. Formulation, toxicity, and antifungal activity *in vitro* of liposome-encapsulated nystatin as therapeutic agent for systemic candidiasis. *Antimicrob Agents Chemother* 1987;31:1897–1900.
25. Arikan S, Rex JH. Lipid-based antifungal agents: Current status. *Curr Pharm Des* 2001;7:395–417.
26. Ng AW, Wasan KM, Lopez-Berestein G. Development of liposomal polyene antibiotics: An historical perspective. *J Pharm Pharm Sci* 2003;6(1):67–83.
27. Silva L, Coutinho A, Fedorov A, et al. Nystatin-induced lipid vesicles permeabilization is strongly dependent on sterol structure. *Bioch Biophys Acta* 2006;1758(4):452–459.
28. Gupta AK, Sauder DN, Shear NH. Antifungal agents: An overview. Part II. *J Am Acad Dermatol* 1994;30:677–698.
29. Oakley KL, Moore CB, Denning DW. Comparison of in vitro activity of liposomal nystatin against *aspergillus* species with those of nystatin, amphotericin B (AB) deoxycholate, AB colloidal dispersion, liposomal AB, AB lipid complex, and itraconazole. *Antimicrob Agents Chemother* 1999;43(5):1264–1266.
30. Kleiberg M. What is the current and future status of conventional amphotericin B? *Int J Antimic Agents* 2006;27(Suppl. 1):12–16.
31. Boswell GW, Buell D, Bekersky I. AmBiosome (liposomal amphotericin B): A comparative review. *J Clin Pharmacol* 1998;38:583–592.
32. Larson JL, Wallace TL, Tyl RW, et al. The reproductive and developmental toxicity of the antifungal drug Nyotran[OR] (liposomal nystatin) in rats and rabbits. *Toxicol Sci* 2000;53:421–429.

33. Peer ET. Case of aspergillosis treated with amphotericin B. *Dis Chest* 1960;38:222–230.

34. Procknow JJ. Treatment of opportunistic fungus infections. *Lab Invest* 1962;11:1217–1230.

35. Plihal V, Jedlickova Z, Viklicky J, et al. Multiple bilateral pulmonary aspergillomata. *Thorax* 1964;19:104–111.

36. Graybill JR, Craven PC, Taylor RL, et al. Treatment of murine cryptococcosis with liposome-associated amphotericin B. *J Infect Dis* 1982;145(5):748–752.

37. Graybill JR. Lipid formulations for amphotericin B: Does the emperor need new clothes? *Ann Int Med* 1996;124(10):921–923.

38. Graybill JR. The future of antifungal therapy. *Clin Infect Dis* 1996;22(Suppl. 2):S166–S178.

39. Boswell GW, Buell D, Bekersky I. AmBisome (liposomal amphotericin B): A comparative review. *J Clin Pharmacol* 1998;38:583–592.

40. Bekersky I, Fielding RM, Dressler DE, et al. Pharmacokinetics, excretion, and mass balance of liposomal amphotericin B (AmBisome) and amphotericin B deoxycholate in humans. *Antimicrob Agents Chemother* 2002;46(3):828–833.

41. Ghannoum MA. Future of antimycotic therapy. *Dermatol Ther* 1997;3:104–111.

42. Maertens JA. History of the development of azole derivatives. *Clin Microbiol Infect* 2004;10(suppl. 1):1–10.

43. Woolley DW. Some biological effects produced by benzimidazole and their reversal by purines. *J Biol Chem* 1944;152:225–232.

44. Jerchel D, Fischer H, Fracht M. Zur darstellung der benzimidazole. *Liebigs Ann Chem* 1952;575:162–173.

45. Holt RJ. Topical pharmacology of imidazole antifungals. *J Cutan Pathol* 1976;3(1):45–59.

46. Herrling S, Sous H, Kruppe W, et al. Experimental studies on a new combination effective against fungi. *Arzneimittelforschung* 1959;9:489–494.

47. Hume AL, Kerkering TM. Ketoconazole. *Drug Intell Clin Pharm* 1983;17(3):169–174.

48. Mendes PR, Negroni R, Bonifaz A, et al. New aspects of some endemic mycoses. *Med Mycol* 2000;38(Suppl. 1):237–241.

49. United States Food and Drug Administration. FDA drug safety communication: FDA limits usage of Nizoral (ketoconazole) oral tablets due to potentially fatal liver injury and risk of drug interactions and adrenal gland problems, 2013. [Online.] https://www.fda.gov/drugs/drugsafety/ucm362415.htm.

50. Gupta AK, Lyons DCA. The rise and fall of oral ketoconazole. *J Cutan Med Surg* 2015;19(4):352–357.

51. Richardson K. Taking a drug to market. *Sci Publ Affairs* 1990;5(3):11–14.

52. Richardson K, Cooper K, Marriott MS, et al. Discovery of fluconazole, a novel antifungal agent. *Rev Infect Dis* 1990;12(Suppl. 3):S267–S271.

53. Sheehan DJ, Hitchcock CA, Sibley CM. Current and emerging azole antifungal agent. *Clin Microbiol Rev* 1999;12:40–79.

54. Coleman JM, Hogg GG, Rosenfeld JV, et al. Invasive central nervous system aspergillosis: Cure with liposomal amphotericin B, itraconazole, and radical surgery—Case report and review of the literature. *Neurosurgery* 1995;36(4):858–863.

55. United States Food and Drug Administration. Hepatotoxicity labelling for sporanox (itraconazole) oral solution, 2002. [Online.] http://www.fda.gov/cder/foi/label/2002/20657s8lbl.pdf.

56. Nolte FS, Parkinson T, Falconer DJ, et al. Isolation and characterization of fluconazole- and amphotericin B-resistant *Candida albicans* from blood of two patients with leukemia. *Antimicrob Agents Chemother* 1997;41(1):196–199.

57. Dismukes WE. Antifungal therapy: Lessons learned over the past 27 years. *Clin Infect Dis* 2006;42:1289–1296.

58. Marriott MS, Richardson K. The discovery and mode of action of fluconazole. In: Formtling RA (Ed.). *Fluconazole, a Significant Advance in the Management of Human Fungal Disease*. Barcelona, Spain: J. R. Prous Science Publishers, 1987:81–92.

59. Pappas PG, Rex JH, Sobel JD, et al. Guidelines for treatment of candidiasis. *Clin Infect Dis* 2004;38:161–189.

60. Lewis RE, Wiederhold NP, Klepser ME. *In vitro* pharmacodynamics of amphotericin B, itraconazole, and voriconazole against *aspergillus*, *fusarium*, and *scedosporium* spp. *Antimicrob Agents Chemother* 2005;49(3):945–951.

61. Walsh TJ, Anaissie EJ, Denning DW, et al. Treatment of aspergillosis: Clinical practice guidelines of the infectious diseases society of America. *Clin Infect Dis* 2008;46:327–360.

62. Consigny S, Dhedin N, Datry A. Successful voriconazole treatment of disseminated *Fusarium* infection in an immunocompromised patient. *Clin Infect Dis* 2003;37:311–313.

63. Marco F, Pfaller MA, Messer S, et al. In vitro activities of voriconazole (UK-109,496) and four other antifungal agents against 394 clinical isolates of *Candida* spp. *Antimicrob Agents Chemother* 1998;42(1):161–163.

64. Farowski F, Vehreschild JJ, Cornely OA. Posaconazole: A next-generation triazole antifungal. *Future Microbiol* 2007;2:231–243.

65. Chiou CC, Groll AH, Walsh TJ. New drugs and novel targets for treatment of invasive fungal infections in patients with cancer. *Oncologist* 2000;5(2):120–135.

66. Sun QN, Fothergill AW, McCarthy DI, et al. In vitro activities of posaconazole, itraconazole, voriconazole, amphotericin B, and fluconazole against 37 clinical isolates of zygomycetes. *Antimicrob Agents Chemother* 2002;46(5):1581–1582.

67. United States Food and Drug Administration. Center for Drug Evaluation and Research: Application Number: 205596Orig1s000 Summary review, 2014. [Online.] https://www.accessdata.fda.gov/drugsatfda_docs/nda/2014/205596Orig1s000SumR.pdf.

68. Mullard A. FDA approvals for the first 6 months of 2015. *Nat Rev Drug Discov* 2015;14:517.

69. Pettit NN, Carver PL. Isavuconazole: A new option for the management of invasive fungal infections. *Ann Pharmacother* 2015;49(7):825–842.

70. Moriyama B, Gordon LA, McCarthy M, et al. Emerging drugs and vaccines for candidemia. *Mycoses* 2014;57(12):718–733.

71. Schell WA, Jones AM, Garvey EP, et al. Fungal CYP51 inhibitors VT-1161 and VT-1129 exhibit strong in vitro activity against *Candida glabrata* and *C. krusei* isolates clinically resistant to azole and echinocandin antifungal compounds. *Antimicrob Agents Chemother* 2017;61(3):e01817–16.

72. Warrilow AG, Parker JE, Price CL, et al. The investigational drug VT-1129 is a highly potent inhibitor of cryptococcus species CYP51 but only weakly inhibits the human enzyme. *Antimicrob Agents Chemother* 2016;60(8):4530–4538.

73. Chang Y, Yu S, Heitman J, et al. New facets of antifungal therapy. *Virulence* 2017;8(2):222–236.

74. Morris MI, Villmann M. Echinocandins in the management of invasive fungal infections, part 2. *Am J of Health Syst Pharm* 2006;63(19):1813–1820.

75. Kim R, Khachikian D, Reboli AC. A comparative evaluation of properties and clinical efficacy of the echinocandins. *Expert Opin Pharmacother* 2007;8(10):1479–1492.

76. Denning DW. Echinocandins: A new class of antifungal. *J Antimicrob Chemother* 2002;49:899–891.

77. Leonard WR Jr, Belyk KM, Conlon DA, et al. Synthesis of the antifungal beta-1,3-glucan synthase inhibitor CANCIDAS (caspofungin acetate) from pneumocandin B0. *J Org Chem* 2007;72(7):2335–2343.

78. Minassian B, Huczko E, Washo T, et al. In vitro activity of ravuconazole against *zygomycetes*, *scedosporium* and *fusarium* isolates. *Clin Micro Infect Dis* 2003;9:1250–1252.

79. Isham N, Ghannoum MA. Determination of MICs of aminocandin for *Candida spp.* and filamentous fungi. *J Clin Microbiol* 2006;44(12):4342–4344.

80. Ernst EJ, Roling EE, Petzold CR, et al. *In vitro* activity of micafungin (FK-463) against *Candida* spp.: Microdilution, time-kill, and postantifungal-effect studies. *Antimicrob Agents Chemother* 2002;46(12):3846–3853.

81. van Burik JH, Ratanatharathorn V, Stepan DE, et al. Micafungin versus fluconazole for prophylaxis against invasive fungal infections during neutropenia in patients undergoing hematopoietic stem cell transplantation. *Clin Infect Dis* 2004;39:1407–1416.

82. Messer A, Diekema DJ, Boyken L, et al. Activities of micafungin against 315 invasive clinical isolates of fluconazole-resistant *Candida* spp. *J Clin Microbiol* 2006;44:324–326.

83. Ghannoum M, D'Angelo M. Anidulafungin, a potent antifungal that target *Candida* and *Aspergillus*. *Infect Dis Clin Pract* 2005;13(4):1–14.

84. Pfaller MA, Messer SA, Rhomberg PR, et al. Activity of a long-acting echinocandin (CD101) and seven comparator antifungal agents tested against a global collection of contemporary invasive fungal isolates in the SENTRY 2014 antifungal surveillance program. *Antimicrob Agents Chemother* 2017;61(3):e02045–16.

85. ClinicalTrials.gov. RADIANT: CD101 vs. Standard of care in subjects with acute vaginal yeast infections, 2016. [Online.] https://clinicaltrials.gov/ct2/show/NCT02733432.

86. ClinicalTrials.gov. CD101 Compared to caspofungin followed by oral step down in subjects with candidemia and/or *Invasive Candidiasis* (STRIVE), 2016. [Online.] https://clinicaltrials.gov/ct2/show/NCT02734862.

87. ClinicalTrials.gov. Open-label study to evaluate efficacy and safety of SCY-078 in patients with refractory or intolerant fungal diseases (FURI), 2017. [Online.] https://clinicaltrials.gov/ct2/show/NCT03059992.

88. Jimenez-Ortigosa C, Perez WB, Angulo D, et al. De novo acquisition of resistance to SCY-078 in *Candida glabrata* involves FKS mutations that both overlap and are distinct from those conferring echinocandin resistance. *Antimicrob Agents Chemother* 2017;61(9):e00833-17.

89. Watanabe N, Miyazaki M, Horii T, et al. E1210, a new broad-spectrum antifungal, suppresses *Candida albicans* hyphal growth through inhibition of glycosylphosphatidylinositol biosynthesis. *Antimicrob Agents Chemother* 2012;56(2):960–971.

90. Hata K, Horii T, Miyazaki M, et al. Efficacy of oral E1210, a new broad-spectrum antifungal with a novel mechanism of action, in murine models of *Candidiasis*, *Aspergillosis*, and fusariosis. *Antimicrob Agents Chemother* 2011;55(10):4543–4551.

91. Wiederhold NP, Najvar LK, Fothergill AW, et al. The investigational agent E1210 is effective in treatment of experimental invasive *Candidiasis* caused by resistant *Candida albicans*. *Antimicrob Agents Chemother* 2015;59(1):690–692.

92. Castanheira M, Duncanson FP, Diekema DJ, et al. Activities of E1210 and comparator agents tested by CLSI and EUCAST broth microdilution methods against *Fusarium and Scedosporium* species identified using molecular methods. *Antimicrob Agents Chemother* 2012;56(1):352–357.

93. Pfaller MA, Duncanson F, Messer SA, et al. In vitro activity of a novel broad-spectrum antifungal, E1210, tested against *Aspergillus spp.* determined by CLSI and EUCAST broth microdilution methods. *Antimicrob Agents Chemother* 2011;55(11):5155–5158.

94. Miyazaki M, Horii T, Hata K, et al. *In vitro* activity of E1210, a novel antifungal, against clinically important yeasts and molds. *Antimicrob Agents Chemother* 2011;55(10):4652–4658.

95. Oliver JD, Sibley GEM, Beckmann N, et al. F901318 represents a novel class of antifungal drug that inhibits dihydroorotate dehydrogenase. *PNAS* 2016;113(45):12809–12814.

96. Buil JB, Rijs AJM, Meis JF, et al. *In vitro* activity of the novel antifungal compound F901318 against difficult-to-treat *Aspergillus* isolates. *J Antimicrob Chemther* 2017;72(9):2548–2552.

97. Wiederhold NP, Law D, Birch M. Dihydroorotate dehydrogenase inhibitor F901318 has potent in vitro activity against *Scedosporium species* and *Lomentospora prolificans*. *J Antimicrob Chemther* 2017;72:1977–1980.

98. Ghannoum MA, Hajjeh RA, Scher R, et al. A large-scale North American study of fungal isolates from nails: The frequency of onychomycosis, fungal distribution, and antifungal susceptibility patterns. *J Am Acad Dermatol* 2000;43(4):641–648.

99. Thomas J, Jacobson GA, Narkowicz CK, et al. Toenail onychomycosis: An important global disease burden. *J Clin Pharm Ther* 2010;35(5):497–519.

100. Katoh T. Guidelines for diagnosis and treatment of mucocutaneous candidiasis. *Jpn J Med Mycol* 2009;50(4):207–212.

101. Iorizzo M, Piraccini BM, Rech G, et al. Treatment of onychomycosis with oral antifungal agents. *Expert Opin Drug Deliv* 2005;2(3):435–440.

102. Bao YQ, Wan Z, Li RY. *In vitro* antifungal activity of micafungin and caspofungin against dermatophytes isolated from China. *Mycopathologia* 2013;175(1–2):141–145.

103. Tauber A, Muller-Goymann CC. Comparison of the antifungal efficacy of terbinafine hydrochloride and ciclopirox olamine containing formulations against the dermatophyte *Trichophyton rubrum* in an infected nail plate model. *Mol Pharm* 2014;11(7):1991–1996.

104. Saunders J, Maki K, Koski R, et al. Tavaborale, efinazconazole, and luliconazole: Three new antimycotic agents for the treatment of dermatophytic fungi. *J Pharm Pract* 2016;30:621–630.

105. Buchwald UK, Pirofski L. Immune therapy for infectious diseases at the dawn of the 21st century: The past, present and future role of antibody therapy, therapeutic vaccination and biological response modifiers. *Curr Pharm Des* 2003;9:945–968.

106. Casadevall A, Scharff MD. Serum therapy revisted: Animal models of infection and development of passive antibody therapy. *Antimicrob Agents Chemother* 1994;38:1695–1702.

107. Heitman J. Cell biology: A fungal Achilles' heel. *Science* 2005;309:2175–2176.

108. Scorzoni L, de Paula e Silva ACA, Marcos CM, et al. Antifungal therapy: New advances in the understanding and treatment of mycosis. *Front Microbiol* 2017;8:36.

109. Casadevall A. The third age of antimicrobial therapy. *Clin Infect Dis* 2006;42:1414–1416.

110. Franco R, Pacheco R, Lluis C, et al. The emergence of neurotransmitters as immune modulators. *Trends Immun* 2007;28(9):400–407.

111. Burnie JP, Carter TL, Hodgetts SJ, et al. Fungal heat shock proteins in human disease. *FEMS Rev* 2006;30(1):53–88.

112. Spellberg B, Ibrahim AS, Yeaman MR, et al. The antifungal vaccine derived from the recombinant N terminus of Als3p protects mice against the bacterium *Staphylococcus aureus*. *Infect Immun* 2008;76:4574–4580.

113. Spellberg BJ, Ibrahim AS, Avanesian V, et al. Efficacy of the anti-*Candida* rAls3p-N or rAls1p-N vaccines against disseminated and mucosal candidiasis. *J Infect Dis* 2006;194:256–260.

114. Torosantucci A, Bromuro C, Chiani P, et al. A novel glycol-congate vaccine against fungal pathogens. *J Exp Med* 2005;202(5):597–606.

115. Torosantucci A, Chiani P, Bromuro C, et al. Protection by anti-beta-glucan antibodies is associated with restricted beta-1,3 glucan binding specificity and inhibition of fungal growth and adherence. *PLoS One* 2009;4(4):e5392.

116. Saito K, Dai Y, Ohtsuka K. Enhanced expression of heat shock proteins in gradually dying cells and their release from necrotically dead cells. *Exp Cell Res* 2005;310:229–236.

117. Matthews R, Burnie J. Antibodies against *Candida*: Potential therapeutics? *Trends Microbiol* 1996;4:354–358.

118. Casadevall A. Antibody immunity and invasive fungal infections. *Infect Immun* 1995;63:4211–4218.

119. Pachl J, Svoboda P, Jacobs F. A randomized, blinded, multicenter trial of lipid-associated amphotericin B alone versus in combination with an antibody-based inhibitor of heat shock protein 90 in patients with *invasive candidiasis*. *Clin Infect Dis* 2006;42(10):1404–1413.

120. Bugli F, Cacai M, Martini C, et al. Human monoclonal antibody-based therapy in the treatment of *invasive candidiasis*. *Clin Dev Immunol* 2013;2013:403121.

121. Matthews RC, Rigg G, Hodgetts S. Preclinical assessment of the efficacy of mycograb, a human recombinant antibody against fungal Hsp90. *Antimicrob Agents Chemother* 2003;47(7):2208–2216.

122. Delgado J, Owens RA, Doyle S, et al. Impact of the antifungal protein PgAFP from *Penicillium chrysogenum* on the protein profile in *Aspergillus flavus*. *Appl Microbiol Biotechnol* 2015;99(20):8701–8715.

123. Wen C, Guo W, Chen X. Purification and identification of a novel antifungal protein secreted by *Penicillium citrinum* from the Southwest Indian Ocean. *J Microbiol Biotechnol* 2014;24(10):1337–45.

124. Ajesh K, Sreejith K. A novel antifungal protein with lysozyme-like activity from seeds of *Clitoria ternatea*. *Appl Biochem Biotechnol* 2014;173(3):682–693.

125. Yasmin N, Saleem M. Biochemical characterization of fruit-specific pathogenesis-related antifungal protein from Basrai banana. *Microbiol Res* 2014;169(5–6):369–377.

2

Epidemiology of fungal infections: What, where, and when

FREDERIC LAMOTH, SYLVIA F. COSTA, AND BARBARA D. ALEXANDER

INTRODUCTION

Fungal infections represent an important cause of morbidity worldwide, including localized cutaneous or subcutaneous diseases (e.g., onycomycosis, tineas, dermatophytoses, eumycetomas, hypho- or phaeo-hyphomycoses, keratitis) and deep-seated or invasive fungal infections (IFIs). While some systemic fungal diseases, referred to as endemic mycoses (e.g., histoplasmosis, blastomycosis, coccidioidomycosis, paracoccidioidomycosis, penicilliosis) are associated with specific geographical areas and have the ability to affect the immunosuppressed as well as immunocompetent host, the majority of IFIs (e.g., *Candida* bloodstream infections,

invasive aspergillosis, invasive mucormycosis, cryptococcosis, and *Pneumocystis* pneumonia) affect the frail or immunosuppressed patient and are associated with the highest mortality. The most common immunosuppressive conditions predisposing to IFIs include neutropenia following anticancer therapies, and prolonged corticostroid therapy or immunosuppressive treatments following allogeneic hematopoietic stem cell transplantation (HSCT) or solid organ transplantation (SOT). IFIs are increasingly reported possibly as a consequence of active screening and improved diagnostic methods, but also due to an ever-enlarging at-risk population [1]. Surveillance data, though not perfect and likely still reflecting underdiagnosis and underreporting of these entities, indicate that over the past several decades, there has been an increasing incidence of IFIs due to yeasts, such as *Candida* spp. and *Cryptococcus* spp., and molds, such as *Aspergillus* spp. and fungi of the order *Mucorales* [2]. Epidemiologic trends also suggest that other filamentous hyphomycetes, such as *Fusarium* spp., *Scedosporium* spp., and *Paecilomyces* spp., are becoming more common [3]. Emergence of these rare fungal pathogens, which often exhibit multiresistance to antifungals, is an increasing concern. This chapter reviews the epidemiology of the most common fungal infections including the typical clinical manifestations associated with each fungal pathogen.

ASPERGILLOSIS

Aspergillus is a ubiquitous hyalohyphomycete (mold with nonpigmented, regularly septate hyphae) found in soil, dust, compost, rotted plants, and other organic debris including foods and spices [4,5]. About 339 species are known [6] and divided into 20 sections, though only a few have been reported as pathogenic to humans. The more commonly reported human pathogens include *Aspergillus* of the section *Fumigati* (*Aspergillus fumigatus*), *Flavi* (*A. flavus*), *Nigri* (*A. niger*), and *Terrei* (*A. terreus*). Of these, *A. fumigatus* is the most common species to cause invasive disease, and *A. flavus* is the second most commonly reported. Though *A. terreus* is less common, it is resistant to amphotericin B and has historically been associated with an exceptionally high mortality [7–10]. *Aspergillus* of section *Usti* (e.g., *A. calidoustus*) with intrinsic pan-azole resistance has emerged as a new opportunistic pathogen in patients receiving azole prophylaxis [11,12]. Other *Aspergillus* species such as *A. versicolor* and *A. nidulans* are occasionnally reported [4]. Moreover, some species belonging to the section *Fumigati* (*A. lentulus*, *A. udagawae*, *N. pseudofischeri*), *Flavi* (*A. alliaceus*), or *Nigri* (*A. tubingensis*) are increasingly recognized and may be misidentified in clinical practice. These cryptic species represent 3%–10% of all *Aspergillus* clinical isolates and some, such as *A. lentulus* or *A. udagawae*, may also exhibit intrinsic resistance to triazoles and other antifungal drug classes [13–15].

Aspergillus grows best at 37°C, forming hyaline hyphae with asexual reproduction by conidia that give each species a distinctive colony color. Conidia are easily aerosolized and, when small airborne conidia (2–3 μm for *A. fumigatus*) are inhaled, they can settle deep in the lungs where colonization and a variety of clinical syndromes may develop. The type of host plays a role in the clinical spectrum of disease, as the host's immune response and the ability of *Aspergillus* to invade and destroy tissue determine the clinical presentation. In patients with asthma, the inflammatory condition of allergic bronchopulmonary aspergillosis (ABPA) may develop. Allergic sinusitis is also a feature of *Aspergillus* that can set up a fungus ball or aspergilloma in lungs with preformed cavities. Those with underlying chronic lung disease can progress to chronic necrotizing aspergillosis or present with tracheobronchitis. In immunocompromised hosts, invasive disease may develop as invasive pulmonary aspergillosis, invasive sinusitis, or dissemination to extrapulmonary sites [4,16].

ABPA arises from a hypersensitivity reaction to *Aspergillus* antigens. Patients with asthma or cystic fibrosis may develop ABPA late in the course of their disease [17–19]. In patients with cystic fibrosis (CF), one study has shown lung function to deteriorate over time in those CF patients with ABPA compared with CF controls [20]. Similarly, patients with bronchiectasis and evidence of ABPA have been shown to have worse lung function when compared to those with bronchiectasis without ABPA [21]. The diagnosis of ABPA is suspected on clinical findings and confirmed by radiologic and serologic results. Impaired mucous clearance, productive cough with mucous plugs or brown specks, mucoid impaction, and episodic bronchial obstruction are characteristics of ABPA. Those with chronic disease may present with bronchiectasis and fibrosis. Imaging with computed tomography (CT) may show pulmonary infiltrates or bronchiectasis, and laboratory findings, such as growth of *Aspergillus* in culture or immunologic response with skin reactivity to *Aspergillus* antigens, support the diagnosis.

Allergic fungal sinusitis tends to arise in patients with atopy, history of allergic rhinitis/sinusitis, nasal polyps, and sometimes, asthma [4,22]. Direct microscopy often reveals thick green mucus or mucopurulent secretions, crusting, or the presence of polyps. Histologic examination of tissue biopsy demonstrates thick allergic mucin, hyaline, septate hyphae without invasion of tissue, and a chronic inflammatory response. Growth in culture of the offending mold and high levels of IgE aid in the diagnosis of this entity.

Aspergilloma, or fungus ball, is the most common form of pulmonary involvement due to *Aspergillus* [4,16]. It usually develops in a preformed pulmonary cavity (e.g., a consequence of prior tuberculosis or bronchiectasis) or in the paranasal sinuses and consists of masses of mycelia, inflammatory cells, debris, and mucus [23]. The aspergilloma can remain asymptomatic for a prolonged period of time, though some patients with pulmonary aspergilloma may experience hemoptysis, ranging from mild to severe, secondary to bleeding from bronchial blood vessels. A fungus ball in the sinus cavity can likewise remain asymptomatic, evolve to cause allergic-type presentation, or invade the contiguous tissue. The latter may occur in patients who are immunosuppressed with hematologic malignancy, diabetes, chronic steroid use, SOT, and AIDS [24]. Invasion of tissue and bone may progress to invasion of adjacent structures, such as the orbit or the brain. The clinical presentation is variable and requires a high index of suspicion, along with imaging, tissue histology, and culture to establish the diagnosis.

Endobronchial fungal infections are being increasingly described with the use of surveillance flexible bronchoscopy [25]. Presentation can range from mild mucosal inflammation to central airway obstruction with invasive disease. In lung transplant recipients, ulcerative or pseudomembranous tracheobronchitis, including infection of the anastomotic site, has been described [26,27].

Chronic necrotizing pulmonary aspergillosis is due to locally destructive invasion of lung parenchyma by *Aspergillus* without distal invasion or dissemination to other organs [4,16]. Patients usually have chronic underlying lung diseases, such as chronic obstructive pulmonary disease (COPD), and present with fever, cough productive of sputum, and weight loss over a period of several months.

In immunocompromised patients (neutropenia, corticosteroid use, transplant recipients, hematologic malignancy, cytotoxic chemotherapy, AIDS), invasive pulmonary aspergillosis (IPA) may develop, remaining largely asymptomatic early on or presenting with non-specific signs, such as fever, cough and dyspnea. Pleuritic chest pain and hemoptysis may also be present, as can altered mental status and respiratory failure. IPA is characterized by being more invasive than chronic necrotizing aspergillosis as it includes invasion of small vessels with hemorrhage and/or infarction and the possibility of dissemination [4,16,28]. Radiologically, alveolar infiltrates, either bilateral or diffuse, nodules, cavitation, and pleural effusion can be present. Review of the baseline chest CT findings from 235 patients with IPA, who participated in the global multicenter trial comparing voriconazole with amphotericin B for treatment of invasive aspergillosis (IA) revealed that, at presentation, most patients (94%) had one or more macronodules [29]. In patients with neutropenia and IPA, the CT scan may have a nodule surrounded by ground glass attenuation, the classic halo sign. As this occurs early, it allows the presumption of IPA diagnosis to be made prior to cavitation. However, this lesion is transitory and by the first week, three-fourths of the CT halo signs disappear. With recovery of the neutrophil count, an air crescent sign (representing early cavitation) may be seen, which is highly indicative of IPA [30]. In addition to radiological signs, serological markers, such as circulating galactomannan or 1,3-β-d-glucan in serum or galactomannan in bronchoalveolar lavage fluid, are important diagnostic tools as microbiological documentation of *Aspergillus* spp. by standard culture methods is often lacking [31,32]. Molecular methods (PCR) targeting ribosomal rRNA (18S) or the internal transcribed spacer (ITS) are also adjunctive tools for the diagnosis of invasive aspergillosis [33]. Pre-emptive strategies that combine screening with these markers coupled with chest CT are common practice for the early diagnosis and management of high-risk onco-hematological patients [34]. Guidelines have been established by the European Organization for Research and Treatment of Cancer (EORTC) and Mycoses Study Group (MSG) to assess the probability of invasive aspergillosis on the basis of host criteria, clinical and radiological signs, and microbiology results [35].

Patients who are immunocompromised can have dissemination of *Aspergillus* to the central nervous system (CNS) [28,36,37]. At-risk immunocompromised individuals are posttransplant and hematologic malignancy patients, but aspergillosis of the CNS has also been reported in AIDS, chronic asthma with steroid use, burn patients, patients with hepatic failure, and infections in the postoperative period. Cultures from non-CNS sites (most of which are from lung) are positive for *Aspergillus* in approximately half the patients with CNS aspergillosis [37]. Pathology reports from a series of CNS aspergillosis cases diagnosed by autopsy described hemorrhagic necrosis, abscesses, large hemorrhages, bland nonhemorrhagic infarctions, myelitis, mycotic aneurysm, basilar meningitis, sino-orbital disease, carotid artery invasion and thrombosis, dural abscesses, as well as findings of minimal inflammation in CNS lesions [37]. Imaging studies of patients with cerebral aspergillosis reveal three general patterns: single or multiple infarcts, ring lesions (single or multiple) consistent with abscess formation after infarction, and dural or vascular infiltration arising from the paranasal sinuses or orbits. Other findings on imaging include mycotic aneurysm and contrast enhancement of affected parenchyma, as well as hemorrhagic transformation of infarcted areas [38]. Galactomannan detection in cerebrospinal may be an important adjunctive tool for the diagnosis of cerebral aspergillosis.

The cumulative incidence of IA in the United States for two of the highest populations at risk, HSCT and SOT recipients, has been reported from the Transplant-Associated Infection Surveillance Network (TRANSNET) multicenter studies [39,40]. In the HSCT population, *Aspergillus* now exceeds *Candida* as the most common invasive fungal pathogen with a cumulative incidence at 12 months of 1.6% and a one-year overall mortality rate of 75% [39]. In the SOT population, the 12-month cumulative incidence of IA was lower (0.7%) as was the mortality rate (41%) [40].

In the Prospective Antifungal Therapy (PATH) Alliance Registry, a cohort of 960 cases of proven/probable invasive aspergillosis reported from 2004 to 2008 in North America, 48.3% of patients had hematologic malignancies and 29.2% were SOT recipients, 33.8% were neutropenic and 27.9% were HSCT recipients [41]. The lung was the most common site of infection (76% of cases). Most common sites of extrapulmonary aspergillosis were the tracheobronchial tree, sinuses, skin/soft tissues and central nervous system. Among patients with a positive culture, *A. fumigatus* accounted for 72.6% of cases, followed by *A. flavus* (9.9%), *A. niger* (8.7%) and *A. terreus* (4.3%). In 25% of cases, the diagnosis of invasive aspergillosis relied on a positive galactomannan and/or histopathologic examination of tissue biopsy without *Aspergillus* growth in culture. The proportion of cases for which a positive galactomannan in serum or bronchoalveolar lavage (BAL) is the only microbiologic diagnostic criterion was as high as 50%–80% in recent cohort studies [42,43].

Studies have also evaluated risk factors for IA in transplant populations [44–46]. Factors associated with development of early IA (≤40 days posttransplant) in the HSCT population included older age at transplant, underlying disease other than chronic myelogenous leukemia in the chronic phase (aplastic anemia, myelodysplastic syndrome, and multiple myeloma), the type of transplant (receipt of T-cell depleted or CD-34–selected stem cell products or cord blood), prolonged neutropenia, cytomegalovirus (CMV) disease, and receipt of corticosteroids for treatment of acute graft-versus-host disease (GvHD). Risk factors for IA following engraftment (days 41–180) in the HSCT population included older age at the time of transplant, receipt of T-cell depleted or CD-34–selected stem cell products, multiple myeloma as an underlying disease, delayed engraftment of T-lymphocytes, neutropenia, lymphopenia, grade II–IV GvHD, treatment with high dose steroids, CMV disease after day 40, and respiratory viral infections (especially parainfluenza 3) [44,47]. In the very late period (>6 months) post HSCT, risk factors for IA included neutropenia, clinically extensive chronic GvHD, CMV disease, and receipt of an unrelated or HLA-mismatched peripheral blood stem cell transplant. The outcome of IA was poor independent of the timing post transplant of IA; survival was approximately 30% at 6 months and 20% at 12 months after the diagnosis of the infection. Different risk factors have been identified for IA among the various SOT populations as well. In general, poor status prior to transplant, severe immunosuppression, colonization with *Aspergillus*, and complicated postoperative course are the common risk factors [48–55].

Invasive aspergillosis is also increasingly reported in other populations, including patients with chronic lung diseases and prolonged corticosteroid therapy, immune diseases, liver cirrhosis, severe Influenza infections, or prolonged ICU stay [56–58]. The disease is often underestimated in these populations and associated with a high mortality.

NON-*ASPERGILLUS* HYALOHYPHOMYCETES

The hyalohyphomycete molds are a heterogeneous group; however, they do have in common septate, hyaline hyphae when visualized in tissue [5]. It is important to remember that fungal hyphae of the various hyalohyphomycetes (including *Aspergillus*) as seen in direct specimen examination and tissue preparation are indistinguishable. Culture of infected tissue or body fluid is, therefore, required to definitively identify the invading pathogen. Over 30 non-*Aspergillus* hyalohyphomycetes have been implicated in human disease including, most commonly, species of *Acremonium*, *Fusarium*, *Paecilomyces*, and *Scedosporium* (Table 2.1) [59]. Several of the non-*Aspergillus* hyalohyphomycetes are unique in their capability of producing adventitial forms that are able to sporulate *in vivo*, which permits release of propagules into the bloodstream and dissemination to other organs [60].

Acremonium

Acremonium is a mold found in soil, decaying vegetation, and food that can be pathogenic to plants, insects, and humans. Human infection has been reported with *Acremonium alabamense*, *A. falciforme*, *A. kiliense*, *A. roseogriseum*, *A. strictum*, *A. potronii*, *A. curvulum*, *A. artrogriseum*, and *A. recifei*.

In immunocompetent individuals, *Acremonium* has been implicated in cases of keratitis and endophthalmitis either following trauma or laser in situ keratomileusis (Lasik) [61–64]. It has also been reported as causing cutaneous and subcutaneous dermal infections, eumycetoma, onychomycosis, osteomyelitis, peritonitis in patients undergoing continuous ambulatory peritoneal dialysis (CAPD), prosthetic valve endocarditis, and CNS infection [65–69]. In immunocompromised patients, dialysis fistula infections, peritonitis, pneumonia, cerebritis, and disseminated infection have been reported [5,60,70–76]. Although rare, *Acremonium* eumycetoma has also been reported in SOT recipients [77]. Given the presence of adventitial forms, *Acremonium* can disseminate through the bloodstream to distant sites [78–82]. The portal of entry may be either the lungs or gastrointestinal tract or skin, with dissemination at times producing endophthalmitis, meningitis, or fungemia with sepsis and end organ damage. Recently, a cluster of *A. kiliense* fungemia in 3 HSCT recipients, possibly related to intravascular catheter infections, has been described in Greece [83].

Fusarium

Members of the genus *Fusarium* are ubiquitous filamentous fungi commonly found as soil saprophytes and plant pathogens. Characterized by canoe-shaped macroconidia, *Fusarium solani* is the most frequent cause of human infections, followed by *F. oxysporum*, *F. verticilloides* and *F. moniliforme*. Human disease ranges from mycotoxicosis, caused by ingestion of fusarial toxins, to infections, which may be superficial, localized, or disseminated [5,70,84]. These infections are particularly difficult to treat because of common resistance to multiple antifungal drug classes. In onco-hematological patients, a cutaneous port of entry, such as onychomycosis or interdigital intertrigo, may precede disseminated infection in as many as 2/3 of cases [85].

In the US, *Fusarium* spp. are responsible for about 3% of IFIs among HSCT recipients, ranking fourth after invasive aspergillosis, candidiasis and mucormycosis [39]. However, in tropical areas, such as Brasil, invasive fusariosis may account to up to 35% of invasive fungal diseases [86]. A particularity of disseminated fusariosis is the high proportion of fungemia, which is observed in about 40% of cases [87,88].

In a multicenter study involving 9 centers, 61 bone marrow transplant (BMT) patients with fusariosis were reported. The overall incidence was 5.97 cases/1000 transplants [88].

Table 2.1 Currently documented agents of hyalohypmycoses

Acremonium spp	Emmonsia Parva	Paecilomyces variotii	Trichoderma spp
A. alabamense	Engyodontium album	Purpureocillium lilacinum	T. harzianum
A. atrogriseum	Fusarium spp	Rasamsonia argillacea	T. longibrachiatum
A. curvulum	F. chlamydosporum	Penicillium spp	Tritirachium oryzae
A. falciforme	F. dimerum	P. chrysagenum	Verticillium serrae
A. kilinse	F. incarnatum	P. citrinum	Volutella cinerescens
A. potronii	F. moniliforme	P. commune	
A. roseogriseum	F. napiforme	P. decumbens	
A. strictum	F. nivale	P. expansum	
Aphanoascus fulvescens	F. nygamai	P. marneffei[a]	
Arthrographis kalrae	F. oxysporum	Phaeoacremonium parasiticum	
Beauveria spp	F. pallidoroserum	P. inflatipes	
B. alba	F. proliferatum	P. rubrigenum	
B. bassiana	F. solani	Phialemonium obovatum	
Cephaliophora irregularis	F. veriticillioides	Phialemonium curvatum	
Chrysonilia sitophila	Gymnascella dankaliensis	Polycytella hominis	
Chrysosporium spp	Lecythophora hoffmannii	Schizophyllum commune	
C. pannicola	Lecythophora mutabilis	Scedosporium spp	
C. zonatum	Metarhizium anisopliae	S. apiospermum	
Coprinus cinereus	Myceliophthora thermophila	Lomentospora prolificans	
Cylindrocarpon spp	Onychocola canadensis	Scopulariopsis spp	
C. destructans	Ovadendron sulphureoochraceum	S. brevicaulis	
C. lichenicola	Neocosmospora vasinfecta	Scytalidium dimidiatum	
C. vaginae			

Source: Munoz, P. et al., *Am. J. Transplant.*, 4, 636–643, 2004.
Note: List not inclusive.
[a] Most authorities refer to disease as penicilliosis.

Fifty-four patients were allogeneic and seven were autologous BMT recipients. Disseminated infection with metastatic skin lesions was the most frequent presentation (75%) followed by fungemia alone (11%). Lung infiltrates were seen in 64% and sinusitis in 36% of the cases. Presenting symptoms included fever (92%) and papular or nodular skin lesions with or without central necrosis [88,89]. At the time of diagnosis, 46% of the patients were neutropenic, and most had acute or chronic GvHD. There was a trimodal distribution of infection: an "early peak" was seen prior to engraftment (median posttransplant day 16), a "second peak" was seen late (median posttransplant day 64), and a "very late" third peak was observed after posttransplant day 360. Mortality was very high at 75%–90%, and median survival after diagnosis was 13 days, with only 13% of patients alive at 90 days [89]. Persistent neutropenia and corticosteroid treatment were significant prognostic factors [88,89]. A recent study identified treatment with antithymocyte globulin, acute myeloid leukemia and hyperglycemia as independent risk factors for invasive fusariosis in the early phase after allogeneic HSCT, while an association with non-myeloblative conditioning regimen, severe GvHD and previous invasive mold disease was found during the later phase [90].

A study of *Fusarium* infection conducted in Israel reported a slightly different clinical scenario, with 76% patients considered immunocompetent [91]. These tended to be older patients who had ischemic heart disease, diabetes, peripheral vascular disease, and chronic renal failure as the underlying disease. Of the mycologic data available, 10 infections were with *Fusarium oxysporum*, 8 were *F. solani*, and 4 were *F. dimerum*. The proportion of disseminated and localized disease was about equal in immunocompetent and immunosuppressed patients, and as in the BMT population, skin ulcerations were a common clinical presentation. Risk factors for infection were hematologic malignancy, immunosuppression, burns, other disseminated infections, and chronic renal failure. Mortality was 11% during hospitalization, significantly lower than that reported in the BMT series.

Isolated outbreaks of *Fusarium* keratitis associated with contact lenses have been reported from several states in the United States [92]. Most outbreaks have been traced to contaminated contact lens fluids [93]. *Fusarium* has also been isolated from a hospital water reservoir during an outbreak of fusariosis [94]. The epidemiologic investigation determined that aerosolization occurring during showers constituted the potential source of infection.

Paecilomyces

Paecilomyces species are isolated from soil and decaying plant matter and are often implicated in decay of food and cosmetics. The two most common species are *Paecilomyces lilacinus*, which has been reassigned to a new genus as *Purpureocillium lilacinum*, and *P. variotii*, both rarely pathogenic for humans. In immunocompetent hosts, these organisms have been reported as the cause of keratitis after corneal implants, endophthalmitis, onychomycosis, skin infections, peritonitis in CAPD patients, pneumonitis, sinusitis, and endocarditis following valve replacement [95–97]. A case of pulmonary fungus ball by *Paecilomyces* in an immunocompetent individual has also been reported [98]. *P. variotii* was also reported as a cause of outbreak of fungal peritonitis in patients undergoing peritoneal dialysis following contamination of fluid bags by dust [99,100]. Immunosuppressed patients may also present with *Paecilomyces* infection. It has been reported as causing infection in patients with chronic granulomatous disease (CGD), including cellulitis, osteomyelitis, pneumonitis, and splenic abscess, and pneumonia, and lung abscess in patients with hairy cell leukemia, CGD, and CF [98,101]. Disseminated disease appears to occur predominantly in immunosuppressed hosts.

Paecilomyces variotii has been reported in a multiple myeloma patient who had undergone autologous HSCT 6 months prior to presentation. Fever was the predominant symptom, and *P. variotii* was isolated from line and peripheral blood cultures [102]. *P. variotii* has also been recovered from the cerebral spinal fluid (CSF) of a patient with metastatic breast cancer and multiple enhancing brain lesions on magnetic resonance imaging (MRI) [103]. CSF parameters were abnormal, and numerous fungal cells and septate hyphae were seen on mycological examination. Importantly, disseminated *P. variotii* infection has also been reported breaking through voriconazole prophylaxis in a neutropenic child with relapsed leukemia [104]. The clinical presentation consisted of persistent fever with a pink macular and nodular rash on the child's forearms and face.

Purpureocillium lilacinum has been isolated from many sites of infection. In a large study from Spain, 119 cases were reported from 1964 to 2004 [105]. Most cases of *P. lilacinum* were onychomycosis (51.3%) followed by cutaneous and subcutaneous infection (35.3%). For cutaneous infections, risk factors included SOT, HSCT, surgery, primary immunodeficiency, and AIDS. Lesions presented as painful red nodules that sometimes progressed to excoriated nodules and draining pustules. Severe onychomycosis, as with *Fusarium* spp., may constitute a risk factor for invasive disease since the toenail may serve as a portal of entry and provide contiguous or lymphangitic spread [106]. Cases of oculomycosis presenting as scleritis, keratitis, and endophthalmitis have also been reported, with lens implantation, diabetes, prior scleritis, surgery, and immunosuppression constituting risk factors [105,107,108].

An outbreak of invasive *P. lilacinum* was reported in severely neutropenic patients due to contaminated skin lotion [109,110]. Neutropenic patients in a laminar flow ward presented with cutaneous lesions that erupted either during the neutropenic period or shortly thereafter. Invasive disease occurred in 36% of patients treated with chemotherapy for leukemia or lymphoma and in 100% of BMT recipients. Moisturizing skin lotion was found to be contaminated with the organism. *P. lilacinum* causing cutaneous lesions have also been reported in SOT, steroid users, and patients with CGD [111]. Lesions may be papular, pustular, nodular, or ulcerated, and located on any part of the skin.

Scedosporium

Species of the genus *Scedosporium* are frequently encountered in soil from rural areas, parks, potted plants, from compost, manure of cattle and fowl, polluted waters and sewage, and occasionally from hospital air during construction [5,70,71,112]. Infections are caused by species of the *Scedosporium apiospermum* complex (including *S. apiospermum*, *S. boydii* and its sexual form *Pseudallescheria boydii*, and *S. auranthiacum*). *S. prolificans*, actually reassigned to a new genus as *Lomentospora prolificans*, has occasionally been designated as a dematiaceous mold and is characterized by resistance to virtually all antifungal classes [113]. The first case of *L. prolificans* infection was reported in 1984 [114]. Since that time, multiple cases have been reported in the literature, with fairly large case series from Spain, Australia, and the United States [115–118]. SOT recipients, especially lung-transplant recipients, seem to be particularly susceptible to *Scedosporium* colonization and infection [119–121]. In one series, approximately 66% of the patients with *L. prolificans* infection were receiving amphotericin B prior to the infection [122]. In a series from a tertiary care cancer center, the incidence of *Scedosporium* infection increased from 0.82 cases per 100,000 patient-inpatient days (1993–1998) to 1.33 cases per 100,000 patient-inpatient days, with all cases of *S. prolificans* presenting as breakthrough infections after the year 2000 [123]. In a series of 162 cases of *L. prolificans* infections, major risk factors were malignancy (45%), cystic fibrosis (11%) and SOT (8%) [124]. Most common clinical presentations were disseminated infections (44%), pulmonary infections (29%) and bone and joint infections (10%). Fungemia was present in 70% of cases of systemic infections and overall mortality was 47%. The increase in *S. prolificans* infections may be linked to the increasing use of antifungal prophylaxis, which in turn may select for this opportunistic pathogen that is notoriously resistant to practically all antifungal agents.

It is important to note that both *S. apiospermum* complex and *L. prolificans* may simply colonize body sites without overt disease, or they may produce a variety of clinical syndromes in a wide range of hosts. For example, *S. apiospermum* has been isolated as a colonizer from the airways of CF patients, and *S. prolificans* has been reported to colonize airways and external auditory canals [116,117,125–129]. Patients in these reports had the organism isolated from culture on multiple occasions; however, they did not appear to have clinical disease, nor did they receive systemic antifungal therapy. On the other hand, both organisms may cause severe infection of the eye, lung, skin and soft tissues, bone, CNS, and bloodstream. In fact, disseminated infection is the most commonly reported presentation of *S. prolificans*, and blood cultures are frequently positive (in 75%–100% of cases) in the setting of disseminated disease [113,115,117,123,130–135]. The high rate of bloodstream infection may be one feature distinctive of infection with *S. prolificans* when compared with *S. apiospermum* infection. In one large review of transplant recipients with scedosporiosis, fungemia occurred in 40% of cases with *S. prolificans* infection versus 4.7% of cases with *S. apiospermum* infection [122]. The overall mortality rate among transplant recipients with scedosporiosis was 58%. Among the HSCT recipients, overall mortality rate was 68% (77.8% for *S. prolificans* and 61.5% for *S. apiospermum*) whereas the mortality for SOT recipients was 54% (77.8% for *S. prolificans* and 54.5% for *S. apiospermum*).

The respiratory tract is a common site of *Scedosporium* infection. This may remain a localized process or be the portal of entry for hematogenous dissemination. Pulmonary scedosporiosis with *S. apiospermum* has been described in patients with CGD, chronic steroid use, hematologic malignancy, and after bone marrow and solid organ transplantation [44,119,122,135–141]. Initial presentation includes fever, cough, sputum production, pleuritic chest pain, tachypnea, and malaise. Imaging of the lung may demonstrate bilateral infiltrates, nodules, abscess, fungus ball, cavitary lesions, effusion, or empyema. Infection of the respiratory tract with *S. prolificans* has been reported most commonly in immunosuppressed patients, including those with malignancy (usually hematologic), post SOT or HSCT, chronic immunosuppressive therapy or chronic corticosteroids, and AIDS [117,122,141]. Pulmonary infection with *S. prolificans* is indistinguishable from *S. apiospermum* based on clinical and radiographic presentation alone. Dissemination from the lungs to multiple organs, including brain and skin, has been described in both BMT and SOT recipients for both organisms [119,122,123,141]. As previously noted, the incidence of dissemination appears to be lower for *S. apiospermum* compared with *S. prolificans* [122]. The large majority of patients with disseminated *S. prolificans* infection have predisposing risk factors, such as immunosuppression, neutropenia, BMT, SOT, malignancy, and AIDS.

Scedosporium apiospermum and *S. prolificans* have also been implicated as the etiologic agent of keratomycosis, with and without overt ocular injury, as well as endophthalmitis [129,133,134,142–151]. Patients with keratomycosis may experience eye pain, photophobia, foreign body sensation, conjunctival or corneal erythema, tearing, and changes in visual acuity. Cases have been reported in patients with a retained contact lens, and in patients who had experienced scleral necrosis after pterygium surgery with adjunctive beta-irradiation. The lesions have ranged from corneal abrasion to frank corneal ulceration or abscess and anterior chamber hypopion. Cases of *Scedosporium* endophthalmitis have occurred in a different setting, many times as part of hematogenously disseminated disease in an immunosuppressed host. Endogenous endophthalmitis presents with eye pain, photosensitivity, and worsening visual acuity. Fundoscopic exam reveals exudates and hazy vitreous. Mortality is almost uniform in patients with *Scedosporium* endophthalmitis in the setting of disseminated disease with either *S. prolificans* or *S. apiospermum* [133,134,147]. Some patients who have *S. apiospermum* endophthalmitis without extra-ocular sites of infection may survive after enucleation or evisceration of the eye (3 of 9 in one series) [146,147].

Scedosporium has been frequently implicated as the cause of CNS infection including meningoencephalitis, encephalitis, and cerebral abscesses. *S. apiospermum* infection of the CNS has been reported after near-drowning episodes, in patients with hematologic malignancy, after BMT, SOT, and penetrating trauma of the foot complicated by osteomyelitis [119,137,152–160]. Central nervous system infection with *S. prolificans* has been reported in the setting of disseminated infection [115,122,130,161]. For both organisms, patients may present with variable neurologic findings, such as headache, confusion, disorientation, agitation, cognitive decline, progressive lethargy, hemiparesis, or tonic–clonic seizures. Although typically present, the absence of ring enhancement has been reported [152,156,158,159].

Scedosporium has been reported presenting as skin lesions following traumatic inoculation and sometimes in the setting of disseminated infection [119,122,158,162–165]. Skin lesions may appear as skin nodules, or as erythematous to purple papulae or papulo-bullae, which may develop a necrotic center and that can have lymphangitic spread. Biopsy of skin nodules reveals an inflammatory granulomatous lesion with abscess, necrotic areas, large multinucleate giant cells, and vascular proliferation. A nodule may even contain a mycetoma, with branched septate fungal hyphae visualized under microscopic examination. Soft tissue infection, arthritis, and osteomyelitis due to *S. apiospermum* and its sexual form, *P. boydii,* as well as *S. prolificans* have also been reported [116,118,137,165–172]. The most frequently reported predisposing event was trauma to the affected extremity. Initial presentations included laceration or cellulitis at the site, with progression to joint effusion with inflammation and tenderness, and low-grade fever.

Scopulariopsis

Scopulariopsis spp. (teleomorph: *Microascus* spp.) belong to the same family as *Scedosporium* spp. (*Microascaceae*) and include both hyaline and dematiaceous species. These fungi are commonly found in the environment, such as soil, wood, paper, and food. They cause localized non-invasive diseases, such as onycomychosis, keratitis, and otomycosis [173]. They are uncommon, but emerging opportunistic pathogens in immunocompromised patients have been causing invasive diseases [174]. The most frequent pathogenic species is *S. brevicaulis*, while many other species (*S. brumptii, S. acremonium, S. candida, S. cirrosus, S. cinereus*) have also been reported as the cause of invasive infection. Pulmonary infections, sinusitis, deep cutaneous infections, endocarditis, brain abscesses, and disseminated infections have been reported in the literature [174]. As these molds commonly exhibit resistance to all antifungal drug classes, they are a concern among the increasing population of patients at risk for invasive fungal disease.

PHAEOHYPHOMYCOSES

The dematiaceous fungi are a heterogeneous group of organisms with darkly pigmented hyphae, conidia, or both owing to dihydroxynaphthalene melanin in their cell walls. Melanin is thought to play a role in pathogenesis as it is a known virulence factor in fungi [175,176]. Though these organisms are molds, several have a pleomorphic appearance, and a yeast or mold form can predominate during different phases of growth. This has led to confusion and frequently changing nomenclature [5]. Dematiaceous molds most often implicated in human infections include species of *Alternaria, Bipolaris, Cladophialophora, Curvularia, Ochroconis/Verruconis (Dactylaria), Exophiala,* and *Phialophora* (Table 2.2). Cutaneous and subcutaneous infections after penetrating injury, such as chromoblastomycosis and keratitis, are seen in immunocompetent patients, whereas disseminated

disease, often referred to as phaeohyphomycosis, may occur in immunosuppressed individuals [113,177–185].

Alternaria

Exposure to *Alternaria* has been associated with both development and severity of asthma [186,187]. Exposure may occur outdoors or in indoor environments, with biologically active moieties consisting of spores, fragments of spores, and dust particles. In one study, practically all (95%–99%) of the dust samples collected in homes contained detectable levels of *Alternaria alternata* antigens, and active asthma was positively associated with the *A. alternata* antigen level in the home [186].

Alternaria keratitis has been reported, usually in association with foreign body removal, Lasik, or due to a keratoprosthesis [188–190]. Alternariosis has also been reported in patients receiving SOTs [191–199]. Interestingly, most of these patients had cutaneous manifestation of infection. Lesions were solitary or multiple and presented as papules, plaques, nodules, recurrent cellulitis with ulceration, and in one report, the cutaneous lesions presented in a sporotrichoid distribution. Invasive fungal infection due to *Alternaria*, including rhinosinusitis and rhinocerebral infection, has been reported in patients with hematologic malignancy and in BMT recipients. A patient with CGD was documented to have *Alternaria* causing dermal induration [200–204].

Bipolaris

Bipolaris spicifera and *B. hawaiiensis* have been reported in human infections, including keratitis, endophthalmitis, and skin and soft tissue infections [205–207]. Prior use of

Table 2.2 Currently reported agents of phaeohyphomycosis

Alternaria spp	*Exophiala* spp	*Piedraia hortae*
A. alternata	*Exophiala dermatitidis* (*Wangiella dermatitidis*)	*Phaeoannellomyces werneckii*
Aureobasidium pullulans	*Exophiala jeanselmei*	*Phaeoacremonium parasiticum*
Bipolaris spp	*Exserohilum* spp	*Phialemonium*
B. spicifera	*E. rostratum*	*Phialophora* spp
B. hawaiiensis	*E. longirostratum*	*P. richardsiae*
Chaetomium spp	*E. mcginnisii*	*P. verrucosa*
Cladophialophora spp	*Fonsecaea* spp	*Pseudoallescheria boydii*
C. bantiana	*F. compacta*	*Phoma*
C. carrionii	*F. pedrosoi*	*Ramichloridium mackenzei*
Curvularia spp	*Hormonema dermatoides*	*Scedosporium prolificans*
C. clavata	*Madurella* spp	*Scytalidium* spp
C. lunata	*M. grisea*	*Ulocladium*
Dactylaria gallopava (formerly Ochroconis gallopavum)	*M. mycetomatis*	*Wangiella (Exophiala) dermatitidis*

Note: List not inclusive.

topical corticosteroids and antibiotics have been associated with the development of a corneal ulcer caused by *Bipolaris*, and cutaneous infections with *Bipolaris* have been reported in patients who either used topical steroids, had atopic or seborrheic dermatitis, or onychomycosis [208]. Cutaneous *Bipolaris* has also been reported in a child with acute lymphoblastic leukemia (ALL) and neutropenia without preceding trauma [209]. A tender erythematous patch with central punctate areas of hemorrhage appeared on the left cheek. A skin biopsy revealed epidermal necrosis and dematiaceous, septate hyphae in an edematous papillary dermis with infiltration of vessel wall. Culture revealed the pathogen to be *B. spicifera*.

Cladophialophora

Cladophialophora bantiana is notoriously associated with CNS infection in immunosuppressed and immunocompetent patients [210–212]. In a large review of 101 cases of CNS phaeohyphomycosis, 48% were caused by *C. bantiana* [213]. Though 37% of the infected patients had some degree of immune dysfunction, over half (52%) of the cases had no known underlying risk factors for infection. Of CNS infections, brain abscesses constituted the most common clinical presentation (87% of cases) with single lesions present in 71%, meningitis 9%, encephalitis 2%, and myelitis 2%. For those in whom histopathology was available, fungal hyphae were noted in 86%; however, granulomatous inflammation was present in only 48% of cases. Overall mortality was 73%, with equivalent mortality between immunocompromised (71%) and immunocompetent individuals (74%). Recipients of SOTs appeared to have lower mortality at 64%, though in most cases, despite antifungal therapy and surgical intervention, the outcome was still fatal [211,213–216].

Extracerebral involvement with *Cladophialophora* has been reported in both immunocompromised and immunocompetent patients as well [217–219]. Cutaneous lesions are the most common extracerebral manifestation. Chromoblastomycosis caused by *Cladophialophora carrionii* is an endemic cutaneous infection presenting with desquamating erythematous papules or squamous plaques [220]. The extremities are mainly involved, and treatment is protracted and may not lead to resolution, leaving deformities and incapacitation.

Curvularia

Curvularia, such as *C. lunata* and *C. clavata*, has been implicated as the cause of infections in both immunocompetent and immunosuppressed hosts. Cases of keratitis, cutaneous and soft tissue infections, sinusitis with and without invasion of the brain, brain abscess, peritonitis, and saline breast implant contamination have all been reported [22,181,185,221–229]. Keratitis due to *Curvularia* may be secondary to trauma or nontrauma, and it appears to vary with the season in the subtropical region, with a higher incidence in late summer and throughout autumn [181].

Verruconis/Ochroconis

Verruconis spp. (also called *Dactylaria* or *Ochroconis*) are ubiquitous dematiaceous molds found in soil, decaying vegetables or cave rocks [230]. Some of the thermophilic and pathogenic species of *Ochroconis* have been reassigned to the new genus *Verruconis*. They cause infections in birds, as well as cats and dogs. In humans, the most frequent species encountered in clinical specimens is *V. gallopava* (68%), followed by *O. mirabilis* (21%) [230]. Invasive infections have been described in SOT recipients with a tropism for the central nervous system [231]. In a review of 12 published cases, *D. gallopavum* affected the lung only in 42% cases and the brain was affected in 50% cases [231]. Cutaneous and joint involvement with *Dactylaria* has also been reported [232]. *V. gallopava* CNS infections may present as single or multiple cerebral abscesses, which on microscopic examination of tissue appear black, with extensive necrosis-containing neutrophils, multinucleated giant cells, and pigmented septate hyphae [233–238]. Disseminated *Dactylaria* infections in other immunocompromised patients such as HIV have also been reported, with CNS involvement similar to that described in SOT patients [239].

Exophiala (Wangiella) dermatitidis and *Exophiala jeanselmei*

Exophiala is a dematiaceous mold that, in certain phases of its development, appears yeast-like, with black creamy colonies and unicellular forms that replicate by budding [240]. Clinically, *Exophiala* can have a wide range of presentations. Infection of the CNS with *Exophiala (Wangiella) dermatitidis* has been reported [213,241–246]. This may present as primary brain abscess, secondary cerebral infections from contiguous or hematogenous spread, and meningitis [242,246]. Though the majority of cases are reported in East Asia, cases in the United States have also been described. *E. dermatitidis* has also been recovered from some European steam baths, where conditions are hot and moist [247]. *E. dermatitidis* has been found to colonize the respiratory tract of 6% of patients with cystic fibrosis [248] and has also been isolated from stool [249].

Exophiala jeanselmei has been implicated in eumycotic mycetoma and in rare cases of chromoblastomycosis [250–253]. Infection of the skin and subcutaneous tissue with *Exophiala* has been reported in SOT recipients and other immunosuppressed individuals [182–184,254]. Trauma typically precedes cutaneous infection, which can present as a necrotic skin lesion with surrounding erythema, nodules, or subcutaneous cysts. Disseminated disease has also been reported involving blood, heart valves, lung, and the CNS [113].

Environmental contamination of products has been implicated in *E. dermatitidis* infections, including peritonitis in patients undergoing CAPD and meningitis from contaminated compounded injectable steroids [246,255,256]. Similarly, *E. jeanselmei* fungemia has been associated with contaminated water products in immunocompromised patients [257]. An outbreak of *E. jeanselmei* fungemia over a 10-month period was ultimately related to contaminated deionized water from a hospital pharmacy. Over half the patients presenting with fungemia had malignancy, mostly hematologic, while the other patients had AIDS, agranulocytosis, and systemic lupus erythematosus (SLE) with thrombotic thrombocytopenic purpura. Invasive *Exophiala* infections also have been recently reported in patients with inherited CARD9 deficiency [258]. The most common presenting clinical sign associated with *Exophilala* infections is fever [257].

Exserohilum

Exserohilum may also cause infections in both immunocompromised and immunocompetent hosts [113,259–262]. Reported cases are mainly from warm tropical and subtropical regions of the world. Patients typically present with infections of the skin and soft tissue, cornea, paranasal sinuses, including allergic fungal sinusitis, lungs, bone, and brain. Before the 2012 outbreak in the United States discussed below, 48 cases of *Exserohilum* infections were reported in the literature and consisted mainly in systemic infections affecting sinuses in half of the cases, followed by localized cutaneous/subcutaneous or corneal infections [263]. *E. rostratum* was the most frequent causal agent (60% of cases), followed by *E. longirostratum* (6%) and *E. mcginnisii* (2%). Immunosuppression was present in only 27% of cases and corneal or cutaneous infections were usually secondary to trauma or surgery. Cutaneous lesions can present as papules, plaques, vesicles, nodules, or ecthyma gangrenosum. Though some skin infections became systemically invasive, most cases of invasive infection were acquired via inhalation, with subsequent dissemination via the bloodstream to other organs mainly in immunosuppressed patients. In 2012, *E. rostratum* was identified as the cause of an outbreak of fungal infections, consisting mainly in meningitis and some cases of arthrtitis, which was associated with contaminated lots of injectable methylprednisolone acetate from a single compounding pharmacy. A total of 749 patients in 20 states of the United States were affected, and 61 of the infected patients died [264].

Fonsecaea

Fonsecaea pedrosoi is one of the leading causes of chromoblastomycosis [177,179]. *F. pedrosoi* and *F. compacta*, which are endemic to various tropical parts of the world, are the most common infecting species [177,179,265]. Males in rural areas are most often affected, with painless nodular or verrucous lesions predominating on the extremities. Lesions tend to appear weeks to months after the initial trauma, which tends to be minor and often passes unnoticed. Examination of skin scrapings or tissue histology reveals the typical muriform or sclerotic bodies, and culture is required for correct identification of the etiologic agent.

Phialophora

Phialophora verrucosa has been reported as a cause of chromoblastomycosis [177,179]. Occurring predominantly in the tropics, chromoblastomycosis occurs after traumatic inoculation, usually to the extremities (lower greater than upper), of mostly male farmers and other rural workers. Lesions are slowly growing, vegetating, nodular, verrucous, or mixed nodular-verrucous. *P. verrucosa* has also been reported in a case of fatal hemorrhage due to invasive tracheal infection in a BMT patient with prolonged neutropenia [266].

Ramichloridium

Ramichloridium mackenzei (previously *Ramichloridium obovoideum*) is a dematiaceous mold that has been reported from the Middle East, where it appears to be endemic and possibly geographically restricted. *Ramichloridium* is also considered neurotropic, and reports of cerebral abscesses in both immunocompetent and immunodeficient patients have described uniformly fatal outcome despite aggressive surgical and antifungal interventions [267–271]. Only one case of nonfatal *R. mackenzei* cerebral abscess, in a kidney transplant recipient, has been reported [272].

MUCORMYCOSIS

The agents of mucormycosis are members either of the order Entomophthorales or of the order Mucorales. These organisms are characterized by sparsely septate hyphae in tissue. The hyphae are broad, variable in diameter, and polymorphic, with irregular branching, and in the case of the Mucorales, may invade blood vessels with thrombosis, tissue infarction, and necrosis [5,70,215,273]. The molds of the order Entomophthorales are usually found in tropical areas, in soil, decaying vegetation, on insects, and as saprobes in the gastrointestinal tract of reptiles, amphibians, and mammals. Of the Entomophthorales, *Basidiobolus* and *Conidiobolus* species are pathogenic to humans, causing subcutaneous infections of the extremities and trunk, and of the nasal submucosa, respectively [274]. Members of the order Mucorales are found in soil, decaying vegetation, fruits, foodstuffs, and animal excreta in a wide geographic distribution. The portal of entry for infection is likely pulmonary with eventual dissemination to other sites, though primary cutaneous infection has been reported [275]. The Mucorales cause the majority of cases of human mucormycosis, with *Rhizopus*, *Mucor*, *Rhizomucor*, *Lichtheimia* (formerly *Absidia*), *Apophysomyces*, and *Cunninghamella*, among others, found in the literature [47,274,276–279]. The most commonly reported cause of human infection is *Rhizopus*.

Risk factors for mucromycosis include diabetes mellitus, malnutrition, malignancy, and use of voriconazole

[47,280–285]. Iron overload and deferoxamine therapy have been associated with a higher risk of mucormycosis [281,286–290]. Iron is an important virulence factor for *Mucorales*, and when deferoxamine binds to iron in the host, it serves as a siderophore for this mold.

In a large series study, 65% of infections occurred in males. Underlying conditions included diabetes in 36%, no underlying condition in 19%, and malignancy in 17% (of which 95% were hematologic). The site of infection varied based on the population, but overall, the most frequent locations were rhinocerebral 48% (particularly in diabetics and intravenous drug users), lung 24% (neutropenic patients, SOT patients), skin 19% (penetrating wounds), gastrointestinal 7%, and disseminated infection 3% (burns, prematurity, diabetes) [281]. Deep extension to bone, tendon, or muscle occurred in 24%, and hematogenous dissemination from skin to other organs in 20%. Overall mortality approached 54% but varied with the site of infection: in disseminated disease mortality was 96%; in rhinocerebral and localized cerebral disease it was 62%; and in gastrointestinal infection it was 85% due to bowel perforation. Survival was 3% with no therapy, approximately 60% for antifungal or surgical treatment alone, and 70% for combination surgical and antifungal therapy.

Data from the Transplant-Associated Infection Surveillance Network show a 12-month cumulative incidence of 0.29% in BMT recipients and 0.07% in SOT [120]. In SOT recipients, mucormycosis is associated with corticosteroid treatment, with 78.9% of infected patients having received a cumulative dose of ≥600 mg of prednisone [283]. Clinical presentations were as mentioned above and were similar among the various organ transplant groups. Interestingly, all kidney transplant recipients had infection of the allograft in one series [283]. The genus most frequently isolated was *Rhizopus* (73%) followed by *Mucor* (13%). In a series of 263 consecutive BMT patients, 1.9% developed invasive zygomycosis over 10 years, 80% thereof >100 days after transplant [286]. Interestingly, no cases of disseminated infection occurred. Iron overload, neutropenia, and GvHD were reported as risk factors for death in BMT recipients. Breakthrough mucormycosis after voriconazole administration (as prophylaxis, empirical, preemptive, and targeted therapy for IA), in patients following allogeneic BMT, and following intensive chemotherapy in patients with hematologic malignancies, has been increasingly reported [47,280,282,284,285,291]. Most of these infections occurred late in the posttransplant/chemotherapy period, and lungs and sinuses were the most frequently affected sites. *Rhizopus* was again the most common genus isolated in culture [47,282]. Overall mortality for mucormycosis breaking through voriconazole therapy was very high, with a 69%–73% attributable mortality reported [282,284]. Infections with *Cunninghamella bertholletiae*, though rare, have been reported in patients following both BMT and SOT [275,276,292–298].

Cutaneous mucormycosis may also be observed in immunocompetent patients following penetrating trauma or burns [299]. A cluster of 13 cases of necrotizing cutaneous mucormycosis due to *Apophysomyces trapeziformis* has been observed after a devastating tornado in Joplin (MO, USA) in 2011 [300].

ENDEMIC MYCOSES

The endemic mycoses are a group of thermally dimorphic fungi characterized by growing as a mycelial form at 25°C but as a yeast or yeast-like form at 37°C. The major etiologic agents of endemic mycoses are *Histoplasma capsulatum*, *Blastomyces dermatitidis*, *Coccidioides immitis*, *Paracoccidioides brasiliensis*, *Sporothrix schenckii*, and *Penicillium marneffei*, each one with a distinct geographic distribution. These fungi are usually present in the soil, and inhalation of conidia may lead to systemic infection, with clinical manifestation of disease varying in relation to the intensity of exposure and the immune status of the host [5]. Disease manifestation may occur on primary exposure or through reactivation of a latent focus when there is a decrease in cell-mediated immunity. In the SOT population, though the overall incidence is low, the most frequent endemic mycosis reported in a prospective study was *Histoplasma capsulatum*, with almost two-thirds presenting as disseminated disease [301]. Most occurred at a median of 13.7 months posttransplant and appeared unrelated to rejection episodes.

Blastomyces

Blastomyces dermatitidis is the dimorphic fungus causing blastomycosis (also called North American blastomycosis). *B. dermatitidis* grows on decaying organic material. In North America, the fungus is found in the south central and southeastern states, states bordering the Mississippi and Ohio River basins, the Canadian provinces and Midwest states that border the Great Lakes, and areas of Canada and New York along the St. Lawrence River, although cases west of the Mississippi River Valley have also been reported [302,303]. Africa is also considered an endemic region for blastomycosis [5]. The portal of entry is via inhalation of conidia; in the alveoli, transformation to the yeast form takes place with an inflammatory response generating granulomata. Specific cell-mediated immunity is the major host defense system to prevent dissemination. Most infected individuals are asymptomatic. The clinical presentation of pulmonary blastomycosis is varied and includes flu-like illness, acute pneumonia, subacute or chronic respiratory illness, or fulminant ARDS; verrucous or ulcerative cutaneous lesions have also been reported [5,304].

In a large case series, the incidence of blastomycosis in an endemic area was 23.88/100,000 admissions or 0.62 cases/100,000 population [305,306]. The average patient age was approximately 40 years, with 75% of the patients in the 25–64 years age group. Approximately 65% of the patients were male. The overall distribution of organ involvement was pulmonary 90%, cutaneous/subcutaneous 20%, osseous

15%, CNS 1%–3%, lymph nodes 3%, and genitourinary 1%. Multiple organs were involved in almost one-third of the cases, and the mortality rate in one Canadian study reached 6.3% [306].

Though the numbers are small, cases of blastomycosis have been reported in SOT recipients [307–309]. One review of cases from 1966 to 1991 found only four definite and one probable report of blastomycosis in transplant recipients [308]. Infection most often originated in the lung then disseminated, with skin lesions present in two patients.

Coccidioides

Coccidioides immitis is the etiologic agent of coccidioidomycosis. This organism is found in the soil in the southwestern United States, Mexico, Central America (Guatemala, Honduras, Nicaragua), and South America (Argentina, Paraguay, Venezuela and Colombia) in areas of arid to semiarid climate [5,310,311]. Environmental conditions that favor its growth are heat, low altitudes, sparse flora, and alkaline soils. The portal of entry is via inhalation of the arthroconidia, and a single arthroconidium is able to produce respiratory infection. Arthroconidia germinate to produce spherules and endospores, which are released when the spherules rupture. The spherules are surrounded by neutrophils and macrophages, leading to granuloma formation. The organism is resistant to killing by neutrophils and macrophages, and a cell-mediated response is essential. Defects in cell-mediated immunity are associated with dissemination. More than half of the *Coccidioides* infections are asymptomatic, with about 40% having a self-limited flu-like illness in the ensuing weeks after exposure [5,311,312]. Other manifestations include pneumonia and disseminated disease to other sites including the blood, meninges, joint, bone, skin, and urogenital tract [310,313–317].

Immunocompetent patients may present with infection after activities or natural events that lead to soil disruption. Between 1998 and 2001, the incidence of coccidioidomycosis in Arizona, an endemic area, was 43/100,000 population, representing an increase of 186% since 1995 [318]. The epidemic was associated with a winter season that followed a prolonged drought, and the presence of hot and dusty conditions likely facilitated aerosolization of spores. Though most patients (85%) presented with mild influenza-like illness, approximately 8% developed severe disease [319]. Risk factors for severe pulmonary disease include diabetes, recent cigarette smoking, and older age, while risk for dissemination include Asian or black race, pregnancy, and immunosuppression.

Miliary coccidioidomycosis is the initial presentation in about 1% of immunocompetent patients [320]. Two distinct patterns of miliary coccidioidomycosis have been noted with equal distribution, one acute with primarily respiratory symptoms lasting ≤1 week, and another chronic with symptoms lasting 5–12 weeks, in patients ethnically predisposed and with multiple sites of involvement. Initial symptoms include cough, dyspnea, fever, chills, and chest pain.

Sixty percent of patients developed dissemination to various organs and 40% died. Therefore, early recognition and prompt treatment are crucial to avoid mortality in miliary coccidioidomycosis, and a high index of suspicion is important because early in the course of illness, skin test results are negative, and serology is unrevealing.

Coccidioides fungemia has been rarely reported, and of 33 adult reported cases, 31 were male and 29 were seropositive for HIV [316]. Seventy-four percent of patients died during the admission or shortly thereafter, with a mean survival of only eight days. Antifungal therapy did not seem to have any effect on survival, probably because in most instances, treatment was instituted late due to technique-related delays in diagnosis. Survival also did not depend on CD4 count, lymphocyte count, age, or other risk factors.

Infections in SOT recipients have an incidence varying from 3.8% to 8.7% in highly endemic areas [310,313–315,321–325]. The clinical presentation in SOT recipients is variable; those with pulmonary involvement may have an acute illness with fever, cough, and dyspnea, whereas others progress to respiratory distress, altered sensorium, dissemination to other organs, and disseminated intravascular coagulation with multiorgan failure [321,322,324–326]. In a review of coccidioidomycosis in transplant recipients, antirejection therapy was associated with an increased risk of disease [315]. The risk after transplant is also increased if there is a prior history of coccidioidomycosis, or there is any positive serologic finding in the period just before transplant. As with histoplasmosis, coccidioidomycosis in SOT recipients may occur as a primary infection following transplant after exposure in endemic areas, or through reactivation of latent infection. Patients who have resided or traveled to endemic areas are at risk for reactivation, which occurs about 4–6 months posttransplant [315,323]. In highly endemic areas, some centers, therefore, test for *C. immitis* and prophylactically treat those with a positive serology or prior history of coccidioidomycosis before transplantation [327,328]. This obviously does not preclude transmission via a donated organ. Such reports describe fulminant infections occurring very early in the posttransplant period, usually within 2–3 weeks [321,322,324]. In a nonendemic area, the absence of clinical suspicion along with lack of detailed information about the donor, such as travel history, may lead to a delay in diagnosis. In contrast to SOT, coccidioidomycosis in BMT recipients has not been widely reported, even in endemic areas. In a retrospective review of autologous recipients, the low incidence was attributed to possible underreporting of disease and possibly reduced sensitivity of coccidioidal serology in patients with malignancy [329].

Histoplasma

Two varieties of *Histoplasma* may cause disease in humans: *Histoplasma capsulatum* var. *capsulatum* and *H. capsulatum* var. *duboisii*. The mycelial form of *Histoplasma* in the environment is found in soils with high nitrogen content; namely, soil contaminated with droppings from fowl, in roosts, caves, and old buildings. In the United States, the areas endemic for *H. capsulatum* var. *capsulatum* include the Ohio, Mississippi, and St. Lawrence River valleys. The organism is found throughout most of Latin America, as well. *H. capsulatum* var. *duboisii* is found in tropical Africa [5]. The portal of entry of infection is via inhalation of microconidia. The transformation into the yeast form takes place intracellularly in neutrophils and macrophages. Circulating yeasts are cleared by the reticuloendothelial system. When a specific cell-mediated response develops, macrophages are then able to kill the organism, and the host develops a granulomatous necrotizing inflammatory response. Most people remain asymptomatic following primary exposure, with more than 50% of the population in endemic areas having a positive skin test indicating exposure [330]. Immunocompromised patients, children, and immunocompetent individuals after exposure to a large inoculum may develop symptoms after primary infection, including acute self-limited pulmonary histoplasmosis, progressive pulmonary histoplasmosis, or progressive disseminated histoplasmosis.

Disruption of the soil (e.g., roto-tiling, construction, or landfill work) leads to aerosolization of topsoil and dust. Areas with bird or bat guano, where soil conditions favor growth of *Histoplasma*, can lead to large outbreaks of histoplasmosis in immunocompetent individuals [331–333]. Symptoms consist of headache, fatigue, fever, cough, myalgias, chills, and chest pain, with the majority of cases having five or more symptoms.

Series of histoplasmosis in SOT and BMT recipients in both nonendemic and endemic areas have been published. It is worth noting that transmission of *Histoplasma capsulatum* through donated organs has been reported [334,335]. In one case, reactivation from donor-transmitted histoplasmosis occurred 4 years after transplantation [335]. However, histoplasmosis is generally not found in transplant patients even in endemic regions, suggesting that, in the absence of an outbreak, histoplasmosis is a rare infection even in the face of immunosuppression [336]. In one study, the estimated incidence of histoplasmosis in a SOT population in a nonendemic area was approximately 0.4% [337]. Most patients presented with a nonspecific febrile illness, and the infections were judged to be due to endogenous reactivation. All patients had concurrent CMV infection or had received augmented immunosuppression prior to histoplasmosis dissemination, suggesting that reactivation in these cases was due to a severely immunosuppressed state. Primary infection due to inhalation of conidia was thought to account for outbreaks of histoplasmosis among kidney transplant patients in endemic areas [338,339]. Fever, cough, and dyspnea or hoarseness were common presenting symptoms, and dissemination occurred in most cases.

Paracoccidioides

Paracoccidioides brasiliensis is the etiologic agent of paracoccidioidomycosis, also referred to as South American blastomycosis. This dimorphic fungus is found in several countries in Latin America from Mexico to Argentina, with Brazil, Colombia, Venezuela, Ecuador, and Argentina reporting the greatest number of cases [5,340]. The precise ecologic niche of *P. brasiliensis* remains undefined though the conditions of endemic regions include mild temperatures, many forests, high humidity with plenty of water, rainy summers, and short winters. The areas are also notable for tobacco and coffee farming [341]. Naturally acquired infection occurs in armadillos; in humans, it is presumed that the portal of entry may be either via inhalation or traumatic inoculation, with most patients involved in farming activities. The organism undergoes conversion to the yeast form in the lung parenchyma from where it can disseminate. The characteristic appearance of the organism is as multiple budding yeasts in a pilot wheel configuration. Polymorphonuclear leukocytes and cell-mediated immunity play a role in host defense against the organism. Most primary infections are self-limited. The organism has the ability to remain dormant for long periods of time and cause clinical disease at a time when host defenses are impaired. In the subacute form (present in young or in immunocompromised individuals), the disease may manifest with minimal pulmonary symptoms, with hypertrophy of the reticuloendothelial system, or with bone marrow dysfunction. In the chronic or adult form, the sole manifestation might be respiratory symptoms, such as cough, sputum production, dyspnea; fever, weight loss, malaise, and asthenia are also reported. Radiographic images are variable, with infiltrates, nodules, cavity, or fibrosis seen; occasionally, a large mass termed paracoccidioma is seen. Extrapulmonary sites include the skin and mucosa (around the mouth and nose as well as lower extremities), reticuloendothelial organs, adrenals, bone, and CNS [340,342–346].

Infections in SOT patients have been reported in endemic areas [347–350]. In one study of 71 renal transplant recipients from an endemic area who died from infectious causes, fungi represented 27.5% of infections, with *P. brasiliensis* representing 4.5% of these [348]. Some case studies report presentation many years after transplant. *Paracoccidioides* infection has also been reported in patients with HIV [345,346,351,352].

Penicillium marneffei

Penicillium marneffei is the only dimorphic fungus in the genus *Penicillium*. Other *Penicillium* species are hyaline, saprophytic molds, which rarely cause infection and are known to contaminate plates in microbiology labs, whereas *Penicillium marneffei* infections are frequently reported in HIV-infected individuals. This fungus is geographically restricted to Southeast Asia and China though reports of infection have come from Europe, Australia, and the United States in HIV-infected and other immunosuppressed travelers [5,70,273,353,354]. *P. marneffei* is isolated from bamboo rats and their burrows; the rodents themselves not only harbor but sometimes succumb to *P. marneffei* [358,359]. However, the question still remains as to whether human disease is zoonotically or environmentally transmitted [354]. The portal of entry is the respiratory tract. Pulmonary macrophages and blood monocytes then take up the organism, where intracellularly, it divides by binary fission, showing a characteristic morphology of septate elliptical yeast with prominent cross-walls. Host response is dependent on polymorphonuclear leukocytes and cell-mediated immunity, and when either or both are lacking, dissemination ensues [357]. Though clinical presentation may resemble other infections, such as histoplasmosis, cryptococcosis, tuberculosis, leishmaniasis, and melioidosis, the diagnosis is not difficult if *P. marneffei* is suspected. The organism may be cultured from specimens of skin lesions, blood, bone marrow, or lymph node biopsy and will grow on conventional media, where it produces a characteristic soluble red pigment that diffuses into the agar.

Penicillium marneffei infections rarely occur in immunocompetent individuals and, prior to the HIV epidemic, penicilliosis was only sporadically reported in the literature. However, between 1991 and 1997, 1173 cases of penicilliosis were reported in HIV-infected patients in Thailand [358]. In HIV patients, the clinical picture is one of fever, weight loss, diarrhea, cough, molluscum-like skin lesions, plus generalized lymphadenopathy and hepatosplenomegaly. Skin lesions typically are papules with central necrosis involving the extremities, trunk, face, and mucocutaneous surfaces. Pulmonary presentation includes pleural effusion, interstitial pneumonia, and diffuse alveolar infiltrates. Lytic bone lesions or arthritis of the large joints and small joints of fingers can occur. Anemia, leukopenia, and thrombocytopenia are often present [354,358–362]. Most patients respond to treatment with itraconazole within one week, with complete resolution of cutaneous lesions after 3 weeks of treatment [362]. Cases of *P. marneffei* have been rarely reported in SOT and BMT recipients, with presentation similar to that in HIV patients [359,363–367].

Emmonsia

Emmonsia spp. are ubiquitous dimorphic fungi. *E. parva* and *E. crescens* cause adiaspiromycosis, a pulmonary disease affecting rodents and occasionally humans [368]. Recently, a disseminated fungal disease due to an *Emmonsia* spp. closely related to *E. pasteuriana* was described among HIV patients with low CD4 counts in South Africa [368]. Similar cases of disseminated infections due to *E. pasteuriana* have also been reported in other parts of the world [370,371].

Sporothrix

Sporothrix schenckii is the agent of sporotrichosis. Direct skin inoculation with contaminated soil or thorn plants such as roses leads to a subacute or chronic cutaneous and subcutaneous infection, with nodular lesions that follow the lymphatics and occasionally ulcerate [372,373]. The lesions have been mistaken for pyoderma gangrenosum [372]. The yeast form of the organism, which may be visualized under microscopic examination, is often cigar-shaped, though some varieties may produce large budding cells [5].

Large series of patients with sporotrichosis have been reported from Brazil and India [374,375]. In these series, both fixed cutaneous lesions and lymphangitic/lymphocutaneous forms are described. In a series of 304 patients with sporotrichosis, 96% of the patients had *S. schenckii* recovered in culture, whereas only 32% of cases from India had growth of the organism [374,375]. Occupational exposure is frequent, particularly in those jobs involving agricultural activities (farming, horticulture, and forestry). Exposure through hobbies such as carpentry, beekeeping, hunting, and fishing were also reported. Interestingly, while in the study from Brazil, males constituted 68.4% of the patients [210/306], in India females predominated. This was probably due to increased agricultural or horticultural exposure in these women. Upper extremities were predominantly affected, followed by the lower limbs. Though cutaneous and lymphangitic/lymphocutaneous are the most common presentations, unusual manifestations have been reported, involving buttock, abdomen, face, neck, presternal, periumbilical, and pubic region, while extracutaneous involvement was noted as osteomyelitis, oral lesions, and primary conjunctival *S. schenckii* infection [376]. In a zoonotic outbreak described between 1998 and 2001, 178 cases of culture-proven sporotrichosis were diagnosed [377]. Females predominated, and professional or domiciliary contact with cats was reported in 90.7% of patients, with many reporting traumatic injury preceding the symptoms. Sporotrichosis has been reported only in isolated cases of SOT patients [378–380].

YEASTS

Candida

Candida is one of the leading causes of nosocomial infection in the United States. In one prospective nationwide surveillance study that included 24,179 cases of bloodstream infections reported between 1995 and 2002, 9.5% were due to *Candida*, thus positioning this organism as the fourth most commonly isolated blood pathogen [381]. More recently, the Extended Prevalence of Infection in Intensive Care (EPIC) study showed that *Candida* was the third most common cause of infection in intensive care units (ICUs) worldwide (and the second cause in the United States) [382]. In the United States, the incidence of candidemia-related hospitalization rose by 49% from 2000 to 2005 (0.28–0.42 cases per 1,000 hospitalizations) [383]. Overall, an increased incidence of candidemia has been reported over the years in most US and European Centers with an epidemiological shift from *C. albicans* to non-*albicans Candida* spp. [384–387]. While *C. albicans* remains the major cause of candidemia, *C. glabrata* represents the second most frequent species. Results of two large multicenter studies, the Prospective Antifungal Therapy (PATH) Alliance (2004–2008) and the SENTRY

Antimicrobial Surveillance Programme (2008–2009) show that *C. albicans* and *C. glabrata* accounted for 42%–50% and 17%–26% of candidemia, while *C. parapsilosis*, *C. tropicalis* and *C. krusei* accounted for most remaining cases (15%–16%, 8%–10%, and 2%–3%, respectively) [387,388]. Epidemiology of candidemia in neonates exhibits a different trend with an overall decrease of incidence during the last decade [384,389]. After *C. albicans*, *C. parapsilosis* is the second most frequent causal agent in this population.

The explanation for the increase in non-*albicans Candida* infections has yet to be fully elucidated, but one of the most likely explanations is the increasing use of antifungal prophylaxis [390,391]. For example, the Transplant Associated Infection Surveillance Network (TRANSNET) prospectively monitored over 32,000 SOT and BMT recipients for invasive fungal infections between 2001 and 2006. *Candida* was the most common invasive fungal infection in the SOT population, and the *Candida* species distribution mirrored that of prior epidemiologic reports. However, in the BMT population where fluconazole prophylaxis is routinely employed, *Aspergillus* has now replaced *Candida* as the most common invasive fungal infection. Further, in BMT recipients, *C. glabrata* was the most common infecting *Candida* species (39%) followed by *C. krusei* (18%) and then *C. albicans* (16%) [392]. The association between *C. parapsilosis* and neonatal candidiasis is less easily explained. It is known that *C. parapsilosis* has the propensity to adhere to foreign material, including intravascular catheters so often used in pediatrics and neonates. In one neonatal study, patients infected with *C. parapsilosis* were more likely to have received >3 days of third-generation cephalosporins compared with those infected with *C. albicans*. [389,393–400]. Exposure of the neonate to *Candida* is vertical and horizontal, and studies have examined the potential link between *C. parapsilosis* infections in neonates and vaginal colonization in the birth mother, as well as skin colonization on the neonate and on the hands of healthcare workers. Though highly suggestive, so far, no definite conclusive link has been established for *C. parapsilosis* [398,399,401–404].

Much effort has been put into defining risk factors associated with the development of invasive candidiasis (IC) in various populations (Table 2.3). For example, in patients admitted to a surgical ICU for more than 48 hours, acute renal failure, total parenteral nutrition, and central venous catheters were significantly associated with the development of candidemia [405]. Other factors that have repeatedly been associated with a risk for invasive candidiasis include receipt of immunosuppressive therapy, cancer and chemotherapy, transplantation, high acuity of illness, increased length of hospital stay, *Candida* colonization at multiple sites, diabetes, and broad-spectrum antibiotics. Unfortunately, using the presence of a single factor to predict infection is not effective since the factors occur frequently in hospitalized patients. A predictive rule for invasive candidiasis in adult ICU patients was developed that consistently identified a population with 9.9% incidence of infection [406]. The definition included patients admitted to a medical or surgical

Table 2.3 Risk factors for invasive candidiasis in adults and neonates

Risk factors for adults and neonates
Acute renal failure/hemodialysis/peritoneal dialysis
Broad spectrum antibiotics
Cancer and chemotherapy
Central venous catheter (CVC)
Colonization with *Candida*
Corticosteroids
Diabetes mellitus
Endotracheal intubation/mechanical ventilation
Immunosuppressive drugs
Neutropenia
Pancreatitis
Prior surgery
Prolonged hospital stay
Total parenteral nutrition (TPN)
Transplant (SOT, HSCT)
Trauma

Additional risk factors for neonates
Age at first enteral feed
DIC/shock
Low APGAR scores Prematurity
Use of H2 blockers
Very low birth weight

Source: Fridkin, S.K. et al., *Pediatrics*, 117, 1680–1687, 2006; Benjamin, D.K. Jr et al., *Pediatrics*, 106, 712–718, 2000; Saiman, L. et al., *Pediatr. Infect Dis. J.*, 20, 1119–1124, 2001; Almirante, B. et al., *J. Clin. Microbiol.*, 44, 1681–1685, 2006; Blumberg, H.M. et al., *Clin. Infect. Dis.*, 33, 177–186, 2001; Ostrosky-Zeichner, L. et al., *Eur. J. Clin. Microbiol. Infect. Dis.*, 26, 271–276, 2007; Colombo, A.L. et al., *J. Clin. Microbiol.*, 44, 2816–2823, 2006; Pappas, P.G. et al., *Clin. Infect. Dis.*, 37(5), 634–643, 2003; Benjamin, D.K. Jr et al. *Pediatrics*, 112, 634–640, 2003; Hajjeh, R.A. et al., *J. Clin. Microbiol.*, 424, 1519–1527, 2004; Ostrosky-Zeichner, L. and Pappas, P.G., *Crit. Care Med.*, 343, 857–863, 2006; Marr, K.A. et al., *J. Infect. Dis.*, 181, 309–316, 2000.

ICU for greater than or equal to 48 hours, and receiving an antibiotic or having a central venous catheter in place during the first 4 days of admission, and found to have any two additional risk factors including: total parenteral nutrition or dialysis on ICU days 1–4, or major surgery, or pancreatitis, or receiving steroids or other immunosuppressive agent within 7 days of ICU admission. Although the definition was highly selective, recruiting only 11% of patients admitted to the ICU, the definition lacked sensitivity (34.1%) for the individual patient [406]. A simpler prediction rule, the "Candida score" has been developed by Leon et al. to guide pre-emptive antifungal therapy in non-neutropenic ICU patients at high-risk of IC [407]. The score is calculated on the basis of the following parameters: surgery, multifocal *Candida* colonization, total parenteral nutrition and severe sepsis. A value equal to or greater than 3 predicted IC with

81% sensitivity and 74% specificity. In further analyses, this score was found to have some interest for its negative predictive value with a 5% incidence of IC for a score <3, but the positive predictive value is relatively low [408].

Other populations at increased risk for candidemia include infants born at 26 weeks, independent of birth weight, and patients who have undergone abdominal surgery [409]. Historically, 80% of HIV-infected patients developed mucosal candidiasis; however, the introduction of highly active antiretroviral therapy (HAART) has resulted in a marked reduction in AIDS-related IC [2].

The clinical presentation of systemic *Candida* infection is variable and nonspecific, and patients with *Candida* infections may or may not appear seriously ill [410]. In a retrospective review of 476 episodes of candidemia, only 7% (37/478) of patients had sepsis syndrome on the date of the first positive blood culture. This was the same for both neutropenic and nonneutropenic patients [411].

Although deep-seated infections such as endocarditis, endophthalmitis, disseminated infection with skin lesions, peritonitis, and chronic disseminated disease have all been well described, fever is the most frequent clinical manifestation (62%, 419/678) [412]. In fact, fever is often the only clinical clue of invasive candidiasis, and in neutropenic patients, fever that persists for 5 days or more despite broad-spectrum antibiotics at adequate doses, and for which a non-infectious cause is not discernible, suggests the presence of invasive candidiasis [418]. Not all patients with candidemia have the same risk of visceral dissemination. Patients with neutropenia have a much higher rate of this complication, and in a review of almost 70 cases of hepatosplenic candidiasis reported in the literature, characteristics include persistent fever in a neutropenic patient whose leukocyte count is returning to normal. The fever is often coupled with abdominal pain, an elevated alkaline phosphatase level, and less commonly, rebound leukocytosis [419]. Characteristic "bull's eye" lesions (target-like abscesses) may be seen with ultrasound, MRI, or CT examination of the liver and spleen, but these lesions are not generally detectable radiographically until neutrophil recovery has occurred.

Although not common, when present, a characteristic macronodular rash may be isolated (extremities, abdomen) or may cover the entire body and is frequently confused with a drug reaction [420]. In a review of 53 documented systemic candidiasis cases, 36% (19/55) had skin lesions. Interestingly, 80% (15/19) of patients that developed skin manifestations were neutropenic [421].

Historically, endophthalmitis was documented to be present in up to 30% of patients with candidemia. Typical lesions of candidal endophthalmitis are whitish chorioretinal spots with filamentous borders protruding into the vitreous and causing vitreal haze. The percent of patients with actual vitreal involvement appears to be decreasing with the earlier initiation of antifungal therapy [422,423]. In a study of 118 patients with candidemia examined within 72 hours of a reported positive blood culture, 9% (11) were documented to have chorioretinal lesions consistent with

fungal chorioretinitis, but no patient had vitreal involvement (endophthalmitis) [424]. Data from a randomized trial comparing fluconazole with amphotericin B for the treatment of candidemia in nonneutropenic patients revealed an incidence of candidal endophthalmitis of only 1% [425]. If a fundoscopic examination is performed at the time that candidemia is either suspected or proven, the majority of patients with positive findings will be asymptomatic [426]. Progressive disease is associated with decreased vision, eye discomfort, foreign body sensation, floaters, and eye redness and pain in cases with advanced iritis [427]. Based on a rabbit model, an appropriate immune response seems to be necessary for *Candida* endophthalmitis to become manifest [428]. Accordingly, neutropenic patients rarely develop clinically apparent candidal endogenous endophthalmitis.

Cryptococcus

Cryptococcus neoformans is an encapsulated yeast that reproduces by multilateral budding [4,429–432]. *C. neoformans* has been isolated from fruit, trees, and soil enriched by bird droppings, whereas *C. gattii* has been found in eucalyptus trees, and possibly firs and oaks as seen in a recent outbreak from British Columbia [433,434]. Aerosolization of infectious particles from disruption of a contaminated environment (soil or trees) leads to inhalation into the respiratory tract as the portal of entry; from here, extrapulmonary spread may ensue. Though the lung and CNS are considered the two primary sites of infection, three other sites frequently involved are skin, prostate, and eye.

Cell-mediated immunity plays a major role in host defenses with granulomatous inflammation essential for containment of the organisms, and conditions that impair cell-mediated immunity render patients more vulnerable to this pathogen. However, it is important to note that in the immunocompetent population, *C. neoformans* and *C. gattii* infections have been reported [434–442].

In the pre-HAART era, cryptococcosis was often seen in HIV-infected individuals, frequently as the presenting AIDS-defining illness. In a population survey conducted in the United States between 1992 and 1994, 86% of *Cryptococcus* cases occurred in HIV-positive individuals [443]. Smoking and outdoor activities, such as building and landscaping, were associated with a higher risk of cryptococcosis, whereas fluconazole in the preceding 3 months conferred protection. Since the advent of HAART, the incidence of cryptococcosis has significantly decreased in developed countries. In the United States, the incidence of cryptococcosis in patients who have HIV/AIDS has decreased from 24 to 66 per 1000 in 1992 to 2–7 per 1000 in 2000 [444]. In France, there was a 46% decrease of the incidence of cryptococcosis during the post-HAART era (1997–2001) [445]. Unfortunately, in developing countries where access to HAART is limited, cryptococcosis continues to be a frequent opportunistic infection [438,446,447].

In immunocompetent hosts, pulmonary and extrapulmonary sites (predominantly the CNS) are affected, and presenting symptoms include cough, fever, chills, dyspnea, anorexia, and possibly night sweats. Pulmonary imaging shows patchy airspace consolidation or nodules, predominantly in the periphery, with cavitation occurring in 40% [439]. Pulmonary and CNS infections are the most common presentations in HIV-positive individuals as well, but other forms such as cutaneous, genitourinary, ocular, and fungemia are also reported [432,448,449]. HIV patients infected with *C. gattii* most often present with symptoms of meningitis although vomiting, cough, dyspnea, and night sweats were also reported [438]. Immune reconstitution inflammatory syndrome (IRIS) occurring after initiating HAART may lead to worsening clinical or radiologic features [432]. Lymphadenitis, CNS findings such as meningitis and mass lesions, and pulmonary cavitation have been reported as part of immune reconstitution in patients with cryptococcosis [450,451].

In SOT recipients, most cryptococcal infections develop late in the posttransplant period compared with other fungal pathogens [452]. In large databases, cryptococcosis accounted for 1%–4% of invasive fungal infections [453–455]. Time to diagnosis after transplant varied from 7 to 21 months, depending on the organ transplanted, and the overall incidence was significantly higher in heart transplant recipients compared to lung, liver, kidney, and small bowel recipients. In one series, 38% of transplant patients with cryptococcosis had isolated pneumonia, 35% had isolated meningitis, and 24% had disseminated disease [453]. In another review, meningitis was the most common presentation (55%) followed by skin and/or osteoarticular involvement (13%) and pneumonia (6%) [454]. The risk for disseminated disease appears to be highest in liver transplant and lowest for lung transplant recipients. In liver transplant recipients, the risk of dissemination was 80% in patients with hepatitis C and 71% in those with alcoholism [456].

Among SOT recipients with cryptococcal pneumonia, dyspnea (95%), cough (76%), and fever (62%) were the predominating symptoms. However, asymptomatic pulmonary cryptococcosis has also been reported in SOT recipients [457]. In such cases, incidental findings on radiographic imaging (ground-glass infiltrates, multiple nodules, or mass with cavitation) led to the histopathological or microbiologic diagnosis. Also of note, up to 25% of SOT recipients with disease limited to the lung had negative serum cryptococcal antigen tests. Positive serum antigen tests were more frequent in disseminated disease (100%) and meningitis (86%) than in isolated pneumonia, suggesting that the latex agglutination test is unreliable for diagnosis of pulmonary cryptococcosis and more invasive methods may be needed [453].

Cryptococcus laurentii is a rare human pathogen in immunocompromised patients. As with *C. neoformans*, this infection is most commonly seen in those with impaired cell-mediated immunity [458]. Based on one review, it appears the presence of an indwelling device confers a significant risk for infection with *C. laurentii*. Infections of the blood and CNS are most frequently reported though infection of lung and other sites have also been described.

Malassezia

The lipophilic yeasts *Malassezia furfur*, *M. pachydermatis*, *M. sympodialis*, and *M. globosa* cause infections such as tinea versicolor, infectious folliculitis, and catheter-related fungemia [459–462]. More invasive infection has been described in immunocompromised hosts, neonates, burn patients, and those receiving intravenous lipids [70,71,112,459,463,464].

Tinea versicolor (pityriasis versicolor) is caused by *Malassezia*, but as taxonomy has evolved, new species have been implicated as the etiologic agent [465]. *M. furfur* was originally claimed to be the etiologic agent, but now *M. globosa* and *M. sympodialis* are also involved, with *M. globosa* occurring in temperate climates [462,466–468]. A distinct presentation was reported in 12 patients with atrophic dermatitis found to have tinea versicolor [460]. The lesions, atrophic plaques and papules, resembled other dermatologic conditions such as mycosis fungoides, SLE, and steroid atrophy. Histology revealed hyphae and spores in an atrophied epidermis and dermis, along with other characteristics that prompted the authors to propose the name atrophying tinea versicolor. *Malassezia* folliculitis, due to *M. furfur* or *M. pachydermatis*, has been reported in heart transplant, kidney transplant, and BMT recipients [469–472]. The rash can present as an acneiform eruption or as folliculitis with a papular or papular-pustular appearance. Fever may precede the rash in BMT recipients [313,471,472].

Malassezia, both *M. furfur* and *M. pachydermatis*, has been implicated in fungemia in adults, children, and infants receiving intravenous lipids or with prolonged catheterization [461,463,464,473,474]. The central venous catheter is most often considered the portal of entry though other sites, such as upper respiratory tract, lung, and urine, may be colonized or infected. Fungemia manifests as fever refractory to antibiotics. Patients may also present with respiratory findings, pulmonary infiltrates, and thrombocytopenia, the latter especially in infants [464,474]. In one series of 3044 BMT recipients, infection with *M. furfur* was reported in 6 patients over a 25-year period. These infections occurred at a median of 59 days posttransplant and the majority of the infections (5/6) were in allogeneic recipients. The spectrum of disease ranged from infection of the mucosal surface and skin (folliculitis) to catheter-related fungemia. No patient in this group had pulmonary involvement [472].

Trichosporon

Trichosporon species are opportunist basidiomycetous yeasts that cause infections in immunocompromised patients [70,71,313]. Distinct subgroups with different morphologic, biochemical, and genetic profiles are members of the genus, which may lead to confusion. The taxonomy of the genus *Trichosporon* has been deeply revised since 1994, including now 50 species, of which about 17 are considered clinically relevant [475]. Notably, the name *Trichosporon beigelii* is no longer in use and has been replaced by several species.

Trichosporon spp., saprophytic yeasts usually found in the soil, can be cultured from human skin, stool, and urine. These organisms have been implicated as the etiologic agent of white piedra, an infection of the distal end of the hair shaft, as well as causing cutaneous infections in immunocompetent patients [476–478]. In immunosuppressed patients, particularly in those with underlying malignancy, it has been implicated as the cause of fungemia, renal insufficiency, pulmonary infiltrates, cutaneous lesions, chorioretinitis, and chronic hepatic trichosporonosis [479–488]. An increasing incidence of trichosporonosis has been reported over the last decade [489,490]. Increasing use of echinocandins, to which *Trichosporon* spp. are intrinsically resistant, may be involved in this changing epidemiology. A recent review of 203 cases of invasive trichosporonosis reported in the literature since 1994 shows that the disease affects mainly patients with hematologic cancers (39%), especially those with neutropenia [490]. Other populations at risk include patients with other immunosuppressive conditions and newborns (21% and 12% of cases, respectively). *T. asahii* was the most frequent pathogenic agent (46.7% of cases), followed by *T. inkin* and *T. mucoides/dermatis*. Fongemia was present in 74% of cases. Other affected organs were skin, lung, liver/spleen, intestinal tract, brain and eye.

Rhodotorula

Rhodotorula spp. are ubiquitous basidiomycetous yeasts and opportunistic human pathogens. Most cases of *Rhodotorula* infections are fungemia (mainly central venous catheter-related) occurring in patients with underlying immunosuppression or cancer [491,492]. *Rhodotorula* spp. are responsible for less than 1% of fungemia, but are, with *Trichosporon* spp., the most frequent non-*Candida* yeasts causing bloodstream infections [493,494]. Eye infections, peritonitis associated with peritoneal dialysis, endocarditis and meningitis have also been reported. *R. mucilaginosa* account for most cases, while *R. glutinis* and *R. minuta* account for the few remaining cases. *Rhodotorula* spp. are intrinsically resistant to azoles and echinocandins and may cause breakthrough infections in onco-hematological patients receiving antifungal prophylaxis [495]. *Rhodotorula* infections are difficult to treat because of the absence of alternative therapy to amphotericin B.

Saccharomyces

Saccharomyces cerevisiae is a yeast used in the food industry for beers, wines and bakery products, and it is also part of the normal flora of the gastrointestinal tract, respiratory tract, and vaginal mucosa. *Saccharomyces boulardii*, which is now considered as a variety of *S. cerevisiae*, is used in probiotics for the prevention or treatment of antibiotic-related diarrhea. *Saccharomyces* fungemia has been increasingly reported during the last decade and has been associated with the use of probiotics [496]. In addition to translocation from the gastrointestinal tract, intravenous cather infection can also be a port of entry. Fungemia may occur in immunocompromised as well as immunocompetent patients. In a review of 60 cases of *S. cerevisiae* fungemia, 60% of patients were in the ICU, 71% were receiving enteral or parenteral nutrition, 93% had a central venous catheter and 88% were receiving broad-spectrum antibacterial therapy and the use of probiotics was reported for 46% [496]. In addition to fungemia, other clinical presentations of *S. cerevisiae* infections include: endocarditis, liver abscess, esophagitis, peritonitis, pneumonia or empyema, urinary tract infection and vaginitis [496,497]. The presence of antibodies to *S. cerevisiae* has also been associated with Crohn disease [498].

Geotrichum

Geotrichum candidum is a filamentous yeast forming arthroconidia that colonizes the gastrointestinal and respiratory tract. Although *G. candidum* is frequently encountered in stool specimens of onco-hematological patients receiving azole prophylaxis [499], it rarely causes invasive disease. In a review of 12 cases of *Geotrichum* disseminated infections reported in the literature from 1971 to 2007, 8 (67%) occurred in patients with underlying malignancies [500]. Fungemia was present in 7 (58%) cases. Other infection sites included lungs, gastro-intestinal tract, liver, spleen, kidney, brain, lymph nodes, bone marrow and skin.

Pneumocystis

Pneumocystis pneumonia (PCP), due to *P. jiroveci* (previously *P. carinii* f. sp. *hominis*), remains one of the most feared complications of immunosuppression due to its significant morbidity and mortality [501,502]. Though the genus *Pneumocystis* has been known for years, taxonomic assignment of *Pneumocystis* has placed it with either fungi or protozoa, with phylogenetic data and characteristics that would lend credence to having it belong to either [503]. Furthermore, DNA sequence analyses have revealed DNA diversity of the organism in different host species. This has led to a renaming of the species that infects humans to *P. jiroveci* [501,504]. The term PCP, however, is still used to refer to *Pneumocystis* pneumonia in humans. The organism has different morphologic forms in its life cycle, including trophozoites, cysts, and intracystic bodies (sporozoites), and the portal of entry appears to be inhalational though the infective form is unknown [505]. The incidence of disease relates to the degree of immunosuppression, with impairment in T-cell–mediated responses lending increased susceptibility. Patients with HIV/AIDS, with CD4 less than 200 cells/mm3, who are not receiving HAART or who do not receive PCP prophy-laxis, and patients iatrogenically immunosuppressed after transplant are especially vulnerable [506,507].

Pneumocystis jiroveci is widespread though its source in nature has not been identified [507]. As the organism is host specific, transmission likely occurs from human to human [508–510]. Exposure seems to occur in early childhood, with antibodies to *Pneumocystis* detected in 85% of children up to 20 months of age [511,512]. Under usual circumstances, little or no respiratory symptoms develop during this primary exposure, though some infants may present with a self-limiting upper respiratory tract infection, and some children have presented with bronchiolitis [513–515]. Adults have also been found to be colonized with *P. jiroveci,* and patients with chronic lung disease may be at an increased risk of colonization [516–519]. Thus, both children and adults may play a role in the epidemiology of *Pneumocystis,* serving as potential reservoirs. Immunosuppressed individuals may be newly exposed to *P. jiroveci* or experience reactivation of latent *Pneumocystis* infection, and disease may result from either recent acquisition or reactivation of longstanding, dormant organisms [520]. Nosocomial transmission of PCP has been reported [510].

PCP was the first AIDS-defining illness, and as the HIV epidemic has evolved, the epidemiology of PCP has also changed, especially after the advent of HAART [502,521]. In patients with HIV/AIDS, PCP usually presents as a subacute onset of dyspnea, nonproductive cough, and occasionally low-grade fever. The patient may present with tachypnea and tachycardia but unremarkable lung exam. Hypoxemia is present in the more severe cases, reflecting a high burden of organism and host inflammatory response. Chest imaging often reveals bilateral perihilar interstitial infiltrates, which can become diffuse, alveolar, or confluent if the disease progresses [507,522]. Imaging with CT scan reveals ground glass opacities in a perihilar, patchy or geographic distribution, with thickening of the interlobular septa. Affected areas may be interspersed with normal parenchyma. Less often, CT of *Pneumocystis* pneumonia will reveal large cystic lesions, often multiple, which carry a high risk of pneumothorax [523]. Other less common imaging findings include mass lesions, nodules, consolidation, pleural effusion, and lymph node involvement [522].

Although PCP has historically presented in patients with HIV/AIDS, it has also been reported in patients with other underlying immunosuppressive conditions such as hematologic malignancies, inflammatory and autoimmune diseases, and in patients receiving cytotoxic drugs or prolonged corticosteroid therapy, particularly after BMT and SOT [502,524–533]. A 2% incidence of PCP has been reported in lung transplant recipients in the absence of prophylaxis [533]. Concomitant conditions, which may play a role in increasing the risk of PCP in both SOT and BMT recipients, include the presence of CMV, rejection (including GvHD), and an increase in immunosuppressive therapy [503,531–535]. The mean time to diagnosis is 20 weeks posttansplantation, with 54% of patients developing PCP within 6 months of transplant. The incidence in the first year posttransplant is 8 times higher than subsequent years. The incidence also varies by transplanted organ, with lung recipients having the highest (22 cases per 1000 patient years) and kidney recipients having the lowest (0.8 cases per 1000 patient years) rates [533]. PCP in transplant patients mirrors the presentation in HIV/AIDS patients, although atypical pneumonias with no infiltrates, unilateral infiltrates, alveolar infiltrates, granulomata, nodules, and cavities, and even asymptomatic infection, have been reported [529,536–538].

In general, PCP rarely develops in patients receiving prophylaxis, and observed cases are mostly attributed to noncompliance [539]. In the rare instances when breakthrough PCP infection in patients on prophylaxis with adequate systemic absorption occurs, the infection may be atypical in presentation and require lung biopsy for diagnosis [503].

REFERENCES

1. Ascioglu S, Rex JH, de Pauw B, et al. Defining opportunistic invasive fungal infections in immunocompromised patients with cancer and hematopoietic stem cell transplants: An international consensus. *Clin Infect Dis.* 2002;34(1):7–14.
2. Warnock DW. Trends in the epidemiology of invasive fungal infections. *Nihon Ishinkin Gakkai Zasshi.* 2007;48(1):1–12.
3. Richardson M, Lass-Florl C. Changing epidemiology of systemic fungal infections. *Clin Microbiol Infect.* 2008;14 Suppl 4:5–24.
4. Marr KA, Patterson T, Denning D. Aspergillosis. Pathogenesis, clinical manifestations, and therapy. *Infect Dis Clin North Am.* 2002;16(4):875–894, vi.
5. Anaissie E, McGinnis MR, Pfaller M. *Clinical Mycology,* 1st ed. Philadelphia, PA: Church Livingstone. 2003.
6. Samson RA, Visagie CM, Houbraken J, et al. Phylogeny, identification and nomenclature of the genus *Aspergillus. Studies in Mycology.* 2014;78:141–173.
7. Hachem RY, Kontoyiannis DP, Boktour MR, et al. *Aspergillus terreus*: An emerging amphotericin B-resistant opportunistic mold in patients with hematologic malignancies. *Cancer.* 2004;101(7):1594–1600.
8. Iwen PC, Rupp ME, Langnas AN, Reed EC, Hinrichs SH. Invasive pulmonary aspergillosis due to *Aspergillus terreus*: 12-year experience and review of the literature. *Clin Infect Dis.* 1998;26(5):1092–1097.
9. Tritz DM, Woods GL. Fatal disseminated infection with *Aspergillus terreus* in immunocompromised hosts. *Clin Infect Dis.* 1993;16(1):118–122.
10. Steinbach WJ, Benjamin DK, Jr., Kontoyiannis DP, et al. Infections due to *Aspergillus terreus*: A multicenter retrospective analysis of 83 cases. *Clin Infect Dis.* 2004;39(2):192–198.

11. Verweij PE, van den Bergh MF, Rath PM, de Pauw BE, Voss A, Meis JF. Invasive aspergillosis caused by *Aspergillus ustus*: Case report and review. *J Clin Microbiol.* 1999;37(5):1606–1609.

12. Pavie J, Lacroix C, Hermoso DG, et al. Breakthrough disseminated *Aspergillus ustus* infection in allogeneic hematopoietic stem cell transplant recipients receiving voriconazole or caspofungin prophylaxis. *J Clin Microbiol.* 2005;43(9):4902–4904.

13. Balajee SA, Kano R, Baddley JW, et al. Molecular identification of *Aspergillus* species collected for the Transplant-Associated Infection Surveillance Network. *J Clin Microbiol.* 2009;47(10):3138–3141.

14. Alastruey-Izquierdo A, Mellado E, Pelaez T, et al. Population-based survey of filamentous fungi and antifungal resistance in Spain (FILPOP Study). *Antimicrob Agents Chemother.* 2013;57(7):3380–3387.

15. Alcazar-Fuoli L, Mellado E, Alastruey-Izquierdo A, Cuenca-Estrella M, Rodriguez-Tudela JL. *Aspergillus* section Fumigati: Antifungal susceptibility patterns and sequence-based identification. *Antimicrob Agents Chemother.* 2008;52(4):1244–1251.

16. Soubani AO, Chandrasekar PH. The clinical spectrum of pulmonary aspergillosis. *Chest.* 2002;121(6):1988–1999.

17. Kumar R. Mild, moderate, and severe forms of allergic bronchopulmonary aspergillosis: A clinical and serologic evaluation. *Chest.* 2003;124(3):890–892.

18. Kumar R, Gaur SN. Prevalence of allergic bronchopulmonary aspergillosis in patients with bronchial asthma. *Asian Pac J Allergy Immunol.* 2000;18(4):181–185.

19. Stevens DA, Moss RB, Kurup VP, et al. Allergic bronchopulmonary aspergillosis in cystic fibrosis— state of the art: Cystic Fibrosis Foundation Consensus Conference. *Clin Infect Dis.* 2003;37 Suppl 3:S225–S264.

20. Kraemer R, Delosea N, Ballinari P, Gallati S, Crameri R. Effect of allergic bronchopulmonary aspergillosis on lung function in children with cystic fibrosis. *Am J Respir Crit Care Med.* 2006;174(11):1211–1220.

21. Kunst H, Wickremasinghe M, Wells A, Wilson R. Nontuberculous mycobacterial disease and *Aspergillus*-related lung disease in bronchiectasis. *Eur Respir J.* 2006;28(2):352–357.

22. Taj-Aldeen SJ, Hilal AA, Schell WA. Allergic fungal rhinosinusitis: A report of 8 cases. *Am J Otolaryngol.* 2004;25(3):213–218.

23. Dufour X, Kauffmann-Lacroix C, Ferrie JC, Goujon JM, Rodier MH, Klossek JM. Paranasal sinus fungus ball: Epidemiology, clinical features and diagnosis— A retrospective analysis of 173 cases from a single medical center in France, 1989–2002. *Med Mycol.* 2006;44(1):61–67.

24. Parikh SL, Venkatraman G, DelGaudio JM. Invasive fungal sinusitis: A 15-year review from a single institution. *Am J Rhinol.* 2004;18(2):75–81.

25. Karnak D, Avery RK, Gildea TR, Sahoo D, Mehta AC. Endobronchial fungal disease: An under-recognized entity. *Respiration.* 2007;74(1):88–104.

26. Mehrad B, Paciocco G, Martinez FJ, Ojo TC, Iannettoni MD, Lynch JP, 3rd Spectrum of *Aspergillus* infection in lung transplant recipients: Case series and review of the literature. *Chest.* 2001;119(1):169–175.

27. Hadjiliadis D, Howell DN, Davis RD, et al. Anastomotic infections in lung transplant recipients. *Ann Transplant.* 2000;5(3):13–19.

28. Trullas JC, Cervera C, Benito N, et al. Invasive pulmonary aspergillosis in solid organ and bone marrow transplant recipients. *Transplant Proc.* 2005;37(9):4091–4093.

29. Greene RE, Schlamm HT, Oestmann JW, et al. Imaging findings in acute invasive pulmonary aspergillosis: Clinical significance of the halo sign. *Clin Infect Dis.* 2007;44(3):373–379.

30. Caillot D, Couaillier JF, Bernard A, et al. Increasing volume and changing characteristics of invasive pulmonary aspergillosis on sequential thoracic computed tomography scans in patients with neutropenia. *J Clin Oncol.* 2001;19(1):253–259.

31. Pfeiffer CD, Fine JP, Safdar N. Diagnosis of invasive aspergillosis using a galactomannan assay: A meta-analysis. *Clin Infect Dis.* 2006;42(10):1417–1427.

32. Lamoth F, Cruciani M, Mengoli C, et al. Beta-Glucan antigenemia assay for the diagnosis of invasive fungal infections in patients with hematological malignancies: A systematic review and meta-analysis of cohort studies from the Third European Conference on Infections in Leukemia (ECIL-3). *Clin Infect Dis.* 2012;54(5):633–643.

33. Mengoli C, Cruciani M, Barnes RA, Loeffler J, Donnelly JP. Use of PCR for diagnosis of invasive aspergillosis: Systematic review and meta-analysis. *Lancet Infect Dis.* 2009;9(2):89–96.

34. Maertens J, Theunissen K, Verhoef G, et al. Galactomannan and computed tomography-based preemptive antifungal therapy in neutropenic patients at high risk for invasive fungal infection: A prospective feasibility study. *Clin Infect Dis.* 2005;41(9):1242–1250.

35. De Pauw B, Walsh TJ, Donnelly JP, et al. Revised definitions of invasive fungal disease from the European Organization for Research and Treatment of Cancer/ Invasive Fungal Infections Cooperative Group and the National Institute of Allergy and Infectious Diseases Mycoses Study Group (EORTC/MSG) Consensus Group. *Clin Infect Dis.* 2008;46(12):1813–1821.

36. Jantunen E, Piilonen A, Volin L, et al. Diagnostic aspects of invasive *Aspergillus* infections in allogeneic BMT recipients. *Bone Marrow Transplant.* 2000;25(8):867–871.

37. Kleinschmidt-DeMasters BK. Central nervous system aspergillosis: A 20-year retrospective series. *Hum Pathol.* 2002;33(1):116–124.

38. Gabelmann A, Klein S, Kern W, et al. Relevant imaging findings of cerebral aspergillosis on MRI: A retrospective case-based study in immunocompromised patients. *Eur J Neurol.* 2007;14(5):548–555.

39. Kontoyiannis DP, Marr KA, Park BJ, et al. Prospective surveillance for invasive fungal infections in hematopoietic stem cell transplant recipients, 2001–2006: Overview of the Transplant-Associated Infection Surveillance Network (TRANSNET) Database. *Clin Infect Dis.* 2010;50(8):1091–1100.

40. Pappas PG. Cryptococcosis in the developing world: An elephant in the parlor. *Clin Infect Dis.* 2010;50(3):345–346.

41. Steinbach WJ, Marr KA, Anaissie EJ, et al. Clinical epidemiology of 960 patients with invasive aspergillosis from the PATH Alliance registry. *J Infect.* 2012;65(5):453–464.

42. Maertens JA, Raad II, Marr KA, et al. Isavuconazole versus voriconazole for primary treatment of invasive mould disease caused by Aspergillus and other filamentous fungi (SECURE): A phase 3, randomised-controlled, non-inferiority trial. *Lancet.* 2016;387(10020):760–769.

43. Marr KA, Schlamm HT, Herbrecht R, et al. Combination antifungal therapy for invasive aspergillosis: A randomized trial. *Ann Intern Med.* 2015;162(2):81–89.

44. Marr KA, Carter RA, Crippa F, Wald A, Corey L. Epidemiology and outcome of mould infections in hematopoietic stem cell transplant recipients. *Clin Infect Dis.* 2002;34(7):909–917.

45. Marr KA, Carter RA, Boeckh M, Martin P, Corey L. Invasive aspergillosis in allogeneic stem cell transplant recipients: Changes in epidemiology and risk factors. *Blood.* 2002;100(13):4358–4366.

46. Wald A, Leisenring W, van Burik JA, Bowden RA. Epidemiology of *Aspergillus* infections in a large cohort of patients undergoing bone marrow transplantation. *J Infect Dis.* 1997;175(6):1459–1466.

47. Kontoyiannis DP, Lionakis MS, Lewis RE, et al. Zygomycosis in a tertiary-care cancer center in the era of *Aspergillus*-active antifungal therapy: A case-control observational study of 27 recent cases. *J Infect Dis.* 2005;191(8):1350–1360.

48. Silveira FP, Husain S. Fungal infections in solid organ transplantation. *Med Mycol.* 2007;45(4):305–320.

49. Singh N, Avery RK, Munoz P, et al. Trends in risk profiles for and mortality associated with invasive aspergillosis among liver transplant recipients. *Clin Infect Dis.* 2003;36(1):46–52.

50. Singh N, Paterson DL. Aspergillus infections in transplant recipients. *Clin Microbiol Rev.* 2005;18(1):44–69.

51. Singh N, Husain S. Aspergillus infections after lung transplantation: Clinical differences in type of transplant and implications for management. *J Heart Lung Transplant.* 2003;22(3):258–266.

52. George MJ, Snydman DR, Werner BG, et al. The independent role of cytomegalovirus as a risk factor for invasive fungal disease in orthotopic liver transplant recipients. Boston Center for Liver Transplantation CMVIG-Study Group. Cytogam, MedImmune, Inc. Gaithersburg, Maryland. *Am J Med.* 1997;103(2):106–113.

53. Osawa M, Ito Y, Hirai T, et al. Risk factors for invasive aspergillosis in living donor liver transplant recipients. *Liver Transpl.* 2007;13(4):566–570.

54. Munoz P, Rodriguez C, Bouza E, et al. Risk factors of invasive aspergillosis after heart transplantation: Protective role of oral itraconazole prophylaxis. *Am J Transplant.* 2004;4(4):636–643.

55. Panackal AA, Dahlman A, Keil KT, et al. Outbreak of invasive aspergillosis among renal transplant recipients. *Transplantation.* 2003;75(7):1050–1053.

56. Meersseman W, Vandecasteele SJ, Wilmer A, Verbeken E, Peetermans WE, Van Wijngaerden E. Invasive aspergillosis in critically ill patients without malignancy. *Am J Respir Crit Care Med.* 2004;170(6):621–625.

57. Cornillet A, Camus C, Nimubona S, et al. Comparison of epidemiological, clinical, and biological features of invasive aspergillosis in neutropenic and nonneutropenic patients: A 6-year survey. *Clin Infect Dis.* 2006;43(5):577–584.

58. Alshabani K, Haq A, Miyakawa R, Palla M, Soubani AO. Invasive pulmonary aspergillosis in patients with influenza infection: Report of two cases and systematic review of the literature. *Expert Rev Respir Med.* 2015;9(1):89–96.

59. Alexander B, Schell W. Hyalohyphomycosis. In: Kauffman CA, Mandell GL, eds. *Atlas of Fungal Infections*, 2nd ed. Philadelphia, PA: Current Medicine Group, Inc. 2006:253–266.

60. Schell WA. New aspects of emerging fungal pathogens: A multifaceted challenge. *Clin Lab Med.* 1995;15(2):365–387.

61. Alfonso JF, Baamonde MB, Santos MJ, Astudillo A, Fernandez-Vega L. Acremonium fungal infection in 4 patients after laser in situ keratomileusis. *J Cataract Refract Surg.* 2004;30(1):262–267.

62. Wang MX, Shen DJ, Liu JC, Pflugfelder SC, Alfonso EC, Forster RK. Recurrent fungal keratitis and endophthalmitis. *Cornea.* 2000;19(4):558–560.

63. Rodriguez-Ares T, De Rojas Silva V, Ferreiros MP, Becerra EP, Tome CC, Sanchez-Salorio M. *Acremonium keratitis* in a patient with herpetic neurotrophic corneal disease. *Acta Ophthalmol Scand.* 2000;78(1):107–109.

64. Read RW, Chuck RS, Rao NA, Smith RE. Traumatic Acremonium atrogriseum keratitis following laser-assisted in situ keratomileusis. *Arch Ophthalmol.* 2000;118(3):418–421.

65. Erbagci Z, Tuncel AA, Erkilic S, Zer Y. Successful treatment of antifungal- and cryotherapy-resistant subcutaneous hyalohyphomycosis in an immuno-competent case with topical 5% imiquimod cream. *Mycopathologia*. 2005;159(4):521–526.

66. Anadolu R, Hilmioglu S, Oskay T, Boyvat A, Peksari Y, Gurgey E. Indolent *Acremonium strictum* infec-tion in an immunocompetent patient. *Int J Dermatol*. 2001;40(7):451–453.

67. Zaitz C, Porto E, Heins-Vaccari EM, et al. Subcutaneous hyalohyphomycosis caused by *Acremonium recifei*: Case report. *Rev Inst Med Trop Sao Paulo*. 1995;37(3):267–270.

68. Negroni R, Lopez Daneri G, Arechavala A, Bianchi MH, Robles AM. Clinical and microbiological study of mycetomas at the Muniz hospital of Buenos Aires between 1989 and 2004. *Rev Argent Microbiol*. 2006;38(1):13–18.

69. Venugopal PV, Venugopal TV. Pale grain eumy-cetomas in Madras. *Australas J Dermatol*. 1995;36(3):149–151.

70. Groll AH, Walsh TJ. Uncommon opportunistic fungi: New nosocomial threats. *Clin Microbiol Infect*. 2001;7 Suppl 2:8–24.

71. Perfect JR, Schell WA. The new fungal opportun-ists are coming. *Clin Infect Dis*. 1996;22 Suppl 2:S112–S118.

72. Schell WA, Perfect JR. Fatal, disseminated *Acremonium strictum* infection in a neutropenic host. *J Clin Microbiol*. 1996;34(5):1333–1336.

73. Miyakis S, Velegraki A, Delikou S, et al. Invasive *Acremonium strictum* infection in a bone mar-row transplant recipient. *Pediatr Infect Dis J*. 2006;25(3):273–275.

74. Novicki TJ, LaFe K, Bui L, et al. Genetic diversity among clinical isolates of *Acremonium strictum* determined during an investigation of a fatal myco-sis. *J Clin Microbiol*. 2003;41(6):2623–2628.

75. Heins-Vaccari EM, Machado CM, Saboya RS, et al. *Phialemonium curvatum* infection after bone mar-row transplantation. *Rev Inst Med Trop Sao Paulo*. 2001;43(3):163–166.

76. Breton P, Germaud P, Morin O, Audouin AF, Milpied N, Harousseau JL. Rare pulmonary mycoses in patients with hematologic diseases. *Rev Pneumol Clin*. 1998;54(5):253–257.

77. Geyer AS, Fox LP, Husain S, Della-Latta P, Grossman ME. *Acremonium* mycetoma in a heart transplant recipient. *J Am Acad Dermatol*. 2006;55(6):1095–1100.

78. Mattei D, Mordini N, Lo Nigro C, et al. Successful treatment of *Acremonium* fungemia with voricon-azole. *Mycoses*. 2003;46(11–12):511–514.

79. Yalaz M, Hilmioglu S, Metin D, et al. Fatal dissemi-nated *Acremonium strictum* infection in a preterm newborn: A very rare cause of neonatal septicaemia. *J Med Microbiol*. 2003;52(Pt 9):835–837.

80. Roilides E, Bibashi E, Acritidou E, et al. *Acremonium fungemia* in two immunocompromised children. *Pediatr Infect Dis J*. 1995;14(6):548–550.

81. Nedret Koc A, Erdem F, Patiroglu T. Case Report. *Acremonium falciforme* fungemia in a patient with acute leukaemia. *Mycoses*. 2002;45(5–6):202–203.

82. Warris A, Wesenberg F, Gaustad P, Verweij PE, Abrahamsen TG. *Acremonium strictum* fungaemia in a paediatric patient with acute leukaemia. *Scand J Infect Dis*. 2000;32(4):442–444.

83. Ioakimidou A, Vyzantiadis TA, Sakellari I, et al. An unusual cluster of *Acremonium kiliense* fungaemias in a haematopoietic cell transplantation unit. *Diagn Microbiol Infect Dis*. 2013;75(3):313–316.

84. Paya CV. Fungal infections in solid-organ transplan-tation. *Clin Infect Dis*. 1993;16(5):677–688.

85. Nucci M, Varon AG, Garnica M, et al. Increased inci-dence of invasive fusariosis with cutaneous portal of entry, Brazil. *Emerg Infect Dis*. 2013;19(10):1567–1572.

86. Nucci M, Garnica M, Gloria AB, et al. Invasive fungal diseases in haematopoietic cell transplant recipi-ents and in patients with acute myeloid leukaemia or myelodysplasia in Brazil. *Clin Microbiol Infect*. 2013;19(8):745–751.

87. Nucci M, Anaissie E. *Fusarium* infections in immu-nocompromised patients. *Clin Microbiol Rev*. 2007;20(4):695–704.

88. Nucci M, Marr KA, Queiroz-Telles F, et al. *Fusarium* infection in hematopoietic stem cell transplant recipients. *Clin Infect Dis*. 2004;38(9):1237–1242.

89. Nucci M, Anaissie EJ, Queiroz-Telles F, et al. Outcome predictors of 84 patients with hemato-logic malignancies and *Fusarium* infection. *Cancer*. 2003;98(2):315–319.

90. Garnica M, da Cunha MO, Portugal R, Maiolino A, Colombo AL, Nucci M. Risk factors for invasive fusa-riosis in patients with acute myeloid leukemia and in hematopoietic cell transplant recipients. *Clin Infect Dis*. 2015;60(6):875–880.

91. Nir-Paz R, Strahilevitz J, Shapiro M, et al. Clinical and epidemiological aspects of infections caused by *Fusarium* species: A collaborative study from Israel. *J Clin Microbiol*. 2004;42(8):3456–3461.

92. Fusarium keratitis—multiple states, 2006. *MMWR Morb Mortal Wkly Rep*. 2006;55(14):400–401.

93. Chang DC, Grant GB, O'Donnell K, et al. Multistate outbreak of *Fusarium keratitis* associated with use of a contact lens solution. *JAMA*. 2006;296(8):953–963.

94. Anaissie EJ, Kuchar RT, Rex JH, et al. Fusariosis asso-ciated with pathogenic *Fusarium* species colonization of a hospital water system: A new paradigm for the epidemiology of opportunistic mold infections. *Clin Infect Dis*. 2001;33(11):1871–1878.

95. Dykewicz MS, Laufer P, Patterson R, Roberts M, Sommers HM. Woodman's disease: Hypersensitivity pneumonitis from cutting live trees. *J Allergy Clin Immunol*. 1988;81(2):455–460.

96. Muller-Wening D, Renck T, Neuhauss M. Wood chip alveolitis. *Pneumologie.* 1999;53(7):364–368.

97. Wright K, Popli S, Gandhi VC, Lentino JR, Reyes CV, Leehey DJ. *Paecilomyces peritonitis:* Case report and review of the literature. *Clin Nephrol.* 2003;59(4):305–310.

98. Gutierrez F, Masia M, Ramos J, Elia M, Mellado E, Cuenca-Estrella M. Pulmonary mycetoma caused by an atypical isolate of *Paecilomyces* species in an immunocompetent individual: Case report and literature review of *Paecilomyces* lung infections. *Eur J Clin Microbiol Infect Dis.* 2005;24(9):607–611.

99. Torres R, Gonzalez M, Sanhueza M, et al. Outbreak of *Paecilomyces variotii* peritonitis in peritoneal dialysis patients after the 2010 Chilean earthquake. *Perit Dial Int.* 2014;34(3):322–325.

100. Marzec A, Heron LG, Pritchard RC, et al. *Paecilomyces variotii* in peritoneal dialysate. *J Clin Microbiol.* 1993;31(9):2392–2395.

101. Wang SM, Shieh CC, Liu CC. Successful treatment of *Paecilomyces variotii* splenic abscesses: A rare complication in a previously unrecognized chronic granulomatous disease child. *Diagn Microbiol Infect Dis.* 2005;53(2):149–152.

102. Salle V, Lecuyer E, Chouaki T, et al. *Paecilomyces variotii* fungemia in a patient with multiple myeloma: Case report and literature review. *J Infect.* 2005;51(3):e93–e95.

103. Kantarcioglu AS, Hatemi G, Yucel A, De Hoog GS, Mandel NM. *Paecilomyces variotii* central nervous system infection in a patient with cancer. *Mycoses.* 2003;46(1–2):45–50.

104. Chamilos G, Kontoyiannis DP. Voriconazole-resistant disseminated *Paecilomyces variotii* infection in a neutropenic patient with leukaemia on voriconazole prophylaxis. *J Infect.* 2005;51(4):e225–e228.

105. Pastor FJ, Guarro J. Clinical manifestations, treatment and outcome of *Paecilomyces lilacinus* infections. *Clin Microbiol Infect.* 2006;12(10):948–960.

106. Safdar A. Progressive cutaneous hyalohyphomycosis due to *Paecilomyces lilacinus:* Rapid response to treatment with caspofungin and itraconazole. *Clin Infect Dis.* 2002;34(10):1415–1417.

107. Garbino J, Ondrusova A, Baglivo E, Lew D, Bouchuiguir-Wafa K, Rohner P. Successful treatment of *Paecilomyces lilacinus* endophthalmitis with voriconazole. *Scand J Infect Dis.* 2002;34(9):701–703.

108. Chung PC, Lin H, Hwang YS, Tsai YJ, Ngan KW, Huang SC, Hsiao CH. *Paecilomyces lilacinus scleritis* with secondary keratitis. *Cornea.* 2007;26(2):232–234.

109. Orth B, Frei R, Itin PH, et al. Outbreak of invasive mycoses caused by *Paecilomyces lilacinus* from a contaminated skin lotion. *Ann Intern Med.* 1996;125(10):799–806.

110. Itin PH, Frei R, Lautenschlager S, et al. Cutaneous manifestations of *Paecilomyces lilacinus* infection induced by a contaminated skin lotion in patients who are severely immunosuppressed. *J Am Acad Dermatol.* 1998;39(3):401–409.

111. Hall VC, Goyal S, Davis MD, Walsh JS. Cutaneous hyalohyphomycosis caused by *Paecilomyces lilacinus:* Report of three cases and review of the literature. *Int J Dermatol.* 2004;43(9):648–653.

112. Jahagirdar BN, Morrison VA. Emerging fungal pathogens in patients with hematologic malignancies and marrow/stem-cell transplant recipients. *Semin Respir Infect.* 2002;17(2):113–120.

113. Revankar SG, Patterson JE, Sutton DA, Pullen R, Rinaldi MG. Disseminated phaeohyphomycosis: Review of an emerging mycosis. *Clin Infect Dis.* 2002;34(4):467–476.

114. Malloch D, Salkin I. A new species of *Scedosporium* associated with osteomyelitis in humans. *Mycotaxon.* 1984;21(October–December):247–255.

115. Berenguer J, Rodriguez-Tudela JL, Richard C, et al. Deep infections caused by *Scedosporium prolificans:* A report on 16 cases in Spain and a review of the literature: Scedosporium Prolificans Spanish Study Group. *Medicine (Baltimore).* 1997;76(4):256–265.

116. Wood GM, McCormack JG, Muir DB, et al. Clinical features of human infection with *Scedosporium inflatum. Clin Infect Dis.* 1992;14(5):1027–1033.

117. Idigoras P, Pérez-Trallero E, Pineiro L, et al. Disseminated infection and colonization by *Scedosporium prolificans:* A review of 18 cases, 1990–1999. *Clin Infect Dis.* 2001;32(11):E158–E165.

118. Wilson CM, O'Rourke EJ, McGinnis MR, et al. *Scedosporium inflatum:* Clinical spectrum of a newly recognized pathogen. *J Infect Dis.* 1990;161(1):102–107.

119. Castiglioni B, Sutton DA, Rinaldi MG, Fung J, Kusne S. *Pseudallescheria boydii* (Anamorph Scedosporium apiospermum): Infection in solid organ transplant recipients in a tertiary medical center and review of the literature. *Medicine (Baltimore).* 2002;81(5):333–348.

120. Park BJ, Pappas PG, Wannemuehler KA, et al. Invasive non-Aspergillus mold infections in transplant recipients, United States, 2001–2006. *Emerg Infect Dis.* 2011;17(10):1855–1864.

121. Johnson LS, Shields RK, Clancy CJ. Epidemiology, clinical manifestations, and outcomes of Scedosporium infections among solid organ transplant recipients. *Transpl Infect Dis.* 2014;16(4):578–587.

122. Husain S, Munoz P, Forrest G, et al. Infections due to *Scedosporium apiospermum* and *Scedosporium prolificans* in transplant recipients: Clinical characteristics and impact of antifungal agent therapy on outcome. *Clin Infect Dis.* 2005;40(1):89–99.

123. Lamaris GA, Chamilos G, Lewis RE, Safdar A, Raad, II, Kontoyiannis DP. *Scedosporium* infection in a tertiary care cancer center: A review of 25 cases from 1989–2006. *Clin Infect Dis.* 2006;43(12):1580–1584.

124. Rodriguez-Tudela JL, Berenguer J, Guarro J, et al. Epidemiology and outcome of *Scedosporium prolificans* infection, a review of 162 cases. *Med Mycol.* 2009;47(4):359–370.

125. Cimon B, Carrere J, Vinatier JF, Chazalette JP, Chabasse D, Bouchara JP. Clinical significance of *Scedosporium apiospermum* in patients with cystic fibrosis. *Eur J Clin Microbiol Infect Dis.* 2000;19(1):53–56.

126. Defontaine A, Zouhair R, Cimon B, et al. Genotyping study of *Scedosporium apiospermum* isolates from patients with cystic fibrosis. *J Clin Microbiol.* 2002;40(6):2108–2114.

127. Symoens F, Knoop C, Schrooyen M, et al. Disseminated *Scedosporium apiospermum* infection in a cystic fibrosis patient after double-lung transplantation. *J Heart Lung Transplant.* 2006;25(5):603–607.

128. Williamson EC, Speers D, Arthur IH, Harnett G, Ryan G, Inglis TJ. Molecular epidemiology of *Scedosporium apiospermum* infection determined by PCR amplification of ribosomal intergenic spacer sequences in patients with chronic lung disease. *J Clin Microbiol.* 2001;39(1):47–50.

129. del Palacio A, Garau M, Amor E, et al. Case reports. Transient colonization with *Scedosporium prolificans*. Report of four cases in Madrid. *Mycoses.* 2001;44(7–8):321–325.

130. Nenoff P, Gutz U, Tintelnot K, et al. Disseminated mycosis due to *Scedosporium prolificans* in an AIDS patient with Burkitt lymphoma. *Mycoses.* 1996;39(11–12):461–465.

131. de Batlle J, Motje M, Balanza R, Guardia R, Ortiz R. Disseminated infection caused by *Scedosporium prolificans* in a patient with acute multilineal leukemia. *J Clin Microbiol.* 2000;38(4):1694–1695.

132. Howden BP, Slavin MA, Schwarer AP, Mijch AM. Successful control of disseminated *Scedosporium prolificans* infection with a combination of voriconazole and terbinafine. *Eur J Clin Microbiol Infect Dis.* 2003;22(2):111–113.

133. Maertens J, Lagrou K, Deweerdt H, et al. Disseminated infection by *Scedosporium prolificans*: An emerging fatality among haematology patients. Case report and review. *Ann Hematol.* 2000;79(6):340–344.

134. McKelvie PA, Wong EY, Chow LP, Hall AJ. *Scedosporium endophthalmitis*: Two fatal disseminated cases of Scedosporium infection presenting with endophthalmitis. *Clin Exp Ophthalmol.* 2001;29(5):330–334.

135. Klopfenstein KJ, Rosselet R, Termuhlen A, Powell D. Successful treatment of *Scedosporium pneumonia* with voriconazole during AML therapy and bone marrow transplantation. *Med Pediatr Oncol.* 2003;41(5):494–495.

136. Jabado N, Casanova JL, Haddad E, et al. Invasive pulmonary infection due to *Scedosporium apiospermum* in two children with chronic granulomatous disease. *Clin Infect Dis.* 1998;27(6):1437–1441.

137. Horre R, Jovanic B, Marklein G, et al. Fatal pulmonary scedosporiosis. *Mycoses.* 2003;46(9–10):418–421.

138. Perlroth J, Choi B, Spellberg B. Nosocomial fungal infections: Epidemiology, diagnosis, and treatment. *Med Mycol.* 2007;45(4):321–346.

139. Talbot TR, Hatcher J, Davis SF, Pierson RN, 3rd, Barton R, Dummer S. *Scedosporium apiospermum* pneumonia and sternal wound infection in a heart transplant recipient. *Transplantation.* 2002;74(11):1645–1647.

140. Tamm M, Malouf M, Glanville A. Pulmonary scedosporium infection following lung transplantation. *Transpl Infect Dis.* 2001;3(4):189–194.

141. Raj R, Frost AE. *Scedosporium apiospermum* fungemia in a lung transplant recipient. *Chest.* 2002;121(5):1714–1716.

142. Diaz-Valle D, Benitez del Castillo JM, Amor E, Toledano N, Carretero MM, Diaz-Valle T. Severe keratomycosis secondary to *Scedosporium apiospermum*. *Cornea.* 2002;21(5):516–518.

143. Nulens E, Eggink C, Rijs AJ, Wesseling P, Verweij PE. Keratitis caused by *Scedosporium apiospermum* successfully treated with a cornea transplant and voriconazole. *J Clin Microbiol.* 2003;41(5):2261–2264.

144. Wu Z, Ying H, Yiu S, Irvine J, Smith R. Fungal keratitis caused by *Scedosporium apiospermum*: Report of two cases and review of treatment. *Cornea.* 2002;21(5):519–523.

145. Arthur S, Steed LL, Apple DJ, Peng Q, Howard G, Escobar-Gomez M. *Scedosporium prolificans* keratouveitis in association with a contact lens retained intraocularly over a long term. *J Clin Microbiol.* 2001;39(12):4579–4582.

146. Figueroa MS, Fortun J, Clement A, De Arevalo BF. Endogenous endophthalmitis caused by *Scedosporium apiospermum* treated with voriconazole. *Retina.* 2004;24(2):319–320.

147. Larocco A, Jr., Barron JB. Endogenous *Scedosporium apiospermum* endophthalmitis. *Retina.* 2005;25(8):1090–1093.

148. Leck A, Matheson M, Tuft S, Waheed K, Lagonowski H. *Scedosporium apiospermum* keratomycosis with secondary endophthalmitis. *Eye (Lond).* 2003;17(7):841–843.

149. Taylor A, Wiffen SJ, Kennedy CJ. Post-traumatic *Scedosporium inflatum* endophthalmitis. *Clin Exp Ophthalmol.* 2002;30(1):47–48.

150. Vagefi MR, Kim ET, Alvarado RG, Duncan JL, Howes EL, Crawford JB. Bilateral endogenous *Scedosporium prolificans* endophthalmitis after lung transplantation. *Am J Ophthalmol.* 2005;139(2):370–373.

151. Hernandez Prats C, Llinares Tello F, Burgos San Jose A, Selva Otaolaurruchi J, Ordovas Baines JP. Voriconazole in fungal keratitis caused by *Scedosporium apiospermum*. *Ann Pharmacother*. 2004;38(3):414–417.

152. Chakraborty A, Workman MR, Bullock PR. *Scedosporium apiospermum* brain abscess treated with surgery and voriconazole. Case report. *J Neurosurg*. 2005;103(1 Suppl):83–87.

153. Kowacs PA, Soares Silvado CE, Monteiro de Almeida S, et al. Infection of the CNS by *Scedosporium apiospermum* after near drowning: Report of a fatal case and analysis of its confounding factors. *J Clin Pathol*. 2004;57(2):205–207.

154. Mursch K, Trnovec S, Ratz H, et al. Successful treatment of multiple Pseudallescheria boydii brain abscesses and ventriculitis/ependymitis in a 2-year-old child after a near-drowning episode. *Childs Nerv Syst*. 2006;22(2):189–192.

155. Baddley JW, Stroud TP, Salzman D, Pappas PG. Invasive mold infections in allogeneic bone marrow transplant recipients. *Clin Infect Dis*. 2001;32(9):1319–1324.

156. Mellinghoff IK, Winston DJ, Mukwaya G, Schiller GJ. Treatment of *Scedosporium apiospermum* brain abscesses with posaconazole. *Clin Infect Dis*. 2002;34(12):1648–1650.

157. Safdar A, Papadopoulos EB, Young JW. Breakthrough *Scedosporium apiospermum* (*Pseudallescheria boydii*) brain abscess during therapy for invasive pulmonary aspergillosis following high-risk allogeneic hematopoietic stem cell transplantation: Scedosporiasis and recent advances in antifungal therapy. *Transpl Infect Dis*. 2002;4(4):212–217.

158. Montejo M, Muniz ML, Zarraga S, et al. Case Reports: Infection due to *Scedosporium apiospermum* in renal transplant recipients—A report of two cases and literature review of central nervous system and cutaneous infections by *Pseudallescheria boydii/Sc. apiospermum*. *Mycoses*. 2002;45(9–10):418–427.

159. Nesky MA, McDougal EC, Peacock JE, Jr. *Pseudallescheria boydii* brain abscess successfully treated with voriconazole and surgical drainage: Case report and literature review of central nervous system pseudallescheriasis. *Clin Infect Dis*. 2000;31(3):673–677.

160. Luu KK, Scott IU, Miller D, Davis JL. Endogenous *Pseudallescheria boydii* endophthalmitis in a patient with ring-enhancing brain lesions. *Ophthalmic Surg Lasers*. 2001;32(4):325–329.

161. Marco de Lucas E, Sadaba P, Lastra Garcia-Baron P, et al. *Cerebral scedosporiosis*: An emerging fungal infection in severe neutropenic patients—CT features and CT pathologic correlation. *Eur Radiol*. 2006;16(2):496–502.

162. Canet JJ, Pagerols X, Sanchez C, Vives P, Garau J. Lymphocutaneous syndrome due to *Scedosporium apiospermum*. *Clin Microbiol Infect*. 2001;7(11):648–650.

163. Girmenia C, Luzi G, Monaco M, Martino P. Use of voriconazole in treatment of *Scedosporium apiospermum* infection: Case report. *J Clin Microbiol*. 1998;36(5):1436–1438.

164. Karaarslan A, Arikan S, Karaarslan F, Cetin ES. Skin infection caused by *Scedosporium apiospermum*. *Mycoses*. 2003;46(11–12):524–526.

165. Schaenman JM, DiGiulio DB, Mirels LF, et al. *Scedosporium apiospermum* soft tissue infection successfully treated with voriconazole: Potential pitfalls in the transition from intravenous to oral therapy. *J Clin Microbiol*. 2005;43(2):973–977.

166. German JW, Kellie SM, Pai MP, Turner PT. Treatment of a chronic *Scedosporium apiospermum* vertebral osteomyelitis: Case report. *Neurosurg Focus*. 2004;17(6):E9.

167. O'Doherty M, Hannan M, Fulcher T. Voriconazole in the treatment of fungal osteomyelitis of the orbit in the immunocompromised host. *Orbit (Amsterdam, Netherlands)*. 2005;24(4):285–289.

168. Levine NB, Kurokawa R, Fichtenbaum CJ, Howington JA, Kuntz C. An immunocompetent patient with primary *Scedosporium apiospermum* vertebral osteomyelitis. *J Spinal Disord Tech*. 2002;15(5):425–430.

169. Kanafani ZA, Comair Y, Kanj SS. *Pseudallescheria boydii* cranial osteomyelitis and subdural empyema successfully treated with voriconazole: A case report and literature review. *Eur J Clin Microbiol Infect Dis*. 2004;23(11):836–840.

170. Lonser RR, Brodke DS, Dailey AT. Vertebral osteomyelitis secondary to *Pseudallescheria boydii*. *J Spinal Disord*. 2001;14(4):361–364.

171. Gosbell IB, Toumasatos V, Yong J, Kuo RS, Ellis DH, Perrie RC. Cure of orthopaedic infection with *Scedosporium prolificans*, using voriconazole plus terbinafine, without the need for radical surgery. *Mycoses*. 2003;46(5–6):233–236.

172. Steinbach WJ, Schell WA, Miller JL, Perfect JR. *Scedosporium prolificans* osteomyelitis in an immunocompetent child treated with voriconazole and caspofungin, as well as locally applied polyhexamethylene biguanide. *J Clin Microbiol*. 2003;41(8):3981–3985.

173. Schinabeck MK, Ghannoum MA. Human hyalohyphomycoses: A review of human infections due to Acremonium spp., Paecilomyces spp., Penicillium spp., and Scopulariopsis spp. *J Chemother*. 2003;15 Suppl 2:5–15.

174. Iwen PC, Schutte SD, Florescu DF, Noel-Hurst RK, Sigler L. Invasive *Scopulariopsis brevicaulis* infection in an immunocompromised patient and review of prior cases caused by *Scopulariopsis* and *Microascus* species. *Med Mycol*. 2012;50(6):561–569.

175. Jacobson ES. Pathogenic roles for fungal melanins. *Clin Microbiol Rev.* 2000;13(4):708–717.

176. Schnitzler N, Peltroche-Llacsahuanga H, Bestier N, Zundorf J, Lutticken R, Haase G. Effect of melanin and carotenoids of Exophiala (Wangiella) dermatitidis on phagocytosis, oxidative burst, and killing by human neutrophils. *Infect Immun.* 1999;67(1):94–101.

177. Bonifaz A, Carrasco-Gerard E, Saul A. *Chromoblastomycosis*: Clinical and mycologic experience of 51 cases. *Mycoses.* 2001;44(1–2):1–7.

178. Lopez Martinez R, Mendez Tovar LJ. *Chromoblastomycosis. Clin Dermatol.* 2007;25(2):188–194.

179. Silva JP, de Souza W, Rozental S. *Chromoblastomycosis*: A retrospective study of 325 cases on Amazonic Region (Brazil). *Mycopathologia.* 1998;143(3):171–175.

180. Garg P, Gopinathan U, Choudhary K, Rao GN. Keratomycosis: Clinical and microbiologic experience with dematiaceous fungi. *Ophthalmology.* 2000;107(3):574–580.

181. Wilhelmus KR. Climatology of dematiaceous fungal keratitis. *Am J Ophthalmol.* 2005;140(6):1156–1157.

182. Agger WA, Andes D, Burgess JW. Exophiala jeanselmei infection in a heart transplant recipient successfully treated with oral terbinafine. *Clin Infect Dis.* 2004;38(11):e112–115.

183. Chua JD, Gordon SM, Banbury J, Hall GS, Procop GW. Relapsing *Exophiala jeanselmei* phaeohyphomycosis in a lung-transplant patient. *Transpl Infect Dis.* 2001;3(4):235–238.

184. Xu X, Low DW, Palevsky HI, Elenitsas R. *Subcutaneous phaeohyphomycotic* cysts caused by Exophiala jeanselmei in a lung transplant patient. *Dermatol Surg.* 2001;27(4):343–346.

185. Tessari G, Forni A, Ferretto R, et al. Lethal systemic dissemination from a cutaneous infection due to *Curvularia lunata* in a heart transplant recipient. *J Eur Acad Dermatol Venereol.* 2003;17(4):440–442.

186. Salo PM, Arbes SJ, Jr., Sever M, et al. Exposure to *Alternaria alternata* in US homes is associated with asthma symptoms. *J Allergy Clin Immunol.* 2006;118(4):892–898.

187. Bush RK, Prochnau JJ. *Alternaria*-induced asthma. *J Allergy Clin Immunol.* 2004;113(2):227–234.

188. Barnes SD, Dohlman CH, Durand ML. Fungal colonization and infection in *Boston keratoprosthesis. Cornea.* 2007;26(1):9–15.

189. Ozbek Z, Kang S, Sivalingam J, Rapuano CJ, Cohen EJ, Hammersmith KM. Voriconazole in the management of *Alternaria keratitis. Cornea.* 2006;25(2):242–244.

190. Verma K, Vajpayee RB, Titiyal JS, Sharma N, Nayak N. Post-LASIK infectious crystalline keratopathy caused by *Alternaria. Cornea.* 2005;24(8):1018–1020.

191. Gilaberte M, Bartralot R, Torres JM, et al. *Cutaneous alternariosis* in transplant recipients: Clinicopathologic review of 9 cases. *J Am Acad Dermatol.* 2005;52(4):653–659.

192. Benito N, Moreno A, Puig J, Rimola A. *Alternariosis* after liver transplantation. *Transplantation.* 2001;72(11):1840–1843.

193. Luque P, Garcia-Gil FA, Larraga J, et al. Treatment of cutaneous infection by *Alternaria alternata* with voriconazole in a liver transplant patient. *Transplant Proc.* 2006;38(8):2514–2515.

194. Vieira R, Veloso J, Afonso A, Rodrigues A. *Cutaneous alternariosis* in a liver transplant recipient. *Revista iberoamericana de micologia.* 2006;23(2):107–109.

195. Gerdsen R, Uerlich M, De Hoog GS, Bieber T, Horre R. *Sporotrichoid phaeohyphomycosis* due to Alternaria infectoria. *Br J Dermatol.* 2001;145(3):484–486.

196. Nulens E, De Laere E, Vandevelde H, et al. *Alternaria infectoria* phaeohyphomycosis in a renal transplant patient. *Med Mycol.* 2006;44(4):379–382.

197. Torres-Rodriguez JM, Gonzalez MP, Corominas JM, Pujol RM. Successful thermotherapy for a subcutaneous infection due to Alternaria alternata in a renal transplant recipient. *Arch Dermatol.* 2005;141(9):1171–1173.

198. Romano C, Vanzi L, Massi D, Difonzo EM. *Subcutaneous alternariosis. Mycoses.* 2005;48(6):408–412.

199. Robertshaw H, Higgins E. Cutaneous infection with *Alternaria tenuissima* in an immunocompromised patient. *Br J Dermatol.* 2005;153(5):1047–1049.

200. Mullane K, Toor AA, Kalnicky C, Rodriguez T, Klein J, Stiff P. *Posaconazole salvage* therapy allows successful allogeneic hematopoietic stem cell transplantation in patients with refractory invasive mold infections. *Transpl Infect Dis.* 2007;9(2):89–96.

201. Park AH, Muntz HR, Smith ME, Afify Z, Pysher T, Pavia A. Pediatric invasive fungal rhinosinusitis in immunocompromised children with cancer. *Otolaryngol Head Neck Surg.* 2005;133(3):411–416.

202. Morrison VA, Haake RJ, Weisdorf DJ. The spectrum of non-Candida fungal infections following bone marrow transplantation. *Medicine (Baltimore).* 1993;72(2):78–89.

203. Sorensen J, Becker M, Porto L, et al. Rhinocerebral zygomycosis in a young girl undergoing allogeneic stem cell transplantation for severe aplastic anaemia. *Mycoses.* 2006;49 Suppl 1:31–36.

204. Uenotsuchi T, Moroi Y, Urabe K, et al. Cutaneous alternariosis with chronic granulomatous disease. *Eur J Dermatol.* 2005;15(5):406–408.

205. Gopalakrishnan K, Daniel E, Jacob R, Ebenezer G, Mathews M. Bilateral Bipolaris keratomycosis in a borderline lepromatous patient. *Int J Lepr Other Mycobact Dis.* 2003;71(1):14–17.

206. Newell CK, Steinmetz RL, Brooks HL, Jr. Chronic postoperative endophthalmitis caused by Bipolaris australiensis. *Retina.* 2006;26(1):109–110.

207. Saha R, Das S. Bipolaris keratomycosis. *Mycoses.* 2005;48(6):453–455.

208. Robb CW, Malouf PJ, Rapini RP. Four cases of dermatomycosis: Superficial cutaneous infection by *Alternaria* or *Bipolaris. Cutis.* 2003;72(4):313–316, 319.

209. Bilu D, Movahedi-Lankarani S, Kazin RA, Shields C, Moresi M. *Cutaneous Bipolaris* infection in a neutropenic patient with acute lymphoblastic leukemia. *J Cutan Med Surg.* 2004;8(6):446–449.

210. Roche M, Redmond RM, O'Neill S, Smyth E. A case of multiple cerebral abscesses due to infection with *Cladophialophora bantiana. J Infect.* 2005;51(5):e285–288.

211. Tunuguntla A, Saad MM, Abdalla J, Myers JW. Multiple brain abscesses caused by *Cladophialophora bantianum:* A challenging case. *Tenn Med.* 2005;98(5):227–228, 235.

212. Lyons MK, Blair JE, Leslie KO. Successful treatment with voriconazole of fungal cerebral abscess due to *Cladophialophora bantiana. Clin Neurol Neurosurg.* 2005;107(6):532–534.

213. Revankar SG, Sutton DA, Rinaldi MG. Primary central nervous system phaeohyphomycosis: A review of 101 cases. *Clin Infect Dis.* 2004;38(2):206–216.

214. Keyser A, Schmid FX, Linde HJ, Merk J, Birnbaum DE. Disseminated *Cladophialophora bantiana* infection in a heart transplant recipient. *J Heart Lung Transplant.* 2002;21(4):503–505.

215. Silveira ER, Resende MA, Mariano VS, et al. Brain abscess caused by *Cladophialophora (Xylohypha) bantiana* in a renal transplant patient. *Transpl Infect Dis.* 2003;5(2):104–107.

216. Levin TP, Baty DE, Fekete T, Truant AL, Suh B. *Cladophialophora bantiana* brain abscess in a solid-organ transplant recipient: Case report and review of the literature. *J Clin Microbiol.* 2004;42(9):4374–4378.

217. Arnoldo BD, Purdue GF, Tchorz K, Hunt JL. A case report of phaeohyphomycosis caused by *Cladophialophora bantiana* treated in a burn unit. *J Burn Care Rehabil.* 2005;26(3):285–287.

218. Howard SJ, Walker SL, Andrew SM, Borman AM, Johnson EM, Denning DW. Sub-cutaneous phaeohyphomycosis caused by *Cladophialophora devriesii* in a United Kingdom resident. *Med Mycol.* 2006;44(6):553–556.

219. Werlinger KD, Yen Moore A. Eumycotic mycetoma caused by *Cladophialophora bantiana* in a patient with systemic lupus erythematosus. *J Am Acad Dermatol.* 2005;52(5 Suppl 1):S114–S117.

220. Perez-Blanco M, Hernandez Valles R, Garcia-Humbria L, Yegres F. Chromoblastomycosis in children and adolescents in the endemic area of the Falcon State, Venezuela. *Med Mycol.* 2006;44(5):467–471.

221. Guarro J, Akiti T, Horta RA, et al. Mycotic keratitis due to *Curvularia senegalensis* and in vitro antifungal susceptibilities of Curvularia spp. *J Clin Microbiol.* 1999;37(12):4170–4173.

222. Boonpasart S, Kasetsuwan N, Puangsricharern V, Pariyakanok L, Jittpoonkusol T. Infectious keratitis at King Chulalongkorn Memorial Hospital: A 12-year retrospective study of 391 cases. *J Med Assoc Thai.* 2002;85 Suppl 1:S217–S230.

223. Bonduel M, Santos P, Turienzo CF, Chantada G, Paganini H. Atypical skin lesions caused by *Curvularia* sp. and *Pseudallescheria boydii* in two patients after allogeneic bone marrow transplantation. *Bone Marrow Transplant.* 2001;27(12):1311–1313.

224. Torda AJ, Jones PD. Necrotizing cutaneous infection caused by *Curvularia brachyspora* in an immunocompetent host. *Australas J Dermatol.* 1997;38(2):85–87.

225. Still JM, Jr., Law EJ, Pereira GI, Singletary E. Invasive burn wound infection due to *Curvularia* species. *Burns.* 1993;19(1):77–79.

226. Ebright JR, Chandrasekar PH, Marks S, Fairfax MR, Aneziokoro A, McGinnis MR. Invasive sinusitis and cerebritis due to *Curvularia clavata* in an immunocompetent adult. *Clin Infect Dis.* 1999;28(3):687–689.

227. Carter E, Boudreaux C. Fatal cerebral phaeohyphomycosis due to Curvularia lunata in an immunocompetent patient. *J Clin Microbiol.* 2004;42(11):5419–5423.

228. Pimentel JD, Mahadevan K, Woodgyer A, et al. Peritonitis due to *Curvularia inaequalis* in an elderly patient undergoing peritoneal dialysis and a review of six cases of peritonitis associated with other *Curvularia* spp. *J Clin Microbiol.* 2005;43(8):4288–4292.

229. Kainer MA, Keshavarz H, Jensen BJ, et al. Saline-filled breast implant contamination with *Curvularia* species among women who underwent cosmetic breast augmentation. *J Infect Dis.* 2005;192(1):170–177.

230. Giraldo A, Sutton DA, Samerpitak K, et al. Occurrence of Ochroconis and Verruconis species in clinical specimens from the United States. *J Clin Microbiol.* 2014;52(12):4189–4201.

231. Shoham S, Pic-Aluas L, Taylor J, et al. Transplant-associated *Ochroconis gallopava* infections. *Transpl Infect Dis.* 2008;10(6):442–448.

232. Mazur JE, Judson MA. A case report of a dactylaria fungal infection in a lung transplant patient. *Chest.* 2001;119(2):651–653.

233. Mancini MC, McGinnis MR. Dactylaria infection of a human being: Pulmonary disease in a heart transplant recipient. *J Heart Lung Transplant.* 1992;11(4 Pt 1):827–830.

234. Kralovic SM, Rhodes JC. Phaeohyphomycosis caused by *Dactylaria* (human dactylariosis): Report of a case with review of the literature. *J Infect.* 1995;31(2):107–113.

235. Malani PN, Bleicher JJ, Kauffman CA, Davenport DS. Disseminated *Dactylaria constricta* infection in a renal transplant recipient. *Transpl Infect Dis.* 2001;3(1):40–43.

236. Vukmir RB, Kusne S, Linden P, et al. Successful therapy for cerebral phaeohyphomycosis due to *Dactylaria gallopava* in a liver transplant recipient. *Clin Infect Dis.* 1994;19(4):714–719.

237. Singh N, Chang FY, Gayowski T, Marino IR. Infections due to dematiaceous fungi in organ transplant recipients: Case report and review. *Clin Infect Dis.* 1997;24(3):369–374.

238. Rossmann SN, Cernoch PL, Davis JR. Dematiaceous fungi are an increasing cause of human disease. *Clin Infect Dis.* 1996;22(1):73–80.

239. Boggild AK, Poutanen SM, Mohan S, Ostrowski MA. Disseminated phaeohyphomycosis due to *Ochroconis gallopavum* in the setting of advanced HIV infection. *Med Mycol.* 2006;44(8):777–782.

240. Garcia-Martos P, Marquez A, Gene J. Human infections by black yeasts of genus *Exophiala*. *Revista iberoamericana de micologia.* 2002;19(2):72–79.

241. Kantarcioglu AS, de Hoog GS. Infections of the central nervous system by melanized fungi: A review of cases presented between 1999 and 2004. *Mycoses.* 2004;47(1–2):4–13.

242. Chang CL, Kim DS, Park DJ, Kim HJ, Lee CH, Shin JH. Acute cerebral phaeohyphomycosis due to *Wangiella dermatitidis* accompanied by cerebrospinal fluid eosinophilia. *J Clin Microbiol.* 2000;38(5):1965–1966.

243. Taj-Aldeen SJ, El Shafie S, Alsoub H, Eldeeb Y, de Hoog GS. Isolation of *Exophiala dermatitidis* from endotracheal aspirate of a cancer patient. *Mycoses.* 2006;49(6):504–509.

244. Hiruma M, Kawada A, Ohata H, et al. Systemic phaeohyphomycosis caused by *Exophiala dermatitidis*. *Mycoses.* 1993;36(1–2):1–7.

245. Matsumoto T, Matsuda T, McGinnis MR, Ajello L. Clinical and mycological spectra of *Wangiella dermatitidis* infections. *Mycoses.* 1993;36(5–6):145–155.

246. Exophiala infection from contaminated injectable steroids prepared by a compounding pharmacy—United States, July–November 2002. *MMWR Morb Mortal Wkly Rep.* 2002;51(49):1109–1112.

247. Matos T, de Hoog GS, de Boer AG, de Crom I, Haase G. High prevalence of the neurotrope *Exophiala dermatitidis* and related oligotrophic black yeasts in sauna facilities. *Mycoses.* 2002;45(9–10):373–377.

248. Horre R, Schaal KP, Siekmeier R, Sterzik B, de Hoog GS, Schnitzler N. Isolation of fungi, especially *Exophiala dermatitidis*, in patients suffering from cystic fibrosis. A prospective study. *Respiration.* 2004;71(4):360–366.

249. de Hoog GS, Matos T, Sudhadham M, Luijsterburg KF, Haase G. Intestinal prevalence of the neurotropic black yeast *Exophiala* (*Wangiella*) dermatitidis in healthy and impaired individuals. *Mycoses.* 2005;48(2):142–145.

250. Neumeister B, Zollner TM, Krieger D, Sterry W, Marre R. Mycetoma due to Exophiala jeanselmei and *Mycobacterium chelonae* in a 73-year-old man with idiopathic CD4+ T lymphocytopenia. *Mycoses.* 1995;38(7–8):271–276.

251. Desnos-Ollivier M, Bretagne S, Dromer F, Lortholary O, Dannaoui E. Molecular identification of black-grain mycetoma agents. *J Clin Microbiol.* 2006;44(10):3517–3523.

252. Kinkead S, Jancic V, Stasko T, Boyd AS. Chromoblastomycosis in a patient with a cardiac transplant. *Cutis.* 1996;58(5):367–370.

253. Kondo M, Hiruma M, Nishioka Y, et al. A case of chromomycosis caused by *Fonsecaea pedrosoi* and a review of reported cases of dematiaceous fungal infection in Japan. *Mycoses.* 2005;48(3):221–225.

254. Heinz T, Perfect J, Schell W, Ritter E, Ruff G, Serafin D. Soft-tissue fungal infections: Surgical management of 12 immunocompromised patients. *Plast Reconstr Surg.* 1996;97(7):1391–1399.

255. Vlassopoulos D, Kouppari G, Arvanitis D, et al. *Wangiella dermatitidis* peritonitis in a CAPD patient. *Perit Dial Int.* 2001;21(1):96–97.

256. Greig J, Harkness M, Taylor P, Hashmi C, Liang S, Kwan J. Peritonitis due to the dermataceous mold *Exophiala dermatitidis* complicating continuous ambulatory peritoneal dialysis. *Clin Microbiol Infect.* 2003;9(7):713–715.

257. Nucci M, Akiti T, Barreiros G, et al. Nosocomial outbreak of *Exophiala jeanselmei* fungemia associated with contamination of hospital water. *Clin Infect Dis.* 2002;34(11):1475–1480.

258. Lanternier F, Barbati E, Meinzer U, et al. Inherited CARD9 deficiency in 2 unrelated patients with invasive *Exophiala* infection. *J Infect Dis.* 2015;211(8):1241–1250.

259. Adler A, Yaniv I, Samra Z, et al. Exserohilum: An emerging human pathogen. *Eur J Clin Microbiol Infect Dis.* 2006;25(4):247–253.

260. Levy I, Stein J, Ashkenazi S, Samra Z, Livni G, Yaniv I. Ecthyma gangrenosum caused by disseminated *Exserohilum* in a child with leukemia: A case report and review of the literature. *Pediatr Dermatol.* 2003;20(6):495–497.

261. Lasala PR, Smith MB, McGinnis MR, Sackey K, Patel JA, Qiu S. Invasive Exserohilum sinusitis in a patient with aplastic anemia. *Pediatr Infect Dis J.* 2005;24(10):939–941.

262. Al-Attar A, Williams CG, Redett RJ. Rare lower extremity invasive fungal infection in an immunosuppressed patient: *Exserohilum longirostratum*. *Plast Reconstr Surg.* 2006;117(3):44e-47e.

263. Katragkou A, Pana ZD, Perlin DS, Kontoyiannis DP, Walsh TJ, Roilides E. *Exserohilum* infections: Review of 48 cases before the 2012 United States outbreak. *Med Mycol.* 2014;52(4):376–386.

264. Smith RM, Schaefer MK, Kainer MA, et al. Fungal infections associated with contaminated methylprednisolone injections. *N Engl J Med.* 2013;369(17):1598–1609.

265. Sharma NL, Sharma RC, Grover PS, Gupta ML, Sharma AK, Mahajan VK. Chromoblastomycosis in India. *Int J Dermatol.* 1999;38(11):846–851.

266. Lundstrom TS, Fairfax MR, Dugan MC, et al. *Phialophora verrucosa* infection in a BMT patient. *Bone Marrow Transplant.* 1997;20(9):789–791.

267. Kanj SS, Amr SS, Roberts GD. Ramichloridium mackenziei brain abscess: Report of two cases and review of the literature. *Med Mycol.* 2001;39(1):97–102.

268. Khan ZU, Lamdhade SJ, Johny M, et al. Additional case of *Ramichloridium mackenziei* cerebral phaeohyphomycosis from the Middle East. *Med Mycol.* 2002;40(4):429–433.

269. Naim-ur-Rahman, Mahgoub ES, Chagla AH. Fatal brain abscesses caused by *Ramichloridium obovoideum*: Report of three cases. *Acta Neurochir (Wien).* 1988;93(3–4):92–95.

270. Podnos YD, Anastasio P, De La Maza L, Kim RB. Cerebral phaeohyphomycosis caused by *Ramichloridium obovoideum* (*Ramichloridium mackenziei*): Case report. *Neurosurgery.* 1999;45(2):372–375.

271. Sutton DA, Slifkin M, Yakulis R, Rinaldi MG. U.S. case report of cerebral phaeohyphomycosis caused by *Ramichloridium obovoideum* (*R. mackenziei*): Criteria for identification, therapy, and review of other known dematiaceous neurotropic taxa. *J Clin Microbiol.* 1998;36(3):708–715.

272. Al-Abdely HM, Alkhunaizi AM, Al-Tawfiq JA, Hassounah M, Rinaldi MG, Sutton DA. Successful therapy of cerebral phaeohyphomycosis due to *Ramichloridium mackenziei* with the new triazole posaconazole. *Med Mycol.* 2005;43(1):91–95.

273. Walsh TJ, Groll AH. Emerging fungal pathogens: Evolving challenges to immunocompromised patients for the twenty-first century. *Transpl Infect Dis.* 1999;1(4):247–261.

274. Ribes JA, Vanover-Sams CL, Baker DJ. Zygomycetes in human disease. *Clin Microbiol Rev.* 2000;13(2):236–301.

275. Quinio D, Karam A, Leroy JP, et al. Zygomycosis caused by *Cunninghamella bertholletiae* in a kidney transplant recipient. *Med Mycol.* 2004;42(2):177–180.

276. Lanternier F, Sun HY, Ribaud P, Singh N, Kontoyiannis DP, Lortholary O. Mucormycosis in organ and stem cell transplant recipients. *Clin Infect Dis.* 2012;54(11):1629–1636.

277. Xhaard A, Lanternier F, Porcher R, et al. Mucormycosis after allogeneic haematopoietic stem cell transplantation: A French Multicentre Cohort Study (2003–2008). *Clin Microbiol Infect.* 2012;18(10):E396–400.

278. Marty FM, Ostrosky-Zeichner L, Cornely OA, et al. Isavuconazole treatment for mucormycosis: A single-arm open-label trial and case-control analysis. *Lancet Infect Dis.* 2016;16(7):828–837.

279. Petrikkos G, Skiada A, Lortholary O, Roilides E, Walsh TJ, Kontoyiannis DP. Epidemiology and clinical manifestations of mucormycosis. *Clin Infect Dis.* 2012;54 Suppl 1:S23–34.

280. Marty FM, Cosimi LA, Baden LR. Breakthrough zygomycosis after voriconazole treatment in recipients of hematopoietic stem-cell transplants. *N Engl J Med.* 2004;350(9):950–952.

281. Roden MM, Zaoutis TE, Buchanan WL, et al. Epidemiology and outcome of zygomycosis: A review of 929 reported cases. *Clin Infect Dis.* 2005;41(5):634–653.

282. Trifilio SM, Bennett CL, Yarnold PR, et al. Breakthrough zygomycosis after voriconazole administration among patients with hematologic malignancies who receive hematopoietic stem-cell transplants or intensive chemotherapy. *Bone Marrow Transplant.* 2007;39(7):425–429.

283. Almyroudis NG, Sutton DA, Linden P, Rinaldi MG, Fung J, Kusne S. Zygomycosis in solid organ transplant recipients in a tertiary transplant center and review of the literature. *Am J Transplant.* 2006;6(10):2365–2374.

284. Imhof A, Balajee SA, Fredricks DN, Englund JA, Marr KA. Breakthrough fungal infections in stem cell transplant recipients receiving voriconazole. *Clin Infect Dis.* 2004;39(5):743–746.

285. Vigouroux S, Morin O, Moreau P, et al. Zygomycosis after prolonged use of voriconazole in immunocompromised patients with hematologic disease: Attention required. *Clin Infect Dis.* 2005;40(4):e35–37.

286. Maertens J, Demuynck H, Verbeken EK, et al. Mucormycosis in allogeneic bone marrow transplant recipients: Report of five cases and review of the role of iron overload in the pathogenesis. *Bone Marrow Transplant.* 1999;24(3):307–312.

287. Prokopowicz GP, Bradley SF, Kauffman CA. Indolent zygomycosis associated with deferoxamine chelation therapy. *Mycoses.* 1994;37(11–12):427–431.

288. Boelaert JR, Van Cutsem J, de Locht M, Schneider YJ, Crichton RR. Deferoxamine augments growth and pathogenicity of Rhizopus, while hydroxypyridinone chelators have no effect. *Kidney Int.* 1994;45(3):667–671.

289. Boelaert JR, de Locht M, Van Cutsem J, et al. Mucormycosis during deferoxamine therapy is a siderophore-mediated infection: In vitro and in vivo animal studies. *J Clin Invest.* 1993;91(5):1979–1986.

290. Boelaert JR, Fenves AZ, Coburn JW. Deferoxamine therapy and mucormycosis in dialysis patients: Report of an international registry. *Am J Kidney Dis.* 1991;18(6):660–667.

291. Marty FM, Lowry CM, Cutler CS, et al. Voriconazole and sirolimus coadministration after allogeneic hematopoietic stem cell transplantation. *Biol Blood Marrow Transplant.* 2006;12(5):552–559.

292. Paul S, Marty FM, Colson YL. Treatment of cavitary pulmonary zygomycosis with surgical resection and posaconazole. *Ann Thorac Surg.* 2006;82(1):338–340.

293. Hampson FG, Ridgway EJ, Feeley K, Reilly JT. A fatal case of disseminated zygomycosis associated with the use of blood glucose self-monitoring equipment. *J Infect.* 2005;51(5):e269–272.

294. Vazquez L, Mateos JJ, Sanz-Rodriguez C, Perez E, Caballero D, San Miguel JF. Successful treatment of rhinocerebral zygomycosis with a combination of caspofungin and liposomal amphotericin B. *Haematologica.* 2005;90(12 Suppl):Ecr39.

295. Rickerts V, Bohme A, Viertel A, et al. Cluster of pulmonary infections caused by *Cunninghamella bertholletiae* in immunocompromised patients. *Clin Infect Dis.* 2000;31(4):910–913.

296. Garey KW, Pendland SL, Huynh VT, Bunch TH, Jensen GM, Pursell KJ. *Cunninghamella bertholletiae* infection in a bone marrow transplant patient: Amphotericin lung penetration, MIC determinations, and review of the literature. *Pharmacotherapy.* 2001;21(7):855–860.

297. Darrisaw L, Hanson G, Vesole DH, Kehl SC. Cunninghamella infection post bone marrow transplant: Case report and review of the literature. *Bone Marrow Transplant.* 2000;25(11):1213–1216.

298. Zhang R, Zhang JW, Szerlip HM. Endocarditis and hemorrhagic stroke caused by *Cunninghamella bertholletiae* infection after kidney transplantation. *Am J Kidney Dis.* 2002;40(4):842–846.

299. Lelievre L, Garcia-Hermoso D, Abdoul H, et al. *Posttraumatic mucormycosis*: A nationwide study in France and review of the literature. *Medicine (Baltimore).* 2014;93(24):395–404.

300. Neblett Fanfair R, Benedict K, Bos J, et al. Necrotizing cutaneous mucormycosis after a tornado in Joplin, Missouri, in 2011. *N Engl J Med.* 2012;367(23):2214–2225.

301. Freifeld A, Kauffman C, Pappas PG. Endemic fungal infections (EFIs) among solid organ transplant recipients (SOTRs). *43rd Annual Meeting of IDSA.* October 6–9, 2005. San Franscico, CA.

302. De Groote MA, Bjerke R, Smith H, Rhodes IL. Expanding epidemiology of blastomycosis: Clinical features and investigation of 2 cases in Colorado. *Clin Infect Dis.* 2000;30(3):582–584.

303. Rudmann DG, Coolman BR, Perez CM, Glickman LT. Evaluation of risk factors for blastomycosis in dogs: 857 cases (1980–1990). *J Am Vet Med Assoc.* 1992;201(11):1754–1759.

304. Bradsher RW, Chapman SW, Pappas PG. Blastomycosis. *Infect Dis Clin North Am.* 2003;17(1):21–40, vii.

305. Lemos LB, Guo M, Baliga M. Blastomycosis: Organ involvement and etiologic diagnosis: A review of 123 patients from Mississippi. *Ann Diagn Pathol.* 2000;4(6):391–406.

306. Crampton TL, Light RB, Berg GM, et al. Epidemiology and clinical spectrum of blastomycosis diagnosed at Manitoba hospitals. *Clin Infect Dis.* 2002;34(10):1310–1316.

307. Butka BJ, Bennett SR, Johnson AC. Disseminated inoculation blastomycosis in a renal transplant recipient. *Am Rev Respir Dis.* 1984;130(6):1180–1183.

308. Serody JS, Mill MR, Detterbeck FC, Harris DT, Cohen MS. Blastomycosis in transplant recipients: Report of a case and review. *Clin Infect Dis.* 1993;16(1):54–58.

309. Winkler S, Stanek G, Hubsch P, et al. Pneumonia due to blastomyces dermatitidis in a European renal transplant recipient. *Nephrol Dial Transplant.* 1996;11(7):1376–1379.

310. Blair JE, Logan JL. Coccidioidomycosis in solid organ transplantation. *Clin Infect Dis.* 2001;33(9):1536–1544.

311. Galgiani JN. Coccidioidomycosis. *West J Med.* 1993;159(2):153–171.

312. Chiller TM, Galgiani JN, Stevens DA. Coccidioidomycosis. *Infect Dis Clin North Am.* 2003;17(1):41–57, viii.

313. Virgili A, Zampino MR, Mantovani L. Fungal skin infections in organ transplant recipients. *Am J Clin Dermatol.* 2002;3(1):19–35.

314. Wise GJ. Genitourinary fungal infections: A therapeutic conundrum. *Expert Opin Pharmacother.* 2001;2(8):1211–1226.

315. Blair JE. Coccidioidal pneumonia, arthritis, and soft-tissue infection after kidney transplantation. *Transpl Infect Dis.* 2004;6(2):74–76.

316. Rempe S, Sachdev MS, Bhakta R, Pineda-Roman M, Vaz A, Carlson RW. Coccidioides immitis fungemia: Clinical features and survival in 33 adult patients. *Heart Lung.* 2007;36(1):64–71.

317. Yurkanin JP, Ahmann F, Dalkin BL. Coccidioidomycosis of the prostate: A determination of incidence, report of 4 cases, and treatment recommendations. *J Infect.* 2006;52(1):e19–25.

318. Increase in coccidioidomycosis—Arizona, 1998–2001. *MMWR Morb Mortal Wkly Rep.* 2003;52(6):109–112.

319. Rosenstein NE, Emery KW, Werner SB, et al. Risk factors for severe pulmonary and disseminated coccidioidomycosis: Kern County, California, 1995–1996. *Clin Infect Dis.* 2001;32(5):708–715.

320. Arsura EL, Kilgore WB. Miliary coccidioidomycosis in the immunocompetent. *Chest.* 2000;117(2):404–409.

321. Miller MB, Hendren R, Gilligan PH. Posttransplantation disseminated coccidioidomycosis acquired from donor lungs. *J Clin Microbiol.* 2004;42(5):2347–2349.

322. Wright PW, Pappagianis D, Wilson M, et al. Donor-related coccidioidomycosis in organ transplant recipients. *Clin Infect Dis.* 2003;37(9):1265–1269.

323. Logan JL, Blair JE, Galgiani JN. Coccidioidomycosis complicating solid organ transplantation. *Semin Respir Infect.* 2001;16(4):251–256.

324. Tripathy U, Yung GL, Kriett JM, Thistlethwaite PA, Kapelanski DP, Jamieson SW. Donor transfer of pulmonary coccidioidomycosis in lung transplantation. *Ann Thorac Surg.* 2002;73(1):306–308.

325. Hall KA, Sethi GK, Rosado LJ, Martinez JD, Huston CL, Copeland JG. Coccidioidomycosis and heart transplantation. *J Heart Lung Transplant.* 1993;12(3):525–526.

326. Cha JM, Jung S, Bahng HS, et al. Multi-organ failure caused by reactivated coccidioidomycosis without dissemination in a patient with renal transplantation. *Respirology.* 2000;5(1):87–90.

327. Blair JE, Douglas DD, Mulligan DC. Early results of targeted prophylaxis for coccidioidomycosis in patients undergoing orthotopic liver transplantation within an endemic area. *Transpl Infect Dis.* 2003;5(1):3–8.

328. Blair JE, Kusne S, Carey EJ, Heilman RL. The prevention of recrudescent coccidioidomycosis after solid organ transplantation. *Transplantation.* 2007;83(9):1182–1187.

329. Glenn TJ, Blair JE, Adams RH. Coccidioidomycosis in hematopoietic stem cell transplant recipients. *Med Mycol.* 2005;43(8):705–710.

330. Wheat LJ. Histoplasmosis in Indianapolis. *Clin Infect Dis.* 1992;14 Suppl 1:S91–S99.

331. Garcia-Vazquez E, Velasco M, Gascon J, Corachan M, Mejias T, Torres-Rodriguez JM. Histoplasma capsulatum infection in a group of travelers to Guatemala. *Enferm Infecc Microbiol Clin.* 2005;23(5):274–276.

332. Chamany S, Mirza SA, Fleming JW, et al. A large histoplasmosis outbreak among high school students in Indiana, 2001. *Pediatr Infect Dis J.* 2004;23(10):909–914.

333. Luby JP, Southern PM, Jr., Haley CE, Vahle KL, Munford RS, Haley RW. Recurrent exposure to *Histoplasma capsulatum* in modern air-conditioned buildings. *Clin Infect Dis.* 2005;41(2):170–176.

334. Limaye AP, Connolly PA, Sagar M, et al. Transmission of *Histoplasma capsulatum* by organ transplantation. *N Engl J Med.* 2000;343(16):1163–1166.

335. Watanabe M, Hotchi M, Nagasaki M. An autopsy case of disseminated histoplasmosis probably due to infection from a renal allograft. *Acta Pathol Jpn.* 1988;38(6):769–780.

336. Vail GM, Young RS, Wheat LJ, Filo RS, Cornetta K, Goldman M. Incidence of histoplasmosis following allogeneic bone marrow transplant or solid organ transplant in a hyperendemic area. *Transpl Infect Dis.* 2002;4(3):148–151.

337. Davies SF, Sarosi GA, Peterson PK, et al. Disseminated histoplasmosis in renal transplant recipients. *Am J Surg.* 1979;137(5):686–691.

338. Wheat LJ, Smith EJ, Sathapatayavongs B, et al. Histoplasmosis in renal allograft recipients: Two large urban outbreaks. *Arch Intern Med.* 1983;143(4):703–707.

339. Peddi VR, Hariharan S, First MR. Disseminated histoplasmosis in renal allograft recipients. *Clin Transplant.* 1996;10(2):160–165.

340. Bethlem EP, Capone D, Maranhao B, Carvalho CR, Wanke B. Paracoccidioidomycosis. *Curr Opin Pulm Med.* 1999;5(5):319–325.

341. Calle D, Rosero DS, Orozco LC, Camargo D, Castaneda E, Restrepo A. Paracoccidioidomycosis in Colombia: An ecological study. *Epidemiol Infect.* 2001;126(2):309–315.

342. de Almeida SM, Queiroz-Telles F, Teive HA, Ribeiro CE, Werneck LC. Central nervous system paracoccidioidomycosis: Clinical features and laboratorial findings. *J Infect.* 2004;48(2):193–198.

343. dos Santos JW, Debiasi RB, Miletho JN, Bertolazi AN, Fagundes AL, Michel GT. Asymptomatic presentation of chronic pulmonary paracoccidioidomycosis: Case report and review. *Mycopathologia.* 2004;157(1):53–57.

344. Godoy H, Reichart PA. Oral manifestations of paracoccidioidomycosis. Report of 21 cases from Argentina. *Mycoses.* 2003;46(9–10):412–417.

345. Goldani LZ, Sugar AM. Paracoccidioidomycosis and AIDS: An overview. *Clin Infect Dis.* 1995;21(5):1275–1281.

346. Marques SA, Conterno LO, Sgarbi LP, et al. Paracoccidioidomycosis associated with acquired immunodeficiency syndrome: Report of seven cases. *Rev Inst Med Trop Sao Paulo.* 1995;37(3):261–265.

347. Zavascki AP, Bienardt JC, Severo LC. Paracoccidioidomycosis in organ transplant recipient: Case report. *Rev Inst Med Trop Sao Paulo.* 2004;46(5):279–281.

348. Reis MA, Costa RS, Ferraz AS. Causes of death in renal transplant recipients: A study of 102 autopsies from 1968 to 1991. *J R Soc Med.* 1995;88(1):24–27.

349. Shikanai-Yasuda MA, Duarte MI, Nunes DF, et al. Paracoccidioidomycosis in a renal transplant recipient. *J Med Vet Mycol.* 1995;33(6):411–414.

350. Sugar AM, Restrepo A, Stevens DA. Paracoccidioidomycosis in the immunosuppressed host: Report of a case and review of the literature. *Am Rev Respir Dis.* 1984;129(2):340–342.

351. Silva-Vergara ML, Teixeira AC, Curi VG, et al. Paracoccidioidomycosis associated with human immunodeficiency virus infection: Report of 10 cases. *Med Mycol.* 2003;41(3):259–263.

352. Paniago AM, de Freitas AC, Aguiar ES, et al. Paracoccidioidomycosis in patients with human immunodeficiency virus: Review of 12 cases observed in an endemic region in Brazil. *J Infect.* 2005;51(3):248–252.

353. Walsh TJ, Groll A, Hiemenz J, Fleming R, Roilides E, Anaissie E. Infections due to emerging and uncommon medically important fungal pathogens. *Clin Microbiol Infect.* 2004;10 Suppl 1:48–66.

354. Vanittanakom N, Cooper CR, Jr., Fisher MC, Sirisanthana T. Penicillium marneffei infection and recent advances in the epidemiology and molecular biology aspects. *Clin Microbiol Rev.* 2006;19(1):95–110.

355. Ajello L, Padhye AA, Sukroongreung S, Nilakul CH, Tantimavanic S. Occurrence of Penicillium marneffei infections among wild bamboo rats in Thailand. *Mycopathologia.* 1995;131(1):1–8.

356. Gugnani H, Fisher MC, Paliwal-Johsi A, Vanittanakom N, Singh I, Yadav PS. Role of Cannomys badius as a natural animal host of Penicillium marneffei in India. *J Clin Microbiol.* 2004;42(11):5070–5075.

357. Kudeken N, Kawakami K, Kusano N, Saito A. Cell-mediated immunity in host resistance against infection caused by Penicillium marneffei. *J Med Vet Mycol.* 1996;34(6):371–378.

358. Sirisanthana T, Supparatpinyo K. Epidemiology and management of penicilliosis in human immunodeficiency virus-infected patients. *Int J Infect Dis.* 1998;3(1):48–53.

359. Liyan X, Changming L, Xianyi Z, Luxia W, Suisheng X. Fifteen cases of penicilliosis in Guangdong, China. *Mycopathologia.* 2004;158(2):151–155.

360. Duong TA. Infection due to Penicillium marneffei, an emerging pathogen: Review of 155 reported cases. *Clin Infect Dis.* 1996;23(1):125–130.

361. Singh PN, Ranjana K, Singh YI, et al. Indigenous disseminated Penicillium marneffei infection in the state of Manipur, India: Report of four autochthonous cases. *J Clin Microbiol.* 1999;37(8):2699–2702.

362. Ranjana KH, Priyokumar K, Singh TJ, et al. Disseminated Penicillium marneffei infection among HIV-infected patients in Manipur state, India. *J Infect.* 2002;45(4):268–271.

363. Chan YH, Wong KM, Lee KC, et al. Pneumonia and mesenteric lymphadenopathy caused by disseminated Penicillium marneffei infection in a cadaveric renal transplant recipient. *Transpl Infect Dis.* 2004;6(1):28–32.

364. Wang JL, Hung CC, Chang SC, Chueh SC, La MK. Disseminated Penicillium marneffei infection in a renal-transplant recipient successfully treated with liposomal amphotericin B. *Transplantation.* 2003;76(7):1136–1137.

365. Hsueh PR, Teng LJ, Hung CC, et al. Molecular evidence for strain dissemination of Penicillium marneffei: An emerging pathogen in Taiwan. *J Infect Dis.* 2000;181(5):1706–1712.

366. Hung CC, Hsueh PR, Chen MY, Hsiao CH, Chang SC, Luh KT. Invasive infection caused by Penicillium marneffei: An emerging pathogen in Taiwan. *Clin Infect Dis.* 1998;26(1):202–203.

367. Woo PC, Lau SK, Lau CC, et al. Penicillium marneffei fungaemia in an allogeneic bone marrow transplant recipient. *Bone Marrow Transplant.* 2005;35(8):831–833.

368. Anstead GM, Sutton DA, Graybill JR. Adiaspiromycosis causing respiratory failure and a review of human infections due to Emmonsia and Chrysosporium spp. *J Clin Microbiol.* 2012;50(4):1346–1354.

369. Kenyon C, Bonorchis K, Corcoran C, et al. A dimorphic fungus causing disseminated infection in South Africa. *N Engl J Med.* 2013;369(15):1416–1424.

370. Malik R, Capoor MR, Vanidassane I, et al. Disseminated Emmonsia pasteuriana infection in India: A case report and a review. *Mycoses.* 2016;59(2):127–132.

371. Pelegrin I, Alastruey-Izquierdo A, Ayats J, Cuenca-Estrella M, Cabellos C. A second look at Emmonsia infection can make the difference. *Transpl Infect Dis.* 2014;16(3):519–520.

372. Byrd DR, El-Azhary RA, Gibson LE, Roberts GD. Sporotrichosis masquerading as pyoderma gangrenosum: Case report and review of 19 cases of sporotrichosis. *J Eur Acad Dermatol Venereol.* 2001;15(6):581–584.

373. Harris LF. Sporotrichosis, a hazard of outdoor work or recreation: Three illustrative cases. *Postgrad Med.* 1985;78(3):199–202.

374. da Rosa AC, Scroferneker ML, Vettorato R, Gervini RL, Vettorato G, Weber A. Epidemiology of sporotrichosis: A study of 304 cases in Brazil. *J Am Acad Dermatol.* 2005;52(3 Pt 1):451–459.

375. Mahajan VK, Sharma NL, Sharma RC, Gupta ML, Garg G, Kanga AK. *Cutaneous sporotrichosis* in Himachal Pradesh, India. *Mycoses.* 2005;48(1):25–31.

376. Schubach A, de Lima Barros MB, Schubach TM, et al. Primary conjunctival sporotrichosis: Two cases from a zoonotic epidemic in Rio de Janeiro, Brazil. *Cornea.* 2005;24(4):491–493.

377. Barros MB, Schubach Ade O, do Valle AC, et al. Cat-transmitted sporotrichosis epidemic in Rio de Janeiro, Brazil: Description of a series of cases. *Clin Infect Dis.* 2004;38(4):529–535.

378. Gullberg RM, Quintanilla A, Levin ML, Williams J, Phair JP. Sporotrichosis: Recurrent cutaneous, articular, and central nervous system infection in a renal transplant recipient. *Rev Infect Dis.* 1987;9(2):369–375.

379. Tambini R, Farina C, Fiocchi R, et al. Possible pathogenic role for *Sporothrix cyanescens* isolated from a lung lesion in a heart transplant patient. *J Med Vet Mycol.* 1996;34(3):195–198.

380. Grossi P, Farina C, Fiocchi R, Dalla Gasperina D. Prevalence and outcome of invasive fungal infections in 1,963 thoracic organ transplant recipients: A multicenter retrospective study—Italian Study Group of Fungal Infections in Thoracic Organ Transplant Recipients. *Transplantation.* 2000;70(1):112–116.

381. Wisplinghoff H, Bischoff T, Tallent SM, Seifert H, Wenzel RP, Edmond MB. Nosocomial bloodstream infections in US hospitals: Analysis of 24,179 cases from a prospective nationwide surveillance study. *Clin Infect Dis.* 2004;39(3):309–317.

382. Vincent JL, Rello J, Marshall J, et al. International study of the prevalence and outcomes of infection in intensive care units. *JAMA.* 2009;302(21):2323–2329.

383. Zilberberg MD, Shorr AF, Kollef MH. Secular trends in candidemia-related hospitalization in the United States, 2000–2005. *Infect Control Hosp Epidemiol.* 2008;29(10):978–980.

384. Cleveland AA, Farley MM, Harrison LH, et al. Changes in incidence and antifungal drug resistance in candidemia: Results from population-based laboratory surveillance in Atlanta and Baltimore, 2008–2011. *Clin Infect Dis.* 2012;55(10):1352–1361.

385. Lockhart SR, Iqbal N, Cleveland AA, et al. Species identification and antifungal susceptibility testing of Candida bloodstream isolates from population-based surveillance studies in two U.S. cities from 2008 to 2011. *J Clin Microbiol.* 2012;50(11):3435–3442.

386. Arendrup MC, Bruun B, Christensen JJ, et al. National surveillance of fungemia in Denmark (2004 to 2009). *J Clin Microbiol.* 2011;49(1):325–334.

387. Pfaller M, Neofytos D, Diekema D, et al. Epidemiology and outcomes of candidemia in 3648 patients: Data from the Prospective Antifungal Therapy (PATH Alliance(R)) registry, 2004–2008. *Diagn Microbiol Infect Dis.* 2012;74(4):323–331.

388. Pfaller MA, Messer SA, Moet GJ, Jones RN, Castanheira M. Candida bloodstream infections: Comparison of species distribution and resistance to echinocandin and azole antifungal agents in Intensive Care Unit (ICU) and non-ICU settings in the SENTRY Antimicrobial Surveillance Program (2008–2009). *Int J Antimicrob Agents.* 2011;38(1):65–69.

389. Fridkin SK, Kaufman D, Edwards JR, Shetty S, Horan T. Changing incidence of Candida bloodstream infections among NICU patients in the United States: 1995–2004. *Pediatrics.* 2006;117(5):1680–1687.

390. Wingard JR, Merz WG, Rinaldi MG, Miller CB, Karp JE, Saral R. Association of *Torulopsis glabrata* infections with fluconazole prophylaxis in neutropenic bone marrow transplant patients. *Antimicrob Agents Chemother.* 1993;37(9):1847–1849.

391. Wingard JR, Merz WG, Rinaldi MG, Johnson TR, Karp JE, Saral R. Increase in *Candida krusei* infection among patients with bone marrow transplantation and neutropenia treated prophylactically with fluconazole. *N Engl J Med.* 1991;325(18):1274–1277.

392. Andes D, Safdar N, Hadley S. Epidemiology of invasive Candida infections in solid and hematologic transplantation: Prospective surveillance results from the TRANSNET database. 44th ICAAC, Washington DC. October 30–November 2, 2004.

393. Weems JJ, Jr. *Candida parapsilosis*: Epidemiology, pathogenicity, clinical manifestations, and antimicrobial susceptibility. *Clin Infect Dis.* 1992;14(3):756–766.

394. Benjamin DK, Jr., Ross K, McKinney RE, Jr., Benjamin DK, Auten R, Fisher RG. When to suspect fungal infection in neonates: A clinical comparison of *Candida albicans* and *Candida parapsilosis* fungemia with coagulase-negative staphylococcal bacteremia. *Pediatrics.* 2000;106(4):712–718.

395. Fairchild KD, Tomkoria S, Sharp EC, Mena FV. Neonatal *Candida glabrata* sepsis: Clinical and laboratory features compared with other *Candida* species. *Pediatr Infect Dis J.* 2002;21(1):39–43.

396. Feja KN, Wu F, Roberts K, et al. Risk factors for candidemia in critically ill infants: A matched case-control study. *J Pediatr.* 2005;147(2):156–161.

397. Lopez Sastre JB, Coto Cotallo GD, Fernandez Colomer B. Neonatal invasive candidiasis: A prospective multicenter study of 118 cases. *Am J Perinatol.* 2003;20(3):153–163.

398. Saiman L, Ludington E, Dawson JD, et al. Risk factors for *Candida* species colonization of neonatal intensive care unit patients. *Pediatr Infect Dis J.* 2001;20(12):1119–1124.

399. Almirante B, Rodriguez D, Cuenca-Estrella M, et al. Epidemiology, risk factors, and prognosis of *Candida parapsilosis* bloodstream infections: Case-control population-based surveillance study of patients in Barcelona, Spain, from 2002 to 2003. *J Clin Microbiol.* 2006;44(5):1681–1685.

400. Brito LR, Guimaraes T, Nucci M, et al. Clinical and microbiological aspects of candidemia due to *Candida parapsilosis* in Brazilian tertiary care hospitals. *Med Mycol.* 2006;44(3):261–266.

401. Huang YC, Lin TY, Leu HS, Peng HL, Wu JH, Chang HY. Outbreak of *Candida parapsilosis* fungemia in neonatal intensive care units: Clinical implications and genotyping analysis. *Infection.* 1999;27(2):97–102.

402. Waggoner-Fountain LA, Walker MW, Hollis RJ, et al. Vertical and horizontal transmission of unique *Candida* species to premature newborns. *Clin Infect Dis.* 1996;22(5):803–808.

403. Barchiesi F, Caggiano G, Falconi Di Francesco L, Montagna MT, Barbuti S, Scalise G. Outbreak of fungemia due to *Candida parapsilosis* in a pediatric oncology unit. *Diagn Microbiol Infect Dis.* 2004;49(4):269–271.

404. Posteraro B, Bruno S, Boccia S, et al. *Candida parapsilosis* bloodstream infection in pediatric oncology patients: Results of an epidemiologic investigation. *Infect Control Hosp Epidemiol.* 2004;25(8):641–645.

405. Blumberg HM, Jarvis WR, Soucie JM, et al. Risk factors for candidal bloodstream infections in surgical intensive care unit patients: The NEMIS prospective multicenter study. The National Epidemiology of Mycosis Survey. *Clin Infect Dis.* 2001;33(2):177–186.

406. Ostrosky-Zeichner L, Sable C, Sobel J, et al. Multicenter retrospective development and validation of a clinical prediction rule for nosocomial invasive candidiasis in the intensive care setting. *Eur J Clin Microbiol Infect Dis.* 2007;26(4):271–276.

407. Leon C, Ruiz-Santana S, Saavedra P, et al. A bedside scoring system ("*Candida* score") for early antifungal treatment in nonneutropenic critically ill patients with *Candida* colonization. *Crit Care Med.* 2006;34(3):730–737.

408. Leon C, Ruiz-Santana S, Saavedra P, et al. Usefulness of the "*Candida* score" for discriminating between *Candida* colonization and invasive candidiasis in nonneutropenic critically ill patients: A prospective multicenter study. *Crit Care Med.* 2009;37(5):1624–1633.

409. Shetty SS, Harrison LH, Hajjeh RA, et al. Determining risk factors for candidemia among newborn infants from population-based surveillance: Baltimore, Maryland, 1998–2000. *Pediatr Infect Dis J.* 2005;24(7):601–604.

410. Solomkin JS. Pathogenesis and management of *Candida* infection syndromes in non-neutropenic patients. *New Horiz.* 1993;1(2):202–213.

411. Anaissie EJ, Rex JH, Uzun O, Vartivarian S. Predictors of adverse outcome in cancer patients with candidemia. *Am J Med.* 1998;104(3):238–245.

412. Colombo AL, Nucci M, Park BJ, et al. Epidemiology of candidemia in Brazil: A nationwide sentinel surveillance of candidemia in eleven medical centers. *J Clin Microbiol.* 2006;44(8):2816–2823.

413. Pappas PG, Rex JH, Lee J, et al. A prospective observational study of candidemia: Epidemiology, therapy, and influences on mortality in hospitalized adult and pediatric patients. *Clin Infect Dis.* 2003;37(5):634–643.

414. Benjamin DK, Jr., Poole C, Steinbach WJ, Rowen JL, Walsh TJ. Neonatal candidemia and end-organ damage: A critical appraisal of the literature using meta-analytic techniques. *Pediatrics.* 2003;112(3 Pt 1):634–640.

415. Hajjeh RA, Sofair AN, Harrison LH, et al. Incidence of bloodstream infections due to *Candida* species and in vitro susceptibilities of isolates collected from 1998 to 2000 in a population-based active surveillance program. *J Clin Microbiol.* 2004;42(4):1519–1527.

416. Ostrosky-Zeichner L, Pappas PG. Invasive candidiasis in the intensive care unit. *Crit Care Med.* 2006;34(3):857–863.

417. Marr KA, Seidel K, White TC, Bowden RA. Candidemia in allogeneic blood and marrow transplant recipients: Evolution of risk factors after the adoption of prophylactic fluconazole. *J Infect Dis.* 2000;181(1):309–316.

418. Hughes WT, Armstrong D, Bodey GP, et al. 2002 guidelines for the use of antimicrobial agents in neutropenic patients with cancer. *Clin Infect Dis.* 2002;34(6):730–751.

419. Thaler M, Pastakia B, Shawker TH, O'Leary T, Pizzo PA. Hepatic candidiasis in cancer patients: The evolving picture of the syndrome. *Ann Intern Med.* 1988;108(1):88–100.

420. Bodey GP, Luna M. Skin lesions associated with disseminated candidiasis. *JAMA.* 1974;229(11):1466–1468.

421. Bae GY, Lee HW, Chang SE, et al. Clinicopathologic review of 19 patients with systemic candidiasis with skin lesions. *Int J Dermatol.* 2005;44(7):550–555.

422. Donahue SP. Intraocular candidiasis in patients with candidemia. *Ophthalmology.* 1998;105(5):759–760.

423. Scherer WJ, Lee K. Implications of early systemic therapy on the incidence of endogenous fungal endophthalmitis. *Ophthalmology.* 1997;104(10):1593–1598.

424. Donahue SP, Greven CM, Zuravleff JJ, et al. Intraocular candidiasis in patients with candidemia: Clinical implications derived from a prospective multicenter study. *Ophthalmology.* 1994;101(7):1302–1309.

425. Rex JH, Bennett JE, Sugar AM, et al. A randomized trial comparing fluconazole with amphotericin B for the treatment of candidemia in patients without neutropenia: Candidemia Study Group and the National Institute. *N Engl J Med.* 1994;331(20):1325–1330.

426. Brooks RG. Prospective study of *Candida* endophthalmitis in hospitalized patients with candidemia. *Arch Intern Med.* 1989;149(10):2226–2228.

427. Edwards JE, Jr., Foos RY, Montgomerie JZ, Guze LB. Ocular manifestations of *Candida* septicemia: Review of seventy-six cases of hematogenous *Candida* endophthalmitis. *Medicine (Baltimore).* 1974;53(1):47–75.

428. Henderson DK, Hockey LJ, Vukalcic LJ, Edwards JE, Jr. Effect of immunosuppression on the development of experimental hematogenous *Candida* endophthalmitis. *Infect Immun.* 1980;27(2):628–631.

429. Perfect JR, Casadevall A. Cryptococcosis. *Infect Dis Clin North Am.* 2002;16(4):837–874, v-vi.

430. Vilchez RA, Fung J, Kusne S. Cryptococcosis in organ transplant recipients: An overview. *Am J Transplant.* 2002;2(7):575–580.

431. Zeluff BJ. Fungal pneumonia in transplant recipients. *Semin Respir Infect.* 1990;5(1):80–89.

432. Chayakulkeeree M, Perfect JR. Cryptococcosis. *Infect Dis Clin North Am.* 2006;20(3):507–544, v–vi.

433. Kidd SE, Bach PJ, Hingston AO, et al. *Cryptococcus gattii* dispersal mechanisms, British Columbia, Canada. *Emerg Infect Dis.* 2007;13(1):51–57.

434. MacDougall L, Kidd SE, Galanis E, et al. Spread of *Cryptococcus gattii* in British Columbia, Canada, and detection in the Pacific Northwest, USA. *Emerg Infect Dis.* 2007;13(1):42–50.

435. Lui G, Lee N, Ip M, et al. Cryptococcosis in apparently immunocompetent patients. *QJM.* 2006;99(3):143–151.

436. Dora JM, Kelbert S, Deutschendorf C, et al. Cutaneous cryptococccosis due to *Cryptococcus gattii* in immunocompetent hosts: Case report and review. *Mycopathologia.* 2006;161(4):235–238.

437. Lindberg J, Hagen F, Laursen A, Stenderup J, Boekhout T. *Cryptococcus gattii* risk for tourists visiting Vancouver Island, Canada. *Emerg Infect Dis.* 2007;13(1):178–179.

438. Morgan J, McCarthy KM, Gould S, et al. *Cryptococcus gattii* infection: Characteristics and epidemiology of cases identified in a South African province with high HIV seroprevalence, 2002–2004. *Clin Infect Dis.* 2006;43(8):1077–1080.

439. Chang WC, Tzao C, Hsu HH, et al. Pulmonary cryptococcosis: Comparison of clinical and radiographic characteristics in immunocompetent and immunocompromised patients. *Chest.* 2006;129(2):333–340.

440. Chang WC, Tzao C, Hsu HH, Chang H, Lo CP, Chen CY. Isolated cryptococcal thoracic empyema with osteomyelitis of the rib in an immunocompetent host. *J Infect.* 2005;51(3):e117–119.

441. Fox DL, Muller NL. Pulmonary cryptococcosis in immunocompetent patients: CT findings in 12 patients. *AJR Am J Roentgenol.* 2005;185(3):622–626.

442. Wise GJ, Shteynshlyuger A. How to diagnose and treat fungal infections in chronic prostatitis. *Current urology reports.* 2006;7(4):320–328.

443. Hajjeh RA, Conn LA, Stephens DS, et al. Cryptococcosis: Population-based multistate active surveillance and risk factors in human immunodeficiency virus-infected persons: Cryptococcal Active Surveillance Group. *J Infect Dis.* 1999;179(2):449–454.

444. Mirza SA, Phelan M, Rimland D, et al. The changing epidemiology of cryptococcosis: An update from population-based active surveillance in 2 large metropolitan areas, 1992–2000. *Clin Infect Dis.* 2003;36(6):789–794.

445. Dromer F, Mathoulin-Pelissier S, Fontanet A, Ronin O, Dupont B, Lortholary O. Epidemiology of HIV-associated cryptococcosis in France (1985–2001): Comparison of the pre- and post-HAART eras. *AIDS.* 2004;18(3):555–562.

446. French N, Gray K, Watera C, et al. Cryptococcal infection in a cohort of HIV-1-infected Ugandan adults. *AIDS.* 2002;16(7):1031–1038.

447. Wong ML, Back P, Candy G, Nelson G, Murray J. Cryptococcal pneumonia in African miners at autopsy. *Int J Tuberc Lung Dis.* 2007;11(5):528–533.

448. Moreira Tde A, Ferreira MS, Ribas RM, Borges AS. Cryptococosis: Clinical epidemiological laboratory study and fungi varieties in 96 patients. *Rev Soc Bras Med Trop.* 2006;39(3):255–258.

449. Garbino J, Kolarova L, Lew D, Hirschel B, Rohner P. Fungemia in HIV-infected patients: A 12-year study in a tertiary care hospital. *AIDS Patient Care STDS.* 2001;15(8):407–410.

450. Broom J, Woods M, 2nd, Allworth A. Immune reconstitution inflammatory syndrome producing atypical presentations of cryptococcal meningitis: Case report and a review of immune reconstitution-associated cryptococcal infections. *Scand J Infect Dis.* 2006;38(3):219–221.

451. Skiest DJ, Hester LJ, Hardy RD. Cryptococcal immune reconstitution inflammatory syndrome: Report of four cases in three patients and review of the literature. *J Infect.* 2005;51(5):e289–297.

452. Fishman JA, Rubin RH. Infection in organ-transplant recipients. *N Engl J Med.* 1998;338(24):1741–1751.

453. Vilchez R, Shapiro R, McCurry K, et al. Longitudinal study of cryptococcosis in adult solid-organ transplant recipients. *Transpl Int.* 2003;16(5):336–340.

454. Husain S, Wagener MM, Singh N. *Cryptococcus neoformans* infection in organ transplant recipients: Variables influencing clinical characteristics and outcome. *Emerg Infect Dis.* 2001;7(3):375–381.

455. Pappas PG, Alexander B, Marr KA, et al. Invasive fungal infections (IFIs) in hematopoietic stem cell (HSCTs) and organ transplant recipients (OTRs): Overview of the TRANSNET database. *42nd Annual Meeting of the Infectious Disease Society of America, Boston, MA.* September 2004:174.

456. Singh N, Alexander BD, Lortholary O, et al. *Cryptococcus neoformans* in organ transplant recipients: Impact of calcineurin-inhibitor agents on mortality. *J Infect Dis.* 2007;195(5):756–764.

457. Mueller NJ, Fishman JA. Asymptomatic pulmonary cryptococcosis in solid organ transplantation: Report of four cases and review of the literature. *Transpl Infect Dis.* 2003;5(3):140–143.

458. Khawcharoenporn T, Apisarnthanarak A, Mundy LM. Non-neoformans cryptococcal infections: A systematic review. *Infection.* 2007;35(2):51–58.

459. Giusiano G, Mangiaterra M, Saito VG, Rojas F, Gomez V, Diaz MC. Etiology of fungaemia and catheter colonisation in Argentinean paediatric patients. *Mycoses.* 2006;49(1):49–54.

460. Crowson AN, Magro CM. Atrophying tinea versicolor: A clinical and histological study of 12 patients. *Int J Dermatol.* 2003;42(12):928–932.

461. Chryssanthou E, Broberger U, Petrini B. *Malassezia pachydermatis* fungaemia in a neonatal intensive care unit. *Acta Paediatr.* 2001;90(3):323–327.

462. Gupta AK, Kohli Y, Faergemann J, Summerbell RC. Epidemiology of *Malassezia* yeasts associated with pityriasis versicolor in Ontario, Canada. *Med Mycol.* 2001;39(2):199–206.

463. Dankner WM, Spector SA, Fierer J, Davis CE. *Malassezia* fungemia in neonates and adults: Complication of hyperalimentation. *Rev Infect Dis.* 1987;9(4):743–753.

464. Redline RW, Redline SS, Boxerbaum B, Dahms BB. Systemic *Malassezia furfur* infections in patients receiving intralipid therapy. *Hum Pathol.* 1985;16(8):815–822.

465. Gueho E, Midgley G, Guillot J. The genus *Malassezia* with description of four new species. *Antonie Van Leeuwenhoek.* 1996;69(4):337–355.

466. Morishita N, Sei Y. Microreview of Pityriasis versicolor and *Malassezia* species. *Mycopathologia.* 2006;162(6):373–376.

467. Crespo-Erchiga V, Florencio VD. Malassezia yeasts and pityriasis versicolor. *Curr Opin Infect Dis.* 2006;19(2):139–147.

468. Gupta AK, Batra R, Bluhm R, Boekhout T, Dawson TL, Jr. Skin diseases associated with *Malassezia* species. *J Am Acad Dermatol.* 2004;51(5):785–798.

469. Rhie S, Turcios R, Buckley H, Suh B. Clinical features and treatment of *Malassezia folliculitis* with fluconazole in orthotopic heart transplant recipients. *J Heart Lung Transplant.* 2000;19(2):215–219.

470. Alves EV, Martins JE, Ribeiro EB, Sotto MN. *Pityrosporum folliculitis*: Renal transplantation case report. *J Dermatol.* 2000;27(1):49–51.

471. Bufill JA, Lum LG, Caya JG, et al. *Pityrosporum folliculitis* after bone marrow transplantation. Clinical observations in five patients. *Ann Intern Med.* 1988;108(4):560–563.

472. Morrison VA, Weisdorf DJ. The spectrum of *Malassezia* infections in the bone marrow transplant population. *Bone Marrow Transplant.* 2000;26(6):645–648.

473. Chang HJ, Miller HL, Watkins N, et al. An epidemic of *Malassezia pachydermatis* in an intensive care nursery associated with colonization of health care workers' pet dogs. *N Engl J Med.* 1998;338(11):706–711.

474. Richet HM, McNeil MM, Edwards MC, Jarvis WR. Cluster of *Malassezia furfur* pulmonary infections in infants in a neonatal intensive-care unit. *J Clin Microbiol.* 1989;27(6):1197–1200.

475. Colombo AL, Padovan AC, Chaves GM. Current knowledge of *Trichosporon* spp. and Trichosporonosis. *Clin Microbiol Rev.* 2011;24(4):682–700.

476. Sugita T, Nishikawa A, Shinoda T, Kume H. Taxonomic position of deep-seated, mucosa-associated, and superficial isolates of *Trichosporon cutaneum* from trichosporonosis patients. *J Clin Microbiol.* 1995;33(5):1368–1370.

477. Gueho E, Improvisi L, de Hoog GS, Dupont B. Trichosporon on humans: A practical account. *Mycoses.* 1994;37(1–2):3–10.

478. Kiken DA, Sekaran A, Antaya RJ, Davis A, Imaeda S, Silverberg NB. White piedra in children. *J Am Acad Dermatol.* 2006;55(6):956–961.

479. Erer B, Galimberti M, Lucarelli G, et al. *Trichosporon beigelii*: A life-threatening pathogen in immuno-compromised hosts. *Bone Marrow Transplant.* 2000;25(7):745–749.

480. Lussier N, Laverdiere M, Delorme J, Weiss K, Dandavino R. *Trichosporon beigelii* funguria in renal transplant recipients. *Clin Infect Dis.* 2000;31(5):1299–1301.

481. Moretti-Branchini ML, Fukushima K, Schreiber AZ, et al. *Trichosporon* species infection in bone marrow transplanted patients. *Diagn Microbiol Infect Dis.* 2001;39(3):161–164.

482. Lowenthal RM, Atkinson K, Challis DR, Tucker RG, Biggs JC. Invasive *Trichosporon cutaneum* infection: An increasing problem in immunosuppressed patients. *Bone Marrow Transplant.* 1987;2(3):321–327.

483. Mirza SH. Disseminated *Trichosporon beigelii* infection causing skin lesions in a renal transplant patient. *J Infect.* 1993;27(1):67–70.

484. Ness MJ, Markin RS, Wood RP, Shaw BW, Jr., Woods GL. Disseminated *Trichosporon beigelii* infection after orthotopic liver transplantation. *Am J Clin Pathol.* 1989;92(1):119–123.

485. Rello J, Brunet S, Ausina V, et al. Disseminated infection caused by *Trichosporon beigelii* in a patient with acute leukemia. *Enferm Infecc Microbiol Clin.* 1990;8(7):443–445.

486. Tashiro T, Nagai H, Nagaoka H, Goto Y, Kamberi P, Nasu M. *Trichosporon beigelii* pneumonia in patients with hematologic malignancies. *Chest.* 1995;108(1):190–195.

487. Vasta S, Menozzi M, Scime R, et al. Central catheter infection by *Trichosporon beigelii* after autologous blood stem cell transplantation: A case report and review of the literature. *Haematologica.* 1993;78(1):64–67.

488. Walsh TJ, Melcher GP, Lee JW, Pizzo PA. Infections due to *Trichosporon* species: New concepts in mycology, pathogenesis, diagnosis and treatment. *Curr Top Med Mycol.* 1993;5:79–113.

489. Liao Y, Lu X, Yang S, Luo Y, Chen Q, Yang R. Epidemiology and outcome of *Trichosporon* fungemia: A review of 185 reported cases from 1975 to 2014. *Open Forum Infect Dis.* 2015;2(4):ofv141.

490. de Almeida Junior JN, Hennequin C. Invasive trichosporon infection: A systematic review on a re-emerging fungal pathogen. *Front Microbiol.* 2016;7:1629.

491. Tuon FF, Costa SF. Rhodotorula infection: A systematic review of 128 cases from literature. *Revista iberoamericana de micologia.* 2008;25(3):135–140.

492. Tuon FF, de Almeida GM, Costa SF. Central venous catheter-associated fungemia due to *Rhodotorula* spp.: A systematic review. *Med Mycol.* 2007;45(5):441–447.

493. Chitasombat MN, Kofteridis DP, Jiang Y, Tarrand J, Lewis RE, Kontoyiannis DP. Rare opportunistic (non-*Candida*, non-*Cryptococcus*) yeast bloodstream infections in patients with cancer. *J Infect.* 2012;64(1):68–75.

494. Fernandez-Ruiz M, Guinea J, Puig-Asensio M, et al. Fungemia due to rare opportunistic yeasts: Data from a population-based surveillance in Spain. *Med Mycol.* 2017;55(2):125–136.

495. Mori T, Nakamura Y, Kato J, et al. Fungemia due to *Rhodotorula mucilaginosa* after allogeneic hematopoietic stem cell transplantation. *Transpl Infect Dis.* 2012;14(1):91–94.

496. Munoz P, Bouza E, Cuenca-Estrella M, et al. *Saccharomyces cerevisiae* fungemia: An emerging infectious disease. *Clin Infect Dis.* 2005;40(11):1625–1634.

497. Enache-Angoulvant A, Hennequin C. Invasive Saccharomyces infection: A comprehensive review. *Clin Infect Dis.* 2005;41(11):1559–1568.

498. Darroch CJ, Barnes RM, Dawson J. Circulating antibodies to *Saccharomyces cerevisiae* (bakers'/brewers' yeast) in gastrointestinal disease. *J Clin Pathol.* 1999;52(1):47–53.

499. Salonen JH, Richardson MD, Gallacher K, et al. Fungal colonization of haematological patients receiving cytotoxic chemotherapy: Emergence of azole-resistant *Saccharomyces cerevisiae*. *J Hosp Infect.* 2000;45(4):293–301.

500. Henrich TJ, Marty FM, Milner DA, Jr., Thorner AR. Disseminated *Geotrichum candidum* infection in a patient with relapsed acute myelogenous leukemia following allogeneic stem cell transplantation and review of the literature. *Transpl Infect Dis.* 2009;11(5):458–462.

501. Stringer JR, Beard CB, Miller RF, Wakefield AE. A new name (*Pneumocystis jiroveci*) for Pneumocystis from humans. *Emerg Infect Dis.* 2002;8(9):891–896.

502. Morris A, Lundgren JD, Masur H, et al. Current epidemiology of Pneumocystis pneumonia. *Emerg Infect Dis.* 2004;10(10):1713–1720.

503. Fishman JA. Prevention of infection caused by *Pneumocystis carinii* in transplant recipients. *Clin Infect Dis.* 2001;33(8):1397–1405.

504. Frenkel JK. *Pneumocystis jiroveci* n. sp. from man: Morphology, physiology, and immunology in relation to pathology. *Natl Cancer Inst Monogr.* 1976;43:13–30.

505. Wakefield AE. *Pneumocystis carinii. Br Med Bull.* 2002;61:175–188.

506. Phair J, Munoz A, Detels R, Kaslow R, Rinaldo C, Saah A. The risk of *Pneumocystis carinii* pneumonia among men infected with human immunodeficiency virus type 1. Multicenter AIDS Cohort Study Group. *N Engl J Med.* 1990;322(3):161–165.

507. Thomas CF, Jr., Limper AH. Pneumocystis pneumonia. *N Engl J Med.* 2004;350(24):2487–2498.

508. Hocker B, Wendt C, Nahimana A, Tonshoff B, Hauser PM. Molecular evidence of Pneumocystis transmission in pediatric transplant unit. *Emerg Infect Dis.* 2005;11(2):330–332.

509. Morris A, Beard CB, Huang L. Update on the epidemiology and transmission of *Pneumocystis carinii. Microb Infect.* 2002;4(1):95–103.

510. Rabodonirina M, Vanhems P, Couray-Targe S, et al. Molecular evidence of interhuman transmission of Pneumocystis pneumonia among renal transplant recipients hospitalized with HIV-infected patients. *Emerg Infect Dis.* 2004;10(10):1766–1773.

511. Pifer LL, Hughes WT, Stagno S, Woods D. *Pneumocystis carinii* infection: Evidence for high prevalence in normal and immunosuppressed children. *Pediatrics.* 1978;61(1):35–41.

512. Vargas SL, Hughes WT, Santolaya ME, et al. Search for primary infection by *Pneumocystis carinii* in a cohort of normal, healthy infants. *Clin Infect Dis.* 2001;32(6):855–861.

513. Nevez G, Totet A, Pautard JC, Raccurt C. *Pneumocystis carinii* detection using nested-PCR in nasopharyngeal aspirates of immunocompetent infants with bronchiolitis. *J Eukaryot Microbiol.* 2001;Suppl:122s–123s.

514. Totet A, Respaldiza N, Pautard JC, Raccurt C, Nevez G. *Pneumocystis jiroveci* genotypes and primary infection. *Clin Infect Dis.* 2003;36(10):1340–1342.

515. Larsen HH, von Linstow ML, Lundgren B, Hogh B, Westh H, Lundgren JD. Primary pneumocystis infection in infants hospitalized with acute respiratory tract infection. *Emerg Infect Dis.* 2007;13(1):66–72.

516. Huang L, Crothers K, Morris A, et al. Pneumocystis colonization in HIV-infected patients. *J Eukaryot Microbiol.* 2003;50 Suppl:616–617.

517. Nevez G, Raccurt C, Jounieaux V, Dei-Cas E, Mazars E. Pneumocystosis versus pulmonary *Pneumocystis carinii* colonization in HIV-negative and HIV-positive patients. *AIDS.* 1999;13(4):535–536.

518. Morris A, Sciurba FC, Lebedeva IP, et al. Association of chronic obstructive pulmonary disease severity and Pneumocystis colonization. *Am J Respir Crit Care Med.* 2004;170(4):408–413.

519. Probst M, Ries H, Schmidt-Wieland T, Serr A. Detection of *Pneumocystis carinii* DNA in patients with chronic lung diseases. *Eur J Clin Microbiol Infect Dis.* 2000;19(8):644–645.

520. Stringer JR. Pneumocystis. *Int J Med Microbiol.* 2002;292(5–6):391–404.

521. Pneumocystis pneumonia—Los Angeles. *MMWR Morb Mortal Wkly Rep.* 1981;30(21):250–252.

522. Franquet T, Gimenez A, Hidalgo A. Imaging of opportunistic fungal infections in immunocompromised patient. *Eur J Radiol.* 2004;51(2):130–138.

523. Chow C, Templeton PA, White CS. Lung cysts associated with *Pneumocystis carinii* pneumonia: Radiographic characteristics, natural history, and complications. *AJR Am J Roentgenol.* 1993;161(3):527–531.

524. De Castro N, Neuville S, Sarfati C, et al. Occurrence of *Pneumocystis jiroveci* pneumonia after allogeneic stem cell transplantation: A 6-year retrospective study. *Bone Marrow Transplant.* 2005;36(10):879–883.

525. Roblot F, Godet C, Le Moal G, et al. Analysis of underlying diseases and prognosis factors associated with *Pneumocystis carinii* pneumonia in immunocompromised HIV-negative patients. *Eur J Clin Microbiol Infect Dis.* 2002;21(7):523–531.

526. Roblot F, Le Moal G, Godet C, et al. *Pneumocystis carinii* pneumonia in patients with hematologic malignancies: A descriptive study. *J Infect.* 2003;47(1):19–27.

527. Roblot F, Imbert S, Godet C, et al. Risk factors analysis for *Pneumocystis jiroveci* pneumonia (PCP) in patients with haematological malignancies and pneumonia. *Scand J Infect Dis.* 2004;36(11–12):848–854.

528. Torres HA, Chemaly RF, Storey R, et al. Influence of type of cancer and hematopoietic stem cell transplantation on clinical presentation of *Pneumocystis jiroveci* pneumonia in cancer patients. *Eur J Clin Microbiol Infect Dis.* 2006;25(6):382–388.

529. Gryzan S, Paradis IL, Zeevi A, et al. Unexpectedly high incidence of *Pneumocystis carinii* infection after lung-heart transplantation: Implications for lung defense and allograft survival. *Am Rev Respir Dis.* 1988;137(6):1268–1274.

530. Joos L, Chhajed PN, Wallner J, et al. Pulmonary infections diagnosed by BAL: A 12-year experience in 1066 immunocompromised patients. *Respir Med.* 2007;101(1):93–97.

531. Kramer MR, Stoehr C, Lewiston NJ, Starnes VA, Theodore J. Trimethoprim-sulfamethoxazole prophylaxis for *Pneumocystis carinii* infections in heart-lung and lung transplantation—how effective and for how long? *Transplantation.* 1992;53(3):586–589.

532. Radisic M, Lattes R, Chapman JF, et al. Risk factors for *Pneumocystis carinii* pneumonia in kidney transplant recipients: A case-control study. *Transpl Infect Dis.* 2003;5(2):84–93.

533. Gordon SM, LaRosa SP, Kalmadi S, et al. Should prophylaxis for *Pneumocystis carinii* pneumonia in solid organ transplant recipients ever be discontinued? *Clin Infect Dis.* 1999;28(2):240–246.

534. Yoo JH, Lee DG, Choi SM, et al. Infectious complications and outcomes after allogeneic hematopoietic stem cell transplantation in Korea. *Bone Marrow Transplant.* 2004;34(6):497–504.

535. Arend SM, Westendorp RG, Kroon FP, et al. Rejection treatment and cytomegalovirus infection as risk factors for *Pneumocystis carinii* pneumonia in renal transplant recipients. *Clin Infect Dis.* 1996;22(6):920–925.

536. Hazzan M, Copin MC, Pruvot FR, et al. Lung granulomatous pneumocystosis after kidney transplantation: An uncommon complication. *Transplant Proc.* 1997;29(5):2409.

537. Leroy X, Copin MC, Ramon P, Jouet JP, Gosselin B. Nodular granulomatous *Pneumocystis carinii* pneumonia in a bone marrow transplant recipient. Case report. *APMIS.* 2000;108(5):363–366.

538. Walzer PD. Pneumocystis carinii. In: Mandell GL, Bennett JE, Dolin R, eds. *Principles and Practice of Infectious Diseases*, 5th ed. Philadelphia, PA: Churchill Livingstone. 2000:2781–2795.

539. Paradis IL, Williams, P. Infection after lung transplantation. *Semin Respir Infect.* 1993;8(3):207–215.

3

Experimental animal models of invasive fungal infections

CHRISTOPHER L. HAGER, LISA LONG, YOSHIFUMI IMAMURA, AND MAHMOUD A. GHANNOUM

INTRODUCTION

Animal models play an important role in antimicrobial drug discovery. The initial standard approach to discovery and development of antimicrobial agents, including antifungals, is to screen activity of a large number of various compounds (e.g., chemical libraries) against reference organisms *in vitro*. This step is known as primary screening. When a potential candidate is identified, antifungal activity against a large panel of clinical isolates is undertaken. Candidate compounds, which demonstrate an appreciable antimicrobial activity in these tests, are selected and their properties characterized further using many different test systems *in vitro* and *in vivo* (e.g., pharmacokinetic properties). The *in vivo* efficacy of a candidate compound can be dramatically affected by pharmacokinetics and pharmacodynamics of the drugs [1]. Hence, no matter how sophisticated drug screening and development may be, an essential step in the discovery and development of new antimicrobial and antifungal therapies, before testing in humans, is evaluation of the drug for its antimicrobial efficacy and toxicity

in animal models. In this regard, showing that a candidate compound is active *in vitro* does not necessarily guarantee that it is active *in vivo*. Importantly, some compounds that possess outstanding activity *in vitro* turn up to be very toxic when introduced into animals. Therefore, evaluation of candidate drugs in animal models is a critical step in predicting the efficacy and toxicity of antifungal agents in humans.

This chapter describes animal models of medically important fungal infections, including candidiasis, aspergillosis, and cryptococcosis, as well as catheter-associated biofilm *in vivo* models developed by our group. This chapter also describes a guinea pig model that is used in evaluating antifungals targeting superficial fungal infections (*dermatophytosis*).

CANDIDIASIS

Hematogenously disseminated models

A suitable animal model is essential to delineate the efficacy of any therapeutic agent, optimize its mode of delivery, and assess drug–drug interactions when combined, in the treatment of candidiasis. Systemic infection models for candidiasis have been established in mice, rats, guinea pigs, and rabbits. Among these animals, the mouse is the most popular species for evaluating the efficacy of antifungal agents followed by rabbit, rat, and guinea pig. The reason why the murine model is often used is: (*i*) mice can be easily infected, (*ii*) disseminated candidiasis in the mouse produces disseminated infection in a manner similar to that developed in immunocompromised patients (e.g., kidney and brain invasion), (*iii*) a large body of literature exists regarding antifungal therapy in this model, (*iv*) the mouse model is the best system for large-scale evaluation of anti-*Candida* agents, (*v*) the mouse is the lowest member of the phylogenic tree in which an infection can be produced that resembles human candidiasis, (*vi*) only small quantities of candidate compounds are needed for initial screening, and (*vii*) the mouse model is more economical with respect to purchase, per diem, and husbandry costs. Finally, a well-known background and variety of strains exist, such as outbred mice, inbred mice, and specific gene mutant mice. Outbred mice, such as CD-1 mice (or ICR mice) [2] and CF1 [3] mice, or inbred mice, including BALB/c [4], C57BL/6 [5], and C3H/He [6], are generally used for evaluating the efficacy of candidate antifungals in the treatment of hematogenously disseminated candidiasis. Moreover, immunocompetent and immunocompromised models have been employed to evaluate the efficacy of antifungal agents. Immunosuppression can be induced with cyclophosphamide [7], 5-fluorouracil [8], or gold sodium thiomalate [9].

Challenge of mice in this model is generally achieved by infecting the animals by intravenous injection (i.v.) through the tail vein. Challenge dose used to infect animals is determined based on the virulence of the *Candida* strain used to challenge them and the susceptibility of the mouse strain to the infection. In general, an i.v. inoculum higher than 10^6 *Candida albicans* is rapidly lethal while an inoculum less than 10^4 gives a low-grade, chronic infection with spontaneous resolution [1]. MacCallum and Odds [10] demonstrated the effect of challenge dose on infection outcomes. They examined the relationship between challenge dose and survival time for two mouse species (BALB/c and DBA/2) and *C. albicans* strain (SC5314) and found the range 2×10^4 to 1×10^5 organisms/g of body weight for BALB/c and 2×10^2 to 1×10^3 organisms/g of body weight for DBA/2 lead to reproducible survival times in the range of 2–10 days (Figure 3.1). In neutropenic mice, the minimal lethal dose may decrease by two logs or more. Low virulent strains require much higher inoculum to cause a lethal infection up to 5×10^7 colony-forming units (CFUs) per mouse [11].

Drugs being evaluated for their efficacy in the treatment of systemic candidiasis are administered via various routes, such as intraperitoneally (i.p.), orally (p.o.), subcutaneously (s.c.) or intravenously. Intraperitoneal route

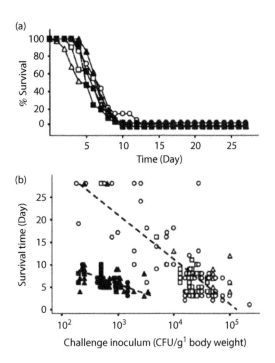

Figure 3.1 **(a)** Kaplan–Meier survival curves and **(b)** survival times (times to termination) of individual mice as a function of challenge inoculum for female BALB/c (open symbols) and DBA/2 (closed symbols) mice inoculated i.v. with *Candida albicans* SC5314 (circles), CAF2–1 (triangles), or CAI-4 + Clp10 (squares). Dashed lines shown are regression lines calculated for each mouse strain without regard to *C. albicans* challenge strain. (From MacCallum, D.M. and Odds, F.C., *Mycoses*, 48, 151–161, 2005.)

is more convenient to use than the i.v. route for repeated administration, since tail veins may collapse, especially when more than once daily dosing is used. Some antifungal agents, such as voriconazole and terbinafine, are rapidly cleared from mice (voriconazole causes autoclearance in rodents). In such cases, alternative guinea pig models have been used [12]. Alternatively, doses of voriconazole can be given two or three times a day to sustain drug levels in the plasma.

Survival rates (Figure 3.1) and tissue fungal burden, particularly the kidneys and also increasingly the brain, are the main endpoints used to assess efficacy of an agent in the treatment of systemic candidiasis. Other read-outs, although used infrequently, include body weight [13] and physiological characteristics of mice (such as blood pressure, heart rate, and body temperature as well as blood chemistry parameters) [14].

Vaginal candidiasis models

Mouse and rat models of vaginal candidiasis have been used for testing the efficacy of topical or systematic antifungal agents. Different kinds of animal strains, such as mice

(BALB/c [15], C57BL/6, CBA/J [16], DBA/2, and C3H/HEN) and rats (Sprague-Dawley [17], CD, Wistar, and Alderley Park), have been used in these models. Calderon et al. reported that differences in host factors influence the susceptibility of the different strains to vaginally administered *C. albicans*. These authors compared BALB/c, CD-1, DBA/2, AKR/j, C3H/HeN, A/J, C57BL/6, and CBA/J mice strains for their susceptibility to *Candida* infections. Of these mouse strains, only CD-1 mice showed resistance to vaginal candidiasis [18]. Therefore, all of the different mouse strains tested, with the exception of CD-1 strain, can be used in *in vivo* screening of potential antifungal agents for treating vaginal candidiasis.

Vaginitis in rodents is inducible only under conditions of a pseudo-estrus [19]. Estradiol valerate is injected subcutaneously to induce and maintain the pseudo-estrus condition [15,17]. Animals are anesthetized and inoculated intravaginally with 1×10^5–2.5×10^8 cells/mouse [15] (DA Stevens J *Antimicrob Chemother* (2002) 50 (3): 361–364 or 10^7 cells/rat [17]). Topical drugs are administrated with a small volume of an oil-based vehicle, such as polyethyleneglycol using a pipetman or a gavage needle, while p.o. treatment is administrated using a gavage needle.

To monitor the course of infection and the efficacy of antifungal agents in the treatment of candidiasis, fungal cells are recovered from lavage fluid or homogenized tissue. Vaginal lavage is obtained by gentle to moderate agitation with phosphate buffered saline (PBS). Alternatively, vaginal infection is monitored by obtaining a swab from the vagina and used for semi-quantitative evaluation. The vaginal lumen is sampled with a sterile cotton swab or a calibrated (1 µL) plastic loop and either plated onto Sabouraud dextrose agar (SDA) plates or collected in PBS for serial dilution and plating.

Oral candidiasis model

Oropharyngeal *Candida* infection is a serious problem for patients with AIDS, diabetes mellitus, those receiving broad-spectrum antibiotics, steroids, or immunosuppressive drugs, as well as radiation for head and neck cancer. There are several clinical variants of oral candidiasis, such as pseudomembranous, erythematous, angular cheilitis, and hyperplastic type [20,22]. Among these variants, pseudomembranous candidiasis (thrush) is the best-known form of mucosal candidiasis and is mainly encountered in HIV-infected patients. *C. albicans* is the predominant species to cause oral candidiasis. However, recent data shows that *C. glabrata* is increasing in incidence particularly in head and neck cancer patients treated with radiation [23].

Rats and mice have been most used to develop oral candidiasis models because of their variety and convenience to manipulate. Since establishing an oral candidal

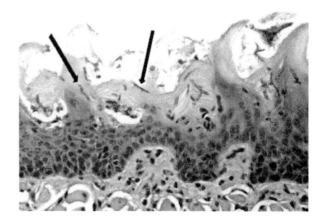

Figure 3.2 Period Acid Schiff stained tongue from a mouse 24 hours post inoculation with *C. albicans* (200×). Fungal hyphae are visible in the epithelium (arrows).

infection is challenging in immunocompetent animals, a variety of approaches have been employed to establish the infection. These approaches include the use of: (*i*) broad-spectrum antibiotic therapy (e.g., tetracycline) [21], (*ii*) carbohydrate-rich diets [24], (*iii*) topical use of corticosteroids [25], (*iv*) corticosteroid inhalation [26], (*v*) estrogen injection [27], (*vi*) trauma [28], (*vii*) iron deficiency [29], (*viii*) diabetes [30], (*ix*) xerostomia [30], and (*x*) immunosuppressive therapy [31]. Oral infection is accomplished by means of a cotton swab rolled over all parts of the mouth [32], or cotton-tipped applicators soaked with inoculum are kept sublingually for at least 90 minutes to consistently induce infection, while drug efficacy is assessed by measuring the number of *C. albicans* CFUs in oral swabs or homogenized tissue. Histopathological examination is also employed to assess the efficacy of drugs [32] (Figure 3.2).

Rabbit *Candida* biofilm model

Central venous catheters infected with *Candida* biofilms are problematic since biofilms are nearly totally resistant to common antifungal agents [33–35]. Therefore, developing and evaluating new drugs against *Candida* biofilms by using animal models is quite valuable. While rabbits and rats have been used to develop catheter-associated *Candida* biofilm models [36], rabbits are more commonly used in evaluating the efficacy of antifungal agents in the treatment of catheter infections caused by candidal biofilms [37]. For example, the author's group showed that using a rabbit model of catheter-associated *C. albicans* biofilm, lipid-based amphotericin B, and echinocandins (anidulafungin, caspofungin, and micafungin) are effective in the treatment of biofilms formed on the internal lumen of

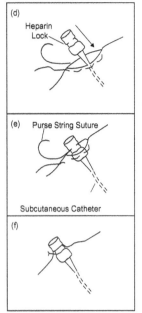
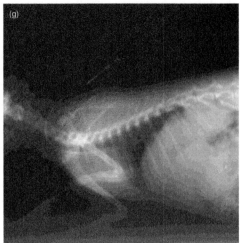

Figure 3.3 Surgical placement of the intravenous catheter. **(a–c)** Catheter insertion into the external jugular vein; **(d–f)** attachment of the heparin lock device to skin; **(g)** postoperative venogram of catheter placement. (From Ghannoum, M.A., Are there antifungals that are effective against *Candida* biofilms? *16th Congress of the International Society for Human and Animal Mycology*, Paris, France, 2006.)

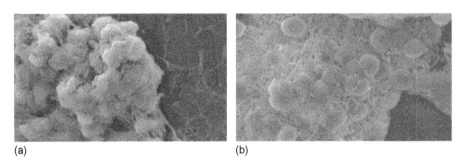

Figure 3.4 Mature *in vivo* biofilm formation during model development. Scanning electron micrographs of *C. albicans* biofilms adherent to the intraluminal surface of catheters showing no difference in biofilm architecture at 7 days postinfection (magnification, ×6500) **(a)** and 3 days postinfection (magnification, ×2500) **(b)**. (From Ghannoum, M.A., Are there antifungals that are effective against *Candida* biofilms? *16th Congress of the International Society for Human and Animal Mycology*, Paris, France, 2006.)

catheters when used as antifungal lock therapy [38]. In brief, the rabbit model involves surgically placing a silicone catheter in the external jugular vein of New Zealand white rabbits under anesthesia (Figure 3.3). To form a biofilm, an inoculum of *Candida* cells are locked in the internal lumen of the catheter, allowed to dwell for 24 hours and then removed. To evaluate the efficacy of a candidate antifungal in the treatment of catheter-associated biofilm, a solution of the agent is locked in the lumen for 2–8 hours/day for 7 days. Upon completion of therapy, blood cultures are obtained and the catheters are removed for quantitative culture (CFU

determination). Additionally, the ability of the agent to eradicate the biofilm is also analyzed using scanning electron microscopy analysis (Figure 3.4).

Mouse subcutaneous *Candida* biofilm model

While using mice to evaluate the ability of lock solutions to treat intraluminal biofilms is challenging, owing to difficulties encountered in placing a catheter in their tiny vein, this animal has utility as a subcutaneous (s.c.) model in evaluating the effectiveness of catheter coating in preventing

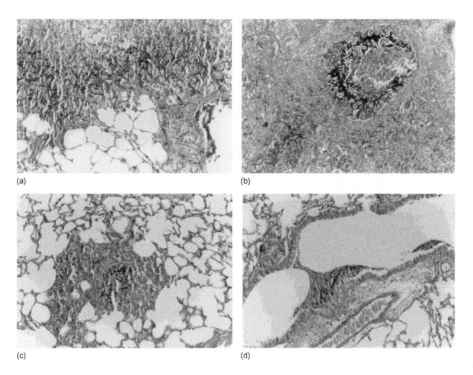

Figure 3.5 Histopathological findings for lung tissues of mice treated with 5% glucose **(a)**, AmBisome at 2.0 mg/kg **(b)**, PEG-L-AmB at 2.0 mg/kg **(c)**, and 34A-PEG-L-AmB at 2.0 mg/kg **(d)** on day 3 after injection. The tissues were stained with periodic acid-Schiff stain. (From Otsubo, T. et al., *Antimicrob. Agents Chemother.*, 42, 40–44, 1998.)

biofilm formation [39]. This model employs BALB/c mice. The mice are anesthetized, their backs shaved, a midline incision is made in the skin above the midthoracic spine, and a pocket is made subcutaneously by blunt dissection. The author's group used this s.c. model and evaluated the ability of amphogel, a dextran-based hydrogel into which amphotericin B is adsorbed, in killing *C. albicans* biofilm. Amphogels or hydrogels without amphotericin B were inoculated with *C. albicans*, implanted subcutaneously in mice and allowed to form a biofilm. Animals were sacrificed and disks were removed for enumeration of cells and microscopic examination. The data showed that no fungal survival was observed with amphogels, whereas dextran hydrogels were heavily colonized. Additionally, SEM analysis showed that amphogel surfaces did not have any *Candida* cells or biofilm attached (Figure 3.5c). In contrast, dextran hydrogels without amphotericin B were covered with *Candida* biofilm (Figure 3.5e), *Candida* blastospores and white blood cells (Figure 3.5f) [39].

ASPERGILLOSIS

To test the efficacy of antifungal agents in the treatment of invasive aspergillosis, some animal models including rabbits [40], guinea pigs [41], rats, and mice were employed. In order to mimic immunocompromised hosts and to facilitate the establishment of infections (as *Aspergillus* tends to be less pathogenic than *C. albicans*), immunosuppressive agents, such as cyclophosphamide and/or a corticosteroid, are given to the animals. To render the animals neutropenic, cyclophosphamide is usually administered before and after challenging them with the fungi [42]. Cortisone acetate is also used to produce an immunocompromised host [43]. To prevent bacterial superinfections, animals receive several broad-spectrum antimicrobial agents before and after fungal challenge [44]. This chapter describes rats and mouse models of invasive pulmonary aspergillosis. For description of aspergillosis in rabbits, refer to the work of Walsh et al. [45].

Rat pulmonary aspergillosis model

Aspergillus fumigatus is delivered to the lung by several methods: (*i*) intratracheal (surgical): the trachea of the animal is surgically opened and then the conidial suspension is injected into the trachea with a tuberculin syringe [46], (*ii*) intratracheal (nonsurgical): a tube is nonsurgically intubated, then a cannula is passed through the tube and conidial suspension is introduced [47] to the lung of the animals, and (*iii*) intranasal: a conidial suspension is delivered with a micropipette to the nares of the rat [42]. Antifungal agents are given to the animals via i.v. [48], p.o. [49], i.p. [48], or inhalation routes. The effect of antifungal treatment is evaluated by survival rate, tissue fungal cell burden, or histopathological examination [42].

Mouse pulmonary aspergillosis model

There are several routes for conidial inoculation in murine models of aspergillosis including: (*i*) intratracheal—a conidial suspension is delivered to the surgically exposed trachea under anesthesia by using a syringe with a small size (25–26 gauge) needle [50], (*ii*) intranasal—a single droplet of a conidial suspension is slowly instilled on both nares [51], and (*iii*) inhalational—mice are exposed to aerosolized conidial suspension (12 mL) for one hour in an inhalational chamber [52]. Antifungal agents are administrated via i.v., i.p., or p.o. route after infection. To evaluate the effects and toxicities of the drugs, several parameters such as survival rate, pulmonary fungal burden, histopathology (Figure 3.5) [53], and drug distribution are examined.

Systemic aspergillosis model

For the systemic aspergillosis model, the conidial suspension is inoculated via the lateral tail vein of immunosuppressed (induced by cyclophosphamide with/without corticosteroid) rats [54] and mice [55]. Guinea pigs have also been used in systemic aspergillosis models [56].

CRYPTOCOCCOSIS

Animal models of cryptococcal meningitis and pneumonia are often examined to assess the efficacy of antifungal agents to these life-threatening diseases. Among the experimental animals, mice have been widely used to assess the efficacy of antifungal agents because their susceptibility to *Cryptococcus* and ability of using a large number of animals allow comparison of a variety of treatment regimens.

MOUSE CRYPTOCOCCAL MENINGITIS MODEL

Murine models of cryptococcal meningitis have been widely used to evaluate the efficacy of antifungal agents in the treatment of this disease. Murine models are used because: (*i*) mice can be easily infected, (*ii*) disseminated cryptococcosis in the mouse produces meningoencephalitis in a manner similar to that developed in AIDS patients (Figure 3.6), (*iii*) a large body of literature exists regarding antifungal therapy in this model, (*iv*) the mouse model is the best system for large-scale evaluation of anticryptococcal agents, (*v*) the mouse is the lowest member of the phylogenic tree in which an infection can be produced that resembles human cryptococcosis, (*vi*) only small quantities of candidate compounds are needed for initial

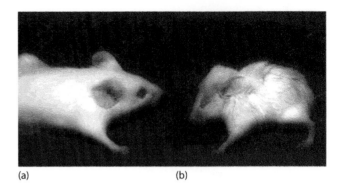

(a)   (b)

Figure 3.6 Intracranial model of Crytococcal infection; **(a)** Healthy Mouse, **(b)** Infected mouse.

screening, and (*vii*) the mouse model is more economical with respect to purchase, per diem, and husbandry costs.

To deliver the cells into the intracranial space, a pericranial approach is employed. Under brief anesthesia, the animals are challenged intracranially with *C. neoformans* using a tuberculin syringe through a 27-gauge needle. The needle is pushed through the skull with a rotating movement into the posterior half of the skull, about 6 mm lateral to the midline in order to avoid the superior sagittal sinus. A sleeve attached to the needle guides the penetration of the needle and prevents too deep penetration of the needle, which could cause death of the animal [57]. Several parameters such as survival rate, fungal burden in the tissues (brain, CSF, lung, etc.), histopathology, and pharmacokinetics are evaluated to assess the efficacy of antifungal agents.

Other animal models for cryptococcal meningitis

Rabbits [58], rats [59], and guinea pigs [60] have also been used to evaluate the efficacy of antifungals in the treatment of cryptococcosis. The advantage of using large animals (e.g., rabbits) include: (*i*) reproducible infection that mimics the human infection in histopathology and response to treatment, (*ii*) ease of drug administration and withdrawal of body fluids, including CSF, which facilitate pharmacokinetics/pharmacodynamic studies, (*iii*) drug pharmacokinetics/pharmacodynamics can be studied concurrently with the efficacy studies, (*iv*) immunosuppression is an important feature of the model that is similar to many human cases of cryptococcal infection, (*v*) a fewer number of animals are required because this model has been relatively consistent and statistical comparison can be made with small numbers, (*vi*) it provides an alternative species for pharmacokinetics analysis, and (*vii*) comparison with most old and new antifungal agents is already available. However, since rabbits and guinea pigs are less susceptible to *C. neoformans*, they are treated by steroids to maintain the infection. *C. neoformans* cell suspension is inoculated intracisternally to these animals. In addition, guinea pigs can be infected via pericranial puncture [60].

Mouse pulmonary cryptococcosis

To establish a cryptococcal infection of the lungs, *C. neoformans* cell suspension is inoculated to the mouse either intratracheally or intranasally. For the intratracheal infection, a 30–50 μL cell suspension is placed in the trachea distal to the vocal cords, using a blunted 25-gauge needle followed by injection of 200 μL of air at the same site to disperse the instilled organisms [61]. For the intranasal infection, a single droplet (50 μL) of yeast cell suspension is instilled on both nares [62]. Gilbert et al. showed the time course of an experimental murine model of cryptococcal pneumonia induced by intranasal fungal inoculation [62]. Although the total number of organisms in the lungs is dependent on the size of the initial inoculum, the greatest increase in growth took place with smaller inocula during the first 7–10 days [62]. Lungs appeared to become saturated with organisms by 2–3 weeks, with most alveoli containing one or more yeast cells when examined histologically [62]. At this time, cryptococcal cells could be found in other organs as well, especially the brain, liver, and kidneys [62]. Over the 4-week period, the level of cryptococcal cells in the lungs, brain, and liver with the two largest inocula used to challenge the animals increased 10- to 100-fold or more [62].

DERMATOPHYTOSIS

Guinea pigs have been used as *in vivo* models to assess the efficacy of antifungals in the treatment of dermatophytosis caused principally by the three fungal genera that belong to the dermatophytes, namely *Trichophyton, Microsporum,* and *Epidermophyton* [63].

Animals are anesthetized intramuscularly and an area of skin on the left side of the guinea pig's back is clipped, shaved, and a 2.5 cm square drawn on the shaved area. The marked area is abraded with sandpaper, and infected with a standardized suspension (1×10^7) of *Trichophyton mentagrophytes* conidia using a sterile pipette-tip and rubbed thoroughly. Animals can be treated topically or systemically. Both clinical and mycological criteria are used to evaluate the efficacy of potential antifungals. Clinical evaluation involves daily monitoring of changes in redness (mild, moderate, or severe), ulceration, scaling, or hair-loss at the site of inoculation. These signs are used in the clinical assessment of efficacy of different treatments and control regimens. Clinical efficacy is scored on a scale from 0 to 5 as follows: 0 = no signs of infection; 1 = few slightly erythematous areas on the skin; 2 = well-defined redness, swelling with bristling hairs, bald patches, scaly areas; 3 = large areas of marked redness, incrustation, scaling, bald patches, ulcerated in places; 4 = partial damage to the integument, loss of hair; and 5 = extensive damage to the integument and complete loss of hair at the site of infection (Figure 3.7).

Mycological evaluation of efficacy (also known as the hair root invasion test) is used to assess mycological cure resulting from antifungal treatment. In brief, following clinical assessment, hairs are removed from each animal in the treatment and control groups, and then planted on the surface of potato dextrose agar plates. Following incubation, hairs showing fungal growth at the hair root are counted (Figure 3.8). Mycological evaluation is based on the number of culture positive hair obtained from each animal.

In addition, the efficacy of an agent is assessed using histopathological analysis, where skin biopsy samples are obtained from a representative animal. Next, the tissue is fixed with 10% neutral buffered formalin, embedded in paraffin, and processed for histopathological examination. Fungal elements are visualized using Grocott Methenamine Silver (GMS) stain. Tissue is examined for the presence of fungal elements, inflammation, and tissue destruction using a light microscope.

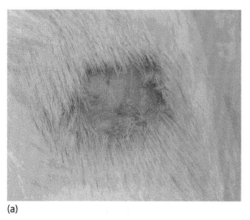
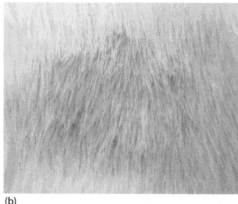

(a)   (b)

Figure 3.7 **(a)** Untreated showing: hair loss, redness, scaling and **(b)** Treatment showing: normal hair growth, no redness, no scaling.

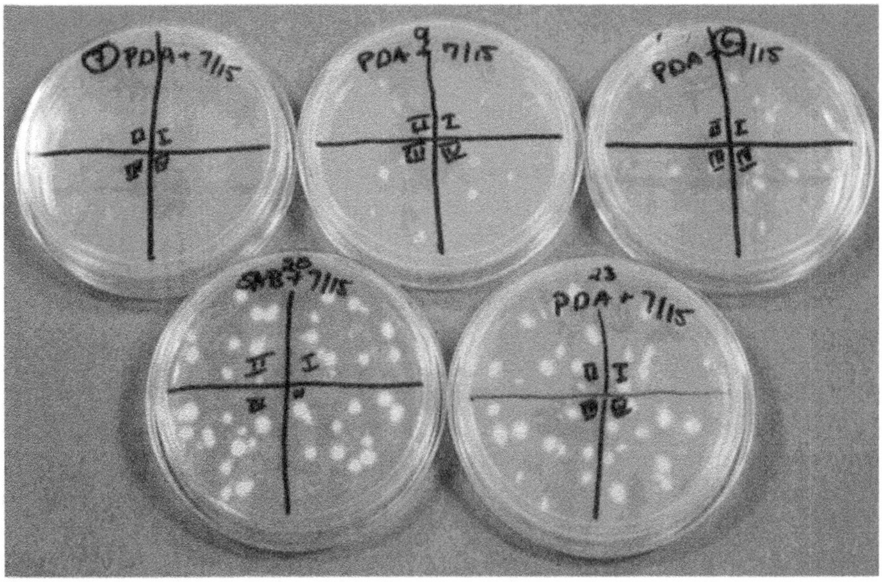

Figure 3.8 Hair root invasion test: Note the reduction of fungal growth in hairs obtained from the treated guinea pigs (top). Untreated controls showed abundant fungal growth (bottom) in the hair root when cultured in PDA plates.

Yeasts can also cause skin infections. *C. albicans* is the primary causative agent on these infections [64]. Therefore, models of cutaneous *Candida* infection are also needed for pharmaceutical development. The above model of guinea pig dermatophytosis has been adapted for the evaluation of antifungal therapies against cutaneous candidiasis [65]. Briefly, guinea pigs receive 30 mg/kg of body weight of prednisolone, subcutaneously, 1 day prior to infection and 1-day postinfection in order to induce immunosuppression. On the day of infection, the guinea pigs are prepared as described above. However, the hair is plucked instead of shaved from the left side of each guinea pig's back. It is important to clear the skin and prevent regrowth of the hair during the study. A 100 µl cell suspension containing 10^7 blastospores of *C. albicans* is applied onto the abraded area. Animals can be treated topically of systemically. On day-7 post inoculation, a clinical assessment of local changes of the infected skin area is performed. In this assessment, each area was scored as follows: 0 for absent, with no erythema and no evidence of crusting; 1 for mild, with the lesion appearing pink, with minimal inflammation and evidence of light crusting; 2 for moderate, with the lesion appearing red with areas of inflammation and medium crusting present over the infected area; and 3 for severe, with the lesion appearing red over the entire infected area and thick crusting appearing over the infected area. The percent efficacy of each treatment is determined based on the average clinical score for the untreated controls. After the clinical evaluations, each guinea pig is sacrificed, and the skin from the infected square is removed for enumeration of colony forming units per gram of tissue. Statistical

comparisons of the clinical assessments and the fungal burden of the sampled skin is performed to determine the antifungal efficacy of the test compounds.

NONINVASIVE MONITORING OF INFECTION IN LIVING ANIMAL MODELS

Animal models commonly used to evaluate efficacy of antimicrobial agents, including antifungals, utilize postmortem recovery of the infected tissue, homogenization, plating on agar plates, and counting CFUs. Such an approach requires a large number of animals to be sacrificed (which is frowned upon by animal review committees), and comparison of data sets from different groups of animals introduces unavoidable large variations. Moreover, these conventional models are expensive, time consuming, and labor intensive. Therefore, alternative models that use noninvasive approaches are encouraged.

One such approach is the use of noninvasive monitoring of infection in living animals using bioluminescent gene-tagged organisms [66,67]. The usefulness of employing such a model with candidiasis has been demonstrated by Doyle et al., who used a *C. albicans* strain that functionally expresses the firefly luciferase gene in infected animals [15]. *C. albicans* clinical isolates, which are stably transformed with a codon-optimized luciferase gene to constitutively express luciferase, are infected systemically or vaginally to mice. Mice infected with this luciferase-expressing strain are imaged following luciferin injection at a number of time points post infection using an IVIS 100TM CCD camera

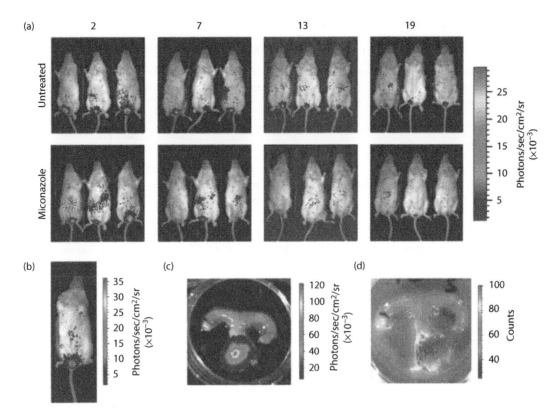

Figure 3.9 Bioluminescent *C. albicans* ATCC 90234 strain in a mouse vulvo-vaginal candidiasis model, with and without antifungal treatment. **(a)** Groups of three pseudo-estrous mice were infected in the vaginal lumen with approximately 5×10^5 CFU of *Candida* and were imaged on subsequent days following anesthesia with 2%–3% v/v isoflurane and vaginal lavage with 50 mL 16 mg/mL luciferin in PBS in the IVIS 100TM Imaging System, and representative images are shown at four different days postinfection. Groups of mice were treated with topical miconazole (lower group) or were left untreated as controls (*Top*). **(b)** Single untreated mouse imaged 30 days postinfection prior to end of experiment. **(c)** Excised vaginal/uterine tissue from mouse in **(b)** removed postmortem, the lumen opened to display the inner surface, and imaged directly after application of a luciferin solution. **(d)** Same vaginal/uterine imaged at high resolution with the close-up attachment lens.

system. The efficacy of the antifungal drug miconazole was tested in this model, and clearance in animals was apparent by both direct imaging and fungal load determination (Figure 3.9) [15].

INVERTEBRATE HOST

Invertebrate organisms have been increasingly used as *in vivo* assays for antifungal drug efficacy studies because of their low cost and simplicity [68] (Table 3.1). For example, *Drosophila melanogaster* have been used as *Aspergillus* [69] and *Candida* [70] infection models. *Drosophila* is infected with fungi either by injection, rolling, or ingestion methods. For injection assay, the dorsal side of the thorax of CO_2-anesthetized *Drosophila* flies is punctured with a thin sterile needle that is dipped in concentrated solutions of fungal cells. For rolling assay, CO_2-anesthetized *Drosophila* flies are rolled for 2 minutes on yeast extract

glucose plates that contain a carpet of fungal cells. For ingestion assay, flies are placed in special fly-food vials containing yeast extract–peptone–dextrose agar medium, on which a lawn of fungal cells grew. Antifungal drug–containing foods are given to the animals for the treatment [70].

Galleria mellonella (the greater wax moth) caterpillar is used for cryptococcal infection. A 10-µL Hamilton syringe is used to inject 10 µL of inoculum into the hemocoel of each caterpillar via the last left proleg. Antifungal drugs are injected using the same technique that was used for fungal challenge [71].

Silkworms have been used to evaluate the efficacy of antifungals in the treatment of *Candida* infections. Suspensions of *C. albicans* or *C. tropicalis* in Sabouraud dextrose medium are injected into the hemolymph through the dorsal surface of the silkworm. Antifungal drugs are injected into the hemolymph or by the intramid-gut route [72].

Table 3.1 Invertebrate animal models for the study of antifungal agents

Invertebrate	Fungus	Infection	Treatment	Evaluation	Reference
Drosophila melanogaster (Oregon R fly, WT and Toll mutant)	*Aspergillus fumigatus*	Injection Rolling Ingestion	VRC via Drug-containing Food	Survival rate Tissue fungal burden (PCR) Tissue Drug Concentration (Bioassay) Histopathological and SEM analysis	67
Drosophila melanogaster (Oregon R fly, WT and Toll mutant)	*C. albicans* *C. parapsilosis* *C. krusei*	Injection Ingestion	FLC via Drug-containing Food	Survival rate Tissue Fungal burden (CFU) Histopathology	68
Galleria mellonella (in the final instar larval stage)	*C. neoformans* *C. laurentii*	Injection	AMB, FLU and 5-FC via Injection	Survival rate Tissue Fungal burden (CFU)	69
Silkworms	*C. albicans* *C. tropicalis*	Injection	AMB and FLU via Drug-containing Food or injection	Survival rate	70

Although these studies provide an alternative to using live animals, these invertebrate models have a number of limitations, which include neither drug levels being measured nor pharmacokinetic analysis undertaken. Although high-performance liquid chromatography (HPLC) analysis and bioassay methods are feasible in invertebrates, such studies are more cumbersome, imprecise, and technically challenging in these models compared with mammal models [68]. Furthermore, little is known regarding the metabolism and elimination pathway of drugs and potential for drug–drug interactions in mini-host models [68]. However, despite these limitations, invertebrates are attractive models for the mass screening of candidate antifungal compounds that require subsequent validation in mammalian systems [68].

CONCLUSION

Animal models for evaluating the efficacy of antifungal agents in the treatment of various mycoses with demonstrated utility are available. Because of ethical concerns (advocating limiting the number of animals in each treatment), new alterative models, such as using bioluminescent pathogens, have been developed. Showing that a compound is effective *in vivo* is an important step in drug discovery since it shows the potential of activity in humans and identifies toxicity issues early. A compound that fails to demonstrate efficacy in animals is unlikely to show potency in humans. However, showing activity *in vivo* does not guarantee success in patients.

ACKNOWLEDGMENTS

The authors would like to thank the National Institutes of Health, funding from various pharmaceuticals and biotech companies, and Bristol Myers Squibb for the Freedom to Discover Award (to MAG) that allowed the authors to develop a number of these models at their Center.

REFERENCES

1. Oto Zak E, Sande MA. *Handbook of Animal Models of Infection: Experimental Models in Antimicro- bial Chemotherapy.* 1st ed. New York: Academic Press, 1999.
2. Matsumoto M, Ishida K, Konagai A, et al. Strong antifungal activity of SS750, a new triazole derivative, is based on its selective binding affinity to cytochrome P450 of fungi. *Antimicrob Agents Chemother* 2002;46(2):308–314.
3. Anaissie E, Hachem R, Tin U, et al. Experimental hematogenous candidiasis caused by *Candida krusei* and *Candida albicans*: Species differences in pathogenicity. *Infect Immun* 1993;61(4):1268–1271.
4. Ghannoum MA, Kim HG, Long L. Efficacy of aminocandin in the treatment of immunocompetent mice with haematogenously disseminated fluconazole-resistant *candidiasis*. *J Antimicrob Chemother* 2007;59(3):556–559.

5. Garcia A, Adler-Moore JP, Proffitt RT. Single-dose AmBisome (Liposomal amphotericin B) as pro-phylaxis for murine systemic candidiasis and histoplasmosis. *Antimicrob Agents Chemother* 2000;44(9):2327–2332.

6. Kuhara T, Uchida K, Yamaguchi H. Therapeutic efficacy of human macrophage colony-stimulating factor, used alone and in combination with anti-fungal agents, in mice with systemic *Candida albicans* infection. *Antimicrob Agents Chemother* 2000;44(1):19–23.

7. Marine M, Serena C, Pastor FJ, et al. Combined antifungal therapy in a murine infection by *Candida glabrata*. *J Antimicrob Chemother* 2006;58(6):1295–1298.

8. Wiederhold NP, Najvar LK, Bocanegra R, et al. *In vivo* efficacy of anidulafungin and caspofungin against *Candida glabrata* and association with *in vitro* potency in the presence of sera. *Antimicrob Agents Chemother* 2007;51(5):1616–1620.

9. Atkinson BA, Bocanegra R, Colombo AL, et al. Treatment of disseminated *Torulopsis glabrata* infection with DO870 and amphotericin B. *Antimicrob Agents Chemother* 1994;38(7):1604–1607.

10. MacCallum DM, Odds FC. Temporal events in the intravenous challenge model for experimental *Candida albicans* infections in female mice. *Mycoses* 2005;48(3):151–161.

11. Graybill JR. The role of murine models in the development of antifungal therapy for systemic mycoses. *Drug Resist Updates* 2000;3(6):364–383.

12. Ghannoum MA, Okogbule-Wonodi I, Bhat N, et al. Antifungal activity of voriconazole (UK-109496), fluconazole and amphotericin B against hematogenous *Candida krusei* infection in neutropenic guinea pig model. *J Chemother* 1999;11(1):34–39.

13. Graybill JR, Najvar LK, Holmberg JD, et al. Fluconazole treatment of *Candida albicans* infection in mice: Does *in vitro* susceptibility predict *in vivo* response? *Antimicrob Agents Chemother* 1995;39(10):2197–2200.

14. Spellberg B, Ibrahim AS, Edwards JE Jr, et al. Mice with disseminated candidiasis die of progressive sepsis. *J Infect Dis* 2005;192(2):336–343.

15. Doyle TC, Nawotka KA, Kawahara CB, et al. Visualizing fungal infections in living mice using bioluminescent pathogenic *Candida albicans* strains transformed with the firefly luciferase gene. *Microb Pathog* 2006;40(2):82–90.

16. Fidel PL Jr, Lynch ME, Sobel JD. Candida-specific Th1-type responsiveness in mice with experimental *vaginal candidiasis*. *Infect Immun* 1993;61(10):4202–4207.

17. Zhang JD, Xu Z, Cao YB, et al. Antifungal activities and action mechanisms of compounds from *Tribulus terrestris* L. *J Ethnopharmacol* 2006;103(1):76–84.

18. Calderon L, Williams R, Martinez M, et al. Genetic susceptibility to *vaginal candidiasis*. *Med Mycol* 2003;41(2):143–147.

19. Ryley JF, McGregor S. Quantification of vaginal *Candida albicans* infections in rodents. *J Med Vet Mycol* 1986;24(6):455–460.

20. Samaranayake YH, Samaranayake LP. Experimental oral *candidiasis* in animal models. *Clin Microbiol Rev* 2001;14(2):398–429.

21. Hata K, Kimura J, Miki H, et al. Efficacy of ER-30346, a novel oral triazole antifungal agent, in experimental models of *aspergillosis, candidiasis,* and *cryptococcosis*. *Antimicrob Agents Chemother* 1996;40(10):2243–2247.

22. Reichart PA. Oral manifestations in HIV infection: Fungal and bacterial infections, *Kaposi's sarcoma*. *Med Microbiol Immunol (Berl)* 2003;192(3):165–169.

23. Redding SW, Dahiya MC, Kirkpatrick WR, et al. *Candida glabrata* is an emerging cause of oropharyngeal candidiasis in patients receiving radiation for head and neck cancer. *Oral Surg Oral Med Oral Pathol Oral Radiol Endod* 2004;97(1):47–52.

24. Hassan OE, Jones JH, Russell C. Experimental oral candidal infection and carriage of oral bacteria in rats subjected to a carbohydrate-rich diet and tetracycline treatment. *J Med Microbiol* 1985;20(3):291–298.

25. Deslauriers N, Coulombe C, Carre B, et al. Topical application of a corticosteroid destabilizes the host-parasite relationship in an experimental model of the oral carrier state of *Candida albicans*. *FEMS Immunol Med Microbiol* 1995;11(1):45–55.

26. Budtz-Jorgensen E. Effects of triamcinolone ace-tonide on experimental oral *candidiasis* in monkeys. *Scand J Dent Res* 1975;83(3):171–178.

27. Rahman D, Mistry M, Thavaraj S, et al. Murine model of concurrent oral and vaginal *Candida albicans* colonization to study epithelial host-pathogen interactions. *Microbes Infect* 2007;9(5):615–622.

28. O'Grady JF, Reade PC. Role of thermal trauma in experimental oral mucosal *Candida* infections in rats. *J Oral Pathol Med* 1993;22(3):132–137.

29. Rennie JS, Hutcheon AW, MacFarlane TW, et al. The role of iron deficiency in experimentally-induced oral candidosis in the rat. *J Med Microbiol* 1983;16(3):363–369.

30. Dourov N, Coremans-Pelseneer J. Experimental chronic lingual candidosis induced in streptozotocin diabetic rats. *Mykosen* 1987;30(4):175–183.

31. Teichert MC, Jones JW, Usacheva MN, et al. Treatment of oral candidiasis with methylene blue-mediated photodynamic therapy in an immunodeficient murine model. *Oral Surg Oral Med Oral Pathol Oral Radiol Endod* 2002;93(2):155–160.

32. Martinez A, Regadera J, Jimenez E, et al. Antifungal efficacy of GM237354, a sordarin derivative, in experimental oral candidiasis in immunosuppressed rats. *Antimicrob Agents Chemother* 2001;45(4):1008–1013.

33. Chandra J, Kuhn DM, Mukherjee PK, et al. Biofilm formation by the fungal pathogen *Candida albicans* development, architecture and drug resistance. *J Bacteriol* 2001;183(18):5385–5394.

34. Chandra J, Mukherjee PK, Leidich SD, et al. Antifungal resistance of candidal biofilms formed on denture acrylic *in vitro*. *J Dent Res* 2001;80(3):903–908.

35. Kuhn DM, Chandra J, Mukherjee PK, et al. Comparison of biofilms formed by *Candida albicans* and *Candida parapsilosis* on bioprosthetic surfaces. *Infect Immun* 2002;70(2):878–888.

36. Andes D, Nett J, Oschel P, et al. Development and characterization of an *in vivo* central venous catheter *Candida albicans* biofilm model. *Infect Immun* 2004;72(10):6023–6031.

37. Shuford JA, Rouse MS, Piper KE, et al. Evaluation of caspofungin and amphotericin B deoxycholate against *Candida albicans* biofilms in an experimental intravascular catheter infection model. *J Infect Dis* 2006;194(5):710–713.

38. Ghannoum MA. Are there antifungals that are effective against *Candida* biofilms? *16th Congress of the International Society for Human and Animal Mycology*, Paris, France, 2006.

39. Zumbuehl A, Ferreira L, Kuhn D, et al. Antifungal hydrogels. *PNAS* 2007;104(32):12994–12998.

40. Petraitiene R, Petraitis V, Lyman CA, et al. Efficacy, safety, and plasma pharmacokinetics of escalating dosages of intravenously administered ravuconazole lysine phosphoester for treatment of experimental pulmonary aspergillosis in persistently neutropenic rabbits. *Antimicrob Agents Chemother* 2004;48(4):1188–1196.

41. Chandrasekar PH, Cutright J, Manavathu E. Efficacy of voriconazole against invasive pulmonary aspergillosis in a guinea-pig model. *J Antimicrob Chemother* 2000;45(5):673–676.

42. Hachem R, Bahna P, Hanna H, et al. EDTA as an adjunct antifungal agent for invasive pulmonary aspergillosis in a rodent model. *Antimicrob Agents Chemother* 2006;50(5):1823–1827.

43. Gavalda J, Martin T, Lopez P, et al. Efficacy of high loading doses of liposomal amphotericin B in the treatment of experimental invasive pulmonary aspergillosis. *Clin Microbiol Infect* 2005;11(12):999–1004.

44. Becker MJ, de Marie S, Willemse D, et al. Quantitative galactomannan detection is superior to PCR in diagnosing and monitoring invasive pulmonary aspergillosis in an experimental rat model. *J Clin Microbiol* 2000;38(4):1434–1438.

45. Walsh TJ, Petraitis V, Petraitiene R, et al. Experimental pulmonary aspergillosis due to *Aspergillus terreus*: Pathogenesis and treatment of an emerging fungal pathogen resistant to amphotericin B. *J Infect Dis* 2003;188(2):305–319.

46. Schmitt HJ, Bernard EM, Hauser M, et al. Aerosol amphotericin B is effective for prophylaxis and therapy in a rat model of pulmonary aspergillosis. *Antimicrob Agents Chemother* 1988;32(11):1676–1679.

47. Leenders AC, de Marie S, ten Kate MT, et al. Liposomal amphotericin B (AmBisome) reduces dissemination of infection as compared with amphotericin B deoxycholate (Fungizone) in a rate model of pulmonary aspergillosis. *J Antimicrob Chemother* 1996;38(2):215–225.

48. van Vianen W. Caspofungin: Antifungal activity *in vitro*, pharmacokinetics, and effects on fungal load and animal survival in neutropenic rats with invasive pulmonary aspergillosis. *J Antimicrob Chemother* 2006;57:732–740.

49. Murphy M, Bernard EM, Ishimaru T, et al. Activity of voriconazole (UK-109496) against clinical isolates of *Aspergillus* species and its effectiveness in an experimental model of invasive pulmonary aspergillosis. *Antimicrob Agents Chemother* 1997;41(3):696–698.

50. Mehrad B, Strieter RM, Moore TA, et al. CXC chemokine receptor-2 ligands are necessary components of neutrophil-mediated host defense in invasive pulmonary aspergillosis. *J Immunol* 1999;163(11):6086–6094.

51. Lewis RE, Chamilos G, Prince RA, et al. Pretreatment with empty liposomes attenuates the immunopathology of invasive pulmonary aspergillosis in corticosteroid-immunosuppressed mice. *Antimicrob Agents Chemother* 2007;51(3):1078–1081.

52. Chiang LY, Ejzykowicz DE, Tian Z-Q, et al. Efficacy of ambruticin analogs in a murine model of invasive pulmonary aspergillosis. *Antimicrob Agents Chemother* 2006;50(10):3464–3466.

53. Otsubo T, Maruyama K, Maesaki S, et al. Long-circulating immunoliposomal amphotericin B against invasive pulmonary aspergillosis in mice. *Antimicrob Agents Chemother* 1998;42(1):40–44.

54. Scotter JM, Chambers ST. Comparison of galacto-mannan detection, PCR-enzyme-linked immuno-sorbent assay, and real-time PCR for diagnosis of invasive aspergillosis in a neutropenic rat model and effect of caspofungin acetate. *Clin Diagn Lab Immunol* 2005;12(11):1322–1327.

55. Abruzzo GK, Gill CJ, Flattery AM, et al. Efficacy of the echinocandin caspofungin against disseminated aspergillosis and candidiasis in cyclophosphamide-induced immunosuppressed mice. *Antimicrob Agents Chemother* 2000;44(9):2310–2318.

56. Kirkpatrick WR, Perea S, Coco BJ, et al. Efficacy of caspofungin alone and in combination with voriconazole in a guinea pig model of invasive aspergillosis. *Antimicrob Agents Chemother* 2002;46(8):2564–2568.

57. Hossain MA, Mukherjee PK, Reyes G, et al. Effects of fluconazole singly and in combination with 5- fluorocytosine or amphotericin B in the treatment of cryptococcal meningoencephalitis in an intracranial murine model. *J Chemother* 2002;14(4):351–360.

58. Cox GM, McDade HC, Chen SC, et al. Extracellular phospholipase activity is a virulence factor for *Cryptococcus neoformans*. *Mol Microbiol* 2001;39(1):166–175.

59. Fries BC, Lee SC, Kennan R, et al. Phenotypic switching of *Cryptococcus neoformans* can produce variants that elicit increased intracranial pressure in a rat model of cryptococcal meningoencephalitis. *Infect Immun* 2005;73(3):1779–1787.

60. Kirkpatrick WR, Najvar LK, Bocanegra R, et al. New guinea pig model of cryptococcal meningitis. *Antimicrob Agents Chemother* 2007;51(8):3011–3013.

61. Kakeya H, Udono H, Ikuno N, et al. A 77-kilodalton protein of *Cryptococcus neoformans*, a member of the heat shock protein 70 family, is a major antigen detected in the sera of mice with pulmonary cryptococcosis. *Infect Immun* 1997;65(5):1653–1658.

62. Gilbert BE, Wyde PR, Wilson SZ. Aerosolized liposomal amphotericin B for treatment of pulmonary and systemic *Cryptococcus neoformans* infections in mice. *Antimicrob Agents Chemother* 1992;36(7):1466–1471.

63. Ghannoum MA, Long L, Pfister WR. Determination of the efficacy of terbinafine hydrochloride nail solution in the topical treatment of dermatophytosis in a guinea pig model. *Mycoses* 2008;52:35–43.

64. Nenoff P, Krüger C, Ginter-Hanselmayer G, et al. Mycology – an update. Part 1: Dermatomycoses: Causative agents, epidemiology and pathogenesis. *J Dtsch Dermatol Ges* 2014;12(3):188–209.

65. Lafleur MD, Sun L, Lister I, et al. Potentiation of azole antifungals by 2-adamantanamine. *Antimicrob Agents Chemother* 2013;57(8):3585–3592.

66. Xiong YQ, Willard J, Kadurugamuwa JL, et al. Real-time *in vivo* bioluminescent imaging for evaluating the efficacy of antibiotics in a rat *Staphylococcus aureus* endocarditis model. *Antimicrob Agents Chemother* 2005;49(1):380–387.

67. Jawhara S, Mordon S. *In vivo* imaging of bioluminescent *Escherichia coli* in a cutaneous wound infection model for evaluation of an antibiotic therapy. *Antimicrob Agents Chemother* 2004;48(9):3436–3441.

68. Chamilos G, Lionakis MS, Lewis RE, et al. Role of mini-host models in the study of medically important fungi. *Lancet Infect Dis* 2007;7(1):42–55.

69. Lionakis MS, Lewis RE, May GS, et al. Toll-deficient drosophila flies as a fast, high-throughput model for the study of antifungal drug efficacy against invasive aspergillosis and *Aspergillus virulence*. *J Infect Dis* 2005;191(7):1188–1195.

70. Chamilos G, Lionakis MS, Lewis RE, et al. *Drosophila melanogaster* as a facile model for large-scale studies of virulence mechanisms and antifungal drug efficacy in *Candida* species. *J Infect Dis* 2006;193(7):1014–1022.

71. Mylonakis E, Moreno R, El Khoury JB, et al. *Galleria mellonella* as a model system to study *Cryptococcus neoformans* pathogenesis. *Infect Immun* 2005;73(7):3842–3850.

72. Hamamoto H, Kurokawa K, Kaito C, et al. Quantitative evaluation of the therapeutic effects of antibiotics using silkworms infected with human pathogenic microorganisms. *Antimicrob Agents Chemother* 2004;48(3):774–779.

4

Antifungal drug resistance: Significance and mechanisms

SHARVARI DHARMAIAH, RANIA A. SHERIF, AND PRANAB K. MUKHERJEE

INTRODUCTION

Resistance to commonly used antifungals (e.g., azoles, polyenes, echinocandins, allylamines) is a significant problem in nosocomial infections (including invasive and superficial mycoses), as well as those associated with indwelling devices like central venous catheters, urinary catheters, and contact lenses (fungal keratitis). Fungal resistance has been reported even for newer antifungals, such as the echinocandins, underscoring the importance of gaining insight into the mechanisms of antifungal resistance. This chapter briefly describes the methods used to evaluate antifungal susceptibility of fungi, reviews the significance of

antifungal resistance, and summarizes recent advances in identification of the underlying mechanisms.

METHODS USED TO EVALUATE ANTIFUNGAL SUSCEPTIBILITY *IN VITRO*

Antifungal agents are broadly categorized as *fungistatic*, which inhibit but do not kill fungi, and *fungicidal*, which kill fungal organisms. Common methods of evaluating *in vitro* antifungal susceptibility of fungi involve determination of the minimum inhibitory concentration (MIC), minimum effective concentration (MEC) or time-kill assay [1,2]. Fungicidal agents are evaluated based on their minimum fungicidal concentration (MFC), which is the drug concentration that results in at least a 3-log (or 99.9%) reduction in colony forming unit (CFU) compared to the starting fungal inoculum.

Minimum inhibitory concentration

MIC of an antifungal agent is defined as the minimum concentration of the drug resulting in inhibition of fungal growth by 80% (or 50%, in some cases, depending on the established cut-off threshold for the tested drug) relative to growth in the absence of the drug. MIC values for antifungal agents can be determined using microdilution, disk diffusion or Epsilometer test (E-test) methods (see Table 4.1 for representative list of recent studies). Agents with low MICs are considered active, while those with higher MICs indicate reduced susceptibility of the organism and/or antifungal resistance (based on existing breakpoint guidelines for a given drug).

MICRODILUTION METHOD

The most commonly used method to determine the MIC of antifungal agents is the microdilution-based method, in which a standardized number of organisms (e.g., 10^4 cells/mL) are exposed to serially diluted concentrations of the test agent in a 96-well format. The drug concentration resulting in 50% or 80% growth inhibition (compared to drug-free control well) represents the MIC of the agent against the tested organism. In studies testing a large number of isolates, antifungal activity is commonly represented by MIC90, or the concentration of drugs that inhibit growth of 90% of the isolates tested. The microdilution-based method is widely used;

Table 4.1 Commonly used methods to determine activities of different antifungal agents

Testing method	Drugs tested	Organism	Study conclusion	Reference
Broth microdilution	Amphotericin B, flucytosine, fluconazole, itraconazole, voriconazole and caspofungin	*Candida* spp.	Caspofungin was active against the majority of isolates	[3]
	Flucytosine, fluconazole, itraconazole, posaconazole, voriconazole and caspofungin	*Candida* spp.	*In vitro* susceptibility of 375 isolates and biofilm production	[4]
	Voriconazole, posaconazole, and fluconazole	*Candida* and *Cryptococcus* spp.	Both voriconazole and posaconazole were more active than fluconazole	[5]
Disk Diffusion	Lemongrass oils and citral (main component of lemongrass oil)	*Candida* spp.	Lemongrass oil and citral have potent *in vitro* activity	[6]
	Fluconazole and voriconazole	*Candida* spp.	Voriconazole was very active *in vitro* against *C. glabrata* and *C. krusei*	[7]
	Fluconazole and voriconazole	*Cryptococcus* spp., *Saccharomyces* spp., *Trichosporon* spp., and *Rhodotorula* spp.	Voriconazole exhibits broad-spectrum against opportunistic yeast pathogens but has reduced activity against less common species	[8]
	Voriconazole	*C. krusei*	No evidence of increasing resistance of *C. krusei* to voriconazole	[9]
	Ciclopirox, terbinafine, griseofulvin, fluconazole, itraconazole, posaconazole, and ravuconazole	*Trichophyton* spp., *Microsporum canis*, *Epidermophyton floccosum*	Correlation between microdilution and disk diffusion methods was variable	[10]

(Continued)

Table 4.1 (*Continued*) Commonly used methods to determine activities of different antifungal agents

Testing method	Drugs tested	Organism	Study conclusion	Reference
	Voriconazole, Posaconazole, Itraconazole, Amphotericin B, and Caspofungin	*Absidia corymbifera*, *Aspergillus* spp., *Alternaria* spp., *Bipolaris spicifera*, *Fusarium* spp., *Mucor* spp., *Paecilomyces lilacinus*, *Rhizopus* spp., and *Scedosporium* spp.	Identified optimal testing conditions for mold disk diffusion testing	[11]
E-test	Ketoconazole and itraconazole	*Candida* spp.	Increase in *Candida* bloodstream infections were due to non-*albicans Candida* species	[12]
	Posaconazole	*Candida* spp.	Posaconazole exhibited excellent *in vitro* activity against *Candida* strains	[13]
	Voriconazole	*Trichophyton rubrum*	Voriconazole was the most and fluconazole was the less-active drug	[14]
	Posaconazole	*Candida* spp.	Disk diffusion zone diameters are highly reproducible and correlate well with both the E-test and the microdilution method	[15]

standardized methods to determine MIC of antifungals against yeasts and moulds (M 27A-3 and M38-A2) have been developed and validated through the Clinical and Laboratory Standards Institute (CLSI) [16,17].

DISK DIFFUSION ASSAY

Disk diffusion assay, available as a standardized CLSI method (M-44A) for fluconazole susceptibility testing [18], involves placing discs that contain different concentrations of drugs on agar media plates (supplemented with 2% glucose and 0.5 µg of methylene blue per mL) seeded with the fungus. The plates are incubated for specific time periods (usually 24–48 hours). Drug activity is indicated by the clearance zone around the discs, and diameter of the zone diameter is measured to calculate the MIC. Disk diffusion method has been used in several studies [10,19–22], including the ARTEMIS DISK Global Antifungal Surveillance Study [19,20], which evaluated *in vitro* susceptibility of fluconazole (using the CLSI M44-A method) against thousands of *Candida* and non-*Candida* yeasts collected worldwide in 40 countries over a 10-year period (1997–2007).

EPSILOMETER STRIP TEST

The Epsilometer test (E-test, AB Biodisk, Solna, Sweden) is also used to determine the *in vitro* activity of antifungal agents. MICs are determined from the point of intersection of a growth inhibition zone with a calibrated strip impregnated with a gradient of antimicrobial concentration and placed on an agar plate containing a lawn of the microbial isolate

being tested. Several studies have demonstrated good correlation between MIC values obtained using the E-test and broth macro/micro-dilution testing methods [13,15,23–27].

Minimum effective concentration

Antifungal susceptibility of *Aspergillus* and other filamentous fungi is often evaluated by determining the MEC, which is defined as the lowest drug concentration causing a morphological effect (e.g., abnormally swollen and highly branched hyphal tips, cells with distended balloon shapes, stubby growth with thick cell walls, etc.) [28]. The minimum effective concentration assay is often related to inhibition of glucan synthase activity *in vitro*, especially for filamentous fungi, and is increasingly being used to determine susceptibilities of filamentous fungi to echinocandins [29–31].

Time-kill assay

Time-kill assays are used to evaluate the effect of an agent on the rate and extent of antifungal activity over time, thus providing a measure of its *in vitro* pharmacodynamics [32–34]. In this method, a standardized cell suspension (usually 5×10^5 cells/mL) is exposed to different concentrations of drug combinations for different time intervals. After a specified treatment time, cells are retrieved, plated onto agar medium, and incubated to allow growth. The number of CFUs for each incubation time are determined (CFUs/mL) and plotted as a function of time, thus generating a "time-kill" curve.

EPIDEMIOLOGY OF ANTIFUNGAL RESISTANCE

Resistance against azoles

Historically, a large body of knowledge exists for resistance against azole antifungals, mainly because these are also the most commonly used antifungal agents. Particularly, the majority of resistance has been reported for fluconazole and itraconazole, while the newer third generation triazoles (voriconazole, posaconazole, etc.) exhibit excellent activities against all *Candida* species. Most cases of azole resistance are associated with prior exposure to the agent or infection with non-*albicans Candida* species. Risk factor analyses have reported that prior surgery and systemic antifungal exposure were significantly associated with candidemia due to non-*albicans Candida* spp. and a potentially fluconazole-resistant *Candida* species [35–37].

AZOLE RESISTANCE AMONG *CANDIDA* SPECIES

Azole resistance among *C. albicans* isolates is uncommon but is known to occur. Li et al. [38] collected 21 *C. albicans* isolates from three HIV-infected patients over a period of 3 years and reported fluconazole resistance in 5 (24%) isolates, while 4 (19%) isolates exhibited dose-dependent susceptibility. Isolates obtained from individual swab samples and at different time points for each patient were identical; thus, suggesting that the observed fluconazole resistance was associated with long-term fluconazole therapy. More recently, Yenisehirli et al. [39] isolated 201 *C. albicans* strains from clinical samples in Turkey and showed that while these isolates exhibited variable resistance to ketoconazole, fluconazole, itraconazole, voriconazole and posaconazole (32%, 34%, 21%, 14% and 14%, respectively).

In contrast to *C. albicans*, prevalence of azole resistance is more common among non-*albicans Candida* species. International surveillance programs conducted in the late 90s, as well as later studies, reported development of azole resistance among *C. glabrata* and *C. krusei* isolates [40–48]. Similar trends in resistance have continued for other non-*albicans Candida* species, e.g. *C. tropicalis* [49–51], *C. dubliniensis* [52], *C. nivariensis* (which is genetically related to *C. glabrata*) [53], *C. haemulonii* [54], *C. guilliermondii* [55]. Zhang et al. [56] reported development of fluconazole resistance in a series of *C. parapsilosis* isolates from a persistent candidemia patient with prolonged antifungal therapy, indicating that prior exposure to an antifungal can induce resistance in *C. parapsilosis*.

Extensive genetic diversity among clinical isolates of *C. glabrata* has been associated with drug resistance [57,58]. In this regard, *C. glabrata* clinical strains with mutations in the DNA mismatch repair gene *MSH2* have been shown to exhibit "mutator" phenotype and increased frequencies of drug-resistant mutants [58]. Moreover, *C. glabrata* isolates exposed to antifungal treatment exhibited chromosomal changes *in vivo*, suggesting a complex population structure comprising long-term genomic changes triggered by adaptation to environmental changes, contributing to antifungal resistance in this species.

Some studies have suggested geographical distribution of antifungal resistance, although a conclusive association remains to be demonstrated. In this regard, Pfaller et al. [41] studied variation in species and strain distribution and antifungal susceptibility of 408 isolates of *Candida* spp. obtained from the National Epidemiology of Mycoses Survey (NEMIS) from sites in sites in New York and Texas and reported variation in susceptibility to itraconazole and fluconazole in these two states. Pfaller et al. [59] also reported that *Candida* isolates from Canada and Latin America were generally more susceptible to triazoles than U.S. isolates. Tortorano et al. [60] performed an analysis of multi-institutional surveys of *Candida* BSIs performed in Europe and reported a low proportion of antifungal resistance in European countries. Yesudhason et al. [61] isolated 112 *Candida* isolates during 2012 from various clinical specimens in a Tertiary Care Hospital in Southern India and identified 61 isolates (54.3%) as *C. tropicalis*. While all the *C. tropicalis* isolates were sensitive to amphotericin B (100%), 23 isolates (37.7%) were reported to be resistant to fluconazole. Although these studies indicate that antifungal resistance may be linked to specific regions or countries, more detailed investigations into this possibility need to be performed.

While development of drug resistance is often associated with fitness costs, experimental models of infection showed enhanced virulence of azole-resistant *C. glabrata* isolates [62].

Among the most alarming non-*albicans Candida* species to be linked to infections has been *C. auris*, with the Centers for Disease Control (CDC) issuing a clinical alert in June 2016 for the healthcare community, and a recent report describing the first seven U.S. cases of *C. auris* infection (as of August 31, 2016) [63]. CDC noted the transmission of this fungus in U.S. health care facilities and underscored the need for infection control measures against *C. auris*. Due to the potential for mis-identification, *C. auris* isolates are positively identified using multilocus sequence typing, matrix-assisted laser desorption ionization time-of-flight mass spectrometry (MALDI-TOF) and amplified fragment length polymorphism (AFLP) methods [64,65]. The first US occurrence of *C. auris* infection was reported by Calvo et al. [66], who characterized a hospital outbreak of *C. auris* candidemia involving 18 critically ill patients (previously exposed to antibiotics and multiple invasive medical procedures) in Venezuela. The isolates obtained from these patients were resistant to azoles, but susceptible to anidulafungin and 50% of isolates exhibited reduced susceptibility to amphotericin B (MIC > 1 mg/L). Schelenz et al. [67] reported the first hospital outbreak of 50 *C. auris* cases in a European hospital between April 2015 and July 2016, of which 44% (n = 22/50) patients developed possible or proven *C. auris* infection with a candidemia rate of 18% (n = 9/50). Genotyping analyses revealed clustering of *C. auris* isolates from the same geographic region. Infection control and prevention measures in this ongoing outbreak led to the implementation of enhanced measures to limit transmission, including isolation of all positive *C. auris* patients, cohorting with their direct patient contacts, as well as ceasing new admissions to the affected rooms. Strict contact precautions were introduced for all healthcare workers, cleaners and visitors upon entering rooms where patients were isolated. Chakrabarti et al. [68] presented the incidence, characteristics and outcome of intensive care unit (ICU)-acquired candidemia in India in a prospective, nationwide, multicenter, observational study, and reported that drug-resistant *C. auris* was prevalent in 3.9%–8.2% of the ICUs. Thus, extreme measures may be necessitated to counter *C. auris* outbreak.

One specific reason for alarm regarding *C. auris* is that, unlike other *Candida* spp., this species is resistant to all clinically available classes of antifungals, thus severely limiting treatment options. Lockhart et al. [69] conducted whole genome sequencing (WGS) and antifungal susceptibility testing of 41 clinical isolates of *C. auris* collected from patients in Pakistan, India, South Africa, and Venezuela during 2012–2015, and showed that 93% of isolates were resistant to fluconazole, 35% to amphotericin B, and 7% to echinocandins. The authors also concluded that antifungal-resistant *C. auris* is likely to have emerged recently, independently, and almost simultaneously on three continents, rather than as a result of worldwide dissemination of a dominant clone. In an editorial (in *Clinical Infectious Diseases*) on this study, Clancy & Hong issued an *International Call to Arms* to address *C. auris* infections [70] and noted that clonal isolates are likely distributed over large distances within countries and continents. They also concluded that *C. auris* infections may differ from invasive candidiasis caused by most other *Candida* species, which is usually sporadic and caused by genetically distinct, endogenous isolates colonizing the gastrointestinal tract, mucosal surfaces, or skin.

AZOLE RESISTANCE AMONG CRYPTOCOCCUS ISOLATES

Several studies have shown that *C. neoformans* can develop resistance against azoles. Brandt et al. [71] used CLSI microdilution and E-test methodologies to determine antifungal susceptibilities of *Cryptococcus neoformans* over a 6-year period 1992–1998, and showed that although MIC ranges of fluconazole, itraconazole, flucytosine and amphotericin B did not change during this time period for a majority of the isolates, isolated incidences of resistance (increase in the MIC by at least 4-fold) were noted. Datta et al. [72] evaluated susceptibility of clinical isolates of *C. neoformans* against fluconazole and itraconazole at a tertiary care center in India using CLSI methodology and showed that MIC90 values for fluconazole and itraconazole were 16 µg/mL and 0.125 µg/mL, respectively, with MIC/MFC ratios for fluconazole and itraconazole ≥1:32, indicating possible azole tolerance.

Development of cross-resistance to itraconazole following fluconazole treatment is an under-reported problem [71,73,74].

Mondon et al. [75] reported isolation of *C. neoformans* isolates that exhibited unusual patterns of resistance ("heteroresistance") to fluconazole and voriconazole from seven isolates from two different geographical regions (Israel and Italy), where most of the cells of each isolate were susceptible, but cells highly resistant to fluconazole (MICs ≥ 64 µg/mL) were recovered at a variable frequency. In a subsequent study, Yamazumi et al. [76] evaluated fluconazole susceptibility among 107 clinical isolates of *C. neoformans* (MIC between 0.25 and 32 µg/mL) and showed that exposure to fluconazole can induce heteroresistance. Other investigators have also reported the development of resistance in *C. neoformans* [77–79]. Taken together, these studies clearly demonstrate that *C. neoformans* isolates can acquire resistance against azoles.

AZOLE RESISTANCE AMONG FILAMENTOUS AND OTHER FUNGI

Although azole resistance is uncommon among *Aspergillus* isolates, several studies with itraconazole, voriconazole and posaconazole suggest this trend may be changing, with cross-resistance against azoles being reported [77,80,81]. More recently, van der Linden et al. [82] investigated azole resistance in clinical *Aspergillus* isolates by conducting prospective multicenter international surveillance in 22 centers from 19 countries (18 European and 4 non-European sites), screened 3788 *Aspergillus* isolates, and reported a 3.2% prevalence of azole-resistant *A. fumigatus*. Vermeulen et al. [83] reported slightly higher prevalence of 5.5% in a 1-year prospective multicenter cohort study among patients with *Aspergillus* disease in 18 hospitals in Belgium. Anecdotal evidence and prospective surveillance of patients suggest a rise in zygomycosis in association with voriconazole use in immunosuppressed patients [84]. However, the new azole, posaconazole, exhibits excellent activity against Zygomycetes. A recent study reported isolation of *F. solani* isolates that showed high azole MICs [85]. Azole resistance has also been reported among other fungi including *Rhodotorula* and *Trichosporon* [86,87].

Resistance against flucytosine

Primary resistance to flucytosine has been reported for *C. albicans*, but more commonly for *C. krusei* or *C. tropicalis* isolates [88]. Pfaller et al. [89] reported that while flucytosine was very active against most of the *Candida* isolates tested (>8000 clinical isolates of 18 *Candida* spp.; 92%–100% of all species were susceptible), *C. krusei* isolates exhibited intrinsic resistance against this agent (MIC90 = 32 µg/mL). In a more recent study describing the results of the ARTEMIS trial, Pfaller et al. [19] used the disk diffusion and broth microdilution methods and showed that while most *C. krusei* isolates were susceptible to voriconazole or echinocandins, they exhibited decreased susceptibilities to amphotericin B (MIC$_{90}$ = 4 µg/mL) and flucytosine (MIC90 = 16 µg/mL). Flucytosine resistance has also been reported for *C. neoformans* [78].

Resistance against polyenes

AMPHOTERICIN B RESISTANCE AMONG *CANDIDA* ISOLATES

Amphotericin B has a wide spectrum of activity against fungi, and resistance is relatively uncommon. However, incidences of resistance against this agent have been reported. Blignaut et al. [88] demonstrated amphotericin B resistance among 8.4% of the oral *C. albicans* isolates belonging to the "SA" clade in South Africa. Pfaller et al. [89] showed that most *C. krusei* isolates tested in their study exhibited reduced susceptibility to amphotericin B (MIC90 = 4 µg/mL). Yang et al. [90] showed that 16 of the 17 amphotericin B-resistant isolates obtained in a 4-year period in Taiwan were non-*albicans* Candida species. Colombo et al. [91] reported resistance to amphotericin B (MIC $\geq$ 2 µg/mL) in 2.5% of isolates (two strains of *C. albicans*, two of *C. parapsilosis* and one of *C. krusei*). In a separate study, Colombo et al. [92] reported amphotericin B resistance in *C. rugosa* isolates obtained from an outbreak in six hospitalized patients from a tertiary care teaching hospital in Sao Paulo, Brazil.

AMPHOTERICIN B RESISTANCE AMONG ASPERGILLUS AND OTHER FUNGI

In recent years, several cases have been reported documenting amphotericin B among *Aspergillus* species. *A. terreus* is intrinsically resistant to amphotericin B, and isolates of *A. ustus* and *A. lentulus* have been noted increasingly as causes of invasive aspergillosis in tertiary care centers in the US [93,94]. Panagopoulou et al. [80] showed that *Aspergillus* isolates obtained from a tertiary care center in Greece over a 12-month period exhibited reduced susceptibility to amphotericin B. Lass-Florl et al. [95] evaluated the epidemiology and outcome of infections due to *A. terreus* in Austria over a 10-year period, and showed that infections due to this fungus were associated with a lower response rate to amphotericin B therapy (20%), compared with 47% for patients with non-*A. terreus* infections (p < 0.05). Hsueh et al. [77] reported that *A. flavus* was less susceptible to amphotericin B, with MIC_{50} of 1 µg/mL and MIC_{90} of 2 µg/mL, which were 2-fold greater than those for *A. fumigatus* and *A. niger*. However, all *Aspergillus* isolates were susceptible to voriconazole, including isolates with reduced susceptibility to amphotericin B and itraconazole. Although less common, amphotericin B resistance has also been reported for other fungi. Hsueh [77] showed in an earlier study that two (3%) isolates of *C. neoformans* were not inhibited by amphotericin B at 1 µg/mL. *Scedosporium prolificans* is intrinsically resistant to amphotericin B, and resistance to this drug has also been demonstrated among *S. apiospermum*, *Fusarium* spp. and *Sporothrix schenckii* [96,97].

Resistance against echinocandins

Although several surveillance studies have shown that echinocandin has broad spectrum activity against most fungi [98–100], smaller-scale studies and case reports have reported the occurrence of echinocandins resistance, especially among *Candida* isolates. One of the earliest reports demonstrating fungal resistance against echinocandins was by Laverdiere et al. [101], who reported progressive loss of cross-echinocandin activity (increased MICs of caspofungin, micafungin, anidulafungin) against four *C. albicans* isolates obtained at the initiation and during micafungin therapy from a patient with advanced HIV infection and chronic oesophagitis. Echinocandin resistance among *C. albicans* isolates is generally associated with esophageal candidiasis/HIV as the underlying disease, while among non-*albicans* isolates, the underlying conditions commonly noted are leukemia, transplants, and endocarditis. In a separate study, Forrest et al. [102] performed a 5-year retrospective review of cases at a tertiary care center and reported significant correlations between increased caspofungin usage and an increased incidence of *C. parapsilosis* candidemia. Similarly, Pasquale et al. [103] recently reported echinocandin resistance in *C. tropicalis* isolates.

Although caspofungin, micafungin, and anidulafungin belong to the same class of compounds (echinocandins), their activity and efficacy potential can vary greatly. For example, Villareal et al. [104] showed that a *C. glabrata* isolate obtained from a patient, who failed caspofungin, was non-susceptible to caspofungin, (MIC = 8 µg/mL) while remaining susceptible to anidulafungin (MIC = 0.125 µg/mL). Other studies have also showed that the three echinocandins are not alike, when tested against *C. krusei* or *C. parapsilosis* [105–107]. In an expanded study, our group [108] assessed *in vitro* activity of the three echinocandins and two triazoles (fluconazole and voriconazole) against 77 *C. parapsilosis* and 13 *C. albicans* isolates (obtained from patients, healthcare workers, and the hospital environment) using the CLSI M27-A2 method. We found that *C. parapsilosis* isolates obtained from burn unit patients were more susceptible to anidulafungin than to caspofungin or micafungin, while isolates obtained from healthcare workers or environmental sources were susceptible to all antifungals examined. *C. albicans* isolates were susceptible to the antifungals tested. Additionally, Forastiero et al. [109] reported acquisition of echinocandin resistance in *C. krusei* isolates obtained from the blood, urine, and soft tissue of an acute lymphocytic leukemia patient, during caspofungin therapy for 10 days.

Wierman et al. [110] reported isolation of a set of clinical *C. glabrata* isolates from a patient with disseminated candidiasis who failed therapy with caspofungin and micafungin but responded to amphotericin B and anidulafungin. Antifungal susceptibility testing showed that the *C. glabrata* isolates were cross-resistant to caspofungin and micafungin but susceptible to anidulafungin. In another study, Cota et al. [111] evaluated the activities of anidulafungin and caspofungin against 18 *C. glabrata* isolates with reduced caspofungin activity and showed that isolates not susceptible to caspofungin were killed by anidulafungin, with MFC values ranging between and 1–128 µg/mL for caspofungin compared to 0.25–8 µg/mL for anidulafungin.

Vallabhaneni et al. [112] analyzed data from the Centers for Disease Control and Prevention's population-based laboratory surveillance for candidemia in four metropolitan areas (7.9 million persons; 80 hospitals) during 2008–2014 to characterize the epidemiology and risk factors for echinocandin nonsusceptible *C. glabrata* bloodstream infections. These investigators reported 1385 *C. glabrata* cases, of which 83 (6.0%) had non-susceptible isolates (19 intermediate and 64 resistant), and that the proportion of non-susceptible *C. glabrata* isolates increased significantly during 2008–2014 (from 4.2% in 2008 to 7.8% in 2014, p < 0.001). Prior echinocandin exposure, previous candidemia episode, hospitalization in the last 90 days, and fluconazole resistance were significantly associated with nonsusceptible *C. glabrata*. These results suggested acquired resistance due to prior drug exposure, as well as transmission of resistant organisms (occurrence of non-susceptible *C. glabrata* without prior echinocandin exposure).

Echinocandin resistance has also been reported for other fungi. *Aspergillus* isolates resistant to echinocandins has been associated with biofilm formation (discussed below) [113]. In one recent study, Suzuki et al. [114] reported breakthrough cryptococcosis in a patient with systemic lupus erythematosus (SLE) receiving micafungin. Moreover, echinocandins have no activity against Zygomycetes or against *Trichosporon, Scedosporium,* and *Fusarium* species. Therefore, resistance against echinocandins, while uncommon, has been reported in several cases, and more careful monitoring of echinocandin susceptibility among fungi is warranted.

Resistance against allylamines

Resistance against terbinafine, the commonly used allylamine, is rare. However, Mukherjee et al. [115] reported the first instance of terbinafine resistance in dermatophytes. The *in vitro* antifungal susceptibilities of six clinical *T. rubrum* isolates obtained sequentially from a single onychomycosis patient who failed oral terbinafine therapy (250 mg/day for 24 weeks) were determined by broth microdilution and macrodilution methodologies. The MICs of terbinafine for these strains were >4 μg/mL, whereas they were <0.0002 μg/mL for the susceptible reference strains, and MFCs for all six strains were >128 μg/mL, and 0.0002 μg/mL for the reference strain. Since PCR amplification analyses did not reveal any differences between the isolates, and the MIC of terbinafine for the baseline strain (cultured at the initial screening visit and before therapy was started) was increased by 4000-fold, this was identified as a case of primary resistance to terbinafine, acquired during the course of therapy. These terbinafine-resistant isolates exhibited normal susceptibilities to clinically available antimycotics, including itraconazole, fluconazole, and Griseofulvin, but were cross-resistant to several other known squalene epoxidase inhibitors, including naftifine, butenafine, tolnaftate, and tolciclate, suggesting a target-specific mechanism of resistance.

MECHANISMS OF RESISTANCE

Fungi can develop resistance against antifungal agents using one or more mechanisms including reduced availability of the drug, alteration, and complementation of drug target (Figure 4.1) [116]. These mechanisms are described briefly below.

Mechanism of azole resistance

Major mechanisms mediating resistance against azoles involve alteration in membrane sterol composition, increased demethylase and sterol levels, reduction of azole permeability, efflux of the drug, modification in the target enzyme, and/or reduced access to the target [52,117].

REDUCED DRUG PERMEABILITY

Changes in membrane lipid composition and/or fatty acids have been suggested as mechanisms mediating azole resistance in *C. albicans* [118–122]. Such changes can be induced by different mechanisms, including altered biosynthesis of membrane lipids like ergosterol and sphingolipid, binding to sterol biosynthesis enzymes (e.g., demethylase, sterol desaturase), and modulation of membrane transporters. The net effect of changes in membrane lipid composition is to alter the membrane permeability, thus restricting the amount of azole that can enter the cell. Mago and Khuller [118] showed that exposure to cerulenin (a specific inhibitor of fatty acid and sterol biosyntheses) inhibited growth and lipid synthesis in *C. albicans*, an effect that was reversed by exogenous addition of fatty acids. These fatty acid-supplemented cells contained altered levels of phospholipids and sterols, and were more resistant to miconazole, showing that alteration in fatty acid composition is a mechanism by which *C. albicans* is rendered resistant to azoles. For example, by replacing membrane ergosterol with fecosterol [119], changes in sterol composition have been observed in azole-resistant *C. albicans* strains and been proposed to be a mechanism of azole resistance in fungal cells. Furthermore, Hitchcock et al. [123] showed that in a *C. albicans* isolate resistant to both polyene and azole groups of antifungals, ergosterol was replaced by methylated sterol (lanosterol, 24-methylene-24,25-dihydrolanosterol and 4-methylergostadiene-3-ol), which results in double resistance by preventing polyene binding and reducing azole permeability. Other studies have also provided evidence that cross-resistance to fluconazole and amphotericin B among *C. albicans* can be explained by similar defects in sterol Δ5,6-desaturation [124]. In a separate study, Kohli et al. [125] showed that *C. albicans* strains serially passed through increasing concentrations of fluconazole led to acquisition of resistance, overexpression of *CDR1* and *CDR2* genes, and alterations in membrane fluidity and asymmetry.

However, changes in membrane sterol composition cannot always explain azole resistance in fungal cells, as shown in several studies [126]. In one such study, Hitchcock et al. [126] demonstrated that although the 14α-sterol demethylase enzyme in an azole-resistant *C. albicans* strain

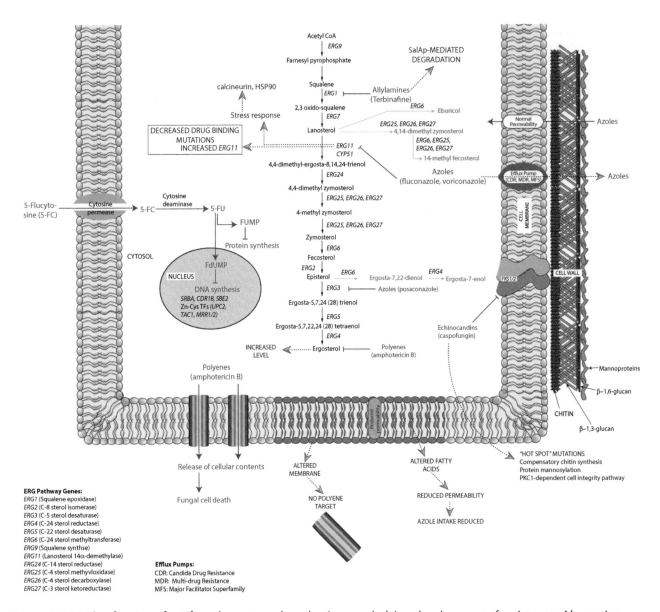

Figure 4.1 Mode of action of antifungal agents and mechanisms underlying development of resistance. Alternative metabolites are indicated in green, targets of antifungal agents are indicated in red, and mechanisms of resistance are indicated in blue (dotted arrows). Fungal cell wall is shown only partially, to indicate the mode of action of echinocandins and their mechanism of resistance.

was less sensitive to a triazole than two azole-sensitive strains, there was no direct correlation between the IC_{50} values for triazole inhibition of the demethylase and IC_{50} values for growth. Lamb et al. [127] separately showed that azole resistance in *C. albicans* strain NCPF 3363 was associated with reduced intracellular accumulation of drug and not reduced affinity for the target site. These results suggest that the basis of azole resistance in some strains may be linked to altered or absent azole targets.

ALTERATION IN TARGET ENZYMES

Azole resistance has also been associated with alteration in activity of cytochrome P450-dependent 14α-demethylase and that of other ergosterol biosynthesis enzymes, like Δ5-6 desaturase [128–131]. In this regard, Vanden Bossche et al.

[132] demonstrated increased microsomal cytochrome P-450 content and subcellular ergosterol synthesis from mevalonate or lanosterol in azole-resistant *C. glabrata*, indicating that the level of P450-dependent 14α-demethylation of lanosterol was higher in these cells, and contributed to resistance. Azole resistance in *C. krusei* has been linked to reduced susceptibility of 14α-demethylase because of reduced binding affinity [133]. Over-expression of CYP51A1 in *C. albicans* and *C. glabrata* may also account for a decreased susceptibility to azole antifungal agents [134].

ACCUMULATION OF TOXIC INTERMEDIATES

Inhibition of sterol biosynthesis pathway can also result in accumulation of intermediates that are toxic to the fungal cells. In this regard, Marichal et al. [121] showed that two azole-resistant

C. albicans isolates (C48 and C56) overexpressed efflux pumps and contained increased intracellular levels (20%–30%) of 14α-methyl-ergosta-8,24(28)-diene-3β,6α-dio 1 (3, 6-diol). Itraconazole treatment of C43 resulted in a dose-dependent inhibition of ergosterol biosynthesis and accumulation of 3,6-diol (up to 60% of the total sterols), eburicol, lanosterol, obtusifoliol, 14α-methyl-ergosta-5,7,22,24(28)-tetraene-3betaol, and 14α-methyl-fecosterol. These investigators also showed that itraconazole exposure led to increased levels of obtusifolione, a toxic 3-ketosteroid earlier shown to accumulate after itraconazole treatment in *C. neoformans* and *Histoplasma capsulatum*, and that obtusifolione accumulation correlated with inhibition of growth of these azole-resistant strains.

Both reduced permeability and activity of demethylase have been suggested to explain azole resistance among *A. fumigatus* isolates [135,136]. Denning et al. [136] demonstrated at least two mechanisms of resistance to be responsible for itraconazole resistance in three clinical isolates of *A. fumigatus* (AF72, AF91 and AF92) obtained from two patients. These investigators showed that isolate AF72 had reduced ergosterol content, greater quantities of sterol intermediates, a similar susceptibility to itraconazole in cell-free ergosterol biosynthesis, and a reduced intracellular itraconazole concentration. In contrast, isolates AF91 and AF92 had slightly higher ergosterol and lower intermediate sterol concentrations, 5-fold increased resistance in cell-free systems to the effect of itraconazole on sterol 14α-demethylation, and intracellular itraconazole concentrations found in susceptible isolates. These studies showed that at least two mechanisms – one involving reduced permeability of itraconazole, the other due to a more direct effect on enzyme activity – were mediating resistance in these isolates. In a subsequent study, Manavathu et al. [135] evaluated itraconazole susceptibility of two resistant *A. fumigatus* isolates and showed that intracellular accumulation of itraconazole in azole-resistant isolates was reduced by up to 80% compared to the susceptible parent, suggesting that the reduced accumulation of itraconazole is more likely associated with diminished drug permeability and not with drug efflux. Moreover, the respiratory inhibitor carbonyl cyanide m-chlorophenyl hydrazone reduced the intracellular accumulation of itraconazole by around 36% the parent and in the mutant strains, demonstrating that uptake of itraconazole in *A. fumigatus* is an energy dependent process.

More recently, Willger et al. [137] showed that azole resistance in *A. fumigatus* is modulated by a sterol-regulatory element binding protein, SrbA. A mutant strain lacking this protein SrbA was hyper-susceptible to fluconazole and voriconazole, suggesting that SrbA plays a role in modulating fungal susceptibility to azoles, most likely by regulating ergosterol biosynthesis.

MODIFICATION OF DRUG TARGET: MUTATION AND OVEREXPRESSION

Mutations in drug target have been associated with azole resistance in several studies. Marichal et al. [138] identified mutations in cytochrome P450 14α-demethylase (Erg11p, Cyp51p), an enzyme involved in ergosterol biosynthesis, play critical roles in azole resistance among fungi. Xu et al. [139] evaluated the relationship between mutations in the *ERG11* gene of 15 fluconazole-resistant and 8 fluconazole-susceptible *C. albicans* isolates obtained from non-AIDS patients and demonstrated 18 silent mutations and 19 missense mutations. These investigators showed that six missense mutations occurred in resistant isolates: G487T (A114S), T916C (Y257H), T541C (Y132H), T1559C (I471T), C1567A (Q474K), and T1493A (F449Y), of which the first four are known to contribute to fluconazole resistance, while the role of the last two have not been investigated. Lockhart et al. [69] used whole genome sequencing and reported that azole resistant clinical isolates of *C. auris* clustered into unique clades based on geographic region, and that different mutations in *ERG11* were associated with resistance in each geographic clade. However, these investigators did not perform functional validation of the role of Erg11p in resistance in *C. auris*.

Modification of the target enzyme is a common mechanism identified for azole resistance in *Aspergillus* species, primarily through amino acid substitutions in the drug target *Cyp51* (encoding 14α-lanosterol demethylase) [140–142]. In azole resistant *A. fumigatus* isolates, the most frequent amino acid substitutions occur at the positions Gly 54, Gly 138, Met 220, and Leu 98, coupled with a tandem repetition in the gene promoter [140,141,143]. Other amino acid substitutions identified in *cyp51* genes of voriconazole-resistant isolates include N22D and M220I in *A. fumigatus* [142]. Among resistant *A. flavus* isolates commonly identifies substitutions include K197N, Y132N, T469S, K197N, D282E, and M288L [144]. Another mechanism by which fungi become resistant is by expressing multiple copies of the drug target. An example of this approach is evident in the study by Osherov et al. [145] who showed that *A. nidulans* and *A. fumigatus* isolates that are resistant to itraconazole induce overexpression of the P-450 14α-demethylase gene.

Recently, a novel azole resistance mechanism has been identified in *A. fumigatus*, where resistance is associated with a 34-bp or 46-bp tandem repeat (TR) in the promoter of *CYP51A*. De Fontbrune et al. [146] reported TR(34)/L98H to be linked to azole resistance in *A. fumigatus* in hematopoietic stem cell transplant patient with invasive aspergillosis. This mutation was also linked to azole resistance of *Aspergillus* in subsequent studies [82,147–150]. In the international surveillance study, van der Linden et al. [82] also determined the full coding sequence of both strands of the *cyp51A* gene and the promoter region by PCR amplification. These investigators reported that among the 46 patients with resistant isolates, 8 patients had azole-resistant *A. fumigatus* sibling isolates, and 38 had a resistant *A. fumigatus* isolate, 19 of which had an isolate that harbored a TR_{34}/L98H or TR_{46}/Y121F/T289A mutation. Overall, the TR_{34}/L98H mutation was the predominant mechanism of resistance (48.9%) in *A. fumigatus* sensu strictu isolates. Recently, Wiederhold et al. [149] became the first to report detection of TR34/L98H and TR46/Y121F

T289A Cyp51 mutations in *A. fumigatus* in the United States. Hagiwara et al. [151] investigated whether an azole-resistant strain with a 46-bp TR (TR46/Y121F/T289A) could be sensitised to azoles by deletion of *srbA*, encoding a direct regulator of cyp51A. The *srbA* deletion strain showed decreased expression of *CYP51A* and hyper-susceptibility to azoles, demonstrating that *srbA* acts as a direct regulator of *CYP51A*-mediated response to azoles in *A. fumigatus*.

Transcriptional regulation of sterol biosynthesis genes plays a critical role in azole resistance and include zinc cluster proteins transcription factors (Zn$_2$-Cys$_6$ TFs) like *TAC1* (transcriptional activator of *CDR* genes), *MRR1/2* (multidrug resistance regulators that regulate *MDR1*), and *UPC2* (activates the expression of related genes in response to sterol depletion through a conserved C-terminal domain) [152–162]. Recently, Hagiwara et al. [163] identified a novel Zn2-Cys6 Transcription Factor *AtrR* that co-regulates *CYP51A* and *CdrlB* expression (by direct binding to both *CYP51A* and *CdrlB* promoters) in *A. fumigatus*, *A. oryzae*, and *A. nidulans*, thus playing a critical role in azole resistance in these *Aspegillus* species. These investigators showed that while *AtrR* was responsible for the expression of *CDR1B*, *SrbA* was not involved in this process. Fluconazole-induced "microevolution" in *C. albicans* has also been suggested as a broader mechanism of resistance and comprises genomic rearrangements that result in gene amplification and loss of heterozygosity for resistance mutations (e.g., in mating type locus MTL), which further increases drug resistance and may also affect extended chromosomal regions with ancillary phenotypic effects [164]. For example, mutations in MTL allows the fungal cells to switch to the mating-competent opaque phenotype, allowing sexual recombination that may result in the generation of highly fluconazole-resistant strains with multiple resistance mechanisms.

TRANSPORTER-MEDIATED DRUG EFFLUX

A major mechanism of azole resistance is induction or over-expression of drug efflux pumps (*Candida* drug resistance, CDR) and transporters (major facilitator superfamily, MFS), which mediate clearance of the drug from fungal cells [165–170]. Different studies have demonstrated that multiple mechanisms can be operative in fungal cells and contribute to azole resistance in *C. albicans* [171–173]. White et al. [171] evaluated mRNA levels in a series of 17 clinical isolates taken from a single HIV-infected patient over 2 years, during which time the levels of fluconazole resistance of the strain increased over 200-fold. These investigators reported increased mRNA levels of *ERG16* (which encodes the 14α-demethylase enzyme), *CDR1*, and *MDR1* in this series, which correlated with increases in fluconazole resistance of the isolates. In a second study, Franz et al. [172] reported the isolation of five *C. albicans* isolates from two AIDS patients with oropharyngeal candidiasis, from recurrent episodes of infection, which became gradually resistant against fluconazole during treatment. Isolates from patient 1 exhibited enhanced expression of *MDR1* and constitutively high expression of *ERG11*, which correlated

with a stepwise development of fluconazole resistance. In the isolates from patient 2, increased *MDR1* mRNA levels and the change from heterozygosity to homozygosity for a mutant form of the *ERG11* gene correlated with continuously decreased drug susceptibility, reduced drug accumulation and increased resistance in activity of sterol 14alpha-demethylase. Exposure of cells to fluconazole can also induce expression of CDR1, which can contribute to development of azole resistance [174].

Sanglard et al. [175] showed that *C. glabrata CDR1* (Cg*CDR1*) is involved in the resistance of clinical isolates to azole antifungal agents [175], while Torelli et al. [176] implicated upregulation of another ATP-binding cassette transporter, CgSNQ2, in azole resistance among *C. glabrata* isolates. Furthermore, Thakur et al. [177] showed that a nuclear receptor-like pathway regulates multidrug resistance in *C. glabrata*.

In a separate study, Katiyar and Edlind [178] showed that in azole resistant *C. krusei* cells, expression of two ATP cassette binding (ABC) transporters (*ABC1* and *ABC2*) increased at stationary phase, which correlated with decreased susceptibility to miconazole. Furthermore, ABC1 was upregulated following brief treatment of *C. krusei* with miconazole and clotrimazole (but not other azoles), and the unrelated compounds albendazole and cycloheximide. The latter two compounds antagonized fluconazole activity versus *C. krusei*, supporting a role for the ABC1 transporter in azole efflux. Finally, miconazole-resistant mutants selected *in vitro* demonstrated increased constitutive expression of ABC1.

Efflux pumps have been shown to contribute to drug resistance in Aspergillus and Cryptococcus species. Overexpression of efflux pumps plays a critical role in itraconazole resistance among *A. fumigatus* isolates, with Afumdr3, Afumdr4, and AtrF playing critical roles, especially in the early stages of resistance acquisition [142,179,180]. Posteraro et al. [181] cloned and sequenced an ABC transporter-encoding gene, *C. neoformans* AntiFungal Resistance 1 (Cn*AFR1*), from a fluconazole-resistant *C. neoformans* isolate, and demonstrated that the isogenic knock-out mutant cnafr1 (in which the Cn*AFR1* gene was disrupted) was highly susceptible to fluconazole, while reintroduction of the functional gene in cnafr1 resulted in restoration of the resistance phenotype. Yang et al. [182] reported that the efflux pump Pdr1p plays a critical role in azole resistance in *C. gattii*.

In a recent study, Zhang et al. [183] reported that Rta2p, a membrane protein with 7 transmembrane domains, is involved in calcineurin-mediated azole resistance and sphingoid long-chain base release in *C. albicans*. These investigators also reported that G234S mutation in Rta4p enhanced the therapeutic efficacy of fluconazole against systemic candidiasis and significantly increased the accumulation of dihydrosphingosine by decreasing its release. In a separate study, Zhang et al. [56] reported overexpression of *MDR1* genes in azole-resistant clinical *C. parapsilosis* isolates, which was associated with L986P mutation.

These studies clearly showed that efflux pumps play important roles in drug resistance among different fungal species.

Mechanism of polyene resistance

ALTERED MEMBRANE LIPID COMPOSITION

Much of amphotericin B resistance is related to changes in sterols in the cell membranes since ergosterol is the molecule interacting with this drug. Such changes include decreased ergosterol production and altered ergosterol products caused by mutation in the sterol biosynthesis pathway.

Walsh et al. [184] showed that amphotericin B resistance in *A. terreus* is linked to decreased levels of membrane ergosterol. These investigators used a persistently neutropenic rabbit model of invasive pulmonary aspergillosis due to *A. terreus* and *A. fumigatus* and investigated possible mechanisms of resistance in *A. terreus* using microbicidal time-kill assays, colorimetric MTT assays of hyphal damage, and sterol composition analysis of the fungal cell membrane by gas-liquid chromatography (GLC). Both time-kill and MTT assays showed that *A. terreus* was resistant to the fungicidal effects of amphotericin B. Membrane sterol composition analysis revealed that the amphotericin B-resistant *A. terreus* contained reduced ergosterol levels (20.3%), and increased levels of zymosterol (17.1%) and squalene (17.5%). These investigators suggested that the depletion of ergosterol in the amphotericin B-resistant *A. terreus* contributes substantially to diminished binding of amphotericin B to the cytoplasmic cell membrane, resulting in polyene resistance. The substituted nonergosterol cytoplasmic membrane sterols and lipids (e.g., zymosterol and squalene) may have further reduced affinity for AmB, resulting in diminished binding. These studies indicated that amphotericin B resistance in *A. terreus* isolates is likely due to reduction in membrane ergosterol levels. In a separate study, defective Δ-8,7 isomerase was found to be associated with decreased intercalation of the drug with the membrane, resulting in amphotericin B resistance in *C. neoformans* [96,185–187].

MODIFICATIONS IN DRUG TARGET

Amphotericin B resistance can also result from alteration in the drug's target. In a recent study, Vandeputte et al. [188] recently reported that a missense mutation in *ERG6* gene (Cys-Phe substitution) correlated with reduced polyene susceptibility (determined using disk diffusion method) of a clinical *C. glabrata* isolate that grew as pseudohyphae. This isolate lacked ergosterol and accumulated late sterol intermediates, indicative of a defect in the final steps of the ergosterol pathway. Functional complementation of the mutation restored susceptibility to polyenes and a classical morphology, demonstrating the role of ERG6 in amphotericin B in *C. glabrata*.

Ikeda et al. [189] suggested that melanin, a virulence factor in *C. neoformans*, also mediates antifungal resistance. These investigators induced melanin formation by growing laccase-active strains of *C. neoformans* and *C. albidus* in L-DOPA and observed no change in MIC of amphotericin B and fluconazole for these cells. However, live cells were detected in wells containing amphotericin B-inhibited cells and contained melanin. In contrast, melanization did not protect *C. albidus* from killing by amphotericin B. Time-kill analysis of the effect of amphotericin B on *C. neoformans* revealed that higher number of melanized cells survived in the first few hours than non-melanized cells. Binding studies suggested that melanin in the cell walls binds amphotericin B, thus reducing its effective concentrations and minimizing exposure of *C. neoformans* cells to this agent.

Zaragoza et al. [190] showed recently that enlargement of the polysaccharide capsule of *C. neoformans* resulted in protection against resistance to reactive oxygen species (ROS) induced by catalase-independent hydrogen peroxide, suggesting that the capsule can act as a scavenger of ROS, thus protecting the cells from phagocytosis. Interestingly, these investigators reported that capsule enlargement also conferred resistance to amphotericin B.

Huang et al. [191] showed that overexpression of *PMP3* gene, encoding the highly-conserved plasma membrane proteolipid 3 protein, contributed to amphotericin B resistance in *S. cerevisiae*. Subsequently, Bari et al. [192] showed that Pmp3p modulates amphotericin B resistance through the sphingolipid biosynthetic pathway and involves phytosphingosine.

Mechanism of flucytosine resistance

Mechanism of flucytosine resistance in fungal cells is well documented and is commonly mediated by modification in cytosine permease and ribosyl transferase activities [193–196]. Additional mechanisms include failure to metabolize flucytosine to 5FUTP and 5FdUMP, or from the loss of feedback control of pyrimidine biosynthesis [134,197]. The homozygous resistant strain *fcy1/fcy1* (lacking functional UMP pyrophosphorylase) was associated with decreased UMP pyrophosphorylase activity that resulted in poor conversion from 5-flucytosine to FUMP, whereas resistance in fcy2/fcy2 strains was associated with decreased cytosine deaminase activity [198,199]. Hope et al. [196] evaluated flucytosine resistance mechanisms in 25 *C. albicans* strains by identifying and sequencing the genes *FCA1* (encoding cytosine deaminase), *FUR1* (encoding uracil phosphoribosyltransferase; UPRT), *FCY21* and *FCY22* (encoding two purine-cytosine permeases). These investigators showed an association between a polymorphic nucleotide and resistance to flucytosine within *FUR1* (with a C301T nucleotide substitution), which resulted in R101C substitution in UPRT. A single resistant isolate, lacking this *FUR1* polymorphism, contained instead a homozygous polymorphism in *FCA1* that resulted in a G28N substitution in cytosine deaminase. Single nucleotide polymorphism has also been linked to clade-specific resistance in *C. albicans* clades. In this regard, Dodgson et al. [200] evaluated flucytosine resistance patterns in *C. albicans* clades and showed that a single nucleotide change (C301T) in *FUR1* can lead to flucytosine resistance in clade I isolates. The flucytosine MICs for strains with no copies, one copy, and two copies of the mutant allele were ≤0.25 µg/mL, >0.5 µg/mL, and >16 µg/mL, respectively. Vlanti and Diallinas [201] recently cloned and characterized the *A. nidulans fcyB*, encoding the closest homologue to the yeast Fcy2p/Fcy21p permeases. A *fcyB* null mutant lacked all known purine transporters and was resistant to flucytosine. These investigators showed FcyBp to be a low-capacity, high-affinity, cytosine-purine transporter, with scavenging of cytosine-purine as its main function. In a recent study, Papon et al. [202] showed that inactivation of the *FCY2*, *FCY1*, and *FUR1* genes in *C. lusitaniae* produced two patterns of resistance to flucytosine. Mutant *fur1* demonstrated resistance to 5-fluorouracil, whereas mutants *fcy1* and *fcy2* demonstrated fluconazole resistance in the presence of sub-inhibitory flucytosine concentrations.

Flucyosine-fluconazole cross-resistance has also been reported [202,203]. In one such study, Noel et al. [203] demonstrated that the cross-resistance involved a fluconazole uptake transporter in purine-cytosine permease-deficient *C. lusitaniae* clinical isolates. Genetic analyses showed that resistance to flucytosine was derived from a recessive mutation in a single gene, whereas cross-resistance to fluconazole seemed to vary like a quantitative trait. Kinetic transport studies with flucytosine showed that flucytosine resistance was due to a defect in the purine-cytosine permease.

Recently, Costa et al. [204] identified cell wall remodeling as a potential mechanism of flucytosine resistance in *C. glabrata* and showed that while arginine supplementation relieved the inhibitory effect of this drug, lyticase susceptibility was increased within the first 30 minutes of 5-flucytosine exposure. Moreover, the aquaglyceroporin encoding genes CgFPS1 and CgFPS2, from *C. glabrata*, were also identified as determinants of 5-flucytosine resistance. The clinical relevance of these mechanisms of resistance remains to be investigated.

Mechanism of allylamine resistance

Resistance against allylamines (e.g., terbinafine) is mostly due to changes in the squalene epoxidase enzyme, which catalyzes the conversion of squalene to epoxysqualenes in the ergosterol biosynthesis pathway [205].

MODIFICATION OF DRUG TARGET: OVEREXPRESSION AND MUTATION

Increased expression of number of copies of squalene epoxidase was shown to lead to terbinafine resistance in *Aspergillus* isolates [206]. Liu et al. [206] identified the gene responsible for terbinafine resistance as the *A. fumigatus* squalene epoxidase gene (*ERG1*). In a separate study, Rocha et al. [207] showed that a F389L substitution in *ergA* confers terbinafine resistance in *Aspergillus*. Osborne et al. [208] characterized a new clinical strain of *T. rubrum* highly resistant to terbinafine and showed that resistance to terbinafine in this strain is caused by a missense mutation in the squalene epoxidase gene leading to the amino acid substitution F397L.

DEGRADATION OF DRUG

Graminha et al. [209] demonstrated that terbinafine resistance in UV-induced *A. nidulans* mutants was mediated by salicylate 1-monooxygenase (salA), a napthalene-degrading enzyme, since transformation of sensitive strain with this gene rendered it resistant. Moreover, salA transcript accumulation analysis showed terbinafine-dependent induction in the wild type strain. These investigators suggested that terbinafine resistance in the resistant isolate could be due to degradation of the naphthalene ring contained in terbinafine.

Mechanism of echinocandin resistance

Echinocandin resistance can be mediated by mutations in the *FKS1* gene, adaptive or lower level drug tolerance and stimulation of chitin synthase gene [210].

MODIFICATION IN DRUG TARGET: MUTATIONS AND ALTERED SUBSTRATE

Mutations in two distinct *FKS1* regions, Hotspot 1 (HS1) and Hotspot 2 (HS2), have been linked to echinocandin resistance. The region around Ser645 (within HS1) is considered to be the major contributor to echinocandin resistance, with the highest frequency of substitution. Amino acid substitutions in HS1 and HS2 were evaluated following DNA sequence analysis of *FKS1* genes from susceptible and resistant *Candida* spp. [211]. In a recent study, Garcia-Effron et al. [212] reported that a naturally occurring Fks1p P600A substitution (immediately distal to the hot spot 1 region) was responsible for reduced echinocandin susceptibility of *C. parapsilosis*, *C. orthopsilosis* and *C. metapsilosis*.

Although mutations in the FKS1 gene are common mechanisms, all cases of echinocandin resistance cannot be explained by this phenomenon. For example, our analysis of echinocandin cross-resistant *C. parapsilosis* isolates [108] showed that although anidulafungin and caspofungin possess equivalent activity against the caspofungin-susceptible *C. parapsilosis* strain, they differed in their ability to damage the caspofungin non-susceptible strain (cellular damage and distortion of morphology was induced by lower concentrations of anidulafungin [1 µg/mL] than that of caspofungin [16 µg/mL]). To determine whether the non-susceptibility of *C. parapsilosis* isolates to caspofungin could be due to mutations in the *FKS1* gene, we compared the sequence of the 493bp portion of this gene associated with echinocandin resistance and found no differences in the amino acid pattern within the targeted region. Therefore, differences in the activity between anidulafungin and the other echinocandins could not be attributed to mutations within the *FKS1* gene, and the observed non-susceptibility to caspofungin was likely due to other mechanism.

Some studies have suggested that modulation of echinocandin susceptibility is associated with differential expression of overlapping set of genes involved in *FKS* regulation, compensatory chitin synthesis, protein mannosylation, and the protein kinase C1 (Pkc1)-dependent cell integrity pathway [213,214]. Osherov et al. [215] proposed over-expression of *SBE2* (which encodes Sbe2p, a Golgi protein involved in the transport of cell wall components) as an adaptive mechanism of resistance against echinocandins. These investigators showed that over-expression of Sbe2p resulted in caspofungin resistance in *S. cerevisiae*, and that deletion of *SBE2* rendered the yeast hypersensitive to caspofungin, thus showing that over-expression of Sbe2p imparts caspofungin resistance. Walker et al. [216] reported that treatment of *C. albicans* with low levels of echinocandins stimulated expression of the gene encoding chitin synthase (CHS), increased activity of this enzyme, elevated chitin content and rendered the cells less susceptible. The role of substrate availability in echinocandin resistance is also underscored by the study performed by Feldmesser et al. [217], who showed that inactivity of caspofungin against *C. neoformans* is largely due to difference in glucan structure in this fungus, which contains both 1,3 β-d-glucan and 1,6 β-d-glucan in the cell wall.

DRUG EFFLUX

Echinocandins are poor substrates for most multidrug efflux transporters, and several studies have argued against the role of drug efflux pumps in echinocandin resistance [218–220]. One study, however, showed that efflux pumps were upregulated in azole-echinocandin cross-resistant isolates [221]. Therefore, it is likely that more than one mechanism of resistance could be operative in such cross-resistant isolates. For example, it is possible that mutation in *FKS1* and overexpression of efflux pumps may be operational in the azole/echinocandin cross-resistant isolates, thereby accounting for the broad cross-resistance.

Biofilm formation as a mechanism of resistance

Fungi including *Candida*, *Cryptococcus*, *Aspergillus*, and *Fusarium* species have been shown to form biofilms on surfaces like catheters, dentures, contact lenses, and wells of microtiter plates [113,222–226]. Biofilms are communities of cells encased in self-produced extracellular matrix (ECM), and are characterized by resistance against commonly used antifungal agents, as well as common biocides [222,223,227], prompting the notion that growth as a biofilm also represents a mechanism by which fungi become drug-resistant. In this section, we will briefly summarize the mechanisms by which fungal biofilms are rendered drug resistant.

PHASE-DEPENDENT MECHANISMS MEDIATE DRUG RESISTANCE IN FUNGAL BIOFILMS

Ramage et al. [228] reported that efflux pumps, including Cdr1p, Cdr2p, and Mdr1p, were not involved in drug resistance associated with mature *C. albicans* biofilms formed on 96-well microtiter plates. In a subsequent study, Mukherjee et al. [229] compared the mechanism of antifungal resistance in biofilms at early and mature phases. These investigators showed that in early phase

biofilms, efflux pumps contributed to antifungal resistance, while in mature phase biofilms, resistance was associated with changes in levels of ergosterol biosynthesis intermediates. The role of efflux pumps in biofilm-associated resistance was confirmed in a separate study by Mateus et al. [230] who showed that expression of *MDR1* and *CDR1* genes was significantly lower in daughter cells from 48-hours biofilms than in firmly adherent cells (2 hours after attachment), demonstrating that efflux pump expression in adherent cultures is transient. These studies clearly demonstrated that antifungal resistance in *Candida* biofilms is due to multiple mechanisms in a phase-dependent manner.

ROLE OF CAPSULE IN BIOFILM RESISTANCE

Recent studies have characterized the role of biofilm formation in drug resistance profile of *C. neoformans* [231,232]. Martin and Casadevall [232] showed that while exposure of *C. neoformans* to amphotericin B or echinocandin prevented biofilm formation, fluconazole or voriconazole did not have any effect on the biofilm-forming ability of this organism. Interestingly, *C. neoformans* biofilms exhibit reduced susceptibility to host antimicrobial peptides, amphotericin B and caspofungin than planktonic cells; the presence of melanin in fungal cells resulted in further reduction of susceptibilities to these drugs [231,232]. *C. neoformans* biofilms were found to be susceptible to amphotericin B and caspofungin at concentrations >2 and 16 μg/mL, respectively, but resistant to fluconazole and voriconazole. It is notable that although amphotericin B and caspofungin reduced biofilm formation by *C. neoformans* cells, the concentrations used were high and were above the levels achievable *in vivo* after systemic administration.

CONCLUSIONS

Antifungal resistance is mediated by a variety of mechanisms, which vary by both species and genera. Therefore, it is critical to identify the organisms under investigation to the species level. With recent advances in technology, such identification is becoming more easily accessible and reliable, and may lead to the better identification of the mechanism of resistance that, in turn, will be an important tool to overcome such resistance. Recent studies have identified some novel mechanisms of resistance and provided deeper insight into already identified mechanisms. The clinical relevance of these mechanisms and the spectrum of their occurrence need to be investigated in further detail.

REFERENCES

1. Mukherjee PK, Sheehan DJ, Hitchcock CA, Ghannoum MA. Combination treatment of invasive fungal infections. *Clinical Microbiology Reviews* 2005;18(1):163–194.
2. Pfaller MA. Antifungal susceptibility testing methods. *Current Drug Targets* 2005;6(8):929–943.

3. Martinez LR, Casadevall A. Susceptibility of *Cryptococcus neoformans* biofilms to antifungal agents *in vitro*. *Antimicrob Agents Chemother* 2006;50(3):1021–1033.

4. Borg-von Zepelin M, Kunz L, Ruchel R, Reichard U, Weig M, Gross U. Epidemiology and antifungal susceptibilities of *Candida* spp. to six antifungal agents: Results from a surveillance study on fungaemia in Germany from July 2004 to August 2005. *J Antimicrob Chemother* 2007;60(2):424–428.

5. Tortorano AM, Prigitano A, Biraghi E, Viviani MA. The European Confederation of Medical Mycology (ECMM) survey of candidaemia in Italy: *In vitro* susceptibility of 375 *Candida albicans* isolates and biofilm production. *J Antimicrob Chemother* 2005;56(4):777–779.

6. Pfaller MA, Messer SA, Boyken L, Hollis RJ, Rice C, Tendolkar S, Diekema DJ. *In vitro* activities of voriconazole, posaconazole, and fluconazole against 4,169 clinical isolates of *Candida* spp. and *Cryptococcus neoformans* collected during 2001 and 2002 in the ARTEMIS global antifungal surveillance program. *Diagn Microbiol Infect Dis* 2004;48(3):201–205.

7. Silva Cde B, Guterres SS, Weisheimer V, Schapoval EE. Antifungal activity of the lemongrass oil and citral against *Candida* spp. *Braz J Infect Dis* 2008;12(1):63–66.

8. Quindos G, Sanchez-Vargas LO, Villar-Vidal M, Eraso E, Alkorta M, Hernandez-Almaraz JL. Activities of fluconazole and voriconazole against bloodstream isolates of *Candida glabrata* and *Candida krusei*: A 14-year study in a Spanish tertiary medical centre. *Int J Antimicrob Agents* 2008;31(3):266–271.

9. Pfaller MA, Diekema DJ, Gibbs DL, Newell VA, Nagy E, Dobiasova S, Rinaldi M, Barton R, Veselov A. *Candida krusei*, a multidrug-resistant opportunistic fungal pathogen: Geographic and temporal trends from the ARTEMIS DISK Antifungal Surveillance Program, 2001 to 2005. *J Clin Microbiol* 2008;46(2):515–521.

10. Singh J, Zaman M, Gupta AK. Evaluation of microdilution and disk diffusion methods for antifungal susceptibility testing of dermatophytes. *Med Mycol* 2007;45(7):595–602.

11. Espinel-Ingroff A, Arthington-Skaggs B, Iqbal N, Ellis D, Pfaller MA, Messer S, Rinaldi M, Fothergill A, Gibbs DL, Wang A. Multicenter evaluation of a new disk agar diffusion method for susceptibility testing of filamentous fungi with voriconazole, posaconazole, itraconazole, amphotericin B, and caspofungin. *J Clin Microbiol* 2007;45(6):1811–1820.

12. Samonis G, Kofteridis DP, Saloustros E, Giannopoulou KP, Ntziora F, Christidou A, Maraki S, Falagas ME. *Candida albicans* versus non-albicans bloodstream infection in patients in a tertiary hospital: An analysis of microbiological data. *Scand J Infect Dis* 2008;40(5):414–419.

13. Soczo G, Kardos G, McNicholas PM, Falusi E, Gergely L, Majoros L. Posaconazole susceptibility testing against *Candida* species: Comparison of broth microdilution and E-test methods. *Mycoses* 2007;50(3):178–182.

14. Pfaller M, Messer S, Boyken L, Rice C, Tendolkar S, Hollis R, Diekema D. *In vitro* survey of triazole cross-resistance among more than 700 clinical isolates of *Aspergillus* species. *J Clin Microbiol* 2008;46(8):2568–2572.

15. Sims CR, Paetznick VL, Rodriguez JR, Chen E, Ostrosky-Zeichner L. Correlation between microdilution, E-test, and disk diffusion methods for antifungal susceptibility testing of posaconazole against *Candida* spp. *J Clin Microbiol* 2006;44(6):2105–2108.

16. Clinical Laboratory Standards Institute. Reference method for broth dilution antifungal susceptibility testing of conidium-forming filamentous fungi: Approved standard M38-A. Wayne, PA: CLSI; 2002.

17. Clinical Laboratory Standards Institute. Reference method for broth dilution antifungal susceptibility testing of yeasts; Approved standard - second edition. CLSI document M27–A3. Wayne, PA: CLSI; 2002.

18. Clinical Laboratory Standards Institute. Methods for antifungal disk diffusion susceptibility testing of yeasts: Approved guideline, CLSI document M44-A. Wayne, PA: National Committee for Clinical Laboratory Standards; 2004.

19. Pfaller MA, Diekema DJ, Gibbs DL, et al. Results from the ARTEMIS DISK Global Antifungal Surveillance Study, 1997 to 2007: 10.5-year analysis of susceptibilities of noncandidal yeast species to fluconazole and voriconazole determined by CLSI standardized disk diffusion testing. *J Clin Microbiol* 2009;47(1):117–123.

20. Pfaller MA, Diekema DJ, Gibbs DL, et al. Geographic variation in the frequency of isolation and fluconazole and voriconazole susceptibilities of *Candida glabrata*: An assessment from the ARTEMIS DISK Global Antifungal Surveillance Program. *Diagn Microbiol Infect Dis* 2010 67(2):162–171.

21. Marchetti O, Moreillon P, Glauser MP, Bille J, Sanglard D. Potent synergism of the combination of fluconazole and cyclosporine in *Candida albicans*. *Antimicrob Agents Chemother* 2000;44(9):2373–2381.

22. Barchiesi F, Spreghini E, Tomassetti S, Giannini D, Scalise G. Caspofungin in combination with amphotericin B against *Candida parapsilosis*. *Antimicrob Agents Chemother* 2007;51(3):941–945.

23. Espinel-Ingroff A. Comparison of three commercial (Etest, YeastOne and Neo-Sensitabs tablet) and disk diffusion (modified M44-A) assays with reference (CLSI M38-A and M27-A2 microdilution) MICs for testing Zygomycetes, *Aspergillus* spp., *Candida* spp., and *Cryptococcus neoformans* with posaconazole and amphotericin B. *J Clin Microbiol* 2006;44(10):3616–3622. doi:10.1128/JCM.01187-06.

24. Pfaller MA, Diekema DJ, Sullivan DJ, et al. Twelve years of fluconazole in clinical practice: Global trends in species distribution and fluconazole susceptibility of bloodstream isolates of *Candida*: Comparison of the epidemiology, drug resistance mechanisms, and virulence of *Candida dubliniensis* and *Candida albicans*. *Clin Microbiol Infect* 2004;10 Suppl 1(4–5):11–23.

25. Lombardi G, Farina C, Andreoni S, Fazii P, Faggi E, Pini G, Manso E, Nanetti A, Mazzoni A. Comparative evaluation of Sensititre YeastOne vs. the NCCLS M27A protocol and E-test for antifungal susceptibility testing of yeasts. *Mycoses* 2004;47(9–10):397–401.

26. Matar MJ, Ostrosky-Zeichner L, Paetznick VL, Rodriguez JR, Chen E, Rex JH. Correlation between E-test, disk diffusion, and microdilution methods for antifungal susceptibility testing of fluconazole and voriconazole. *Antimicrob Agents Chemother* 2003;47(5):1647–1651.

27. Luber P, Bartelt E, Genschow E, Wagner J, Hahn H. Comparison of broth microdilution, E Test, and agar dilution methods for antibiotic susceptibility testing of *Campylobacter jejuni* and *Campylobacter coli*. *J Clin Microbiol* 2003;41(3):1062–1068.

28. Kurtz MB, Heath IB, Marrinan J, Dreikorn S, Onishi J, Douglas C. Morphological effects of lipopeptides against *Aspergillus fumigatus* correlate with activities against (1,3)-á-D-glucan synthase. *Antimicrob Agents Chemother* 1994;38(7):1480–1489.

29. Hof H, Dietz A. Antifungal activity of anidulafungin, a product of *Aspergillus nidulans*, against *Aspergillus nidulans*. *Int J Antimicrob Agents* 2008;33(3):285–286.

30. Espinel-Ingroff A, Fothergill A, Ghannoum M, Manavathu E, Ostrosky-Zeichner L, Pfaller MA, Rinaldi MG, Schell W, Walsh TJ. Quality control and reference guidelines for CLSI broth microdilution susceptibility testing (M38-A document) of anidulafungin against moulds. *J Clin Microbiol* 2007;45(7):2180–2182.

31. Ghannoum MA, D'Angelo M. Anidulafungin: A potent antifungal that targets *Candida* and *Aspergillus*. *Infect Dis Clin Pract* 2005;13(4):165–178.

32. Manavathu EK, Cutright JL, Chandrasekar PH. Organism-dependent fungicidal activities of azoles. *Antimicrob Agents Chemother* 1998;42(11):3018–3021.

33. Hammer KA, Carson CF, Riley TV. Antifungal activity of the components of *Melaleuca alternifolia* (tea tree) oil. *J Appl Microbiol* 2003;95(4):853–860.

34. Espinel-Ingroff A. *In vitro* antifungal activities of anidulafungin and micafungin, licensed agents and the investigational triazole posaconazole as determined by NCCLS methods for 12,052 fungal isolates: Review of the literature. *Rev Iberoam Micol* 2003;20(4):121–136.

35. Ruhnke M. Epidemiology of *Candida albicans* infections and role of non-Candida-albicans yeasts. *Curr Drug Targets* 2006;7(4):495–504.

36. Playford EG, Marriott D, Nguyen Q, Chen S, Ellis D, Slavin M, Sorrell TC. Candidemia in nonneutropenic critically ill patients: Risk factors for non-albicans *Candida* spp. *Crit Care Med* 2008;36(7):2034–2039.

37. Hachem R, Hanna H, Kontoyiannis D, Jiang Y, Raad I. The changing epidemiology of invasive candidiasis: *Candida glabrata* and *Candida krusei* as the leading causes of candidemia in hematologic malignancy. *Cancer* 2008;112(11):2493–2499.

38. Li SY, Yang YL, Chen KW, Cheng HH, Chiou CS, Wang TH, Lauderdale TL, Hung CC, Lo HJ. Molecular epidemiology of long-term colonization of *Candida albicans* strains from HIV-infected patients. *Epidemiol Infect* 2006;134(2):265–269.

39. Yenisehirli G, Bulut N, Yenisehirli A, Bulut Y. *In vitro* susceptibilities of *Candida albicans* isolates to antifungal agents in Tokat, Turkey. *Jundishapur J Microbiol* 2015;8(9):e28057.

40. Pfaller MA, Jones RN, Doern GV, Sader HS, Hollis RJ, Messer SA. International surveillance of bloodstream infections due to *Candida* species: Frequency of occurrence and antifungal susceptibilities of isolates collected in 1997 in the United States, Canada, and South America for the SENTRY Program. The SENTRY Participant Group. *J Clin Microbiol* 1998;36(7):1886–1889.

41. Pfaller MA, Messer SA, Houston A, et al. National epidemiology of mycoses survey: A multicenter study of strain variation and antifungal susceptibility among isolates of *Candida* species. *Diagn Microbiol Infect Dis* 1998;31(1):289–296.

42. Pfaller MA, Jones RN, Doern GV, Fluit AC, Verhoef J, Sader HS, Messer SA, Houston A, Coffman S, Hollis RJ. International surveillance of blood stream infections due to *Candida* species in the European SENTRY Program: Species distribution and antifungal susceptibility including the investigational triazole and echinocandin agents. SENTRY Participant Group (Europe). *Diagn Microbiol Infect Dis* 1999;35(1):19–25.

43. Odds FC, Hanson MF, Davidson AD, Jacobsen MD, Wright P, Whyte JA, Gow NA, Jones BL. One year prospective survey of *Candida* bloodstream infections in Scotland. *J Med Microbiol* 2007;56(Pt 8):1066–1075.

44. Metwally L, Walker MJ, Coyle PV, Hay RJ, Hedderwick S, McCloskey BV, O'Neill HJ, Webb CH, McMullan R. Trends in candidemia and antifungal susceptibility in a university hospital in Northern Ireland 2001–2006. *J Infect* 2007;55(2):174–178.

45. Li L, Redding S, Dongari-Bagtzoglou A. *Candida glabrata*, an emerging oral opportunistic pathogen. *J Dent Res* 2007;86(3):204–215.

46. Lagrou K, Verhaegen J, Peetermans WE, De Rijdt T, Maertens J, Van Wijngaerden E. Fungemia at a tertiary care hospital: Incidence, therapy, and distribution and antifungal susceptibility of causative species. *Eur J Clin Microbiol Infect Dis* 2007;26(8):541–547.

47. Chong PP, Abdul Hadi SR, Lee YL, Phan CL, Tan BC, Ng KP, Seow HF. Genotyping and drug resistance profile of *Candida* spp. in recurrent and one-off vaginitis, and high association of non-albicans species with non-pregnant status. *Infect Genet Evol* 2007;7(4):449–456.

48. Richter SS, Galask RP, Messer SA, Hollis RJ, Diekema DJ, Pfaller MA. Antifungal susceptibilities of *Candida* species causing vulvovaginitis and epidemiology of recurrent cases. *J Clin Microbiol* 2005;43(5):2155–2162.

49. Wang JS, Li SY, Yang YL, Chou HH, Lo HJ. Association between fluconazole susceptibility and genetic relatedness among *Candida tropicalis* isolates in Taiwan. *J Med Microbiol* 2007;56(Pt 5):650–653.

50. Xess I, Jain N, Hasan F, Mandal P, Banerjee U. Epidemiology of candidemia in a tertiary care centre of north India: 5-year study. *Infection* 2007;35(4):256–259.

51. Chou HH, Lo HJ, Chen KW, Liao MH, Li SY. Multilocus sequence typing of *Candida tropicalis* shows clonal cluster enriched in isolates with resistance or trailing growth of fluconazole. *Diagn Microbiol Infect Dis* 2007;58(4):427–433.

52. Pinjon E, Jackson CJ, Kelly SL, Sanglard D, Moran G, Coleman DC, Sullivan DJ. Reduced azole susceptibility in genotype 3 *Candida dubliniensis* isolates associated with increased CdCDR1 and CdCDR2 expression. *Antimicrob Agents Chemother* 2005;49(4):1312–1318.

53. Borman AM, Petch R, Linton CJ, Palmer MD, Bridge PD, Johnson EM. *Candida nivariensis*, an emerging pathogenic fungus with multidrug resistance to antifungal agents. *J Clin Microbiol* 2008;46(3):933–938.

54. Khan ZU, Al-Sweih NA, Ahmad S, Al-Kazemi N, Khan S, Joseph L, Chandy R. Outbreak of fungemia among neonates caused by *Candida haemulonii* resistant to amphotericin B, itraconazole, and fluconazole. *J Clin Microbiol* 2007;45(6):2025–2027.

55. Pfaller MA, Diekema DJ, Mendez M, Kibbler C, Erzsebet P, Chang SC, Gibbs DL, Newell VA. *Candida guilliermondii*, an opportunistic fungal pathogen with decreased susceptibility to fluconazole: Geographic and temporal trends from the ARTEMIS DISK antifungal surveillance program. *J Clin Microbiol* 2006;44(10):3551–3556.

56. Zhang L, Xiao M, Watts MR, Wang H, Fan X, Kong F, Xu YC. Development of fluconazole resistance in a series of *Candida parapsilosis* isolates from a persistent candidemia patient with prolonged antifungal therapy. *BMC Infect Dis* 2015;15:340.

57. Healey KR, Zhao Y, Perez WB, et al. Prevalent mutator genotype identified in fungal pathogen *Candida glabrata* promotes multi-drug resistance. *Nat Commun* 2016;7:11128.

58. Healey KR, Jimenez Ortigosa C, Shor E, Perlin DS. Genetic drivers of multidrug resistance in *Candida glabrata*. *Front Microbiol* 2016;7:1995.

59. Pfaller MA, Jones RN, Doern GV, Sader HS, Messer SA, Houston A, Coffman S, Hollis RJ. Bloodstream infections due to *Candida* species: SENTRY antimicrobial surveillance program in North America and Latin America, 1997–1998. *Antimicrob Agents Chemother* 2000;44(3):747–751.

60. Tortorano AM, Kibbler C, Peman J, Bernhardt H, Klingspor L, Grillot R. Candidaemia in Europe: Epidemiology and resistance. *Int J Antimicrob Agents* 2006;27(5):359–366.

61. Yesudhason BL, Mohanram K. *Candida tropicalis* as a predominant isolate from clinical specimens and its antifungal susceptibility pattern in a tertiary care hospital in southern India. *J Clin Diagn Res* 2015;9(7):DC14–16.

62. Vale-Silva LA, Sanglard D. Tipping the balance both ways: Drug resistance and virulence in *Candida glabrata*. *FEMS Yeast Res* 2015;15(4):fov025.

63. Vallabhaneni S, Kallen A, Tsay S, et al. Investigation of the first seven reported cases of *Candida auris*, a globally emerging invasive, multidrug-resistant fungus - United States, May 2013-August 2016. *MMWR Morb Mortal Wkly Rep* 2016;65(44):1234–1237.

64. Prakash A, Sharma C, Singh A, Kumar Singh P, Kumar A, Hagen F, Govender NP, Colombo AL, Meis JF, Chowdhary A. Evidence of genotypic diversity among *Candida auris* isolates by multilocus sequence typing, matrix-assisted laser desorption ionization time-of-flight mass spectrometry and amplified fragment length polymorphism. *Clin Microbiol Infect* 2016;22(3):277 e271–279.

65. Girard V, Mailler S, Chetry M, Vidal C, Durand G, van Belkum A, Colombo AL, Hagen F, Meis JF, Chowdhary A. Identification and typing of the emerging pathogen *Candida auris* by matrix-assisted laser desorption ionisation time of flight mass spectrometry. *Mycoses* 2016;59(8):535–538.

66. Calvo B, Melo AS, Perozo-Mena A, Hernandez M, Francisco EC, Hagen F, Meis JF, Colombo AL. First report of *Candida auris* in America: Clinical and microbiological aspects of 18 episodes of candidemia. *J Infect* 2016;73(4):369–374.

67. Schelenz S, Hagen F, Rhodes JL, et al. First hospital outbreak of the globally emerging *Candida auris* in a European hospital. *Antimicrob Resist Infect Control* 2016;5:35.

68. Chakrabarti A, Sood P, Rudramurthy SM, et al. Incidence, characteristics and outcome of ICU-acquired candidemia in India. *Intensive Care Med* 2015;41(2):285–295.

69. Lockhart SR, Etienne KA, Vallabhaneni S, et al. Simultaneous emergence of multidrug-resistant *Candida auris* on 3 continents confirmed by whole-genome sequencing and epidemiological analyses. *Clin Infect Dis* 2017;64(2):134–140.

70. Clancy CJ, Nguyen MH. Emergence of *Candida auris*: An international call to arms. *Clin Infect Dis* 2017;64(2):141–143.

71. Brandt ME, Pfaller MA, Hajjeh RA, Hamill RJ, Pappas PG, Reingold AL, Rimland D, Warnock DW, Cryptococcal Disease Active Surveillance G. Trends in antifungal drug susceptibility of *Cryptococcus neoformans* isolates in the United States: 1992 to 1994 and 1996 to 1998. *Antimicrobial Agents and Chemotherapy* 2001;45(11):3065–3069.

72. Datta K, Jain N, Sethi S, Rattan A, Casadevall A, Banerjee U. Fluconazole and itraconazole susceptibility of clinical isolates of *Cryptococcus neoformans* at a tertiary care centre in India: A need for care. *J Antimicrob Chemother* 2003;52(4):683–686.

73. Perkins A, Gomez-Lopez A, Mellado E, Rodriguez-Tudela JL, Cuenca-Estrella M. Rates of antifungal resistance among Spanish clinical isolates of *Cryptococcus neoformans* var. neoformans. *J Antimicrob Chemother* 2005;56(6):1144–1147.

74. Trpkovic A, Pekmezovic M, Barac A, Crncevic Radovic L, Arsic Arsenijevic V. *In vitro* antifungal activities of amphotericin B, 5-fluorocytosine, fluconazole and itraconazole against *Cryptococcus neoformans* isolated from cerebrospinal fluid and blood from patients in Serbia. *J Mycol Med* 2012;22(3):243–248.

75. Mondon P, Petter R, Amalfitano G, Luzzati R, Concia E, Polacheck I, Kwon-Chung KJ. Heteroresistance to fluconazole and voriconazole in *Cryptococcus neoformans*. *Antimicrob Agents Chemother* 1999;43(8):1856–1861.

76. Yamazumi T, Pfaller MA, Messer SA, Houston AK, Boyken L, Hollis RJ, Furuta I, Jones RN. Characterization of heteroresistance to fluconazole among clinical isolates of *Cryptococcus neoformans*. *J Clin Microbiol* 2003;41(1):267–272.

77. Hsueh PR, Lau YJ, Chuang YC, et al. Antifungal susceptibilities of clinical isolates of *Candida* species, *Cryptococcus neoformans*, and *Aspergillus* species from Taiwan: Surveillance of multicenter antimicrobial resistance in Taiwan program data from 2003. *Antimicrob Agents Chemother* 2005;49(2):512–517.

78. Bii CC, Makimura K, Abe S, Taguchi H, Mugasia OM, Revathi G, Wamae NC, Kamiya S. Antifungal drug susceptibility of *Cryptococcus neoformans* from clinical sources in Nairobi, Kenya. *Mycoses* 2007;50(1):25–30.

79. Sar B, Monchy D, Vann M, Keo C, Sarthou JL, Buisson Y. Increasing *in vitro* resistance to fluconazole in *Cryptococcus neoformans* Cambodian isolates: April 2000 to March 2002. *J Antimicrob Chemother* 2004;54(2):563–565.

80. Panagopoulou P, Filioti J, Farmaki E, Maloukou A, Roilides E. Filamentous fungi in a tertiary care hospital: Environmental surveillance and susceptibility to antifungal drugs. *Infect Control Hosp Epidemiol* 2007;28(1):60–67.

81. Rodriguez-Tudela JL, Alcazar-Fuoli L, Mellado E, Alastruey-Izquierdo A, Monzon A, Cuenca-Estrella M. Epidemiological cut-offs and cross-resistance to azole drugs in *Aspergillus fumigatus*. *Antimicrob Agents Chemother* 2008;52(7):2468–2472.

82. van der Linden JW, Arendrup MC, Warris A, et al. Prospective multicenter international surveillance of azole resistance in *Aspergillus fumigatus*. *Emerg Infect Dis* 2015;21(6):1041–1044.

83. Vermeulen E, Maertens J, De Bel A, Nulens E, Boelens J, Surmont I, Mertens A, Boel A, Lagrou K. Nationwide surveillance of azole resistance in *Aspergillus* diseases. *Antimicrob Agents Chemother* 2015;59(8):4569–4576.

84. Kontoyiannis DP, Lionakis MS, Lewis RE, et al. Zygomycosis in a tertiary-care cancer center in the era of Aspergillus-active antifungal therapy: A case-control observational study of 27 recent cases. *J Infect Dis* 2005;191(8):1350–1359.

85. Tortorano AM, Prigitano A, Dho G, Esposto MC, Gianni C, Grancini A, Ossi C, Viviani MA. Species distribution and *in vitro* antifungal susceptibility patterns of 75 clinical isolates of *Fusarium* spp. from northern Italy. *Antimicrob Agents Chemother* 2008;52(7):2683–2685.

86. Diekema DJ, Petroelje B, Messer SA, Hollis RJ, Pfaller MA. Activities of available and investigational antifungal agents against rhodotorula species. *J Clin Microbiol* 2005;43(1):476–478.

87. Netsvyetayeva I, Swoboda-Kopec E, Sikora M, Jaworska-Zaremba M, Blachnio S, Luczak M. *Trichosporon asahii* as a prospective pathogen in solid organ transplant recipients. *Mycoses* 2008;52:263–265.

88. Blignaut E, Molepo J, Pujol C, Soll DR, Pfaller MA. Clade-related amphotericin B resistance among South African *Candida albicans* isolates. *Diagn Microbiol Infect Dis* 2005;53(1):29–31.

89. Pfaller MA, Messer SA, Boyken L, Huynh H, Hollis RJ, Diekema DJ. *In vitro* activities of 5-fluorocytosine against 8,803 clinical isolates of *Candida* spp.: Global assessment of primary resistance using National Committee for Clinical Laboratory Standards susceptibility testing methods. *Antimicrob Agents Chemother* 2002;46(11):3518–3521.

90. Yang YL, Wang AH, Wang CW, Cheng WT, Li SY, Lo HJ. Susceptibilities to amphotericin B and fluconazole of *Candida* species in Taiwan Surveillance of Antimicrobial Resistance of Yeasts 2006. *Diagn Microbiol Infect Dis* 2008;61(2):175–180.

91. Colombo AL, Nakagawa Z, Valdetaro F, Branchini ML, Kussano EJ, Nucci M. Susceptibility profile of 200 bloodstream isolates of Candida spp. collected from Brazilian tertiary care hospitals. Med Mycol 2003;41(3):235–239.

92. Colombo AL, Azevedo Melo AS, Crespo Rosas RF, Salomao R, Briones M, Hollis RJ, Messer SA, Pfaller MA. Outbreak of Candida rugosa candidemia: An emerging pathogen that may be refractory to amphotericin B therapy. Diagn Microbiol Infect Dis 2003;46(4):253–257.

93. Malani AN, Kauffman CA. Changing epidemiology of rare mould infections: Implications for therapy. Drugs 2007;67(13):1803–1812.

94. Masia Canuto M, Gutierrez Rodero F. Antifungal drug resistance to azoles and polyenes. Lancet Infect Dis 2002;2(9):550–563.

95. Lass-Florl C, Griff K, Mayr A, Petzer A, Gastl G, Bonatti H, Freund M, Kropshofer G, Dierich MP, Nachbaur D. Epidemiology and outcome of infections due to Aspergillus terreus: 10-year single centre experience. Br J Haematol 2005;131(2):201–207.

96. Ellis D. Amphotericin B: Spectrum and resistance. J Antimicrob Chemother 2002;49 Suppl A:7–10.

97. Colombo AL, Thompson L, Graybill JR. The north and south of candidemia: Issues for Latin America. Drugs Today (Barc) 2008;44 Suppl A:1–34.

98. Pfaller MA, Boyken L, Hollis RJ, Messer SA, Tendolkar S, Diekema DJ. In vitro susceptibilities of Candida spp. to Caspofungin: Four years of global surveillance. J Clin Microbiol 2006;44(3):760–763.

99. Pfaller MA, Boyken L, Hollis RJ, Messer SA, Tendolkar S, Diekema DJ. Global surveillance of in vitro activity of micafungin against Candida: A comparison with caspofungin by CLSI-recommended methods. J Clin Microbiol 2006;44(10):3533–3538.

100. Pfaller MA, Boyken L, Hollis RJ, Kroeger J, Messer SA, Tendolkar S, Diekema DJ. In vitro susceptibility of invasive isolates of Candida spp. to anidulafungin, caspofungin, and micafungin: Six years of global surveillance. J Clin Microbiol 2008;46(1):150–156.

101. Laverdiere M, Lalonde RG, Baril JG, Sheppard DC, Park S, Perlin DS. Progressive loss of echinocandin activity following prolonged use for treatment of Candida albicans oesophagitis. J Antimicrob Chemother 2006;57(4):705–708.

102. Forrest GN, Weekes E, Johnson JK. Increasing incidence of Candida parapsilosis candidemia with caspofungin usage. J Infect 2008;56(2):126–129.

103. Pasquale T, Tomada JR, Ghannoum M, Dipersio J, Bonilla H. Emergence of Candida tropicalis resistant to caspofungin. J Antimicrob Chemother 2008;61(1):219.

104. Villareal NC, Fothergill AW, Kelly C, et al. Candida glabrata resistance to caspofungin during therapy. In: 44th Interscience Conference on Antimicrob Agents Chemother. Washington, DC: American Society for Microbiology; 2004.

105. Hakki M, Staab JF, Marr KA. Emergence of a Candida krusei isolate with reduced susceptibility to caspofungin during therapy. Antimicrob Agents Chemother 2006;50(7):2522–2524.

106. Kahn JN, Garcia-Effron G, Hsu M-J, Park S, Marr KA, Perlin DS. Acquired echinocandin resistance in a Candida krusei isolate due to modification of glucan synthase. Antimicrob Agents Chemother 2007;51(5):1876–1878.

107. Moudgal V, Little T, Boikov D, Vazquez JA. Multiechinocandin- and multiazole-resistant Candida parapsilosis isolates serially obtained during therapy for prosthetic valve endocarditis. Antimicrob Agents Chemother 2005;49(2):767–769.

108. Ghannoum MA, Chen A, Buhari M, Chandra J, Mukherjee PK, Baxa D, Golembieski A, Vazquez JA. Differential in vitro activity of anidulafungin, caspofungin and micafungin against Candida parapsilosis isolates recovered from a burn unit. Clin Microbiol Infect 2009;15(3):274–279.

109. Forastiero A, Garcia-Gil V, Rivero-Menendez O, Garcia-Rubio R, Monteiro MC, Alastruey-Izquierdo A, Jordan R, Agorio I, Mellado E. Rapid development of Candida krusei echinocandin resistance during caspofungin therapy. Antimicrob Agents Chemother 2015;59(11):6975–6982.

110. Wierman M, et al. Emergence of Candida glabrata isolates with reduced susceptibility to caspofungin and micafungin, but not anidulafungin. In: 47th Interscience Conference on Antimicriobial Agens and Chemotherapy. Chicago, IL: American Society for Microbiology; 2007.

111. Cota J, Carden M, Graybill JR, Najvar LK, Burgess DS, Wiederhold NP. In vitro pharmacodynamics of anidulafungin and caspofungin against Candida glabrata isolates, including strains with decreased caspofungin susceptibility. Antimicrob Agents Chemother 2006;50(11):3926–3928.

112. Vallabhaneni S, Cleveland AA, Farley MM, Harrison LH, Schaffner W, Beldavs ZG, Derado G, Pham CD, Lockhart SR, Smith RM. Epidemiology and risk factors for echinocandin nonsusceptible Candida glabrata bloodstream infections: Data from a large multisite population-based candidemia surveillance program, 2008–2014. Open Forum Infect Dis 2015;2(4):ofv163.

113. Mowat E, Williams C, Jones B, McChlery S, Ramage G. The characteristics of Aspergillus fumigatus mycetoma development: Is this a biofilm? Med Mycol 2009;47(Suppl 1):s120–s126.

114. Suzuki K, Nakase K, Ino K, Sugawara Y, Sekine T, Katayama N. Breakthrough cryptococcosis in a patient with systemic lupus erythematosus (SLE) receiving micafungin. *J Infect Chemother* 2008;14(4):311–314.

115. Mukherjee PK, Leidich SD, Isham N, Leitner I, Ryder NS, Ghannoum MA. Clinical *Trichophyton rubrum* strain exhibiting primary resistance to terbinafine. *Antimicrob Agents Chemother* 2003;47(1):82–86.

116. da Silva Barros ME, de Assis Santos D, Soares Hamdan J. Antifungal susceptibility testing of Trichophyton rubrum by E-test. *Arch Dermatol Res* 2007;299(2):107–109.

117. Pinjon E, Moran GP, Coleman DC, Sullivan DJ. Azole susceptibility and resistance in *Candida dubliniensis*. *Biochem Soc Trans* 2005;33(Pt 5):1210–1214.

118. Mago N, Khuller GK. Influence of lipid composition on the sensitivity of *Candida albicans* to antifungal agents. *Indian J Biochem Biophys* 1989;26(1):30–33.

119. Howell SA, Mallet AI, Noble WC. A comparison of the sterol content of multiple isolates of the *Candida albicans* Darlington strain with other clinically azole-sensitive and - resistant strains. *J Appl Bacteriol* 1990;69(5):692–696.

120. Mishra P, Bolard J, Prasad R. Emerging role of lipids of *Candida albicans*, a pathogenic dimorphic yeast. *Biochimica et Biophysica Acta* 1992;1127(1):1–14.

121. Marichal P, Gorrens J, Laurijssens L, et al. Accumulation of 3-ketosteroids induced by itraconazole in azole-resistant clinical *Candida albicans* isolates. *Antimicrob Agents Chemother* 1999;43(11):2663–2670.

122. Loffler J, Einsele H, Hebart H, Schumacher U, Hrastnik C, Daum G. Phospholipid and sterol analysis of plasma membranes of azole-resistant *Candida albicans* strains. *FEMS Microbiol Lett* 2000;185(1):59–63.

123. Hitchcock CA, Barrett-Bee KJ, Russell NJ. The lipid composition and permeability to azole of an azole- and polyene-resistant mutant of *Candida albicans*. *J Med Vet Mycol* 1987;25(1):29–37.

124. Ghannoum MA, Rice LB. Antifungal agents: Mode of action, mechanisms of resistance, and correlation of these mechanisms with bacterial resistance. *Clin Microbiol Rev* 1999;12(4):501–517.

125. Kelly SL, Lamb DC, Kelly DE, Manning NJ, Loeffler J, Hebart H, Schumacher U, Einsele H. Resistance to fluconazole and cross-resistance to amphotericin B in *Candida albicans* from AIDS patients caused by defective sterol delta5,6- desaturation. *FEBS Lett* 1997;400(1):80–82.

126. Kohli A, Smriti NFN, Mukhopadhyay K, Rattan A, Prasad R. *In vitro* low-level resistance to azoles in *Candida albicans* is associated with changes in membrane lipid fluidity and asymmetry *Antimicrob Agents Chemother* 2002;46(4):1046–1052.

127. Hitchcock CA, Barrett-Bee KJ, Russell NJ. Inhibition of 14 alpha-sterol demethylase activity in *Candida albicans* Darlington does not correlate with resistance to azole. *J Med Vet Mycol* 1987;25(5):329–333.

128. Lamb DC, Kelly DE, Manning NJ, Kelly SL. Reduced intracellular accumulation of azole antifungal results in resistance in *Candida albicans* isolate NCPF 3363. *FEMS Microbiol Lett* 1997;147(2):189–193.

129. Joseph-Horne T, Hollomon D, Loeffler RS, Kelly SL. Altered P450 activity associated with direct selection for fungal azole resistance. *FEBS Lett* 1995;374(2):174–178.

130. Joseph-Horne T, Hollomon D, Loeffler RS, Kelly SL. Cross-resistance to polyene and azole drugs in *Cryptococcus neoformans*. *Antimicrob Agents Chemother* 1995;39(7):1526–1529.

131. Marichal P, Vanden Bossche H. Mechanisms of resistance to azole antifungals. *Acta Biochim Pol* 1995;42(4):509–516.

132. Aoyama Y, Kudo M, Asai K, Okonogi K, Horiuchi T, Gotoh O, Yoshida Y. Emergence of fluconazole-resistant sterol 14-demethylase P450 (CYP51) in *Candida albicans* is a model demonstrating the diversification mechanism of P450. *Arch Biochem Biophys* 2000;379(1):170–171.

133. Vanden Bossche H, Marichal P, Odds FC, Le Jeune L, Coene MC. Characterization of an azole-resistant *Candida glabrata* isolate. *Antimicrob Agents Chemother* 1992;36(12):2602–2610.

134. Orozco AS, Higginbotham LM, Hitchcock CA, Parkinson T, Falconer D, Ibrahim AS, Ghannoum MA, Filler SG. Mechanism of fluconazole resistance in *Candida krusei*. *Antimicrob Agents Chemother* 1998;42(10):2645–2649.

135. Vanden Bossche H, Dromer F, Improvisi I, Lozano-Chiu M, Rex JH, Sanglard D. Antifungal drug resistance in pathogenic fungi. *Med Mycol* 1998;36 Suppl 1(2):119–128.

136. Manavathu EK, Vazquez JA, Chandrasekar PH. Reduced susceptibility in laboratory-selected mutants of *Aspergillus fumigatus* to itraconazole due to decreased intracellular accumulation of the antifungal agent. *Int J Antimicrob Agents* 1999;12(3):213–219.

137. Denning DW, Venkateswarlu K, Oakley KL, Anderson MJ, Manning NJ, Stevens DA, Warnock DW, Kelly SL. Itraconazole resistance in *Aspergillus fumigatus*. *Antimicrob Agents Chemother* 1997;41(6):1364–1368.

138. Willger SD, Puttikamonkul S, Kim KH, Burritt JB, Grahl N, Metzler LJ, Barbuch R, Bard M, Lawrence CB, Cramer RA, Jr. A sterol-regulatory element binding protein is required for cell polarity, hypoxia adaptation, azole drug resistance, and virulence in *Aspergillus fumigatus*. *PLoS Pathog* 2008;4(11):e1000200.

139. Marichal P, Koymans L, Willemsens S, Bellens D, Verhasselt P, Luyten W, Borgers M, Ramaekers FC, Odds FC, Bossche HV. Contribution of mutations in the cytochrome P450 14alpha-demethylase (Erg11p, Cyp51p) to azole resistance in *Candida albicans*. *Microbiology* 1999;145 (Pt 10):2701–2713.

140. Xu Y, Chen L, Li C. Susceptibility of clinical isolates of *Candida* species to fluconazole and detection of *Candida albicans* ERG11 mutations. *J Antimicrob Chemother* 2008;61(4):798–804.

141. Garcia-Effron G, Dilger A, Alcazar-Fuoli L, Park S, Mellado E, Perlin DS. Rapid detection of triazole antifungal resistance in *Aspergillus fumigatus*. *J Clin Microbiol* 2008;46(4):1200–1206.

142. Mellado E, Garcia-Effron G, Alcazar-Fuoli L, Melchers WJ, Verweij PE, Cuenca-Estrella M, Rodriguez-Tudela JL. A new *Aspergillus fumigatus* resistance mechanism conferring *in vitro* cross-resistance to azole antifungals involves a combination of cyp51A alterations. *Antimicrob Agents Chemother* 2007;51(6):1897–1904.

143. da Silva Ferreira ME, Capellaro JL, dos Reis Marques E, et al. *In vitro* evolution of itraconazole resistance in *Aspergillus fumigatus* involves multiple mechanisms of resistance. *Antimicrob Agents Chemother* 2004;48(11):4405–4413.

144. Alastruey-Izquierdo A, Cuenca-Estrella M, Monzon A, Mellado E, Rodriguez-Tudela JL. Antifungal susceptibility profile of clinical *Fusarium* spp. isolates identified by molecular methods. *J Antimicrob Chemother* 2008;61(4):805–809. doi:10.1093/jac/dkn022.

145. Krishnan-Natesan S, Chandrasekar PH, Alangaden GJ, Manavathu EK. Molecular characterisation of cyp51A and cyp51B genes coding for P450 14alpha-lanosterol demethylases A (CYP51Ap) and B (CYP51Bp) from voriconazole-resistant laboratory isolates of *Aspergillus flavus*. *Int J Antimicrob Agents* 2008;32(6):519–524.

146. Osherov N, Kontoyiannis DP, Romans A, May GS. Resistance to itraconazole in *Aspergillus nidulans* and *Aspergillus fumigatus* is conferred by extra copies of the *A. nidulans* P-450 14alpha-demethylase gene, pdmA. *J Antimicrob Chemother* 2001;48(1):75–81.

147. de Fontbrune FS, Denis B, Meunier M, Garcia-Hermoso D, Bretagne S, Alanio A. Iterative break-through invasive aspergillosis due to TR(34)/L98H azole-resistant *Aspergillus fumigatus* and *Emericella sublata* in a single hematopoietic stem cell transplant patient. *Transpl Infect Dis* 2014;16(4):687–691.

148. Alanio A, Denis B, Hamane S, Raffoux E, Peffault de Latour R, Menotti J, Amorim S, Touratier S, Bergeron A, Bretagne S. Azole resistance of *Aspergillus fumigatus* in immunocompromised patients with invasive aspergillosis. *Emerg Infect Dis* 2016;22(1):157–158.

149. Wu CJ, Wang HC, Lee JC, Lo HJ, Dai CT, Chou PH, Ko WC, Chen YC. Azole-resistant *Aspergillus fumigatus* isolates carrying TR(3)(4)/L98H mutations in Taiwan. *Mycoses* 2015;58(9):544–549.

150. Wiederhold NP, Gil VG, Gutierrez F, Lindner JR, Albataineh MT, McCarthy DI, Sanders C, Fan H, Fothergill AW, Sutton DA. First detection of TR34 L98H and TR46 Y121F T289A Cyp51 mutations in *Aspergillus fumigatus* isolates in the United States. *J Clin Microbiol* 2016;54(1):168–171.

151. Snelders E, Camps SM, Karawajczyk A, Rijs AJ, Zoll J, Verweij PE, Melchers WJ. Genotype-phenotype complexity of the TR46/Y121F/T289A cyp51A azole resistance mechanism in *Aspergillus fumigatus*. *Fungal Genet Biol* 2015;82:129–135.

152. Hagiwara D, Watanabe A, Kamei K. Sensitisation of an Azole-Resistant *Aspergillus fumigatus* Strain containing the Cyp51A-Related Mutation by Deleting the SrbA Gene. *Sci Rep* 2016;6:38833.

153. Coste A, Turner V, Ischer F, Morschhauser J, Forche A, Selmecki A, Berman J, Bille J, Sanglard D. A mutation in Tac1p, a transcription factor regulating CDR1 and CDR2, is coupled with loss of heterozygosity at chromosome 5 to mediate antifungal resistance in *Candida albicans*. *Genetics* 2006;172(4):2139–2156.

154. Coste A, Selmecki A, Forche A, Diogo D, Bougnoux ME, d'Enfert C, Berman J, Sanglard D. Genotypic evolution of azole resistance mechanisms in sequential *Candida albicans* isolates. *Eukaryot Cell* 2007;6(10):1889–1904.

155. Coste AT, Crittin J, Bauser C, Rohde B, Sanglard D. Functional analysis of cis- and trans-acting elements of the *Candida albicans* CDR2 promoter with a novel promoter reporter system. *Eukaryot Cell* 2009;8(8):1250–1267.

156. Morschhauser J, Barker KS, Liu TT, Bla BWJ, Homayouni R, Rogers PD. The transcription factor Mrr1p controls expression of the MDR1 efflux pump and mediates multidrug resistance in *Candida albicans*. *PLoS Pathog* 2007;3(11):e164.

157. Liu TT, Znaidi S, Barker KS, Xu L, Homayouni R, Saidane S, Morschhauser J, Nantel A, Raymond M, Rogers PD. Genome-wide expression and location analyses of the *Candida albicans* Tac1p regulon. *Eukaryot Cell* 2007;6(11):2122–2138.

158. Dunkel N, Liu TT, Barker KS, Homayouni R, Morschhauser J, Rogers PD. A gain-of-function mutation in the transcription factor Upc2p causes upregulation of ergosterol biosynthesis genes and increased fluconazole resistance in a clinical *Candida albicans* isolate. *Eukaryot Cell* 2008;7(7):1180–1190.

159. Dunkel N, Blass J, Rogers PD, Morschhauser J. Mutations in the multi-drug resistance regulator MRR1, followed by loss of heterozygosity, are the

main cause of MDR1 overexpression in fluconazole-resistant *Candida albicans* strains. *Mol Microbiol* 2008;69(4):827–840.

160. Heilmann CJ, Schneider S, Barker KS, Rogers PD, Morschhauser J. An A643T mutation in the transcription factor Upc2p causes constitutive ERG11 upregulation and increased fluconazole resistance in *Candida albicans*. *Antimicrob Agents Chemother* 2010;54(1):353–359.

161. Wang Y, Liu JY, Shi C, Li WJ, Zhao Y, Yan L, Xiang MJ. Mutations in transcription factor Mrr2p contribute to fluconazole resistance in clinical isolates of *Candida albicans*. *Int J Antimicrob Agents* 2015;46(5):552–559.

162. Yang H, Tong J, Lee CW, Ha S, Eom SH, Im YJ. Structural mechanism of ergosterol regulation by fungal sterol transcription factor Upc2. *Nat Commun* 2015;6:6129.

163. Vasicek EM, Berkow EL, Flowers SA, Barker KS, Rogers PD. UPC2 is universally essential for azole antifungal resistance in *Candida albicans*. *Eukaryot Cell* 2014;13(7):933–946.

164. Hagiwara D, Miura D, Shimizu K, et al. A Novel Zn2-Cys6 Transcription Factor AtrR Plays a Key Role in an Azole Resistance Mechanism of *Aspergillus fumigatus* by Co-regulating *cyp51A* and *cdr1B* Expressions. *PLoS Pathog* 2017;13(1):e1006096.

165. Morschhauser J. The development of fluconazole resistance in *Candida albicans*–an example of microevolution of a fungal pathogen. *J Microbiol* 2016;54(3):192–201.

166. Prasad R, De Wergifosse P, Goffeau A, Balzi E. Molecular cloning and characterization of a novel gene of *Candida albicans*, CDR1, conferring multiple resistance to drugs and antifungals. *Curr Genet* 1995;27(4):320–329.

167. Parkinson T, Falconer DJ, Hitchcock CA. Fluconazole resistance due to energy-dependent drug efflux in *Candida glabrata*. *Antimicrob Agents Chemother* 1995;39(8):1696–1699.

168. Sanglard D, Kuchler K, Ischer F, Pagani JL, Monod M, Bille J. Mechanisms of resistance to azole antifungal agents in *Candida albicans* isolates from AIDS patients involve specific multidrug transporters. *Antimicrob Agents Chemother* 1995;39(11):2378–2386.

169. Clark FS, Parkinson T, Hitchcock CA, Gow NA. Correlation between rhodamine 123 accumulation and azole sensitivity in *Candida* species: Possible role for drug efflux in drug resistance. *Antimicrob Agents Chemother* 1996;40(2):419–425.

170. Kohli A, Gupta V, Krishnamurthy S, Hasnain SE, Prasad R. Specificity of drug transport mediated by CaMDR1: A major facilitator of *Candida albicans*. *J Biosci* 2001;26(3):333–339.

171. Albertson GD, Niimi M, Cannon RD, Jenkinson HF. Multiple efflux mechanisms are involved in *Candida albicans* fluconazole resistance. *Antimicrob Agents Chemother* 1996;40(12):2835–2841.

172. White TC. Increased mRNA levels of *ERG16*, *CDR*, and *MDR1* correlate with increases in azole resistance in *Candida albicans* isolates from a patient infected with human immunodeficiency virus. *Antimicrob Agents Chemother* 1997;41(7):1482–1487.

173. Franz R, Kelly SL, Lamb DC, Kelly DE, Ruhnke M, Morschhauser J. Multiple molecular mechanisms contribute to a stepwise development of fluconazole resistance in clinical *Candida albicans* strains. *Antimicrob Agents Chemother* 1998;42(12):3065–3072.

174. Lopez-Ribot JL, McAtee RK, Lee LN, Kirkpatrick WR, White TC, Sanglard D, Patterson TF. Distinct patterns of gene expression associated with development of fluconazole resistance in serial *Candida albicans* isolates from human immunodeficiency virus-infected patients with oropharyngeal candidiasis. *Antimicrob Agents Chemother* 1998;42(11):2932–2937.

175. Hernaez ML, Gil C, Pla J, Nombela C. Induced expression of the *Candida albicans* multidrug resistance gene CDR1 in response to fluconazole and other antifungals. *Yeast* 1998;14(6):517–526.

176. Sanglard D, Ischer F, Calabrese D, Majcherczyk PA, Bille J. The ATP binding cassette transporter gene *CgCDR1* from *Candida glabrata* is involved in the resistance of clinical isolates to azole antifungal agents. *Antimicrob Agents Chemother* 1999;43(11):2753–2765.

177. Torelli R, Posteraro B, Ferrari S, La Sorda M, Fadda G, Sanglard D, Sanguinetti M. The ATP-binding cassette transporter-encoding gene CgSNQ2 is contributing to the *CgPDR1*-dependent azole resistance of *Candida glabrata*. *Mol Microbiol* 2008;68(1):186–201.

178. Thakur JK, Arthanari H, Yang F, et al. A nuclear receptor-like pathway regulating multidrug resistance in fungi. *Nature* 2008;452(7187):604–609.

179. Katiyar SK, Edlind TD. Identification and expression of multidrug resistance-related ABC transporter genes in *Candida krusei*. *Med Mycol* 2001;39(1):109–116.

180. Slaven JW, Anderson MJ, Sanglard D, Dixon GK, Bille J, Roberts IS, Denning DW. Increased expression of a novel *Aspergillus fumigatus* ABC transporter gene, *atrF*, in the presence of itraconazole in an itraconazole resistant clinical isolate. *Fungal Genet Biol* 2002;36(3):199–206.

181. Nascimento AM, Goldman GH, Park S, Marras SA, Delmas G, Oza U, Lolans K, Dudley MN, Mann PA, Perlin DS. Multiple resistance mechanisms among Aspergillus fumigatus mutants with high-level resistance to itraconazole. *Antimicrob Agents Chemother* 2003;47(5):1719–1726.

182. Posteraro B, Sanguinetti M, Sanglard D, La Sorda M, Boccia S, Romano L, Morace G, Fadda G. Identification and characterization of a Cryptococcus neoformans ATP binding cassette (ABC) transporter-encoding gene, CnAFR1, involved in the resistance to fluconazole. Mol Microbiol 2003;47(2):357–371.

183. Yang ML, Uhrig J, Vu K, Singapuri A, Dennis M, Gelli A, Thompson GR, 3rd. Fluconazole susceptibility in Cryptococcus gattii is dependent on the ABC transporter Pdr11. Antimicrob Agents Chemother 2015;60(3):1202–1207.

184. Zhang SQ, Miao Q, Li LP, Zhang LL, Yan L, Jia Y, Cao YB, Jiang YY. Mutation of G234 amino acid residue in Candida albicans drug-resistance-related protein Rta2p is associated with fluconazole resistance and dihydrosphingosine transport. Virulence 2015;6(6):599–607.

185. Walsh TJ, Petraitis V, Petraitiene R, et al. Experimental pulmonary aspergillosis due to Aspergillus terreus: Pathogenesis and treatment of an emerging fungal pathogen resistant to amphotericin B. J Infect Dis 2003;188(2):305–319.

186. Dick JD, Merz WG, Saral R. Incidence of polyene-resistant yeasts recovered from clinical specimens. Antimicrob Agents Chemother 1980;18(1):158–163.

187. Karyotakis NC, Anaissie EJ, Hachem R, Dignani MC, Samonis G. Comparison of the efficacy of polyenes and triazoles against hematogenous Candida krusei infection in neutropenic mice. J Infect Dis 1993;168(5):1311–1313.

188. Perfect JR, Cox GM. Drug resistance in Cryptococcus neoformans. Drug Resist Updat 1999;2(4):259–269.

189. Vandeputte P, Tronchin G, Berges T, Hennequin C, Chabasse D, Bouchara JP. Reduced susceptibility to polyenes associated with a missense mutation in the ERG6 gene in a clinical isolate of Candida glabrata with pseudohyphal growth. Antimicrob Agents Chemother 2007;51(3):982–990.

190. Ikeda R, Sugita T, Jacobson ES, Shinoda T. Effects of melanin upon susceptibility of Cryptococcus to antifungals. Microbiol Immunol 2003;47(4):271–277.

191. Zaragoza O, Chrisman CJ, Castelli MV, Frases S, Cuenca-Estrella M, Rodriguez-Tudela JL, Casadevall A. Capsule enlargement in Cryptococcus neoformans confers resistance to oxidative stress suggesting a mechanism for intracellular survival. Cell Microbiol 2008;10(10):2043–2057.

192. Huang Z, Chen K, Zhang J, et al. A functional variomics tool for discovering drug-resistance genes and drug targets. Cell Reports 2013;3(2):577–585.

193. Bari VK, Sharma S, Alfatah M, Mondal AK, Ganesan K. Plasma Membrane Proteolipid 3 Protein Modulates Amphotericin B Resistance through Sphingolipid Biosynthetic Pathway. Sci Rep 2015;5:9685.

194. Block ER, Jennings AE, Bennett JE. 5-fluorocytosine resistance in Cryptococcus neoformans. Antimicrob Agents Chemother 1973;3(6):649–656.

195. Polak A, Scholer HJ. Mode of action of 5-fluorocytosine and mechanisms of resistance. Chemotherapy 1975;21(3–4):113–130.

196. Vermes A, Guchelaar HJ, Dankert J. Flucytosine: A review of its pharmacology, clinical indications, pharmacokinetics, toxicity and drug interactions. J Antimicrob Chemother 2000;46(2):171–179.

197. Hope WW, Tabernero L, Denning DW, Anderson MJ. Molecular mechanisms of primary resistance to flucytosine in Candida albicans. Antimicrob Agents Chemother 2004;48(11):4377–4386.

198. Balkis MM, Leidich SD, Mukherjee PK, Ghannoum MA. Mechanisms of fungal resistance: An overview. Drugs 2002;62(7):1025–1040.

199. Whelan WL. The genetic basis of resistance to 5-fluorocytosine in Candida species and Cryptococcus neoformans. Crit Rev Microbiol 1987;15(1):45–56.

200. Whelan WL, Kerridge D. Decreased activity of UMP pyrophosphorylase associated with resistance to 5-fluorocytosine in Candida albicans. Antimicrob Agents Chemother 1984;26(4):570–574.

201. Dodgson AR, Dodgson KJ, Pujol C, Pfaller MA, Soll DR. Clade-specific flucytosine resistance is due to a single nucleotide change in the FUR1 gene of Candida albicans. Antimicrob Agents Chemother 2004;48(6):2223–2227.

202. Vlanti A, Diallinas G. The Aspergillus nidulans FcyB cytosine-purine scavenger is highly expressed during germination and in reproductive compartments and is downregulated by endocytosis. Mol Microbiol 2008;68(4):959–977.

203. Papon N, Noel T, Florent M, Gibot-Leclerc S, Jean D, Chastin C, Villard J, Chapeland-Leclerc F. Molecular mechanism of flucytosine resistance in Candida lusitaniae: Contribution of the FCY2, FCY1, and FUR1 genes to 5-fluorouracil and fluconazole cross-resistance. Antimicrob Agents Chemother 2007;51(1):369–371.

204. Noel T, Francois F, Paumard P, Chastin C, Brethes D, Villard J. Flucytosine-fluconazole cross-resistance in purine-cytosine permease-deficient Candida lusitaniae clinical isolates: Indirect evidence of a fluconazole uptake transporter. Antimicrob Agents Chemother 2003;47(4):1275–1284.

205. Costa C, Ponte A, Pais P, Santos R, Cavalheiro M, Yaguchi T, Chibana H, Teixeira MC. New mechanisms of flucytosine resistance in *C. glabrata* unveiled by a chemogenomics analysis in S. cerevisiae. *PLoS One* 2015;10(8):e0135110.

206. Favre B, Ryder NS. Cloning and expression of squalene epoxidase from the pathogenic yeast *Candida albicans. Gene* 1997;189(1):119–126.

207. Liu W, May GS, Lionakis MS, Lewis RE, Kontoyiannis DP. Extra copies of the *Aspergillus fumigatus* squalene epoxidase gene confer resistance to terbinafine: Genetic approach to studying gene dose-dependent resistance to antifungals in *A. fumigatus. Antimicrob Agents Chemother* 2004;48(7):2490–2496.

208. Rocha EM, Gardiner RE, Park S, Martinez-Rossi NM, Perlin DS. A *Phe389Leu* substitution in *ergA* confers terbinafine resistance in *Aspergillus fumigatus. Antimicrob Agents Chemother* 2006;50(7):2533–2536.

209. Osborne CS, Leitner I, Hofbauer B, Fielding CA, Favre B, Ryder NS. Biological, biochemical, and molecular characterization of a new clinical *Trichophyton rubrum* isolate resistant to terbinafine. *Antimicrob Agents Chemother* 2006;50(6):2234–2236.

210. Graminha MAS, Rocha EMF, Prade RA, Martinez-Rossi NM. Terbinafine resistance mediated by salicylate 1-monooxygenase in *Aspergillus nidulans.Antimicrob Agents Chemother* 2004;48(9):3530–3535.

211. Perlin DS. Resistance to echinocandin-class antifungal drugs. *Drug Resist Updat* 2007;10(3):121–130.

212. Park S, Kelly R, Kahn JN, et al. Specific substitutions in the echinocandin target Fks1p account for reduced susceptibility of rare laboratory and clinical *Candida* sp. isolates. *Antimicrob Agents Chemother* 2005;49(8):3264–3273.

213. Garcia-Effron G, Katiyar SK, Park S, Edlind TD, Perlin DS. A naturally-occurring Fks1p proline to alanine amino acid change in *Candida parapsilosis, Candida orthopsilosis* and *Candida metapsilosis* accounts for reduced echinocandin susceptibility. *Antimicrob Agents Chemother* 2008;52(7):2305–2312.

214. Stevens DA, Espiritu M, Parmar R. Paradoxical effect of caspofungin: Reduced activity against *Candida albicans* at high drug concentrations. *Antimicrob Agents Chemother* 2004;48(9):3407–3411.

215. Stevens DA, White TC, Perlin DS, Selitrennikoff CP. Studies of the paradoxical effect of caspofungin at high drug concentrations. *Diagn Microbiol Infect Dis* 2005;51(3):173–178.

216. Osherov N, May GS, Albert ND, Kontoyiannis DP. Overexpression of *Sbe2p*, a Golgi protein, results in resistance to caspofungin in *Saccharomyces cerevisiae. Antimicrob Agents Chemother* 2002;46(8):2462–2469.

217. Walker LA, Munro CA, de Bruijn I, Lenardon MD, McKinnon A, Gow NAR. Stimulation of chitin synthesis rescues *Candida albicans* from echinocandins. *PLoS Pathogens* 2008;4(4):e1000040.

218. Feldmesser M, Kress Y, Mednick A, Casadevall A. The effect of the echinocandin analogue caspofungin on cell wall glucan synthesis by *Cryptococcus neoformans. J Infect Dis* 2000;182(6):1791–1795.

219. Niimi K, Maki K, Ikeda F, Holmes AR, Lamping E, Niimi M, Monk BC, Cannon RD. Overexpression of *Candida albicans CDR1, CDR2,* or *MDR1* does not produce significant changes in echinocandin susceptibility. *Antimicrob Agents Chemother* 2006;50(4):1148–1155.

220. Bachmann SP, Patterson TF, Lopez-Ribot JL. *In vitro* activity of caspofungin (MK-0991) against *Candida albicans* clinical isolates displaying different mechanisms of azole resistance. *J Clin Microbiol* 2002;40(6):2228–2230.

221. Pfaller MA, Messer SA, Boyken L, Rice C, Tendolkar S, Hollis RJ, Diekema DJ. Caspofungin activity against clinical isolates of fluconazole-resistant Candida. *J Clin Microbiol* 2003;41(12):5729–5731.

222. Schuetzer-Muehlbauer M, Willinger B, Krapf G, Enzinger S, Presterl E, Kuchler K. The *Candida albicans Cdr2p* ATP-binding cassette (ABC) transporter confers resistance to caspofungin. *Mol Microbiol* 2003;48(1):225–235.

223. Chandra J, Kuhn DM, Mukherjee PK, Hoyer LL, McCormick T, Ghannoum MA. Biofilm formation by the fungal pathogen *Candida albicans* - development, architecture and drug resistance. *J Bacteriol* 2001;183(18):5385–5394.

224. Chandra J, Mukherjee PK, Leidich SD, Faddoul FF, Hoyer LL, Douglas LJ, Ghannoum MA. Antifungal resistance of candidal biofilms formed on denture acrylic *in vitro. J Dent Res* 2001;80(3):903–908.

225. Seidler MJ, Salvenmoser S, Muller FM. Aspergillus fumigatus forms biofilms with reduced antifungal drug susceptibility on bronchial epithelial cells. *Antimicrob Agents Chemother* 2008;52(11):4130–4136.

226. Imamura Y, Chandra J, Mukherjee PK, Abdul Lattif A, Szczotka-Flynn LB, Pearlman E, Lass JH, O'Donnell K, Ghannoum MA. *Fusarium* and *Candida albicans* biofilms on soft contact lenses: Model development, influence of lens type and susceptibility to lens care solutions. *Antimicrob Agents Chemother* 2008;52(1):171–182.

227. Thomas JG, Ramage G, Lopez-Ribot JL. Biofilms and implant infections. In: Ghannoum MA, O'Toole GA (Eds.). *Microbial Biofilms.* Washington, DC: ASM Press, 2005:269–293.

228. Nett JE, Guite KM, Ringeisen A, Holoyda KA, Andes DR. Reduced biocide susceptibility in *Candida albicans* biofilms. *Antimicrob Agents Chemother* 2008;52(9):3411–3413.

229. Ramage G, Bachmann S, Patterson TF, Wickes BL, Lopez-Ribot JL. Investigation of multidrug efflux pumps in relation to fluconazole resistance in *Candida albicans* biofilms. *J Antimicrob Chemother* 2002;49(6):973–980.

230. Mukherjee PK, Chandra J, Kuhn DM, Ghannoum MA. Mechanism of fluconazole resistance in *Candida albicans* biofilms: Phase-specific role of efflux pumps and membrane sterols. *Infect Immun* 2003;71(8):4333–4340.

231. Mateus C, Crow SA, Jr., Ahearn DG. Adherence of *Candida albicans* to silicone induces immediate enhanced tolerance to fluconazole. *Antimicrob Agents Chemother* 2004;48(9):3358–3366.

232. Martinez LR, Casadevall A. *Cryptococcus neoformans* cells in biofilms are less susceptible than planktonic cells to antimicrobial molecules produced by the innate immune system. *Infect Immun* 2006;74(11):6118–6123.

Antifungal prophylaxis: An ounce of prevention is worth a pound of cure

AIMEE K. ZAAS

INTRODUCTION

Given the difficulties inherent in diagnosing and treating invasive fungal infections (IFIs), much attention has been given to the role of prophylaxis against fungal infections. Prophylaxis is one of the principal uses of antifungal agents and is defined as administration of antifungal agents in patients without proven or suspected fungal infection (i.e., absence of microbiological or radiological evidence) but with risk factors for its development (e.g., patients treated with broad spectrum antibiotics, presence of a central venous catheter, under parenteral nutrition or who underwent major abdominal surgery) [1]. Key components of a successful prophylactic strategy include the following: identification of appropriate high-risk patients, identification of which fungi are most likely to cause infection, effort to decrease risk of infection through nonpharmacologic mechanisms (e.g., laminar air flow rooms to decrease risk of invasive mold infections in hematopoietic stem cell transplant recipients), and selection of the appropriate drug at the appropriate dose to provide effective prophylaxis while minimizing side effects and adverse drug reactions. This chapter will provide evidence for prophylaxis against both yeast and mold infections in high-risk settings.

CANDIDA PROPHYLAXIS

Prophylaxis against *Candida* infections is a key component of patient care in certain high-risk situations, particularly in patients hospitalized in intensive care unit (ICU) settings, preterm infants, those receiving hematopoietic stem cell transplantation, and those with certain hematologic malignancies (i.e., acute myelogenous leukemia and myelodysplastic syndromes) and solid organ transplant recipients. In addition to the major risk groups mentioned above, risk factors for the development of invasive candidiasis (IC) also include receipt of broad-spectrum antibacterial agents, disruption of gastrointestinal integrity, mucositis, gastrointestinal surgery or perforation, administration of total parenteral nutrition, presence of central venous catheters, burns, and mechanical ventilation [2,3]. Colonization with *Candida* species at multiple sites remains a somewhat controversial risk factor; however, many studies have noted that while the positive predictive value of *Candida* colonization for development of IC may be low, the negative predictive value is quite high [2,4–6]. Thus, one should note *Candida* colonization but not institute routine surveillance cultures of stool or the oropharynx to document colonization.

In addition to prophylaxis against IC, notable additional issues include the inclusion of mold-active agents in prophylaxis (as opposed to fluconazole prophylaxis) and, for allogeneic stem cell transplant recipients, the extension of prophylaxis to the post-engraftment period during the time of acute and chronic graft-versus-host disease (GvHD) prophylaxis or treatment. As the clinical situation differs markedly for each group mentioned above, prophylactic strategies are typically evaluated in a risk-group-specific fashion.

Risk groups

INTENSIVE CARE UNIT

Due to evidence of increased risk of developing IC amongst persons hospitalized in ICUs, the concept of prophylaxis in this setting has received considerable attention. The greatest difficulty in addressing the role of prophylaxis in the ICU is identification of the appropriate patients to receive prophylaxis. Additional key issues relating to ICU antifungal prophylaxis include the choice of agent and route of administration (if applicable, i.e., azoles). Goals of prophylaxis in this setting also vary with the most obvious goal being reduction of episodes of IC, and with secondary goals being reduction of overall mortality avoidance of toxicity and avoidance of induction of drug resistance [7]. Although the concept that *Candida* colonization precedes and, thus, predicts disease is somewhat controversial [1,2]; some studies of antifungal prophylaxis in the ICU also express the goal of reducing *Candida* colonization. In some settings, investigators have attempted to calculate a "colonization index (CI)" (ratio of the number of culture-positive surveillance sites for *Candida* spp. to the number of sites cultured) for each patient. Typically, patients undergo culture of the nose, throat, stool, urine, and/or protected tracheal aspirate on admission to the ICU and then weekly. Once data is obtained, then a threshold CI of >0.4 or 0.5 is used as an indication to institute prophylaxis [8,9]. While this approach identifies patients who are at potentially high risk for developing IC, it is also labor-intensive and costly.

Many studies evaluating the role of anti-*Candida* prophylaxis in the ICU are single-center studies, although several multi-center studies have been published more recently. Key early trials were conducted in surgical ICUs with considerably high rates of IC. An early study enrolled 43 extremely high-risk patients with refractory gastrointestinal perforation or leakage in a randomized, prospective, double-blind placebo-controlled trial of fluconazole 400 mg IV per day versus placebo [10]. The observed rate of *Candida* peritonitis was reduced from 35% in the placebo group to 4% in the fluconazole group (p = 0.02), highlighting the potential for fluconazole prophylaxis in a highly select group of patients. Subsequently, a larger randomized, double-blind, placebo-controlled trial was performed in a large academic surgical ICU [11]. Inclusion criteria for this study were broad and included any patient predicted to have an ICU stay of at least 3 days. Patients were randomized to receive fluconazole 400 mg/day or placebo. Receipt of fluconazole prophylaxis decreased the rate of IC from 15.3% in the placebo group to 8.5% in the fluconazole group (p = 0.07). Other endpoints included time to onset of fungal infection, which showed marked benefit with fluconazole versus placebo (p = 0.01). Adjusted overall risk of IFI reduced by 55% with fluconazole compared with placebo (RR 0.45; 95% CI = 0.21–0.98). A follow up to this study analyzed the rate of infection and species type in the pre- and post-fluconazole prophylaxis era. This study found that the infection rate in the time period prior to initiation of universal prophylaxis was 1.94/1000 patient days versus in the post prophylaxis era, infection rate was 0.76/1000 patient days (OR 0.44; 95% CI = 0.25–0.78; p = 0.004). Importantly, this retrospective look at *Candida* epidemiology revealed a change in predominant flora to azole-resistant isolates in this ICU [12]. This evaluation occurred in the 2 years following the institution of fluconazole prophylaxis as a standard of care in this particular ICU and would bear repeating after a longer duration as well. Finally, a large randomized trial involving 220 patients evaluated fluconazole 100 mg/day versus placebo in medical or surgical ICU patients, who were on or greater than day 3 of ICU hospitalization [13]. Patients in this study were all mechanically ventilated and had undergone selective digestive decontamination. Although administration of low dose fluconazole as prophylaxis in this study reduced the absolute number of episodes of IC (8.9% of placebo group versus 3.9% of fluconazole group, p = 0.2), reductions in frequency and intensity of candidal colonization was also found in the fluconazole group as compared to the placebo group [13]. The major detraction from the findings in the above-mentioned trials is that each was conducted at a single center. In one particularly high-risk group, patients with anastomotic leakage or necrotizing pancreatitis, a small 19-person non-comparative study showed that caspofungin prophylaxis prevented invasive candidiasis in 18/19 subjects and decreased the *Candida* colonization index in all subjects [14].

As the incidence and epidemiology of IC varies greatly between institutions, prophylactic measures deemed successful in one setting may not be applicable to other institutions. One multicenter, randomized, double-blind, placebo-controlled trial compared caspofungin as antifungal prophylaxis to placebo in 222 adults, who were in the ICU for at least 3 days, were ventilated, received antibiotics, had a central line, and had 1 additional risk factor (parenteral nutrition, dialysis, surgery, pancreatitis, systemic steroids, or other immunosuppressants). Subjects' (1,3)-β-d-glucan levels were monitored twice weekly. The primary endpoint was the incidence of proven or probable invasive candidiasis by European Organization for Research and Treatment of Cancer/Mycoses Study Group (EORTC/MSG) criteria in patients who did not have disease at baseline. This well-constructed study did not show efficacy of prophylaxis as the incidence of proven/probable invasive candidiasis in the placebo and caspofungin arms was 16.7% (14/84) and 9.8% (10/102), respectively, for prophylaxis (p = 0.14) [15]. The multicenter, double-blind, placebo-controlled EMPIRICUS (Empirical Antifungal Treatment in ICUS) trial evaluated whether micafungin, as compared with placebo, increases 28-day invasive fungal infection–free survival among patients with ICU-acquired sepsis, *Candida* colonization at multiple sites, and multiple organ failure. This trial incorporated the pan-fungal marker 1-3-β-D glucan monitoring into the study design. Ultimately, empiric micafungin for nonneutropenic critically ill patients with ICU-acquired sepsis, *Candida* species colonization at multiple sites, and multiple organ failure, empirical treatment with micafungin, compared with placebo, did not increase fungal infection–free survival at day 28. However, this study did provide important information regarding micafungin kinetics in critically ill patients, and perhaps shed light on the question regarding use of 1-3-β-D glucan monitoring for de-escalation of antifungal therapy in known infection as kinetics were not changed by therapy [16]. In addition to this multi-center trial, meta-analyses of well-constructed, randomized, controlled trials provide a broader insight into the role of *Candida* prophylaxis in the ICU setting. A meta-analysis of 12 trials evaluating either fluconazole or ketoconazole versus placebo as prophylaxis in high-risk ICU patients showed that when combined, fluconazole/ketoconazole reduced total mortality by one-quarter (relative risk 0.76, 95% CI = 0.59–0.97) and invasive fungal infections by about one-half (relative risk 0.46, 95% CI = 0.31–0.68) [17,18]. An additional meta-analysis of six randomized, controlled trials of either fluconazole (four), itraconazole (one), or ketoconazole (one) versus placebo concluded that the use of an azole reduced the risk of IC by 75% amongst nonneutropenic adults hospitalized in an ICU [19]. For the purposes of the meta-analysis, the risk factors for IC were defined as having three or more of the following: fungal colonization, diabetes mellitus, solid tumor, abdominal surgery, presence of a central venous catheter for more than 3 days, antibacterial exposure, intubation, or receipt of a solid organ transplant with anticipated more than 5 days ICU postoperative stay. Additionally, fewer fungal infections (816 patients, 0.20, 0.13–0.32), fewer episodes of candidemia (604 patients OR 0.28, 95% CI = 0.09–0.86), non-bloodstream IFIs (OR 0.26, 0.12–0.53), and superficial fungal infections (0.22, 0.11–0.43) were noted in the group receiving prophylaxis versus the placebo group. Overall mortality reduction was similar between groups receiving prophylaxis versus those receiving placebo (0.74, 0.52–1.05), as were adverse events (1.28, 0.82–1.98). As stated in the editorial for the above-discussed meta-analysis, "focused studies in selected high-risk groups have shown that meaningful prophylaxis is possible, but generalizing the idea has not yet been possible" [20]. Despite the availability of multiple meta-analyses of prophylaxis trials, identification of the appropriate patients for prophylaxis and which agent is optimal are the key issues for development of effective IC prophylactic strategies for the ICU.

As not every ICU is a particularly "high risk unit" where universal prophylaxis may be the best option, other authors advocate the use of a "*Candida* score" incorporating known risk factors for IC to predict which patients may benefit from fl from fo prophylaxis [21,22]. The *Candida* prediction score developed by Ostrosky-Zeichner and colleagues [22] was based on data generated from reviewing 2890 patients, who were hospitalized for 4 or more days in an ICU (medical or surgical). Persons were excluded if they were on antifungal agents at the time of admission to the ICU or if the status of antifungal therapy was unknown. This dataset recorded an incidence of IC of 3% (88/2890). Evaluation of multiple predictors derived a prediction rule that predicted 34% of cases (rate of 9.9%, RR 4.36, sensitivity 0.34, specificity 0.9, PPV 0.01, NPV 0.97).

A patient defined as "high risk" using this rule would meet the following criteria:

- Major criteria: Abx days 1–3 OR central venous catheter (CVC) days 1–3
- Need 2 minor criteria: total parenteral nutrition (TPN) days 1–3, surgery days –7 to 0, pancreatitis days –7 to 0, steroids days –7 to 3, immunosuppression days –7 to 0

This rule requires prospective validation, but provides framework for clinical trial design, and has helped clinicians and researchers understand the risk factors and burdens of invasive candidiasis in the intensive care unit setting [23,24].

At this time, practice guidelines for prophylaxis in the ICU are still being defined, but are classified as being weak recommendations with low to moderate quality evidence in the most recent Infectious Diseases Society of America guidelines for the management of *Candida* infections [25]. A recent Cochrane review of antifungal prophylaxis found moderate grade evidence that untargeted antifungal treatment did not significantly reduce or increase total (all-cause) mortality (RR 0.93, 95% CI 0.79–1.09, P value = 0.36; participants = 24; studies = 19 and low grade evidence that untargeted antifungal treatment significantly reduced the risk of proven invasive fungal infections (RR 0.57, 95% CI 0.39–0.83, P value = 0.0001; participants = 2024; studies = 17) [26].

SOLID ORGAN TRANSPLANTATION

Additional situations where prophylaxis against candidal infections is utilized are in abdominal organ transplant recipients (liver, pancreas, small bowel). For a full discussion of the role of prophylaxis against IC and other fungal infections in solid organ transplant recipients, see Chapter 25, "Prophylaxis and treatment of invasive fungal infections in neutropenic cancer and hematopoietic cell transplant patients."

PRETERM INFANTS

Low birth weight and very low birth weight infants represent a high-risk group for the development of IC. For a full discussion of the epidemiology, prophylaxis, and treatment of IC in preterm infants, see Chapter 27, "Infants: Yeasts are beasts in early life."

CANDIDA AND MOLD PROPHYLAXIS

Certain clinical situations, specifically patients with acute leukemia/hematologic malignancies or those who undergo hematopoietic stem cell transplantation, expose patients to risk of both IC and invasive mold infections. Clinicians caring for these patients must consider risk for both types of infection, as portals of entry differ (gastrointestinal tract or IV catheter for yeast versus inhalation for molds), as do the susceptibility to various potential prophylactic agents. Guidelines for who should receive prophylaxis are more established for these clinical situations as compared to ICU prophylaxis; however, much still remains to be learned regarding the optimal agent, dose, and duration.

Risk groups

HEMATOLOGIC MALIGNANCIES

Risk factors for development of invasive fungal infections differ amongst persons with hematologic malignancies, with the lowest risk being those persons undergoing autologous transplantation (Table 5.1). Patients at highest risk for IFI include those with profound and persistent neutropenia ($<0.1 \times 10^9$/L for over 3 weeks), those undergoing allogeneic unrelated or mismatched unrelated transplant, those colonized by *C. tropicalis,* and those receiving high dose corticosteroids or certain types of chemotherapy (high-dose Ara-C) [27]. Of all hematologic malignancies, acute myelogenous leukemia and myelodysplastic syndrome are amongst the highest risk for development of IFIs, including both candidiasis and mold infections [27]. This is likely due to intrinsic defects in myeloid cells, as well as decreased numbers of functional myeloid cells and mucositis.

Current recommendations from the Infectious Diseases Society of America state that Prophylaxis against *Candida* infections is recommended in patient groups in whom the risk of invasive candidal infections is substantial, such as allogeneic hematopoietic stem cell transplantation (HSCT) recipients or those undergoing intensive remission-induction or salvage induction chemotherapy for acute leukemia, and these recommendations receive an A-I grading. Taking together all available evidence, the Infectious Diseases

Society of America (IDSA) states that fluconazole, itraconazole, voriconazole, posaconazole, micafungin, and caspofungin are all acceptable choices for prophylaxis in this setting [25].

Many of the trials leading to prophylaxis recommendations are discussed below. Expert opinions from the IDSA, the National Comprehensive Cancer Network, and the EORTC conclude the following:

1. For patients with acute leukemia undergoing remission-induction or salvage-induction chemotherapy who are expected to develop severe oral and/or gastrointestinal mucositis, we recommend prophylaxis against *Candida* infections. We prefer *fluconazole* (200 or 400 mg orally once daily), but alternative agents may be given. Alternative agents include *itraconazole, voriconazole, posaconazole, micafungin, caspofungin,* and *anidulafungin* [25,28,29].
2. For selected patients who will experience prolonged neutropenia due to intensive chemotherapy for acute myelogenous leukemia or advanced myelodysplastic syndrome, prophylaxis against invasive mold infections and *Candida* spp. with either *posaconazole* or *voriconazole* rather than targeted anti-*Candida* prophylaxis with *fluconazole* is recommended. Therapeutic drug monitoring is recommended if using mold-active azoles to ensure absorption [30].

A meta-analysis of antifungal prophylaxis trials demonstrated the efficacy of prophylaxis in key subgroups of patients along several parameters. This comprehensive analysis included 38 trials (total 7014 patients; study agents, 3515 patients; control patients, 3499 patients). Overall, when comparing patients receiving prophylaxis to patients receiving placebo, there were reductions in the use of parenteral antifungal therapy (prophylaxis success: odds ratio [OR], 0.57; 95% CI = 0.48–0.68; relative risk reduction [RRR], 19%; number requiring treatment for this outcome [NNT], 10 patients), superficial fungal infection (OR, 0.29; 95% CI = 0.20–0.43; RRR, 61%; NNT, 12 patients), invasive fungal infection (OR, 0.44; 95% CI = 0.35–0.55; RRR, 56%; NNT, 22 patients), and fungal infection–related mortality (OR, 0.58; 95% CI = 0.41–0.82; RRR, 47%; NNT, 52 patients). As expected in these highly complex patients, overall mortality was not reduced based on use of antifungal prophylaxis (OR, 0.87; 95% CI = 0.74–1.03). However, subgroup analyses showed reduced mortality in studies of patients who had prolonged neutropenia (OR, 0.72; 95% CI = 0.55–0.95) or were HSCT recipients (OR, 0.77; 95% CI = 0.59–0.99). From the multivariate meta-regression analyses performed, key predictors of treatment effect identified were HSCT, prolonged neutropenia, acute leukemia with prolonged neutropenia, and higher azole dose [31]. A key point learned from the prophylaxis data in these patients is that need is not universal in all patients with hematologic malignancies who undergo cytotoxic chemotherapy, but that certain subsets of patients benefit greatly.

Table 5.1 Risk stratification scheme for invasive fungal infections in patients with hematologic malignancies or hematopoietic stem cell transplantation

- Low risk
  - Autologous transplant
  - Childhood ALL (except for *Pneumocystic carinii pneumonia*) Lymphoma
- Intermediate risk Low-intermediate
  - Moderate neutropenia ($0.1 – 0.5 \times 10^8$/L <3 wk, lymphocytes $<0.5 \times 10^8$/L + antibiotics)
  - Older age
  - Central venous catheter High-intermediate
  - Colonized >1 site or heavy at one site
  - Neutropenia <0.5 to $>0.1 \times 10^8$/L >3–5 wk AML
  - TBI
  - Allogeneic matched sibling donor BMT High risk
  - Neutrophils $<0.1 \times 10^8$/L >3 wk
  - Colonized by *Candida tropicalis*
  - Allogeneic unrelated or mismatched donor BMT GvHD
  - Neutropenia $<0.5 \times 10^8$/L >5 wk
  - Corticosteroids >1 mg/kg and neutrophils $<1 \times 10^8$/L >1 wk Corticosteroids >2 mg/kg >2 wk
  - High-dose Ara-C Fludarabine

Abbreviations: ALL, acute lymphocytic leukemia; AML, acute myelogenous leukemia; TBL, total body irradiation BMT, bone marrow transplant; GvHD, graft-vs-host disease.

Posaconazole, a broad-spectrum triazole, has recently been demonstrated to reduce IFI and mortality in patients with newly diagnosed or relapsed acute myelogenous leukemia (AML) or myelodysplastic syndrome (MDS), who were treated with intensive chemotherapy [24]. Notably, this study enrolled only the highest risk patients (MDS or AML). Patients enrolled in this study received posaconazole, 200 mg thrice daily ($n = 304$) or a standard azole regimen (either fluconazole, 400 mg once daily [$n = 240$] or itraconazole, 200 mg twice daily [$n = 58$], choice determined by the investigative site) with each cycle of chemotherapy until complete remission or for up to 12 weeks. Use of posaconazole as compared to use of fluconazole or itraconazole was associated with fewer total IFI during the treatment phase (2% vs. 8%; $p = 0.0009$) and fewer episodes of invasive aspergillosis (1% vs. 7%; $p = 0.0001$) [32]. In addition to the efficacy of posaconazole for prevention of IFIs in this group of patients, a mortality benefit was found as well. At 100 days post randomization, there was a survival benefit in favor of posaconazole in terms of all cause (15% vs. 22%; $p = 0.0354$) and IFI-related death (2% vs. 5%; $p = 0.0209$). The rates of adverse events were similar between the two treatment groups. While these studies used the oral suspension formulation of posaconazole, the now available tablet is recommended as this formulation does not require a high-fat meal or acidic environment for absorption [33,34].

HEMATOPOIETIC STEM CELL TRANSPLANTATION

Owing to overt immune suppression, as well as disruption of gastrointestinal integrity during intensive chemotherapy, persons undergoing hematopoietic stem cell transplantation (HSCT) are at risk for developing IFIs during the pre-engraftment phase of transplantation. Typically, the risk for IC is highest during the pre-engraftment period. An additional risk period for invasive mold infections occurs during the time of acute GvHD, as the disease itself, as well as the agents used for prophylaxis and/or treatment induce immune suppression.

Several large trials have demonstrated the efficacy of fluconazole versus placebo for the prophylaxis against IC during the period of neutropenia following conditioning for allogeneic and autologous stem cell transplantation. Given the overwhelming evidence from multiple well-constructed clinical trials, a large report cosponsored by the Center for International Blood and Marrow Transplant Research (CIBMTR), National Marrow Donor Program (NMDP), European Blood and Marrow Transplant Group (EBMT), American Society for Blood and Marrow Transplant (ASBMT), Canadian Blood and Marrow Transplant Group (CBMTG), Infectious Diseases Society of America (IDSA), Society for Healthcare Epidemiology of America (SHEA), Association of Medical Microbiology and Infectious Diseases (AMMI), the Center for Disease Control and Prevention (CDC), and the Health Resources and Services Administration recommends fluconazole is the drug of choice for the prophylaxis of invasive candidiasis before engraftment in allogeneic HCT recipients, and may be started from the beginning or just after the end of the conditioning regimen [35]. This report makes several important advances from prior guidelines, including distinguishing between the engraftment period and the GvHD/post engraftment period and the inclusion of micafungin as an alternative to fluconazole for prophylaxis during the time of engraftment. Thus, the report reconciles the question of whether fluconazole is truly appropriate in patients who remain at high-risk for mould infections by proposing these phase-specific guidelines for HSCT recipients: (1) fluconazole is highly recommended in the initial phase, but only when combined with a mould-directed diagnostic approach (for example, galactomannan-based or CT-scan-based) or a mould-directed therapeutic approach (for example, empirical antifungal therapy) for centers not having HEPA-filtered rooms and/or having a high baseline incidence of invasive mould infections. (2) Posaconazole is the drug of choice at onset of acute or chronic GvHD. However, the working group recommended therapeutic drug monitoring, especially in patients with intestinal GvHD. During GvHD, fluconazole becomes less relevant (CI), because of the high risk of mould disease [35,36].

The specific data that led to micafungin's Untied States Food and Drug Administration (US FDA) approval as an agent for prophylaxis during the engraftment period came from a randomized, controlled trial of prophylaxis with micafungin (50 mg/day) versus fluconazole (400 mg IV/day). In this trial, micafungin was found to be superior to fluconazole for prophylaxis during the neutropenic period in patients undergoing allogeneic HSCT (proportion free of IFI at 4 weeks 80% in micafungin group vs. 73.5% in fluconazole group, 95% CI = 0.9%–12%, $p = 0.03$) [37].

Extension of prophylaxis through day +75 has been shown to have global benefit for HSCT recipients, with benefits continuing through long-term follow up. Despite the spectrum limitations of fluconazole, extension of prophylaxis through the post-engraftment period provided benefit in reduction of IFIs in a group of both autologous and allogeneic HSCT recipients. During prophylaxis, systemic fungal infections occurred in 10 (7%) of 152 fluconazole-treated patients compared with 26 (18%) of 148 placebo-treated patients ($p = 0.004$). The probability of survival at day 110 following transplantation was improved in fluconazole recipients, in whom 31 deaths occurred as compared with 52 deaths in placebo recipients ($p = 0.004$) [38]. Eight-year follow up of these patients found that extension of fluconazole prophylaxis (400 mg PO qd) for IC for 75 days following allogeneic stem cell transplantation not only decreased subsequent IC (30 of 148 placebo vs. 4 of 152 fluconazole, $p < 0.001$), but also had a positive impact on eight-year mortality (68 of 152 fluconazole vs. 41 of 148 placebo, $p = 0.0001$). This decrease in mortality was likely as a result of decreased development of gastrointestinal GvHD (20 of 143 placebos vs. 8 of 145 fluconazole, $p = 0.02$) in addition to decreased IC [39]. As a result of this trial, many centers have instituted prolonged fluconazole prophylaxis (through day +75) for allogeneic stem cell transplant recipients.

In addition to IC, invasive mold infections remain a predominant cause of morbidity and mortality in HSCT recipients. Given the limitations of fluconazole coverage, multiple trials have evaluated antifungal agents with activity against yeasts and molds as prophylaxis in hematopoietic stem cell transplant recipients. Risk in autologous transplant recipients is low, particularly compared to allogeneic transplant recipients, due to decreased length of neutropenia and absence of GvHD. Many antifungal doses and agents have been studied as prophylactic agents in HSCT recipients; however, the results of a double-blind, randomized controlled trial evaluating posaconazole versus oral fluconazole for prophylaxis against fungal infections during the period of severe acute GvHD in allogeneic HSCT recipients [24] has positioned posaconazole as the first line prophylaxis against IFI in allogeneic stem cell transplant recipients with GvHD [40].

In this study of 600 allogeneic stem cell transplant recipients with GvHD, patients were randomized to receive posaconazole, 200 mg thrice daily ($n = 301$) or fluconazole, 400 mg once daily ($n = 299$) for up to 16 weeks [24]. Although the incidence of total IFI during the 16-week study period was similar in the posaconazole and fluconazole groups (5% vs. 9%; p = 0.0740), there were fewer total breakthrough IFIs in the posaconazole arm (2% vs. 8%; p = 0.0038). Notably, *Aspergillus* infections were significantly reduced among patients receiving posaconazole during the study period (2% vs. 7%; p = 0.0059). The overall mortality rates were similar in the two arms (25% in the posaconazole arm vs. 28% in the fluconazole arm). Mortality due to IFI was lower in the posaconazole group (1%) versus 4% in the fluconazole group (p = 0.046). The side-effect profiles of the two agents were similar.

To address the role of prophylaxis in the context of a structured screening protocol, the Blood and Marrow Transplant Clinical Trials Network conducted a multicenter, randomized, double-blind trial comparing fluconazole (n = 295) versus voriconazole (n = 305) for the prevention of IFI in patients who were screened regularly for invasive aspergillosis using serum Galactomannan testing. Patients undergoing myeloablative allogeneic HCT were randomized before HCT to receive study drugs for 100 days, or for 180 days in higher-risk patients. Serum galactomannan was assayed twice weekly for 60 days, then at least weekly until day 100. Positive galactomannan or suggestive signs triggered mandatory evaluation for IFI. The primary endpoint was freedom from IFI or death (fungal-free survival [FFS]) at 180 days. Despite trends to fewer IFIs (7.3% vs. 11.2%; p = 0.12), *Aspergillus* infections (9 vs. 17; p = 0.09), and less frequent empiric antifungal therapy (24.1% vs. 30.2%, p = 0.11) with voriconazole, FFS rates (75% vs. 78%; p = 0.49) at 180 days were similar with fluconazole and voriconazole, respectively. By 180 days post-HCT, 55 patients developed IFIs (14 proven, 24 probable, and 17 presumptive IFIs); by year-one post-HCT, 79 patients developed IFIs (28 proven, 33 probable, and 18 presumptive IFIs). *Aspergillus* was the most frequent pathogen, accounting for 26 (47%) and 38 (48%) IFIs at 180 and 365 days, respectively. There

were 4 and 9 patients with Zygomycetes infections at 180 and 365 days, respectively. In addition, there were 70 and 75 patients with possible IFIs at 180 and 365 days post-HCT, respectively [41]. This study showed that in the context of a structured screening program, voriconazole prophylaxis did not offer additional benefit as compared to fluconazole for prophylaxis in this setting.

A meta-analysis evaluated trials considering either voriconazole or micafungin for prophylaxis in hematopoietic stem cell transplant recipients. Data from 13 randomized clinical trials evaluating the effect of antifungal prophylaxis in 3767 patients undergoing hematological stem cell transplantation were included. This meta-analysis indicated that use of primary antifungal prophylaxis with either micafungin or voriconazole in the highest risk patients is beneficial for preventing morbidity and mortality due to IFIs as compared to use of fluconazole or itraconazole. Voriconazole prophylaxis also reduced the mortality from IFIs with less renal-related adverse events or gastrointestinal side effects than amphotericin B or itraconazole [42].

Many options exist for IFI prophylaxis in high-risk stem cell transplant recipients. Comparison of efficacy, toxicity, and cost can be used to determine the appropriate prophylaxis pro-gram for individual patients and centers. As prophylaxis regimens become broader spectrum in scope, clinicians must consider new strategies for empiric therapy when patients develop febrile episodes or pulmonary infiltrates while taking prophylaxis. Many experts believe that empiric regimens for febrile neutropenia will evolve to more "watchful waiting" as prophylactic regimens broaden [43], although trials evaluating this strategy are indicated.

OTHER SITUATIONS

Human immunodeficiency virus/acquired immune deficiency syndrome (HIV/AIDS)

Based on overall CD4 count or percentage, persons infected with the HIV virus are at risk for a myriad of fungal infections, including *Pneumocystis jirovecii* pneumonia and oro-esophageal candidiasis. Geographic location imparts additional risk for infections, such as cryptococcosis, histoplasmosis, coccidioidomycosis, and infection with *Penicillium marneffei*. Recommendations for prophylaxis against fungal infections in HIV-infected persons are based on both degree of immune suppression and geography. Major prophylactic recommendations from the United States Public Health Service and the Infectious Diseases Society of America haven not changed fundamentally since the advent of highly active antiretroviral therapy [51]. Major recommendations include prophylaxis against *Pneumocystis* pneumonia in individuals with CD4 counts <200 cells/uL or oropharyngeal thrush, against *Histoplasma capsulatum* in individuals with CD4 counts <100 cells/uL who live in hyperendemic areas (Ohio River Valley or Puerto Rico) [52,53], and against *Penicillium marneffei* in individuals with CD4 counts <100 cells/uL who live in hyperendemic areas (Chiang Mai province of Thailand) [54–56]. Prophylaxis against oropharyngeal candidiasis is not generally recommended [42,44–50].

CONCLUSIONS

Given the significant morbidity and mortality associated with invasive fungal infections, many situations are suitable for the use of antifungal prophylaxis. While prophylactic regimens have many goals, the foremost is to prevent invasive fungal infections. Preventing colonization, avoiding drug resistance, and avoiding toxicity are secondary goals to consider. As diagnostics for fungal infections improve, the role of prophylaxis will undoubtedly evolve.

REFERENCES

1. Cornely OA, Bassetti M, Calandra T, et al. ESCMID* guideline for the diagnosis and management of *Candida* diseases 2012: Non-neutropenic adult patients. *Clin Microbiol Infec* 2012; 18(7):19–37.

2. Blumberg HM, Jarvis WR, Soucie JM, et al. Risk factors for candidal bloodstream infections in surgical intensive care unit patients: The NEMIS prospective multicenter study. The National Epidemiology of Mycosis Survey. *Clin Infect Dis* 2001;33(2):177–186.

3. Pfaller MA, Diekema DJ. Epidemiology of invasive candidiasis: A persistent public health problem. *Clin Microbiol Rev* 2007;20(1):133–163.

4. Vardakas KZ, Michalopoulos A, Kiriakidou KG, et al. Candidaemia: Incidence, risk factors, characteristics and outcomes in immunocompetent critically ill patients. *Clin Microbiol Infect* 2009;15(3):289–292. doi:10.1111/j.1469-0691.2008.02653.x.

5. Meersseman W, Lagrou K, Spriet I, et al. Significance of the isolation of *Candida* species from airway samples in critically ill patients: A prospective, autopsy study. *Intensive Care Med* 2009;35(9):1526–1531. doi:10.1007/s00134-009-1482-8.

6. Lau AF, Kabir M, Chen SC, et al. *Candida* colonization as a risk marker for invasive candidiasis in mixed medical-surgical intensive care units: Development and evaluation of a simple, standard protocol. *J Clin Microbiol* 2015;53(4):1324–1330. doi:10.1128/JCM.03239-14.

7. Lipsett PA. Clinical trials of antifungal prophylaxis among patients in surgical intensive care units: Concepts and considerations. *Clin Infect Dis* 2004;39(Suppl 4):S193–S199.

8. Charles PE, Dalle F, Aube H, et al. *Candida* spp. colonization significance in critically ill medical patients: A prospective study. *Intensive Care Med* 2005;31(3):393–400.

9. Piarroux R, Grenouillet F, Balvay P, et al. Assessment of preemptive treatment to prevent severe candidiasis in critically ill surgical patients. *Crit Care Med* 2004;32(12):2443–2449.

10. Eggimann P, Francioli P, Bille J, et al. Fluconazole prophylaxis prevents intra-abdominal candidiasis in high-risk surgical patients. *Crit Care Med* 1999;27(6):1066–1072.

11. Pelz RK, Hendrix CW, Swoboda SM, et al. Double-blind placebo-controlled trial of fluconazole to prevent candidal infections in critically ill surgical patients. *Ann Surg* 2001;233(4):542–548.

12. Swoboda SM, Merz WG, Lipsett PA. Candidemia: The impact of antifungal prophylaxis in a surgical intensive care unit. *Surg Infect (Larchmt)* 2003;4(4):345–354.

13. Garbino J, Lew DP, Romand JA, et al. Prevention of severe *Candida* infections in nonneutropenic, high-risk, critically ill patients: A randomized, double-blind, placebo-controlled trial in patients treated by selective digestive decontamination. *Intensive Care Med* 2002;28(12):1708–1717.

14. Senn L, Eggimann P, Ksontini R, et al. Caspofungin for prevention of intra-abdominal candidiasis in high-risk surgical patients. *Intensive Care Med* 2009;35(5):903–908. doi:10.1007/s00134-009-1405-8.

15. Ostrosky-Zeichner L, Shoham S, Vazquez J, et al. MSG-01: A randomized, double-blind, placebo-controlled trial of caspofungin prophylaxis followed by preemptive therapy for invasive candidiasis in high-risk adults in the critical care setting. *Clin Infect Dis* 2014;58(9):1219–1226. doi:10.1093/cid/ciu074.

16. Timsit J-L, Azoulay E, Schwebel, E, et al. Empirical micafungin treatment and survival without invasive fungal infection in adults with ICU-acquired sepsis, *Candida* colonization, and multiple organ failure: The EMPIRICUS randomized clinical trial. *JAMA* 2016;316(15):1555–1564. doi:10.1001/jama.2016.14655.

17. Playford EG, Webster AC, Sorrell TC, et al. Antifungal agents for preventing fungal infections in non-neutropenic critically ill and surgical patients: Systematic review and meta-analysis of randomized clinical trials. *J Antimicrob Chemother* 2006;57(4):628–638.

18. Playford EG, Webster AC, Sorrell TC, et al. Antifungal agents for preventing fungal infections in non-neutropenic critically ill patients. *Cochrane Database Syst Rev* 2006;(1):CD004920.

19. Vardakas KZ, Samonis G, Michalopoulos A, et al. Antifungal prophylaxis with azoles in high-risk, surgical intensive care unit patients: A meta-analysis of randomized, placebo-controlled trials. *Crit Care Med* 2006;34(4):1216–1224.

20. Rex JH. Antifungal prophylaxis in the intensive care unit: Who should get it? *Crit Care Med* 2006;34(4):1286–1287.

21. Leon C, Ruiz-Santana S, Saavedra P, et al. A bedside scoring system ("*Candida* score") for early antifungal treatment in nonneutropenic critically ill patients with *Candida* colonization. *Crit Care Med* 2006;34(3):730–737.

22. Ostrosky-Zeichner L, Sable C, Sobel J, et al. Multicenter retrospective development and validation of a clinical prediction rule for nosocomial invasive candidiasis in the intensive care setting. *Eur J Clin Microbiol Infect Dis* 2007;26(4):271–276.

23. Eggimann P, Que Y-A, Revelly JP, et al. Preventing invasive *Candida* infections. Where could we do better? *J Hosp Infect* 2015;89(4):302–308.

24. Eggimann P, Pittet D. *Candida* colonization index and subsequent infection in critically ill surgical patients: 20 years later. *Intensive Care Med* 2014;40(10):1429–1448. doi:10.1007/s00134-014-3355-z.

25. Pappas PG, Kauffman CA, Andes DR, et al. Executive summary: Clinical practice guideline for the management of candidiasis: 2016 update by the Infectious Diseases Society of America. *Clin Infect Dis* 2016;62(4):409–417. doi:10.1093/cid/civ1194.

26. Cortegiani A, Russotto V, Maggiore A, et al. Antifungal agents for preventing fungal infections in non-neutropenic critically ill patients. *Cochrane Database Syst Rev* 2016;(1):CD004920. doi:10.1002/14651858.CD004920.pub3.

27. Wenzel RP, Gennings C. Bloodstream infections due to *Candida* species in the intensive care unit: Identifying especially high-risk patients to determine prevention strategies. *Clin Infect Dis* 2005;41(Suppl 6):S389–S393.

28. Cornely OA, Gachot B, Akan H, et al. Epidemiology and outcome of fungemia in a cancer Cohort of the Infectious Diseases Group (IDG) of the European Organization for Research and Treatment of Cancer (EORTC 65031). *Clin Infect Dis* 2015;61(3):324–331. doi:10.1093/cid/civ293.

29. Ethier MC, Science M, Beyene J, et al. Mould-active compared with fluconazole prophylaxis to prevent invasive fungal diseases in cancer patients receiving chemotherapy or haematopoietic stem-cell transplantation: A systematic review and meta-analysis of randomised controlled trials. *Br J Cancer* 2012;106(10):1626–1637. doi:10.1038/bjc.2012.147.

30. Patterson TF, Thompson III GR, Denning DW, et al. Executive summary: Practice guidelines for the diagnosis and management of aspergillosis: 2016 update by the Infectious Diseases Society of America. *Clin Infect Dis* 2016;63(4):433–442. doi:10.1093/cid/ciw444.

31. Bow EJ, Laverdiere M, Lussier N, et al. Antifungal prophylaxis for severely neutropenic chemotherapy recipients: A meta analysis of randomized-controlled clinical trials. *Cancer* 2002;94(12):3230–3246.

32. Cornely OA, Maertens J, Winston DJ, et al. Posaconazole vs. fluconazole or itraconazole prophylaxis in patients with neutropenia. *N Engl J Med* 2007;356(4):348–359.

33. Jung DS, Tverdek FP, Kontoyiannis DP. Switching from posaconazole suspension to tablets increases serum drug levels in leukemia patients without clinically relevant hepatotoxicity. *Antimicrob Agents Chemother* 2014;58(11):6993–6995. doi:10.1128/AAC.04035-14.

34. Cumpston A, Caddell R, Shillingburg A, et al. superior serum concentrations with posaconazole delayed-release tablets compared to suspension formulation in hematological malignancies. *Antimicrob Agents Chemother* 2015;59(8):4424–4428. doi:10.1128/AAC.00581-15.

35. Tomblyn M, Chiller T, Einsele H, et al. Center for International Blood and Marrow Research; National Marrow Donor program; European Blood and Marrow Transplant Group; American Society of Blood and Marrow Transplantation; Canadian Blood and Marrow Transplant Group; Infectious Diseases Society of America; Society for Healthcare Epidemiology of America; Association of Medical Microbiology and Infectious Disease Canada; Centers for Disease Control and Prevention. *Biol Blood Marrow Trans* 2009;15(10):1143–1238. doi: 10.1016/j.bbmt.2009.06.019.

36. Maertens J, Marchetti O, Herbrecht R, et al. European guidelines for antifungal management in leukemia and hematopoietic stem cell transplant recipients: Summary of the ECIL 3—2009 update. *Bone Marrow Transpl* 2011;46:709–718.

37. van Burik JA, Ratanatharathorn V, Stepan DE, et al. Micafungin versus fluconazole for prophylaxis against invasive fungal infections during neutropenia in patients undergoing hematopoietic stem cell transplantation. *Clin Infect Dis* 2004;39(10):1407–1416.

38. Slavin MA, Osborne B, Adams R, et al. Efficacy and safety of fluconazole prophylaxis for fungal infections after marrow transplantation—A prospective, randomized, double-blind study. *J Infect Dis* 1995;171(6):1545–1552.

39. Marr KA, Seidel K, Slavin MA, et al. Prolonged fluconazole prophylaxis is associated with persistent protection against candidiasis-related death in allogeneic marrow transplant recipients: Long-term follow-up of a randomized, placebo-controlled trial. *Blood* 2000;96(6):2055–2061.

40. Ullmann AJ, Lipton JH, Vesole DH, et al. Posaconazole or fluconazole for prophylaxis in severe graft-versus-host disease. *N Engl J Med* 2007;356(4):335–347.

41. Wingard JR, Carter SL, Walsh TJ, et al. Randomized, double-blind trial of fluconazole versus voriconazole for prevention of invasive fungal infection after allogeneic hematopoietic cell transplantation. *Blood* 2010;116(24):5111–5118.

42. Xu SX, Shen JL, Tang XF, et al. Newer antifungal agents micafungin and voriconazole for fungal infection prevention during hematopoietic cell transplantation: A meta-analysis. *Eur Rev Med Pharmacol Sci* 2016;20(2):381–390.

43. Segal BH, Almyroudis NG, Battiwalla M, et al. Prevention and early treatment of invasive fungal infection in patients with cancer and neutropenia and in stem cell transplant recipients in the era of newer broad-spectrum antifungal agents and diagnostic adjuncts. *Clin Infect Dis* 2007;44(3):402–409.

44. Guidelines for prophylaxis against *Pneumocystis carinii* pneumonia for persons infected with human immunodeficiency virus. *MMWR Morb Mortal Wkly Rep* 1989;38(Suppl 5):1–9.

45. 2001 USPHS/IDSA guidelines for the prevention of opportunistic infections in persons infected with human immunodeficiency virus. *HIV Clin Trials* 2001;2(6):493–554.

46. Furrer H, Egger M, Opravil M, et al. Discontinuation of primary prophylaxis against *Pneumocystis carinii* pneumonia in HIV-1-infected adults treated with combination antiretroviral therapy. Swiss HIV Cohort Study. *N Engl J Med* 1999;340(17):1301–1306.

47. Kaplan JE, Masur H, Holmes KK, et al. USPHS/IDSA guidelines for the prevention of opportunistic infections in persons infected with human immunodeficiency virus: An overview. USPHS/IDSA Prevention of Opportunistic Infections Working Group. *Clin Infect Dis* 1995;21(Suppl 1):S12–S31.

48. Weverling GJ, Mocroft A, Ledergerber B, et al. Discontinuation of *Pneumocystis carinii* pneumonia prophylaxis after start of highly active antiretroviral therapy in HIV-1 infection. EuroSIDA Study Group. *Lancet* 1999;353(9161):1293–1298.

49. Yangco BG, Von Bargen JC, Moorman AC, et al. Discontinuation of chemoprophylaxis against *Pneumocystis carinii* pneumonia in patients with HIV infection. HIV Outpatient Study (HOPS) Investigators. *Ann Intern Med* 2000;132(3):201–205.

50. Goldman M, Cloud GA, Wade KD, et al. A randomized study of the use of fluconazole in continuous versus episodic therapy in patients with advanced HIV infection and a history of oropharyngeal candidiasis: AIDS Clinical Trials Group Study 323/Mycoses Study Group Study 40. *Clin Infect Dis* 2005;41(10):1473–1480.

51. 2018 USPHS/IDSA guidelines for the prevention of opportunistic infections in persons infected with human immunodeficiency virus. US Public Health Service (USPHS) and Infectious Diseases Society of America (IDSA). Downloaded from https://aidsinfo.nih.gov/guidelines on 7/10/2018.

52. Hajjeh RA, Pappas PG, Henderson H, et al. Multicenter case-control study of risk factors for histoplasmosis in human immunodeficiency virus-infected persons. *Clin Infect Dis* 2001;32(8):1215–1220.

53. McKinsey DS, Wheat LJ, Cloud GA, et al. Itraconazole prophylaxis for fungal infections in patients with advanced human immunodeficiency virus infection: Randomized, placebo-controlled, double-blind study. National Institute of Allergy and Infectious Diseases Mycoses Study Group. *Clin Infect Dis* 1999;28(5):1049–1056.

54. Chaiwarith R, Charoenyos N, Sirisanthana T, et al. Discontinuation of secondary prophylaxis against penicilliosis marneffei in AIDS patients after HAART. *Aids* 2007;21(3):365–367.

55. Chariyalertsak S, Supparatpinyo K, Sirisanthana T, et al. A controlled trial of itraconazole as primary prophylaxis for systemic fungal infections in patients with advanced human immunodeficiency virus infection in Thailand. *Clin Infect Dis* 2002;34(2):277–284.

56. Supparatpinyo K, Perriens J, Nelson KE, et al. A controlled trial of itraconazole to prevent relapse of *Penicillium marneffei* infection in patients infected with the human immunodeficiency virus. *N Engl J Med* 1998;339(24):1739–1743.

6

Preemptive antifungal therapy: Do diagnostics help?

VIDYA JAGADEESAN, MARGARET POWERS-FLETCHER, AND KIMBERLY E. HANSON

INTRODUCTION

Despite the availability of broad-spectrum antifungal drugs, invasive fungal infection (IFI) remains a major cause of morbidity and mortality in immunosuppressed hosts, as well as among critically ill patients in the Intensive Care Unit (ICU). Early initiation of appropriate antifungal therapy is essential to improve outcomes, especially in neutropenic and septic patients.

Unfortunately, clinical risk assessment in conjunction with physical examination and diagnostic imaging are often neither sensitive, nor specific enough to make a rapid diagnosis of IFI. The clinical utility of fungal culture is also limited. Cultures frequently remain negative or only become positive in the advanced stages of infection. Furthermore, deciphering colonization from invasive infection can be difficult when samples are obtained from non-sterile sites. Histopathologic examination of infected tissue has historically been the diagnostic gold standard for invasive disease, but invasive testing may not be feasible in critically ill patients or in those with underlying coagulopathy.

Given the potentially devastating effects of IFI, prevention of overt disease is preferable. Current strategies for the prevention and management of IFI include: (1) antifungal prophylaxis, (2) preemptive therapy, (3) empiric treatment, and (4) treatment of established infection. Definitions, in addition to the advantages and disadvantages of each approach, are outlined in Table 6.1.

Improved biomarker tests, including *Aspergillus* galactomannan, (1,3)-β-D-glucan, and the detection of fungal DNA, have the potential to facilitate identification of IFI and to better inform early antifungal treatment decisions. These tests can be useful as adjuncts to culture and imaging

Table 6.1 Strategies for the prevention and treatment in invasive fungal infection (IFI)

Strategy	Definition	Advantages	Disadvantages
Universal prophylaxis	Administration of antifungal therapy during a defined period to prevent IFI	Effective and logistically easy	1. Drug toxicity 2. Development of antimicrobial resistance 3. Cost incurred by patients who would never develop IFI
Preemptive therapy	Initiation of therapy based on serial monitoring with laboratory biomarkers, radiographic studies, or both, to treat early IFI	1. Targets those patients most likely to benefit from antifungal therapy 2. Facilitates early initiation of antifungal therapy, which may improve outcomes 3. Blood monitoring is non-invasive	1. Effectiveness is based on the performance of the screening strategy in different patient populations 2. Difficult to incorporate into outpatient management 3. Cost of the screening test(s) 4. Not yet shown to improve IFI morbidity or mortality
Empiric treatment	Initiation of therapy to treat suspected IFI based on clinical features. (Example: Antifungal therapy for patients with persistent fever in the setting of neutropenia, without a known source, and despite appropriate antibiotic therapy.)	Improved outcomes documented in the setting of neutropenic fever of unknown origin	Waiting until signs or symptoms of IFI are present delays potentially effective therapy
Treatment of established IFI	Treatment of patients who meet criteria for proven or probable IFI	Currently available antifungal agents are effective in some patients	Waiting until signs or symptoms of IFI are present delays potentially effective therapy

for diagnosis, but their effectiveness as a trigger for preemptive antifungal therapy has not been definitively established.

For the purposes of evaluating a novel diagnostic test, it is essential that a correct diagnosis be made by the comparator or gold standard method. Unfortunately, establishing a diagnosis of IFI remains a major obstacle in studies evaluating fungal diagnostics [1]. The European Organization for Research on the Treatment of Cancer/Mycoses Study Group (EORTC/MSG) has developed standardized definitions for IFI that are intended for use in the context of cancer research [2,3]. The system employs a combination of clinical and microbiological criteria for the classification of "proven", "probable", or "possible" cases of IFI. Diagnoses other than proven disease, however, are often subjective. Furthermore, the EORTC/MSG criteria categorize positive fungal cell-wall biomarkers (i.e., galactomannan and [1,3]-β-D glucan) as microbiologic evidence for probable IFI even in the absence of culture confirmation. Inclusion of biomarker test results in the definition of IFI is a potential source of bias in clinical

studies assessing the utility of the non-culture-based tests that are the subject of this review. Lastly, the definitions were developed for cancer patients and may not be as applicable to other risk groups. Recognizing these limitations, this chapter will review the current literature on non-culture based fungal diagnostic techniques and examine the evidence for their use in clinical practice.

GALACTOMANNAN

Assay principles

Galactomannan (GM) is a polysaccharide cell wall component released primarily by the growing hyphae of *Aspergillus* and *Penicillium* species (sp.). The GM molecule is comprised of a non-immunogenic mannan core with immunoreactive galactofuranosyl (gal*f*) containing side chains of varying lengths [4]. GM was first identified as a potential biomarker of invasive aspergillosis (IA) by Reiss and Lehman [5].

Commercially available GM assays utilize a rat monoclonal antibody (EB-A2) directed against the β (1,5)-linked galactofuranoside side chain-residues [6]. Four or more epitopes are typically required for antibody binding and multiple immunoreactive epitopes are present on each GM molecule [7]. In addition to GM, other fungal glycoproteins, including phospolipase C and phytase, have been shown to react with EB-A2 antibodies [4,8]. It is likely that the "GM antigen" is really a family of molecules whose expression is modulated by the localized fungal microenviroment [9], but the actual galf antigens that circulate *in vivo* have not been fully characterized.

A sandwich enzyme-linked immunosorbent assay (EIA) (Platelia™ BioRad, Marnes-La-Coquette, France) and a latex agglutination test (Pastorex Sanofi Diagnostics Pasteur, Marnes-La-Coquette, France) are commercially available for the detection of GM in *vivo*. An immunochromatographic lateral flow assay (LFA) coupled to a monoclonal antibody specific to an extracellular *Aspergillus* glycoprotein has also been developed [10]. The EIA has a reported limit of detection of 0.5–1.0 ng/mL, which is 10–15 times lower than the latex agglutination test [7,11]. For this reason, and because the EIA is commercially available, it is currently the method of choice in most clinical laboratories that perform GM testing and will be the focus of this review. The Platelia EIA assay (Figure 6.1) has been available in Europe for several decades and was cleared by the US Food and Drug Administration (FDA) in May of 2003 as a serum diagnostic for use in cancer patients. Laboratory test turnaround time is approximately 3–3.5 hours, which marks a significant advance over standard culture techniques.

Kinetics

The kinetics of GM production, release, and systemic circulation *in vivo* are incompletely understood. Multiple groups have shown that GM production is proportional to the tissue fungal burden using both animal models and models of the human alveolus [13–15]. GM levels also appear to have prognostic value, with persistently high or rising concentrations portending a poor prognosis [16–18]. Administration of effective antifungal therapy typically reduces circulating GM levels. However, clinical improvement without a concomitant decline in GM has been described with protracted neutropenia and echinocandin therapy [19–21]. Similarly, GM has been reported to remain elevated in successfully treated patients with underlying renal failure [22]. It had been hypothesized that GM is metabolized by a combination of renal excretion, hepatic clearance, and uptake by macrophage mannose receptors [23,24]. A feature lending to the potential utility of GM as a screening test is that circulating GM can be detected 1–2 weeks before the development of clinical signs or symptoms of IA in some patients [18,25,26]. Furthermore, GM may also precede abnormalities on high-resolution CT scan in individuals with suspected pulmonary IA [27]. Not all studies, however, have demonstrated the development GM antigenemia before a conventional diagnosis of IA was made [26,28,29].

Defining a positive result

The optimal optical density index (ODI) readout used to define a positive GM EIA result has been the focus of many studies. The ODI is defined as the OD value of the specimen divided by the mean OD of the wells containing control serum. The manufacturer initially recommended interpreting an index of ≥1.5 as a positive test, with <1.0 defining a negative result, and the 1.0–1.5 range being intermediate. A reduced threshold for negative (ODI ≤ 0.8) and for positive samples (ODI > 1.0) was suggested in the original evaluation of the inter-laboratory reproducibility of the test [30]. In practice, many European centers actually implemented lower ODI thresholds to classify positive results [31,32] and an index of ≥0.5 has been adopted as the positive test cut-off in the US [33].

Lower ODI cut-offs improve the sensitivity of the test, but also leads to some reduction in specificity. The ODI threshold also influences the timing of positive test results

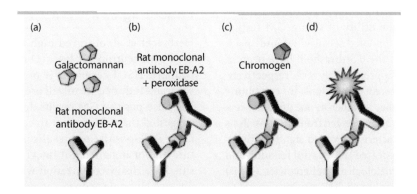

Figure 6.1 Platelia Glatactomannan EIA Test. The assay uses rat EB-A2 monoclonal antibodies directed against *Aspergillus* galactomannan. **(a)** Monoclonal antibodies are used to coat the wells of a microplate. **(b)** Monoclonal antibodies capture the galactomannan antigens and a peroxidase-labled conjugate is added to bind the antigen-antibody-complex. **(c)** A substrate solution is added that reacts with peroxidase. **(d)** Antigen detection via enzymatic color reaction. (Reproduced from Mennink-Kersten, M.A. et al., *Lancet Infect Dis*, 4, 349–57, 2004.)

in relation to the development of signs and/or symptoms of IA. GM antigenemia was detected in the week preceding or coinciding with a conventional diagnosis of IA in 72% of cases of proven or probable disease ($n = 29$) when a cut-off ≥ 0.5 was applied as compared to 41% of the time using the conventional cut-off of 1.5 [32]. This finding was reproduced in 78% of episodes of proven or probable IA when the lower cut-off was used to define a positive test [34]. The primary benefit of the lower threshold, therefore, may actually be the earlier detection of cases of IA.

To maximize accuracy the manufacturer recommends re-testing a second fresh aliquot from all GM positive specimens in addition to collecting a new sample for confirmatory testing from all GM positive patients. Requiring 2 consecutive samples with an OD threshold ≥ 0.5 to define a positive test has been demonstrated to improve test accuracy [32,34]. However, even with consecutive positive samples, the false-positive rate has remained problematic (rate as high as 23%) in some studies [25,35–39].

Frequency of sample collection

The optimal sample collection strategy for IA surveillance has not been rigorously defined. Once or twice weekly determination has generally been used in the published reports to date. In theory, the frequency of monitoring may affect sensitivity, with sporadic testing missing periods of transient antigenemia. Some experts have also recommended assessing GM levels immediately in patients with clinical features suggestive of IA to assist in making a definitive diagnosis [40]. The test performance of GM in a non-surveillance setting, however, is less certain than it is for monitoring high-risk patients.

Test characteristics using serum

Most GM monitoring studies have been conducted in patients receiving cancer chemotherapy or following hematopoietic stem cell transplantation (HSCT), with fewer investigations focused specifically on solid organ transplant (SOT) populations. Three large meta-analyses have attempted to summarize the utility of serum GM testing [41–43] (Table 6.2). Overall, pooled sensitivities and specificities for serum testing at the 0.5 threshold have been in the order of 79%–89% and approximately 85%, respectively.

Although there are inherent limitations in combining multiple heterogeneous studies together in one analysis, several important observations have emerged from meta-analysis studies. First, GM test characteristics varied significantly by host risk group. The assay appeared most useful for adult and pediatric patients with hematological malignancies (HMs) or following HSCT, but was much less sensitive for SOT recipients. This difference may be related to the impact of neutropenia on circulating antigenemia levels. Next, the use of test cut-off values higher than 0.5 reproducibly improved specificity but potentially at the expense of assay sensitivity and studies that used the EORTC/MSG criteria as the reference

Table 6.2 Non-*Aspergillus* species that cross-react with the galactomannan EIA test

Fungus
Acremonium species [44]
Alternaria altenaria [44]
Botrytis tuliae [6]
Blastomyces dermatitidis [45]
Cladosporium cladosporiodes [6]
Cladosporium herbarum [44]
Cryptococcus neoformans [46]
Cryptococcus laurenti [46]
Fusarium oxysporum (not *F. solani*) [6,44]
Geotrichum capitatum [47]
Paecilomyces variotii [39]
Histoplasma capsulatum [48]
Penicillium chrysogenum [6,44]
Penicillium digitatum [6,39]
Penicillium marneffei [6]
Penicillium lilacinus [45]
Nigrospora oryzal [45]
Rhodotorula rubra [6,44]
Phialophora americana [17]
Trichophyton interdigitalis [6]
Trichophyton rubbrum [6]
Wallemia sebi [6]
Wangiella dermatitidis [44]

standard tended to report lower overall sensitivity than did those applying alternative definitions.

Factors affecting serum test performance

GM performance has also been shown to vary based on patient age and as a result of concomitant administration of antibiotics, antifungals, and/or the use of nutritional supplements.

Patient age

Herbrecht et al. observed high false-positive rates in children with neutropenic fever (11 of 25 patients [44%]) and in pediatric HSCT recipients (9 of 12 patients [75%]) [31]. In a separate study of critically ill premature infants, 5 of 6 (83%) had false-positive GM results documented [49]. It has been suggested that GM present in certain milk formulas could cause false-positive test results in children owing to immature and/or impaired gut integrity in the setting of mucositis [50]. Heavy colonization with bifidobacteria, which is observed in some neonates and young infants, has also been implicated as a possible cause of false-positive tests [51].

Differences between adult allogeneic HSCT recipients as compared to autologous HSCT or non-transplant patients have also been reported, with the majority of false-positive tests occurring in the first month after auto-transplant [31].

Similarly, false-positive reactions were more frequent within the first 2 weeks following cytotoxic chemotherapy [7,25,37] or after lung transplantation [52], as well as during periods of graft versus host disease (GvHD) [53,54]. Potential explanations have included dietary absorption of GM [55] due to impaired mucosal barriers after cytotoxic chemotherapy or from GvHD and the presence of interfering substances, such as cyclophosphamide metabolites [56], antibiotics, or auto-antibodies [53,57] that are present during these periods.

Beta lactam antibiotics

The administration of β-lactam antibiotics, including piperacillin-tazobactam, amoxicillin-clavulanate, amoxicillin, ampicillin, and phenoxymethylpenicllin, has all been associated with false-positive GM tests [58–63]. This is not surprising since the mold *Penicillium* is used in the production of these drugs and this organism is known to release GM antigen.

More recent investigations suggest that the newer preparations of piperacillin/tazobactam (PTZ) no longer have the same GM contamination issues. A comparison of blood samples from patients not receiving PTZ ($n = 1606$) to specimens obtained from patients treated with standard doses of the drug ($n = 304$) reported that 1.6% of the non-PTZ specimens tested positive for GM compared to 2.5% of those drawn on PTZ treatment (p = 0.18) [64]. The median GM ODI of the samples drawn in the absence of PTZ was slightly lower than that of those from patients on treatment (0.12 versus 0.14, p < 0.001), but all were below the threshold to define a positive test [64]. In another study, 32 new lots of PTZ and 27 serum specimens obtained from patients receiving PTZ were tested. GM was not detected in any of the PTZ lots and only 1 serum specimen (3.7%) tested positive [65].

Cross reacting microorganisms

Multiple fungi including several human pathogens, common commensals, and potential laboratory contaminants have been shown to cross-react with licensed GM assays (Table 6.3). As a result, positive GM results may also be useful for diagnosing fusariosis, histoplasmosis, and other rarer pathogens, such as *Pacilomyces*. The magnitude of GM release by fungi other than *Aspergillus* or *Penicillium*, however, appears to be significantly lower than is seen with either of the two primary genera [39,44]. One concern has been that patients colonized with *Aspergillus* or *Penicillium* would have false-positive serum GM tests. This has not been observed in the serum studies reporting on colonization among hematology-oncology patients [18], lung transplant recipients [52], and children with cystic fibrosis [38].

False-positive GM tests have also been reported in neutropenic patients with bacteremia [27,39]. However, when the bacterial isolates from these patients were tested directly, no reactivity with the GM EIA was seen [27,39]. Others have failed to confirm false-positive tests in bacteremic patients [37], which suggests that the false-positives may be related to antibiotic usage or another confounder. Only Bifidobacteria (except *B. infantis* and *B. adolescentis*) and *Eggerthella lenta* have been shown to possess reactivity with the GM EIA by virtue of cross-reactive lipoglycan epitopes in the cell wall [51]. Translocation of these organisms into the systemic circulation, therefore, remains a feasible explanation for false-positive tests in some patients.

Antifungal therapy

Marr et al. reported an overall GM sensitivity of 54% with specificity of 98% in 67 adult and pediatric HSCT patients with proven/probably IA using a positive cut off of ≥1.0 [14].

Table 6.3 Meta-analyses of galactomannan serum test performance

Author (No. of studies)	Host risk group	ODI cut-off	Proven IA % (95% CI) Sensitivity	Specificity	Proven/Probable IA % (95% CI) Sensitivity	Specificity	Reference Standard
Pfieffer 2006 [41] (n = 27)	HM	0.5	27 (6–61)	79 (74–83)	79 (69–87)	86 (83–89)	EORTC/MSG or similar criteria
	HSCT	1.0	79 (71–87)	87 (85–88)	65 (57–72)	94 (92–95)	
	SOT NOS	1.5	68 (58–76)	92 (91–93)	48 (41–56)	95 (93–96)	
Leeflang 2015 [42] (n = 50)	HM	0.5	89 (79–99)	72 (62–82)	78 (70–85)	85 (78–91)	EORTC/MSG
	HSCT	1.0	79 (70–89)	83 (78–88)	71 (63–78)	90 (86–93)	
	SOT OTHER	1.5	65 (48–83)	91 (86–96)	63 (49–77)	93 (89–97)	
[a]Lehrnbecher 2016 [43] (n = 25)	HM HSCT	0.5	NR	NR	89 (79–95)	85 (51–97)	EORTC/MSG

Abbreviations: No., number; HM, Hematological malignancies; HSCT, Hematopoietic Stem Cell Transplant recipient; SOT, Solid Organ Transplant recipient; NOS, Not specified; ODI, Optical Density Index; EORTC/MSG, European Organization for Research and Treatment of Cancer/Mycoses Study Group; NR, Not Reported.

[a] Pediatrics only meta-analysis.

Test performance was then recalculated after stratifying for receipt of antifungal therapy (i.e., itraconazole for prophylaxis and Amphotericin B for therapeutic purposes) in the 2 weeks preceding diagnosis of IA. Test sensitivity was significantly lower in those receiving antifungal compounds as compared to those that were not (18% versus 85%) [14]. Similarly, a separate analysis (cut-off value of 0.5) of hematology patients with proven/probable IA found that serum samples from those not on antifungal agents had a GM sensitivity of 89% (95% CI, 65%–97%) as compared to 52% (95% CI, 41%–71%) among samples obtained during antifungal treatment or prophylaxis (i.e., fluconazole or itraconazole prophylaxis and Amphotericin B for antifungal treatment) [66].

A large cohort study of 121 adult hematology patients also evaluated GM test performance in patients on posaconazole prophylaxis [67]. Serum GM was measured twice weekly for surveillance in afebrile patients and as part of a diagnostic algorithm for patients with clinical suspicion for IFI (a positive test was defined as ODI $\geq$0.7 in one sample or $\geq$0.5 in 2 consecutive samples). Overall, GM sensitivity was 100% and specificity 85.5%. The test had 100% NPV and 11.8% PPV when the prevalence of IA was low (i.e., 1.9%) during effective prophylaxis. However, when testing was done for diagnosis due to a high clinical suspicion of IFI (prevalence 55.5%), the NPV remained at 100% but the PPV increased to 89.6% [67]. Taken together, studies have observed a variable impact of antifungal therapy on test sensitivity and false-positive results appear to be more common when prevalence is low due to effective prophylaxis.

Underlying disease

False-negative serum GM results have been reported in a variety of clinical settings, including SOT and patients with congenital immune deficiencies. Examples of immunodeficiencies include a report of false-negative results in a 4 year old with chronic granulomatous disease (CGD) and

progressive pulmonary aspergillosis [68]. Similarly, Walsh et al. reported reduced expression of GM antigenemia in patients with IA and CGD or Job's syndrome [69]. It is hypothesized that angioinvasion might be lower in this host group, thus limiting the amount of circulating GM.

Anti-*Aspergillus* antibodies

One study evaluated the impact that anti-*Aspergillus* antibodies may have on the sensitivity of the GM EIA [31]. Serologic testing for antibodies was performed using an in-house developed assay at the onset of infection in 150 episodes of IA. Anti-*Aspergillus* antibodies were detected in 36% of patients with IA despite their immunocompromised status [31], which is similar to separate study of hematology patients with proven IA (33% seroprevalence) [70]. The sensitivity of the GM test was lower in patients with detectable anti-*Aspergillus* antibodies as compared to patients with negative *Aspergillus* serology (p = 0.0001) [31].

Test characteristics using bronchoalveolar lavage fluid

Two separate meta-analyses (Table 6.4) have evaluated GM testing for the diagnosis of invasive pulmonary aspergillosis (IPA) using bronchoalveolar lavage (BAL) fluid specimens [71,72]. Like serum testing, the majority of BAL studies have focused on adult HM or HSCT patients. Unlike serum testing, however, a single BAL specimen is typically collected for the diagnosis of IPA as opposed to serial monitoring during a defined period of risk. BAL assay sensitivity is approximately 84%–86%, which is equal to or more sensitive than serum testing, and test specificity (89%) has generally been higher with BAL. GM performs best when bronchoscopy is performed in response to CT findings that are suggestive of an IFI resulting in a better prediction for the early detection of IPA in untreated patients.

Table 6.4 Meta-analysis of galactomannan bronchoalveolar lavage fluid test performance

Author (No. of studies)	Host risk group	ODI cut-off	Proven IA % (95% CI) Sensitivity	Specificity	Proven and/or probable IA % (95% CI) Sensitivity	Specificity	Reference standard
Guo 2010 [71] (n = 13)	HM	0.5	NR	NR	86 (70–94)	94 (90–96)	EORTC/MSG or similar criteria
	HSCT	1.0	NR	NR	85 (72–93)	94 (89–97)	
	SOT	1.5	NR	NR	70 (49–85)	96 (93–98)	
	OTHER	2.0	NR	NR	61 (38–80)	96 (92–98)	
Zuo 2012 [72] (n = 30)	HM	0.5	100 (55–100)	77 (64–86)	87 (79–92)	89 (85–92)	EORTC/MSG or similar criteria
	HSCT	1.0	97 (71–100)	83 (75–88)	86 (76–92)	95 (91–97)	
	OTHER	1.5	90 (42–99)	93 (86–97)	85 (71–96)	95 (90–97)	
		2.0	79 (39–96)	93 (89–96)	84 (65–94)	95 (93–96)	
		2.5	45 (15–79)	93 (90–96)	80 (50–94)	95 (93–97)	

Abbreviations: No., number; HM, Hematological malignancies; HSCT, Hematopoietic Stem Cell Transplant recipient; SOT, Solid Organ Transplant recipient; ODI, Optical Density Index; NR, not reported; EORTC/MSG, European Organization for Research and Treatment of Cancer/Mycoses Study Group.

The optimal ODI threshold for BAL samples remains somewhat controversial. In 2011 the US FDA cleared the Platelia EIA for BAL fluids at a cut-off of 0.5 [73]. However, some reports have suggested that a cut-off of ≥1.0 may maximize specificity (low false positivity) with minimal effect on the sensitivity in BAL fluids [74].

Factors affecting performance

AIRWAY COLONIZATION

Aspergillus can be a part of the microbiome found in the upper airways of patients with underlying lung disease. Colonization is especially common in lung transplant recipients, in patients with cystic fibrosis and/or in those with COPD. In a retrospective cohort study of 81 SOT recipients who had BAL testing performed for a variety reasons, 17 (20.9%) were found to have at least one BAL GM result ≥0.5 but only 5 of these patients were diagnosed with proven or probable IPA [75]. False-positive results were disproportionately noted among samples that were culture positive for *Aspergillus* or *Penicillium* and/or had hyphal elements seen on cytology. The level of GM positivity did not differ for patients with IPA versus those that were colonized [75].

ANTIBIOTICS

Few studies have assessed the impact that systemic antibiotics may have on BAL GM values. In one report, 52 patients with a positive BAL GM (≥0.5) were identified and 25 (7%) of these were deemed to be false-positive results [76]. Statistical analysis revealed that treatment with older preparations of PTZ or ampicillin-sulbactam was associated with false-positive BAL GM results.

MOLD ACTIVE ANTIFUNGAL THERAPY

Data regarding the effects of prophylactic or empiric mold active antifungal therapy on BAL GM sensitivity is also conflicting. One recent study found that minimal drug exposure (≥2 days) significantly reduced assay sensitivity (decrease from 100 to 42.9% after treatment) [77]. Two other studies, however, found no differences in sensitivity [78] or GM indices [79] between patients who received no or short duration (mean 3–5 days of treatment) anti-mold therapy.

(1,3)-β-D GLUCAN ASSAY

Assay principles

(1,3)-β-D-Glucan (BDG) is a cell wall polysaccharide found in many fungi; notable exceptions are *Cryptococcus*, the *Mucorales*, and the yeast form of *Blastomyces* [80–82]. All available BDG tests are predicated on the ability of the glucan molecule to induce clot formation in the hemolymph of horseshoe crabs (Figure 6.2). The commercially available chromogenic assays include FungiTec-G (Seikagaku Kogyo Corporation, Tokyo, Japan) and Fungitell (Associates of Cape Cod, Falmouth, MA). Fungitell, previously called Glucatell, is FDA cleared in the US. For the remainder of this review, the Associates of Cape Cod test will be referred to by its current name Fungitell. The Wako test is a turbidimetric based assay manufactured by Wako Pure Chemical Industries (Osaka, Japan).

Kinetics

Little is known about the release and metabolism of BDG *in vivo*. Like gal*f* antigens, BDG is released during the

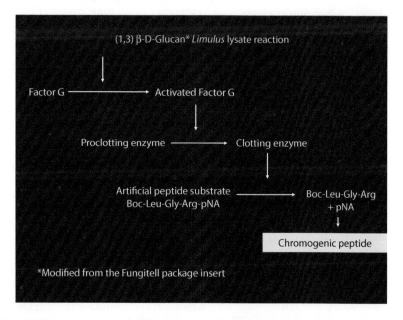

Figure 6.2 Fungitell (1,3)-β-D-Glucan Assay. (1,3)-β-D-Glucan* activates factor G, a serine protease zymogen in the *Limulus* (horseshoe crab) coagulation cascade. Activated factor G converts the inactive pro-clotting enzyme to the active form, which in turn cleaves pNA from the artificial chromogenic peptide substrate Boc-Leu-Gly-Arg-pNA, creating a chromophore that absorbs at 405 nm.

logarithmic growth phase of *Aspergillus fumigatus in vitro* [83]. BDG concentrations then begin to decrease after 24 hours in culture potentially due to the activity of *Aspergillus* cell wall associated glucanases [83]. Similar evaluations with other medically important species (e.g., *Candida* sp., *Fusarium* sp., *Pneumocystis*) have not been published.

Defining a positive result

The BDG level defining a positive test varies by assay. A provisional cut-off for the Fungitell test was determined using stored serum samples collected from 30 non-neutropenic subjects with candidemia [84]. These results were then compared to samples collected from 30 healthy adults. Sera obtained from the candidemic subjects contained a mean BDG concentration of 2999 pg/mL (range, 36–22,263 pg/mL) as compared to 17 pg/mL (range, 0–86 pg/mL) in blood of healthy volunteers. A positive cut-off value of ≥60 pg/mL was selected in this study because it appeared to optimize both the sensitivity (97%) and specificity (93%) of the test [84].

The FDA cleared protocol for Fungitell defines a single positive value of ≥80 pg/mL as positive, and levels from 60 to 79 pg/mL as "equivocal" results. The ≥80 pg/mL was established in a multicenter validation study [85]. It is important to note that optimal thresholds may be different for children and that these have not been extensively defined [86]. Additionally, the Fungitell cut-off is higher than the values established for the Fungitec-G and Wako assays. A 20 pg/mL threshold was set for Fungitec-G test based on the observation that plasma BDG levels in 60 healthy adult controls

were all <10 pg/mL and 37 of 41 patients with autopsy-verified or microbiologically documented fungal infections had concentrations above this level (sensitivity 90% [95% CI; 77%–97%]) [87]. At a concentration >20 pg/mL, the Fungitec-G test also showed 100% specificity when analyzing 59 samples from subjects with non-fungal infection or fever of non-infectious origin [87]. The dissimilarity of cut-off values among chromogenic test kits may be related to differences in the affinity/reactivity of reagents used in each assay. Reagents utilized in the test Fungitell are extracted from *Limulus polyphemus,* a different genera of horseshoe crab than is used in Fungitec-GT (*Tachypleus tridentatus*) [84].

Test characteristics

Several recent meta-analyses have attempted to summarize BDG test characteristics (Table 6.5) [88–95]. BDG test performance has differed (to varying degrees) based on patient population, assay brand name, and the reference standard used to adjudicate IFI diagnoses. Pooled estimates of assay sensitivity and specificity values for IFI have ranged widely from 62% to 89% and 76% to 93%, respectively.

When the sensitivity of the test for individual organism groups was evaluated, BDG performed best for the diagnosis of *Pneumocystis jirovecii* pneumonia (PJP), with consistently high sensitivity (91%–95%) and low negative likelihood ratios (0.06–0.12) for both HIV and non-HIV patient populations [89,92,93]. In comparison, BDG sensitivity for the diagnosis of IC is approximately 80% and IA is 75%.

Table 6.5 Meta-analysis of (1,3)-β-D glucan test performance

Author (No. of studies)	Sub-group analyses		Sensitivity % (95% CI)	Specificity % (95% CI)	Reference standard
Karageorgopoulos 2011 [88] (n = 16)		Fungitell/ Glucatell	71(60–81)	82(70–90)	EORTC/MSG
Onishi 2012 [89] (n = 31)	Assay	Fungitell	75(71–79)	77(75–79)	EORTC/MSG or similar criteria
		Fungitec G	89(83–93)	90(88–92)	
		Wako	84(77–90)	90(87–92)	
	Mycosis	Candidiasis	81(77–85)	81(80–83)	
		Aspergillosis	77(71–82)	83(82–85)	
		PJP	96(92–98)	84(83–86)	
He 2015 [90] (n = 28)	Assay	Fungitell	75(71–79)	76(74–78)	EORTC/MSG or similar criteria
		Fungitec G	86(79–91)	93(90–95)	
		Wako	83(76–89)	90(88–93)	
Hou 2015 [91] (n = 11)	Assay	Fungitell	82(68–90)	86(77–92)	EORTC/MSG
	Mycosis	Candidiasis	80(67–90)	77(67–89)	
		Aspergillosis	73(62–86)	81(64–85)	
Lu 2011 [94] (n = 12)	Assay	Fungitell	75(67–82)	79(61–90)	EORTC/MSG
[a]Lamoth 2012 [95] (n = 6)	Assay	NR	62(48–73)	91(83–95)	EORTC/MSG

Abbreviations: No., number; IFI: Invasive Fungal infection; PJP: Pneumocystis jiroveci; EORTC/MSG: European Organization for Research and Treatment of Cancer/Mycoses Study Group.

[a] Hematology/oncology patients only.

Additional studies have focused on the diagnostic utility of BDG testing specifically in the adult surgical and/or medical ICU. These are clinical settings where mortality attributable to IC remains high, in part due to difficulties and delays in making a culture based diagnosis. In meta-analyses subgroup analyses, the sensitivity and specificity of BDG for IC in the ICU population was approximately 75% and 80%, respectively. Sequential sampling has helped increase specificity in some individual reports [96,97], but PPVs and specificities were generally lower in the critical care setting than in hematology/oncology. Several studies evaluating serial surveillance have also reported earlier identification of IC using BDG (3–6 days sooner) as compared to culture [97,98].

The BDG assay has also been compared to other diagnostic modalities used in critical care. The *Candida* score is a risk assessment tool that aids in differentiation between colonization and invasive infection for non-neutropenic ICU patients. Multifocal *Candida* colonization, total parenteral nutrition, surgery as the reason for ICU admission, and/or clinical symptoms of severe sepsis have been identified as independent predictors of systemic candidiasis in this population. To calculate the *Candida* score, each risk factor is assigned a value of 1 except severe sepsis, which is assigned a value of 2. Scores > 2.5 had a sensitivity of 81% and specificity of 74% for IC [99]. The *Candida* colonization index is defined as the ratio of the number of culture-positive sites to the number of sites cultured, with a threshold of 0.4–0.5 used to potentially initiate preemptive treatment. On the whole, BDG testing has been shown to be more sensitive than either the *Candida* score or the *Candida* colonization index. In two of the larger comparative studies, the sensitivity of BDG testing ranged from 93% to 100% compared to 50%–86% and 64%–75% for the *Candida* score and index, respectively [98,100]

Mannan antigen (Ag) and anti-mannan antibody (Ab) assays (Platelia BioRad; Marnes-la-Coquette France) along with the *Candida albicans* germ tube antibody (CAGTA) test (Vircell kit; Granada Spain) are widely used in Europe. In a meta-analysis, mannan and anti-mannan test sensitivities/specifies were 58%/93% and 59%/83%, respectively. When combined, the assays had 83% sensitivity and 86% sensitivity [101]. A large single center prospective study recently compared all available *Candida* cell wall biomarkers [102]. The study included twice weekly biomarker surveillance in 233 ICU patients with severe abdominal conditions. BDG was the most sensitive (76.7% [95% CI; 57.7%–90.1%]) and least specific (57.2% [95% CI; 49.9%–64.3%]) test. In comparison, mannan Ag, mannan Ab, and CAGTA test had sensitivities/specificities of 43.3%/67.3%, 25.8%/89.0%, and 53.3%/64.3%, respectively. The combination of BDG positivity plus CAGTA showed the greatest sensitivity (90.3%) with high NPV (96.6%), although the specificity was only 42.1% [102]. Similarly, Martinez-Jimenez et al. [103] also observed that sequential positive BDGs plus CAGTAs had a high sensitivity (96.7%) and NPV (97.1%).

The impact of infection prevalence

Figure 6.3 illustrates the impact that IC prevalence has on BDG predictive values, assuming an assay sensitivity of 75% and specificity of 80% for candidiasis in the ICU setting. These calculations are useful for assessing the magnitude of uncertainty around BDG results, but the precise determination of an individual patient's pre-test probability for IC may be difficult to estimate in real-time clinical practice.

As is illustrated in the figure, low pre-test probability (i.e., 3% prevalence in a general ICU population) with a negative BDG result makes candidiasis highly unlikely. In patients with moderate risk (i.e., 10% prevalence as identified by prediction rules [104]) there is about a 3%–4% chance that a negative test is a false-negative result. In those with higher risk (i.e., 30% prevalence), the chance of missing IC with a negative result is 12%. Thus, using BDG results to stop or withhold antifungals may be best deployed in the 3%–10% prevalence range. Below 3% prevalence, the test is unlikely to add much. The optimal pre-test probability to use positive BDG results to initiate preemptive therapy is more difficult to estimate and may be on the order of 15%–35% based on observations that prophylaxis can be beneficial in ICUs with baseline IFI rates in this range [105]. For extremely high-risk patients, such as those with complicated gastrointestinal surgeries, prophylaxis may be preferred.

Factors associated with false-positive results

A variety of different interferences are known to affect BDG results and many of these are common in the ICU and on hematology-oncology wards. False-positive BDG results have been associated with immunoglobulin therapy (e.g., IVIg), albumin supplementation, and other blood products that are filtered through cellulose filters [106–109]. One study suggested BDG may remain positive for up to 3 days after discontinuation of IVIg therapy [106]. Likewise,

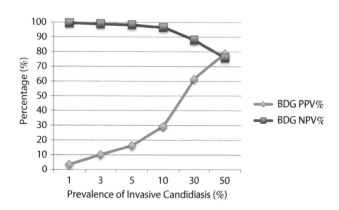

Figure 6.3 (1,3)-Beta-D-Glucan (BDG) predictive values. Abbreviations: PPV, positive predictive value; NPV, negative predictive value.

cellulose containing dialysis membranes are known to cause false-positive BDG tests in some patients [110] and the dialysis procedure, irrespective of filter type, may interfere with the BDG test [96,111]. It has been hypothesized that transient hypoperfusion occurs during hemodialysis and this potentially promotes translocation of gut microbes into the bloodstream, which in turn results in a false-positive BDG test. Awareness of a patient's surgical history is also essential. Serosal exposure to glucan containing gauze products has resulted in positive BDG tests in the immediate postoperative period [112] and factors associated with lung transplantations can be problematic [111]. Lastly, laboratory contamination of samples is possible if glucan free glassware and/or plastics are not used when performing the test.

Marty et al. also tested 44 different antimicrobials for the presence of BDG [113]. Colistin, ertapenem, cefazolin, trimethoprim-sulfamethoxazole, cefotaxime, cefepime, and ampicillin-sulbactam were all positive for BDG at the reconstituted vial concentrations but not when diluted to maximal plasma concentrations. Interestingly, none of the lots of PTZ tested in this study were positive for BDG. Other investigators have also correlated false-positive results with receipt of amoxicillin-clavulanic acid, and BDG has been directly detected in the batches of this antibiotic [111,114,115]. Lastly, there has also been a report of false-positive BDG result in patients with Gram-positive bacteremia [115], as well as with *Alcaligenes faecalis*.

MOLECULAR DIAGNOSTICS

Nucleic acid amplification technologies have been increasingly applied for the detection and identification of fungal pathogens directly from clinical specimens. The majority of these assays are laboratory-developed tests (LDTs) based on polymerase chain reaction (PCR) techniques that amplify gene targets specific to a suspected pathogen or group of pathogens. Well-designed PCR assays have the potential to be highly sensitive and specific, and are amendable to preemptive surveillance strategies.

Aspergillus PCR

Aspergillus LDTs have been developed using a variety of gene targets, specimen types (e.g., whole blood versus plasma or serum), nucleic acid extraction methods, and PCR chemistries. As a result, these assays have varied significantly in terms of their clinical performance. In a meta-analysis of 16 studies that combined results from more than 10,000 serum, plasma, or whole blood samples the overall sensitivity of a single positive *Aspergillus* PCR was 88% and specificity 75% for proven/probable IA [116]. Requiring two sequential positive PCR results to define a positive test increased specificity without affecting sensitivity [116].

The European *Aspergillus* PCR Initiative (EAPCRI) has systematically evaluated and compared different protocols in an attempt to better define the critical components of blood-based *Aspergillus* PCR assays [117]. Using whole blood specimens spiked with *Aspergillus* conidia, extraction variables, including specimen volume, use of a mechanical fungal cell wall disruption step, lysis of white cells, and elution volume all had a significant impact on assay sensitivity. This work resulted in recommendations for optimal *Aspergillus* nucleic acid extraction from whole blood [117].

The optimal fraction of blood to test for IA surveillance purposes, however, has not been defined. From the clinical laboratory perspective plasma or serum are easier to work with than is whole blood. Serum also has the added advantage of allowing simultaneous GM testing from the same specimen. Springer et al. recently compared the three blood fractions using the recommended EAPCRI protocol [118]. Plasma PCR had the highest sensitivity (91%), followed by serum (80%) and then whole blood pellets (55%); but specificity was highest using whole blood pellets (96%) compared to either serum (69%; $p = 0.024$) or plasma (53%; $p = 0.0002$). When two or more specimens with detectable DNA were required to define positive test, the specificity of plasma increased to 91.7% with only a small decline in sensitivity to 81.8%. These findings, along with an additional study [119], suggested that plasma might be optimal for preemptive protocols.

Aspergillus PCR testing has also been applied to lower respiratory tract specimens. A meta-analysis of 15 different BAL studies reported a pooled sensitivity and specificity of 79% and 94%, respectively, for proven/probable IPA [120]. Performing PCR and GM together may further enhance sensitivity. In a meta-analysis comparing the two diagnostic modalities, PCR test performance was similar to that of GM in BAL fluid using an ODI of 0.5 [121]. However, if either PCR or GM was used to define a positive result, the pooled sensitivity was higher than for either test alone without affecting specificity [121]. Additionally, while higher fungal burdens determined by quantitative PCR test may be more suggestive of tissue invasion there is significant overlap between fungal loads measured in cases of airway colonization as compared to invasive disease.

Candida PCR

Multiple studies have evaluated the performance of *Candida* PCR (largely LDTs) applied to different fractions of blood for the diagnosis of IC. A recent meta-analysis combined 54 *Candida* PCR studies with data for 4694 patients and 963 had proven/probable or possible IC [122]. Pooled sensitivity and specificity for the diagnosis of candidemia was 95% (95% CI; 88%–98%) and 92% (88%–95%), respectively. PCR positivity rates among patients with proven or probable IC was 85% (78%–91%), while blood cultures were comparatively positive for only 38% (29%–46%) of subjects. The use of whole-blood samples, rDNA, or P450 gene targets and a PCR detection limit of ≤ 10 CFU/mL were associated with optimal test performance [122].

A prospective case control study also compared a *Candida* PCR to the Fungitell BDG assay for the diagnosis of IC. The sensitivity and specificity of PCR versus BDG was 80% versus 56% ($p = 0.03$) and 70% versus 73% ($p = 0.31$), respectively.

Among 24 patients with deep-seated candidiasis, both PCR (88%) and BDG (62%) were more sensitive than blood cultures (17%). PCR was statistically most sensitive for all forms of IC while both PCR and BDG were both more sensitive than a blood culture in cases of deep-seated candidiasis. The authors concluded that PCR combined with BDG testing was a valuable tool for diagnosing IC [123].

PCR limitations

There are multiple important limitations associated with fungal molecular testing. Because molds are ubiquitous in the environment and *Candida* may be present on the skin, fungal DNA contamination of reagents and collection devices must be monitored and along with careful attention to specimen collection procedures. Knowledge of the assay's gene target(s) is also critical. *Aspergillus* assays targeting ribosomal DNA will likely cross-react with *Penicillium* sp. due to sequence similarities across these genera. This potential cross-reactivity is not as important for blood testing as it is for respiratory tract sampling from potentially colonized patients. Furthermore, *Aspergillus fumigatus* specific assay designs or PCRs designed to identify only the most common *Candida* species will miss infections caused by other pathogenic species. Ultimately, commercially available assays are needed to increase uptake of molecular testing in the US.

PREEMPTIVE ANTIFUNGAL APPROACHES FOR HIGH RISK PATIENTS

The overarching goals of a preemptive therapeutic strategy are potentially two-fold. The first aim is to safely limit use of antifungal treatment for patients that are unlikely to benefit and next is to initiate treatment early for patients with pre-symptomatic infection. As such, the ideal diagnostic should be both sensitive and specific and applied in a setting where the NPV (for withholding or stopping antifungal therapy) and/or PPV (for initiating preemptive treatment) are high. This section reviews the larger prospective intervention studies and a recent meta-analysis of preemptive approaches for IA and IC.

Preemptive studies focused on invasive aspergillosis

The first study to evaluate the feasibility and safety of a preemptive approach for IA used GM testing with defined triggers for high resolution CT (HRCT) scans in patients with cancer and prolonged neutropenia [124]. This observational study evaluated 136 neutropenic episodes in 88 patients. Most study subjects had AML and all received fluconazole prophylaxis. IFI was suspected when there was neutropenic fever despite appropriate broad spectrum antibiotics, other clinical signs/symptoms of IFI, new pulmonary infiltrates, isolation of mold or hyphal elements in a respiratory specimen, and/or two consecutive GM EIAs with an ODI ≥0.5.

Follow-up testing included HRCT guided bronchoscopy with BAL and possible endoscopic biopsies. Patients with ≥2 consecutive positive GM tests or those who had suggestive CT findings with a positive fungal culture or microscopic evaluation received preemptive liposomal amphotericin.

In all, only 9 febrile neutropenia episodes (8%) were treated based on the preemptive algorithm though 41 (35%) would have qualified for empiric treatment using a fever-driven empiric approach. The algorithm led to an estimated 27% reduction in antifungal use, without impacting overall mortality. Of note, one case of mucormycosis and two cases of invasive candidiasis were not detected by the GM strategy, which targets *Aspergillus* [124].

This pilot study was then followed up with the first prospective, randomized, multicenter trial of preemptive therapy that included 403 HSCT recipients receiving fluconazole or amphotericin prophylaxis [125]. Subjects were randomized to *Aspergillus* PCR driven preemptive therapy ($n = 196$) or fever-based empiric therapy ($n = 207$). Whole blood PCR testing was performed twice a week during the first 30 days and then once weekly for up to 90 days after transplant. Antifungal treatment was initiated following one positive PCR result (preemptive group only) or for febrile neutropenia for more than 5 days despite broad-spectrum antibacterial therapy. Subjects could have also received targeted treatment if there was other clinical suspicion for IFI, regardless of group assignment.

A total of 112 (57.1%) patients in preemptive group and 76 (36.7%) in empiric group received antifungal treatment. Excess antifungal use in the preemptive arm was mostly driven by PCR negative cases that had persistent fever. The incidence of IFI did not differ significantly between the groups (14.3% versus 15.8% in the empiric group), but all-cause mortality was lower in the preemptive arm at 30 days (1.5% versus 6.3%; p = 0.015). A possible survival benefit with preemptive therapy, however, was not evident at day 100 [125].

A second randomized multicenter trial also compared fever-driven empiric treatment to a preemptive approach [126]. Preemptive therapy was initiated for patients with clinical and radiographic features of IFI or for a positive GM EIA test (ODI ≥ 1.5). In this study, subjects received antifungal prophylaxis per institution specific protocols and an amphotericin product was first line treatment for suspected IFIs.

A total of 293 adult neutropenic patients were recruited, with 150 randomized to the empiric arm and 143 in preemptive arm. The groups were well balanced with regard to the duration of neutropenia and survival. However, IFI incidence was higher in the preemptive group compared to the empiric group (9.1% versus 2.7%, respectively). Most IFIs occurred during induction chemotherapy as opposed to consolidation treatments or following HSCT and many breakthrough infections were with *Candida* sp. [126].

Fung et al. then combined 9 studies that compared empiric to preemptive treatment in adult HM patients [127]. Empiric antifungal therapy was typically triggered by febrile neutropenia despite broad-spectrum antibiotics while preemptive strategies included a combination of cell wall biomarker, molecular, and imaging findings. Duration and exposure to antifungals was found to be significantly lower with the preemptive approaches (RR 0.48, 95% CI; 0.27–0.85) without increase in IFI related mortality (RR 0.82, 95% CI; 0.36–1.87) or overall mortality (RR 0.95, 95% CI; 0.46–1.99). Cost comparisons showed that preemptive approaches saved $324 per febrile episode [127].

Combination biomarker testing for *Aspergillus*

The optimal test or combination of tests to use for *Aspergillus* surveillance has also been a topic of substantial interest. In a multicenter randomized controlled trial standard microbiologic testing (i.e., fungal culture and histology) was compared to standard testing plus biomarker surveillance using *Aspergillus* PCR combined with GM (ODI $\geq$ 0.5) [128]. Biomarkers were performed twice weekly for inpatients and once a week for outpatients. A single positive GM and/or PCR as well as serially negative GM and PCR in patients with persistent neutropenic fever were followed by HRCT. Subjects with a scan suggestive of IFI were treated with antifungal therapy. Of note, the reference standard used to define probable or possible IA varied between groups because biomarker results were factored in to the composite IFI definition in the surveillance arm.

A total of 240 patients with HM or HSCT were recruited, with 122 assigned to the standard diagnostic strategy and 118 to the biomarker-based approach. During the 26-week follow-up period the total number of antifungal treatment courses was significantly greater in the standard diagnosis group as compared to the biomarker group (113 [21%] versus 47 [9%] treatment courses; p < 0.0001). The incidence of histologically proven IA was similar between groups, but the number of probable IFIs was higher in the biomarker group (16 [14%] versus 0; p < 0.0001) likely because a positive biomarker result was included in the final adjudication of disease. Additionally, more probable cases in the biomarker group were diagnosed by PCR than by GM (11 versus 5). All-cause mortality did not significantly different across group and no patient with serially negative biomarkers had IA diagnosed by standard methods. Retrospective application of biomarkers to the standard diagnostics group would also have decreased time to diagnosis by 4–7 days [128].

A second group of investigators conducted a randomized control trial comparing the utility of serum GM alone ($\geq$2 consecutive samples with ODI indices between 0.5 and 0.7 or a single determination $\geq$0.7) to serum *Aspergillus* PCR plus GM (PCR+GM) in high-risk hematology patients [129]. Positivity in either assay triggered a HRCT and initiation of antifungal therapy was based on the results. No anti-mold prophylaxis was used in the study. A total of 219 subjects were randomized, 114 to the GM only and 105 to the GM + PCR group. The incidence of proven or probable IA was lower in the GM+PCR group (4.2% versus 13.1%; p = 0.028) as was the use of empiric antifungal therapy (16.7% versus 29.0%; p = 0.038). In addition, the median time to diagnosis of IA was shorter in the molecular arm (13 days versus 20 days for GM only; p = 0.02). Patients in the GM+PCR group had higher proven or probable IA–free survival (p = 0.03), but all-cause mortality did not significantly differ between groups (13.5% versus 15.9% in the GM only group; p = 0.695) [129].

Preemptive studies focused on invasive candidiasis in the ICU

The first proof-of-concept study assessing a preemptive approach in the ICU was a single center pilot study that compared preemptive anidulafungin driven by a single positive BDG result ($\geq$60 pg/mL) to empiric therapy [96]. Sixty-four general ICU patients were randomized, with 1 proven IFI case in the empiric group and 5 probable cases identified (2 in the empiric group and 3 in the preemptive group). Although the study was small, several important observations were made. First, more subjects in the preemptive arm received antifungal therapy (53% versus 29%; p = 0.16) and 55% of subjects had at least 1 positive BDG during the ICU admission. Changing the diagnostic algorithm to require at least 2 sequential results $\geq$80 pg/mL, however, would have increased specificity (PPV 30%) and reduced the number of patients preemptively treated without compromising sensitivity [96].

The first randomized, multicenter, double-blind placebo controlled trial of echinocandin prophylaxis in the ICU also included twice weekly BDG surveillance with results reported to clinicians [130]. The incidence of proven/probable IC among 219 at-risk patients receiving prophylaxis or placebo was evaluated and there was no statistical difference noted between groups (9.8% of IC cases in the prophylaxis arm versus 16.7% with placebo; p = 0.14). There were also no differences in secondary end-points, including systemic antifungal use, all-cause mortality, or lengths of hospital and ICU stay between groups. Seven of the 8 (87.5%) proven IC cases had at least 1 positive BDG value and probable cases were adjudicated based on the basis of 2 positive BDG results with clinical signs/symptoms. The number of subjects in the placebo group treated on the basis of BDG surveillance was not reported, but the authors concluded that a preemptive approach deserves further study [130].

A more recent study evaluated the use of BDG ($\geq$80 pg/mL) to direct antifungal therapy for 198 critically ill adult patients with signs and symptoms of sepsis and a *Candiada* score $\geq$3 [131]. There were 47 cases of candidemia and all had a positive BDG. A total of 63 patients tested positive for BDG and were treated, with antifungal therapy eventually stopped for the 16 false-positive cases once IC was ruled out. Antifungal therapy was avoided in approximately 73% of potentially treatable patients based in part on negative BDG results and treatment was shortened in another 20% of cases. Overall, the BDG negative group received less antifungal therapy than did the positive group (10 days versus 5 days; p = 0.04) without impacting outcomes [131].

CONCLUSIONS AND FUTURE DIRECTIONS

Preemptive treatment strategies that incorporate biomarker tests are an attractive approach for the management of IFI because they offer an opportunity to serially monitor at-risk patients and potentially identify infection early, at a point where treatment may be more effective. Additionally, patients without surrogate markers of infection could then be spared the potential toxicity and cost associated with unnecessary empiric or prophylactic treatment. The current literature on biomarker test performance is limited by heterogeneity in study designs, differences in reference standards, and variable test cut-offs used to signal a positive result. Despite this variability, however, most prospective studies have shown that biomarker surveillance can reduce antifungal use relative to empiric therapy without affecting microbiologic or clinical outcomes. It should be noted that individual studies were not necessarily powered to detect a mortality difference and that false-positive biomarker results remain problematic.

Deciding whether or not to deploy a preemptive approach will likely depend on the pretest probability of IFI in a given setting combined with laboratory resources. In-house biomarker testing that is performed at least once or twice weekly is ideally required to inform preemptive treatment decisions in a clinically meaningful timeframe. For *Aspergillus*, the combination of GM testing with PCR as surveillance looks to be superior to either test alone and to routine microbiologic testing with empiric therapy. Fungi other than *Aspergillus* have caused most breakthrough infections. Therefore, future studies should evaluate a preemptive IA strategy combined with *Candida* prophylaxis as compared to universal prophylaxis with a broad-spectrum agent, such as posaconazole or isavuconazole.

Preemptive approaches for IC also appear feasible and there have been no safety concerns raised when testing is combined with routine microbiology and clinical judgment in moderate-risk ICU settings. The possibility that false-positive BDG results would drive unnecessary antifungal use have not necessarily been observed, especially when sequential testing and/or higher cut-offs were employed. Future preemptive studies should seek to identify the optimal test or combination of tests for IC and the role that these can play in preemptive management.

In conclusion, laboratory screening strategies that include single or multiple fungal biomarkers is preferred to empiric treatment for the early detection of IFI, but the optimal testing algorithms have not been determined. When used judiciously in combination with other findings, biomarkers may identify more IFI patents at earlier stages of disease. Randomized intervention trials are ultimately required to assess the potential impact of preemptive strategies on morbidity and mortality as well as to determine the cost effectiveness of diagnostic-based surveillance as compared to usual care.

REFERENCES

1. Marr KA, Leisenring W. Design issues in studies evaluating diagnostic tests for aspergillosis. *Clin Infect Dis* 2005;41 Suppl 6:S381–386.
2. Ascioglu S, et al. Defining opportunistic invasive fungal infections in immunocompromised patients with cancer and hematopoietic stem cell transplants: an international consensus. *Clin Infect Dis* 2002;34(1):7–14.
3. De Pauw B, et al. Revised Definitions of Invasive Fungal Disease from the European Organization for Research and Treatment of Cancer/Invasive Fungal Infections Cooperative Group and the National Institute of Allergy and Infectious Diseases Mycoses Study Group (EORTC/MSG) Consensus Group. *Clinical Infectious Diseases* 2008;46(12):1813–1821.
4. Latge JP, et al. Chemical and immunological characterization of the extracellular galactomannan of *Aspergillus fumigatus*. *Infect Immun* 1994;62(12):5424–5433.
5. Reiss E, Lehmann PF. Galactomannan antigenemia in invasive aspergillosis. *Infection and Immunity* 1979;25(1):357–365.
6. Stynen D, et al. Rat monoclonal antibodies against *Aspergillus galactomannan*. *Infect Immun* 1992;60(6):2237–2245.
7. Stynen D, et al. A new sensitive sandwich enzyme-linked immunosorbent assay to detect galactofuran in patients with invasive aspergillosis. *J Clin Microbiol* 1995;33(2):497–500.
8. Sarfati J, Boucias DG, Latge JP. Antigens of *Aspergillus fumigatus* produced *in vivo*. *J Med Vet Mycol* 1995;33(1):9–14.
9. Morelle W, et al. Galactomannoproteins of *Aspergillus fumigatus*. *Eukaryot Cell* 2005;4(7):1308–1316.
10. Thornton CR. Development of an immunochromatographic lateral-flow device for rapid serodiagnosis of invasive aspergillosis. *Clinical and Vaccine Immunology* 2008;15(7):1095–1105.
11. Verweij PE, et al. Sandwich enzyme-linked immunosorbent assay compared with Pastorex latex agglutination test for diagnosing invasive aspergillosis in immunocompromised patients. *J Clin Microbiol* 1995;33(7):1912–1914.
12. Mennink-Kersten MA, Donnelly JP, Verweij PE. Detection of circulating galactomannan for the diagnosis and management of invasive aspergillosis. *Lancet Infect Dis* 2004;4(6):349–357.
13. Hope WW, et al. Pathogenesis of *Aspergillus fumigatus* and the kinetics of galactomannan in an *in vitro* model of early invasive pulmonary aspergillosis: implications for antifungal therapy. *J Infect Dis* 2007;195(3):455–466.

14. Marr KA, et al. Detection of galactomannan antigenemia by enzyme immunoassay for the diagnosis of invasive aspergillosis: Variables that affect performance. *J Infect Dis* 2004;190(3):641–649.

15. Sheppard DC, et al. Comparison of three methodologies for the determination of pulmonary fungal burden in experimental murine aspergillosis. *Clin Microbiol Infect* 2006;12(4):376–380.

16. Boutboul F, et al. Invasive aspergillosis in allogeneic stem cell transplant recipients: Increasing antigenemia is associated with progressive disease. *Clin Infect Dis* 2002;34(7):939–943.

17. Bretagne S, et al. Serum *Aspergillus galactomannan* antigen testing by sandwich ELISA: Practical use in neutropenic patients. *J Infect* 1997;35(1):7–15.

18. Maertens J, et al. Screening for circulating galactomannan as a noninvasive diagnostic tool for invasive aspergillosis in prolonged neutropenic patients and stem cell transplantation recipients: A prospective validation. *Blood* 2001;97(6):1604–1610.

19. Klont RR, et al. Paradoxical increase in circulating *Aspergillus* antigen during treatment with caspofungin in a patient with pulmonary aspergillosis. *Clin Infect Dis* 2006;43(3):e23–25.

20. Miceli MH, Anaissie EJ. When a paradoxical increase in serum galactomannan antigen during caspofungin therapy is not paradoxical after all. *Clin Infect Dis* 2007;44(5):757–760; author reply 760–761.

21. Petraitiene R, et al. Antifungal efficacy of caspofungin (MK-0991) in experimental pulmonary aspergillosis in persistently neutropenic rabbits: Pharmacokinetics, drug disposition, and relationship to galactomannan antigenemia. *Antimicrob Agents Chemother* 2002;46(1):12–23.

22. El Saleeby CM, et al. Discordant rise in galactomannan antigenemia in a patient with resolving Aspergillosis, renal failure, and ongoing hemodialysis. *J Clin Microbiol* 2005;43(7):3560–3563.

23. Bennett JE, Friedman MM, Dupont B. Receptor-mediated clearance of *Aspergillus galactomannan*. J Infect Dis 1987;155(5):1005–1010.

24. Dupont B, et al. Galactomannan antigenemia and antigenuria in aspergillosis: Studies in patients and experimentally infected rabbits. *J Infect Dis* 1987;155(1):1–11.

25. Sulahian A, et al. Value of antigen detection using an enzyme immunoassay in the diagnosis and prediction of invasive aspergillosis in two adult and pediatric hematology units during a 4-year prospective study. *Cancer* 2001;91(2):311–318.

26. Williamson EC, et al. *Aspergillus* antigen testing in bone marrow transplant recipients. *J Clin Pathol* 2000;53(5):362–366.

27. Pazos C, Ponton J, Del Palacio A. Contribution of (1->3)-beta-D-glucan chromogenic assay to diagnosis and therapeutic monitoring of invasive aspergillosis in neutropenic adult patients: A comparison with serial screening for circulating galactomannan. *J Clin Microbiol* 2005;43(1):299–305.

28. Bretagne S, Costa JM. Towards a molecular diagnosis of invasive aspergillosis and disseminated candidosis. *FEMS Immunol Med Microbiol* 2005;45(3):361–368.

29. Weisser M, et al. Galactomannan does not precede major signs on a pulmonary computerized tomographic scan suggestive of invasive aspergillosis in patients with hematological malignancies. *Clin Infect Dis* 2005;41(8):1143–1149.

30. Verweij PE, et al. Detection of antigen in sera of patients with invasive aspergillosis: Intra- and interlaboratory reproducibility. The Dutch Interuniversity Working Party for Invasive Mycoses. *J Clin Microbiol* 1998;36(6):1612–1616.

31. Herbrecht R, et al. *Aspergillus galactomannan* detection in the diagnosis of invasive aspergillosis in cancer patients. *J Clin Oncol* 2002;20(7):1898–1906.

32. Maertens J, et al. Prospective clinical evaluation of lower cut-offs for galactomannan detection in adult neutropenic cancer patients and haematological stem cell transplant recipients. *Br J Haematol* 2004;126(6):852–860.

33. Wheat LJ. Rapid diagnosis of invasive aspergillosis by antigen detection. *Transpl Infect Dis* 2003;5(4):158–166.

34. Maertens JA, et al. Optimization of the cut-off value for the *Aspergillus* double-sandwich enzyme immunoassay. *Clinical Infectious Diseases* 2007;44(10):1329–1336.

35. Maertens J, et al. Use of circulating galactomannan screening for early diagnosis of invasive aspergillosis in allogeneic stem cell transplant recipients. *J Infect Dis* 186(9):1297–1306.

36. Pinel C, et al. Detection of circulating *Aspergillus fumigatus* Galactomannan: Value and limits of the platelia test for diagnosing invasive Aspergillosis. *J Clin Microbiol* 2003;41(5):2184–2186.

37. Maertens J, et al. Autopsy-controlled prospective evaluation of serial screening for circulating Galactomannan by a sandwich enzyme-linked immunosorbent assay for hematological patients at risk for invasive aspergillosis. *J Clin Microbiol* 1999;37(10):3223–3228.

38. Rohrlich P, et al. Prospective sandwich enzyme-linked immunosorbent assay for serum galactomannan: Early predictive value and clinical use in invasive aspergillosis. *Pediatr Infect Dis J* 1996;15(3):232–237.

39. Swanink CM, et al. Specificity of a sandwich enzyme-linked immunosorbent assay for detecting *Aspergillus galactomannan*. *Journal of Clinical Microbiology* 1997;35(1):257–260.

40. Hope WW, Walsh TJ, Denning DW. Laboratory diagnosis of invasive aspergillosis. *Lancet Infect Dis* 2005;5(10):609–622.

41. Pfeiffer CD, Fine JP, Safdar N. Diagnosis of invasive aspergillosis using a galactomannan assay: A meta-analysis. *Clin Infect Dis* 2006;42(10):1417–1427.

42. Leeflang MM, et al. Galactomannan detection for invasive aspergillosis in immunocompromised patients. *Cochrane Database Syst Rev* 2015;12:Cd007394.

43. Lehrnbecher T, et al. Galactomannan, Beta-D-Glucan and PCR-Based Assays for the Diagnosis of Invasive Fungal Disease in Pediatric Cancer and Hematopoietic Stem Cell Transplantation: A Systematic Review and Meta-Analysis. Clinical Infectious Diseases 2016.

44. Kappe R, Schulze-Berge A. New cause for false-positive results with the Pastorex *Aspergillus* antigen latex agglutination test. *J Clin Microbiol* 1993;31(9):2489–2490.

45. Cummings JR, et al. Cross-reactivity of non-Aspergillus fungal species in the *Aspergillus galactomannan* enzyme immunoassay. *Diagn Microbiol Infect Dis* 2007;59(1):113–115.

46. Dalle F, et al. *Cryptococcus neoformans* Galactoxylomannan contains an epitope(s) that is cross-reactive with *Aspergillus galactomannan*. *J Clin Microbiol* 2005;43(6):2929–2931.

47. Giacchino M, et al. *Aspergillus galactomannan* enzyme-linked immunosorbent assay cross-reactivity caused by invasive *Geotrichum capitatum*. *J Clin Microbiol* 2006;44(9):3432–3434.

48. Wheat LJ, et al. Histoplasmosis-associated cross-reactivity in the BioRad Platelia *Aspergillus* enzyme immunoassay. *Clin Vaccine Immunol* 2007;14(5):638–640.

49. Siemann M, Koch-Dörfler M, Gaude M. False-positive results in premature infants with the Platelia®*Aspergillus* sandwich enzyme-linked immunosorbent assay. *Mycoses* 1998;41(9–10):373–377.

50. Gangneux JP, et al. Transient aspergillus antigenaemia: Think of milk. *The Lancet* 2002;359(9313):1251.

51. Mennink-Kersten MASH, et al. Bifidobacterial lipoglycan as a new cause for false-positive platelia *Aspergillus* enzyme-linked immunosorbent assay reactivity. *Journal of Clinical Microbiology* 2005;43(8):3925–3931.

52. Husain S, et al. Prospective assessment of Platelia™ *Aspergillus galactomannan* antigen for the diagnosis of invasive Aspergillosis in lung transplant recipients. *American Journal of Transplantation* 2004;4(5):796–802.

53. Hamaki T, et al. False-positive results of *Aspergillus* enzyme-linked immunosorbent assay in a patient with chronic graft-versus-host disease after allogeneic bone marrow transplantation. *Bone Marrow Transplant* 2001;28(6):633–634.

54. Murashige N, et al. False-positive results of *Aspergillus* enzyme-linked immunosorbent assays for a patient with gastrointestinal graft-versus-host disease taking a nutrient containing soybean protein. *Clin Infect Dis* 2005;40(2):333–334.

55. Ansorg R, van den Boom R, Rath PM. Detection of *Aspergillus galactomannan* antigen in foods and antibiotics. *Mycoses* 1997;40(9–10):353–357.

56. Hashiguchi K, Niki Y, Soejima R. Cyclophosphamide induces false-positive results in detection of aspergillus antigen in urine. *Chest* 1994;105(3):975–976.

57. Kwak EJ, et al. Efficacy of galactomannan antigen in the platelia *Aspergillus* enzyme immunoassay for diagnosis of invasive Aspergillosis in liver transplant recipients. *J Clin Microbiol* 2004;42(1):435–438.

58. Bart-Delabesse E, et al. Detection of *Aspergillus galactomannan* antigenemia to determine biological and clinical implications of beta-lactam treatments. *J Clin Microbiol* 2005;43(10):5214–5220.

59. Adam O, et al. Treatment with piperacillin-tazobactam and false-positive *Aspergillus galactomannan* antigen test results for patients with hematological malignancies. *Clin Infect Dis* 2004;38(6):917–920.

60. Machetti M, et al. Kinetics of galactomannan in surgical patients receiving perioperative piperacillin/tazobactam prophylaxis. *J Antimicrob Chemother* 2006;58(4):806–810.

61. Viscoli C, et al. False-positive galactomannan platelia *Aspergillus* test results for patients receiving piperacillin-tazobactam. *Clin Infect Dis* 2004;38(6):913–916.

62. Maertens J, et al. False-Positive *Aspergillus galactomannan* Antigen Test Results. *Clinical Infectious Diseases* 2004;39(2):289–290.

63. Walsh TJ, et al. Detection of galactomannan antigenemia in patients receiving piperacillin-tazobactam and correlations between *in vitro*, *in vivo*, and clinical properties of the drug-antigen interaction. *J Clin Microbiol* 2004;42(10):4744–4748.

64. Mikulska M, et al. Piperacillin/tazobactam (Tazocin) seems to be no longer responsible for false-positive results of the galactomannan assay. *J Antimicrob Chemother* 2012;67(7):1746–1748.

65. Vergidis P, et al. Reduction in false-positive *Aspergillus* serum galactomannan enzyme immunoassay results associated with use of piperacillin-tazobactam in the United States. *J Clin Microbiol* 2014;52(6):2199–2201.

66. Marr KA, et al. Antifungal therapy decreases sensitivity of the *Aspergillus galactomannan* enzyme immunoassay. *Clin Infect Dis* 2005;40(12):1762–1769.

67. Duarte RF, et al. Serum galactomannan-based early detection of invasive aspergillosis in hematology patients receiving effective antimold prophylaxis. *Clin Infect Dis* 2014;59(12):1696–1702.

68. Verweij PE, et al. Failure to detect circulating *Aspergillus* markers in a patient with chronic granulomatous disease and invasive Aspergillosis. *J Clin Microbiol* 2000;38(10):3900–3901.

69. Walsh T, et al. Reduced expression of galactomannan antigenemia in patients with invasive aspergillosis and chronic granulomatous disease or Job's syndrome. in *Infectious Disease Society of America 40th annual meeting*. 2002.

70. Chan C, et al. Detection of antibodies specific to an antigenic cell wall galactomannoprotein for serodiagnosis of *Aspergillus fumigatus* aspergillosis. *J Clin Microbiol* 2002;40(6):2041–2045.

71. Guo YL, et al. Accuracy of BAL galactomannan in diagnosing invasive aspergillosis: A bivariate metaanalysis and systematic review. *Chest* 2010;138(4):817–824.

72. Zou M, et al. Systematic review and meta-analysis of detecting galactomannan in bronchoalveolar lavage fluid for diagnosing invasive aspergillosis. *PLoS One* 2012;7(8):e43347.

73. *Platelia Aspergillus EIA package insert* B. Laboratories, Editor. 2009.

74. Maertens J, et al. Bronchoalveolar lavage fluid galactomannan for the diagnosis of invasive pulmonary Aspergillosis in patients with hematologic diseases. *Clin Infect Dis* 2009;49(11):1688–1693.

75. Clancy C, et al. Bronchoalveolar lavage galactomannan in diagnosis of invasive pulmonary aspergillosis among solid-organ transplant recipients. *J Clin Microbiol* 2007;45(6):1759–1765.

76. Park SY, et al. *Aspergillus galactomannan* antigen assay in bronchoalveolar lavage fluid for diagnosis of invasive pulmonary aspergillosis. *J Infect* 2010;61(6):492–498.

77. Racil Z, et al. Galactomannan detection in bronchoalveolar lavage fluid for the diagnosis of invasive aspergillosis in patients with hematological diseases-the role of factors affecting assay performance. *Int J Infect Dis* 2011;15(12):e874–881.

78. Fisher CE, et al. Independent contribution of bronchoalveolar lavage and serum galactomannan in the diagnosis of invasive pulmonary aspergillosis. *Transpl Infect Dis* 2014;16(3):505–510.

79. Nguyen MH, et al. Galactomannan testing in bronchoalveolar lavage fluid facilitates the diagnosis of invasive pulmonary aspergillosis in patients with hematologic malignancies and stem cell transplant recipients. *Biol Blood Marrow Transplant* 2011;17(7):1043–1050.

80. Miyazaki T, et al. Plasma (1-->3)-beta-D-glucan and fungal antigenemia in patients with candidemia, aspergillosis, and cryptococcosis. *J Clin Microbiol* 1995;33(12):3115–3118.

81. Odabasi Z, et al. Differences in beta-glucan levels in culture supernatants of a variety of fungi. *Med Mycol* 2006;44(3):267–272.

82. Yoshida M, et al. Detection of plasma (1 --> 3)-beta-D-glucan in patients with *Fusarium, Trichosporon, Saccharomyces* and *Acremonium* fungaemias. *J Med Vet Mycol* 1997;35(5):371–374.

83. Mennink-Kersten M, et al. *In Vitro* Release by *Aspergillus* fumigatus of Galactofuranose Antigens, 1,3-β-d-Glucan, and DNA, Surrogate Markers Used for Diagnosis of Invasive Aspergillosis. *J Clin Microbiol* 2006;44(5):1711–1718.

84. Odabasi Z, et al. β-d-Glucan as a diagnostic adjunct for invasive fungal infections: Validation, cutoff development, and performance in patients with acute myelogenous leukemia and myelodysplastic syndrome. *Clin Infect Dis* 2004;39(2):199–205.

85. Ostrosky-Zeichner L, et al. Multicenter clinical evaluation of the (1→3) β-D-Glucan assay as an aid to diagnosis of fungal infections in humans. *Clin Infect Dis* 2005;41(5):654–659.

86. Smith PB, et al. Quantification of 1,3-β-d-Glucan levels in children: Preliminary data for diagnostic use of the β-Glucan assay in a pediatric setting. *Clin Vaccine Immunol* 2007;14(7):924–925.

87. Obayashi T, et al. Plasma (1-->3)-beta-D-glucan measurement in diagnosis of invasive deep mycosis and fungal febrile episodes. *Lancet* 1995;345(8941):17–20.

88. Karageorgopoulos DE, et al. beta-D-glucan assay for the diagnosis of invasive fungal infections: A meta-analysis. *Clin Infect Dis* 2011;52(6):750–770.

89. Onishi A, et al. Diagnostic accuracy of serum 1,3-beta-D-glucan for pneumocystis jiroveci pneumonia, invasive candidiasis, and invasive aspergillosis: Systematic review and meta-analysis. *J Clin Microbiol* 2012;50(1):7–15.

90. He S, et al. A systematic review and meta-analysis of diagnostic accuracy of serum 1,3-beta-D-glucan for invasive fungal infection: Focus on cutoff levels. *J Microbiol Immunol Infect* 2015;48(4):351–361.

91. Hou TY, et al. The Screening performance of serum 1,3-Beta-D-Glucan in patients with invasive fungal diseases: A meta-analysis of prospective cohort studies. *PLoS One* 2015;10(7):e0131602.

92. Karageorgopoulos DE, et al. Accuracy of beta-D-glucan for the diagnosis of *Pneumocystis jirovecii* pneumonia: A meta-analysis. *Clin Microbiol Infect* 2013;19(1):39–49.

93. Li WJ, et al. Diagnosis of pneumocystis pneumonia using serum (1-3)-beta-D-Glucan: A bivariate meta-analysis and systematic review. *J Thorac Dis* 2015;7(12):2214–2225.

94. Lu Y, et al. Diagnosis of invasive fungal disease using serum (1-->3)-beta-D-glucan: A bivariate meta-analysis. *Intern Med* 2011;50(22):2783–2791.

95. Lamoth F, et al. beta-Glucan antigenemia assay for the diagnosis of invasive fungal infections in patients with hematological malignancies: A systematic review and meta-analysis of cohort

studies from the Third European Conference on Infections in Leukemia (ECIL-3). *Clin Infect Dis* 2012;54(5):633–643.

96. Hanson KE, et al. beta-D-glucan surveillance with preemptive anidulafungin for invasive candidiasis in intensive care unit patients: A randomized pilot study. *PLoS One* 2012;7(8):e42282.

97. Mohr JF, et al. Prospective survey of (1-->3)-beta-D-glucan and its relationship to invasive candidiasis in the surgical intensive care unit setting. *J Clin Microbiol* 2011;49(1):58–61.

98. Posteraro B, et al. Early diagnosis of candidemia in intensive care unit patients with sepsis: A prospective comparison of (1-->3)-beta-D-glucan assay, *Candida* score, and colonization index. *Crit Care* 2011;15(5):R249.

99. Leon C, et al. A bedside scoring system ("*Candida* score") for early antifungal treatment in nonneutropenic critically ill patients with *Candida* colonization. *Crit Care Med* 2006;34(3):730–737.

100. Liew YX, et al. *Candida* Surveillance in Surgical Intensive Care Unit (SICU) in a Tertiary Institution. *BMC Infect Dis* 2015;15:256.

101. Mikulska M, et al. The use of mannan antigen and anti-mannan antibodies in the diagnosis of invasive candidiasis: Recommendations from the Third European Conference on Infections in Leukemia. *Crit Care* 2010;14(6):R222.

102. Leon C, et al. Contribution of *Candida* biomarkers and DNA detection for the diagnosis of invasive candidiasis in ICU patients with severe abdominal conditions. *Crit Care* 2016;20(1):149.

103. Martinez-Jimenez MC, et al. Potential role of *Candida albicans* germ tube antibody in the diagnosis of deep-seated candidemia. *Med Mycol* 2014;52(3):270–275.

104. Ostrosky-Zeichner L, et al. Multicenter retrospective development and validation of a clinical prediction rule for nosocomial invasive candidiasis in the intensive care setting. *Eur J Clin Microbiol Infect Dis* 2007;26(4):271–276.

105. Clancy CJ, Nguyen MH. Undiagnosed invasive candidiasis: Incorporating non-culture diagnostics into rational prophylactic and preemptive antifungal strategies. *Expert Rev Anti Infect Ther* 2014;12(7):731–734.

106. Ikemura K, et al. False-positive result in Limulus test caused by Limulus amebocyte lysate-reactive material in immunoglobulin products. *J Clin Microbiol* 1989;27(9):1965–1968.

107. Nagasawa K, et al. Experimental proof of contamination of blood components by (1-->3)-beta-D-glucan caused by filtration with cellulose filters in the manufacturing process. *J Artif Organs* 2003;6(1):49–54.

108. Ogawa M, et al. False-positive plasma (1-->3)-beta-D-glucan test following immunoglobulin product replacement in an adult bone marrow recipient. *Int J Hematol* 2004;80(1):97–98.

109. Usami M, et al. Positive (1-->3)-beta-D-glucan in blood components and release of (1-->3)-beta-D-glucan from depth-type membrane filters for blood processing. *Transfusion* 2002;42(9):1189–1195.

110. Kanda H, et al. Influence of various hemodialysis membranes on the plasma (1-->3)-beta-D-glucan level. *Kidney Int* 2001;60(1):319–323.

111. Alexander BD, et al. The (1,3)β-d-Glucan test as an aid to early diagnosis of invasive fungal infections following lung transplantation. *Journal of Clinical Microbiology* 2010;48(11):4083–4088.

112. Kimura Y, et al. Clinical and experimental studies of the limulus test after digestive surgery. *Surg Today* 1995;25(9):790–794.

113. Marty FM, et al. Reactivity of (1→3)-β-d-Glucan assay with commonly used intravenous anti-microbials. *Antimicrob Agents Chemother* 2006;50(10):3450–3453.

114. Mennink-Kersten MA, Warris A, Verweij PE. 1,3-beta-D-glucan in patients receiving intravenous amoxicillin-clavulanic acid. *N Engl J Med* 2006;354(26):2834–2835.

115. Pickering JW, et al. Evaluation of a (1->3)-beta-D-glucan assay for diagnosis of invasive fungal infections. *J Clin Microbiol* 2005;43(12):5957–5962.

116. Mengoli C, et al. Use of PCR for diagnosis of invasive aspergillosis: Systematic review and meta-analysis. *Lancet Infect Dis* 2009;9(2):89–96.

117. White PL, et al. Critical stages of extracting DNA from *Aspergillus fumigatus* in whole-blood specimens. *Journal of Clinical Microbiology* 2010;48(10):3753–3755.

118. Springer J, et al. Comparison of performance characteristics of *Aspergillus* PCR in testing a range of blood-based samples in accordance with international methodological recommendations. *J Clin Microbiol* 2016;54(3):705–711.

119. White PL, et al. Clinical performance of *Aspergillus* PCR for testing serum and plasma: A study by the European *Aspergillus* PCR initiative. *J Clin Microbiol* 2015;53(9):2832–2837.

120. Tuon FF. A systematic literature review on the diagnosis of invasive aspergillosis using polymerase chain reaction (PCR) from bronchoalveolar lavage clinical samples. *Rev Iberoam Micol* 2007;24(2):89–94.

121. Avni T, et al. Diagnostic accuracy of PCR alone compared to galactomannan in bronchoalveolar lavage fluid for diagnosis of invasive pulmonary aspergillosis: A systematic review. *J Clin Microbiol* 2012;50(11):3652–3658.

122. Avni T, Leibovici L, Paul M. PCR diagnosis of invasive candidiasis: Systematic review and meta-analysis. *Journal of Clinical Microbiology* 2011;49(2):665–670.

123. Nguyen MH, et al. Performance of *Candida* real-time polymerase chain reaction, β-D-glucan assay, and blood cultures in the diagnosis of invasive candidiasis. *Clinical Infectious Diseases* 2012;54(9):1240–1248.

124. Maertens J, et al. Galactomannan and computed tomography–based preemptive antifungal therapy in neutropenic patients at high risk for invasive fungal infection: A prospective feasibility study. *Clinical Infectious Diseases* 2005;41(9):1242–1250.

125. Hebart H, et al. A prospective randomized controlled trial comparing PCR-based and empirical treatment with liposomal amphotericin B in patients after allo-SCT. *Bone Marrow Transplant* 2009;43(7):553–561.

126. Cordonnier C, et al. Empirical versus preemptive antifungal therapy for high-risk, febrile, neutropenic patients: A randomized, controlled trial. *Clin Infect Dis* 2009;48(8):1042–1051.

127. Fung M, et al. Meta-analysis and cost comparison of empirical versus pre-emptive antifungal strategies in hematologic malignancy patients with high-risk febrile neutropenia. *PLoS One* 2015;10(11):e0140930.

128. Morrissey CO, et al. Galactomannan and PCR versus culture and histology for directing use of antifungal treatment for invasive aspergillosis in high-risk haematology patients: a randomised controlled trial. *Lancet Infect Dis* 2013;13(6):519–528.

129. Aguado JM, et al. Serum galactomannan versus a combination of galactomannan and polymerase chain reaction-based *Aspergillus* DNA detection for early therapy of invasive aspergillosis in high-risk hematological patients: a randomized controlled trial. *Clin Infect Dis* 2015;60(3):405–414.

130. Ostrosky-Zeichner L, et al. MSG-01: A randomized, double-blind, placebo-controlled trial of caspofungin prophylaxis followed by preemptive therapy for invasive candidiasis in high-risk adults in the critical care setting. *Clin Infect Dis* 2014;58(9):1219–1226.

131. Posteraro B, et al. (1,3)-beta-d-Glucan-based antifungal treatment in critically ill adults at high risk of candidaemia: An observational study. *J Antimicrob Chemother* 2016.

7

The immune response to fungal challenge

JEFFERY HU AND JEFFERY J. AULETTA

INTRODUCTION

Fungal infections are a leading cause of morbidity and mortality in immunocompromised patients. Nearly half a century ago, Bodey and colleagues made the critical observation that profound and prolonged neutropenia increased the risk for disseminated fungal infection [1]. Since this critical observation, understanding for the mammalian immune response in defending the host against fungal disease has dramatically increased [2]. Along with an enhanced understanding for fungal host defense has been the expansion in synthetic immunomodulatory and antifungal agents [3], which have altered the ability to treat invasive fungal infections (IFIs) in immunocompromised patients. Despite pharmaceutical advances in antifungal therapy, the fundamental requirement for surviving an IFI in the context of immunosuppression remains recovery in host immune function [4] (Figure 7.1). Thus, the quest continues to define the host immune response to fungal pathogen and to understand the ability of fungi to evade immune detection and elimination.

This chapter will define the known mammalian immune response to fungal disease and how deficiencies in host immunity predispose to fungal infections with the following caveats. First, review of fungal immunity will be limited to providing an overview of immune responses with specific examples of certain pathogens, as a comprehensive review of immunity relevant to all fungal pathogens is beyond the scope of this chapter. Second, immunomodulatory agents and their influence on fungal immunity and immune restoration will be introduced, but more detailed explanation for their use as treatment for fungal disease will be reserved for the chapter dedicated to antifungal immunotherapy. Lastly, contributions to the antifungal response beyond immune effector cells [5] will not be addressed in this chapter.

OVERVIEW OF THE MAMMALIAN IMMUNE RESPONSE TO FUNGAL CHALLENGE

Immunity is a coordinated and redundant response designed to discriminate between self and non-self. However, healthy individuals coexist with diverse group of organisms, including fungal species, as part of the normal commensal colonies [6]. Thus, the immune system discriminates additionally between pathogenic strains and normal flora (consisting of fungal and bacterial communities referred to as mycobiome [7] and bacteriome [8], respectively) with the overall goal of host preservation, particularly with respect to infectious challenge. To this end, the immune response has classically been divided into the innate and adaptive effector arms. These distinct, but not mutually exclusive, cellular responses are complemented by the production of soluble factors, including cytokines,

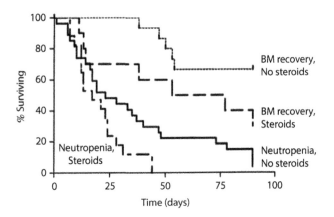

Figure 7.1 Recovery in immune function is imperative to surviving an invasive fungal infection. Percent survival of 84 patients with hematologic malignancies and Fusarium infection. The highest survival rate was seen in those patients with bone marrow ("BM") recovery and who were no longer receiving immunosuppressive therapy ("No steroids"). (From Nucci, M. et al., *Cancer*, 98, 315–319. 2003. Copyright Wiley-Liss, Inc., a subsidiary of John Wiley & Sons. Reproduced with permission.)

chemokines, and complement, which serve to eliminate (i.e., antimicrobial) and to modify (i.e., immunomodulatory) the immune response to pathogen. Furthermore, the microenvironment comprised of these soluble factors directly influences both innate and adaptive immune cell activation, differentiation, and function. The immune response also establishes memory to the pathogen in order to respond rapidly to future infectious challenges. Finally, regulation and tolerance (nonresponse to self) are critical to prevent aberrant autoimmune damage to the host.

Pathogen recognition receptors

Fungi are eukaryotic cells and, thus, share similar features with mammalian cells. The major distinguishing feature between fungi and mammalian cells is that fungi possess a rigid cell wall, containing unique pathogen-associated molecular patterns (PAMPs) including β-glucans, chitins, and mannoproteins. Initiation of the immune response to fungal challenge involves recognition of these PAMPs by pathogen recognition receptors (PRRs), such as Toll-like receptors (TLRs), mannose receptors, and β-glucan receptors [9,10].

Toll-like receptors (TLRs) are type I integral membrane glycoproteins that belong to the Toll/interleukin-1 receptor (TIR) superfamily. The majority of TLRs are expressed on the cellular surface of immune cells (TLR 1, 2, 4–6, 11), while TLR 3, 7/8, and 9 are located in endosomal compartments [11]. TLRs use a conserved TIR domain in the cytosolic region to activate one of four adaptor proteins: the death-domain containing myeloid differentiation factor 88

(MyD88), TIRAP (TIR-adaptor containing adaptor protein, also known as MyD88-adaptor-like protein, MAL), TRIF (TIR-domain-containing adaptor protein inducing IFN-β), and TRAM (TRIF-adaptor molecule). Differential use of these adaptor proteins confers specificity to the TLR signaling pathways [12]. The majority of TLRs utilize MyD88 signal adaptor proteins to activate IRAKs and TRAF6, which ultimately activate NF-κB and mitogen-activated protein (MAP) kinases to synthesize inflammatory cytokines like IL-6 and TNF-α [13]. In contrast, TLR3-mediated signaling utilizes TRIF and IRF3 in producing type I interferons in a MyD88-independent manner [14]. TLR4 activation uniquely leads to both MyD88-dependent, early phase NF-κB transcription of proinflammatory cytokines (IL-1β, TNF-α, and IL-6) and MyD88-independent, late phase NF-κB transcription of IFN-β [13].

Plasticity and redundancy in innate-mediated cytokine responses directly reflect TLR expression and signaling utilized by effector cells [15]. For example, plasmacytoid dendritic cells (pDCs) are the principal producers of type I IFN following viral (TLR-7) and bacterial (TLR-9) challenge [16], while myeloid DCs produce smaller amounts of IFN-α in response to viral challenge (TLR-3) [17]. Finally, tight regulation of TLR signaling cascades is needed to avoid detrimental allo- and autoimmune inflammatory responses [18,19].

Additional PRRs relevant to fungal pathogens include C-type lectin receptors (CLR) [20], including β-glucan (Dectin-1) [21,22] and mannose receptors (MRs) [23], and complement receptors (CRs). Like TLRs, these PRRs are located on the surface of phagocytes, including macrophages, DCs, and neutrophils, and can modulate immune cell function [24]. Dectin 1 (also known as CLEC7A) is the most well-studied CLR expressed on monocytes and macrophages. Ligation of Dectin-1 and MRs initiates phagocytosis in the absence of opsonization (see sections on phagocytosis and complement below), whereas dual ligation of complement receptors, like CR3 (CD11b/CD18 or Mac-1), with receptors for the Fc portion of immunoglobulins (FcRs) dramatically enhance microbial phagocytosis [25]. Additionally, dectin-1 is involved in inducing cytokine production and amplification of response from TLR2 or TLR4 pathway [26,27]. Dectin-1 accomplishes this task via two intracellular signaling: the spleen tyrosine kinase (SYK), caspase activation and recruitment domain containing 9 (CARD9), and protein kinase Cδ pathway [28–32] and the RAF1 kinase signaling pathway [33]. Polymorphisms in the Dectin 1 gene are associated with colonization of the genitourinary tract by *Candida* species, recurrent vulvovaginal candidiasis, and other fungal infection [34–37] whereas CARD9 deficiency showed more severe phenotype demonstrating increased susceptibility to invasive candidiasis [31]. While many other PRRs exist such as NOD-like receptors (NLR), the overall goal of PRRs serves to initially detect infection and coordinate the appropriate response through cross-talk and synergism between PRR and their downstream adaptor protein.

Innate immunity

Key features of innate immunity include PRR activation via recognition of PAMPs [38], induction of antimicrobial effector cell cytokines and chemokines [39], and modulation of adaptive immunity [40]. Innate immune cells functioning as phagocytes in the antifungal immune response include dendritic cells (DCs), macrophages/monocytes, and polymorphonuclear (PMN) cells. These phagocytes are primarily responsible for eliminating fungal pathogens via oxidative and non-oxidative intracellular killing. Specifically, PMN cells ingest and package fungi into phagosomes to which intracellular granules fuse and then discharge their antimicrobial contents [41]. Non-oxidative killing is mediated largely through the content of specific and gelatinase granules, which release lactoferrin, lysozyme, gelatinase, and peroxidase-positive granules including α-defensins. Oxygen-dependent mechanisms include generation of reactive oxygen species (ROS) via the NADPH-oxidase complex in combination with superoxide dismutase and myeloperoxidase. Of note, soluble factors including complement and antibodies promote phagocytosis, enhancing intracellular elimination of fungal pathogens. Finally, PMNs also eliminate fungi via extracellular mechanisms, such as neutrophil extracellular traps (NETs), which bind and kill fungal pathogens, particularly *Candida albicans* [42]. This provides a mechanism to combat hyphae too large to be phagocytosed [43]. Composed of DNA and associated histones, NETs also contain granule proteins from azurophilic, specific and gelatinase granules. These processes literally grab and capture fungal elements, concentrating and preventing their spreading from the site of infection.

Macrophages are another key effector cell in the defense against fungal infection. They have a particular role in controlling disseminated fungal infection and are recruited to site of infection through chemokine receptors. Polymorphism in genes that decrease CX_3C chemokine receptor 1 function found on monocytes revealed increased susceptibility to disseminated infection but not mucosal infection [44,45]. Additionally, deficiency in CC-chemokine receptor 2 in murine models also demonstrated increased susceptibility to disseminated infection. [46]. Monocytes and macrophages play an important role in "innate immunity" or "trained immunity." This has been demonstrated in studies performed in which mice previously exposed to attenuated strains of *C. albicans* were protected from invasive candidiasis in subsequent fungal challenge [47]. Such immunity was thought to have been mediated by epigenetic reprogramming of innate immune cells allowing for enhanced production

of proinflammatory cytokines [48]. Clinical relevance of trained immunity has been suggested by reports of defective trained immunity in patients with chronic mucocutaneous candidiasis and points to new therapeutic approaches to vaccinations [49].

Innate immune cells also serve as antigen-presenting cells (APCs) to adaptive immune cells, namely T cells. In so doing, innate APCs provide two critical signals to activate T-cells – antigen in the context of MHC (major histocompatibility complex) class I or II molecules and co-stimulation. Antigen processing differs depending upon the location of antigen [50]. Intracellular proteins (e.g., viral peptides) in the cytosol are degraded into peptides in proteasomes and presented with class I MHC to $CD8^+$ T-cells. In contrast, extracellular peptides (e.g., fungal proteins) are taken up by endocytosis, sequestered into endosomes, and degraded by lysosomal enzymes and presented with class II MHC to $CD4^+$ T-cells. In addition to endocytosis, other intracellular pathways exist to deliver antigen for lysosomal degradation and MHC II presentation, through a process known as autophagy (reviewed in [51]).

The physical location where cellular exchange of information and molecular interaction among innate APCs and T-cells occurs is known as the "immunologic synapse" [52]. Here, T-cell receptor (TCR)-MHC-peptide cognate interactions in the context of co-stimulation (CD28-CD80/86, CD40-CD40L) activate receptor signaling cascades in T-cells resulting in their activation and cytokine production. Given its critical role in T-cell activation, the immunologic synapse and its associated molecules are ripe targets for immunotherapy directed at modulating T-cell function [53].

Innate APCs function to recruit adaptive cells through production of soluble immunomodulatory factors, including cytokines and chemokines. For example, TLR-stimulated phagocytes produce IL-23, which then expands the IL-17-producing Th-17 population (discussed further in section on adaptive immunity) [54]. IL-17, in turn, induces proinflammatory cytokines and chemokines [55], as well as matures and recruits phagocytes to the site of infection [56].

Dendritic cells (DCs) are the most potent APC for naïve T-cell activation and are critically poised to bridge innate and adaptive immune responses following PRR activation by fungal pathogens [57]. For example, activation of TLR4 causes maturation of peripheral DCs, increasing their surface expression of adhesion and costimulatory molecules, altering their function from antigen-capturing to antigen-processing cells, and promoting their interaction with naïve T-cells by enhancing expression of CCR7 and migration to secondary lymph nodes [58]. In addition, DCs cross talk with other innate effector cells, particularly NK cells [59], is common and such exchange modulates function in each effector cell [60,61]. Finally, DCs are highly plastic effector cells [62], a reflection of the TLRs they possess (as discussed above) as well as the pathogens they encounter [63].

Human DCs include plasmacytoid (pDC) and myeloid (mDC) subtypes, whereas mice have an additional lymphoid DC phenotype [64]. Whether from man or mouse, DC subtypes have distinct surface markers [65], unique TLR [66], chemokine [67], and cytokine [68] profiles, and diverse effects on the immune response [69,70]. In humans, mDCs are the primary producers of IL-12 [71], and pDCs are the chief producers of type I interferon [72], a key mediator of antiviral [73] and antitumor [74] immunity and of immunomodulation [75,76].

Adaptive immunity

B and T-cell lymphocytes comprise the adaptive immune response to fungal pathogens. In general, B-cells produce antibodies, while T cells produce immunomodulatory and antimicrobial cytokines in response to fungal challenge. Both lymphoid effector cells have memory subsets that are activated during fungal re-challenge.

The humoral immune response to fungal pathogens is multi-functional. First, B-cells serve as critical APCs to T cells, and the latter also provide a reciprocal helper function to promote antibody production (though antibody production can occur in the absence of T-helper cells [77]). Of note, B cells themselves can also influence innate cells [78]. Once activated, differentiated B cells (plasma cells) produce antibodies that have direct antifungal and immunomodulatory effects. For example, IgG-coated fungal pathogens bind to FcγR on phagocytes to initiate antibody-dependent cellular cytotoxicity (ADCC) [79]. Cellular processes such as phagocytosis and soluble processes like the classic pathway of complement (antibody-dependent complement opsonization) are also activated by antibodies. Finally, antibodies are involved in the memory response to fungal infection [80]. Given these roles in antifungal immunity, antibodies are the focus of intense study for successful immunotherapy against fungi [81]. Currently, the development of vaccination is being explored as a viable strategy for improving resistance amongst high-risk patients [82–84].

T-cell phenotypes are classically divided into CD4$^+$ and CD8$^+$ subsets, and each is responsible for different immune functions. Within the CD4$^+$ genre are the T-regulatory (T$_{reg}$) cells, Th-17 cells, Th-1, and Th-2 cells, each with its own unique ontogeny and immune function. For example, Th-cells originate from peripheral naïve CD4$^+$ T-cell precursors. In contrast, T-regulatory cell ontogeny is more complex; as subsets arise from both peripheral Th-1 precursors, including induced T$_{reg}$ cells (CD4$^+$CD25$^+$FoxP3$^+$), Tr1 cells, and Th3 cells, and directly from thymic precursors (naturally-occurring T$_{reg}$ cells). Differentiation of CD4$^+$ subsets is mediated by cytokines inducing transcription factor activation within T-cell precursors. For example, TGF-β alone induces FoxP3 expression in naïve T-cells to promote

inducible T$_{reg}$ cells [85], while TGF-β in combination with IL-6 results in Th-17 cell differentiation [86]. Finally, CD8$^+$ T-cells can be divided into effector (primarily cytolytic or cytokine-producing in function) and memory subsets [87]. Sustained CD8$^+$ T-cells memory requires priming from CD4$^+$ T-cells [88,89].

Despite their common ontogeny from the CD4$^+$ precursor, Th-17 and T$_{reg}$ cells have divergent functions in the context of inflammation. Th-17 cells promote inflammation via IL-17 production [90,91], while T$_{reg}$ cells counteract inflammation through IL-10 and TGF-β production [92,93] in order to prevent deleterious chronic inflammation. Like DCs, CD4$^+$ cells regulate the balance between autoimmunity and tolerance within the host [94].

Soluble factors: Complement, cytokines, and chemokines

Complement activation has typically been associated with the innate immune response, but complement pathways also function to influence adaptive immune responses [25]. For example, complement augments antibody responses and enhances immunologic memory, in addition to enhancing phagocytosis (opsonization) and mediating immune cell activation and migration. Three activation pathways culminate to activate C3 convertase, which is instrumental in initiating development of the terminal membrane attack complex, whose formation is usually blocked by the fungal cell wall [95]. The classical pathway is initiated by immune complexes, specifically C1 complex binding to antigen-antibody complexes on the surface of pathogens. The alternative pathway is initiated by C3b binding to various hydroxyl groups on proteins and carbohydrates on cell surfaces. Finally, the mannose-binding lectin (MBL) pathway is activated by the binding of the MBL-MASP (MBL-associated serine protease) complex to mannose groups contained within pathogens such as *Candida albicans* [96,97]. Interestingly, low levels of circulating MBL have been associated with increased susceptibility to fungal infections [98,99], so recombinant MBL could potentially be used as immunotherapy against IFI [100].

Inducible cytokine profiles in response to fungal challenge are a direct reflection of the form of fungal element encountered, as well as the types of PRR and intracellular signaling pathways activated (reviewed in following section). In addition, cytokines function as direct fungicidal agents mediating immune cell activation and modulating immune cell function. Proinflammatory (Th-1) cytokines, including IL-6, IL-12, TNF-α, and IFN-γ, provide antifungal immunity. It has long been shown that IFN-γ production and IL-18, (through induction of Th-1 subtype) are important in increasing the fungicidal activity of neutrophils and macrophages [101–103]. In a recent proof-of-principle trial, treatment of patients with systemic candidiasis showed improvement with recombinant IFN-γ [104]. Th-17 cells also provide antifungal protection via production of proinflammatory IL-17 involved in the recruitment and activation of neutrophil [105,106]. IL-17's importance in mucosal fungal defense is highlighted by increased number of *Candida* infection in psoriatic patients treated with IL-17A-targeted antibodies [107].

Anti-inflammatory (Th-2) cytokines, including IL-4, IL-5, IL-10, and TGF-β, confer susceptibility to and progression of fungal disease [2,108,109]. However, the distinction between pro- and antifungal cytokines is ambiguous for several reasons. First, without anti-inflammatory cytokines, pro-inflammation following fungal challenge is deleterious to the host [110]. Second, anti-inflammatory cytokines can protect the host against fungal infections in certain settings [111]. Thus, effects of cytokines like IL-4 [112], IL-10, and TGF-β [113] are highly context-dependent, much like effects of suppressor cell populations themselves [114]. This is highlighted currently in mouse models that demonstrated early IL-10 production that contributed to development of protective Th-1 cell response in IL-12 deficient mice [115]. Additionally, IL-4 has also been shown to be necessary for the development of protective Th-1 response to *Candida* infection [116]. As such, further investigation is needed to elucidate the highly complex cytokine environment needed for appropriate antifungal defense. In addition to these pro- and anti-inflammatory cytokines, cytokine growth factors, including granulocyte stimulating factor (G-CSF) and granulocyte-macrophage stimulating factor (GM-CSF), have dual roles as stimulators of myeloid proliferation and differentiation and as immunomodulatory agents, enhancing phagocyte fungicidal activity and antigen presenting capacity, and potentially regulating Th-1 responses (reviewed in [117]).

Like cytokines, chemokines have critical roles in immune cell activation and recruitment in the context of fungal infection [118] and inflammation [119]. For example, macrophage inflammatory protein-1 alpha (MIP-1α)/CCL3 and monocyte chemoattractant protein-1 (MCP-1)/CCL2 mediate phagocyte recruitment to sites of infection [120]. Likewise, chemokines such as Epstein-Barr I1 ligand chemokine (ELC)/CCL19 and secondary lymphoid-tissue chemokine (SLC)/CCL21 form gradients to facilitate DC trafficking and antigen presentation within secondary lymph nodes and link innate and adaptive responses [121]. Cytokines, like TNF-α, can also induce chemokine production from immune cells, further driving effector cell recruitment to sites of infection and inflammation [122]. Finally, chemokines like thymus and activation-regulated chemokine (TARC)/CCL17 directly modulate antifungal responses [123].

Other soluble factors relevant to the fungal immune response include collectins, defensins, and heat shock proteins (HSPs). In general, these factors function to enhance phagocytosis (collectins) or to mediate direct antimicrobial effects (defensins), the latter of which is induced by Th-17 production of IL-22 and stimulation of epithelial cells to release antifungal β-defensins [106]. Specifically, HSPs are intracellular molecular chaperones, which normally shuttle peptides during steady-state hemostasis, and function as danger signals during cell stress responses [124]. Interestingly, antibodies to HSP90 protect against *Candida albicans* [125], enhance effects of antifungal agents [126], and potentially decrease resistance of fungal pathogens [127,128].

Regulation

Intracellular signaling cascades of pathogen-recognition receptors like TLRs [13] ultimately converge to activate nuclear factor κB (NF-κB), which mediates gene transcription of proinflammatory factors that holistically comprise the protective antifungal immune response. In contrast, cytokine receptors signal through either Janus kinase (JAK)-signal transducers and activators of transcription (STAT) pathways [129] or mitogen-activated protein (MAP) kinase cascades [130]. Left unchecked, acute inflammation progresses to chronic inflammation and causes host damage [131]. Therefore, the inflammatory response is regulated to preserve host integrity [132]. Such regulation occurs at multiple levels, including at the level of TLR [19] and cytokine [133] receptor activation and signaling, at the level of NF-κB gene transcription [134], and at the level of MAP kinase activation [135]. In addition to these signaling regulators, cytokines (as reviewed above) and regulator cell populations down modulate the host immune response. Examples of suppressor populations include hematopoietic (e.g., myeloid suppressor cells [114], regulatory T cells [136], NKT cells [137]) and non-hematopoietic (e.g., mesenchymal stem cells [138]) cells. Roles for these regulatory signaling and cellular factors in modulating the immune response to fungal challenge remain largely undefined. Furthermore, these soluble and cellular factors are also likely involved in immune evasion by fungal pathogens, and so may be important targets to enhance antifungal immune responses [139].

PUTTING IT ALL TOGETHER: IMMUNE RESPONSES TO *CANDIDA ALBICANS* AND *ASPERGILLUS FUMIGATUS*

The host response to fungal pathogens is a complex and coordinated interaction among innate, adaptive and complement effector arms and their associated soluble factors that combine to eliminate the pathogen and to create long-lasting immunity against the fungal pathogen encountered (Figure 7.2). The antifungal response to *Candida albicans*

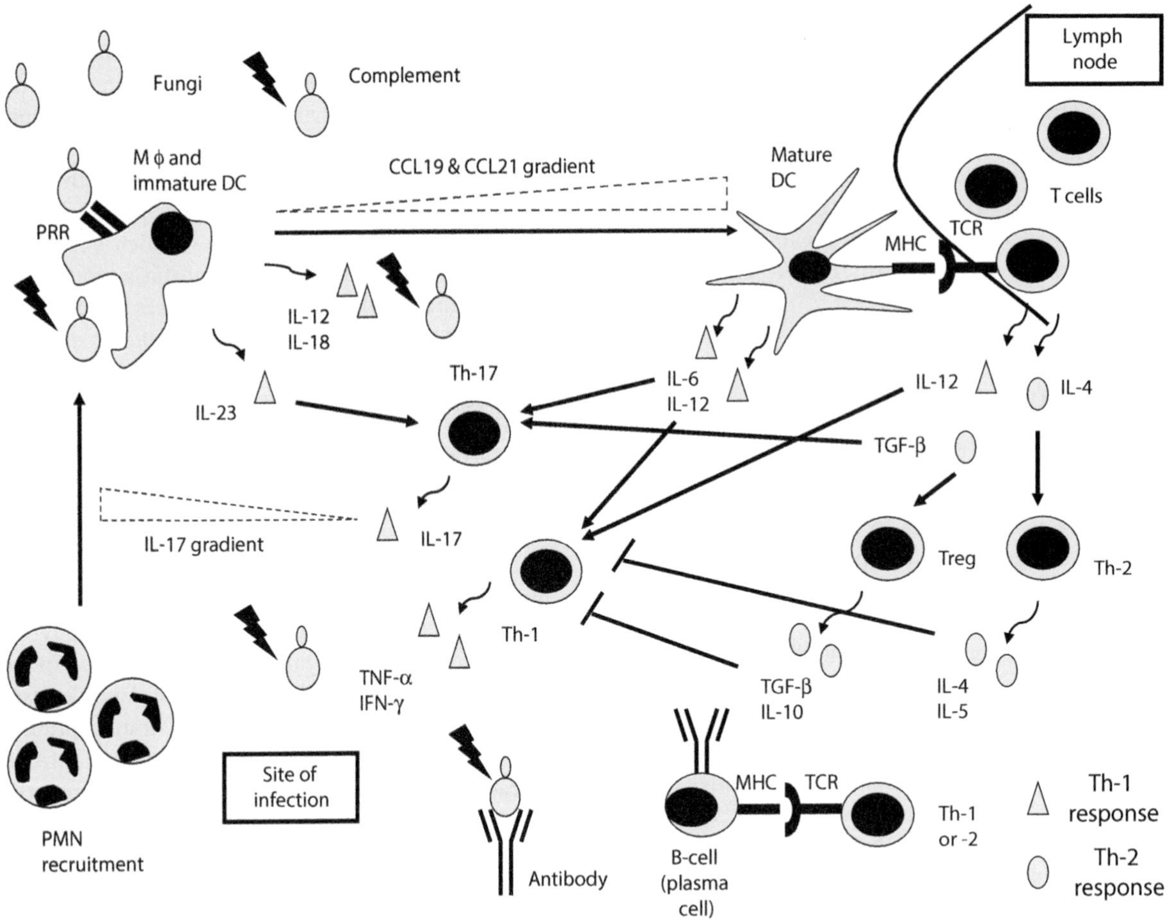

Figure 7.2 The immune response to fungal challenge. The host immune response to fungal challenge involves coordination among the innate and adaptive effector arms as well as activation of complement cascades. In brief, phagocytes (macrophages, Mφ, and dendritic cells, DCs) are activated through pathogen recognition receptors (PRR) to produce antimicrobial and immunomodulatory cytokines and chemokines. In addition, phagocytes serve as antigen-presenting cells, processing antigen in the context of major histocompatibility complex (MHC) class I and class II molecules, which are recognized by the T-cell receptor (TCR) on naïve T-cells in lymph nodes. Activation of T-cells requires antigen-presentation and co-stimulation through cognate interactions (CD28-CD80/86) and soluble factors (IL-12, IL-4). Activation then drives proliferation of distinct CD4 subsets, including IL-17 producing Th-17 cells, inducible T regulatory cells (T$_{reg}$), proinflammatory Th-1 cells, and anti-inflammatory Th-2 cells. Th-2 cells are also important for humoral immunity, including B-cell production of antibodies. Cytokine and chemokine gradients drive immune cell differentiation and expansion, migration to secondary lymph nodes, and recruitment to the site of infection. Secreted soluble factors are shown with curved arrows, while effects on immune cell activation, differentiation, and migration are shown with straight arrows.

and *Aspergillus fumigatus* will be highlighted as representative immune responses against yeasts and molds, respectively. Table 7.1 provides a summary to the key elements of the host immune response to these clinically-important fungi, while the following text provides more details highlighting the complex interactions among immune cells and soluble factors responding to fungal challenge.

Detection, activation, elimination, and regulation

Toll-like receptors (TLRs) 2 and 4 have established roles in detecting fungal elements [140], whether alone or in combination with other PRRs such as dectin-1 [141,142].

Interestingly, fungal dimorphism results in distinct TLR activation, ultimately leading to contrasting cellular and cytokine responses [143,144]. For example, *C. albicans* budding yeast is recognized by both TLR2 and TLR4 receptors, with the latter responsible for proinflammatory cytokine release. However, hyphal forms of *C. albicans* were unrecognized by TLR4 receptors inducing larger amounts of IL-10 through TLR2 receptors [145]. Furthermore, differential activation of TLRs during germination of *A. fumigatus* from conidia (TLR2 and 4) to hyphae (TLR2 only) results in IL-10 induction and, thus, may contribute to the mold's ability to escape immune surveillance [146,147]. Such differential recognition of PRR is thought to be due to the shielding of immunogenic β-D glucan by surface mannan in the

Table 7.1 Host immune responses to *Candida albicans* and *Aspergillus fumigatus*

	Candida albicans	**Aspergillus fumigatus**
Acquisition	Colonization (breach in integrity of intestine mucosa)	Inhalation (breach in pulmonary host defense)
Detection	Yeast & PLM (TLR2), Pseudohyphae & hyphae (TLR4/CD14), β-glucan (Dectin-1/TLR2), mannose (MR)	Conidia (TLR2) Hyphae (TLR2 & TLR4/CD14)
Cellular activation & migration	TLR-inducible cytokine production; PMN and DC migration via chemokine gradients	TLR-inducible cytokine production; PMN and DC migration via chemokine gradients
Cellular phagocytosis	PMN, DC, macrophage Oxidative & non-oxidative killing	Alveolar macrophages (conidia), PMN (hyphae), and DC (conidia & hyphae) Oxidative and non-oxidative killing
Chemokines	IL-8, KC, MCP-1, MIP-1α/β, MIP-2, RANTES	IL-8, MCP-1, MIP-/2
Fungicidal cytokines	IL-1β, IL-6, IL-12, IL-15, IL-18, IFN-γ, TNF-α	IL-1β, IL-6, IL-12, IFN-γ, TNF-α
Regulatory cytokines	IL-4, IL-10, TGF-β	IL-4, IL-10
Memory	Antibody	Antibody
Immune risk factors	T-cell dysfunction (predominant), neutropenia	Neutropenia or aberrant PMN function (predominant)
Acquired risk factors	Broad-spectrum antibiotics, CVAD, recent GI surgery, HAL, extreme ages, prolonged ICU stay, steroids	Steroids, broad-spectrum antibiotics, infliximab therapy
Associated diseases	AIDS, HSCT/SOT, Malignancy	Chronic granulomatous disease, GvHD, HSCT/SOT

Abbreviations: CVAD: central venous access device; DCs: dendritic cells; HAL: hyperalimentation; HSCT/SOT: hematopoietic stem cell/solid organ transplant; ICU: intensive care unit; KC: keratinocyte-derived; MIP: macrophage inhibitory protein; MCP: monocyte chemoattractant protein; MR: mannose receptor; PLM: phospholipomannan; PMN: polymorphonuclear; RANTES: regulated upon activation, normal T-cell expressed and secreted; TLR: Toll-like receptor.

hyphal form in *Candida* species [145]. Finally, multiple elements of the same fungi can activate different PRRs, resulting in different downstream effects. For example, *Candida* mannan activates TLR4, resulting in proinflammatory cytokine and chemokine release and PMN recruitment (protective response) [148] while *Candida* glucan activates TLR2 and induces IL-10 (susceptibility response) [149].

Similar to PRR activation, phagocytosis is complex and is affected by different recognition receptors, resulting in unique fungicidal and immunomodulatory responses [150,151]. The different forms of phagocytosis likely reflect the plasticity in phagocyte function conferred by possessing different PRRs. For example, *Candida* yeasts and *Aspergillus* conidia undergo "coiling" phagocytosis and induce IL-12 production, resulting in protective Th-1 responses. In contrast, *Candida* and *Aspergillus* hyphae are internalized by "zipper-type" phagocytosis and induce IL-4 and IL-10 production, resulting in non-protective Th-2 responses (reviewed in ref [2]). Furthermore, coiling and zipper-type phagocytosis are TLR-independent but involve different PRRs, in particular MRs and CR3-FcγR cooperation, respectively. In similar fashion, chemokine receptor expression [152] and chemokine induction profiles

[120,153] differ depending upon the internalized fungal form, which may ultimately impact immune cell migration and function.

Once initiated, the pro-inflammatory Th-1 response undergoes down modulation. Established mechanisms responsible for immune attenuation in the context of fungal infections include myeloid suppressor cells and regulatory cytokines (both reviewed in previous sections). Interestingly, the role of suppressor cells such as T_{reg} cells is still being defined; as these cells are likely involved in regulating the proinflammatory response and in suppressing the immune response at the site of infection (similar to their proposed effects in tumor beds [154]).

Immune escape mechanisms

Despite the redundancy and complexity of the antifungal immune response, fungal pathogens cause infection, even in the immunocompetent host. Fungal pathogenesis directly reflects both virulence factors [155] and immune escape mechanisms. The very nature of dimorphism is perhaps the most obvious tool used by fungi to obviate the

Table 7.2 Synthetic immunomodulatory agents

Class	Agent	Effect
Corticosteroids	Prednisone, Methylprednisolone	General immune suppression
Antiproliferation	Azathioprine	Induction of thioguanine derivatives, inhibit DNA synthesis
	Mycophenolate mofetil	Blocks purine synthesis, preventing B/T cell proliferation
Calcineurin inhibitors	Cyclosporin A, Tacrolimus (FK506)	Inhibit IL-2 production, T-cell activation
Target of rapamycin (TOR) inhibitors	Sirolimus, Everolimus	Inhibit T-cell cell cycle, proliferation
Cell depletion	Rituxumab (anti-CD20)	B-cell depletion
	Gemtuzumab (anti-CD33)	Myeloid cell depletion
	Alemtuzumab (anti-CD52)	Mononuclear & B/T-cell depletion
	OKT3 (anti-CD3)	T-cell depletion
Soluble factor blockade	Daclizumab (human), Basiliximab (chimeric)	Soluble IL-2 receptor blockade
	Infliximab	TNF-α receptor blockade
	Etanercept	TNF-α blockade
	Adalimumab	TNF-α blockade
	Fontolizumab	IFN-γ blockade
	Anti-p40	IL-12 and IL-23 blockade
	Secukinumab	IL-17A blockade
Activation blockade	Adaptacept	CD28-B7 blockade
	Belatacept	CTLA-4-Ig blocking CD28-B7

immune response [156]. In addition to undergoing morphologic changes, fungi possess virulent structures (capsule of *Cryptococcus neoformans*) and toxins (gliotoxin of *Aspergillus fumigatus*), which inhibit immune cell activation and function and induce immune cell apoptosis [157,158]. Other forms of fungal immune evasion include: PRR escape [144]; loss of TLR signaling [146]; preferential PRR ligation leading to intracellular survival within phagocytes [143]; and induction of suppressor cell populations and soluble factors as previously discussed. Finally, the intrinsic ability of fungi to evade and/or to suppress immunosurveillance is often complemented by iatrogenic suppression in host immune function, as synthetic agents targeting immune cells and soluble factors have dual roles in ameliorating deleterious allo- or auto-immunity and in inhibiting protective antifungal immunity [53,159] (Table 7.2).

HOST DEFENSE: AN IMMUNOMODULATORY INTERFACE BETWEEN HOST AND PATHOGEN

Host defense is an immunomodulatory interface between host and fungal pathogen. The potential for fungal infection reflects the immune status of the host and the cumulative attributes of the pathogen to cause infection (Figure 7.3). With respect to the patient, the more immunosuppressed,

the higher the incidence of clinical infection and the risk for disseminated disease. In contrast, immune restoration within the patient dramatically decreases the risk for disseminated disease and improves the likelihood for complete eradication of fungal pathogen. With respect to the fungal pathogen, its overall prevalence, its intrinsic and acquired resistance, and its virulence factors directly influence the type of host it will infect and the type of disease it will cause (colonization, infection or dissemination).

Several factors influence the net immunosuppressive state of the host including the presence of co-morbid conditions, such as diabetes mellitus, prematurity, or advanced age, and concomitant infection, particularly with immunomodulatory viruses like HIV, Epstein Barr Virus (EBV), Cytomegalovirus (CMV), and Human herpes virus (HHV)-6 [160]. Primary underlying disease and its treatment also affect the immune status of the host. For example, cancer and its associated therapies (chemotherapy and radiation) affect all arms of the immune system [161,162], whereas chronic granulomatous disease is a selective qualitative deficiency in neutrophil function [163]. Finally, exposure to hospital environments, to antifungal chemotherapy, and to high glucose (hyperalimentation) affects the susceptibility of the host to fungal disease [164].

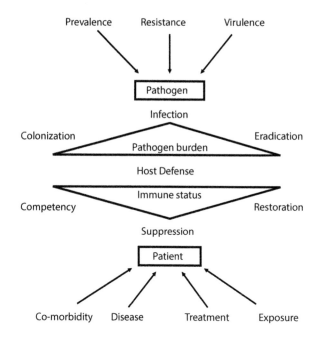

Figure 7.3 Host defense is the immunomodulatory interface between fungal pathogen and host (patient). Factors which affect the ability of fungal pathogen to overcome host defense and to cause infection include its overall prevalence, its resistance, and its virulence factors. With respect to the patient, factors which influence level of immunosuppression include the presence of co-morbid states (e.g., age extremes, diabetes mellitus, infection), the patient's underlying disease (e.g., malignancy, HIV/AIDS) and its associated treatment (e.g., chemotherapy, radiation, antibiotics) and patient exposure (e.g., nosocomial exposure, environmental exposure). Increases in pathogen burden associate with level of immunosuppression, and resolution in pathogen burden associates with immune restoration.

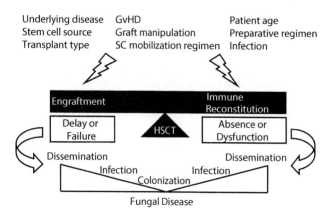

Figure 7.4 Successful outcome following hematopoietic stem cell transplantation (HSCT) requires a balance between donor-derived hematopoiesis (engraftment) and immune reconstitution. Delays and/or failures in HSC engraftment result in cytopenias that predispose the HSCT patient to fungal infection and dissemination. Similarly, absent and/or dysfunctional immune reconstitution also predisposes the HSCT patient to fungal disease. Multiple factors summarily upset this precarious balance, most notably graft-versus-host disease (GvHD), but also underlying disease (malignant versus non-malignant), stem cell source (bone marrow, peripheral blood, umbilical cord blood), stem cell (SC) mobilization regimen (G/GM-CSF versus flt3 ligand), graft manipulation (CD34+-selection, T-cell depletion, tumor purging), transplant type (matched-sibling donor versus matched-unrelated donor), patient age (young versus older patient), preparative regimen (myeloablative versus non-myeloablative), and infection (bacterial, fungal, viral).

Hematopoietic stem cell transplantation (HSCT) serves as the extreme clinical example in which the host's defense is severely compromised. Thus, HSCT patients often develop [165] and succumb [166] to IFI due to innate and adaptive cytopenia and dysfunction. HSCT involves replacement of malignant or non-malignant disease in the transplant host with normal donor-derived hematopoiesis and immunity (Figure 7.4). However, donor-derived HSC engraftment and immune reconstitution are influenced by a variety of factors, which upset their precarious balance and recovery. For example, prophylactic and empiric antifungal therapies have dramatically changed the epidemiology of fungal pathogens in HSCT recipients [167,168]. Furthermore, immunosuppressive agents targeting deleterious alloreactivity in the HSCT patient (i.e., graft versus host disease, GvHD) also increase the risk for IFI [169]. Cellular and soluble factor immunotherapies targeting immune restoration in the HSCT host are currently being explored to augment host defense against infection [170].

CONCLUSION

An enhanced understanding of fungal pathogenesis and immunity has occurred over the last 20 years. Paralleling this understanding has been the increase in pharmaceutical antifungal agents, as well as *ex vivo* expanded and manipulated cellular and synthetic soluble therapies. Thus, the advent of a "third age of antimicrobial therapy" is truly emerging [171]. However, success in using immunotherapy will require a thorough mechanistic understanding for the underlying cellular interactions and soluble mediators involved in the desired clinical response [170].

ACKNOWLEDGMENTS

The author would like to acknowledge those significant contributions to the field of fungal immunity that were not included in this chapter due to space limitations.

REFERENCES

1. Bodey GP, Buckley M, Sathe YS, et al. Quantitative relationships between circulating leukocytes and infection in patients with acute leukemia. *Ann Intern Med* 1966;64(2):328–340.

2. Romani L. Immunity to fungal infections. *Nat Rev Immunol* 2004;4(1):1–23.

3. Wiederhold NP, Patterson TF. What's new in anti-fungals: An update on the in-vitro activity and in-vivo efficacy of new and investigational antifungal agents. *Curr Opin Infect Dis* 2015;28(6):539–545.

4. Nucci M, Anaissie EJ, Queiroz-Telles F, et al. Outcome predictors of 84 patients with hemato-logic malignancies and *Fusarium* infection. *Cancer* 2003;98(2):315–319.

5. BitMansour A, Burns SM, Traver D, et al. Myeloid progenitors protect against invasive aspergillosis and *Pseudomonas aeruginosa* infection following hematopoietic stem cell transplantation. *Blood* 2002;100(13):4660–4667.

6. Sardi JCO, et al. *Candida* species: Current epide-miology, pathogenicity, biofilm formation, natural antifungal products and new therapeutic options. *J Med Microbiol* 2013;62:10–24.

7. Hager CL, Ghannoum MA. The mycobiome: Role in health and disease, and as a potential probiotic target in gastrointestinal disease. *Dig Liver Dis* 2017;49(11):1171–1176.

8. Young VB. The role of microbiome in human health and disease: An introduction for clinicians. *BMJ* 2017;356:j831.

9. Roeder A, Kirschning CJ, Rupec RA, et al. Toll-like receptors as key mediators in innate antifungal immunity. *Med Mycol* 2004;42(6):485–498.

10. Bellocchio S, Montagnoli C, Bozza S, et al. The con-tribution of the Toll-like/IL-1 receptor superfamily to innate and adaptive immunity to fungal patho-gens *in vivo. J Immunol* 2004;172(5):3059–3069.

11. Kawai T, Akira S. Pathogen recognition with Toll-like receptors. *Curr Opin Immunol* 2005;17(4):338–344.

12. Yamamoto M, Takeda K Akira S. TIR domain-containing adaptors define the specificity of TLR signaling. *Mol Immunol* 2004;40(12):861–868.

13. Akira S, Takeda K. Toll-like receptor signalling. *Nat Rev Immunol* 2004;4(7):499–511.

14. Platanias LC. Mechanisms of type-I- and type-II-interferon-mediated signalling. *Nat Rev Immunol* 2005;5(5):375–386.

15. Pulendran B, Smith JL, Caspary G, et al. Distinct dendritic cell subsets differentially regulate the class of immune response *in vivo. Proc Natl Acad Sci U S A* 1999;96(3):1036–1041.

16. Colonna M, Trinchieri G, Liu YJ. Plasmacytoid dendritic cells in immunity. *Nat Immunol* 2004;5(12):1219–1226.

17. Edwards AD, Diebold SS, Slack EM, et al. Toll-like receptor expression in murine DC subsets: Lack of TLR7 expression by CD8 alpha+ DC correlates with unresponsiveness to imidazoquinolines. *Eur J Immunol* 2003;33(4):827–833.

18. Han J, Ulevitch RJ. Limiting inflammatory responses during activation of innate immunity. *Nat Immunol* 2005;6(12):1198–1205.

19. Liew FY, Xu D, Brint EK, et al. Negative regulation of toll-like receptor-mediated immune responses. *Nat Rev Immunol* 2005;5(6):446–458.

20. Dambuza IM, Brown GD. C-type lectins in immu-nity: Recent developments. *Curr Opin Immunol* 2015;32:21–27.

21. Herre J, Marshall AS, Caron E, et al. Dectin-1 uses novel mechanisms for yeast phagocytosis in macro-phages. *Blood* 2004;104(13):4038–4045.

22. Brown GD, Taylor PR, Reid DM, et al. Dectin-1 is a major beta-glucan receptor on macrophages. *J Exp Med* 2002;196(3):407–412.

23. Allavena P, Chieppa M, Monti P, et al. From pattern recognition receptor to regulator of homeostasis: The double-faced macrophage mannose receptor. *Crit Rev Immunol* 2004;24(3):179–192.

24. Lavigne LM, Albina JE, Reichner JS. Beta-glucan is a fungal determinant for adhesion-dependent human neutrophil functions. *J Immunol* 2006;177(12):8667–8675.

25. Walport MJ. Complement. First of two parts. *N Engl J Med* 2001;344(14):1058–1066.

26. Brown GD, Gordon S. Immune recognition. A new receptor for β-glucans. *Nature* 2001;413(6851):36–37.

27. Goodridge HS, et al. Activation of the innate immune receptor Dectin-1 upon for-mation of a 'phagocytic synapse'. *Nature* 2011;472(7344):471–475.

28. Whitney PG, et al. Syk signaling in dendritic cells orchestrates innate resistance to systemic fungal infection. *PLoS Pathog* 2014, 10 (7) e1004276.

29. Bishu S, et al. The adaptor CARD9 is required for adaptive but not innate immunity to oral muco-sal *Candida albicans* infections. *Infect Immun* 2014;82(3):1173–1180.

30. Gross O, et al. Card9 controls a non-TLR signalling pathway for innate anti-fungal immunity. *Nature* 2006, 442, 651–656.

31. Glocker EO, et al. A homozygous CARD9 mutation in a family with susceptibility to fungal infections. *N Engl J Med* 2009;361(18):1727–1735.

32. Strasser D, et al. Syk kinase-coupled C-type lectin receptors engage protein kinase C-σ to elicit Card9 adaptor-mediated innate immunity. *Immunity* 2012. 36 (1), 32–42.

33. Gringhuis SI, et al. Dectin-1 directs T helper cell differentiation by controlling noncanonical NF-κB activation through Raf-1 and Syk. *Nat Immunol* 2009;10(2):203–213.

34. Cunha C, Aversa F, Romani L, Carvalho A. Human genetic susceptibility to invasive aspergillosis. *PLoS Pathog* 2013;9(8):e1003434.

35. Smeekens SP, van de Veerdonk FL, Kullberg BJ, Netea MG. Genetic susceptibility to *Candida* infections. *EMBO Mol Med* 2013;5(6):805–813.

36. Ferwerda B, et al. Human dectin-1 deficiency and mucocutaneous fungal infections. *N Engl J Med* 2009;361(18):1760–1767.

37. De Luca A, et al. IL-22 and IDO1 affect immunity and tolerance to murine and human vaginal candidiasis. *PLoS Pathog* 2013;9(7):e1003486.

38. Janeway CA, Jr. Medzhitov R. Innate immune recognition. *Annu Rev Immunol* 2002;20:197–216.

39. Seder RA, Gazzinelli RT. Cytokines are critical in linking the innate and adaptive immune responses to bacterial, fungal, and parasitic infection. *Adv Intern Med* 1999;44:353–388.

40. Hoebe K, Janssen E, Beutler B. The interface between innate and adaptive immunity. *Nat Immunol* 2004;5(10):971–974.

41. Nathan C. Neutrophils and immunity: Challenges and opportunities. *Nat Rev Immunol* 2006;6(3):173–182.

42. Urban CF, Reichard U, Brinkmann V, et al. Neutrophil extracellular traps capture and kill *Candida albicans* yeast and hyphal forms. *Cell Microbiol* 2006;8(4):668–676.

43. Menegazzi R, Decleva E, Dri P. Killing by neutrophil extracellular traps: Fact or folklore? *Blood* 2012;119(5):1214–1216.

44. Lionakis MS, et al. CX3CR1-dependent renal macrophage survival promotes *Candida* control and host survival. *J Clin Invest* 2013;123(12):5035–5051.

45. Break TJ, et al. CX3CR1 is dispensable for control of mucosal *Candida albicans* infections in mice and humans. *Infect Immun* 2015;83:958–965.

46. Ngo LY, et al. Inflammatory monocytes mediate early and organ-specific innate defense during systemic candidiasis. *J Infect Dis* 2014;209(1):109–119.

47. Bistoni F, et al. Evidence for macrophage-mediated protection against lethal *Candida albicans* infection. *Infect Immun* 1986;51(2):668–674.

48. Bistoni F, et al. Immunomodulation by a low-virulence, agerminative variant of *Candida albicans*. Further evidence for macrophage activation as one of the effector mechanisms of nonspecific anti-infectious protection. *J Med Vet Mycol* 1988;26:285–299.

49. Ifrim DC, et al. Defective trained immunity in patients with STAT1-dependent chronic mucocutaneaous candidiasis. *Clin Exp Immunol* 2015;181(3):434–440.

50. Trombetta ES, Mellman I. Cell biology of antigen processing *in vitro* and *in vivo*. *Annu Rev Immunol* 2005;23:975–1028.

51. Munz C. Autophagy and antigen presentation. *Cell Microbiol* 2006;8(6):891–898.

52. Friedl P, den Boer AT, Gunzer M. Tuning immune responses: Diversity and adaptation of the immunological synapse. *Nat Rev Immunol* 2005;5(7):532–545.

53. Liu EH, Siegel RM, Harlan DM, et al. T cell-directed therapies: Lessons learned and future prospects. *Nat Immunol* 2007;8(1):25–30.

54. McKenzie BS, Kastelein RA, Cua DJ. Understanding the IL-23-IL-17 immune pathway. *Trends Immunol* 2006;27(1):17–23.

55. Fossiez F, Djossou O, Chomarat P, et al. T cell interleukin-17 induces stromal cells to produce proinflammatory and hematopoietic cytokines. *J Exp Med* 1996;183(6):2593–2603.

56. Iwakura Y, Ishigame H. The IL-23/IL-17 axis in inflammation. *J Clin Invest* 2006;116(5):1218–1222.

57. Romani L, Montagnoli C, Bozza S, et al. The exploitation of distinct recognition receptors in dendritic cells determines the full range of host immune relationships with *Candida albicans*. *Int Immunol* 2004;16(1):149–161.

58. Sallusto F, Palermo B, Hoy A, et al. The role of chemokine receptors in directing traffic of naive, type 1 and type 2 T cells. *Curr Top Microbiol Immunol* 1999;246:123–128; discussion 129.

59. Walzer T, Dalod M, Robbins SH, et al. Natural-killer cells and dendritic cells: "l'union fait la force". *Blood* 2005;106(7):2252–2258.

60. Gerosa F, Gobbi A, Zorzi P, et al. The reciprocal interaction of NK cells with plasmacytoid or myeloid dendritic cells profoundly affects innate resistance functions. *J Immunol* 2005;174(2):727–734.

61. Andrews DM, Andoniou CE, Scalzo AA, et al. Crosstalk between dendritic cells and natural killer cells in viral infection. *Mol Immunol* 2005;42(4):547–555.

62. Liu YJ, Kanzler H, Soumelis V, et al. Dendritic cell lineage, plasticity and cross-regulation. *Nat Immunol* 2001;2(7):585–589.

63. Zuniga EI, McGavern DB, Pruneda-Paz JL, et al. Bone marrow plasmacytoid dendritic cells can differentiate into myeloid dendritic cells upon virus infection. *Nat Immunol* 2004;5(12):1227–1234.

64. Shortman K, Liu YJ. Mouse and human dendritic cell subtypes. *Nat Rev Immunol* 2002;2(3):151–161.

65. Dzionek A, Fuchs A, Schmidt P, et al. BDCA-2, BDCA-3, and BDCA-4: Three markers for distinct subsets of dendritic cells in human peripheral blood. *J Immunol* 2000;165(11):6037–6046.

66. Kadowaki N, Ho S, Antonenko S, et al. Subsets of human dendritic cell precursors express different toll-like receptors and respond to different microbial antigens. *J Exp Med* 2001;194(6):863–869.

67. Penna G, Vulcano M, Roncari A, et al. Cutting edge: Differential chemokine production by myeloid and plasmacytoid dendritic cells. *J Immunol* 2002;169(12):6673–6676.

68. Hochrein H, Shortman K, Vremec D, et al. Differential production of IL-12, IFN-alpha, and IFN-gamma by mouse dendritic cell subsets. *J Immunol* 2001;166(9):5448–5455.

69. Steinman RM, Hawiger D Nussenzweig MC. Tolerogenic dendritic cells. *Annu Rev Immunol* 2003;21:685–711.

70. Kalinski P, Hilkens CM, Wierenga EA, et al. T-cell priming by type-1 and type-2 polarized dendritic cells: The concept of a third signal. *Immunol Today* 1999;20(12):561–567.

71. Heufler C, Koch F, Stanzl U, et al. Interleukin-12 is produced by dendritic cells and mediates T helper 1 development as well as interferon-gamma production by T helper 1 cells. *Eur J Immunol* 1996;26(3):659–668.

72. Asselin-Paturel C, Trinchieri G. Production of type I interferons: Plasmacytoid dendritic cells and beyond. *J Exp Med* 2005;202(4):461–465.

73. Bogdan C. The function of type I interferons in antimicrobial immunity. *Curr Opin Immunol* 2000;12(4):419–424.

74. Belardelli F, Ferrantini M, Proietti E, et al. Interferon-alpha in tumor immunity and immunotherapy. *Cytokine Growth Factor Rev* 2002;13(2):119–134.

75. Biron CA. Interferons alpha and beta as immune regulators—a new look. *Immunity* 2001;14(6):661–664.

76. Akbar AN, Lord JM, Salmon M. IFN-alpha and IFN-beta: A link between immune memory and chronic inflammation. *Immunol Today* 2000;21(7):337–342.

77. Poeck H, Wagner M, Battiany J, et al. Plasmacytoid dendritic cells, antigen, and CpG-C license human B cells for plasma cell differentiation and immunoglobulin production in the absence of T-cell help. *Blood* 2004;103(8):3058–3064.

78. Moulin V, Andris F, Thielemans K, et al. B lymphocytes regulate dendritic cell (DC) function *in vivo*: Increased interleukin 12 production by DCs from B cell-deficient mice results in T helper cell type 1 deviation. *J Exp Med* 2000;192(4):475–482.

79. Delves PJ, Roitt IM. The immune system. Second of two parts. *N Engl J Med* 2000;343(2):108–117.

80. Montagnoli C, Bozza S, Bacci A, et al. A role for antibodies in the generation of memory antifungal immunity. *Eur J Immunol* 2003;33(5):1193–1204.

81. Cutler JE, Deepe GS, Jr. Klein BS. Advances in combating fungal diseases: Vaccines on the threshold. *Nat Rev Microbiol* 2007;5(1):13–28.

82. Medici NP, Del Poeta M. New insights on the development of fungal vaccines: From immunity to recent challenges. *Mem Inst Oswaldo Cruz* 2015;110(8):966–973.

83. Sandini S, et al. A highly immunogenic recombinant and truncated protein of the secreted aspartic proteases family (rSap2t) of *Candida albicans* as a mucosal anticandidal vaccine. *FEMS Immunol Med Microbiol* 2011;62(2):215–224.

84. Torosantucci A, et al. Protection by anti-β-glucan antibodies is associated with restricted β-1,3 glucan binding specificity and inhibition of fungal growth and adherence. *PLoS ONE* 2009;4(4):e5392.

85. Wan YY, Flavell RA. The roles for cytokines in the generation and maintenance of regulatory T cells. *Immunol Rev* 2006;212:114–130.

86. Bettelli E, Carrier Y, Gao W, et al. Reciprocal developmental pathways for the generation of pathogenic effector TH17 and regulatory T cells. *Nature* 2006;441(7090):235–238.

87. Seder RA, Ahmed R. Similarities and differences in CD4+ and CD8+ effector and memory T cell generation. *Nat Immunol* 2003;4(9):835–842.

88. Sun JC, Bevan MJ. Defective CD8 T cell memory following acute infection without CD4 T cell help. *Science* 2003;300(5617):339–342.

89. Northrop JK, Shen H. CD8+ T-cell memory: Only the good ones last. *Curr Opin Immunol* 2004;16(4):451–455.

90. Bettelli E, Oukka M, Kuchroo VK. T(H)-17 cells in the circle of immunity and autoimmunity. *Nat Immunol* 2007;8(4):345–350.

91. Aggarwal S, Gurney AL. IL-17: Prototype member of an emerging cytokine family. *J Leukoc Biol* 2002;71(1):1–8.

92. Maloy KJ, Powrie F. Regulatory T cells in the control of immune pathology. *Nat Immunol* 2001;2(9):816–822.

93. Jiang H, Chess L. Regulation of immune responses by T cells. *N Engl J Med* 2006;354(11):1166–1176.

94. Kamradt T, Mitchison NA. Tolerance and autoimmunity. *N Engl J Med* 2001;344(9):655–664.

95. Kozel TR. Activation of the complement system by pathogenic fungi. *Clin Microbiol Rev* 1996;9(1):34–46.

96. Lillegard JB, Sim RB, Thorkildson P, et al. Recognition of *Candida albicans* by mannan-binding lectin *in vitro* and *in vivo*. *J Infect Dis* 2006;193(11):1589–1597.

97. Ip WK, Lau YL. Role of mannose-binding lectin in the innate defense against *Candida albicans*: Enhancement of complement activation, but lack of opsonic function, in phagocytosis by human dendritic cells. *J Infect Dis* 2004;190(3):632–640.

98. Eisen DP, Minchinton RM. Impact of mannose-binding lectin on susceptibility to infectious diseases. *Clin Infect Dis* 2003;37(11):1496–1505.

99. Granell M, Urbano-Ispizua A, Suarez B, et al. Mannan-binding lectin pathway deficiencies and invasive fungal infections following allogeneic stem cell transplantation. *Exp Hematol* 2006;34(10):1435–1441.

100. Petersen KA, Matthiesen F, Agger T, et al. Phase I safety, tolerability, and pharmacokinetic study of recombinant human mannan-binding lectin. *J Clin Immunol* 2006;26(5):465–475.

101. Shalaby MR, et al. Activation of human polymor-phonuclear neutrophil functions by interferon-gamma and tumor necrosis factors. *J Immunol* 1985;135(3):2069–2073.

102. Nathan CF, Murray HW, Wiebe ME, Rubin BY. Identification of interferon-γ as the lymphokine that activates human macrophage oxidative metabolism and antimicrobial activity. *J Exp Med* 1983;158(3):670–689.

103. Netea MG, et al. Differential role of IL-18 and IL-12 in the host defense against disseminated *Candida albicans* infection. *Eur J Immunol* 2003;33(12):3409–3417.

104. van de Veerdonk FL, Kullberg BJ, Netea MG. Adjunctive immunotherapy with recombinant cyto-kines for the treatment of disseminated candidiasis. *Clin Microbiol Infect* 2012;18(2):112–119.

105. Eyerich S, et al. IL-22 and TNF-α represent a key cytokine combination for epidermal integrity dur-ing infection with *Candida albicans*. *Eur J Immunol* 2011;41(7):1894–1901.

106. Tomalka J, et al. β-defensin 1 plays a role in acute mucosal defense against *Candida albicans*. *J Immunol* 2015;194(4):1788–1795.

107. Langley RG, et al. Secukinumab in plaque psoriasis—results of two phase 3 trials. *N Engl J Med* 2014;371(4):326–338.

108. Spellberg B, Edwards JE. Jr. Type 1/Type 2 immunity in infectious diseases. *Clin Infect Dis* 2001;32(1):76–102.

109. Shoham S, Levitz SM. The immune response to fun-gal infections. *Br J Haematol* 2005;129(5):569–582.

110. Karin M, Lawrence T, Nizet V. Innate immunity gone awry: Linking microbial infections to chronic inflam-mation and cancer. *Cell* 2006;124(4):823–835.

111. Mencacci A, Cenci E, Del Sero G, et al. IL-10 is required for development of protective Th1 responses in IL-12-deficient mice upon *Candida albi-cans* infection. *J Immunol* 1998;161(11):6228–6237.

112. Mencacci A, Del Sero G, Cenci E, et al. Endogenous interleukin 4 is required for development of protec-tive CD4+ T helper type 1 cell responses to *Candida albicans*. *J Exp Med* 1998;187(3):307–317.

113. van de Veerdonk FL, Netea MG. T-cell subsets and antifungal host defenses. *Curr Fungal Infect Resp* 2010;4(4):238–243.

114. Mencacci A, Montagnoli C, Bacci A, et al. CD80+Gr-1+ myeloid cells inhibit development of antifungal Th1 immunity in mice with candidiasis. *J Immunol* 2002;169(6):3180–3190.

115. Mencacci A., et al. Endogenous interleukin 4 is required for development of protective CD4+ T helper type 1 cell responses to *Candida albicans*. *J Exp Med* 1998;187:307–317.

116. Spits H., et al. Innate lymphoid cells—a proposal for uniform nomenclature. *Nat Rev Immunol* 2013;13(2):145–14.

117. Antachopoulos C, Roilides E. Cytokines and fungal infections. *Br J Haematol* 2005;129(5):583–596.

118. Traynor TR, Huffnagle GB. Role of chemokines in fungal infections. *Med Mycol* 2001;39(1):41–50.

119. Charo IF, Ransohoff RM. The many roles of chemo-kines and chemokine receptors in inflammation. *N Engl J Med* 2006;354(6):610–621.

120. Mehrad B, Strieter RM, Moore TA, et al. CXC chemokine receptor-2 ligands are necessary components of neutrophil-mediated host defense in invasive pulmonary aspergillosis. *J Immunol* 1999;163(11):6086–6094.

121. Cyster JG. Lymphoid organ development and cell migration. *Immunol Rev* 2003;195:5–14.

122. Mehrad B, Strieter RM, Standiford TJ. Role of TNF-alpha in pulmonary host defense in murine invasive aspergillosis. *J Immunol* 1999;162(3):1633–1640.

123. Carpenter KJ, Hogaboam CM. Immunosuppressive effects of CCL17 on pulmonary antifungal responses during pulmonary invasive aspergillosis. *Infect Immun* 2005;73(11):7198–7207.

124. Wallin RP, Lundqvist A, More SH, et al. Heat-shock proteins as activators of the innate immune system. *Trends Immunol* 2002;23(3):130–135.

125. Matthews R, Burnie J. Antifungal antibodies: A new approach to the treatment of systemic candidiasis. *Curr Opin Investig Drugs* 2001;2(4):472–476.

126. Pachl J, Svoboda P, Jacobs F, et al. A random-ized, blinded, multicenter trial of lipid-associated amphotericin B alone versus in combination with an antibody-based inhibitor of heat shock protein 90 in patients with invasive candidiasis. *Clin Infect Dis* 2006;42(10):1404–1413.

127. Cowen LE, Lindquist S. Hsp90 potentiates the rapid evolution of new traits: Drug resistance in diverse fungi. *Science* 2005;309(5744):2185–2189.

128. Heitman J. Cell biology. A fungal Achilles' heel. *Science* 2005;309(5744):2175–2176.

129. Murray PJ. The JAK-STAT signaling path-way: Input and output integration. *J Immunol* 2007;178(5):2623–2629.

130. Arbabi S, Maier RV. Mitogen-activated protein kinases. *Crit Care Med* 2002;30(1 Suppl):S74–79.

131. Karin M, Greten FR. NF-kappaB: Linking inflam-mation and immunity to cancer development and progression. *Nat Rev Immunol* 2005;5(10):749–759.

132. Nathan C. Points of control in inflammation. *Nature* 2002;420(6917):846–852.

133. Alexander WS. Suppressors of cytokine signalling (SOCS) in the immune system. *Nat Rev Immunol* 2002;2(6):410–416.

134. Li Q, Verma IM. NF-kappaB regulation in the immune system. *Nat Rev Immunol* 2002;2(10):725–734.

135. Liu Y, Shepherd EG, Nelin LD. MAPK phosphatases-regulating the immune response. *Nat Rev Immunol* 2007;7(3):202–212.

136. Belkaid Y, Rouse BT. Natural regulatory T cells in infectious disease. *Nat Immunol* 2005;6(4):353–360.

137. La Cava A, Van Kaer L, Fu Dong S. CD4+CD25+ Tregs and NKT cells: Regulators regulating regulators. *Trends Immunol* 2006;27(7):322–327.

138. Rasmusson I. Immune modulation by mesenchymal stem cells. *Exp Cell Res* 2006;312(12):2169–2179.

139. Lizee G, Radvanyi LG, Overwijk WW, et al. Improving antitumor immune responses by circumventing immunoregulatory cells and mechanisms. *Clin Cancer Res* 2006;12(16):4794–4803.

140. Levitz SM. Interactions of Toll-like receptors with fungi. *Microbes Infect* 2004;6(15):1351–1355.

141. Gantner BN, Simmons RM, Canavera SJ, et al. Collaborative induction of inflammatory responses by dectin-1 and Toll-like receptor 2. *J Exp Med* 2003;197(9):1107–1117.

142. Dillon S, Agrawal S, Banerjee K, et al. Yeast zymosan, a stimulus for TLR2 and dectin-1, induces regulatory antigen-presenting cells and immunological tolerance. *J Clin Invest* 2006;116(4):916–928.

143. Romani L, Bistoni F, Puccetti P. Fungi, dendritic cells and receptors: A host perspective of fungal virulence. *Trends Microbiol* 2002;10(11):508–514.

144. Gantner BN, Simmons RM, Underhill DM. Dectin-1 mediates macrophage recognition of *Candida albicans* yeast but not filaments. *Embo J* 2005;24(6):1277–1286.

145. Van der Graaf CA, et al. Differential cytokine production and Toll-like receptor signaling pathways by *Candida albicans* blastoconidia and hyphae. *Infect Immun* 2005;73(11):7458–7464.

146. Netea MG, Warris A, Van der Meer JW, et al. Aspergillus fumigatus evades immune recognition during germination through loss of toll-like receptor-4-mediated signal transduction. *J Infect Dis* 2003;188(2):320–326.

147. Braedel S, Radsak M, Einsele H, et al. Aspergillus fumigatus antigens activate innate immune cells via toll-like receptors 2 and 4. *Br J Haematol* 2004;125(3):392–399.

148. Netea MG, Van Der Graaf CA, Vonk AG, et al. The role of toll-like receptor (TLR) 2 and TLR4 in the host defense against disseminated candidiasis. *J Infect Dis* 2002;185(10):1483–1489.

149. Netea MG, Sutmuller R, Hermann C, et al. Toll-like receptor 2 suppresses immunity against *Candida albicans* through induction of IL-10 and regulatory T cells. *J Immunol* 2004;172(6):3712–3718.

150. d'Ostiani CF, Del Sero G, Bacci A, et al. Dendritic cells discriminate between yeasts and hyphae of the fungus *Candida albicans*. Implications for initiation of T helper cell immunity *in vitro* and *in vivo*. *J Exp Med* 2000;191(10):1661–1674.

151. Claudia M, Bacci A, Silvia B, et al. The interaction of fungi with dendritic cells: Implications for Th immunity and vaccination. *Curr Mol Med* 2002;2(6):507–524.

152. Gafa V, Lande R, Gagliardi MC, et al. Human dendritic cells following Aspergillus fumigatus infection express the CCR7 receptor and a differential pattern of interleukin-12 (IL-12), IL-23, and IL-27 cytokines, which lead to a Th1 response. *Infect Immun* 2006;74(3):1480–1489.

153. Mehrad B, Moore TA, Standiford TJ. Macrophage inflammatory protein-1 alpha is a critical mediator of host defense against invasive pulmonary aspergillosis in neutropenic hosts. *J Immunol* 2000;165(2):962–968.

154. Beyer M, Schultze JL. Regulatory T cells in cancer. *Blood* 2006;108(3):804–811.

155. Hogan LH, Klein BS, Levitz SM. Virulence factors of medically important fungi. *Clin Microbiol Rev* 1996;9(4):469–488.

156. Romani L, Bistoni F, Puccetti P. Adaptation of *Candida albicans* to the host environment: The role of morphogenesis in virulence and survival in mammalian hosts. *Curr Opin Microbiol* 2003;6(4):338–343.

157. Stanzani M, Orciuolo E, Lewis R, et al. Aspergillus fumigatus suppresses the human cellular immune response via gliotoxin-mediated apoptosis of monocytes. *Blood* 2005;105(6):2258–2265.

158. Urban CF, Lourido S, Zychlinsky A. How do microbes evade neutrophil killing? *Cell Microbiol* 2006;8(11):1687–1696.

159. Brummer E, Kamberi M, Stevens DA. Regulation by granulocyte-macrophage colony-stimulating factor and/or steroids given *in vivo* of proinflammatory cytokine and chemokine production by bronchoalveolar macrophages in response to Aspergillus conidia. *J Infect Dis* 2003;187(4):705–709.

160. Boeckh M, Nichols WG. Immunosuppressive effects of beta-herpesviruses. *Herpes* 2003;10(1):12–16.

161. Lehrnbecher T, Foster C, Vazquez N, et al. Therapy-induced alterations in host defense in children receiving therapy for cancer. *J Pediatr Hematol Oncol* 1997;19(5):399–417.

162. Gerson SL, Talbot GH, Hurwitz S, et al. Prolonged granulocytopenia: The major risk factor for invasive pulmonary aspergillosis in patients with acute leukemia. *Ann Intern Med* 1984;100(3):345–351.

163. Lekstrom-Himes JA, Gallin JI. Immunodeficiency diseases caused by defects in phagocytes. *N Engl J Med* 2000;343(23):1703–1714.

164. Pfaller MA, Diekema DJ. Epidemiology of invasive candidiasis: A persistent public health problem. *Clin Microbiol Rev* 2007;20(1):133–163.

165. Martino R, Subira M, Rovira M, et al. Invasive fungal infections after allogeneic peripheral blood stem cell transplantation: Incidence and risk factors in 395 patients. *Br J Haematol* 2002;116(2):475–482.

166. Marr KA, Carter RA, Crippa F, et al. Epidemiology and outcome of mould infections in hematopoietic stem cell transplant recipients. *Clin Infect Dis* 2002;34(7):909–917.

167. Marr KA, Seidel K, White TC, et al. Candidemia in allogeneic blood and marrow transplant recipients: Evolution of risk factors after the adoption of prophylactic fluconazole. *J Infect Dis* 2000;181(1):309–316.

168. Kontoyiannis DP, Lionakis MS, Lewis RE, et al. Zygomycosis in a tertiary-care cancer center in the era of *Aspergillus*-active antifungal therapy: A case-control observational study of 27 recent cases. *J Infect Dis* 2005;191(8):1350–1360.

169. Marty FM, Lee SJ, Fahey MM, et al. Infliximab use in patients with severe graft-versus-host disease and other emerging risk factors of non-*Candida* invasive fungal infections in allogeneic hematopoietic stem cell transplant recipients: A cohort study. *Blood* 2003;102(8):2768–2776.

170. Auletta JJ, Lazarus HM. Immune restoration following hematopoietic stem cell transplantation: An evolving target. *Bone Marrow Transplant* 2005;35(9):835–857.

171. Casadevall A. The third age of antimicrobial therapy. *Clin Infect Dis* 2006;42(10):1414–1416.

8

Immunomodulators: What is the evidence for use in mycoses?

J. ANDREW ALSPAUGH

INTRODUCTION

Alterations in immunity are the major risk factor for developing invasive mycoses. Therefore, clinicians and scientific investigators have tried to devise immune-based strategies as adjunctive therapy in these infections. For example, in neutropenic patients, efforts to increase neutrophil number and function include the use of granulocyte transfusions and colony-stimulating factors. Investigators have also studied the role of cytokine administration to enhance the antifungal immune response in immunocompromised patients. For several decades, the administration of nonspecific immunoglobulin has been used in the treatment of infections. However, recent advances in this technology suggest that the passive administration of specific antibodies directed against fungal pathogens may be clinically relevant. As the immune status of the patient improves, clinicians must be aware of the risk of damage due to excessive inflammation, such as the immune reconstitution inflammatory syndrome (IRIS). Although often a sign of clinical improvement, the symptoms associated with this syndrome may mimic worsening infection.

ALTERED IMMUNITY AND INVASIVE FUNGAL INFECTIONS

Invasive fungal infections (IFIs) are most frequently encountered in patients with altered immune function. Most often, these infections occur in the setting of profound defects in immunity, such as chemotherapy-induced neutropenia or advanced HIV infection. The direct correlation between immunosuppression and systemic mycoses has prompted clinicians to explore adjunctive immune therapy for the treatment of these diseases. If a compromised immune system is the main risk factor for developing invasive fungal infections, perhaps therapy directed against these infections should include an attempt to restore or augment the immune response.

Rarely, invasive fungal infections occur in patients with innate disorders of immune function. For example, the impaired neutrophil oxidative burst in chronic granulomatous disease places affected patients at risk for invasive aspergillosis [1]. Chronic mucocutaneous candidiasis, causing recurrent and disfiguring *Candida* infections, results from various T-cell abnormalities such as mutations in the autoimmune regulator (AIRE) gene [2]. Also, *Coccidioides immitis* more frequently disseminates in patients of African or Filipino ethnic backgrounds, presumably due to uncharacterized genetic determinants [3].

However, most invasive fungal infections are directly attributable to acquired immune defects, such as those resulting from AIDS, solid organ transplantation, and antineoplastic therapy. Immune restoration using antiretroviral therapy in AIDS has resulted in a dramatic improvement in treating and preventing the opportunistic infections associated with this syndrome. Similar strategies are being explored to manipulate the immune system to better treat mycoses in other immunosuppressed patient populations.

GRANULOCYTE TRANSFUSION

Prolonged neutropenia after cytotoxic chemotherapy poses an important period of risk for the development of infections. In 1994, Morrison evaluated 1186 consecutive patients undergoing bone marrow transplantation at a university hospital [4]. Of these patients, 10% (123 patients) developed an invasive infection by a fungus other than *Candida*. This high rate of fungal infection was associated with accelerated mortality, with only 17% of infected patients surviving greater than 180 days. Among this cohort, risk factors for developing invasive fungal infections included age greater than 18, prior cytomegalovirus (CMV) exposure, graft-versus-host disease, and delayed engraftment. Of these, delayed engraftment carried the greatest relative risk for subsequent fungal infections, underscoring the importance of neutrophil restoration in the prevention and cure of fungal infections. In fact, recovery of neutrophil function is the most important factor in patient survival from severe infections associated with neutropenia [5].

Granulocyte transfusions would appear to be logical therapy for neutropenic patients with infections, restoring functional neutrophils to patients during this period of highest infectious risk. However, several challenges have limited the widespread use of this therapy. Normal healthy adults make approximately 10^{11} neutrophils each day, and these cells have an active life span of 9–10 days [6]. Therefore, harvesting and infusing adequate numbers of neutrophils have historically been technically challenging. Additionally, multiple granulocyte infusions might be required to support patients during the entire period of neutropenia.

Early case reports of granulocyte transfusions in neutropenic patients with active infections lead to an initial enthusiasm for this therapy [7–9]. However, subsequent studies failed to demonstrate a clinical benefit to neutropenic patients for the routine, prophylactic administration of granulocyte transfusions during periods of neutropenia. For example, Strauss evaluated 102 patients with neutropenia resulting from therapy for acute myelogenous leukemia. The patients were randomized to receive daily granulocyte transfusions or placebo. No reduction was observed in the survival or incidence of infection between the two study groups. Moreover, the granulocyte transfusion-treated group had significantly more pulmonary infiltrates than the control patients [10].

Several studies were specifically designed to evaluate the role of granulocyte transfusion in neutropenic patients with fungal infections, and many of these studies failed to demonstrate any measurable benefit from this therapy. A retrospective analysis was performed of 87 patients with invasive fungal infections during the first 100 days after bone marrow transplantation [11]. Fifty patients received both granulocyte transfusions and targeted antifungal therapy, and 37 patients received antifungal therapy alone. Although the transfusions were well-tolerated, no clinical benefit was observed for those patients who received granulocyte transfusions.

Of great concern, other studies during this time suggested that patients treated with granulocyte transfusions seemed to develop more pulmonary infiltrates compared to control patients, especially when the neutrophils were co-administered with amphotericin B, resulting in serious pulmonary damage due to alveolar hemorrhage. In one such study, acute respiratory decompensation occurred in 64% of patients in which amphotericin B and granulocyte infusions were administered together, as opposed to 6% among patients who only received the cell infusion [12]. Subsequent studies failed to confirm this association, including a retrospective analysis of 144 patients in which no excess pulmonary toxicity was attributable to granulocyte transfusions [13]. Nonetheless, largely due to concerns for toxicity and unproven efficacy, granulocyte transfusions were infrequently performed for several years. Also, improvements in the supportive care of neutropenic patients have made life-threatening bacterial and fungal infections less common in this patient group.

There was a renewed enthusiasm for granulocyte infusions with advances in neutrophil harvesting techniques. Because of the concern for inadequate dosing of neutrophils in early studies of granulocyte infusions, newer neutrophil acquisition methods involve pre-treating neutrophil donors with granulocyte colony-stimulating factor (G-CSF) and steroids. This intervention allowed the harvesting and infusion of large numbers of functional granulocytes. Using this strategy, Peters et al. demonstrated that the transfusion of granulocytes in neutropenic patients was well-tolerated and resulted in measurable increases in peripheral leukocyte counts [14]. In this study, seven granulocyte transfusions were required on average for each patient to support them until bone marrow recovery, and these multiple granulocyte infusions were well-tolerated.

A later study used community neutrophil donors stimulated with a single dose of G-CSF plus oral dexamethasone to maximize neutrophil recovery [7]. In this study 19 patients were treated with a mean of 8.6 transfusions.

Granulocyte transfusion therapy resulted in restoration of the peripheral neutrophil count to normal values in 17 of 19 patients. Also, function of the infused neutrophils was confirmed by a buccal neutrophil infiltration response. Transfusion-associated symptoms were observed in 7% of patients, but these symptoms were not enough to limit therapy. Eight of the 11 patients with bacterial or fungal infection resolved their infections with combination antimicrobial therapy and granulocyte infusions [7].

Several more recent trials have also attempted to study the efficacy of granulocyte transfusions in adult patients using modern neutrophil harvesting techniques. Most of these trials found that multiple granulocyte transfusions were well-tolerated. One uncontrolled, observational trial evaluated granulocyte transfusions in 25 neutropenic patients with active infections, concluding that patients with infections due to fungi or gram-negative bacilli may experience more clinical benefit from this intervention than patients with infections due to gram-positive cocci [15]. Three additional trials suggested that granulocyte transfusions may have their greatest effectiveness not during current episodes of neutropenia but as secondary prophylaxis for patients undergoing repeat stem cell transplantation, preventing infections during subsequent periods of neutropenia [16–18].

In 2006, Sachs et al. published one of the most striking studies demonstrating the clinical benefit of pediatric granulocyte infusion therapy, describing their experience with early granulocyte transfusions in neutropenic children [19]. In contrast to prior studies, the 27 patients in this prospective Phase II trial received early granulocyte transfusions, administered a median of 7.5 days after the onset of neutropenia. All patients tolerated the infusions well, and the mean absolute neutrophil count remained greater than 1×10^9 cells/mL for 8 days after granulocyte transfusion. Of the 27 total patients in this study, 25 (92.6%) cleared their initial infection and 81.5% were alive 1 month after infection. All six children with invasive aspergillosis cleared their infection. The authors concluded that early granulocyte transfusions were feasible and safe in immunocompromised children with neutropenia [19].

Published case reports also described the potential efficacy of granulocyte infusions in neutropenic patients with life-threatening invasive fungal infections. For example, the combination of antifungal therapy and granulocyte transfusions was used in three children undergoing stem cell transplantation with life-threatening fungal infections. The infections in this case series included a cerebral mold infection, disseminated candidiasis, and nasopharyngeal mucormycosis. All three children were cured of the fungal infections, and the anticancer therapy was pursued without delay [20].

In addition to the administration of larger numbers of neutrophils to neutropenic patients, other novel variations of granulocyte transfusions have also been pursued. The co-administration of granulocyte transfusions and interferon-gamma-1b was safely performed in 20 patients with neutropenia and active infections [21]. This cytokine enhances the immune response against a number of intracellular pathogens. Also, immortalized phagocytic cells from culture have been administered to neutropenic animals and demonstrated to protect them from otherwise lethal *Candida* infections [22]. In non-neutropenic patients with serious mycoses, immune augmentation with granulocyte transfusions has been suggested but never studied in large clinical trials.

Well-controlled and adequately powered trials would allow clinicians to evaluate the relative risks and benefits of granulocyte transfusions in neutropenic patients with life-threatening infections. In fact, the Resolving Infections in people with Neutropenia with Granulocytes (RING) trial was a randomized, controlled clinical trial designed specifically for this purpose [23]. However, the RING investigators were unable to recruit adequate numbers of patients willing to undergo randomization to treatment (granulocyte transfusion) versus no treatment in this life-threatening situation. Therefore, anecdotal experience will likely define this therapy for the foreseeable future. Additionally, although defining exact cost-of-therapy is quite challenging, the resources required to support granulocyte transfusions (donor G-CSF therapy, granulocyte harvesting by apheresis, cell storage and transfusion) are considerable [24–27].

Summary

Although theoretically promising, granulocyte infusion therapy has not demonstrated a consistent benefit to adult neutropenic patients with invasive fungal infections. One historical limitation of this therapy has been administering sufficient functional neutrophils to offer a sustained antimicrobial effect until patients can make their own granulocytes. This may explain why granulocyte transfusions in pediatric populations appear to be more efficacious than in adults, given a more favorable dose relative to body weight. Modern granulocyte harvesting techniques have improved the effective number of cells that can be administered [7,14].

Currently, granulocyte transfusions are not recommended for routine administration or prophylaxis in neutropenic patients. Even in the absence of evidence-based data, they are used most frequently in patients with prolonged neutropenia (absolute neutrophil count <500 cells/microliter) who have life-threatening infections, especially those failing to respond to antimicrobial therapy. Although alloimmunization and delayed engraftment are potential side effects of granulocyte transfusions, recent studies suggest that granulocyte transfusions are well-tolerated in neutropenic patients (Table 8.1).

Table 8.1 Selected clinical trials of granulocyte transfusions (GTx) in neutropenic patients

References	Study description	Patients	Conclusions
[11]	Retrospective study of GTx in patients with neutropenia and fungal infections	87 patients; 50 received GTx and antifungal therapy; 37 received antifungal therapy alone	GTx was well-tolerated, but no clinical benefit was observed with this therapy over antifungals alone
[28]	Pilot study of GTx in patients with hematological malignancies and serious fungal infections	15 patients	(1) 11/15 patients with GTx had a favorable clinical response (2) 8/15 patients were free of infection 3 weeks after therapy
[14]	Prospective Phase I/II trial of GTx in neutropenic patients with serious bacterial or fungal infections	30 patients; median of 7 GTx per patient	GTx was well-tolerated; 20/30 patients were alive with complete clinical resolution 100 days after GTx
[7]	Prospective Phase I/II trial of GTx in neutropenic patients with serious bacterial or fungal infections	19 patients receiving GTx from G-CSF/dexamethasone-treated community leukocyte donors	(1) Restoration of normal neutrophil counts in 17/19 patients (2) Normal buccal neutrophil response in most patients (3) Resolution of infection in 8/11 patients with invasive bacterial or Candida infections
[15]	GTx in neutropenic patients with active infections	25 patients	Favorable clinical response in 8/11 patients with fungal infections, 9/15 patients with gram-negative bacilli infections, and 5/16 with gram-positive cocci infections
[16]	GTx in patients with neutropenia-related infections; evaluating this therapy as treatment as well as secondary prophylaxis for infections	42 patients received GTx, 18 with active infection (treatment group) and 8 with severe prior infection (prophylaxis group)	(1) 12/18 patients with improved or resolved active infection (2) 0/8 patients with recurrence of severe prior infection
[17]	GTx in patients with prior invasive aspergillosis (IA) or high risk for developing IA	8 patients with IA (or high risk for IA), 18 controls (similar conditioning regimens but no prior IA)	Compared to controls, GTx-treated patients had decrease duration of fevers and fewer days of neutropenia; 4/7 GTx-treated patients had improved chest radiographs
[18]	Observational trial of GTx in patients undergoing stem cell transplantation with active infections or recent serious fungal infections	67 patients; 44 with active infections, and 23 with recent serious fungal infections	(1) No reactivation of fungal infections (0/23) in GTx-treated patients (2) Control of active infections in 36/44 patients
[19]	Prospective Phase II trial of early-onset GTx in neutropenic children with severe infections	27 pediatric patients with neutropenia-related infected refractory to standard therapy	(1) 92.6% of patients resolved initial infection (2) 81.5% of patients alive without signs of infection at 1 month (3) 6/6 children with IA resolved their infection

Abbreviations: GTx: granulocyte transfusion; IA: invasive aspergillosis.

CYTOKINE THERAPY

Colony stimulating factors

Mature human leukocytes differentiate from precursor cells in response to colony stimulating factors (CSFs). Granulocyte colony-stimulating factor (G-CSF) increases the number of mature neutrophils by increasing the production of these cells and by inhibiting apoptosis [29]. Clinically, G-CSF has played a major role in the treatment of many hematological disorders. This cytokine reduces the period of neutropenia after chemotherapy, resulting in reduced hospitalizations and antimicrobial use [30,31]. Also, G-CSF therapy has allowed the transplantation of hematopoietic stem cells instead of bone marrow cells for recovery after marrow ablative therapy. Similarly, GM-CSF (granulocyte-macrophage colony-stimulating factor) and M-CSF (macrophage colony-stimulating factor) promote the maturation of granulocytes/macrophages or macrophages, respectively [32].

Numerous *in vitro* studies have suggested that G-CSF may enhance fungal killing by antimicrobials and leukocytes [33–35]. For example, G-CSF enhances the antifungal effect of voriconazole and neutrophils against *Candida albicans in vitro* [36]. This cytokine was also demonstrated to increase the antifungal effects of neutrophils by promoting an increased oxidative burst [37,38]. G-CSF treatments in neutropenic AIDS patients resulted in an increased number of circulating neutrophils as well as an augmentation of the *in vitro* fungicidal effects of these cells [39].

In other studies, the administration of colony-stimulating factors protected animals from death due to experimental infections with *Aspergillus*, *Candida*, and *Cryptococcus* [40–43]. For example, although G-CSF had no beneficial effect alone in a murine neutropenic model of disseminated candidiasis, it did improve the survival of fluconazole-treated animals more than drug therapy alone [44]. Also, in mouse models of systemic aspergillosis, the addition of G-CSF to various combinations of antifungal drugs improved survival in neutropenic animals [45,46].

Despite the effectiveness of colony-stimulating factors in promoting hematopoietic cell recovery, clinical trials have been less consistent in demonstrating a clear survival benefit for the routine use of G-CSF or GM-CSF as prophylactic therapy in neutropenic patients with infections. For example, Crawford et al. demonstrated that prophylactic use of G-CSF in neutropenic patients receiving therapy for small-cell lung cancer resulted in reduced duration of neutropenia and fewer episodes of fever. However, no reduction in mortality was demonstrated in the G-CSF-treated patients [31]. Similarly, in a randomized, double-blind, placebo-controlled trial, G-CSF administration for chemotherapy-induced neutropenia resulted in reduced median days of neutropenia and time to resolution of febrile neutropenia; the trial was not designed to evaluate a mortality difference [47]. There were insufficient numbers of fungal infections in these trials to determine whether this cytokine contributed to the prevention of invasive mycoses.

Cytokine therapy in neutropenic patients was associated with increased survival in one study in which 124 patients aged 55–70 were randomized to receive either GM-CSF or placebo after induction therapy for acute myelogenous leukemia (AML). Compared to the placebo-arm, the GM-CSF-treated patients experienced reduced periods of neutropenia, improved survival, and decreased mortality due to invasive fungal infections [32]. Therefore, in this neutropenic subpopulation of patients, prophylactic therapy with GM-CSF, and not G-CSF, has been demonstrated to offer a survival benefit. The authors postulate that the macrophage-stimulatory activity of GM-CSF may be important in preventing the growth of pathogenic microorganisms in the lungs and on mucosal surfaces.

It is important to note that GM-CSF therapy is often associated with more patient-reported symptoms (myalgias, fatigue) than treatment with G-CSF. G-CSF is rarely associated with allergic reactions, and the most commonly reported side-effect is mild bone pain in 20%–30% of patients [48]. Most patients tolerate this medication well. In contrast, the most frequent side-effect associated with GM-CSF is fever in 20% of patients, which can complicate the clinical assessment of neutropenic patients. Also, influenza-like symptoms have also been associated with GM-CSF administration, and high doses may contribute to a capillary-leak syndrome [49].

Because of the enhancement of leukocyte antifungal effects by G-CSF, this cytokine has also been used in non-neutropenic patients with various infections. For example, a phase II trial of recombinant G-CSF in hospitalized patients with pneumonia failed to demonstrate a survival benefit in patients treated with G-CSF compared to placebo-treated patients. However, adverse secondary end-points, such as development of empyema and progression to acute respiratory distress syndrome (ARDS), were less common in patients in the G-CSF arm of the study [50].

Interferon-gamma

Interferon-gamma (INF-gamma) activates macrophages and other immune cells. Although it induces only a modest antiviral activity, its effect on macrophages and T-cells is associated with a marked increase in the antifungal action of these cells.

INF-gamma therapy has been studied extensively in patients with chronic granulomatous disease (CGD). The neutrophils of these patients have impaired respiratory burst and a resulting inability to produce antimicrobial reactive oxygen species. Therefore, patients with CGD are at risk for developing a number of bacterial and fungal diseases, often presenting with recurrent staphylococcal infections as well as invasive aspergillosis [1].

In 1991, a large clinical trial in patients with CGD demonstrated that INF-gamma therapy resulted in substantially fewer serious infections compared to placebo [51]. Interestingly, there was no measurable effect of this therapy on superoxide production by the immune cells.

Among treated patients, INF-gamma therapy was well-tolerated [51]. The combination of early recognition of CGD, aggressive management of infections, antimicrobial prophylaxis, and interferon-gamma therapy in selected patients has resulted in significant improvement in the clinical outcomes of this disease.

In addition to its use as prophylactic therapy, case reports have demonstrated that INF-gamma may be helpful in the treatment of invasive fungal infections in patients with CGD [52,53]. However, no large clinical trials have yet indicated that routine use of INF-gamma is beneficial in other immunosuppressed patient populations. Of note, increased levels of endogenous INF-gamma are associated with increased risk of rejection in transplant patients [54,55]. Therefore, careful study of this agent in clinical trials is warranted before its more general use can be recommended in immunosuppressed patients.

INF-gamma has been studied as adjunctive therapy in cryptococcosis. A phase II, double blind trial of INF-gamma versus placebo in AIDS-associated cryptococcal meningitis revealed that this intervention was well-tolerated. Also, the patients in this study who were treated with INF-gamma demonstrated a trend toward improved clinical and microbiological outcomes [56]. INF-gamma has also been used in patients with *C. neoformans* meningitis refractory to aggressive medical therapy [55]. A trial of INF-gamma in aspergillosis was planned but terminated prior to patient recruitment.

Interleukin-12 (IL-12)

Expression of the interleukin-12 cytokine is associated with an enhanced Th-1 immune response. Th-1 immunity is often required for effective clearance of many systemic fungal infections. Therefore, IL-12 therapy has been studied as a way to help resolve invasive fungal infections in experimental animals. For example, two studies demonstrated that IL-12 given to mice infected with *Cryptococcus neoformans* resulted in increased survival and reduced fungal burden [57,58]. Similarly, the early administration of IL-12 in a model of disseminated histoplasmosis resulted in improved survival compared to untreated animals [59].

Importantly, high doses of IL-12 in non-neutropenic animals resulted in an excessive immune response and poorer clinical outcomes in an animal model of aspergillosis [60]. It is unclear if the excessive inflammation could be avoided with a reduced dose of IL-12, or if this therapy should only be considered for profoundly immune-deficient subjects.

There are numerous clinical trials of IL-12 as adjunctive therapy in treating patients with various malignancies. However, there is no substantial, published clinical experience describing IL-12 therapy in human mycoses.

Interleukin-2

IL-2 plays a major role in promoting the graft-versus-tumor effect after stem cell transplantation. Since this is often a desirable outcome after myeloablative therapy, investigators in Israel conducted a trial to determine whether routine administration of this cytokine would improve clinical outcomes in patients undergoing stem cell transplantation. The investigators noted that 2 of the first 12 patients treated with IL-2 therapy developed invasive fungal infections; this was a much higher incidence of systemic mycoses than would be expected from historic data. Therefore, the trial was terminated prematurely [61]. However, subsequent published studies of low-dose IL-2 administration in stem cell transplantation reported an overall beneficial effect, and no significant increases in observed infections [62]. The potential for unexpected, dose-related effects of cytokine therapy on invasive fungal infections underscores that novel therapy should be conducted in the setting of monitored clinical trials that are designed to identify adverse events.

PASSIVE ANTIBODY THERAPY

The use of non-specific antibody therapy in immunocompromised patients was studied in a series of patients undergoing bone marrow transplantation [63]. Forty-five patients received intravenous immunoglobulin (IVIG) weekly for three months after transplantation. Although the IVIG-treated patients received less amphotericin B than controls, the untreated controls were less likely to experience fatal veno-occlusive disease of the liver. No difference was noted in other transplant-related complications or in two-year survival between the two groups, suggesting that no overall clinical benefit derived from routine IVIG therapy in this patient population [63]. In contrast, liver transplant patients receiving IVIG for CMV prophylaxis experienced significantly fewer fungal infections than untreated controls [64].

Pathogen-specific passive antibody therapy has demonstrated efficacy in models of human fungal infections, even when humoral immunity does not seem to play a major role in the clearance of natural infections. For example, a monoclonal antibody directed against the polysaccharide capsule of *Cryptococcus neoformans* helped to prevent death due to cryptococcosis in experimentally infected mice [65]. Such studies have prompted human trials of antibody therapy for cryptococcosis. An anticryptococcal antibody preparation was well-tolerated in treated patients, and it was associated with more rapid clearance of serum cryptococcal antigen than untreated controls. However, inadequate sample size prevented clear answers about efficacy [66]. Monoclonal antibodies directed against the *C. neoformans* capsule are also in human trials [67].

Similarly, monoclonal antibodies have been developed against the *Candida albicans* hsp90 heat shock protein and various surface polysaccharides. Several of these antibodies protect mice in experimental models of lethal candidiasis [68–70].

In addition to pathogen-specific antibody therapy, investigators have recently reported developing antibodies against microbial features that are common to diverse bacterial, fungal, and parasite pathogens. One such feature is the PNAG surface capsule (ß-[1,6]-linked poly-N-acetyl-D-glucosamine) found in *S. aureus*, various gram-negative bacteria, *Candida* species, and *Plasmodium* species [71]. Polyclonal antibodies against the acetylated and de-acetylated forms of this molecule were passively administered in several animal models of infection, demonstrating protective and therapeutic efficacy in many cases [71]. Therefore, broadly reactive antibodies against common microbial targets may have clinical utility in recalcitrant infections.

IMMUNE RECONSTITUTION INFLAMMATORY SYNDROME (IRIS)

The specific restoration of defective immune function offers significant promise in treating and preventing infections in immunocompromised patients. However, this same intervention may also result in unexpected worsening symptoms of infections. This observation has been frequently observed in patients with AIDS who undergo immune recovery in response to highly active antiretroviral therapy. With increased immune system function, these patients can paradoxically develop symptomatic infections with various pathogens, presumably due to a reawakening immune system with a renewed ability to respond to resident microbes. For example, as their CD4 counts increase in response to antiretroviral therapy, newly treated HIV-infected patients may experience worsening retinal or colonic inflammation due to previously subclinical CMV disease at these anatomic sites.

Similarly, other instances are clearly described in which increasing immune function might paradoxically result in increased symptoms of fungal infections. Pulmonary aspergillosis is frequently identified during the period of neutrophil recovery after prolonged neutropenia, presumably due to the renewed ability of the infected patient to mount an inflammatory response to this pathogen [72]. Moreover, it is clear that much of the host damage in many fungal infections of the central nervous system is often due to the host immune response. A recent clinical trial attempted to address this issue by treating patients with HIV-associated cryptococcal meningitis with adjunctive corticosteroids in addition to standard antifungal therapy. In contrast to the initial hypothesis, the steroid-treated patients had worse clinical outcomes than the untreated controls, prompting early discontinuation of the trial [73]. Although more targeted immune suppressive therapies may actually benefit these patients, high-dose dexamethasone is clearly not routinely indicated in this infection.

In contrast, immune suppression is beneficial in other types of immune pathology associated with invasive fungal infections. In a retrospective analysis of Immune Reconstitution Inflammatory Syndrome (IRIS) associated with invasive fungal diseases, Singh et al. described that AIDS patients with cryptococcal meningitis developed IRIS

Table 8.2 Suggested diagnostic criteria for Immune Reconstitution Inflammatory Syndrome (IRIS) associated with opportunistic mycoses

1. New appearance or worsening of:
   a. Clinical or radiographic manifestations consistent with increased inflammation
   b. CSF pleocytosis
   c. Increased intracranial pressure
   d. Histopathology showing granulomatous inflammation
   e. Unexplained hypercalcemia
2. Symptoms occurring during receipt of appropriate antifungal therapy, and symptoms not consistent with newly acquired infection
3. Negative cultures for initial fungal pathogen, or stable/reduced biomarkers of initial infection

Source: Singh, N. and Perfect, J.R., *Lancet Infect Dis*, 7, 395–401, 2007.

in 30%–33% of cases when antiretroviral therapy was initiated soon after diagnosis of the infection [74]. IRIS was also reported in 5% of solid-organ transplant patients within 5.5 weeks of initiating antifungal therapy for an invasive mycosis [74,75]. Singh and Perfect also proposed diagnostic criteria for defining IRIS associated with opportunistic fungal infections (Table 8.2). As this syndrome is distinguished from uncontrolled fungal infections, most patients with IRIS benefit from antimicrobial therapy combined with immune suppression.

For clinicians who care for highly immunosuppressed patients with invasive fungal infections, it will be important to develop an ever-increasing sophistication concerning the interplay between two types of host damage: (1) that due to the microbe itself in the setting of poor immune reactivity and (2) that due to a dysregulated or excessive immune response. Future advances in the management of infectious diseases will require improved definition and quantification of immune function in individual patients. While some patients may benefit from more rapid recovery from drug-induced neutropenia, others may benefit from targeted immune suppression, in the case of IRIS of other states of accelerated immune responses. As this occurs, we will be able to more directly confront the excessive morbidity and mortality due to infectious diseases in our most vulnerable patients.

CONCLUSION

The rising incidence of invasive fungal infections is directly correlated with advances in medical therapies, and associated alterations in innate immune barriers and adaptive immune responses. Many patients with these infections have identifiable, specific defects in immunity. Therefore, investigators in many clinical disciplines are exploring whether the specific modulation of the immune system can improve patient outcomes in the setting of invasive mycoses.

REFERENCES

1. Winkelstein JA, Marino MC, Johnston RB, Jr., Boyle J, Curnutte J, Gallin JI, Malech HL, Holland SM, Ochs H, Quie P, et al. Chronic granulomatous disease. Report on a national registry of 368 patients. *Medicine (Baltimore)*. 2000;79(3):155–169.

2. Kirkpatrick CH. Chronic mucocutaneous candidiasis. *Pediatr Infect Dis J* 2001;20(2):197–206.

3. Louie L, Ng S, Hajjeh R, Johnson R, Vugia D, Werner SB, Talbot R, Klitz W. Influence of host genetics on the severity of coccidioidomycosis. *Emerg Infect Dis* 1999;5(5):672–680.

4. Morrison VA, Haake RJ, Weisdorf DJ. Non-*Candida* fungal infections after bone marrow transplantation: Risk factors and outcome. *Am J Med* 1994;96(6):497–503.

5. Gerson SL, Talbot GH, Hurwitz S, Strom BL, Lusk EJ, Cassileth PA. Prolonged granulocytopenia: The major risk factor for invasive pulmonary aspergillosis in patients with acute leukemia. *Ann Intern Med* 1984;100(3):345–351.

6. Boggs DR. Transfusion of neutrophils as prevention or treatment of infection in patients with neutropenia. *N Engl J Med* 1974;290(19):1055–1062.

7. Price TH, Bowden RA, Boeckh M, Bux J, Nelson K, Liles WC, Dale DC. Phase I/II trial of neutrophil transfusions from donors stimulated with G-CSF and dexamethasone for treatment of patients with infections in hematopoietic stem cell transplantation. *Blood* 2000;95(11):3302–3309.

8. Alavi JB, Root RK, Djerassi I, Evans AE, Gluckman SJ, MacGregor RR, Guerry D, Schreiber AD, Shaw JM, Koch P, et al. A randomized clinical trial of granulocyte transfusions for infection in acute leukemia. *N Engl J Med* 1977;296(13):706–711.

9. Vogler WR, Winton EF. A controlled study of the efficacy of granulocyte transfusions in patients with neutropenia. *Am J Med* 1977;63(4):548–555.

10. Strauss RG, Connett JE, Gale RP, Bloomfield CD, Herzig GP, McCullough J, Maguire LC, Winston DJ, Ho W, Stump DC, et al. A controlled trial of prophylactic granulocyte transfusions during initial induction chemotherapy for acute myelogenous leukemia. *N Engl J Med* 1981;305(11):597–603.

11. Bhatia S, McCullough J, Perry EH, Clay M, Ramsay NK, Neglia JP. Granulocyte transfusions: Efficacy in treating fungal infections in neutropenic patients following bone marrow transplantation. *Transfusion* 1994;34(3):226–232.

12. Wright DG, Robichaud KJ, Pizzo PA, Deisseroth AB. Lethal pulmonary reactions associated with the combined use of amphotericin B and leukocyte transfusions. *N Engl J Med* 1981;304(20):1185–1189.

13. Dana BW, Durie BG, White RF, Huestis DW. Concomitant administration of granulocyte transfusions and amphotericin B in neutropenic patients: Absence of significant pulmonary toxicity. *Blood* 1981;57(1):90–94.

14. Peters C, Minkov M, Matthes-Martin S, Potschger U, Witt V, Mann G, Hocker P, Worel N, Stary J, Klingebiel T, et al. Leucocyte transfusions from rhG-CSF or prednisolone stimulated donors for treatment of severe infections in immunocompromised neutropenic patients. *Br J Haematol* 1999;106(3):689–696.

15. Lee JJ, Chung IJ, Park MR, Kook H, Hwang TJ, Ryang DW, Kim HJ. Clinical efficacy of granulocyte transfusion therapy in patients with neutropenia-related infections. *Leukemia* 2001;15(2):203–207.

16. Illerhaus G, Wirth K, Dwenger A, Waller CF, Garbe A, Brass V, Lang H, Lange W. Treatment and prophylaxis of severe infections in neutropenic patients by granulocyte transfusions. *Ann Hematol* 2002;81(5):273–281.

17. Kerr JP, Liakopolou E, Brown J, Cornish JM, Fleming D, Massey E, Oakhill A, Pamphilon DH, Robinson SP, Totem A, et al. The use of stimulated granulocyte transfusions to prevent recurrence of past severe infections after allogeneic stem cell transplantation. *Br J Haematol* 2003;123(1):114–118.

18. Mousset S, Hermann S, Klein SA, Bialleck H, Duchscherer M, Bomke B, Wassmann B, Bohme A, Hoelzer D, Martin H. Prophylactic and interventional granulocyte transfusions in patients with haematological malignancies and life-threatening infections during neutropenia. *Ann Hematol* 2005;84(11):734–741.

19. Sachs UJ, Reiter A, Walter T, Bein G, Woessmann W. Safety and efficacy of therapeutic early onset granulocyte transfusions in pediatric patients with neutropenia and severe infections. *Transfusion* 2006;46(11):1909–1914.

20. Grigull L, Beilken A, Schmid H, Kirschner P, Sykora KW, Linderkamp C, Donnerstag F, Goudeva L, Heuft HG, Welte K. Secondary prophylaxis of invasive fungal infections with combination antifungal therapy and G-CSF-mobilized granulocyte transfusions in three children with hematological malignancies. *Support Care Cancer* 2006;14(7):783–786.

21. Safdar A, Rodriguez GH, Lichtiger B, Dickey BF, Kontoyiannis DP, Freireich EJ, Shpall EJ, Raad, II, Kantarjian HM, Champlin RE. Recombinant interferon gamma1b immune enhancement in 20 patients with hematologic malignancies and systemic opportunistic infections treated with donor granulocyte transfusions. *Cancer* 2006;106(12):2664–2671.

22. Spellberg BJ, Collins M, Avanesian V, Gomez M, Edwards JE, Jr., Cogle C, Applebaum D, Fu Y, Ibrahim AS. Optimization of a myeloid cell transfusion strategy for infected neutropenic hosts. *J Leukoc Biol* 2007;81(3):632–641.

23. Price TH, Boeckh M, Harrison RW, McCullough J, Ness PM, Strauss RG, Nichols WG, Hamza TH, Cushing MM, King KE, et al. Efficacy of transfusion with granulocytes from G-CSF/dexamethasone-treated donors in neutropenic patients with infection. *Blood* 2015;126(18):2153–2161.

24. Quillen K, Byrne P, Yau YY, Leitman SF. Ten-year follow-up of unrelated volunteer granulocyte donors who have received multiple cycles of granulocyte-colony-stimulating factor and dexamethasone. *Transfusion* 2009;49(3):513–518.

25. Adkins D, Spitzer G, Johnston M, Velasquez W, Dunphy F, Petruska P. Transfusions of granulocyte-colony-stimulating factor-mobilized granulocyte components to allogeneic transplant recipients: Analysis of kinetics and factors determining posttransfusion neutrophil and platelet counts. *Transfusion* 1997;37(7):737–748.

26. Hubel K, Carter RA, Liles WC, Dale DC, Price TH, Bowden RA, Rowley SD, Chauncey TR, Bensinger WI, Boeckh M. Granulocyte transfusion therapy for infections in candidates and recipients of HPC transplantation: A comparative analysis of feasibility and outcome for community donors versus related donors. *Transfusion* 2002;42(11):1414–1421.

27. Hubel K, Rodger E, Gaviria JM, Price TH, Dale DC, Liles WC. Effective storage of granulocytes collected by centrifugation leukapheresis from donors stimulated with granulocyte-colony-stimulating factor. *Transfusion* 2005;45(12):1876–1889.

28. Dignani MC, Anaissie EJ, Hester JP, O'Brien S, Vartivarian SE, Rex JH, Kantarjian H, Jendiroba DB, Lichtiger B, Andersson BS, et al. Treatment of neutropenia-related fungal infections with granulocyte colony-stimulating factor-elicited white blood cell transfusions: A pilot study. *Leukemia* 1997;11(10):1621–1630.

29. Dale DC, Liles WC, Llewellyn C, Price TH. Effects of granulocyte-macrophage colony-stimulating factor (GM-CSF) on neutrophil kinetics and function in normal human volunteers. *Am J Hematol* 1998;57(1):7–15.

30. Antman KS, Griffin JD, Elias A, Socinski MA, Ryan L, Cannistra SA, Oette D, Whitley M, Frei E, 3rd, Schnipper LE. Effect of recombinant human granulocyte-macrophage colony-stimulating factor on chemotherapy-induced myelosuppression. *N Engl J Med* 1988;319(10):593–598.

31. Crawford J, Ozer H, Stoller R, Johnson D, Lyman G, Tabbara I, Kris M, Grous J, Picozzi V, Rausch G, et al. Reduction by granulocyte colony-stimulating factor of fever and neutropenia induced by chemotherapy in patients with small-cell lung cancer. *N Engl J Med* 1991;325(3):164–170.

32. Rowe JM, Andersen JW, Mazza JJ, Bennett JM, Paietta E, Hayes FA, Oette D, Cassileth PA, Stadtmauer EA, Wiernik PH. A randomized placebo-controlled phase III study of granulocyte-macrophage colony-stimulating factor in adult patients (>55 to 70 years of age) with acute myelogenous leukemia: A study of the Eastern Cooperative Oncology Group (E1490). *Blood* 1995;86(2):457–462.

33. Gaviria JM, van Burik JA, Dale DC, Root RK, Liles WC. Comparison of interferon-gamma, granulocyte colony-stimulating factor, and granulocyte-macrophage colony-stimulating factor for priming leukocyte-mediated hyphal damage of opportunistic fungal pathogens. *J Infect Dis* 1999;179(4):1038–1041.

34. Gaviria JM, van Burik JA, Dale DC, Root RK, Liles WC. Modulation of neutrophil-mediated activity against the pseudohyphal form of *Candida albicans* by granulocyte colony-stimulating factor (G-CSF) administered *in vivo*. *J Infect Dis* 1999;179(5):1301–1304.

35. Liles WC, Huang JE, van Burik JA, Bowden RA, Dale DC. Granulocyte colony-stimulating factor administered *in vivo* augments neutrophil-mediated activity against opportunistic fungal pathogens. *J Infect Dis* 1997;175(4):1012–1015.

36. Vora S, Purimetla N, Brummer E, Stevens DA. Activity of voriconazole, a new triazole, combined with neutrophils or monocytes against *Candida albicans*: Effect of granulocyte colony-stimulating factor and granulocyte-macrophage colony-stimulating factor. *Antimicrob Agents Chemother* 1998;42(4):907–910.

37. Roilides E, Uhlig K, Venzon D, Pizzo PA, Walsh TJ. Enhancement of oxidative response and damage caused by human neutrophils to *Aspergillus fumigatus* hyphae by granulocyte colony-stimulating factor and gamma interferon. *Infect Immun* 1993;61(4):1185–1193.

38. Roilides E, Holmes A, Blake C, Pizzo PA, Walsh TJ. Effects of granulocyte colony-stimulating factor and interferon-gamma on antifungal activity of human polymorphonuclear neutrophils against pseudohyphae of different medically important *Candida* species. *J Leukoc Biol* 1995;57(4):651–656.

39. Vecchiarelli A, Monari C, Baldelli F, Pietrella D, Retini C, Tascini C, Francisci D, Bistoni F. Beneficial effect of recombinant human granulocyte colony-stimulating factor on fungicidal activity of polymorphonuclear leukocytes from patients with AIDS. *J Infect Dis* 1995;171(6):1448–1454.

40. Hamood M, Bluche PF, De Vroey C, Corazza F, Bujan W, Fondu P. Effects of recombinant human granulocyte-colony stimulating factor on neutropenic mice infected with *Candida albicans*: Acceleration of recovery from neutropenia and potentiation of anti-C. *albicans* resistance. *Mycoses* 1994;37(3–4):93–99.

41. Kullberg BJ, Netea MG, Curfs JH, Keuter M, Meis JF, van der Meer JW. Recombinant murine granulocyte colony-stimulating factor protects against acute disseminated *Candida albicans* infection in nonneutropenic mice. *J Infect Dis* 1998;177(1):175–181.

42. Polak-Wyss A. Protective effect of human granulocyte colony stimulating factor (hG-CSF) on *Candida* infections in normal and immunosuppressed mice. *Mycoses* 1991;34(3–4):109–118.

43. Polak-Wyss A. Protective effect of human granulocyte colony-stimulating factor (hG-CSF) on *Cryptococcus* and *Aspergillus* infections in normal and immunosuppressed mice. *Mycoses* 1991;34(5–6):205–215.

44. Graybill JR, Bocanegra R, Luther M. Antifungal combination therapy with granulocyte colony-stimulating factor and fluconazole in experimental disseminated candidiasis. *Eur J Clin Microbiol Infect Dis* 1995;14(8):700–703.

45. Sionov E, Mendlovic S, Segal E. Experimental systemic murine aspergillosis: Treatment with polyene and caspofungin combination and G-CSF. *J Antimicrob Chemother* 2005;56(3):594–597.

46. Graybill JR, Bocanegra R, Najvar LK, Loebenberg D, Luther MF. Granulocyte colony-stimulating factor and azole antifungal therapy in murine aspergillosis: Role of immune suppression. *Antimicrob Agents Chemother* 1998;42(10):2467–2473.

47. Maher DW, Lieschke GJ, Green M, Bishop J, Stuart-Harris R, Wolf M, Sheridan WP, Kefford RF, Cebon J, Olver I, et al. Filgrastim in patients with chemotherapy-induced febrile neutropenia. A double-blind, placebo-controlled trial. *Ann Intern Med* 1994;121(7):492–501.

48. Frampton JE, Lee CR, Faulds D. Filgrastim. A review of its pharmacological properties and therapeutic efficacy in neutropenia. *Drugs* 1994;48(5):731–760.

49. Root RK, Dale DC. Granulocyte colony-stimulating factor and granulocyte-macrophage colony-stimulating factor: Comparisons and potential for use in the treatment of infections in nonneutropenic patients. *J Infect Dis* 1999;179 Suppl 2:S342–S352.

50. Nelson S, Belknap SM, Carlson RW, Dale D, DeBoisblanc B, Farkas S, Fotheringham N, Ho H, Marrie T, Movahhed H, et al. A randomized controlled trial of filgrastim as an adjunct to antibiotics for treatment of hospitalized patients with community-acquired pneumonia. CAP Study Group. *J Infect Dis* 1998;178(4):1075–1080.

51. A controlled trial of interferon gamma to prevent infection in chronic granulomatous disease. The International Chronic Granulomatous Disease Cooperative Study Group. *N Engl J Med* 1991;324(8):509–516.

52. Williamson PR, Kwon-Chung KJ, Gallin JI. Successful treatment of Paecilomyces varioti infection in a patient with chronic granulomatous disease and a review of Paecilomyces species infections. *Clin Infect Dis* 1992;14(5):1023–1026.

53. Phillips P, Forbes JC, Speert DP. Disseminated infection with *Pseudallescheria boydii* in a patient with chronic granulomatous disease: Response to gamma-interferon plus antifungal chemotherapy. *Pediatr Infect Dis J* 1991;10(7):536–539.

54. D'Elios MM, Josien R, Manghetti M, Amedei A, de Carli M, Cuturi MC, Blancho G, Buzelin F, del Prete G, Soulillou JP. Predominant Th1 cell infiltration in acute rejection episodes of human kidney grafts. *Kidney Int* 1997;51(6):1876–1884.

55. Netea MG, Brouwer AE, Hoogendoorn EH, Van der Meer JW, Koolen M, Verweij PE, Kullberg BJ. Two patients with cryptococcal meningitis and idiopathic CD4 lymphopenia: Defective cytokine production and reversal by recombinant interferon- gamma therapy. *Clin Infect Dis* 2004;39(9):e83–e87.

56. Pappas PG, Bustamante B, Ticona E, Hamill RJ, Johnson PC, Reboli A, Aberg J, Hasbun R, Hsu HH. Recombinant interferon- gamma 1b as adjunctive therapy for AIDS-related acute cryptococcal meningitis. *J Infect Dis* 2004;189(12):2185–2191.

57. Kawakami K, Tohyama M, Xie Q, Saito A. IL-12 protects mice against pulmonary and disseminated infection caused by *Cryptococcus neoformans. Clin Exp Immunol* 1996;104(2):208–214.

58. Clemons KV, Brummer E, Stevens DA. Cytokine treatment of central nervous system infection: Efficacy of interleukin-12 alone and synergy with conventional antifungal therapy in experimental cryptococcosis. *Antimicrob Agents Chemother* 1994;38(3):460–464.

59. Zhou P, Sieve MC, Tewari RP, Seder RA. Interleukin-12 modulates the protective immune response in SCID mice infected with Histoplasma capsulatum. *Infect Immun* 1997;65(3):936–942.

60. Romani L, Puccetti P, Bistoni F. Interleukin-12 in infectious diseases. *Clin Microbiol Rev* 1997;10(4):611–636.

61. Toren A, Or R, Ackerstein A, Nagler A. Invasive fungal infections in lymphoma patients receiving immunotherapy following autologous bone marrow transplantation (ABMT). *Bone Marrow Transplant* 1997;20(1):67–69.

62. Rizzieri DA, Crout C, Storms R, Golob J, Long GD, Gasparetto C, Sullivan KM, Horwitz M, Chute J, Lagoo AS, et al. Feasibility of low-dose interleukin-2 therapy following T-cell-depleted nonmyeloablative allogeneic hematopoietic stem cell transplantation from HLA-matched or -mismatched family member donors. *Cancer Invest* 2011;29(1):56–61.

63. Klaesson S, Ringden O, Ljungman P, Aschan J, Hagglund H, Winiarski J. Does high-dose intravenous immune globulin treatment after bone marrow transplantation increase mortality in veno-occlusive disease of the liver? *Transplantation* 1995;60(11):1225–1230.

64. Stratta RJ, Shaefer MS, Cushing KA, Markin RS, Reed EC, Langnas AN, Pillen TJ, Shaw BW, Jr. A randomized prospective trial of acyclovir and immune globulin prophylaxis in liver transplant recipients receiving OKT3 therapy. *Arch Surg* 1992;127(1):55–63; discussion 63–64.

65. Dromer F, Charreire J, Contrepois A, Carbon C, Yeni P. Protection of mice against experimental crypto-coccosis by anti-*Cryptococcus neoformans* monoclonal antibody. *Infect Immun* 1987;55(3):749–752.

66. Gordon MA, Casadevall A. Serum therapy for Cryptococcal meningitis. *Clin Infect Dis* 1995;21(6):1477–1479.

67. Casadevall A, Cleare W, Feldmesser M, Glatman-Freedman A, Goldman DL, Kozel TR, Lendvai N, Mukherjee J, Pirofski LA, Rivera J, et al. Characterization of a murine monoclonal antibody to *Cryptococcus neoformans* polysaccharide that is a candidate for human therapeutic studies. *Antimicrob Agents Chemother* 1998;42(6):1437–1446.

68. Matthews R, Hodgetts S, Burnie J. Preliminary assessment of a human recombinant antibody fragment to hsp90 in murine invasive candidiasis. *J Infect Dis* 1995;171(6):1668–1671.

69. Han Y, Kanbe T, Cherniak R, Cutler JE. Biochemical characterization of *Candida albicans* epitopes that can elicit protective and nonprotective antibodies. *Infect Immun* 1997;65(10):4100–4107.

70. Han Y, Ulrich MA, Cutler JE. *Candida albicans* mannan extract-protein conjugates induce a protective immune response against experimental candidiasis. *J Infect Dis* 1999;179(6):1477–1484.

71. Cywes-Bentley C, Skurnik D, Zaidi T, Roux D, Deoliveira RB, Garrett WS, Lu X, O'Malley J, Kinzel K, Zaidi T, et al. Antibody to a conserved antigenic target is protective against diverse prokaryotic and eukaryotic pathogens. *Proc Natl Acad Sci U S A* 2013;110(24):E2209–E2218.

72. Todeschini G, Murari C, Bonesi R, Pizzolo G, Verlato G, Tecchio C, Meneghini V, Franchini M, Giuffrida C, Perona G, et al. Invasive aspergillosis in neutropenic patients: Rapid neutrophil recovery is a risk factor for severe pulmonary complications. *Eur J Clin Invest* 1999;29(5):453–457.

73. Beardsley J, Wolbers M, Kibengo FM, Ggayi AB, Kamali A, Cuc NT, Binh TQ, Chau NV, Farrar J, Merson L, et al. Adjunctive Dexamethasone in HIV-Associated Cryptococcal Meningitis. *N Engl J Med* 2016;374(6):542–554.

74. Singh N. Acute lung injury and acute respiratory distress syndrome. *Lancet* 2007;370(9585):383–384; author reply 4–5.

75. Singh N, Lortholary O, Alexander BD, Gupta KL, John GT, Pursell K, Munoz P, Klintmalm GB, Stosor V, del Busto R, et al. An immune reconstitution syndrome-like illness associated with *Cryptococcus neoformans* infection in organ transplant recipients. *Clin Infect Dis* 2005;40(12):1756–1761.

76. Singh N, Perfect JR. Immune reconstitution syndrome associated with opportunistic mycoses. *Lancet Infect Dis* 2007;7(6):395–401.

9

Fungal biofilms and catheter-associated infections

JYOTSNA CHANDRA AND MAHMOUD A. GHANNOUM

INTRODUCTION

The use of indwelling medical devices (e.g., central venous catheters [CVCs]) in current therapeutic practice has been found to be responsible for more than 80%–90% of hospital-acquired bloodstream and deep tissue infections [1]. Transplantation procedures, immunosuppression, and prolonged intensive care unit stays have also increased the prevalence of nosocomial, especially fungal infections. *Candida* species are the most commonly associated fungal organisms with such nosocomial infections, with *Candida albicans* being the predominant species causing systemic disease. Even with current antifungal therapy, mortality associated with invasive candidiasis due to nosocomial infections can be as high as 40% in adults [2,3], and up to 30% in the neonate population [4]. In a multicenter study of 427 consecutive patients with candidemia, the mortality rate for patients with catheter-related candidemia was found to be 41% [5]. *Candida* infections are often associated with indwelling medical devices, such as dental implants, catheters, heart valves, vascular bypass grafts, ocular lenses, artificial joints, and central nervous system shunts, that commonly involve biofilm formation. These are all suitable devices for microbial colonization, mostly by *C. albicans*, but also by other non-*albicans Candida* species, such as *C. parapsilosis, C. glabrata, C. tropicalis, or C. kruzei*. The expanded clinical importance of fungal biofilms is reflected by a growing number of reports associating biofilms with other yeasts and filamentous fungi, including *Cryptococcus neoformans, Candida lusitaniae, Aspergillus fumigatus*, and *Fusarium species* [6]. For example, *Aspergillus* species have been implicated in infections of cardiac pacemakers, joint replacements, and breast augmentation implants [6]. Forty percent of patients with microbial colonization of intravenous catheters develop occult fungemia, with consequences ranging from focal disease to severe sepsis and death [5,7]. The tenacity with which *Candida* infects indwelling biomedical devices necessitates their removal to affect a cure. For candidemia-associated non-tunneled CVCs, initial management includes exchanging of catheter and performing semi-quantitative or quantitative catheter cultures [8]. The Infectious Diseases Society of America (IDSA) guidelines suggest that antifungal therapy is necessary in all cases of vascular catheter-related candidemia [9].

Catheter-related bloodstream infections (CRBSIs) commonly involve colonization of microorganisms on catheter surfaces where they eventually become embedded in a biofilm [10]. Biofilms are defined as extensive communities of sessile organisms irreversibly associated with a surface, encased within a polysaccharide-rich extracellular matrix (ECM), exhibiting enhanced resistance to antimicrobial drugs [10]. Since *C. albicans* is the most common fungus associated with CRBSIs, biofilms formed by this pathogenic fungus can be used as a model to investigate the biology and pathogenesis of biofilm-associated infections. Recent studies have provided revealing insight into the effect of different variables (including growth time, nutrients, and physiological conditions) on fungal biofilm formation, morphology, and architecture.

This chapter provides an update on biofilms and discusses major recent advances achieved in the clinically relevant area of catheter-associated fungal biofilms.

BIOFILM FORMATION UNDER *IN VITRO*, *IN VIVO*, AND CLINICAL CONDITIONS

In vitro studies: Biofilm models, microscopic evaluation, resistance mechanisms, and microarray/proteomic metabolic pathway studies

IN VITRO BIOFILM MODELS

In the last decade, various model systems have been used to investigate the properties of *Candida* biofilms *in vitro* [11]. These models range from simple assays with catheter discs to more complex flow systems, such as the perfused biofilm fermenter [12]. Subsequent *in vitro* model systems have included a variety of different plastics, microtiter plates, glass slides, microporous cellulose filters, acrylic strips, voice prostheses, catheter discs, contact lenses, and tissue culture flasks [13–19]. Although a variety of substrates support formation of biofilms, those formed on clinically relevant substrates such as catheters, denture acrylic strips, and contact lenses under physiological conditions are likely to be closer to the clinical setting than those formed on non-physiologically relevant substrates. The biodiversity and abundance of biofilm-associated microorganisms in polymicrobial communities is detected using a combination of molecular diagnostics based on PCR, sequencing technologies, and advanced mathematical algorithms to identify the presence of biofilm-producing microorganisms and analyze the copy number of each organism relative to the total number of copies for all organisms [20].

Initial characterization of *C. albicans* biofilms by Hawser and Douglas [15] involved growing adherent *C. albicans* populations on the surface of small disks cut from a variety of catheters [15], including latex urinary catheters, polyvinyl chloride CVCs, silicone elastomer-coated latex urinary Foley catheters, silicone urinary Foley catheters, and polyurethane CVCs. In this model, growth was quantified using a colorimetric assay on the basis of reduction of a tetrazolium salt (3-[4,5-dimethylthiazol-2-yl]-2,5-diphenyltetrazolium bromide [MTT]) or incorporation of 3H-leucine [15]. This study showed an increase in MTT values and 3H-leucine incorporation levels with the maturation of biofilms and showed that both methods resulted in strong correlation with biofilm dry weight [15].

Our initial work on fungal biofilms involved development and characterization of *C. albicans* biofilms formed on common bioprosthetic material: silicone elastomer (SE), a model material used for indwelling devices including catheters [14]. Measurement of biofilm growth was performed using two quantitative methods: (*i*) colorimetric assays that involved the reduction of 2,3-bis(2-methoxy-4-nitro-5-sulfophenyl)-5-[(phenyl amino) carbonyl]-2*H*-tetrazolium hydroxide (XTT) by mitochondrial dehydrogenase in the living cells, into a colored water-soluble product measured spectrophotometrically, and (*ii*) dry weight determination, in which biofilms were scraped off the substrate surface and filtered through a pre-weighed membrane filter under vacuum [13–15]. Dry weight and XTT values increased with the formation of biofilms [14]. Garcia-Sanchez et al. [21] utilized disks to form biofilms and quantified biofilm formation using XTT and showed an increase in XTT values with the formation of biofilm. Ramage et al. [22], using a 96-well microtiter plate model, performed a series of experiments to assess the variability between *C. albicans* biofilms formed in independent wells of the same microtiter plate. All biofilms formed on the microtiter plates over a 24-hour time period displayed consistent XTT readings when the intensity of the colorimetric product was measured [22]. In general, formation of biofilm is associated with increase in metabolic activity and dry weight [13–15]. However, some later studies showed that there were some limitations of the XTT assay, especially when using metabolic activities to compare biofilm formation between *C. albicans* and *C. parapsilosis* isolates [23,24]. Additionally, increase in dry weight of biofilms may not always correlate with increase in metabolic activity with biofilm development, since these assays characterize different properties within the biofilm (biomass and metabolic state, respectively) [23,24]. Therefore, careful interpretation is critical while assessing results obtained using these *in vitro* models.

Recently, Simitsopoulou et al. [6], described methods involving quantification of biofilm extracellular DNA (e-DNA) and protein associated with extracellular matrix, by EDTA-based disaggregation followed by recovering the supernatant after high-speed centrifugation. The e-DNA was isolated from supernatants using a DNA extraction kit following manufacturer's instructions. These investigators also quantified the protein content of the extracellular matrix with the Bradford procedure using a commercial kit [6]. Roilides et al. [20] used quantitative measurement of biofilm growth using different methods, such as dry cell weight assays and XTT reduction assays and assessed the colony forming unit (CFU) by plating on solid media and DNA quantification methods. Nascimento et al. [25] used a DNA checkerboard method (which enables the simultaneous identification of distinct microorganisms in a large number of samples) to quantify *Candida* biofilms. Iturrieta-Gonzalez et al. [26] used crystal violet staining to quantify *Trichosporon* biofilms, where biofilms were washed twice with phosphate buffered saline, stained with 0.4% aqueous crystal violet solution for 45 minutes and absorbance was measured at 570 nm.

Development of these *in vitro* models/techniques have allowed detailed investigation, microscopic evaluation, and gene/protein profiling of *Candida* biofilms.

MICROSCOPIC EVALUATION: FUNGAL BIOFILM EXHIBIT PHASE-DEPENDENT GROWTH AND HETEROGENEOUS ARCHITECTURE

Various microscopic techniques, including scanning electron microscopy (SEM), fluorescence microscopy (FM), and confocal scanning laser microscopy (CSLM), have been used to visualize the structure of biofilms. Fluorescence microscopy analysis allows visualization of gross biofilm morphology and the appearance of extracellular matrix during biofilm formation, while SEM enables evaluation of detailed surface topography and morphology at very high resolutions. However, sample processing for SEM involves fixation and dehydration steps, which degrade the native hydrated structural features. In contrast, confocal microscopy is a nondestructive technology that can visualize the intact structure of live biofilms at lower resolutions [27] and allows researchers to overcome some drawbacks of SEM.

Hawser and Douglas [15] used SEM to show that *C. albicans* biofilms comprise a network of yeasts, hyphae,

pseudohyphae, and extracellular polymeric material visible on the surface of some of these morphological forms. Similar structures were seen by Chandra et al. [13], where they showed amorphous granular material (Figure 9.1b, *arrow*) covering yeast and hyphal forms (Figure 9.1a, b). Using a 96-well plate model, Ramage et al. [28] also showed that mature *C. albicans* biofilms consisted of a dense network of yeast cells and hyphal elements embedded within exopolymeric material. Hawser and Douglas [15] showed that after 1 hour of incubation, cell population consisted of all budding yeast cells adhering to the catheter. After 3–6 hours, some cells had developed into germ-tubes, and biofilms grown to 24–48 hours consisted of a mixed population of yeast, hyphae, pseudohyphae, and extracellular matrix [15].

Owing to the limitations of SEM, FM and CSLM were used to visualize intact structures of biofilm and the developmental phases associated with the biofilm growth were identified (Figure 9.2). FM studies showed that biofilm develops in three distinct phases: early (0–11 hours), intermediate (~12–24 hours), and mature phase (24–48 hours) [14]. CSLM allows the visualization of three-dimensional (3D) architecture at different depths of biofilms and the measurement of biofilm thickness without distortion of the native biofilm structure. In CSLM studies, two stains were utilized: Concanavalin A (Con A) Alexa Fluor™, which binds polysaccharides and gives a green fluorescence, and FUN-1, which stains metabolic active yeast cells as red fluorescence. In the 3D reconstructed images of *C. albicans* biofilms, at the early phase, only adhered yeast cells were attached to the catheter surface and lacked any extracellular material, while mature biofilms consisted of *C. albicans* cells at the basal layer and hyphae encased in a dense extracellular matrix (Figure 9.2) [14]. Our study and those of other showed that biofilms have two distinct morphological

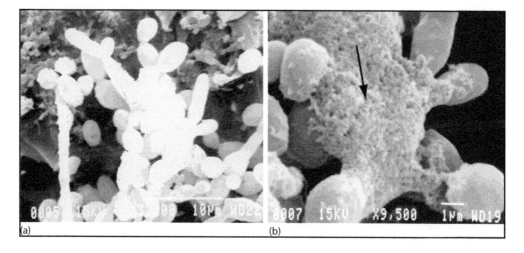

Figure 9.1 **(a)** Scanning electron microscopy (SEM) of a *C. albicans* biofilm showing fungal cells covered with biofilm matrix. Some hyphal forms are also seen (magnification 3300×). **(b)** *C. albicans* cells observed embedded in extracellular polymeric material that had an amorphous granular appearance (as shown by arrow) (magnification 9500×).

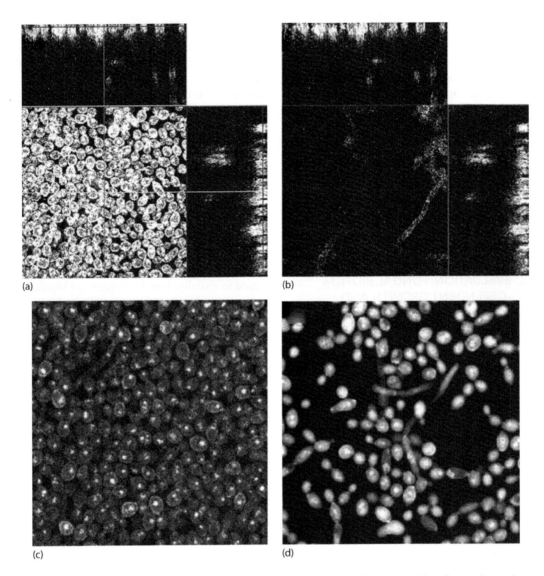

Figure 9.2 Confocal scanning laser microscopy (CSLM) images of mature *C. albicans* biofilms formed on silicone elastomer surface. Orthogonal images of the basal (10–12 μm thick) **(a)** and upper layers (450 μm thick) of *C. albicans* mature biofilm **(b)**. The ECM-derived haziness seen in mature biofilm **(c)** is absent when the extracellular material is removed **(d)** (magnification 20×).

layers: a thin, basal yeast layer that anchors the biofilm to the surface and a thicker, more open hyphal layer surrounded by an extracellular matrix [14,29]. These microscopic evaluations of catheter-related *Candida* biofilms also showed that biofilms are formed in three distinct developmental phases and exhibit a highly heterogeneous structure.

Shukla et al. [30] reported that biofilm formation by *Aspergillus nidulans* involved depolymerization of microtubules (MT), modulated by MT +end-binding proteins (+TIPS) and SrbA hypoxic transcription factor, revealing a potentially new mode of MT regulation in response to changing gaseous biofilm microenvironments, which could contribute to the unique characteristics of fungal biofilms in medical and industrial settings [30].

The polysaccharide capsule of *Cryptococcus neoformans*, a human pathogenic fungus, promotes the attachment process to prosthetic medical devices, whereas cell-surface glycoproteins facilitate adhesion of *C. albicans* and *C. glabrata* [6]. Attachment is promoted by several environmental signals, such as changes in nutrient concentrations, pH, flow velocity of surrounding body fluids (urine, blood, saliva), temperature, oxygen concentration, osmolality, and iron [20].

Another way to trap both nutrients and planktonic cells once a critical biofilm mass has been achieved is the production and secretion of extracellular matrix predominantly composed of polysaccharides, proteins, and extracellular DNA. Biofilm matrix promotes initial cell adhesion, triggers polysaccharide formation, and serves as a support that links molecules together in the biofilm matrix, thus influencing the structure and organization of mature biofilms. Extracellular DNA is an important component of *A. fumigatus* biofilms that originates from either fungal autolysis [31] or is externally supplied from human neutrophils attracted to the infected site and is important for protection from environmental stresses, including antifungal therapy [31].

ANTIFUNGAL RESISTANCE IN BIOFILMS IS MEDIATED BY MULTIPLE MECHANISMS, IN A PHASE-DEPENDENT MANNER

Biofilm lifestyle confers numerous advantages to pathogens, including a high tolerance to environmental stresses such as antimicrobials and host immune responses [32]. The development of various models has helped detailed characterization of *C. albicans* biofilms and gaining insight into biofilm resistance and underlying mechanisms. Hawser and Douglas [33] initially showed that fungal biofilms grown on catheter material for 48 hours become resistant to a variety of antifungals including amphotericin B, flucytosine (5-fluorocytosine), fluconazole, itraconazole, and ketoconazole. Ramage et al. [22] using 96-well microtiter plate model studied antifungal susceptibility testing of several *C. albicans* strains grown as biofilms against amphotericin B and fluconazole, and the increased resistance of *C. albicans* biofilms against these antifungal agents was demonstrated. Chandra et al. [14] showed a similar resistance pattern with a silicone elastomer model where minimum inhibitory concentrations (MICs) of fluconazole were 1 and >128 μg/mL for planktonic and biofilm-grown *C. albicans* cultures, respectively. Since it is possible that antifungal resistance evolves as the biofilm grows to maturation, Chandra et al. [14] investigated correlations between biofilm development and antifungal susceptibility. MICs of amphotericin B, nystatin, fluconazole, and chlorhexidine were determined for early, intermediate, or mature biofilm phases. *C. albicans* exhibited low MICs at the early biofilm phase. MICs during this phase were 0.5, 1, 8, and 16 μg/mL for amphotericin B, fluconazole, nystatin, and chlorhexidine, respectively. Moreover, as the biofilms developed, MICs progressively increased. By 72 hours, *C. albicans* cells were highly resistant, with MICs of 8, 128, 32, and 256 μg/mL for amphotericin B, fluconazole, nystatin, and chlorhexidine, respectively [14]. The progression of drug resistance was associated with the concomitant increase in metabolic activity of developing biofilms [14]. This indicated that the observed increase in drug resistance was not simply a reflection of higher metabolic activity of cells in maturing biofilms but that drug resistance develops over time, coincident with biofilm maturation [14].

To further evaluate drug resistance mechanisms involved with *C. albicans* biofilms, studies were conducted at the biochemical and molecular levels. Earlier studies showed that antifungal resistance of planktonically grown *C. albicans* are linked to the expression of efflux pumps, such as Cdr1p,

Cdr2p, and Mdr1p [34]. In this regard, using a 96-well microtiter plate model of biofilm formation, Ramage et al. [35] reported that efflux pumps, including Cdr1p, Cdr2p, and Mdr1p, were not involved in drug resistance associated with mature *C. albicans* biofilms. In a subsequent study, Mukherjee et al. [36] compared the mechanism of antifungal resistance in biofilms at early and mature phases. These investigators showed that in early phase biofilms, efflux pumps contributed to antifungal resistance, while in mature phase biofilms, resistance was associated with changes in levels of ergosterol biosynthesis intermediates [36]. The role of efflux pumps in biofilm-associated resistance was confirmed in a separate study by Mateus et al. [37]. Adherence of *C. albicans* to silicone induces immediate enhanced tolerance to fluconazole [37] and they showed that expression of *MDR1* and *CDR1* genes was significantly lower in daughter cells from 48-hour biofilms than in firmly adherent cells (2 hours after attachment), suggesting that efflux pump expression in adherent cultures is transient. These studies clearly demonstrated that antifungal resistance in *Candida* biofilms is due to multiple mechanisms that are phase dependent.

BIOFILM FORMATION IS ASSOCIATED WITH DIFFERENTIAL EXPRESSION OF METABOLIC PATHWAYS

Evidence from gene expression and microarray studies

Since biofilms are very complex structures and highly resistant to antifungals, it was necessary to identify detailed molecular mechanisms involved with biofilm formation. Initial studies involved investigating biofilm-specific expression profile of genes known to be associated with adhesion (e.g., *ALS* family genes) and germination of *C. albicans* cells. Chandra et al. [14] showed that there was a differential expression of *ALS* family of genes between biofilm and planktonic cultures with additional gene(s) expressed in biofilms. Higher expression of *ALS* genes in biofilms suggested that adhesion phase plays an important role in biofilm formation.

Microarray analyses have been used in two different studies to identify biofilm-specific gene expression patterns in *C. albicans* [21,38]. Garcia-Sanchez et al. [21] identified a cluster of 325 differentially expressed genes, using different sets of biofilm models. In agreement with the overrepresentation of amino acid biosynthesis genes in this cluster, Gcn4p, a regulator of amino acid metabolism, was shown to be required for normal biofilm growth [21]. To identify biofilm-related genes that are independent of mycelial development, Garcia-Sanchez et al. [21] also studied the transcriptome of biofilms produced by a wild-type, hypha-producing strain and a *cph1/cph1 efg1/efg1* strain defective for hypha production. This analysis identified a cluster of 317 genes expressed independently of hyphal formation, whereas 86 genes were dependent on mycelial development [21]. Both sets revealed the activation of the sulfur-amino acid biosynthesis pathway as a feature of *C. albicans* biofilms [21]. In a separate study, Yeater et al. [38] used microarrays to identify changes in gene expression patterns associated with different developmental phases of biofilms formed by two different clinical isolates of *C. albicans* (one associated with denture stomatitis, the other with invasive candidiasis) on two different substrates (denture strips and catheter discs, respectively). They showed that 243 genes were differentially expressed over the experimental time-course in either biofilm or planktonic cells, of which the majority (191 genes) was differentially expressed only during biofilm development. Genes involved in cellular processes such as glycolytic and non-glycolytic carbohydrate assimilation, amino acid metabolism, and intracellular transport mechanisms were upregulated during the early phase of biofilm formation (Figure 9.3). These early events increased intracellular pools of pyruvate, pentoses, and amino acids

and upregulated genes involved with these processes. These intermediate processes prepared the biofilm for the large biomass increase that begins around 12 hours of development [38]. This developmental stage also demands energy and utilizes specific transporters for amino acids, sugars, ions, oligopeptides, and lactate/pyruvate. At mature phase (48 hours), few genes were differentially expressed compared with the 12-hour time point, suggesting a lack of initiation of new metabolic activity (Figure 9.3) [38].

Despite differences in experimental design and focus, data from these microarray studies compared favorably with each other [21,38]. The fact that similar gene upregulation can be found between disparate datasets suggests that processes fundamental to biofilm development are conserved across various models. These varied experimental approaches have contributed to a better understanding of gene expression associated with biofilm development.

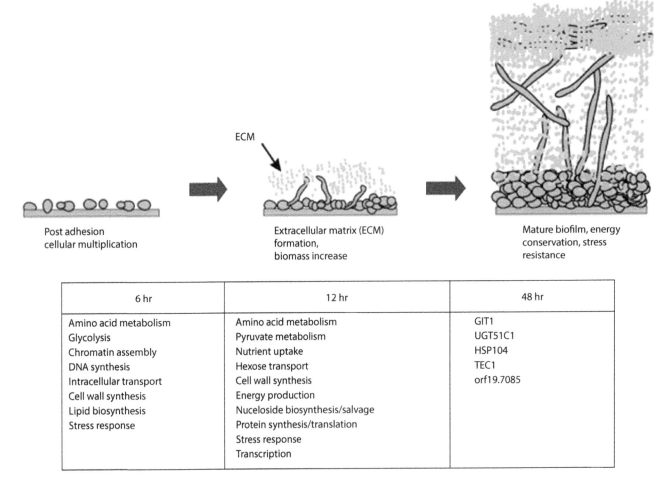

6 hr	12 hr	48 hr
Amino acid metabolism	Amino acid metabolism	GIT1
Glycolysis	Pyruvate metabolism	UGT51C1
Chromatin assembly	Nutrient uptake	HSP104
DNA synthesis	Hexose transport	TEC1
Intracellular transport	Cell wall synthesis	orf19.7085
Cell wall synthesis	Energy production	
Lipid biosynthesis	Nucleoside biosynthesis/salvage	
Stress response	Protein synthesis/translation	
	Stress response	
	Transcription	

Figure 9.3 Summary of the cellular processes that are associated with genes upregulated at the different time points during *C. albicans* biofilm development. The time-course of biofilm development is shown highlighting the time points (6, 12, and 48 hours) studied by microarray analysis. Descriptions of cellular processes are summarized. Categories of genes upregulated at 6 hours versus 12 hours are summarized under the 6-hour heading. Data from both the 12 hours versus 6 hours and 12 hours versus 48 hours comparisons are placed under the 12-hour heading. Few genes are upregulated at 48 hours compared to 12 hours, suggesting that initiation of new metabolic activity is relatively low in the mature biofilm. The individual genes upregulated at 48 hours versus 12 hours are listed.

EVIDENCE FROM PROTEOMICS AND METABOLIC PATHWAY MAPPING STUDIES

Although microarray and other gene expression studies have identified a number of differentially expressed genes in *Candida* biofilms, such expression is not always correlated at the functional protein level. Moreover, redundant gene expression profiles likely compensate for any loss of function in the biofilms. Therefore, it is necessary to evaluate global protein profile of biofilms and identify protein/s that are specifically produced in biofilms, since such proteins represent novel drug targets. Initial studies by Mukherjee et al. [39] involving proteomic screening of early phase *C. albicans* catheter-related biofilms showed differential expression of 24 proteins. One of the proteins that was downregulated was alcohol dehydrogenase (Adh1p) [39]. Targeted disruption of *ADH1* or inhibition of the enzyme using specific inhibitors resulted in thicker biofilm *in vitro* than those of the parent and revertant strains [39]. As it is known that Adh1p catalyzes the reversible conversion of acetaldehyde to ethanol, Mukherjee et al. also showed that deletion of the *C. albicans ADH1* gene resulted in a decrease in ethanol and an increase in acetaldehyde levels [39]. These results suggested that the effect of Adh1p on biofilm formation was mediated by its enzymatic activity and not by a general change in cellular metabolism.

In another study, proteomic analyses of the carbohydrate-rich extracellular matrix (ECM) and cell wall proteins of catheter-associated biofilms at early phase (6 hours) and mature phase (48 hours) showed differential expression of 151 proteins (107 proteins to be differentially expressed in ECM, while 44 were differentially expressed in cell walls), compared to planktonically grown cells [40]. Among these differentially expressed proteins, 95% (102/107) and 68% (30/44) were upregulated in ECM and cell walls of biofilms, respectively [40]. To narrow down the list of targeted proteins, these investigators mapped differentially expressed proteins based on their putative functions to known pathways. Such pathway mapping analyses revealed that the majority of these differentially expressed proteins were associated with metabolic pathways, in a phase-dependent manner [40]. Among ECM-associated proteins, proteins within 18 pathways were differentially expressed, with two pathways (glutamate and nitrogen metabolism) unique to early phase, and four pathways (purine, Gly/Ser/Thr, inositol metabolism, and carbon fixation) unique to mature phase biofilms [40] (Table 9.1). Differences in proteins were also observed in cell wall associated proteins, where proteins associated with 14 specific pathways were differentially regulated (Table 9.1). Lattif et al. [40] also showed that glycolytic enzymes, including the key enzyme glyceraldehyde-3-phosphate dehydrogenase (GAPDH), were overexpressed in biofilms at both early and mature phases, compared to planktonic controls [40]. These results suggested that glycolytic pathway and GAPDH play critical roles in *Candida* biofilm formation.

The difference between microarray and proteomic data [38,40] may be due to the fact that cellular processes in *Candida* cells are known to be regulated differently at the transcriptional and translational levels, and similar differential regulation of pathways involved in cell wall biogenesis, general metabolism, and signaling events is likely to occur in mature *Candida* biofilms. Studying these pathways and associated proteins helped tremendously in understanding the critical roles played by them in *Candida* biofilm formation. Importantly, these proteins represent potential targets for designing antibiofilm drugs, as well as for early diagnosis of infections associated with *Candida* biofilms.

In vivo studies: Biofilm models and antifungal therapy

IN VIVO BIOFILM MODELS

Most of the studies involving fungal biofilms are performed using *in vitro* systems. It is important to validate the *in vitro* results using *in vivo* biofilm models that mimic the clinical environment. Use of *in vivo* models involving *C. albicans* biofilms have been conducted mainly in vascular catheter models. Additionally, a murine model of subcutaneous catheter-associated *C. albicans* biofilms was also developed [41, 42]. In this model, catheters were inserted subcutaneously by making a mid-line incision on BALB/c mice backs, and formation of biofilms on catheters was confirmed using QCC assays and SEM. The data revealed abundant *Candida* hyphal elements and blastospores embedded in thick ECM and showed that 1×10^3 CFU/mL grew on cultured catheters. This data correlates well with clinical catheter-associated infections where growth of 1×10^3 CFU/mL from catheter indicates catheter-associated infection [42].

Nett and Andes in their review reported that *in vivo* biofilms are structurally similar to those formed under laboratory conditions with the exception that *in vivo* biofilms have numerous host cells including red blood cells, macrophages, neutrophils, and platelets that are embedded within the matrix [43]. Using a rat central venous catheter model, Andes et al. [44] characterized *in vivo C. albicans* biofilm development. Time-course quantitative culture demonstrated a progressive increase in the burden of viable cells for the first 24 hours of development. Fluorescence and SEM examination revealed a bilayered architecture on the catheter surface with yeast cells and hyphal forms densely embedded in an extracellular matrix and were similar to those described for *in vitro* models [44]. Andes et al. [44] using their *in vivo* model determined drug susceptibility and demonstrated a biofilm-associated drug resistance phenotype. They also showed a differential gene expression associated with *in vivo* biofilm growth and in this regard two fluconazole efflux pumps, *CDR1* and *CDR2*, were upregulated in the *in vivo* biofilm-associated cells [44]. However, transcription of *ERG11* (14-alpha demethylase) and MDR1 (major facilitator efflux pump) did not appear to be effected by biofilm growth *in vivo* when compared to planktonic cells [43].

Table 9.1 Differentially expressed pathways in matrix and cell walls isolated from *C. albicans* biofilms grown to early and mature developmental phases

Protein sample	Early phase (6 hours)	Mature phase (48 hours)
Matrix	Purine metabolism	Fructose and mannose metabolism
	Fructose and mannose metabolism	Purine metabolism
	Pentose phosphate pathway	Glycolysis/gluconeogenesis
	Glycine, serine, and threonine metabolism	Pentose phosphate pathway
	Glycolysis/gluconeogenesis	Glycine, serine, and threonine metabolism
	Biosynthesis of steroids	Carbon fixation
	Urea cycle and metabolism of amino groups	Inositol metabolism
	Glutamate metabolism	Biosynthesis of steroids
	Methionine metabolism	Urea cycle and metabolism of amino groups
	Valine, leucine, and isoleucine biosynthesis	Methionine metabolism
	Lysine biosynthesis	Valine, leucine, and isoleucine biosynthesis
	β-Alanine metabolism	Lysine biosynthesis
	Glycerolipid metabolism	β-Alanine metabolism
	Glycerophospholipid metabolism	Glycerolipid metabolism
	Pantothenate and CoA biosynthesis	Glycerophospholipid metabolism
	Terpenoid biosynthesis	Pantothenate and CoA biosynthesis
	Nitrogen metabolism	Terpenoid biosynthesis
	Calcium signaling pathway	Calcium signaling pathway
Cell walls	Glycolysis/gluconeogenesis	Glycolysis/gluconeogenesis
	Fructose and mannose metabolism	Fructose and mannose metabolism
	Inositol metabolism	Fatty acid metabolism
	Fatty acid metabolism	Oxidative phosphorylation
	Bile acid biosynthesis	Carbon fixation
	Oxidative phosphorylation	Inositol metabolism
	Valine, leucine, and isoleucine degradation	Aminoacyl-tRNA biosynthesis
	Valine, leucine, and isoleucine biosynthesis	PPAR signaling pathway
	Lysine biosynthesis Lysine degradation Tyrosine metabolism	Citrate cycle (TCA cycle)
	Phenylalanine, tyrosine, and tryptophan biosynthesis	Pentose phosphate pathway
	Glycerolipid metabolism	Bile acid biosynthesis
	1- and 2-methylnaphthalene degradation	Glycine, serine, and threonine metabolism
	3-Chloroacrylic acid degradation	Methionine metabolism
	Carbon fixation	Cysteine metabolism
	Pantothenate and CoA biosynthesis	Valine, leucine, and isoleucine degradation
		Valine, leucine, and isoleucine biosynthesis
		Lysine biosynthesis
		Arginine and proline metabolism
		Tyrosine metabolism
		Phenylalanine, tyrosine, and tryptophan biosynthesis
		Glycerolipid metabolism
		β-Linolenic acid metabolism
		Pyruvate metabolism
		1- and 2-methylnaphthalene degradation
		3-Chloroacrylic acid degradation
		Pantothenate and CoA biosynthesis
		Metabolism of xenobiotics by cyt-P450
		Polyunsaturated fatty acid biosynthesis
		Proteasome
		Type III secretion system
		Calcium signaling pathway

Schinabeck et al. [45] for the first time described development of a rabbit model of catheter-associated infection with *C. albicans* biofilms [45]. These authors used two types of CVCs, polyurethane and silicone CVCs, and placed them surgically in the jugular vein of female white rabbits [45]. They showed using quantitative catheter culture (QCC) and SEM analyses that mature biofilms were formed equally on both catheters with abundant hyphal elements and blastospores embedded in thick extracellular matrix [45].

These *in vivo* models have provided some understanding of fungal biofilms, their resistance, and genes involved with these processes.

ANTIFUNGAL THERAPY *IN VIVO*

Evaluation of the efficacy of a number of antifungal agents using many *in vivo* models has been conducted. Lazzell et al. developed a mouse catheter model to examine the efficacy of caspofungin to treat and prevent *C. albicans* biofilms [46]. Their data showed that locking caspofungin in catheters for 24-hours dwell time led to a reduction of fungal burden in both catheters and kidneys when used for either treatment or prevention of catheter-related infection compared to untreated controls.

Schinabeck et al. [45] described development of a rabbit model of catheter-associated infection with *C. albicans* biofilms and showed that antifungal lock therapy with liposomal amphotericin B was an effective treatment strategy for these infections [45].

Mukherjee et al. [47] studied the utility of amphotericin B lipid complex as a lock strategy against *C. albicans* biofilms in a rabbit silicone catheter model. All catheters retrieved from treated animals were sterilized, while none of the catheters obtained from untreated control animals were [47]. In a different rabbit catheter model, Shuford et al. compared amphotericin B deoxycholate to caspofungin for the treatment of *C. albicans* catheter infection following a 7-day lock therapy [48]. Of the 16 animals in each arm, 16 catheters were sterilized in the caspofungin arm, 13 catheters were sterilized in the amphotericin B deoxycholate arm, and none in the control arm.

Overall, these results suggest that lipid formulations of amphotericin or an echinocandin may be a promising approach as an antifungal lock therapy to prevent and treat catheter-associated biofilm infections.

CLINICAL STUDIES INVOLVING BIOFILMS

Catheter-related bloodstream infections (CRBSIs) commonly involve colonization of microorganisms on catheter surfaces where they eventually become embedded in a biofilm [10]. Over the past two decades, the use of intravascular devices, such as central venous and hemodialysis catheters, has paralleled the increasing incidence of CRBSIs [49], and studies involving CRBSIs caused by *Candida* or other fungal species have become important. In addition to systematic efforts to reduce the incidence of CRBSIs through a range of infection

control approaches and new technologies, such as antibiotic-coated CVCs, clinicians have attempted antifungal lock therapy with significant interest and promise as a strategy to treat CRBSIs in situations where the need for catheter salvage in *Candida*-related CRBSIs appears to outweigh the risks [49]. Walraven et al. [49] reported the most promising antifungal lock therapy strategies, including the use of amphotericin, ethanol, or echinocandins. There are a limited number of case reports published describing the use of antifungal lock therapy in various patient populations. The majority of case reports describe antilock therapy experience in pediatric patients, ranging from infants to 18 years of age, but there are a few cases in adult patients [49]. Among the case reports, the most commonly isolated fungi was *C. albicans* (9 of the 22 cases) followed by *C. parapsilosis* (4 of 22 cases). *C. glabrata* (2 cases), *C. tropicalis* (1 case), *Candida guillermondii* (1 case), and *Candida lipolytica* (1 case) were isolated less frequently [49].

The most commonly employed antifungal lock was amphotericin B deoxycholate, with a combined catheter salvage rate of 76.9% (10 of 13 cases) [50]. Krzywda et al. [50] reported using a significantly lower dose of amphotericin B deoxycholate (0.33 mg/mL) compared to those used in other studies, which may have contributed to unsuccessful catheter salvage in all five episodes of fungemia in two patients [50]. In contrast, Liposomal amphotericin antifungal lock approach was associated with a 60% (3 of 5 cases) salvage rate [50]. In the only report of echinocandin lock therapy, caspofungin (3.33 mg/mL) combined with systemic caspofungin for 14 days was used to successfully treat *C. lipolytica* CR-BSIs [51]. Blackwood et al. reported the successful use of a 70% EtOH lock solution for catheter salvage in three pediatric patients with invasive candidiasis [52].

Recently, it has been demonstrated that trisodium citrate (TSC) has superior antimicrobial effects over heparin for catheter locking. In this randomized controlled trial, Bosma et al. [53], compared the influence of catheter locking with heparin and TSC on the intraluminal biofilm formation in hemodialysis catheters. Six patients were studied from the time of catheter insertion for hemodialysis treatment. They were randomly assigned to TSC 30% or heparin 5000 U/mL for catheter locking for the duration of 1 month [53]. After elective guidewire exchange of the catheter, the locking solution was also changed. Following removal, catheters were dissected into three segments and examined by SEM to assess quantitative biofilm formation [53]. Furthermore, standardized cultures of all segments were performed to identify any microorganisms present on the catheters. Data showed that catheters filled with TSC, the average coverage by biofilm was 16% versus 63% in the heparin group (p < 0.001) [53]. A total of eight sub-segments were associated with local catheter infection in patients who were randomized to heparin locking versus three sub-segments who were assigned to TSC (p < 0.05) [53]. Thus, using TSC 30% for catheter locking reduces the formation of microbial biofilm in catheters and culture-positive colonization in hemodialysis patients [53]. Randomized clinical trials of the most promising antifungal lock combined with systemic therapy is warranted to evaluate the safety and efficacy of antifungal lock therapy.

Another study by do Nascimento (37) evaluated the ability of *Candida* to adhere to machined or cast titanium and zirconia (Zc) abutment substrates [54]. Six healthy subjects were enrolled in this randomized crossover clinical investigation. The study was conducted in three phases. Participants were advised to use an intraoral splint containing four discs of the same tested substrate for 24 hours. Two discs were located in the anterior region and two in the posterior region. DNA checkerboard hybridization method was used to detect and quantify five different *Candida* species [54]. Data on the surface roughness and the total area of discs covered by formed biofilm were also provided to correlate the species and biofilm found between different substrates. Zirconia presented the highest means of surface roughness. Total area of the biofilm covering was not different in the tested groups. Moderate to high levels of target microorganisms were recorded for all the tested substrates. Zirconia showed the lowest indices, followed by machined pure titanium (MPT) and cast and polished titanium (CPT) [54]. *C. albicans* and *C. krusei* were not detected in the Zc group. The region of disc placement did not show differences in relation to *Candida* adhesion. There was a significant difference in the total cell count between the three groups. CPT presented the highest mean counts, followed by MPT and Zc. There was no positive correlation between the cell counts recorded and the surface roughness or total area of formed biofilm [54].

Another study analyzed biofilms formed on the inner side of endotracheal tubes (ETT) in critically ill, mechanically ventilated patients [55]. Measurement of the ETT inner volume was first performed before extubation using the acoustic reflection method. After extubation, the biofilm was studied by means of optical and atomic force microscopy [55]. Twenty-four subjects were enrolled in this study. Duration of intubation lasted from 2 to 79 d (mean ± SD: 11 ± 15 d). The mean percentage of ETT volume loss evaluated *in situ* ($n = 21$) was 7.1% and was not linked with the duration of intubation [55]. Analyses with atomic force microscopy ($n = 6$) showed a full coverage of the inner part of the tube with biofilm, even after saline rinse. Its thickness ranged from 0.8 to 5 µm. *C. albicans* and *Pseudomonas aeruginosa* were among the most frequent microorganisms present [55].

MIXED SPECIES BIOFILMS

Mixed-species biofilms have been associated with significant mortality and morbidity in adults and children, and *Staphylococcus epidermidis* and *Candida albicans* are the most frequent combination of organisms isolated from such polymicrobial infections [56]. Using *in vitro* and *in vivo* (subcutaneous catheter) infection models, Pammi et al. [56] showed that mixed species biofilms were increased compared to single species biofilms of either *S. epidermidis* or *C. albicans in vitro*, and increased catheter infection and

dissemination of *S. epidermidis* in mice. Microarray analyses showed that 2.7% of *S. epidermidis* genes were upregulated and 6% were down regulated in mixed species biofilms, compared to single species *S. epidermidis* biofilms. Moreover, staphylococcal autolysis repressors *lrgA* and *lrgB* were down regulated 36-fold and 27-fold respectively. These investigators also reported that *S. epidermidis*-specific eDNA was increased in mixed species biofilms. These results indicated that enhancement and systemic dissemination of *S. epidermidis* may explain adverse outcomes after clinical polymicrobial infections of *S. epidermidis* and *C. albicans* [56].

P. aeruginosa and *C. albicans* are frequently coexisting opportunistic pathogens, responsible for colonization and infection in predisposed patients [57]. Study showed that they share a virulence specificity relying on auto-inducing, cell density-dependent molecules named quorum-sensing (QS) [57]. *C. albicans* virulence depends on its QS that influences morphological switch from yeast to filamentous form. Similarly, the production of *P. aeruginosa* virulence factors depends partly on QS molecules. Interactions have been investigated and demonstrated *in vitro*. *P. aeruginosa* may kill *C. albicans* either by producing toxins, such as pyocyanin, or by direct contact on its biofilm-dependent filamentous form [57]. Cross-kingdom communication is a subtler interaction: *C. albicans* can adapt its morphology in the presence of *P. aeruginosa* QS molecules and inhibit *P. aeruginosa* QS-dependent virulence factor secretion through farnesol, one of its QS molecules [57].

ACKNOWLEDGMENTS

Studies by our group were supported by funds from NIH grants 5R01AI035097-13 and 5R01DE017486-03 to M.A.G and the NIH Grant R01DE024228 to MAG and PKM. We acknowledge support from the Swagelok Center for Surface Analysis of Materials, Case Western Reserve University, for SEM analyses and from the NIH-funded Skin Diseases Research Center (NIAMS P30 AR039750). We also like to acknowledge the CSLM Core, Genetics Department, Case Western Reserve University.

REFERENCES

1. Nicastri E, Petrosillo N, Viale P, Ippolito G. Catheter-related bloodstream infections in HIV-infected patients. *Ann N Y Acad Sci* 2001;946:274–290.
2. Wenzel RP. Nosocomial candidemia: Risk factors and attributable mortality. *Clin Infect Dis* 1995;20:1531–1534.
3. Hollenbach E. Invasive candidiasis in the ICU: Evidence based and on the edge of evidence. *Mycoses* 2008;51:25–45.
4. Ganesan K, Harigopal S, Neal T, Yoxall CW. Prophylactic oral nystatin for preterm babies under 33 weeks' gestation decreases fungal colonisation and invasive fungaemia. *Arch Dis Child Fetal Neonatal Ed.* 2009;94:F275–278.

5. Nguyen MH, Peacock JE, Jr., Tanner DC, et al. Therapeutic approaches in patients with candidemia. Evaluation in a multicenter, prospective, observational study. *Arch Intern Med* 1995;155:2429–2435.

6. Simitsopoulou M, Chatzimoschou A, Roilides E. Biofilms and antifungal susceptibility testing. *Methods in molecular biology* 2016;1356:183–197.

7. Anaissie EJ, Rex JH, Uzun O, Vartivarian S. Predictors of adverse outcome in cancer patients with candidemia. *Am J Med* 1998;104:238–245.

8. Mermel LA, Farr BM, Sherertz RJ, et al. Guidelines for the management of intravascular catheter-related infections. *J Intraven Nurs* 2001;24:180–205.

9. Pappas PG, Rex JH, Sobel JD, et al. Guidelines for treatment of candidiasis. *Clin Infect Dis* 2004;38:161–189.

10. Donlan RM. Biofilms: Microbial life on surfaces. *Emerg Infect Dis* 2002;8:881–890.

11. Douglas LJ. *Candida* biofilms and their role in infection. *Trends Microbiol* 2003;11:30–36.

12. Baillie GS, Douglas LJ. *Candida* biofilms and their susceptibility to antifungal agents. *Methods Enzymol* 1999;310:644–656.

13. Chandra J, Mukherjee PK, Leidich SD, et al. Antifungal resistance of candidal biofilms formed on denture acrylic *in vitro*. *J Dent Res* 2001;80:903–908.

14. Chandra J, Kuhn DM, Mukherjee PK, Hoyer LL, McCormick T, Ghannoum MA. Biofilm formation by the fungal pathogen *Candida albicans*: Development, architecture, and drug resistance. *J Bacteriol* 2001;183:5385–5394.

15. Hawser SP, Douglas LJ. Biofilm formation by *Candida* species on the surface of catheter materials *in vitro*. *Infect Immun* 1994;62:915–921.

16. Ramage G, Vande Walle K, Wickes BL, Lopez-Robot JL. Biofilm formation by *Candida dubliniensis*. *J Clin Microbiol* 2001;39:3234–3240.

17. Samaranayake YH, Ye J, Yau JY, Cheung BP, Samaranayake LP. *In vitro* method to study antifungal perfusion in *Candida* biofilms. *J Clin Microbiol* 2005;43:818–825.

18. van der Mei HC, Free RH, Elving GJ, Van Weissenbruch R, Albers FW, Busscher HJ. Effect of probiotic bacteria on prevalence of yeasts in oropharyngeal biofilms on silicone rubber voice prostheses *in vitro*. *J Med Microbiol* 2000;49:713–718.

19. Imamura Y, Chandra J, Mukherjee PK, et al. *Fusarium* and *Candida albicans* biofilms on soft contact lenses: Model development, influence of lens type, and susceptibility to lens care solutions. *Antimicrob Agents Chemother* 2008;52:171–182.

20. Roilides E, Simitsopoulou M, Katragkou A, Walsh TJ. How biofilms evade host defenses. *Microbiol Spectr*. 2015;3.

21. Garcia-Sanchez S, Aubert S, Iraqui I, Janbon G, Ghigo JM, d'Enfert C. *Candida albicans* biofilms: A developmental state associated with specific and stable gene expression patterns. *Eukaryotic Cell* 2004;3:536–545.

22. Ramage G, Vande Walle K, Wickes BL, Lopez-Robot JL. Standardized method for *in vitro* antifungal susceptibility testing of *Candida albicans* biofilms. *Antimicrob Agents Chemother* 2001;45:2475–2479.

23. Chandra J, Mukherjee PK, Ghannoum MA. *In vitro* growth and analysis of *Candida* biofilms. *Nat Protoc* 2008;3:1909–1924.

24. Kuhn DM, Balkis M, Chandra J, Mukherjee PK, Ghannoum MA. Uses and limitations of the XTT assay in studies of *Candida* growth and metabolism. *J Clin Microbiol* 2003;41:506–508.

25. do Nascimento C, Ferreira de Albuquerque Junior R, Issa JP, et al. Use of the DNA Checkerboard hybridization method for detection and quantitation of *Candida* species in oral microbiota. *Can J Microbiol* 2009;55:622–626.

26. Iturrieta-Gonzalez IA, Padovan AC, Bizerra FC, Hahn RC, Colombo AL. Multiple species of Trichosporon produce biofilms highly resistant to triazoles and amphotericin B. *PLoS One*. 2014;9:e109553.

27. White JG, Amos WB, Fordham M. An evaluation of confocal versus conventional imaging of biological structures by fluorescence light microscopy. *J Cell Biol* 1987;105:41–48.

28. Ramage G, Vandewalle K, Wickes BL, Lopez-Robot JL. Characteristics of biofilm formation by *Candida albicans*. *Rev Iberoam Micol* 2001;18:163–170.

29. Baillie GS, Douglas LJ. Role of dimorphism in the development of *Candida albicans* biofilms. *J Med Microbiol* 1999;48:671–679.

30. Shukla N, Osmani AH, Osmani SA. Microtubules are reversibly depolymerized in response to changing gaseous microenvironments within *Aspergillus nidulans* biofilms. *Mol Biol Cell*. 2017;28(5):634–644.

31. Rajendran R, Williams C, Lappin DF, Millington O, Martins M, Ramage G. Extracellular DNA release acts as an antifungal resistance mechanism in mature *Aspergillus fumigatus* biofilms. *Eukaryot Cell* 2013;12:420–429.

32. de Mello TP, de Souza Ramos L, Braga-Silva LA, Branquinha MH, Dos Santos AL. Fungal biofilm - a real obstacle against an efficient therapy: Lessons from Candida. *Current Top Med Chem*. 2017.

33. Hawser SP, Douglas LJ. Resistance of *Candida albicans* biofilms to antifungal agents *in vitro*. *Antimicrob Agents Chemother* 1995;39:2128–2131.

34. Albertson GD, Niimi M, Cannon RD, Jenkinson HF. Multiple efflux mechanisms are involved in *Candida albicans* fluconazole resistance. *Antimicrob Agents Chemother* 1996;40:2835–2841.

35. Ramage G, Bachmann S, Patterson TF, Wickes BL, Lopez-Ribot JL. Investigation of multidrug efflux pumps in relation to fluconazole resistance in *Candida albicans* biofilms. *J Antimicrob Chemother* 2002;49:973–980.

36. Mukherjee PK, Chandra J, Kuhn DM, Ghannoum MA. Mechanism of fluconazole resistance in *Candida albicans* biofilms: Phase-specific role of efflux pumps and membrane sterols. *Infect Immun* 2003;71:4333–4340.

37. Mateus C, Crow SA, Jr., Ahearn DG. Adherence of *Candida albicans* to silicone induces immediate enhanced tolerance to fluconazole. *Antimicrob Agents Chemother* 2004;48:3358–3366.

38. Yeater KM, Chandra J, Cheng G, et al. Temporal analysis of *Candida albicans* gene expression during biofilm development. *Microbiology* 2007;153:2373–2385.

39. Mukherjee PK, Mohamed S, Chandra J, et al. Alcohol dehydrogenase restricts the ability of the pathogen *Candida albicans* to form a biofilm on catheter surfaces through an ethanol-based mechanism. *Infect Immun* 2006;74:3804–3816.

40. Lattif AA, Jyotsna C, Chang J, Liu S, et al. Proteomics and pathway mapping analyses reveal phase-dependent over-expression of proteins associated with carbohydrate metabolic pathways in *Candida albicans* biofilms. *Open Proteomics J* 2008;1:5–26.

41. Zumbuehl A, Ferreira L, Kuhn D, et al. Antifungal hydrogels. *Proc Natl Acad Sci U S A* 2007;104:12994–12998.

42. Cleri DJ, Corrado ML, Seligman SJ. Quantitative culture of intravenous catheters and other intravascular inserts. *J Infect Dis* 1980;141:781–786.

43. Nett J, Andes D. *Candida albicans* biofilm development, modeling a host-pathogen interaction. *Curr Opin Microbiol* 2006;9:340–345.

44. Andes D, Nett J, Oschel P, Albrecht R, Marchillo K, Pitula A. Development and characterization of an *in vivo* central venous catheter *Candida albicans* biofilm model. *Infect Immun* 2004;72:6023–6031.

45. Schinabeck MK, Long LA, Hossain MA, et al. Rabbit model of *Candida albicans* biofilm infection: Liposomal amphotericin B antifungal lock therapy. *Antimicrob Agents Chemother* 2004;48:1727–1732.

46. Lazzell AL, Chaturvedi AK, Pierce CG, Prasad D, Uppuluri P, Lopez-Ribot JL. Treatment and prevention of *Candida albicans* biofilms with caspofungin in a novel central venous catheter murine model of candidiasis. *J Antimicrob Chemother* 2009;64:567–570.

47. Mukherjee PK, Long L, Kim HG, Ghannoum MA. Amphotericin B lipid complex is efficacious in the treatment of *Candida albicans* biofilms using a model of catheter-associated *Candida* biofilms. *Int J Antimicrob A* 2009;33:149–153.

48. Shuford JA, Rouse MS, Piper KE, Steckelberg JM, Patel R. Evaluation of caspofungin and amphotericin B deoxycholate against *Candida albicans* biofilms in an experimental intravascular catheter infection model. *J Infect Dis* 2006;194:710–713.

49. Walraven CJ, Lee SA. Antifungal lock therapy. *Antimicrob Agents Chemother* 2013;57:1–8.

50. Krzywda EA, Andris DA, Edmiston CE, Jr., Quebbeman EJ. Treatment of Hickman catheter sepsis using antibiotic lock technique. *Infect Control Hosp Epidemiol* 1995;16:596–598.

51. Ozdemir H, Karbuz A, Ciftci E, et al. Successful treatment of central venous catheter infection due to *Candida lipolytica* by caspofungin-lock therapy. *Mycoses.* 2011;54:e647–649.

52. Blackwood RA, Klein KC, Micel LN, et al. Ethanol locks therapy for resolution of fungal catheter infections. *Pediatr Infect Dis J* 2011;30:1105–1107.

53. Bosma JW, Siegert CE, Peerbooms PG, Weijmer MC. Reduction of biofilm formation with trisodium citrate in haemodialysis catheters: A randomized controlled trial. *Nephrol Dial Transplant* 2010;25:1213–1217.

54. do Nascimento C, Pita MS, Pedrazzi V, de Albuquerque Junior RF, Ribeiro RF. *In vivo* evaluation of *Candida spp.* adhesion on titanium or zirconia abutment surfaces. *Arch Oral Biol* 2013;58:853–861.

55. Danin PE, Girou E, Legrand P, et al. Description and microbiology of endotracheal tube biofilm in mechanically ventilated subjects. *Respir Care* 2015;60:21–29.

56. Pammi M, Liang R, Hicks J, Mistretta TA, Versalovic J. Biofilm extracellular DNA enhances mixed species biofilms of *Staphylococcus epidermidis* and *Candida albicans.BMC Microbiol.* 2013;13:257.

57. Mear JB, Kipnis E, Faure E, et al. *Candida albicans* and *Pseudomonas aeruginosa* interactions: More than an opportunistic criminal association? *Med Mal Infect* 2013;43:146–151.

10

Polyenes for prevention and treatment of invasive fungal infections

RICHARD H. DREW

INTRODUCTION

Polyene antifungals, notably amphotericin B, have been mainstays for the prevention and treatment of invasive fungal infections (IFIs). Because nystatin is restricted to topical (nonsystemic) administration, its application (even as prophylaxis against IFI in select high-risk patients) has largely been replaced by alternate strategies. In contrast, amphotericin B (administered intravenously as either amphotericin B deoxycholate [AmBd] or one of three lipid-based formulations [LBFAmB]) has been a mainstay for the prevention and treatment of select invasive IFIs since 1957 [1–10].

This chapter will review the clinical use of polyenes for the prevention and treatment of IFIs. Because of the limited indications for nystatin, the discussion will focus on amphotericin B unless otherwise stated.

MECHANISM OF ACTION

Polyenes interact with sterols in the fungal cell membrane [11,12]. The result is the production of pores that allow concentration-dependent leakage of intracellular cations (such as potassium and magnesium) and other cell components [11,12]. This leads to loss of membrane potential and subsequent fungal cell collapse [11,12]. Other mechanisms proposed include cell damage resulting from oxidative reactions linked to lipoperoxidation of the cell membrane [13]. While polyenes demonstrate a greater affinity for ergosterol (the primary sterol of the fungal cell membrane), the nonselective binding to cholesterol (the primary sterol in human cell membranes) may contribute to polyene-related adverse events.

Although *in vitro* activity can vary between test conditions and isolates tested, studies have generally documented that amphotericin B's activity is rapidly fungicidal against susceptible organisms [14–16]. Fungicidal concentrations *in vitro* are generally 1–3 dilutions higher than that required for inhibition [17].

The immunomodulatory effect of amphotericin B has been examined by numerous investigations [18–21] and summarized in detail elsewhere [22]. These effects include stimulation of pro-inflammatory cytokines: tumor necrosis factor (TNF)α, interleukin (IL)-1 and IL-6, the chemokines IL-8, MCP-1, MIP1β, nitric oxide, prostaglandins, and ICAM-1 from murine and human immune cells *in vitro* and *in vivo* [18–22]. The cytokine release resulting from amphotericin B administration may also be responsible (in part) for infusion-related reactions, and differences may exist between preparations [21–23]. Other proposed mechanisms for such reactions include the release of prostaglandins [24]. Finally, the antifungal activity of pulmonary alveolar macrophages and polymorphonuclear leukocytes against *A. fumigatus* may be augmented by the administration of amphotericin B [13].

In addition to its rapidly fungicidal activity, amphotericin B has demonstrated prolonged post-antifungal effect (PAFE) against both *Candida* [25,26] and *Cryptococcus* spp [26]. The PAFE for *Aspergillus*, however, may be species-dependent with significantly shorter PAFEs, or lack of PAFE, observed for *A. terreus, A. ustus,* and *A. nidulans* [27].

In contrast to their activity against planktonic fungal cells, the *in vitro* activity of antifungals (including polyenes) can vary significantly in biofilms [28–31]. While AmBd's activity *in vitro* against *Candida* spp. in biofilms is markedly reduced, both liposomal amphotericin B (LAmB) and amphotericin B lipid complex (ABLC) exhibited similar inhibitory activity *in vitro* against *Candida* biofilms in one report [29]. Similar findings were seen for ABLC in a rabbit model [32].

Numerous *in vitro* and animal model studies have been performed to assess the interaction of amphotericin B with other antifungals (such as flucytosine, azoles and echinocandins) against a variety of fungal pathogens (see *Drug Interactions* below). Review of such data may be found elsewhere [33–37] and is beyond the scope of this chapter. However, the lack of standards for synergy and antagonism testing may limit the utility of such information, and data may differ with the agents tested, model, test conditions and endpoint(s). The potential for amphotericin B in combination with nonantifungals has also been explored. Examples include combinations with azithromycin (against *Fusarium* [38] and Aspergillus spp. [39]) rifabutin (for both *Fusarium* and *Aspergillus* [40]), tacrolimus against *Trichosporon* [41] and rifampin (against *Fusarium* and *Aspergillus* spp [42]). However, the clinical significance of such interactions has not been established.

MECHANISMS OF FUNGAL RESISTANCE

While infrequently encountered in clinical practice, intrinsic polyene resistance has been demonstrated in *Candida lusitaniae, Aspergillus terreus,* and *Scedosporium* spp [12,43–45]. Likewise, reports of acquired polyene resistance during therapy are rare. Proposed mechanisms of resistance include depletion of ergosterol in the cell membrane [46] or other sterol-independent modifications of the cell membrane [47]. Alternate mechanisms include elevations in catalase levels, enhancing resistance against oxidative damage to the fungal cell by amphotericin B [45,48].

While incomplete, the potential for significant *in vitro* cross-resistance in yeasts between amphotericin B and nystatin exists [49]. *In vitro* resistance of molds to nystatin has not been reported [49].

PHARMACODYNAMICS

The majority of studies investigating the pharmacodynamics of polyenes have involved AmBd [50–53]. Existing *in vivo* and *in vitro* models for both *Candida* spp. and *Aspergillus* spp. suggest the rate and extent of amphotericin B's activity increases as the concentration of drug is increased [14,16,25,54–56]. Similar findings have been observed with LFAmB [57,58]. However, the limited drug solubility, reversible binding in tissues, and dose-dependent drug clearance of amphotericin B may limit the benefit of dose-escalation in attempts at increasing the antifungal activity [58–60]. (see *Pharmacokinetics* and *Dosing and Administration*)

Data in humans to examine relationship between pharmacodynamics and outcomes are limited [61]. Subset analysis of data obtained in 10 pediatric oncology patients treated with liposomal amphotericin B (LAmB) for whom pharmacokinetic and susceptibility data were available suggested that a peak serum concentration: minimium inhibitory concentration (C_{max}/MIC) ratio exceeding 40 were more likely to achieve a complete versus partial clinical response [62]. However, while such information might be important in the empiric selection and dosing of antifungal therapy, neither amphotericin B serum concentrations nor *in vitro* susceptibility information is routinely available in clinical situations.

SPECTRUM OF ACTIVITY

Nystatin has demonstrated activity against a variety of fungal isolates in various *in vitro* and *in vivo* models [48]. This includes a variety of *Candida* spp, *Cryptococcus neoformans* [63], *Aspergillus fumigatus, Histoplasma capsulatum,* and *Coccidioides immitis.* However, the clinical usefulness of such activity is significantly limited by lack of a preparation for systemic administration.

Amphotericin B possesses a broad-spectrum of antifungal activity against a variety of yeasts and molds [64]. Potency differences *in vitro* are consistently observed between AmBd and the three lipid-based formulations: amphotericin B lipid complex (ABLC), amphotericin B colloidal dispersion (ABCD), and liposomal amphotericin B (LAmB). LBFAmB generally exhibit a 5-fold reduction in potency *in vitro* (when expressed as mg/kg) relative to AmBd [57]. The relevance of these *in vitro* differences remains uncertain, since higher MICs for LFAmB may not account for release from the lipid carrier. In contrast, data from the European Committee on Antimicrobial Susceptibility Testing (EUCAST) reported increased potency for LAmB (relative to AmBd) for several strains of *Candida* spp [17]. The reasons for such findings, however, were not clear.

While Clinical Laboratory Standards Institute (CLSI) standards exist for susceptibility testing of amphotericin B against yeasts by both macrodilution and microdilution methods, no breakpoints have been approved [65,66]. CLSI-recommended disk diffusion methods for susceptibility testing of yeasts do not include amphotericin B [65]. In addition, the utility of *in vitro* testing may be limited by the general lack of correlation between *in vitro* susceptibility and treatment outcome in patients with IFIs [61,67].

Amphotericin B is highly active *in vitro* against most *Candida* spp. (including *C. albicans, C. glabrata, C. tropicalis, C. parapsilosis,* and *C. auris*), with MIC's generally ranging between 0.25 and 1 μg/mL when tested by CSLI-based microdilution techniques [17,66,68–70]. While some report *C. lusitaniae* to be intrinsically resistant to amphotericin B, *in vitro* data are often conflicting and the clinical significance of this resistance is questionable [17,71,72]. In general, MICs of *C. lusitaniae* to amphotericin B may be higher than seen with most other *Candida* spp, but most within 2 mcg/mL [66].

Amphotericin B also displays favorable activity *in vitro* against *Cryptococcus* spp. [73], *Malassezia* spp., *Rhodotorula*, *Blastoschizomyces* spp., and *Saccharomyces* spp. [74]. While most *Trichosporon* spp would be considered susceptible, *T. beigelii* and *T. asahii* display variable susceptibility to amphotericin B *in vitro* [75].

Amphotericin B is highly active *in vitro* against fungi responsible for endemic mycoses, such as *Coccidioides* spp., *Blastomyces* spp., *Histoplasma capsulatum*, and *Paracoccidioides brasiliensis* [76–78]. It also exhibits activity *in vitro* against most *Sporothrix schenkii,* although strain-dependent resistance has been reported [79].

In addition to its activity against yeasts, amphotericin B has also demonstrated significant activity against a variety of molds, including most *Aspergillus* spp. (with the exception of *A. terreus*) [17,64,69,80,81]. Other non-*fumigatis* spp of *Aspergillus* may also be less susceptible to amphotericin (notably *A. flavis* in one report) [69]. Amphotericin B is active *in vitro* against the Zygomycetes [82]. While *Scedosporium apiospermum* may be susceptible to polyenes, *Scedosporium prolificans* is generally resistant [3,12]. Although amphotericin B may be active against *Fusarium* spp., MICs of 0.25–8 mcg/mL have been reported for *F. solani,* and, therefore, some strains of this species are considered resistant [12]. *Cladophialophora* isolates have demonstrated variable susceptibility to amphotericin B. Finally, intrinsic resistance has been reported in both *Malassezia furfur* [3] and *Paecilomyces lilacinus* [12].

PHARMACOKINETICS

Nystatin is not significantly absorbed following oral or topical administration [49]. Therefore, metabolism, distribution, and elimination of nystatin are largely unknown.

While alternate delivery systems may significantly enhance the oral absorption of amphotericin B in the future [83], amphotericin B (as presently formulated) demonstrates limited and erratic absorption following oral exposure. Low (yet detectable) serum concentrations of amphotericin B have been reported following oral administration [84,85]. While such absorption may be altered in the setting of mucositis, it is generally considered insufficient to treat systemic infections, but has been used (in combination with nonabsorbable antibacterials) for selective gut decontamination [86–88].

The dose, frequency, infusion rate, formulation of amphotericin B and patient population can influence plasma concentrations. Peak plasma concentrations following IV infusion of 1 mg/kg of AmBd have been reported to be approximately 2 mcg/mL [4]. The high protein binding of amphotericin B (in excess of 90%) to serum albumin and α-1-acid glycoprotein is directly related to concentration [59,60]. Distribution has been described using a three-compartment model [59,60,89] with the resulting volume of distribution approximately 4 L/kg [89]. Penetration of amphotericin B into the central nervous system is thought to be minimal, with cerebrospinal fluid (CSF) concentrations 0%–4% of simultaneous serum concentrations [90]. However, such CSF concentrations are not likely to reflect higher concentrations in the meninges.

Metabolism plays a minor role in elimination of amphotericin B [61,62]. Elimination of amphotericin B is also poorly understood. For example, only 3% of the total dose is excreted as unchanged drug [61,62]. Clearance from plasma is slow and dose-dependent, with a terminal half-life of >15 days [61,62]. Concentrations in blood have been detected up to 4 weeks after an amphotericin B treatment course and in urine for 4–8 weeks following completion of therapy.

The pharmacokinetic differences between preparations of amphotericin B have been reviewed in detail elsewhere [57,59,60,91–93]. In general, LFAmB exhibit a range of serum concentrations, with ABLC and ABCD demonstrating similar C_{max} values to AmBd when given at recommended dosages. In contrast, LAmB exhibits both a higher C_{max} and area under the time-concentration curve (AUC) relative to AmBd, ABLC, and ABCD at comparable doses likely due to significant reduction in LAmB's volume of distribution and total body clearance [93]. Reductions in unbound amphotericin B have been reported with LFAmB relative to AmBd [59,60]. LAmB may produce lower tissue concentrations in liver, spleen, lung and kidney [2]. In contrast, LAmB achieves higher concentrations in brain tissue [91]. ABLC achieves higher lung concentrations [57,92].

Studies have examined the pharmacokinetics of amphotericin B (including LFAmB) in a variety of special populations, including patients with renal dysfunction [94,95] (see *Dosing and Administration*) and in patients undergoing hematopoetic stem cell transplantation [96]. Amphotericin is poorly removed by dialysis [97]. Studies have also been conducted to examine the pharmacokinetic profile of AmBd [98–100], LAmB [62,101], and ABLC [102] in pediatrics. In general, significant differences between adult and pediatric patients justifying alterations in weight-based dosing ranges have not been observed.

ADVERSE EFFECTS

It is perhaps the adverse event profile that most limits the current use of amphotericin B. These consist primarily of electrolyte disturbances, infusion-related reactions, hepatic dysfunction and hematologic reactions.

Electrolyte disturbances. A variety of electrolyte abnormalities have been associated with amphotericin B administration, most commonly hypokalemia and hypomagnesemia [103]. More recent clinical studies report hypokalemia in approximately 10%–20% of patients receiving various amphotericin B formulations [104–107]. Hyperkalemia is less frequently reported, and has been more frequently associated with rapid infusions [108].

Infusion-related reactions. Infusion-related reactions related to intravenous administration of amphotericin B occur frequently, ranging from 20% to 90% (depending largely upon population, preparation, administration and the use of premedications) [109,110]. Such effects usually occur during the infusion or within 1–3 hours following therapy. These include headache, fever, chills, and rigors. Gastrointestinal complaints (such as nausea, vomiting, and abdominal discomfort.) may also occur during or directly following administration. Less common reactions during or immediately following infusion include bronchospasm, hypotension, thrombophlebitis, and cardiac arrhythmias. Hypertension has also been reported [111–113]. Anaphylaxis associated with amphotericin B administration has rarely been reported [114].

Rapid infusion of AmBd (i.e., less than 4–6 hours) may increase the incidence of infusion-related reactions [115,116]. In addition, the formulation of amphotericin B may also influence the frequency of infusion-related reactions [21,110]. For example, infusion-related reactions on day 1 of empiric therapy without premedications were reported in 88.5% of febrile neutropenic patients receiving ABLC 5 mg/kg/day compared to 52% and 48% of those receiving LAmB 3 mg/kg/day or 5 mg/kg/day, respectively (p < 0.001) [110]. Infusion-related reactions have also been reported more frequently among subjects receiving ABCD than those receiving AmBd [117,118]. Select reactions have been reported to occur more frequently with certain formulations. For example, a triad of hypoxia, back pain, and chest pain has been reported following administration of LAmB [119–121]. A prospective analysis found a 20% mean overall frequency (range 0%–100%) of acute infusion-related reactions among 84 patients at 64 centers [121]. While these reactions rarely required discontinuation of therapy, slowing the infusion rate had no effect on the infusion-related reactions described. ABCD administration has been associated with hypoxia, dyspnea, and respiratory distress, which may necessitate cessation of therapy and the need for supportive care [122,123]. Reactions in individual patients may also be formulation-specific and not necessarily recur upon rechallenge with a different formulation.

Nephrotoxicity. Renal dysfunction secondary to amphotericin B administration is often the treatment-limiting adverse effect of amphotericin B. Proposed mechanisms include direct interaction with epithelial cell membranes (causing cellular disruption) and renal vasoconstriction (with resulting reductions in renal blood flow) [124,125]. Manifestations may include renal tubular acidosis, casts in the urine, azotemia, oliguria, and magnesium and potassium wasting [124,125]. The incidence of amphotericin B-induced nephrotoxicity varies widely between studies because of differences in definition, study population, underlying risk factors, duration of therapy, formulation and use

of premedications. However, such reactions (often described as a doubling of the baseline creatinine value) have been reported up to 50% of patients receiving AmBd [126–131]. Risk factors include underlying renal dysfunction, formulation, concomitant nephrotoxins, and dosing (daily and cumulative) [128,132–135]. Significant economic and clinical consequences can result [129,136,137].

Numerous strategies have been employed in attempts to reduce the incidence and severity of amphotericin B-induced renal dysfunction. This includes careful patient selection and (whenever possible) minimizing concomitant nephrotoxins. Use of saline loading [125,138–140], aggressive fluid resuscitation [141], and continuous infusions [142,143] have also been investigated. (see *Dosing and Administration*). More common today in patients at increased risk or experiencing AmBd-related nephrotoxicity is the use of LBFAmB, which all exhibit a reduced incidence of nephrotoxicity when compared to AmBd [110,118,144–146]. For example, ABLC-associated nephrotoxicity (defined as a doubling of baseline serum creainine) was observed in 13% of 3,514 patients with suspected or proven IFI in an multicenter, open-label retrospective study [144]. Studies comparing the incidence of nephrotoxicity between preparations has also been evaluated. For example, doubling of serum creatinine was significantly less frequent with LAmB 3 mg/kg/day than with AmBd 0.6 mg/kg/day, when given as empiric therapy in persistently febrile neutropenic patients (18.7% vs. 33.7%, respectively, p < 0.001) [126]. LAmB (3 or 5 mg/kg/day) has also been compared to ABLC (5 mg/kg/day) in this patient population, with rates of doubling of serum creatinine from baseline observed in 29.4%, 25.9%, and 42%, respectively [110]. Other reports comparing LAmB and ABLC for a variety of indications and ranges of doses for both agents (i.e., between 3 and 5 mg/kg/d) failed to detect significant differences between these preparations [145]. ABCD 6 mg/kg/day demonstrated a reduced incidence of nephrotoxicity relative to AmBd 1–1.5 mg/kg/day in patients with invasive aspergillosis (12.5% vs. 38.4%, respectively) [118].

Hematologic. Hematologic toxicities associated with the administration of amphotericin B most commonly include anemia, leukopenia, and/or thrombocytopenia [147]. Anemia (usually normochromic, normocytic) has been reported secondary to amphotericin B administration, and may be a consequence either of direct inhibition of erythropoietin [148] or secondary to renal toxicity. In one study, patients with underlying human immunodeficiency virus (HIV) infection were at increased risk of severe anemia, while severe leukopenia was more common in patients receiving ABLC and with an underlying hematologic cancer [147]. Hematological cancer was also a risk factor for severe thrombocytopenia in patients receiving amphotericin B.

Other. Elevations in liver function tests have less frequently been associated with amphotericin B administration [149].

Overview of Clinical Applications *(Note: THESE ARE NOT INTENDED TO BE COMPREHENSIVE. REFER TO OTHER CHAPTERS FOR COMPREHENSIVE DISCUSSION)*

Amphotericin B's status as the "gold standard" for the prevention and treatment of IFIs has been put into question by the recent introduction of new options, namely extended-spectrum triazoles and echinocandins [2,3]. Despite these new alternatives, amphotericin B is continually cited by numerous consensus guidelines as an option for serious and treatment-refractory IFIs [4–10]. With few exceptions, AmBd is often replaced by LBFAmB, largely based on the potential for increased safety rather than improvement in efficacy [146]. However, relative to AmBd, controlled studies examining LFAmB as primary therapy for IFIs are limited. In addition, while ABCD may be associated with increased infusion-related reactions [117,118], clinically-significant differences between other LBFAmB (i.e., LAmB and ABLC) may be less clear [150].

Candidiasis. Nystatin for the treatment of infections due to *Candida* spp. is restricted to the treatment of mucocutaneous forms. This may include oropharyngeal, cutaneous, mucocutaneous, and vulvovaginal infections.

The efficacy of AmBd caused by many *Candida* spp has been established in invasive candidiasis, including candidemia, osteomyelitis, disseminated candidiasis, endophthalmitis and endocarditis [5,151–153]. Use in candidemia is generally restricted to settings where drug intolerance or resistance has been demonstrated to alternate treatments [5]. Extensive experience with AmBd has also been documented for invasive candidiasis in the neonatal population [154,155]. A comparative trial of AmBd with fluconazole in non-neutropenic patients with candidemia have failed to demonstrate differences in efficacy between the two treatments [151]. More recently, AmBd has been used as the comparative agent against both caspofungin [105] and voriconazole [156]. In general, efficacy for AmBd is comparable to these new agents. However, newer agents are generally better tolerated than AmBd. In the case of voriconazole, an alternative exists for continued oral therapy once the patient is stable.

LBFAmB have also been used in the treatment of invasive candidiasis. The efficacy of ABLC has been reported in open-label studies [157,158]. For example, cure (30%) or improvement (30%) was noted in the treatment of invasive candidiasis in ABLC-treated patients in a retrospective observational trial [158]. Use of LAmB for the treatment of invasive candidiasis has also been reported in pediatric patients [159,160]. Published experience with ABCD is somewhat limited. It has been studied in an open label, phase-I [118] and

retrospective analysis of open-labeled trials. Early trials comparing ABCD with azoles (fluconazole) demonstrated comparable efficacy, but the ABCD was less well tolerated [152]. More recently, LAmB was demonstrated to be equally effective but less well tolerated than micafungin for candidemia and invasive candidiasis in adults [104]. ABLC and LAmB are FDA-approved as second-line therapy for use in proven candidiasis in patients intolerant or refractory to AmBd.

The potential role of AmBd as part of combination therapy (with fluconazole) was examined in a randomized study in non-neutropenic patients with candidemia [161]. In this trial, 30-day success rates were not different between subjects receiving fluconazole plus placebo (57%) or fluconazole in combination with AmBd (69%, p = 0.08).

The availability of equally efficacious and better-tolerated agents limits the role of amphotericin B for invasive candidiasis. Current expert guidelines for the treatment of invasive candidiasis limit the role of amphotericin B in severe, refractory infections, CNS infections and in pregnant patients [5]. In addition to its continued role in severe disease [162], some authorities [163] recognize the potential for a continued role in the treatment of neonatal infections. However, studies reporting both the safety and efficacy of alternate agents (i.e., azoles and echinocandins) in this patient population make continued justification for this indication problematic.

Aspergillosis. For many years, AmBd represented the standard of care for the treatment of invasive aspergillosis [4,164]. Overall efficacy rates varied with preparation, population, site of infection, and confirmation (possible, probable, definite). Since higher doses of AmBd (1–1.4 mg/kg/day) and longer durations of therapy were required, LBFAmB assumed a growing role. Published data included experience with LAmB [121,165–167], ABCD [118], and ABLC [157,168,169].

Based on trials demonstrating superiority of voriconazole over AmBd [4,170,171] and improved mortality [172], AmBd and LBFAmB (including ABLC and LAmB) are now used as alternative or salvage therapy in settings were voriconazole cannot be used [4]. Other options for refractory infections (i.e., echinocandins) also exist.

Cryptococcal infections. While mild-moderate forms of cryptococcosis outside the central nervous system (CNS) may be managed by an azole such as fluconazole or itraconazole, amphotericin B has become the standard of care for the initial therapy of severe, disseminated disease and those involving the CNS [6]. The efficacy of AmBd for the treatment of cryptococcal meningitis has been established by randomized controlled trials in both HIV and non-HIV patient populations [173–178]. Combination therapy of AmBd with flucytosine has improved clinical efficacy, time to sterilization of the CSF and the reduction in relapse rates [174]. In HIV-infected patients, AmBd (0.7 mg/kg/day) combined with flucytosine 100 mg/kg/day for two weeks followed by azole maintenance therapy was superior to AmBd + placebo, but more prolonged courses of flucytosine were of no additional benefit [176]. More recently, two different studies in patients with HIV infection reported a combination of amphotericin B plus flucytosine improved survival among patients with cryptococcal meningitis [179], but did not improve CSF clearance of organism [180] when compared to patients receiving amphotericin B monotherapy.

Current expert treatment guidelines recommend that AmBd be combined with flucytosine as initial "induction therapy" for cryptococcal meningitis in both HIV-infected and non-HIV-infected persons [6]. However, the optimal dose of AmBd for this indication is unknown. The potential role of AmBd dose escalation for induction therapy of cryptococcal meningitis was recently examined in HIV-postive patients [181]. Initial doses of 0.7–1.0 mg/kg/d (plus 5FC) × 2 weeks were followed by fluconazole. In this study, increasing doses demonstrated more rapid fungicidal activity.

There is less published experience with LBFAmB for cryptococcal infections. A comparison of LAmB 4 mg/kg/day and AmBd 0.7 mg/kg/day as induction therapy in HIV-infected patients (n = 28) concluded that LAmB was more effective than AmBd in sterilizing the cerebrospinal fluid (p < 0.05) [182]. However, overall clinical response was similar between the two treatments. The efficacy of ABLC has also been reported for cryptoccocosis [183] and cryptococcal meningitis [184]. In patients with HIV-associated cryptococcal meningitis (n = 21), successful treatment was reported in 86% of subjects receiving ABLC 5 mg/kg/day [184]. However, rates of CSF sterilization at 6 weeks were only 58%. The current IDSA treatment guidelines recommend LAmB 4 mg/kg/d be used as the LBFAmB, although such treatment is not currently FDA-approved [6]. In addition, while initial treatment of serious cryptococcal disease in solid organ transplant recipients has not been evaluated by prospective controlled clinical trials, LBFAmB (either LAmB or ABLC) may also be considered over AmBd in this population due to the frequent coadministration of nephrotoxic calcineurin inhibitors [185].

Zygomycoses. Limited options exist for the treatment of invasive zygomycoses. While amphotericin B maintains activity *in vitro* against zygomycetes, treatment outcomes (especially in the immunocompromised host) remain poor [186,187]. AmBd [188] or lipid-based formulations [188,189] of amphotericin B are frequently prescribed in this clinical setting, especially as initial therapy and frequently in combination with surgical intervention [187,188]. The introduction of newer agents (i.e., posaconazole and isavuconazole) may impact the role of amphotericin B in the future to use for initial management of severe infections [187,190].

Visceral Leishmaniasis. Published data have reported the clinical applications of AmBd [191], ABCD [192], ABLC [193], and LAmB [194,195] for visceral leishmaniasis. Of these treatment options, LAmB has received FDA approval. Investigations with LAmB have also reported efficacy of single-dose therapy for this infection [196,197].

Endemic Mycoses. Current expert treatment guidelines for histoplasmosis identify AmBd as initial management of severe infections (such as pulmonary and CNS infections, mediastinitis and disseminated disease) [7]. It is rarely used today, except in severe cases [198]. In general, higher doses of AmBd (i.e., 0.7–1 mg/kg/d) have been employed as initial therapy, with reduced doses (i.e., 0.5–0.6 mg/kg/d) for patients unable to tolerate higher doses. Patients improved or with stable disease following initial AmBd therapy (usually two weeks) can often be transitioned to azole therapy. LBFAmB may also have a role, especially for patients intolerant to AmBd [7]. ABLC was evaluated in 25 patients, with efficacy (cure + improvement) observed in 84% [189]. In a randomized, double-blind multicenter study for disseminated histoplasmosis comparing AmBd (0.7 mg/kg/day) to LAmB (3 mg/kg/day) as initial (i.e., 2 week) induction therapy for moderate-severe disease in AIDS patients, clinical success rates were 64% and 88% (respectively, p = 0.014) [199]. Fewer deaths and improved treatment tolerability were reported in patients receiving LAmB. However, no difference in time to defervescence, rate of blood culture conversion, or change in *Histoplasma capsulatum* antigen levels was observed.

Similar to its role in histoplasmosis and despite lack of published data from large controlled clinical trials, AmBd is considered as primary therapy for pulmonary, disseminated and CNS blastomycosis based on published guidelines [8]. AmBd is also the preferred therapy for immunocompromised or pregnant patients [8,200]. Cure rates for AmBd have been reported to range between 70% and 91% [8,200] with LBFAmB 3–5 mg/kg per day or AmBd 0.7–1 mg/kg per day and can be administered for 1–2 weeks or until improvement, followed by a transition to an oral agent [8]. Low relapse rates have been reported when cumulative doses of AmBd greater than 1 g have been employed. Similar to histoplamosis, higher doses of AmBd (0.7–1.0 mg/kg/d) should be considered for disseminated disease with blastomycosis, in which cumulative doses of 1.5–2.5 g or higher (at least 2 g) for CNS disease are used. Published experience with LBFAmB are limited. Some open-label experience exists with ABLC, with cure or improvement in 9/14 (64%) of cases [189]. Despite this relative lack of published data, LBFAmB are generally recommended for CNS disease [8].

In general, the use of amphotericin B for the treatment of sporotrichosis is restricted to pregnant patients or those with osteoarticular, pulmonary, or disseminated infections [9]. LBFAmB 3–5 mg/kg daily or AmBd 0.7–1.0 mg/kg daily can be used in such settings [9]. Similar to other guidelines, LBFAmB have been preferred by some clinicians for CNS disease. In a similar circumstance, fluconazole and itraconazole have largely replaced the need for the use of amphotericin B in the treatment of coccidioidomycosis [10,201]. AmBd 0.5–1.5 mg/kg IV daily or on alternating days may be considered in patients with rapidly-progressing disease, hypoxia and/or respiratory failure, or pregnant women. Experience with LBFAmB for the treatment of coccidioidomycosis is largely limited to case reports [157,189].

Emerging mycoses. Due to lack of drugs active against many of the emerging mycoses, limited positive clinical experience (primarily case reports or case series) and/or *in vitro* data has been reported for amphotericin B against *Exophiala oligosperma* [202] and rare molds [203].

Neutropenic Fever. Numerous studies have examined the efficacy and safety of amphotericin B in the treatment of fever in neutropenic oncology patients. Early published experience with AmBd helped establish a role of antifungal therapy in empiric regimens for patients persistently (>7 days) febrile despite broad-spectrum antibacterials [204,205]. More recently, AMBd has been compared to voriconazole [206], fluconazole [207,208], and caspofungin [106] in this patient population.

LBFAmB have also been evaluated for persistent fever in neutropenics. LAmB (3 mg/kg/day) was compared to AmBd (0.6 m/kg/day) among 660 patients in a large, double-blind, multicenter, randomized trial [126]. Similar rates of success (based on a composite endpoint of defervescence, survival, treatment of baseline infection, and absence of breakthrough IFI or toxicity requiring treatment discontinuation) of 50% (172/343) for LAmB vs. 49% (170/344) for AmBd were reported. However, LAmB-treated patients experienced fewer proven breakthrough fungal infections (3.2% [11/343] vs. 7.8% [27/344], p = 0.009). In addition, a reduction in infusion-related reactions (including fever [17% vs. 44%] and chills or rigors [18% vs. 54%]) was observed in LAmB vs. AmBd-treatments. Other studies have compared LAmB to AmBd [126,209] and voriconazole [210]. ABCD (4 mg/kg/day)therapy has also been compared to AmBd (0.8 mg/kg/day) in a prospective, randomized, double-blind study among neutropenic adults and children [117]. Success rates were 50% (49/98) and 43.2% (41/95), respectively (p = 0.31), while documented or suspected breakthrough fungal infection were reported is 14.3% and 14.7%, respectively. Although ABLC has been compared to both LAmB [110,145] and AmB [211], in this patient population, such evaluations were designed primarily to evaluate the safety and tolerability rather than efficacy.

Recent systematic comparisons of amphotericin B to fluconazole [212] and voriconazole [213] have been performed in the setting of suspected or documented IFIs in cancer patients. Amphotericin B was favored

over fluconazole due to its mortality benefit [212], and LAmB was favored over voriconazole [213]. However, given the expanded options of alternative therapies and the underlying risks for toxicities associated with amphotericin B, published guidelines for the empiric management of fever in neutropenic oncology patients recommend limiting the role of amphotericin B in this patient population [214,215]. Examples include empiric treatment of patients for whom alternate (i.e., azole or echinocandin) therapies are inappropriate. These may include patients at highest risk and/or with clinical evidence or radiologic evidence for invasive fungal infections (such as aspergillosis or mucormycosis) or those receiving prior azole therapy at risk of invasive mold infections. In these cases, either LAmB or ABLC should be considered [214,215].

Prophylaxis. Numerous investigations have involved use of polyenes orally (in the case of nystatin and AmBd), parenterally and via aerosol (amphotericin B formulations) in attempts to reduce IFIs in selected high-risk patient populations in the prevention of fungal infections in high-risk patient populations. Detailed discussions regarding this indication can be found elsewhere [216].

Orally-administered nystatin has been examined as an antifungal prophylaxis in a variety of populations, including low birthweight infants [217], oncology [218], and solid organ transplant recipients [216,219]. While some of these investigations reported the effectiveness of nystatin (relative to placebo) in the reduction of mucocutaneous disease, its role in the prevention of IFIs is not well-established [216]. In select patient populations (such as solid organ transplant recipients), use of nystatin has largely been replaced by azoles [216,219]. Similar investigations have used oral AmBd. In addition to its lack of superiority over other options (such as azoles), combined with a lack of a commercially-available oral formulation and definitive studies demonstrating success, the use of orally-administered AmBd as a popular strategy to prevent IFIs is also very limited.

In patients with hematologic malignancy, the application of AmBd as prophylaxis has been examined in a variety of studies, including comparisons between AmBd and LFAmB [220], fluconazole [207], and voriconazole [206]. LBFAmB have also been studied in this patient population [122,221–224]. Studies of the LBFAmB generally reflect the use of alternate dosing strategies (i.e., ABLC 2.5 mg/kg three times weekly prophylaxis and LAmB 3 mg/kg three times weekly) [223]. There is less experience with ABCD, since a study evaluating it as prophylaxis in neutropenic patients was discontinued prematurely because of severe infusion-related adverse events [122].

For patients undergoing hematologic stem cell transplant (HSCT), AmBd has been compared to placebo [225,226] and fluconazole [227,228]. Reduced doses of AmBd (i.e., 0.1–0.2 mg/kg/d) are more commonly studied in these settings.

Use of LBFAmB have also studied in this patient population, including LAmB [221,229,230] and ABLC [223,230].

Current published guidelines for the prevention of invasive fungal infections in cancer patients reflect that the toxicities of amphotericin B, along with the expanding options for alternate strategies, limit the routine use of amphotericin B in this setting [214,215]. However, amphotericin B (preferably either LAmB or ABLC) should be considered as an option for prophylaxis in patients at intermediate-or high-risk of invasive mold infections (such as those with allogeneic stem cell transplant recipients, myelodysplastic syndrome, acute myelogenous leukemia, or graft-versus-host disease).

Amphotericin B has also been examined as an antifungal prophylaxis in select solid organ transplant recipients [231–234]. A randomized, placebo-controlled trial evaluated LAmB 1 mg/kg/d × 7 in liver transplant recipients (compared to fluconazole or placebo) [233]. Active treatments demonstrated superior infection- and colonization-free rates when compared with placebo (40.6%, 34.9% and 2.3% for LAmB, fluconazole, and placebo, respectively. p < 0.01) Comparisons LAmB 50 mg/d to AmBd 15 mg/d have also been conducted in this population [235]. IFIs occurred in 4/44 (9%) and 3/48 (6%) patients, respectively. A statistically significant survival benefit was attributable to LAmB in this study (79.6% vs. 59.5%; p = 0.038). Alternate dosing strategies have also been investigated for the administration of amphotericin B as prophylaxis, including weekly administration of higher doses of LAmB in patients undergoing liver transplantation [236].

Prophylactic strategies for solid organ transplant recipients vary widely between transplant centers and patient populations. However, use of amphotericin B (in the form of LFAmB) as a prophylaxis against IFI in this setting may be restricted primarily to patients at significant risk of invasive candidiasis (such as pancreas, small bowel or liver transplant recipients) unable to receive azole prophylaxis (either due to increased risk of intolerance or azole resistance) or select patients at increased risk of aspergillosis (such as lung transplant recipients) [234].

Secondary prevention against recurrence of some fungal infections is needed in select patients with HIV [237]. Such infections may include cryptococcosis, histoplasmosis, and coccidiodomycosis. However, due to the availability of alternate agents (such as fluconazole and itraconazole), amphotericin B plays a limited role in such prevention.

Use of systemic administration of amphotericin B formulations may be problematic, mostly due to tolerability issues. As reviewed extensively elsewhere [238], aerosol administration of various formulations of amphotericin B as a prophylactic strategy has been studied in a variety of patient populations, including AmBd in neutropenic cancer patients, HSCT and lung transplantation patients [239–246]. Animal models suggest that aerosolized lipid formulations of amphotericin B achieve higher tissue penetration (relative to AmBd) [247–251]. Despite this, several issues regarding aerosol therapy persist, including (but not limited to) determination of the optimal agent, dose, frequency, duration and nebulizer [252–254].

DOSING AND ADMINISTRATION

Nystatin. As previously described, treatment with nystatin is restricted to cutaneous and mucocutaneous forms of candidiasis. Doses of nystatin used for prophylaxis varied by population, with the usual range in adult patients of 300,000–7.5 million international units per day in divided doses [216–219].

Amphotericin B. The optimal dose, frequency of administration and duration of amphotericin B is unknown. Considerations generally include the indication and formulation. For AmBd, the recommended dosing for most treatment indications range from 0.5 to 1.5 mg/kg/day, administered as a single daily dose. Doses of 1.5 mg/kg/d are generally reserved for infections with severe, life-threatening invasive infections and less-responsive organisms (such as *Aspergillus* spp or for treatment of mucormycosis). Studies examining AmBd for prophylaxis have employed lower doses and/or alternate day (sometimes three times weekly) administration. FDA-approved doses for LFAmB generally range from 3 to 5 mg/kg/d. The use of alternate administration schedules (including intermittent and weekly dosing) have been examined for LAmB and for AmBd [10,236,255].

Because of its concentration-dependent pharmacodynamic profile, dose-escalation has been proposed as a potential strategy to improve efficacy [236,255]. However, limited drug solubility and reversible binding of AmB in tissues, however, may limit the benefit of dose-escalation [59–61]. (see *Pharmacokinetics*) Existing studies involving LAmB, which compared initial therapy at either 3 mg/kg/d and 10 mg/kg/d × 14 days followed by 3 mg/kg/d for suspected or documented invasive mold infections, observed increased toxicity without improvements in efficacy at higher doses [135]. More recently, investigations of higher doses of LFAmB have also been reported for LAmB (up to 10 mg/kg/d) for mucormycosis [256], a single 15 mg/kg dose of LAmB for prevention in patients with AML [257], two consecutive daily doses of LAmB 15 mg/kg for leishmaniasis [195], and the use of ABLC 7.5 mg/kg weekly as prophylaxis for HSCT patients [258].

Dosage modification is unnecessary for patients with underlying renal dysfunction. For those experiencing AmB-induced nephrotoxicity, dose reductions or the use of twice the daily dose administered on alternate days has been described, but data to support this practice is lacking [259,260]. Such strategies are now largely replaced by substitution of AmBd with a LBFAmB or (in some cases) alternate therapies (such as echinocandins or extended-spectrum azoles). Amphotericin B is poorly removed by hemodialysis [94,95]. Pharmacokinetic data are lacking for patients with hepatic insufficiency, and currently no adjustments are recommended in this population.

Several issues surround the administration of amphotericin B, including the use of test doses, premedications, infusion rate, and various strategies to reduce nephrotoxicity and electrolyte abnormalities. Administration of a 1 mg test dose (without premeds) has been recommended to screen for anaphylaxis. This practice is of questionable clinical value, and will not rule-out subsequent adverse events (including infusion-related reactions). If performed, administration of a test dose should not delay institution of therapy. An alternate solution is to deliver a 1 mg aliquot from first dose, observe for several hours, and then complete the infusion.

For the prevention of select infusion-related reactions, administration of acetaminophen and/or diphenhydramine prior to the infusion may reduce the frequency and/or severity [109]. Pretreatment with corticosteroids in this setting has been described [261] but is less desirable. Heparin has been recommended by some to treat phlebitis, although controlled trials are lacking to support this practice. When possible, use of a central line may assist in reducing phlebitis. Meperidine has been reported to treat the rigors, but is less frequently employed as a prophylactic strategy [262]. Ibuprofen may significantly decrease the reaction [261].

Measures to reduce the frequency and/or severity of nephrotoxocity include careful patient selection, minimizing concomitant nephrotoxins, "saline loading", alternate day therapy, continuous infusion, combination of AmBd with Intralipids, use of acetylcysteine, and use of LFAmB [141]. Administration of normal saline prior and/or subsequent to the infusion is thought to reduce AmBd-related nephrotoxicity, but controlled clinical data to support is lacking [125,138,139,263]. The optimal method of saline administration is unknown, but often described as 500 mL normal saline before and following infusion. Aggressive fluid resuscitation has also been explored [141]. Caution should be used in patients with heart failure and renal dysfunction. It is also unknown if saline loading is necessary as a routine practice in patients receiving LFAmB, since such practices are not usually described in clinical studies. In all cases, assuring eunatremia and euvolemia prior to AmB administration is desirable. The safety and tolerability of combining AmBd with Intralipids has also been reported [264–268]. However, efficacy, toxicity, and quality control data are generally lacking with such preparations and, therefore, cannot be recommended [269]. More recently, administration of N-acetylcysteine has been investigated as a strategy to minimize amphotericin B-related toxicities, but failed to demonstrate a reduction of either nephrotoxicity or electrolyte imbalances [270,271].

Currently, LBFAmB would be selected for patients requiring continued therapy with amphotericin B and at risk or experiencing nephrotoxicity.

The rate of infusion may also impact toxicity. Therefore, rapid infusions should be avoided [272]. Despite pharmacodynamic studies that illustrate the concentration-dependent nature of AmBd's fungicidal activity [14,50], continuous infusion of the daily dose over 24 hours as a strategy to reduce nephrotoxicity has been investigated [142,143,273,274]. For AmBd, continuous infusion has decreased infusion-related reactions, nephrotoxicity, and mortality relative to a 4-hours infusion [142]. Other open-labeled trials have also documented the reductions in nephrotoxicity [143]. It is unknown, however, whether such data applies to LBFAmB, since these preparations were not studied. Models accounting for human serum albumin fail to show significant pharmacodyanmic differences between methods of administration [14]. In addition, such a method of administration cannot be recommended due to lack of efficacy data in patients with documented infections.

In addition to clinical monitoring for efficacy and adverse effects, patients receiving amphotericin B should receive close laboratory monitoring, including baseline blood counts, hepatic and renal function, and serum chemistries. In addition to serum creatinine, serum electrolytes (most notably potassium) should be monitored frequently in patients receiving amphotericin B preparations. For patients experiencing hypokalemia, judicious monitoring and replacement of potassium should occur. Successful coadministration of agents to prevent potassium wasting have been described, including amiloride [275–277] and spironolactone [278]. Currently, there is no clinical role for monitoring amphotericin B serum concentrations in attempts to improve either safety or efficacy [51].

DRUG INTERACTIONS

Reports of pharmacokinetic drug interactions with amphotericin B are largely a consequence of its nephrotoxic effects [1]. Declines in renal dysfunction as a result of amphotericin B administration may alter the elimination of agents that undergo significant renal clearance. An increased incidence of nephrotoxicity may be seen with concomitant use of other nephrotoxins. Electrolyte abnormalities secondary to amphotericin B administration may be enhanced by other agents known to produce such imbalances (such as corticosteroids). Amphotericin B-induced hypokalemia may enhance the activity of agents such as nondepolarizing skeletal muscle relaxants and cardiac glycosides.

Data and interpretation regarding the combination of amphotericin B with other antifungals is highly dependent upon test conditions, and is hindered by the lack of standardized testing methods. Perhaps the interaction best studied clinically is the favorable combinations of amphotericin B with flucytosine in the initial management of patients with cryptococcal meningitis [6]. However, it should be noted that declines in renal function secondary to amphotericin B may necessitate flucytosine dosage reductions.

Potential antagonism between azoles (which inhibit ergosterol synthesis) and polyenes (which bind directly to ergosterol in cell membranes) has been hypothesized in patients receiving sequential azole-polyene treatment. However, no impact on mortality could be detected during analysis of patients receiving LAmB with or without prior azole therapy (predominantly voriconazole) [279]. While antagonistic effects were noted previously when combined with the azole class *in vitro*, no antagonism was noted in a clinical trial of patients with candidemia [161]. More recently, interactions between amphotericin B and voriconazole have been investigated in an *in vitro* model, with results (both synergy and antagonism) depended upon dosing of the two agents [280]. Amphotericin B is currently recommended to be combined with fluconazole as an alternative induction therapy in HIV patients with cryptococcal meningitis unable to receive flucytosine therapy [6]. *In vitro* data regarding the combination of amphotericin with echinocandins (notably micafungin) against clinical isolates of *C. glabrata* demonstrated antagonism in over 50% of the isolates tested [37]. Clinical data regarding the potential interaction between amphotericin B and echinocandins are lacking, although case reports and historically-controlled studies suggest a potential role in treatment-refractory patients [36]. No pharmacokinetic interaction was observed in one trial when amphotericin B was coadministered with micafungin, although the combination was associated with more adverse effects [281]. Similarly, LAmB does not appear to alter the pharmacokinetics of caspofungin [279].

SUMMARY

Nystatin, while continuing to represent a treatment option for selected forms of cutaneous and mucocutaneous forms of candidiasis, currently plays a limited role in the prevention and treatment of IFIs due primarily to its lack of systemic absorption after oral administration and the lack of a commercially-available parenteral formulation.

Amphotericin B continues to be the broadest-spectrum antifungal with cidal activity against many pathogens and a very low potential for treatment-emergent resistance. It's efficacy has been established for numerous IFIs in a variety of patient populations. Despite the recent introduction of new options for prevention and treatment of IFIs, amphotericin B is still prominent in numerous treatment guidelines for severe, life-threatening infections [4–6,10].

Requirements for parenteral administration, along with treatment-related adverse effects, restrict the widespread use of amphotericin B. Of particular note is the significant clinical and economic impact of AmB-induced nephrotoxicity [129]. The introduction of LBFAmB have expanded the population who can safely receive the drug [93,282]. However, increased efficacy with LBFAmB is less clear [283]. Increases in LBFAmB drug acquisition cost (relative to AmBd) may be offset by reductions in costs associated with amphotericin B nephrotoxicity [129,136,137]. Despite these advantages, AmBd may continue to play a role in select uses and patient populations, such as neonates and children, intrathecal use in patients

with *Coccidiodes immitis* meningitis, or in patients otherwise at low risk of amphotericin B nephrotoxicity [2,141,284,285] or in azole/echinocandin-resistant fungal strains.

REFERENCES

1. Gallis HA, Drew RH, Pickard WW. Amphotericin B: 30 years of clinical experience. *Rev Infect Dis* 1990;12(2):308–329.
2. Ostrosky-Zeichner L, Marr KA, Rex JH, Cohen SH. Amphotericin B: Time for a new "gold standard". *Clin Infect Dis* 2003;37(3):415–425.
3. Kleinberg M. What is the current and future status of conventional amphotericin B? *Int J Antimicrob Agents* 2006;27 Suppl 1:12–16.
4. Patterson TF, Thompson GR, 3rd, Denning DW, et al. Practice guidelines for the diagnosis and management of aspergillosis: 2016 Update by the Infectious Diseases Society of America. *Clin Infect Dis* 2016;63(4):e1–e60.
5. Pappas PG, Kauffman CA, Andes DR, et al. Clinical practice guideline for the management of candidiasis: 2016 Update by the Infectious Diseases Society of America. *Clin Infect Dis* 2016;62(4):e1–50.
6. Perfect JR, Dismukes WE, Dromer F, et al. Clinical practice guidelines for the management of cryptococcal disease: 2010 update by the infectious diseases society of america. *Clin Infect Dis* 2010;50(3):291–322.
7. Wheat LJ, Freifeld AG, Kleiman MB, et al. Clinical practice guidelines for the management of patients with histoplasmosis: 2007 update by the Infectious Diseases Society of America. *Clin Infect Dis* 2007;45(7):807–825.
8. Chapman SW, Dismukes WE, Proia LA, et al. Clinical practice guidelines for the management of blastomycosis: 2008 update by the Infectious Diseases Society of America. *Clin Infect Dis* 2008;46(12):1801–1812.
9. Kauffman CA, Bustamante B, Chapman SW, Pappas PG. Clinical practice guidelines for the management of sporotrichosis: 2007 update by the Infectious Diseases Society of America. *Clin Infect Dis* 2007;45(10):1255–1265.
10. Galgiani JN, Ampel NM, Blair JE, et al. 2016 Infectious Diseases Society of America (IDSA) clinical practice guideline for the treatment of coccidioidomycosis. *Clin Infect Dis* 2016;63(6):e112–146.
11. Ramos H, Valdivieso E, Gamargo M, Dagger F, Cohen BE. Amphotericin B kills unicellular leishmanias by forming aqueous pores permeable to small cations and anions. *J Membrane Biol* 1996;152(1):65–75.
12. Kanafani ZA, Perfect JR. Resistance to antifungal agents: Mechanisms and clinical impact. *Clin Infect Dis* 2008;46(1):120–128.

13. Roilides E, Lyman CA, Filioti J, et al. Amphotericin B formulations exert additive antifungal activity in combination with pulmonary alveolar macrophages and polymorphonuclear leukocytes against *Aspergillus fumigatus*. *Antimicrob Agents Chemother* 2002;46(6):1974–1976.

14. Lewis RE, Wiederhold NP, Prince RA, et al. *In vitro* pharmacodynamics of rapid versus continuous infusion of amphotericin B deoxycholate against *Candida* species in the presence of human serum albumin. *J Antimicrob Chemother* 2006;57(2):288–293.

15. Lewis RE, Wiederhold NP, Klepser ME, Lewis RE, Wiederhold NP, Klepser ME. In *vitro* pharmacodynamics of amphotericin B, itraconazole, and voriconazole against *Aspergillus*, *Fusarium*, and *Scedosporium* spp. *Antimicrob Agents Chemother* 2005;49(3):945–951.

16. Wiederhold NP, Tam VH, Chi JD, Prince RA, Kontoyiannis DP, Lewis RE. Pharmacodynamic activity of amphotericin B deoxycholate is associated with peak plasma concentrations in a neutropenic murine model of invasive pulmonary aspergillosis. *Antimicrob Agents Chemother* 2006;50(2):469–473.

17. Lass-Florl C, Mayr A, Perkhofer S, et al. Activities of antifungal agents against yeasts and filamentous fungi: Assessment according to the methodology of the European Committee on Antimicrobial Susceptibility Testing. *Antimicrob Agents Chemother* 2008;52(10):3637–3641.

18. Rogers PD, Pearson MM, Cleary JD, Sullivan DC, Chapman SW. Differential expression of genes encoding immunomodulatory proteins in response to amphotericin B in human mononuclear cells identified by cDNA microarray analysis. *J Antimicrob Chemother* 2002;50(6):811–817.

19. Vonk AG, Netea MG, Denecker NEJ, Verschueren ICMM, van der Meer JWM, Kullberg BJ. Modulation of the pro- and anti-inflammatory cytokine balance by amphotericin B. *J Antimicrob Chemother* 1998;42(4):469–474.

20. Sau K, Mambula SS, Latz E, et al. The antifungal drug amphotericin B promotes inflammatory cytokine release by a Toll-like receptor- and CD14-dependent mechanism. *J Biol Chem* 2003;278(39):37561–37568.

21. Arning M, Kliche KO, Heer-Sonderhoff AH, et al. Infusion-related toxicity of three different amphotericin B formulations and its relation to cytokine plasma levels. *Mycoses* 1995;38(11–12):459–465.

22. Ben Ami R, Lewis RE, Kontoyiannis DP. Immunocompromised hosts: Immunopharmacology of modern antifungals. *Clin Infect Dis* 2008;47(2):226–235.

23. Reyes E, Cardona J, Prieto A, et al. Liposomal amphotericin B and amphotericin B-deoxycholate show different immunoregulatory effects on human peripheral blood mononuclear cells. *J Infect Dis* 2000;181(6):2003–2010.

24. Gigliotti F, Shenep JL, Lott L, Thornton D. Induction of prostaglandin synthesis as the mechanism responsible for the chills and fever produced by infusing amphotericin B. *J Infect Dis* 1987;156(5):784–789.

25. Andes D, Stamsted T, Conklin R, Andes D, Stamsted T, Conklin R. Pharmacodynamics of amphotericin B in a neutropenic-mouse disseminated-candidiasis model. *Antimicrob Agents Chemother* 2001;45(3):922–926.

26. Ernst EJ, Klepser ME, Pfaller MA, Ernst EJ, Klepser ME, Pfaller MA. Postantifungal effects of echinocandin, azole, and polyene antifungal agents against *Candida albicans* and *Cryptococcus neoformans*. *Antimicrob Agents Chemother* 2000;44(4):1108–1111.

27. Vitale RG, Meis JF, Mouton JW, et al. Evaluation of the post-antifungal effect (PAFE) of amphotericin B and nystatin against 30 zygomycetes using two different media. *J Antimicrob Chemother* 2003;52(1):65–70.

28. Al Dhaheri RS, Douglas LJ. Absence of amphotericin B-Tolerant persister cells in biofilms of some *Candida* species. *Antimicrob Agents Chemother* 2008;52(5):1884–1887.

29. Kuhn DM, George T, Chandra J, et al. Antifungal susceptibility of *Candida* biofilms: Unique efficacy of amphotericin B lipid formulations and echinocandins. *Antimicrob Agents Chemother* 2002;46(6):1773–1780.

30. Al Fattani MA, Douglas LJ. Penetration of *Candida* biofilms by antifungal agents. *Antimicrob Agents Chemother* 2004;48(9):3291–3297.

31. Marcos-Zambrano LJ, Escribano P, Bouza E, Guinea J. Comparison of the antifungal activity of micafungin and amphotericin B against *Candida tropicalis* biofilms. *J Antimicrob Chemother* 2016;71(9):2498–2501.

32. Mukherjee PK, Long L, Kim HG, Ghannoum M. Amphotericin B lipid complex is efficacious in the treatment of *Candida albicans* biofilms using a model of catheter-associated *Candida* biofilms. *Int J Antimicrob Agents* 2008;doi:10.1016/j.ijantimicag.2008.07.030.

33. Ostrosky-Zeichner L. Combination antifungal therapy: A critical review of the evidence. *Clin Microbiol Infect* 2008;14 Suppl 4:65–70.

34. Vazquez JA, Vazquez JA. Clinical practice: Combination antifungal therapy for mold infections: Much ado about nothing? *Clin Infect Dis* 2008;46(12):1889–1901.

35. Baddley JW, Pappas PG. Combination antifungal therapy for the treatment of invasive yeast and mold infections. *Curr Inf Dis Reports* 2007;9(6):448–456.

36. Johnson MD, MacDougall C, Ostrosky-Zeichner L, Perfect JR, Rex JH. Combination antifungal therapy. *Antimicrob Agents Chemother* 2004;48(3):693–715.

37. Denardi LB, Keller JT, Oliveira V, Mario DAN, Santurio JM, Alves SH. Activity of combined antifungal agents against multidrug-resistant

Candida glabrata strains. *Mycopathologia* 2017;182(9–10):819–828. doi:10.1007/ s11046-11017-10141-11049.

38. Clancy CJ, Nguyen MH, Clancy CJ, Nguyen MH. The combination of amphotericin B and azithromycin as a potential new therapeutic approach to fusariosis. *J Antimicrob Chemother* 1998;41(1):127–130.

39. Nguyen MH, Clancy CJ, Yu YC, et al. Potentiation of antifungal activity of amphotericin B by azithromycin against *Aspergillus* species. *Eur J Clin Micro Infect Dis* 1997;16(11):846–848.

40. Clancy CJ, Yu YC, Lewin A, et al. Inhibition of RNA synthesis as a therapeutic strategy against *Aspergillus* and *Fusarium*: Demonstration of *in vitro* synergy between rifabutin and amphotericin B. *Antimicrob Agents Chemother* 1998;42(3):509–513.

41. Kubica TF, Denardi LB, Azevedo MI, et al. Antifungal activities of tacrolimus in combination with antifungal agents against fluconazole-susceptible and fluconazole-resistant *Trichosporon asahii* isolates. *Braz J Infect Dis* 2016;20(6):539–545.

42. He Y, Zhou L, Gao C, Han L, Xu Y. Rifampin enhances the activity of amphotericin B against *Fusarium solani* species complex and *Aspergillus flavus* species complex isolates from Keratitis patients. *Antimicrob Agents Chemother* 2017;61(4).

43. Rogers TR. Antifungal drug resistance: Limited data, dramatic impact? *Int J Antimicrob Agents* 2006;27 Suppl 1:7–11.

44. Klepser ME. *Candida* resistance and its clinical relevance. *Pharmacother* 2006;26(6):68S–75S.

45. Blum G, Hortnagl C, Jukic E, et al. New insight into amphotericin B resistance in *Aspergillus terreus*. *Antimicrob Agents Chemother* 2013;57(4):1583–1588.

46. Athar MA, Winner HI. Development of resistance by *Candida* species to polyene antibiotics *in vitro*. *J Med Microbiol* 1971;4(4):505–517.

47. Broughton MC, Bard M, Lees ND. Polyene resistance in ergosterol producing strains of *Candida albicans*. *Mycoses* 1991;34(1–2):75–83.

48. Sokol-Anderson M, Sligh JE, Elberg S, Brajtburg J, Kobayashi GS, Medoff G. Role of cell defense against oxidative damage in the resistance of *Candida albicans* to the killing effect of amphotericin-B. *Antimicrob Agents Chemother* 1988;32(5):702–705.

49. Mohr JF, Ostrosky-Zeichner L. Nystatin. In: Yu VI, Edwards G, McKinnon PS, Peloquin C, Morse GD, (Eds.). *Antimicrobial Therapy and Vaccines*, 2nd ed. Pittsburg, PA: ESun Technologies, LLC, 2005:669–677.

50. Dodds ES, Drew RH, Perfect JR, Dodds ES, Drew RH, Perfect JR. Antifungal pharmacodynamics: Review of the literature and clinical applications. *Pharmacother* 2000;20(11):1335–1355.

51. Smith D, Andes D. Therapeutic drug monitoring of antifungals: Pharmacokinetic and pharmacodynamic considerations. *Ther Drug Monit* 2008;30(2):167–172.

52. Lepak AJ, Andes DR. Antifungal pharmacokinetics and pharmacodynamics. *Cold Spring Harb Perspect Med* 2014;5(5):a019653.

53. Nett JE, Andes DR. Antifungal agents: Spectrum of activity, pharmacology, and clinical indications. *Infect Dis Clin North Am* 2016;30(1):51–83.

54. Burgess DS, Hastings RW, Summers KK, et al. Pharmacodynamics of fluconazole, itraconazole, and amphotericin B against *Candida albicans*. *Diagn Microbiol Infect Dis* 2000;36(1):13–18.

55. Andes D, Safdar N, Marchillo K, et al. Pharmacokinetic-pharmacodynamic comparison of amphotericin B (AMB) and two lipid-associated AMB preparations, liposomal AMB and AMB lipid complex, in murine candidiasis models. *Antimicrob Agents Chemother* 2006;50(2):674–684.

56. Stone NR, Bicanic T, Salim R, Hope W. Liposomal amphotericin B (AmBisome(®)): A review of the pharmacokinetics, pharmacodynamics, clinical experience and future directions. *Drugs* 2016;76(4):485–500.

57. Lewis RE, Liao G, Hou J, Chamilos G, Prince RA, Kontoyiannis DP. Comparative analysis of amphotericin B lipid complex and liposomal amphotericin B kinetics of lung accumulation and fungal clearance in a murine model of acute invasive pulmonary aspergillosis. *Antimicrob Agents Chemother* 2007;51(4):1253–1258.

58. Bekersky I, Fielding RM, Dressler DE, Kline S, Buell DN, Walsh TJ. Pharmacokinetics, excretion, and mass balance of 14C after administration of 14C-cholesterol-labeled AmBisome to healthy volunteers. *J Clin Pharmacol* 2001;41(9):963–971.

59. Bekersky I, Fielding RM, Dressler DE, et al. Plasma protein binding of amphotericin B and pharmacokinetics of bound versus unbound amphotericin B after administration of intravenous liposomal amphotericin B (AmBisome) and amphotericin B deoxycholate. *Antimicrob Agents Chemother* 2002;46(3):834–840.

60. Bekersky I, Fielding RM, Dressler DE, et al. Pharmacokinetics, excretion, and mass balance of liposomal amphotericin B (AmBisome) and amphotericin B deoxycholate in humans. *Antimicrob Agents Chemother* 2002;46(3):828–833.

61. Park BJ, Arthington-Skaggs BA, Hajjeh RA, et al. Evaluation of amphotericin B interpretive breakpoints for *Candida* bloodstream isolates by correlation with therapeutic outcome. *Antimicrob Agents Chemother* 2006;50(4):1287–1292.

62. Hong Y, Shaw PJ, Nath CE, et al. Population pharmacokinetics of liposomal amphotericin B in pediatric patients with malignant diseases. *Antimicrob Agents Chemother* 2006;50(3):935–942.

63. Smith KD, Achan B, Hullsiek KH, et al. Increased antifungal drug resistance in clinical isolates of *Cryptococcus neoformans* in Uganda. *Antimicrob Agents Chemother* 2015;59(12):7197–7204.

64. Sabatelli F, Patel R, Mann PA, et al. *In vitro* activities of posaconazole, fluconazole, itraconazole, voriconazole, and amphotericin B against a large collection of clinically important molds and yeasts. *Antimicrob Agents Chemother* 2006;50(6):2009–2015.

65. Clinical and Laboratory Standards Institute. *Reference Method for Broth Dilution Antifungal Susceptibilty Testing of Yeasts.* Fourth Informational Supplement M-27 S-4. Wayne, PA: Clinical and Laboratory Standards Institute, 2012.

66. Pfaller MA, Espinel-Ingroff A, Canton E, et al. Wild-type MIC distributions and epidemiological cutoff values for amphotericin B, flucytosine, and itraconazole and *Candida* spp. as determined by CLSI broth microdilution. *J Clin Microbiol* 2012;50(6):2040–2046.

67. Hawkins JL, Baddour LM. *Candida lusitaniae* infections in the era of fluconazole availability. *Clin Infect Dis* 2003;36(2):E14–E18.

68. Ellis D. Amphotericin B: Spectrum and resistance. *J Antimicrob Chemother* 2002;49:7–10.

69. Espinel-Ingroff A, Arendrup M, Canton E, et al. A multi-center study of method-dependent epidemiological cutoff values (ECVs.) for resistance detection in *Candida* spp. and *Aspergillus* spp. to amphotericin B and echinocandins for the Etest agar diffusion method. *Antimicrob Agents Chemother.* 2016;61(1).

70. Arendrup MC, Prakash A, Meletiadis J, Sharma C, Chowdhary A. *Candida auris*: Comparison of the EUCAST and CLSI reference microdilution MICs for eight antifungal compounds and associated tentative ECOFFs. *Antimicrob Agents Chemother.* 2017;61(1).

71. Hadfield TL, Smith MB, Winn RE, Rinaldi MG, Guerra C. Mycoses caused by *Candida lusitaniae*. *Rev Infect Dis* 1987;9(5):1006–1012.

72. Christenson JC, Guruswamy A, Mukwaya G, Rettig PJ. *Candida lusitaniae* - an emerging human pathogen. *Pediatr Infect Dis J* 1987;6(8):755–757.

73. Barchiesi F, Schimizzi AM, Caselli F, et al. Interactions between triazoles and amphotericin B against *Cryptococcus neoformans*. *Antimicrob Agents Chemother* 2000;44(9):2435–2441.

74. Marcon MJ, Durrell DE, Powell DA, Buesching WJ. *In vitro* activity of systemic antifungal agents against *Malassezia furfur*. *Antimicrob Agents Chemother* 1987;31(6):951–953.

75. Walsh TJ, Melcher GP, Rinaldi MG, et al. *Trichosporon beigelii*, an emerging pathogen resistant to amphotericin-B. *J Clin Microbiol* 1990;28(7):1616–1622.

76. Li RK, Ciblak MA, Nordoff N, et al. *In vitro* activities of voriconazole, itraconazole, and amphotericin B against *Blastomyces dermatitidis*, *Coccidioides immitis*, and *Histoplasma capsulatum*. *Antimicrob Agents Chemother* 2000;44(6):1734–1736.

77. Kauffman CA. Endemic mycoses: Blastomycosis, histoplasmosis, and sporotrichosis. *Infect Dis Clin North Am* 2006;20(3):645–662, vii.

78. Thompson GR, 3rd, Barker BM, Wiederhold NP. Large-scale evaluation of *in vitro* amphotericin B, triazole, and echinocandin activity against *Coccidioides* species from U.S. institutions. *Antimicrob Agents Chemother* 2017;61(4).

79. McGinnis MR, Nordoff N, Li RK, Pasarell L, Warnock DW. *Sporothrix schenckii* sensitivity to voriconazole, itraconazole and amphotericin B. *Med Mycol* 2001;39(4):369–371.

80. Diekema DJ, Messer SA, Hollis RJ, et al. Activities of caspofungin, itraconazole, posaconazole, ravuconazole, voriconazole, and amphotericin B against 448 recent clinical isolates of filamentous fungi. *J Clin Microbiol* 2003;41(8):3623–3626.

81. Sutton DA, Sanche SE, Revankar SG, et al. *In vitro* amphotericin B resistance in clinical isolates of *Aspergillus terreus,* with a head-to-head comparison to voriconazole. *J Clin Microbiol* 1999;37(7):2343–2345.

82. Sun QN, Fothergill AW, McCarthy DI, et al. *In vitro* activities of posaconazole, itraconazole, voriconazole, amphotericin B, and fluconazole against 37 clinical isolates of zygomycetes. *Antimicrob Agents Chemother* 2002;46(5):1581–1582.

83. Liu M, Chen M, Yang Z. Design of amphotericin B oral formulation for antifungal therapy. *Drug Deliv* 2017;24(1):1–9.

84. Hofstra W, Vries-Hospers H, van der WD. Concentrations of amphotericin B in faeces and blood of healthy volunteers after the oral administration of various doses. *Infection* 1982;10(4):223–227.

85. Ching M, Raymond K, Bury R, Mashford M, Morgan D. Absorption of orally administered amphotericin B lozenges. *Br J Clin Pharmacol* 1983;16(1):106–108.

86. Oostdijk EA, de Smet AM, Bonten MJ. Effects of decontamination of the digestive tract and oropharynx in intensive care unit patients on 1-year survival. *Am J Respir Crit Care Med* 2013;188(1):117–120.

87. Roos D, Dijksman LM, Oudemans-van Straaten HM, de Wit LT, Gouma DJ, Gerhards MF. Randomized clinical trial of perioperative selective decontamination of the digestive tract versus placebo in elective gastrointestinal surgery. *Br J Surg* 2011;98(10):1365–1372.

88. de Smet AM, Kluytmans JA, Cooper BS, et al. Decontamination of the digestive tract and oropharynx in ICU patients. *N Engl J Med* 2009;360(1):20–31.

89. Atkinson AJ, Bennett JE. Amphotericin-B pharmacokinetics in humans. *Antimicrob Agents Chemother* 1978;13(2):271–276.

90. Perfect JR, Durack DT. Comparison of amphotericin-B and N-D-ornithyl amphotericin B methyl ester in experimental cryptococcal meningitis and *Candida albicans* endocarditis with pyelonephritis. *Antimicrob Agents Chemother* 1985;28(6):751–755.

91. Groll AH, Giri N, Petraitis V, et al. Comparative efficacy and distribution of lipid formulations of amphotericin B in experimental *Candida albicans* infection of the central nervous system. *J Infect Dis* 2000;182(1):274–282.

92. Groll AH, Lyman CA, Petraitis V, et al. Compartmentalized intrapulmonary pharmacokinetics of amphotericin B and its lipid formulations. *Antimicrob Agents Chemother* 2006;50(10):3418–3423.

93. Gibbs WJ, Drew RH, Perfect JR. Liposomal amphotericin B: Clinical experience and perspectives. *Exp Rev Anti Infect Ther* 2005;3(2):167–181.

94. Morgan DJ, Ching MS, Raymond K, et al. Elimination of amphotericin B in impaired renal function. *Clin Pharmacol Ther* 1983;34(2):248–253.

95. Bellmann R, Egger P, Djanani A, et al. Pharmacokinetics of amphotericin B lipid complex in critically ill patients on continuous veno-venous haemofiltration. *Int J Antimicrob Agents* 2004;23(1):80–83.

96. Wurthwein G, Young C, Lanvers-Kaminsky C, et al. Population pharmacokinetics of liposomal amphotericin B and caspofungin in allogeneic hematopoietic stem cell recipients. *Antimicrob Agents Chemother* 2012;56(1):536–543.

97. Tomlin M, Priestley GS, Tomlin M, Priestley GS. Elimination of liposomal amphotericin by hemodiafiltration. *Intensive Care Med* 1995;21(8):699–700.

98. Nath CE, McLachlan AJ, Shaw PJ, Coakley JC, Earl JW. Amphotericin B dose optimization in children with malignant diseases. *Chemother* 2007;53(2):142–147.

99. Nath CE, McLachlan AJ, Shaw PJ, Gunning R, Earl JW. Population pharmacokinetics of amphotericin B in children with malignant diseases. *Br J Clin Pharmacol* 2001;52(6):671–680.

100. Nath CE, Shaw PJ, Gunning R, McLachlan AJ, Earl JW. Amphotericin B in children with malignant disease: A comparison of the toxicities and pharmacokinetics of amphotericin B administered in dextrose versus lipid emulsion. *Antimicrob Agents Chemother* 1999;43(6):1417–1423.

101. Walsh TJ, SHAD A, Bekersky I, et al. Safety, tolerability and pharmacokinetics of liposomal amphotericin B in immunocompromised pediatric patients (abstract). *Proceedings of the 48th Interscience Conference on Antimicrobial Agents and Chemotherapy and the Infectious Diseases Society of America 46th Annual Meeting Washington, DC October 25–28, 2008.* 2008.

102. Wurthwein G, Groll AH, Hempel G, et al. Population pharmacokinetics of amphotericin B lipid complex in neonates. *Antimicrob Agents Chemother* 2005;49(12):5092–5098.

103. Barton CH, Pahl M, Vaziri ND, Cesario T. Renal magnesium wasting associated with amphotericin B therapy. *Am J Med* 1984;77(3):471–474.

104. Kuse ER, Chetchotisakd P, da Cunha CA, et al. Micafungin versus liposomal amphotericin B for candidaemia and invasive candidosis: A phase III randomised double-blind trial. *Lancet* 2007;369(9572):1519–1527.

105. Mora-Duarte J, Betts R, Rotstein C, et al. Comparison of caspofungin and amphotericin B for invasive candidiasis. *N Engl J Med* 2002;347(25):2020–2029.

106. Walsh TJ, Teppler H, Donowitz G, et al. Caspofungin versus liposomal amphotericin B for empirical antifungal therapy in patients with persistent fever and neutropenia. *N Engl J Med* 2004;351(14):1391–1402.

107. Queiroz-Telles F, Berezin E, Leverger G, et al. Micafungin versus liposomal amphotericin B for pediatric patients with invasive candidiasis: Substudy of a randomized double-blind trial. *Pediatr Infect Dis J* 2008;27(9):820–826.

108. Barcia JP. Hyperkalemia associated with rapid infusion of conventional and lipid complex formulations of amphotericin B. *Pharmacother* 1998;18(4):874–876.

109. Goodwin SD, Cleary JD, Walawander CA, Taylor JW, Grasela TH. Pretreatment regimens for adverse events related to infusion of amphotericin B. *Clin Infect Dis* 1995;20(4):755–761.

110. Wingard J, White M, Anaissie E, Raffalli J, Goodman J, Arrieta A. A randomized, double-blind comparative trial evaluating the safety of liposomal amphotericin B versus amphotericin B lipid complex in the empirical treatment of febrile neutropenia. *Clin Infect Dis* 2000;31(5):1155–1163.

111. Wiwanitkit V. Severe hypertension associated with the use of amphotericin B: An appraisal on the reported cases. *J Hyperten* 2006;24(7):1445–1445.

112. Ferreira E, Perreault MM. Hypertension exacerbated by amphotericin B administration. *Ann Pharmacother* 1997;31(11):1407–1408.

113. Rowles DM, Fraser SL. Amphotericin B lipid complex (ABLC)-associated hypertension: Case report and review. *Clin Infect Dis* 1999;29(6):1564–1565.

114. Maddux MS, Barriere SL. A review of complications of amphotericin B therapy - recommendations for prevention and management. *Drug Intell Clin Pharm* 1980;14(3):177–181.

115. Oldfield EC, III, Garst PD, Hostettler C, White M, Samuelson D. Randomized, double-blind trial of 1- versus 4-hour amphotericin B infusion durations. *Antimicrob Agents Chemother* 1990;34(7):1402–1406.

116. Ellis ME, Alhokail AA, Clink HM, et al. Double-blind randomized study of the effect of infusion rates on toxicity of amphotericin-B. *Antimicrob Agents Chemother* 1992;36(1):172–179.

117. White MH, Bowden RA, Sandler ES, et al. Randomized, double-blind clinical trial of amphotericin B colloidal dispersion vs. amphotericin B in the empirical treatment of fever and neutropenia. *Clin Infect Dis* 1998;27(2):296–302.

118. Bowden R, Chandrasekar P, White MH, et al. A double-blind, randomized, controlled trial of amphotericin B colloidal dispersion versus amphotericin B for treatment of invasive aspergillosis in immunocompromised patients. *Clin Infect Dis* 2002;35(4):359–366.

119. Roden MM, Nelson LD, Knudsen TA, et al. Triad of acute infusion-related reactions associated with liposomal amphotericin B: Analysis of clinical and epidemiological characteristics. *Clin Infect Dis* 2003;36(10):1213–1220.

120. Johnson MD, Drew RH, Perfect JR. Chest discomfort associated with liposomal amphotericin B: Report of three cases and review of the literature. *Pharmacother* 1998;18(5):1053–1061.

121. Walsh TJ, Goodman JL, Pappas P, et al. Safety, tolerance, and pharmacokinetics of high-dose liposomal amphotericin B (AmBisome) in patients infected with *Aspergillus* species and other filamentous fungi: Maximum tolerated dose study. *Antimicrob Agents Chemother* 2001;45(12):3487–3496.

122. Timmers GJ, Zweegman S, Simoons-Smit AM, van Loenen AC, Touw D, Huijgens PC. Amphotericin B colloidal dispersion (Amphocil) vs. fluconazole for the prevention of fungal infections in neutropenic patients: Data of a prematurely stopped clinical trial. *Bone Marrow Transplant* 2000;25(8):879–884.

123. Sanders SW, Buchi KN, Goddard MS, Lang JK, Tolman KG. Single-dose pharmacokinetics and tolerance of a cholesteryl sulfate complex of amphotericin B administered to healthy volunteers. *Antimicrob Agents Chemother* 1991;35(6):1029–1034.

124. Sabra R, Branch RA. Amphotericin B nephrotoxicity. *Drug Saf* 1990;5(2):94–108.

125. Sawaya BP, Briggs JP, Schnermann J. Amphotericin B nephrotoxicity: The adverse consequences of altered membrane properties. *J Am Soc Nephrol* 1995;6(2):154–164.

126. Walsh TJ, Finberg RW, Arndt C, et al. Liposomal amphotericin B for empirical therapy in patients with persistent fever and neutropenia. National Institute of Allergy and Infectious Diseases Mycoses Study Group. *N Engl J Med* 1999;340(10):764–771.

127. Wingard J, Kubilis P, Lee L, et al. Clinical significance of nephrotoxicity in patients treated with amphotericin B for suspected or proven aspergillosis. *Clin Infect Dis* 1999;29(6):1402–1407.

128. Harbarth S, Pestotnik SL, Lloyd JF, et al. The epidemiology of nephrotoxicity associated with conventional amphotericin B therapy. *Am J Med* 2001;111(7):528–534.

129. Bates DW, Su L, Yu DT, et al. Mortality and costs of acute renal failure associated with amphotericin B therapy. *Clin Infect Dis* 2001;32(5):686–693.

130. Fanos V, Cataldi L. Amphotericin B-induced nephrotoxicity: A review. *J Chemother* 2000;12(6):463–470.

131. Rocha PN, Kobayashi CD, de Carvalho Almeida L, de Oliveira Dos Reis C, Santos BM, Glesby MJ. Incidence, predictors, and impact on hospital mortality of amphotericin B nephrotoxicity defined using newer acute kidney injury diagnostic criteria. *Antimicrob Agents Chemother* 2015;59(8):4759–4769.

132. Ullmann AJ, Sanz MA, Tramarin A, et al. Prospective study of amphotericin B formulations in immunocompromised patients in 4 European countries. *Clin Infect Dis* 2006;43(4):e29–e38.

133. Luber AD, Maa L, Lam M, et al. Risk factors for amphotericin B-induced nephrotoxicity. *J Antimicrob Chemother* 1999;43(2):267–271.

134. Fisher MA, Talbot GH, Maislin G, Mckeon BP, Tynan KP, Strom BL. Risk factors for amphotericin B-associated nephrotoxicity. *Am J Med* 1989;87(5):547–552.

135. Cornely OA, Maertens J, Bresnik M, et al. Liposomal amphotericin B as initial therapy for invasive mold infection: A randomized trial comparing a high-loading dose regimen with standard dosing (AmBiLoad trial). *Clin Infect Dis* 2007;44(10):1289–1297.

136. Harbarth S, Burke JP, Lloyd JF, Evans RS, Pestotnik SL, Samore MH. Clinical and economic outcomes of conventional amphotericin B-associated nephrotoxicity. *Clin Infect Dis* 2002;35(12):e120–e127.

137. Cagnoni PJ, Walsh TJ, Prendergast MM, et al. Pharmacoeconomic analysis of liposomal amphotericin B versus conventional amphotericin B in the empirical treatment of persistently febrile neutropenic patients. *J Clin Oncol* 2000;18(12):2476–2483.

138. Stein RS, Alexander JA. Sodium protects against nephrotoxicity in patients receiving amphotericin B. *Am J Med Sci* 1989;298(5):299–304.

139. Branch RA. Prevention of amphotericin B-induced renal impairment. A review on the use of sodium supplementation. *Arch Intern Med* 1988;148(11):2389–2394.

140. Bicanic T, Bottomley C, Loyse A, et al. Toxicity of amphotericin B deoxycholate-based induction therapy in patients with HIV-associated cryptococcal meningitis. *Antimicrob Agents Chemother* 2015;59(12):7224–7231.

141. Mayer J, Doubek M, Doubek J, et al. Reduced nephrotoxicity of conventional amphotericin B therapy after minimal nephroprotective measures: Animal experiments and clinical study. *J Infect Dis* 2002;186(3):379–388.

142. Eriksson U, Seifert B, Schaffner A, Eriksson U, Seifert B, Schaffner A. Comparison of effects of amphotericin B deoxycholate infused over 4 or 24 hours: Randomised controlled trial. *BMJ* 2001;322(7286):579–582.

143. Imhof A, Walter RB, Schaffner A. Continuous infusion of escalated doses of amphotericin B deoxycholate: An open-label observational study. *Clin Infect Dis* 2003;36(8):943–951.

144. Alexander BD, Wingard JR, Alexander BD, Wingard JR. Study of renal safety in amphotericin B lipid complex-treated patients. *Clin Infect Dis* 2005;40 Suppl 6:S414–S421.

145. Fleming RV, Kantarjian HM, Husni R, et al. Comparison of amphotericin B lipid complex (ABLC) vs. ambisome in the treatment of suspected or documented fungal infections in patients with leukemia. *Leuk Lymphoma* 2001;40(5–6):511–520.

146. Steimbach LM, Tonin FS, Virtuoso S, et al. Efficacy and safety of amphotericin B lipid-based formulations-A systematic review and meta-analysis. *Mycoses* 2017;60(3):146–154.

147. Falci DR, da Rosa FB, Pasqualotto AC. Hematological toxicities associated with amphotericin B formulations. *Leuk Lymphoma* 2015;56(10):2889–2894.

148. MacGregor RR, Bennett JE, Erslev AJ. Erythropoietin concentration in amphotericin B-induced anemia. *Antimicrob Agents Chemother* 1978;14(2):270–273.

149. Fischer MA, Winkelmayer WC, Rubin RH, Avorn J. The hepatotoxicity of antifungal medications in bone marrow transplant recipients. *Clin Infect Dis* 2005;41(3):301–307.

150. Wingard JR. Lipid formulations of amphotericins: Are you a lumper or a splitter? *Clin Infect Dis* 2002;35(7):891–895.

151. Rex JH, Bennett JE, Sugar AM, et al. A randomized trial comparing fluconazole with amphotericin B for the treatment of candidemia in patients without neutropenia. Candidemia Study Group and the National Institute of Health. *N Engl J Med* 1994;331(20):1325–1330.

152. Anaissie EJ, Darouiche RO, Abi-Said D, et al. Management of invasive candidal infections: Results of a prospective, randomized, multicenter study of fluconazole versus amphotericin B and review of the literature. *Clin Infect Dis* 1996;23(5):964–972.

153. Phillips P, Shafran S, Garber G, et al. Multicenter randomized trial of fluconazole versus amphotericin B for treatment of candidemia in non-neutropenic patients. Canadian Candidemia Study Group. *Eur J Clin Micro Infect Dis* 1997;16(5):337–345.

154. Zaoutis T, Walsh TJ. Antifungal therapy for neonatal candidiasis. *Curr Opin Infect Dis* 2007;20(6):592–597.

155. Filioti J, Spiroglou K, Panteliadis CP, Roilides E. Invasive candidiasis in pediatric intensive care patients: Epidemiology, risk factors, management, and outcome. *Intensive Care Med* 2007;33(7):1272–1283.

156. Kullberg BJ, Sobel JD, Ruhnke M, et al. Voriconazole versus a regimen of amphotericin B followed by fluconazole for candidaemia in non-neutropenic patients: A randomised non-inferiority trial. *Lancet* 2005;366(9495):1435–1442.

157. Walsh TJ, Hiemenz JW, Seibel NL, et al. Amphotericin B lipid complex for invasive fungal infections: Analysis of safety and efficacy in 556 cases. *Clin Infect Dis* 1998;26(6):1383–1396.

158. Ito JI, Hooshmand-Rad R. Treatment of *Candida* infections with amphotericin B lipid complex. *Clin Infect Dis* 2005;40:S384–S391.

159. Juster-Reicher A, Leibovitz E, Linder N, et al. Liposomal amphotericin B (AmBisome) in the treatment of neonatal candidiasis in very low birth weight infants. *Infection* 2000;28(4):223–226.

160. Juster-Reicher A, Flidel-Rimon O, Amitay M, Even-Tov S, Shinwell E, Leibovitz E. High-dose liposomal amphotericin B in the therapy of systemic candidiasis in neonates. *Eur J Clin Micro Infect Dis* 2003;22(10):603–607.

161. Rex JH, Pappas PG, Karchmer AW, et al. A randomized and blinded multicenter trial of high-dose fluconazole plus placebo versus fluconazole plus amphotericin B as therapy for candidemia and its consequences in nonneutropenic subjects. *Clin Infect Dis* 2003;36(10):1221–1228.

162. Ostrosky-Zeichner L, Pappas PG. Invasive candidiasis in the intensive care unit. *Crit Care Med* 2006;34(3):857–863.

163. Tiffany KF, Smith PB, Benjamin DK, Jr. Neonatal candidiasis: Prophylaxis and treatment. *Exp Opin Pharmacother* 2005;6(10):1647–1655.

164. Patterson TF, Kirkpatrick WR, White M, et al. Invasive aspergillosis - disease spectrum, treatment practices, and outcomes. *Medicine (Baltimore)* 2000;79(4):250–260.

165. Cordonnier C, Bresnik M, Ebrahimi R, Cordonnier C, Bresnik M, Ebrahimi R. Liposomal amphotericin B (AmBisome) efficacy in confirmed invasive aspergillosis and other filamentous fungal infections in immunocompromised hosts: A pooled analysis. *Mycoses* 2007;50(3):205–209.

166. Ellis M, Spence D, de Pauw B, et al. An EORTC international multicenter randomized trial (EORTC number 19923) comparing two dosages of liposomal amphotericin B for treatment of invasive aspergillosis. *Clin Infect Dis* 1998;27(6):1406–1412.

167. Ringden O, Meunier F, Tollemar J, et al. Efficacy of amphotericin B encapsulated in liposomes (AmBisome) in the treatment of invasive fungal infections in immunocompromised patients. *J Antimicrob Chemother* 1991;28 Suppl B:73–82.

168. Chandrasekar PH, Ito JI, Chandrasekar PH, Ito JI. Amphotericin B lipid complex in the management of invasive aspergillosis in immunocompromised patients. *Clin Infect Dis* 2005;40 Suppl 6:S392–S400.

169. Linden PK, Coley K, Fontes P, Fung JJ, Kusne S. Invasive aspergillosis in liver transplant recipients: Outcome comparison of therapy with amphotericin B lipid complex and a historical cohort treated with conventional amphotericin B. *Clin Infect Dis* 2003;37(1):17–25.

170. Herbrecht R, Denning DW, Patterson TF, et al. Voriconazole versus amphotericin B for primary therapy of invasive aspergillosis. *N Engl J Med* 2002;347(6):408–415.

171. Herbrecht R, Patterson TF, Slavin MA, et al. Application of the 2008 definitions for invasive fungal diseases to the trial comparing voriconazole versus amphotericin B for therapy of invasive aspergillosis: A collaborative study of the Mycoses Study Group (MSG 05) and the European Organization for Research and Treatment of Cancer Infectious Diseases Group. *Clin Infect Dis* 2015;60(5):713–720.

172. Nivoix Y, Velten M, Letscher-Bru V, et al. Factors associated with overall and attributable mortality in invasive aspergillosis. *Clin Infect Dis* 2008;47(9):1176–1184.

173. De Lalla F, Pellizzer G, Vaglia A, et al. Amphotericin B as primary therapy for cryptococcosis in patients with AIDS - reliability of relatively high doses administered over a relatively short period. *Clin Infect Dis* 1995;20(2):263–266.

174. Bennett JE, Dismukes WE, Duma RJ, et al. Comparison of amphotericin B alone and combined with flucytosine in the treatment of cryptoccal meningitis. *N Engl J Med* 1979;301(3):126–131.

175. Dismukes WE, Cloud G, Gallis HA, et al. Treatment of cryptococcal meningitis with combination amphotericin B and flucytosine for 4 as compared with 6 weeks. *N Engl J Med* 1987;317(6):334–341.

176. van der Horst CM, Saag MS, Cloud GA, et al. Treatment of cryptococcal meningitis associated with the acquired immunodeficiency syndrome. National Institute of Allergy and Infectious Diseases Mycoses Study Group and AIDS Clinical Trials Group. *N Engl J Med* 1997;337(1):15–21.

177. Saag MS, Powderly WG, Cloud GA, et al. Comparison of amphotericin B with fluconazole in the treatment of acute AIDS-associated cryptococcal meningitis. The NIAID Mycoses Study Group and the AIDS Clinical Trials Group. *N Engl J Med* 1992;326(2):83–89.

178. Powderly WG, Saag MS, Cloud GA, et al. A controlled trial of fluconazole or amphotericin B to prevent relapse of cryptococcal meningitis in patients with the acquired immunodeficiency syndrome. The NIAID AIDS Clinical Trials Group and Mycoses Study Group. *N Engl J Med* 1992;326(12):793–798.

179. Day JN, Chau TT, Wolbers M, et al. Combination antifungal therapy for cryptococcal meningitis. *N Engl J Med* 2013;368(14):1291–1302.

180. Loyse A, Wilson D, Meintjes G, et al. Comparison of the early fungicidal activity of high-dose fluconazole, voriconazole, and flucytosine as second-line drugs given in combination with amphotericin B for the treatment of HIV-associated cryptococcal meningitis. *Clin Infect Dis* 2012;54(1):121–128.

181. Bicanic T, Wood R, Meintjes G, et al. High-dose amphotericin B with flucytosine for the treatment of cryptococcal meningitis in HIV-infected patients: A randomized trial. *Clin Infect Dis* 2008;47(1):123–130.

182. Leenders AC, Reiss P, Portegies P, et al. Liposomal amphotericin B (AmBisome) compared with amphotericin B both followed by oral fluconazole in the treatment of AIDS-associated cryptococcal meningitis. *AIDS* 1997;11(12):1463–1471.

183. Baddour LM, Perfect JR, Ostrosky-Zeichner L. Successful use of amphotericin B lipid complex in the treatment of cryptococcosis. *Clin Infect Dis* 2005;40 Suppl 6:S409–S413.

184. Sharkey PK, Graybill JR, Johnson ES, et al. Amphotericin B lipid complex compared with amphotericin B in the treatment of cryptococcal meningitis in patients with AIDS. *Clin Infect Dis* 1996;22(2):315–321.

185. Singh N, Dromer F, Perfect JR, Lortholary O. Cryptococcosis in solid organ transplant recipients: Current state of the science. *Clin Infect Dis* 2008;47(10):1321–1327.

186. Almyroudis NG, Sutton DA, Linden P, et al. Zygomycosis in solid organ transplant recipients in a tertiary transplant center and review of the literature. *Am J Transplant* 2006;6(10):2365–2374.

187. Chayakulkeeree M, Ghannoum MA, Perfect JR. Zygomycosis: The re-emerging fungal infection. *Eur J Clin Micro Infect Dis* 2006;25(4):215–229.

188. Roden MM, Zaoutis TE, Buchanan WL, et al. Epidemiology and outcome of zygomycosis: A review of 929 reported cases. *Clin Infect Dis* 2005;41(5):634–653.

189. Perfect JR. Treatment of non-Aspergillus moulds in immunocompromised patients, with amphotericin B lipid complex. *Clin Infect Dis* 2005;40:S401–S408.

190. Wilson DT, Dimondi VP, Johnson SW, Jones TM, Drew RH. Role of isavuconazole in the treatment of invasive fungal infections. *Ther Clin Risk Manag* 2016;12:1197–1206.

191. Mishra M, Biswas UK, Jha AM, Khan AB. Amphotericin versus sodium stibogluconate in first-line treatment of Indian kala-azar. *Lancet* 1994;344(8937):1599–1600.

192. Dietze R, Milan EP, Berman JD, et al. Treatment of Brazilian kala-azar with a short-course of amphocil (amphotericin-B cholesterol dispersion). *Clin Infect Dis* 1993;17(6):981–986.

193. Sundar S, Agrawal NK, Sinha PR, Horwith GS, Murray HW. Short-course, low-dose amphotericin B lipid complex therapy for visceral leishmaniasis unresponsive to antimony. *Ann Intern Med* 1997;127(2):133–137.

194. Meyerhoff A. U.S. Food and Drug Administration approval of AmBisome (liposomal amphotericin B) for treatment of visceral leishmaniasis. *Clin Infect Dis* 1999;28(1):42–48.

195. Goswami RP, Goswami RP, Das S, Satpati A, Rahman M. Short-course treatment regimen of Indian visceral leishmaniasis with an Indian liposomal amphotericin B preparation (Fungisome™). *Am J Trop Med Hyg* 2016;94(1):93–98.

196. Sundar S, Agrawal G, Rai M, Makharia MK, Murray HW. Treatment of Indian visceral leishmaniasis with single or daily infusions of low dose liposomal amphotericin B: Randomised trial. *BMJ* 2001;323(7310):419–422.

197. Sundar S, Jha TK, Thakur CP, Mishra M, Singh VP, Buffels R. Single-dose liposomal amphotericin B in the treatment of visceral leishmaniasis in India: A multicenter study. *Clin Infect Dis* 2003;37(6):800–804.

198. Kauffman CA, Kauffman CA. Histoplasmosis: A clinical and laboratory update. *Clin Microbiol Rev* 2007;20(1):115–132.

199. Johnson PC, Wheat LJ, Cloud GA, et al. Safety and efficacy of liposomal amphotericin B compared with conventional amphotericin B for induction therapy of histoplasmosis in patients with AIDS. *Ann Intern Med* 2002;137(2):105–109.

200. Bradsher RW, Chapman SW, Pappas PG. Blastomycosis. *Infect Dis Clin North Am* 2003;17(1):21–28.

201. Anstead GM, Graybill JR, Anstead GM, Graybill JR. Coccidioidomycosis. *Infect Dis Clin North Am* 2006;20(3):621–643.

202. Al Obaid I, Ahmad S, Khan ZU, et al. Catheter-associated fungemia due to *Exophiala oligosperma* in a leukemic child and review of fungemia cases caused by *Exophiala* species. *Eur J Clin Micro Infect Dis* 2006;25(11):729–732.

203. Malani AN, Kauffman CA. Changing epidemiology of rare mould infections: Implications for therapy. *Drugs* 2007;67(13):1803–1812.

204. Pizzo PA, Robichaud KJ, Gill FA, Witebsky FG. Empiric antibiotic and antifungal therapy for cancer patients with frolonged fever and granulocytopenia. *Am J Med* 1982;72(1):101–111.

205. Meunier F. Empiric antifungal therapy in febrile granulocytopenic patients. *Am J Med* 1989;86(6):668–672.

206. Jorgensen KJ, Gotzsche PC, Johansen HK. Voriconazole versus amphotericin B in cancer patients with neutropenia. *Cochrane Database Syst Rev* 2006(1):CD004707.

207. Johansen HK, Gotzsche PC, Johansen HK, Gotzsche PC. Amphotericin B versus fluconazole for controlling fungal infections in neutropenic cancer patients. *Cochrane Database Syst Rev* 2002(2):CD000239.

208. Malik IA, Moid I, Aziz Z, et al. A randomized comparison of fluconazole with amphotericin B as empiric anti-fungal agents in cancer patients with prolonged fever and neutropenia. *Am J Med* 1998;105(6):478–483.

209. Prentice HG, Hann IM, Herbrecht R, et al. A randomized comparison of liposomal versus conventional amphotericin B for the treatment of pyrexia of unknown origin in neutropenic patients. *Br J Haematol* 1997;98(3):711–718.

210. Walsh TJ, Pappas P, Winston DJ, et al. Voriconazole compared with liposomal amphotericin B for empirical antifungal therapy in patients with neutropenia and persistent fever. *N Engl J Med* 2002;346(4):225–234.

211. Subira M, Martino R, Gomez L, Marti JM, Estany C, Sierra J. Low-dose amphotericin b lipid complex vs. conventional amphotericin B for empirical antifungal therapy of neutropenic fever in patients with hematologic malignancies - a randomized, controlled trial. *Eur J Haematol* 2004;72(5):342–347.

212. Johansen HK, Gotzsche PC. Amphotericin B versus fluconazole for controlling fungal infections in neutropenic cancer patients. *Cochrane Database Syst Rev* 2014(9):Cd000239.

213. Jorgensen KJ, Gotzsche PC, Dalboge CS, Johansen HK. Voriconazole versus amphotericin B or fluconazole in cancer patients with neutropenia. *Cochrane Database Syst Rev* 2014(2):Cd004707.

214. Klastersky J, de Naurois J, Rolston K, et al. Management of febrile neutropaenia: ESMO Clinical Practice Guidelines. *Annal Oncol* 2016;27(Suppl 5):v111–v118.

215. National Comprehensive Cancer Network. Prevention and Treatment of Cancer-Related Infections (version 1.2017, December 21, 2016). Available 2016; https://www.nccn.org/professionals/physician_gls/pdf/infections.pdf.

216. Drew R. Polyenes for prevention of invasive fungal infections. *Infect Med* 2006;23(10S):12–24.

217. Austin NC, Darlow B, Austin NC, Darlow B. Prophylactic oral antifungal agents to prevent systemic *Candida* infection in preterm infants. *Cochrane Database Syst Rev* 2004(1):CD003478.

218. Gotzsche PC, Johansen HK. Nystatin prophylaxis and treatment in severely immunodepressed patients. *Cochrane Database Syst Rev* 2002(2):CD002033.

219. Lumbreras C, Cuervas-Mons V, Jara P, et al. Randomized trial of fluconazole versus nystatin for the prophylaxis of *Candida* infection following liver transplantation. *J Infect Dis* 1996;174(3):583–588.

220. Johansen HK, Gotzsche PC. Amphotericin B lipid soluble formulations vs. amphotericin B in cancer patients with neutropenia. *Cochrane Database Syst Rev* 2000(3):CD000969.

221. Kelsey SM, Goldman JM, McCann S, et al. Liposomal amphotericin (AmBisome) in the prophylaxis of fungal infections in neutropenic patients: A randomised, double-blind, placebo-controlled study. *Bone Marrow Transplant* 1999;23(2):163–168.

222. Mattiuzzi GN, Estey E, Raad I, et al. Liposomal amphotericin B versus the combination of fluconazole and itraconazole as prophylaxis for invasive fungal infections during induction chemotherapy for patients with acute myelogenous leukemia and myelodysplastic syndrome. *Cancer* 2003;97(2):450–456.

223. Mattiuzzi GN, Kantarjian H, Faderl S, et al. Amphotericin B lipid complex as prophylaxis of invasive fungal infections in patients with acute myelogenous leukemia and myelodysplastic syndrome undergoing induction chemotherapy. *Cancer* 2004;100(3):581–589.

224. Tollemar J, Hockerstedt K, Ericzon BG, Sundberg B, Ringden O. Fungal prophylaxis with AmBisome in liver and bone marrow transplant recipients: Results of two randomized double-blind studies. *Transplant Proc* 1994;26(3):1833.

225. Riley DK, Pavia AT, Beatty PG, et al. The prophylactic use of low-dose amphotericin B in bone marrow transplant patients. *Am J Med* 1994;97(6):509–514.

226. Perfect JR, Klotman ME, Gilbert CC, et al. Prophylactic intravenous amphotericin B in neutropenic autologous bone marrow transplant recipients. *J Infect Dis* 1992;165(5):891–897.

227. Wolff SN, Fay J, Stevens D, et al. Fluconazole vs. low-dose amphotericin B for the prevention of fungal infections in patients undergoing bone marrow transplantation: A study of the North American Marrow Transplant Group. *Bone Marrow Transplant* 2000;25(8):853–859.

228. Koh LP, Kurup A, Goh YT, Fook-Chong SM, Tan PH. Randomized trial of fluconazole versus low-dose amphotericin B in prophylaxis against fungal infections in patients undergoing hematopoietic stem cell transplantation. *Am J Hematol* 2002;71(4):260–267.

229. Tollemar J, Ringden O, Andersson S, Sundberg B, Ljungman P, Tyden G. Randomized double-blind study of liposomal amphotericin B (Ambisome) prophylaxis of invasive fungal infections in bone marrow transplant recipients. *Bone Marrow Transplant* 1993;12(6):577–582.

230. Fortun J, Martin-Davila P, Moreno S, et al. Prevention of invasive fungal infections in liver transplant recipients: The role of prophylaxis with lipid formulations of amphotericin B in high-risk patients. *J Antimicrob Chemother* 2003;52(5):813–819.

231. (anon). Fungal infections. *Am J Transplant* 2004;4(s10):110–134.

232. Tollemar J, Hockerstedt K, Ericzon BG, Jalanko H, Ringden O. Prophylaxis with liposomal amphotericin B (AmBisome) prevents fungal infections in liver transplant recipients: Long-term results of a randomized, placebo-controlled trial. *Transplant Proc* 1995;27(1):1195–1198.

233. Biancofiore G, Bindi ML, Baldassarri R, et al. Antifungal prophylaxis in liver transplant recipients: A randomized placebo-controlled study. *Transpl Int* 2002;15(7):341–347.

234. Playford EG, Webster AC, Sorell TC, Craig JC. Antifungal agents for preventing fungal infections in solid organ transplant recipients. *Cochrane Database Syst Rev* 2004;(3):Cd004291.

235. Shah T, Lai WK, Gow P, et al. Low-dose amphotericin for prevention of serious fungal infection following liver transplantation. *Transpl Infect Dis* 2005;7(3–4):126–132.

236. Giannella M, Ercolani G, Cristini F, et al. High-dose weekly liposomal amphotericin b antifungal prophylaxis in patients undergoing liver transplantation: A prospective phase II trial. *Transplantation* 2015;99(4):848–854.

237. (anon). Guidelines for Prevention and Treatment of Opportunistic Infections in HIV-Infected Adults and Adolescents. *Recommendations of the National Institutes of Health (NIH), the Centers for Disease Control and Prevention (CDC), and the HIV Medicine Association of the Infectious Diseases Society of America (HIVMA/IDSA) Available at http://AIDSinfo nih gov* 2008.

238. Drew R. Potential role of aerosolized amphotericin B formulations in the prevention and adjunctive treatment of invasive fungal infections. *Int J Antimicrob Agents* 2006;27 Suppl 1:36–44.

239. Behre GF, Schwartz S, Lenz K, et al. Aerosol amphotericin B inhalations for prevention of invasive pulmonary aspergillosis in neutropenic cancer patients. *Ann Hematol* 1995;71(6):287–291.

240. Conneally E, Cafferkey M, Daly P, Keane C, McCann S. Nebulized amphotericin B as prophylaxis against invasive aspergillosis in granulocytopenic patients. *Bone Marrow Transplant* 1990;5(6):403–406.

241. Erjavec Z, Woolthuis G, Vries-Hospers H, et al. Tolerance and efficacy of Amphotericin B inhalations for prevention of invasive pulmonary aspergillosis in haematological patients. *Eur J Clin Microbiol* 1997;16(5):364–368.

242. Schwartz S, Behre G, Heinemann V, et al. Aerosolized amphotericin B inhalations as prophylaxis of invasive *Aspergillus* infections during prolonged neutropenia: Results of a prospective randomized multicenter trial. *Blood* 1999;93(11):3654–3661.

243. Drew RH, Dodds AE, Benjamin DK, Jr., Duane DR, Palmer SM, Perfect JR. Comparative safety of amphotericin B lipid complex and amphotericin B deoxycholate as aerosolized antifungal prophylaxis in lung-transplant recipients. *Transplantation* 2004;77(2):232–237.

244. Palmer S, Drew R, Whitehouse J, et al. Safety of aerosolized amphotericin B lipid complex in lung transplant recipients. *Transplantation* 2001;72(3):545–548.

245. Calvo V, Borro J, Morales P, et al. Antifungal prophylaxis during the early postoperative period of lung transplantation. Valencia Lung Transplant Group. *Chest* 1999;115(5):1301–1304.

246. Reichenspurner H, Gamberg P, Nitschke M, et al. Significant reduction in the number of fungal infections after lung-, heart-lung, and heart transplantation using aerosolized amphotericin B prophylaxis. *Transplant Proc* 1997;29(1–2):627–628.

247. Allen SD, Sorensen KN, Nejdl MJ, Durrant C, Proffit RT. Prophylactic efficacy of aerosolized liposomal (AmBisome) and non-liposomal (Fungizone) amphotericin B in murine pulmonary aspergillosis. *J Antimicrob Chemother* 1994;34(6):1001–1013.

248. Allen SD, Sorensen KN, Nejdl MJ, Proffitt RT. Efficacy of aerosolized liposomal amphotericin b (Ambisome) as a prophylactic treatment in an immune compromised murine model of pulmonary aspergillosis. *J Control Release* 1994;28(1–3):348–349.

249. Cicogna CE, White MH, Bernard EM, et al. Efficacy of prophylactic aerosol amphotericin B lipid complex in a rat model of pulmonary aspergillosis. *Antimicrob Agents Chemother* 1997;41(2):259–261.

250. Ruijgrok EJ, Vulto AG, Van Etten EW. Efficacy of aerosolized amphotericin B desoxycholate and liposomal amphotericin B in the treatment of invasive pulmonary aspergillosis in severely immunocompromised rats. *J Antimicrob Chemother* 2001;48(1):89–95.

251. Vyas SP, Quraishi S, Gupta S, Jaganathan KS. Aerosolized liposome-based delivery of amphotericin B to alveolar macrophages. *Int J Pharm* 2005;296(1–2):12–25.

252. Perfect JR, Dodds AE, Drew R. Design of aerosolized amphotericin b formulations for prophylaxis trials among lung transplant recipients. *Clin Infect Dis* 2004;39 Suppl 4:S207–S210.

253. Peghin M, Monforte V, Martin-Gomez MT, et al. 10 years of prophylaxis with nebulized liposomal amphotericin B and the changing epidemiology of *Aspergillus* spp. infection in lung transplantation. *Transpl Int* 2016;29(1):51–62.

254. Xia D, Sun WK, Tan MM, et al. Aerosolized amphotericin B as prophylaxis for invasive pulmonary aspergillosis: A meta-analysis. *Int J Infect Dis* 2015;30:78–84.

255. Hope WW, Goodwin J, Felton TW, Ellis M, Stevens DA. Population pharmacokinetics of conventional and intermittent dosing of liposomal amphotericin B in adults: A first critical step for rational design of innovative regimens. *Antimicrob Agents Chemother* 2012;56(10):5303–5308.

256. Lanternier F, Poiree S, Elie C, et al. Prospective pilot study of high-dose (10 mg/kg/day) liposomal amphotericin B (L-AMB) for the initial treatment of mucormycosis. *J Antimicrob Chemother* 2015;70(11):3116–3123.

257. Annino L, Chierichini A, Anaclerico B, et al. Prospective phase II single-center study of the safety of a single very high dose of liposomal amphotericin B for antifungal prophylaxis in patients with acute myeloid leukemia. *Antimicrob Agents Chemother* 2013;57(6):2596–2602.

258. Chaftari AM, Hachem RY, Ramos E, et al. Comparison of posaconazole versus weekly amphotericin B lipid complex for the prevention of invasive fungal infections in hematopoietic stem-cell transplantation. *Transplantation* 2012;94(3):302–308.

259. Bindschadler D, Bennett J. A pharmacologic guide to the clinical use of amphotericin B. *J Infect Dis* 1969;120(4):427–436.

260. Nagata MP, Gentry CA, Hampton EM, Nagata MP, Gentry CA, Hampton EM. Is there a therapeutic or pharmacokinetic rationale for amphotericin B dosing in systemic *Candida* infections? *Ann Pharmacother* 1996;30(7–8):811–818.

261. Tynes BS, Utz JP, Bennett JE, Alling DW. Reducing amphotericin B reactions - a double-blind study. *Am Rev Respir Dis* 1963;87(2):264–8.

262. Burks LC, Aisner J, Fortner CL, Wiernik PH. Meperidine for the treatment of shaking chills and fever. *Arch Intern Med* 1980;140(4):483–484.

263. Anderson CM. Sodium chloride treatment of amphotericin B nephrotoxicity. Standard of care? *West J Med* 1995;162(4):313–317.

264. Moreau P, Milpied N, Fayette N, Ramee JF, Harousseau JL. Reduced renal toxicity and improved clinical tolerance of amphotericin B mixed with intralipid compared with conventional amphotericin B in neutropenic patients. *J Antimicrob Chemother* 1992;30(4):535–541.

265. Petit N, Parola P, Dhiver C, Gastaut JA. Efficacy and tolerance of amphotericin B in a lipid emulsion in the treatment of visceral leishmaniasis in AIDS patients. *J Antimicrob Chemother* 1996;38(1):154–157.

266. Egito ES, Araujo IB, Damasceno BP, et al. Amphotericin B/emulsion admixture interactions: An approach concerning the reduction of amphotericin B toxicity. *J Pharm Sci* 2002;91(11):2354–2366.

267. Nucci M, Loureiro M, Silveira F, et al. Comparison of the toxicity of amphotericin B in 5% dextrose with that of amphotericin B in fat emulsion in a randomized trial with cancer patients. *Antimicrob Agents Chemother* 1999;43(6):1445–1448.

268. Sorkine P, Nagar H, Weinbroum A, et al. Administration of amphotericin B in lipid emulsion decreases nephrotoxicity: Results of a prospective, randomized, controlled study in critically ill patients. *Crit Care Med* 1996;24(8):1311–1315.

269. Herbrecht R, Letscher V, Andres E, Cavalier A. Safety and efficacy of amphotericin B colloidal dispersion. An overview. *Chemother* 1999;45 Suppl 1:67–76.

270. Karimzadeh I, Khalili H, Sagheb MM, Farsaei S. A double-blinded, placebo-controlled, multicenter clinical trial of N-acetylcysteine for preventing amphotericin B-induced nephrotoxicity. *Expert Opin Drug Metab Toxicol* 2015;11(9):1345–1355.

271. Karimzadeh I, Khalili H, Dashti-Khavidaki S, et al. N-acetyl cysteine in prevention of amphotericin-induced electrolytes imbalances: A randomized, double-blinded, placebo-controlled, clinical trial. *Eur J Clin Pharmacol* 2014;70(4):399–408.

272. Gales MA, Gales BJ. Rapid infusion of amphotericin B in dextrose. *Ann Pharmacother* 1995;29(5):523–529.

273. Peleg AY, Woods ML. Continuous and 4h infusion of amphotericin B: A comparative study involving high-risk haematology patients. *J Antimicrob Chemother* 2004;54(4):803–808.

274. de Rosa FG, Bargiacchi O, Audagnotto S, Garazzino S, Ranieri VM, di Perri G. Continuous infusion of amphotericin B deoxycholate: Does decreased nephrotoxicity couple with time-dependent pharmacodynamics? *Leuk Lymphoma* 2006;47(9):1964–1966.

275. Bearden DT, Muncey LA, Bearden DT, Muncey LA. The effect of amiloride on amphotericin B-induced hypokalaemia. *J Antimicrob Chemother* 2001;48(1):109–111.

276. Goldman RD, Koren G. Amphotericin B nephrotoxicity in children. *J Ped Hematol Oncol* 2004;26(7):421–426.

277. Wazny LD, Brophy DF. Amiloride for the prevention of amphotericin B-induced hypokalemia and hypomagnesemia. *Ann Pharmacother* 2000;34(1):94–97.

278. Ural AU, Avcu F, Cetin T, et al. Spironolactone: Is it a novel drug for the prevention of amphotericin B-related hypokalemia in cancer patients? *Eur J Clin Pharmacol* 2002;57(11):771–773.

279. Groll AH, Silling G, Young C, et al. Randomized comparison of safety and pharmacokinetics of caspofungin, liposomal amphotericin B, and the combination of both in allogeneic hematopoietic stem cell recipients. *Antimicrob Agents Chemother* 2010;54(10):4143–4149.

280. Siopi M, Siafakas N, Vourli S, Zerva L, Meletiadis J. Optimization of polyene-azole combination therapy against aspergillosis using an *in vitro* pharmacokinetic-pharmacodynamic model. *Antimicrob Agents Chemother* 2015;59(7):3973–3983.

281. Undre NA, Stevenson P, Wilbraham D. Pharmacokinetic profile of micafungin when co-administered with amphotericin B in healthy male subjects. *Int J Clin Pharmacol Ther* 2014;52(3):237–244.

282. Adler-Moore JP, Proffitt RT. Amphotericin B lipid preparations: What are the differences? *Clin Microbiol Infect* 2008;14 Suppl 4:25–36.

283. Barrett JP, Vardulaki KA, Conlon C, et al. A systematic review of the antifungal effectiveness and tolerability of amphotericin B formulations. *Clin Ther* 2003;25(5):1295–1320.

284. Bates DW, Su L, Yu DT, et al. Correlates of acute renal failure in patients receiving parenteral amphotericin B. *Kidney Int* 2001;60(4):1452–1459.

285. Goldstein EJC, Ho J, Fowler P, Heidari A, Johnson RH. Intrathecal amphotericin B: A 60-year experience in treating coccidioidal meningitis. *Clin Infect Dis* 2017;64(4):519–524.

Flucytosine

RICHARD H. DREW

OVERVIEW

Originally developed as a treatment for leukemia, flucytosine (5-fluorocytosine, 5FC) is an antifungal with restricted use in present-day therapy. Use as a monotherapy is significantly limited by concerns for both primary and secondary resistance, and is restricted for systemic use in modern-day therapy to the use in select cases of *Candida cystitis/pyelonephritis* [1]. In contrast, combination therapy of flucytosine with amphotericin B has been proven to improve treatment outcomes in patients with cryptococcal meningitis when used as the initial part of therapy [2–7]. Its role in combination with azole antifungals for the treatment of disseminated cryptococcal infections is less clear [7]. Combination therapy (usually with amphotericin B) is also used in select cases of invasive *Candida* infections [1]. In addition to concerns regarding resistance, flucytosine use is also limited by its toxicities (primarily hematologic), lack of a parenteral preparation in the United States (US), limited availability worldwide, and cost. Serum concentration monitoring and dose adjustment in patients with renal insufficiency should be employed in an attempt to achieve target serum concentrations while reducing the potential for serum concentration-related side effects.

MECHANISM OF ACTION

Flucytosine penetrates the fungal cell wall with the aid of cytosine permease [8] and is then deaminated to 5-fluorouracil (5-FU) by cytosine deaminase [9] (an enzyme absent in mammalian cells). Fluorouracil then incorporates into fungal RNA (in place of uracil), interrupting protein synthesis [10,11]. The 5-FU is then converted to 5-fluorodeoxyuridylic acid monophosphate, a noncompetitive inhibitor of thymidylate synthetase, which interferes with DNA synthesis [12–14]. Depending upon test conditions and organism, the resulting antifungal activity may be either fungistatic or fungicidal [15].

Post-antifungal effect (PAFE) exhibited by flucytosine *in vitro* is dependent on organism, concentration and test conditions [16,17]. Against *C. albicans*, PAFEs ranged from 0 to 4.2 hours after a 0.5-hour exposure and extended beyond 10 hours after the exposure was increased to 1–2 hours [17]. When concentrations exceeded the MIC by fourfold, the rate and extent of fungistatic activity was limited [17]. Similar findings have been reported in other *Candida* spp. and *Cryptococcus neoformans*, with PAFEs ranging from 0.8 to 7.4 hours and 2.4 to 5.4 hours, respectively [18]. Prolongation of PAFE has been observed against *C. albicans* with the combination therapy of flucytosine with either fluconazole [19–21] or amphotericin B [22].

The effects of flucytosine on immunity have been investigated using both *in vitro* and animal models. In a guinea pig model, flucytosine had no effect on cellular immunity [23,24]. Exposure of *C. albicans* to amphotericin B and flucytosine significantly enhanced neutrophils killing [25]. Combination with immunoglobulin therapy (i.e., an IgG1 monoclonal antibody to *C. neoformans* capsular glucuronoxylomannan) has also been investigated *in vitro* and in a murine animal model of cryptococcal infection.

The combination was found to be more effective than agent alone in reducing the numbers of *C. neoformans* colony-forming units (CFUs) [26]. The clinical relevance of these findings, however, is unknown.

RESISTANCE

Flucytosine resistance (both innate and acquired) may be due to several mechanisms, including alterations in cytosine permease, cytosine deaminase, and uracil phosphoribosyl transferase [8,13,14,27–30]. The exact mechanism may depend upon the isolate. For example, use of cytosine as a nitrogen source has been proposed as a mechanism of resistance in *Aspergillus* spp. [14]. In contrast, *C. albicans* isolates have demonstrated both decreased uridylic acid monophosphate (UMPP) activity and decreased cytosine deaminase activity [28].

The genetic basis of susceptibility to flucytosine has been described in *C. albicans* [28,31]. While isolates possessing heterozygous resistance traits (FCY1 and FCY2) exhibit minimal elevations in minimum inhibitory concentrations (MICs), they may occur at a significant frequency among clinical strains. It has been proposed that single-step mutation promoted by drug exposure selects for homozygous isolates, resulting in significant elevations in MIC that contribute to treatment failure [28]. However, high-level resistance has also been reported in isolates with heterozygous resistance [31].

PHARMACODYNAMICS

Pharmacodynamic studies with flucytosine are lacking in humans [32]. However, animal models have investigated the pharmacodynamic parameters that best correlate to the outcome. For example, in a neutropenic murine model of invasive candidiasis, concentration-independent killing was observed [33]. A dose-dependent suppression of growth was reported, and regrowth occurred after serum concentration fell below the MIC. Increasing dosing intervals resulted in increases in the dose necessary for fungistatic activity. Based on existing animal models for invasive candidiasis, a time above MIC best predicted outcome, with maximal efficacy observed when concentrations exceeded the MIC for approximately 40% of the dosing interval [33,34]. In contrast to these findings, AUC/MIC was the pharmacodynamic parameter best correlated with survival in a nonneutropenic mouse model of aspergillosis [35].

SPECTRUM OF ACTIVITY

Results of *in vitro* susceptibility testing of flucytosine vary with culture media, serum, pH, buffering agents, inoculum, temperature, and incubation time [36–43]. As a result, significant interlaboratory variability has been reported [38]. Standards have been approved by the Committee for Laboratory Standards Institute (CLSI) using macrodilution broth techniques [44,45]. E-testing of yeasts for flucytosine susceptibility has also received FDA approval. Minimum inhibitory concentrations (MICs) of <4 μg/mL,

8.0–16 μg/mL, and >32 μg/mL for *Candida* spp. are considered susceptible, intermediate, and resistant (respectively).

Most common clinical isolates of *Candida* spp. (with the exception of *C. krusei*) are considered susceptible to flucytosine *in vitro* [46,47]. In one report, only 3% of 5,208 isolates of *C. albicans* were reported as resistant [48]. However, results are dependent on geographic location, serotype, and species [49]. Serotype B is much less susceptible to flucytosine [49]. *C. glabrata* is also highly susceptible *in vitro* to flucytosine [48,50,51], with 99% of 1267 isolates susceptible in one report [48]. For 27 clinical isolates of *C. lusitaniae*, the MIC$_{90}$ reported in one study was <0.125 μg/mL [52], while others reported that 93% susceptible at breakpoints <4 μg/mL [48]. In contrast, the MIC$_{50}$ and MIC$_{90}$ for *C. krusei* to flucytosine were reported to be 16 and 32 μg/mL, respectively [48,53]. Therefore, only 5% of the isolates were considered susceptible according to CLSI breakpoints [48]. Similar findings have been reported by other investigators [54,55].

The *in vitro* activity of flucytosine against *Cryptococcus* spp. varies significantly between reports. Primary resistance rates have reported to range between 1 and 24.5% of *C. neoformans* isolates [41,56–58]. The influence of serotypes on susceptibility, however, is less clear. Lower susceptibilities in B/C serotypes in one report [57] were not observed by others [59]. Higher MICs have been observed in non-*neoformans* strains of *Cryptococcus* [60].

In vitro susceptibilities of flucytosine have been reported for pathogens causing chromomycoses. *Cladosporium* spp. and *Phialophora* spp. appear sensitive [61,62]. For 31 isolates of *Saccharomyces cerevisiae*, an MIC$_{90}$ of 0.2 μg/mL was reported [63]. Dimorphic fungi (i.e., *Blastomyces dermatitidis, Paracoccidioides brasiliensis, Sporothrix schenckii, Histoplasma capsulatum,* and *Coccidioides immitis*) and most dermatophytes are also considered resistant [41]. Flucytosine also lacks significant activity *in vitro* against *Fusarium* [64], zygomycetes [65–68], and *Aspergillus* spp. [37].

In vitro evaluation of antifungal combinations is complex, and standards for methodology and interpretation of results are generally lacking [69–73]. When tested in combination with amphotericin B against *Candida* spp., some form of positive interaction was reported in 35 of 40 (85%) of isolates [74]. Synergy with amphotericin B may be more common in flucytosine-sensitive organisms [75]. However, antagonism of amphotericin B with flucytosine for *Candida* spp. is infrequent. Against cryptococcal isolates, conflicting data has been reported with *in vitro* combinations of flucytosine and amphotericin B. Synergistic, additive, neutral, or antagonistic effects have all been reported with this combination [70,76,77]. As was seen is *Candida* spp., pre-treatment sensitivity to flucytosine may influence such results, since flucytosine-sensitive isolates more frequently demonstrate at least additive effects [75]. In contrast, antagonism was more common in isolates resistant to flucytosine. There are extensive studies with flucytosine and fluconazole against *Cryptococcus neoformans* [78–82]. In combination with fluconazole against *Cryptococcus* spp., synergy was observed in 62% of the 50 clinical strains isolated, while no antagonism was observed [78]. In the presence of fluconazole, flucytosine MICs for cryptococcal isolates were markedly reduced. However, flucytosine did not improve the *in vitro* activity of fluconazole against fluconazole-resistant isolates. Itraconazole in combination with flucytosine has also been studied against *C. neoformans*, and synergistic (63%) and additive (31%) effects were reported [83]. Finally, amphotericin B and flucytosine combinations against *Aspergillus* spp. have resulted in additive [84] or indifferent [85,86] activity.

PHARMACOKINETICS

Flucytosine is highly absorbed after oral administration (approximately 80%–90%), with peak serum concentrations (C_{max}) of 30–45 µg/mL 1–2 hours after a single 150 mg/kg dose [87,88]. A significant increase in serum concentrations of flucytosine was noted in one report when the drug was administered in a lipophilic vehicle [89]. In contrast, reductions in serum concentrations after oral administration have been reported in a pediatric patient with Schwachmann syndrome [89] and in patients with advanced HIV infection [90]. Intraperitoneal administration may also result in significant systemic absorption [91–93].

The protein binding of flucytosine is low (approximately 4%) [94]. As a result, it is widely distributed in body water, with a volume of distribution ranging between 0.6 and 0.9 L/kg [94,95]. Flucytosine penetrates highly into bone [96], vertebral disks [96], and synovial fluid [97,98]. Based on a rabbit model, flucytosine also achieves high concentrations in both the vitreous and aqueous humor [99,100]. Concentrations in spleen, heart, liver, kidney, and lung also have been reported to be comparable to simultaneous serum concentrations [94]. Concentrations in the cerebrospinal fluid (CSF) are approximately 80% of simultaneous serum concentrations [101,102] Significant peritoneal fluid concentrations have been reported following oral administration [103]. In patients with chronic respiratory disease, mean peak concentrations in bronchial secretions of 7.76 ± 7 µg/mL were reported following a single 25-mg/kg intravenous dose [104]. Serum and bronchoalveolar lavage (BAL) fluid concentrations ranged from <0.2 to 9.3 µg/mL and <0.4 to 1.5 µg/mL, respectively, after oral administration of 4.5–6.0 g/day [105]. Concentrations of flucytosine in the urine generally exceed that of serum by severalfold [87]. It may also cross the placental barrier, with one report in amniotic fluid of 168 µg/mL 4 hours after a 2 gm dose [106].

As much as 96% of the total flucytosine dose may be eliminated as unchanged drug [107]. For the small metabolized fraction, several metabolites have been reported. Intestinal microflora may deaminate flucytosine to 5-fluorouracil (5-FU) [12,14,108–110]. Deamination to 5-FU may be influenced by either chronic flucytosine exposure [108] or by use of broad-spectrum antibacterials [109]. Other metabolites include 5-fluorodeoxyuridine monophosphate (5-FC-UMP) and fluor-oorotic acid [14]. Fluoro-p-alanine (FBAL), 5-hydroxy-5-fluorocytosine, 0-2P-glucuronide, 6-hydroxy-5-fluorocytosine (60HFC), and fluoride ion (F-) have been reported in urine [107,111,112]. Flucytosine undergoes a high degree of renal elimination, with 60%–95% of the dose eliminated by glomerular filtration [87,107,113]. The serum half-life in patients with normal renal function ranges between 3 and 8 hours [87,114] and may be prolonged (i.e., 60–250 hours) in patients with significant renal disease [87,114].

There are limited pharmacokinetic data for flucytosine in patients undergoing concomitant dialysis. Intermittent hemodialysis may remove a significant quantity of flucytosine [115]. A dialysate clearance ratio of approximately 70% has been reported [115,116]. Peritoneal dialysis may also enhance flucytosine elimination [92,117]. Limited data also exist for patients receiving flucytosine and undergoing concomitant continuous hemofiltration [95,118,119]. Serum half-lives ranging between 15.9 and 37.2 hours following an intravenous dose of 2.5 gm have been reported [95]. Removal may vary with ultrafiltration flow rate, serum concentration, and hemofilter type [95,118,119]. Mean clearance of 77.0% ± 15.6% (SD) and 51.0% ± 5.7% (SD) of the ultrafiltrate flow rate were observed with polysulfone and polyacrylonitrile membranes, respectively [118]. Therefore, continuous hemofiltration can remove an appreciable quantity of flucytosine.

Pharmacokinetic data for flucytosine in children are also sparse [120–122]. In one report, 13 neonates (mean birth weight 1.2 ± 0.8 kg) underwent serum concentration monitoring following the first dose and after 5 days flucytosine 25–100 mg/kg/day) [120]. Extreme interindividual variability for half-life, volume of distribution, and clearance was reported. Peak serum concentrations comparable to those reported in adults despite a two-fold increase in half-life (up to 35 hours). Serum concentrations are often excessive in newborns. A retrospective study of 391 pediatric patients reported that, in children 1–30 days, 65% of flucytosine trough concentrations exceeded the target range [121]. Therefore, dose reductions in children appear warranted [122].

Published data for the pharmacokinetics of flucytosine in patients with obesity is limited to a single case report [123]. A morbidly obese female receiving 2500 mg orally 4 times/day. When ideal body weight (IBW) was employed for the pharmacokinetic estimates, both the volume of distribution and drug clearance were comparable to population estimates previously published. However, it is presently unknown whether IBW or an adjusted body weight should be utilized in this patient population for life-threatening infections until further data can be obtained in this patient population.

ADVERSE EVENTS

Hematologic, gastrointestinal, and hepatic toxicities are considered the most frequent and clinically-relevant side effects of flucytosine [124]. Conversion of flucytosine to 5-fluorouracil *in vivo* is thought to be responsible for most toxicities [108,125]. The incidence of reactions directly attributable to flucytosine is often difficult to quantify because of the underlying infection, comorbidities, and concomitant therapies of patients receiving flucytosine.

The hematologic toxicity resulting from flucytosine may be treatment-limiting, especially in patients at increased risk. Leukopenia and thrombocytopenia are thought to occur more frequently in patients with serum flucytosine concentrations exceeding 100 µg/mL [5,124,126–128]. In patients receiving concomitant amphotericin B, neutropenia was more common in one study [129] but not in others [130]. Rarely, bone marrow aplasia thought due to flucytosine has been reported [131,132]. Hematologic effects are especially common in patients with advanced HIV infection receiving high doses (i.e., up to 150 mg/kg/day) [82,133].

Gastrointestinal complaints (most commonly nausea, vomiting and diarrhea) may result from flucytosine therapy. However, the relationship between such events and serum concentrations is not clear [124]. Hepatotoxicity (including hepatic necrosis) may result from flucytosine administration [134–137]. In one report, approximately 5% of patients receiving flucytosine experienced elevations in hepatic transaminases and/or alkaline phosphatase [41].

Less frequent side effects associated with flucytosine include photosensitivity reaction [138], anaphylaxis [139], and CNS abnormalities (such as headache, drowsiness, vertigo, confusion, and hallucinations). Flucytosine is generally not considered nephrotoxic [140]. Early reports of nephrotoxicity were likely due to interference with selected laboratory methods used to determine serum creatinine [141] or to the concomitant administration of nephrotoxic agents.

CLINICAL APPLICATIONS

Cryptococcus

Current clinical trials with flucytosine for serious cryptococcal infections utilize combination therapy, and in most settings with amphotericin B [7]. Therefore, published clinical experience with flucytosine monotherapy of cryptococcosis is limited. While the failure rate in 27 patients with invasive infection was 57%, it was not associated with drug resistance in most cases [142]. Flucytosine monotherapy has also been reported for the treatment of pulmonary cryptococcosis [143,144].

Flucytosine treatment of cryptococcal infections in humans is best studied in the treatment of central nervous system (CNS) infections. Amphotericin B (0.3 mg/kg/day) plus flucytosine (150 mg/kg/day) was compared with monotherapy with amphotericin B (0.4 mg/kg/day) for cryptococcal meningitis in patients without AIDS [2]. Combination therapy for 6 weeks reduced the time to CSF sterilization, had similar efficacy and fewer failures/relapses and less nephrotoxicity than amphotericin B monotherapy administered for 10 weeks.

While retrospective evaluations of patients with AIDS and cryptococcal meningitis failed to detect a survival benefit of combination therapy over monotherapy [133],

prospective studies in this population were subsequently performed in this patient population [3]. Amphotericin B (0.7 mg/kg/day) with or without flucytosine (100 mg/kg/day) for 2 weeks was followed by either itraconazole or fluconazole therapy for 8 weeks in a randomized trial [3]. At 2 weeks, 51% and 60% of patients had sterile CSF cultures receiving monotherapy and combination therapy, respectively. While clinical outcomes were similar between treatment groups, addition of flucytosine was associated with improved rates of sterilization at 2 weeks. Subsequent investigations comparing maintenance therapy with either fluconazole or itraconazole in this population detected an increased risk of relapse in patients not receiving initial therapy with flucytosine (relative risk = 5.88; 95% confidence interval, 1.27–27.14; p = 0.04) [6]. Further supporting data for the combination comes from a small randomized comparative study comparing initial combination therapy with amphotericin B 0.7 mg/kg/day plus flucytosine 150 mg/kg/day to oral fluconazole (400 mg/day) [4]. In contrast to the 57% of the 14 patients who failed fluconazole therapy, none of the 6 patients receiving the combination regimen failed. Similar to previous studies, a shorter time to negative CSF cultures (15.6 ± 6.6 days) was observed in the combination therapy group. Similar observations were made when the combination was compared to itraconazole [145]. Most recently, an open-label trial in patients with HIV and cryptococcal meningitis were randomized to receive amphotericin 1 mg/kg/day × 4 weeks, amphotericin 1 mg/kg/day × 2 weeks + flucytosine 100 mg/kg/d × 2 weeks, or amphotericin 1 mg/kg/day × 2 weeks + fluconazole 400 mg twice daily × 2 weeks [129]. Amphotericin B plus flucytosine was associated with significantly increased rates of yeast clearance from cerebrospinal fluid and improved survival relative to amphotericin B monotherapy. A similar survival benefit was not demonstrated in the fluconazole combination arm.

Recent studies of HIV-associated cryptococcal meningitis have begun to question the role of flucytosine in the treatment of this infection, due largely to its restricted access in Asia and Africa. In one such study, 80 HIV-positive patients with cryptococcal meningitis receiving amphotericin B 0.7–1 mg/kg/day were randomized to receive a 2-week course of either flucytosine 25 mg/kg 4 times daily, fluconazole 800 mg daily, fluconazole 600 mg twice daily, or voriconazole 300 mg twice daily [146]. No statistically significant differences in rates of CSF clearance or mortality could be detected between the groups. In contrast, an unblinded evaluation comparing amphotericin B alone or with flucytosine reported a quicker decline of CSF cryptococcal colony count but no difference in mortality at 2 or 10 weeks [147]. A meta-analysis of studies comparing survival benefit of the addition of either flucytosine or fluconazole to amphotericin B have also been performed and reported that mortality was lower and clearance of Cryptococcus earlier in patients who were given flucytosine at 2 weeks [148]. However, mortality was no different at 3 months.

In contrast to studies evaluating the benefits of flucytosine in combination with amphotericin B, limited data are available evaluating the potential benefit of combining flucytosine with triazoles (e.g., fluconazole or itraconazole) in the treatment of cryptococcal meningitis in patients without AIDS [149,150]. For patients with AIDS and acute cryptococcal meningitis, higher failure rates were reported in patients receiving fluconazole monotherapy when compared with the combination of fluconazole with flucytosine in a retrospective study (n = 76) [151]. A significant increase in the 6 month survival was reported in patients receiving in short-course combination therapy (2 weeks) of flucytosine (150 mg/kg/day) plus fluconazole compared to fluconazole monotherapy in a randomized trial of 58 patients with AIDS-associated cryptococcal meningitis [152]. Most recently, flucytosine improved fluconazole treatment outcomes for cryptococcal meningitis in HIV-positive patients [153–155].

Data regarding the use of flucytosine-containing regimens used to treat disseminated forms of other cryptococcal infections (including osteomyelitis, pneumonia, and prostatitis) are restricted to case reports and case series. Since most of these reports involve treatment-refractory cases with prior and/or concomitant antifungal therapy, the contribution of flucytosine to the treatment outcome is difficult to assess [7].

Candida

Mucocutaneous forms of candidiasis have been successfully treated with flucytosine, administered either systemically or locally. Topical creams have been successfully used in the treatment of vulvovaginal candidiasis [1,46,156–162]. Treatment of esophageal candidiasis has also been investigated. Flucytosine 100 mg/kg/daily was compared with fluconazole and placebo in the treatment of the first episode of esophageal candidiasis in 60 patients with AIDS in a double-blind crossover study [163]. Endoscopic cure was reported in 9 (70%) and 9 patients (33%) in the fluconazole and flucytosine groups, respectively. Currently, use of flucytosine for mucocutaneous disease is restricted primarily to the topical treatment of recalcitrant vulvovaginal candidiasis due to the availability of alternate therapies [1].

Investigations of flucytosine monotherapy for invasive candidal infections in humans is infrequent (due primarily to concerns regarding the rapid development of resistance). Candidal cystitis or pyelonephritis is the best-studied use for flucytosine monotherapy in humans [1,164–168]. While initial clinical success was reported in 94% of 225 patients with genitourinary candidiasis caused by sensitive strains in vitro, 6% subsequently received supplemental therapy with systemic or bladder irrigations of amphotericin B due to failure or relapse [164]. Other investigators have also reported similar experience in treating candidal urinary tract infections with flucytosine [165,169]. In one of these reports, patients received 20–150 mg/kg/day for the treatment of Candida (n = 51) or T. beigelii (n = 6) [169]. Overall,

89.5% of the organisms were eradicated. Currently, treatment guidelines identify monotherapy with flucytosine 25 mg/kg dosed four times daily as an option for candiduria cystitis or pyelonephritis in cases involving azole-resistant Candida, notably C. glabrata [1].

With high concentrations achieved in peritoneal fluid following oral administration [103], flucytosine had potential as adjunctive therapy for treatment of fungal peritonitis. Case reports and case series described the use of flucytosine (both orally and intraperitoneal), often as part of combination therapy, for the treatment of patients with Candida peritonitis [91,92,170,171]. Some investigators reported high rates of relapse after intraperitoneal flucytosine administration despite initial response [91,172].

Combination with amphotericin B is generally considered in the more invasive candidal infections because of the potential synergism and protection against primary and secondary flucytosine resistance [1,173,174]. Flucytosine may be used (in combination with amphotericin B) for the treatment of conditions such as Candida endophthalmitis, implantable cardiac devices, endocarditis, pericarditis, and meningitis [1,46,175–177]. However, treatment outcomes in immunocompromised patients may remain poor despite flucytosine-containing combination therapy. For example, combination therapy of amphotericin B with flucytosine failed to demonstrate a benefit over amphotericin B monotherapy in a randomized study in persistently neutropenic patients with microbiologically- and/or histologically-documented systemic mycoses in patients with advanced disease [178]. In contrast to these findings, in a retrospective study of neutropenic patients with C. tropicalis fungemia, success was reported in 5 of 9 patients receiving a combination of amphotericin plus flucytosine (5 of 9) compared to 4 of 25 patients receiving amphotericin B monotherapy [179].

Combinations of flucytosine with azoles, such as fluconazole [180] and itraconazole [163], have been reported for select invasive forms of candidiasis. While the efficacy of flucytosine use in combination with fluconazole has been reported in HIV patients [82,152], such combinations are not considered optimal as initial therapy for CNS disease [181] and have been associated with significant toxicity in this patient population [82]. In general, such combinations in HIV-infected patients are generally restricted to those with mild-moderate pulmonary infections [181]. Published reports on flucytosine-containing combinations with echinocandins are sparse. One case report described the use of flucytosine in combination with caspofungin for the treatment of a prosthetic joint infection due to C. glabrata [182].

Aspergillus

Animal models of infection evaluating flucytosine in combination with azoles [183] and amphotericin B [183,184] generally report either no effect, weakly additive or indifferent effect against Aspergillus with this combination. Prior to the availability of newer agents for the prevention and treatment of aspergillosis, secondary prevention utilizing amphotericin B plus flucytosine was reported in 9 patients received 13 subsequent courses of myelosuppressive chemotherapy for leukemia [185]. Radiographic findings suggestive of invasive aspergillosis occurred during 2 of the 13 courses.

Similar to other fungal pathogens, only observational and uncontrolled data are available to describe flucytosine's use in the treatment of disseminated aspergillosis, including meningitis, pulmonary infections, and endocarditis. Availability of newer treatment options (such as voriconazole, posaconazole, and echinocandins) and the relative lack of data demonstrating flucytosine's effectiveness have significantly limited its usefulness in the treatment of invasive aspergillosis [186,187]. Once exception may be for consideration in the treatment of azole-resistant CNS infections (in combination with amphotericin B) [188].

Chromomycoses

In addition to extended-spectrum azoles, flucytosine is considered a treatment option for certain chromomycoses [189–192]. Susceptibility testing of isolates prior to therapy was recommended by one investigator due to the potential for drug-resistant relapse [193]. However, similar to the treatment of other invasive fungal infections, availability of safer, alternative therapy options for these infections (such as itraconazole, voriconazole, and posaconazole) limit the clinical application of flucytosine for this indication.

Amebiasis

The use of flucytosine (in combination with other therapies, including pentamidine, fluconazole, and sulfadiazine) was reported in five AIDS patients with disseminated acanthamebiasis without CNS involvement [194]. However, the contribution of flucytosine to the outcome cannot be determined by this report.

DOSING AND ADMINISTRATION

While pharmacodynamic modeling has suggested doses as low as 25 mg/kg/day may be sufficient to treatment patients with disseminated candidiasis [195], published recommended ranges for oral dosing of flucytosine in adult patients with normal renal function are generally between 100–150 mg/kg/day in four equally divided doses [46,181]. In most situations, 25 mg/kg orally four times daily should be used [46,181]. Higher amounts (i.e., up to 150 mg/kg/day in 4 equal doses) may be associated with higher incidences of dose-related toxicities in patients already at increased risk of adverse events. Because 250 and 500 mg capsules are commercially available, individual oral doses are usually rounded to the nearest 250 mg increments in adult patients.

In patients with renal dysfunction, the dose of flucytosine should be modified based on estimates of creatinine

Table 11.1 Dosage adjustment of 5-flucytosine in patients with renal insufficiency

Creatinine clearance (mL/min)	Dose
>40	25 mg/kg q6h
>20–40	25 mg/kg q12
10–20	25 mg/kg q24h
<10	25 mg/kg q48h
Intermittent hemodialysis	25 mg/kg q48–72h administered after dialysis

Source: Panel on Opportunistic Infections in HIV-Infected Adults and Adolescents. Guidelines for the prevention and treatment of opportunistic infections in HIV-infected adults and adolescents: Recommendations from the Centers for Disease Control and Prevention, the National Institutes of Health, and the HIV Medicine Association of the Infectious Diseases Society of America. Available at http://aidsinfo.nih.gov/contentfiles/lvguidelines/adult_oi.pdf (accessed 5/17/17). 2017.

clearance [41,87,88,113,124] (see Table 11.1). Since flucytosine is most often administered in combination with amphotericin B (which may produce renal dysfunction), careful monitoring of renal function is required in order to optimize the dose. For patients undergoing either hemo- or peritoneal dialysis, supplemental doses of 25–50 mg/kg after dialysis have been recommended [115]. Further adjustments may be indicated based on results of serum concentration monitoring [116,118]. Dosing guidelines have also been proposed in patients undergoing continuous hemofiltration based on filtration rate [95,196]. Dosing adjustment has not been recommended in patients with hepatic insufficiency [197].

Data supporting the optimal dosing of flucytosine in children are limited [120–122]. In general, the oral pediatric dose of flucytosine is the same as the adult dose [120,199]. However, extreme variability in half-life, volume of distribution, and clearance has been reported in pediatric patients (especially low birthweight neonates) [120]. Therefore, doses of 100 mg/kg/day may be excessive in some children, and serum concentration monitoring should be employed in this patient population [121]. For patients who are morbidly obese, ideal body weight may be best for dosing (based on limited information) [123].

Availability of flucytosine varies by geography, and is significantly impacted by country-specific approval and cost [200–205] Alternate formulations and routes of administration for flucytosine have been described in the literature. Intravenous preparations are available in select countries outside the United States [199]. The advantages of the intravenous formulation are unclear, and similar dosing to oral administration (i.e., 100 mg/kg/day) may be excessive [90]. A liquid formulation for oral administration has been described [206,207]. Intraperitoneal administration has been reported in patients with peritonitis undergoing peritoneal dialysis [92], and topical administration has been described in the treatment of *Candida vaginitis* [156,157].

Because flucytosine may be converted in the gut to 5-fluorouracil (a teratogen as demonstrated in animal models), use is considered contraindicated in pregnancy unless benefit is considered to exceed risk. Despite such recommendations, isolated reports of flucytosine use during pregnancy have indicated normal pregnancy with delivery of normal infants [208–213].

THERAPEUTIC SERUM CONCENTRATION MONITORING

The role of serum drug concentration for antifungals has been reviewed in detail elsewhere [214]. Monitoring flucytosine serum drug concentrations aid in individualizing therapy by avoiding excessive serum concentrations (associated with increased risks of hematologic toxicity) while obtaining "target concentrations" recommended for the effective of select invasive fungal infections [215]. Bioassay [25,88] fluorometric [216], high pressure liquid chromatography (HPLC) [217–219], enzymatic [220–222], and gas chromatography [223] methods for analysis have been reported. Clinical studies have established association of flucytosine toxicity and peak serum flucytosine concentrations >100 μg/mL or more during 2 or more weeks of therapy [5,124,126–128,199,224]. While some authors recommend determining serum levels 2 hours after and immediately before a dose [174,225], others have found minimal difference between such levels [124]. Routine monitoring should include obtaining a sample for analysis 2 hours post-dose after 3–5 doses. For efficacy, target serum concentrations of 40–60 mcg/mL have been identified for invasive candidiasis [46] while a 2 hours post-dose range of 30–80 mcg/mL has been recommended for the treatment of cryptococcosis [181]. Monitoring may be repeated on a weekly basis or earlier if alterations in renal function indicate the potential for altered flucytosine clearance when timely drug concentration data are unavailable [127]. Frequent blood counts should also be performed and may be particularly useful in the absence of available serum concentration assays to predict the need for dose modification and reduce the potential for serious hematologic toxicities.

DRUG INTERACTIONS

Aluminum hydroxide/magnesium hydroxide, when administered concomitantly with flucytosine, may delay its absorption [94]. However, effects of other agents altering gastric pH (such as other antacids, histamine 2 antagonists, or proton pump inhibitors) have not been reported. While the FDA-approved product information states that cytarabine may inactivate the antifungal activity of flucytosine [199], there are no published data studies to support this statement [199,226]. Concomitant administration of flucytosine with agents possessing similar toxicities (most notably hematologic, hepatic, or gastrointestinal) should be done with caution.

REFERENCES

1. Pappas PG, Kauffman CA, Andes DR, et al. Clinical practice guideline for the management of Candidiasis: 2016 update by the Infectious Diseases Society of America. *Clin Infect Dis* 2016;62(4):e1–e50.

2. Bennett JE, Dismukes WE, Duma RJ, et al. A comparison of amphotericin B alone and combined with flucytosine in the treatment of cryptoccal meningitis. *N Engl J Med* 1979;301(3):126–131.

3. van der Horst CM, Saag MS, Cloud GA, et al. Treatment of cryptococcal meningitis associated with the acquired immunodeficiency syndrome. National Institute of Allergy and Infectious Diseases Mycoses Study Group and AIDS Clinical Trials Group. *N Engl J Med* 1997;337(1):15–21.

4. Larsen RA, Leal MA, Chan LS. Fluconazole compared with amphotericin B plus flucytosine for cryptococcal meningitis in AIDS. A randomized trial. *Ann Intern Med* 1990;113(3):183–187.

5. Dismukes WE, Cloud G, Gallis HA, et al. Treatment of cryptococcal meningitis with combination amphotericin B and flucytosine for four as compared with six weeks. *N Engl J Med* 1987;317(6):334–341.

6. Saag MS, Cloud GA, Graybill JR, et al. A comparison of itraconazole versus fluconazole as maintenance therapy for AIDS-associated cryptococcal meningitis. *Clin Infect Dis* 1999;28(2):291–296.

7. Perfect JR, Dismukes WE, Dromer F, et al. Clinical practice guidelines for the management of cryptococcal disease: 2010 update by the Infectious Diseases Society of America. *Clin Infect Dis* 2010;50(3):291–322.

8. Montplaisir S, Drouhet E, Mercier-Soucy L. Sensitivity and resistance of pathogenic yeasts to 5-fluoropyrimidines. II.–Mechanisms of resistance to 5-fluorocytosine (5-FC) and 5-fluorouracil (5-FU). *Ann Microbiol (Paris)* 1975;126B(1):41–49.

9. Wei K, Huber BE. Cytosine deaminase gene as a positive selection marker. *J Biol Chem* 1996;271(7):3812–3816.

10. Polak A. Mode of action of 5-fluorocytosine and 5-fluorouracil in dematiaceous fungi. *Sabouraudia* 1983;21(1):15–25.

11. Wain WH, Polak A. The effect of flucytosine on the germination of *Candida albicans*. *Postgrad Med J* 1979;55(647):671–673.

12. Diasio RB, Lakings DE, Bennett JE. Evidence for conversion of 5-fluorocytosine to 5-fluorouracil in humans: Possible factor in 5-fluorocytosine clinical toxicity. *Antimicrob Agents Chemother* 1978;14(6):903–908.

13. Polak A, Scholer HJ. Mode of action of 5-fluorocytosine and mechanisms of resistance. *Chemotherapy* 1975;21(3–4):113–130.

14. Wagner GE, Shadomy S. Studies on the mode of action of 5-fluorocytosine in *Aspergillus* species. *Chemotherapy* 1979;25(2):61–69.

15. Medoff G, Kobayashi GS. Strategies in the treatment of systemic fungal infections. *N Engl J Med* 1980;302(3):145–155.

16. Scalarone GM, Mikami Y, Kurita N, Yazawa K, Miyaji M. The postantifungal effect of 5-fluorocytosine on *Candida albicans*. *J Antimicrob Chemother* 1992;29(2):129–136.

17. Lewis RE, Klepser ME, Pfaller MA. *In vitro* pharmacodynamic characteristics of flucytosine determined by time-kill methods. *Diagn Microbiol Infect Dis* 2000;36(2):101–105.

18. Turnidge JD, Gudmundsson S, Vogelman B, Craig WA. The postantibiotic effect of antifungal agents against common pathogenic yeasts. *J Antimicrob Chemother* 1994;34(1):83–92.

19. Mikami Y, Scalarone GM, Kurita N, Yazawa K, Uno J, Miyaji M. Synergistic postantifungal effect of flucytosine and fluconazole on *Candida albicans*. *J Med Vet Mycol* 1992;30(3):197–206.

20. Arai T, Mikami Y, Yokoyama K, Kawata T, Masuda K. Morphological changes in yeasts as a result of the action of 5-fluorocytosine. *Antimicrob Agents Chemother* 1977;12(2):255–260.

21. Scalarone GM, Mikami Y, Kurita N, Yazawa K, Uno J, Miyaji M. *In vitro* comparative evaluations of the postantifungal effect: Synergistic interaction between flucytosine and fluconazole against *Candida albicans*. *Mycoses* 1991;34(9–10):405–410.

22. Scalarone GM, Mikami Y, Kurita N, Yazawa K, Miyaji M. Comparative studies on the postantifungal effect produced by the synergistic interaction of flucytosine and amphotericin B on *Candida albicans*. *Mycopathologia* 1992;120(3):133–138.

23. Berenbaum MC. The immunosuppressive effects of 5-fluorocytosine and 5-fluorouracil. *Chemotherapy* 1979;25(1):54–59.

24. Roselle GA, Kauffman CA. Amphotericin B and 5-fluorocytosine: Effects on cell-mediated immunity. *Clin Exp Immunol* 1980;40(1):186–192.

25. Richardson MD, Paton M, Shankland GS. Intracellular killing of *Candida albicans* by human neutrophils is potentiated by exposure to combinations of amphotericin B and 5-fluorocytosine. *Mycoses* 1991;34(5–6):201–204.

26. Feldmesser M, Mukherjee J, Casadevall A. Combination of 5-flucytosine and capsule-binding monoclonal antibody in the treatment of murine *Cryptococcus neoformans* infections and *in vitro*. *J Antimicrob Chemother* 1996;37(3):617–622.

27. Hoeprich PD, Ingraham JL, Kleker E, Winship MJ. Development of resistance to 5-fluorocytosine in *Candida parapsilosis* during therapy. *J Infect Dis* 1974;130(2):112–118.

28. Whelan WL. The genetic basis of resistance to 5-fluorocytosine in *Candida* species and *Cryptococcus neoformans*. *Crit Rev Microbiol* 1987;15(1):45–56.

29. Papon N, Noel T, Florent M, et al. Molecular mechanism of flucytosine resistance in *Candida lusitaniae*: Contribution of the FCY2, FCY1, and FUR1 genes to 5-fluorouracil and fluconazole cross-resistance. *Antimicrob Agents Chemother* 2007;51(1):369–371.

30. Chapeland-Leclerc F, Bouchoux J, Goumar A, Chastin C, Villard J, Noel T. Inactivation of the FCY2 gene encoding purine-cytosine permease promotes cross-resistance to flucytosine and fluconazole in *Candida lusitaniae*. *Antimicrob Agents Chemother* 2005;49(8):3101–3108.

31. Defever KS, Whelan WL, Rogers AL, Beneke ES, Veselenak JM, Soll DR. *Candida albicans* resistance to 5-fluorocytosine: Frequency of partially resistant strains among clinical isolates. *Antimicrob Agents Chemother* 1982;22(5):810–815.

32. Lepak AJ, Andes DR. Antifungal pharmacokinetics and pharmacodynamics. *Cold Spring Harb Perspect Med* 2014;5(5):a019653.

33. Andes D, van Ogtrop M. *In vivo* characterization of the pharmacodynamics of flucytosine in a neutropenic murine disseminated candidiasis model. *Antimicrob Agents Chemother* 2000;44(4):938–942.

34. Hope WW, Warn PA, Sharp A, et al. Derivation of an *in vivo* drug exposure breakpoint for flucytosine against *Candida albicans* and Impact of the MIC, growth rate, and resistance genotype on the antifungal effect. *Antimicrob Agents Chemother* 2006;50(11):3680–3688.

35. Te Dorsthorst DT, Verweij PE, Meis JF, Mouton JW. Efficacy and pharmacodynamics of flucytosine monotherapy in a nonneutropenic murine model of invasive aspergillosis. *Antimicrob Agents Chemother* 2005;49(10):4220–4226.

36. Te Dorsthorst DT, Verweij PE, Meis JF, Mouton JW. Relationship between *in vitro* activities of amphotericin B and flucytosine and pH for clinical yeast and mold isolates. *Antimicrob Agents Chemother* 2005;49(8):3341–3346.

37. Te Dorsthorst DT, Mouton JW, van den Beukel CJ, van der Lee HA, Meis JF, Verweij PE. Effect of pH on the *in vitro* activities of amphotericin B, itraconazole, and flucytosine against *Aspergillus* isolates. *Antimicrob Agents Chemother* 2004;48(8):3147–3150.

38. Calhoun DL, Roberts GD, Galgiani JN, et al. Results of a survey of antifungal susceptibility tests in the United States and interlaboratory comparison of broth dilution testing of flucytosine and amphotericin B. *J Clin Microbiol* 1986;23(2):298–301.

39. Gehrt A, Peter J, Pizzo PA, Walsh TJ. Effect of increasing inoculum sizes of pathogenic filamentous fungi on MICs of antifungal agents by broth microdilution method. *J Clin Microbiol* 1995;33(5):1302–1307.

40. Martin E, Maier F, Bhakdi S. Antagonistic effects of fluconazole and 5-fluorocytosine on candidacidal action of amphotericin B in human serum. *Antimicrob Agents Chemother* 1994;38(6):1331–1338.

41. Bennet JE. Flucytosine. *Ann Intern Med* 1977;86(3):319–321.

42. Garcia MT, Llorente MT, Minguez F, Prieto J. Influence of pH and concentration on the postantifungal effect and on the effects of sub-MIC concentrations of 4 antifungal agents on previously treated *Candida* spp. *Scand J Infect Dis* 2000;32(6):669–673.

43. Rex JH, Pfaller MA. Has antifungal susceptibility testing come of age? *Clin Infect Dis* 2002;35(8):982–989.

44. (anon). (M27-A3) *Reference Method for Broth Dilution Antifungal Susceptibility Testing of Yeasts; Approved Standard - Third Edition*. Clinical Laboratory Standards Institute, Wayne, PA *2008*. 2008;28(14).

45. (anon). Clinical and Laboratory Standards Institute. Method for antifungal disk diffusion susceptibility testing of yeasts; Approved guideline. CLSI document M44-A, Clinical and Laboratory Standards Institute, Wayne, PA 2004. 2004.

46. Pappas PG, Rex JH, Sobel JD, et al. Guidelines for treatment of candidiasis. *Clin Infect Dis* 2004;38(2):161–189.

47. Pfaller MA, Diekema DJ, Gibbs DL, et al. *Candida krusei*, a multidrug-resistant opportunistic fungal pathogen: Geographic and temporal trends from the ARTEMIS DISK Antifungal Surveillance Program, 2001 to 2005. *J Clin Microbiol* 2008;46(2):515–521.

48. Pfaller MA. *In vitro* activities of 5-fluorocytosine against 8,803 clinical isolates of *Candida* spp.: Global assessment of primary resistance using National Committee for Clinical Laboratory Standards susceptibility testing methods. *Antimicrob Agents Chemother* 2002;46(11):3518–3521.

49. Auger P, Dumas C, Joly J. A study of 666 strains of *Candida albicans*: Correlation between serotype and susceptibility to 5-fluorocytosine. *J Infect Dis* 1979;139(5):590–594.

50. Schonebeck J, Ansehn S. 5-Fluorocytosine resistance in *Candida* spp. and *Torulopsis glabrata*. *Sabouraudia* 1973;11(1):10–20.

51. Wingard JR, Merz WG, Rinaldi MG, Miller CB, Karp JE, Saral R. Association of *Torulopsis glabrata* infections with fluconazole prophylaxis in neutropenic bone marrow transplant patients. *Antimicrob Agents Chemother* 1993;37(9):1847–1849.

52. Diagnani MC, Karyotakis NC, Paetznick V, Anaissie E. *Candida lusitaniae: In vitro* susceptibility and *in vivo* correlation in experimental murine candidiasis

(abstract A23). *Programs and Abstracts of the Conference on candida and Candidiasis: Biology, Pathogenesis and Management (Baltimore)*. 1993.

53. Berenguer J, Fernandez-Baca V, Sanchez R, Bouza E. *In vitro* activity of amphotericin B, flucytosine and fluconazole against yeasts causing bloodstream infections. *Eur J Clin Microbiol Infect Dis* 1995;14(4):362–365.

54. Lee J, Cooper I, Postelnick M, Stosor V, Weitzman S, Peterson LR. Nosocomial transmission of *Candida krusei* between oncology patients. *36th Interscience Conference on Antimicrobial Agents and Chemotherapy*. 1996.

55. Odds FC, Vranckx L, Woestenborghs F. Antifungal susceptibility testing of yeasts - evaluation of technical variables for test automation. *Antimicrob Agents Chemother* 1995;39(9):2051–2060.

56. Chin CS, Cheong YM, Wong YH. 5-Fluorocytosine resistance in clinical isolates of *Cryptococcus neoformans*. *Med J Malaysia* 1989;44(3):194–198.

57. Shadomy HJ, Wood-Helie S, Shadomy S, Dismukes WE, Chau RY. Biochemical serogrouping of clinical isolates of *Cryptococcus neoformans*. *Diagn Microbiol Infect Dis* 1987;6(2):131–138.

58. Franzot SP, Hamdan JS. *In vitro* susceptibilities of clinical and environmental isolates of *Cryptococcus neoformans* to five antifungal drugs. *Antimicrob Agents Chemother* 1996;40(3):822–824.

59. Fromtling RA, Abruzzo GK, Bulmer GS. *Cryptococcus neoformans*: Comparisons of *in vitro* antifungal susceptibilities of serotypes AD and BC. *Mycopathologia* 1986;94(1):27–30.

60. Bava AJ, Negroni R. *In vitro* susceptibility of *Cryptococcus* strains to 5 antifungal drugs. *Rev Inst Med Trop Sao Paulo* 1989;31(5):346–350.

61. Block ER, Jennings AE, Bennett JE. Experimental therapy of cladosporiosis and sporotrichosis with 5-fluorocytosine. *Antimicrob Agents Chemother* 1973;3(1):95–98.

62. Mauceri AA, Cullen SI, Vandevelde AG, Johnson JE, 3d. Flucytosine. An effective oral treatment for chromomycosis. *Arch Dermatol* 1974;109(6):873–876.

63. Tiballi RN, Spiegel JE, Zarins LT, Kauffman CA. *Saccharomyces cevevisiae* infections and antifungal susceptibility studies by colorimetric and broth macrodilution methods. *Diagn Microbiol Infect Dis* 1995;23(4):135–140.

64. Pujol I, Guarro J, Gene J, Sala J. *In vitro* antifungal susceptibility of clinical and environmental *Fusarium* spp. strains. *J Antimicrob Chemother* 1997;39(2):163–167.

65. Dannaoui EA. *In vitro* susceptibilities of zygomycetes to combinations of antimicrobial agents. *Antimicrob Agents Chemother* 2002;46(8):2708–2711.

66. Medoff G, Brajtburg J, Kobayashi GS, Bolard J. Antifungal agents useful in therapy of systemic fungal infections. *Annu Rev Pharmacol Toxicol* 1983;23:303–330.

67. Gomez-Lopez A, Cuenca-Estrella M, Monzon A, Rodriguez-Tudela JL. *In vitro* susceptibility of clinical isolates of *Zygomycota* to amphotericin B, flucytosine, itraconazole and voriconazole. *J Antimicrob Chemother* 2001;48(6):919–921.

68. Almyroudis NG, Sutton DA, Fothergill AW, Rinaldi MG, Kusne S. *In vitro* susceptibilities of 217 clinical isolates of zygomycetes to conventional and new antifungal agents. *Antimicrob Agents Chemother* 2007;51(7):2587–2590.

69. Ghannoum MA, Fu Y, Ibrahim AS, Mortara LA, Shafiq MC, Edwards JE. *In vitro* determination of optimal antifungal combinations against *Cryptococcus neoformans* and *Candida albicans*. *Antimicrob Agents Chemother* 1995;39(11):2459–2465.

70. Te Dorsthorst DT, Verweij PE, Meletiadis T. *In vitro* interaction of flucytosine combined with amphotericin B or fluconazole against thirty-five yeast isolates determined by both the fractional inhibitory concentration index and the response surface approach. *Antimicrob Agents Chemother* 2002;46(9):2982–2989.

71. Ernst EJ, Yodoi K, Roling EE, Klepser ME. Rates and extents of antifungal activities of amphotericin B, flucytosine, fluconazole, and voriconazole against *Candida lusitaniae* determined by microdilution, Etest, and time-kill methods. *Antimicrob Agents Chemother* 2002;46(2):578–581.

72. Ostrosky-Zeichner L. Combination antifungal therapy: A critical review of the evidence. *Clin Microbiol Infect* 2008;14 Suppl 4:65–70.

73. Vazquez JA. Clinical practice: Combination antifungal therapy for mold infections: Much ado about nothing? *Clin Infect Dis* 2008;46(12):1889–1901.

74. Montgomerie JZ, Edwards JE, Jr., Guze LB. Synergism of amphotericin B and 5-fluorocytosine for *Candida* species. *J Infect Dis* 1975;132(1):82–86.

75. Hamilton JD, Elliott DM. Combined activity of amphotericin B and 5-fluorocytosine against *Cryptococcus neoformans in vitro* and *in vivo* in mice. *J Infect Dis* 1975;131(2):129–137.

76. Schwarz P, Janbon G, Dromer F, et al. Combination of amphotericin B with flucytosine is active *in vitro* against flucytosine-resistant isolates of *Cryptococcus neoformans*. *Antimicrob Agents Chemother* 2007;51(1):383–385.

77. Schwarz P, Dromer F, Lortholary O, et al. Efficacy of amphotericin B in combination with flucytosine against flucytosine-susceptible or flucytosine-resistant isolates of *Cryptococcus neoformans* during disseminated murine cryptococcosis. *Antimicrob Agents Chemother* 2006;50(1):113–120.

78. Nguyen MH, Najvar LK, Yu CY, Graybill JR. Combination therapy with fluconazole and flucytosine in the murine model of cryptococcal meningitis. *Antimicrob Agents Chemother* 1997;41(5):1120–1123.

79. Larsen RA, Bauer M, Weiner JM, et al. Effect of fluconazole on fungicidal activity of flucytosine in murine cryptococcal meningitis. *Antimicrob Agents Chemother* 1996;40(9):2178–2182.

80. Naito K, Murate T, Hotta T, et al. [A comparative clinical study on flucytosine alone and in combination with fluconazole in hematological malignancies: A multicenter study using the envelope method]. [Japanese]. *Jpn J Antibiot* 1994;47(10):1413–1420.

81. Pappas PG, Hamill RJ, Kauffman CA, et al. Treatment of cryptococcal meningitis in non-HIV infected patients-a randomized comparative trial. *34th Infectious Diseases Society of America* 1996.

82. Larsen RA, Bozzette SA, Jones BE, et al. Fluconazole combined with flucytosine for treatment of cryptococcal meningitis in patients with AIDS. *Clin Infect Dis* 1994;19(4):741–745.

83. Barchiesi F, Gallo D, Caselli F, et al. In-vitro interactions of itraconazole with flucytosine against clinical isolates of *Cryptococcus neoformans*. *J Antimicrob Chemother* 1999;44(1):65–70.

84. Odds FC. Interactions among amphotericin B, 5-fluorocytosine, ketoconazole, and miconazole against pathogenic fungi *in vitro*. *Antimicrob Agents Chemother* 1982;22(5):763–770.

85. Hughes CE, Harris C, Moody JA, Peterson LR, Gerding DN. *In vitro* activities of amphotericin B in combination with four antifungal agents and rifampin against *Aspergillus* spp. *Antimicrob Agents Chemother* 1984;25(5):560–562.

86. Lauer BA, Reller LB, Schroter GP. Susceptibility of *Aspergillus* to 5-fluorocytosine and amphotericin B alone and in combination. *J Antimicrob Chemother* 1978;4(4):375–380.

87. Dawborn JK, Page MD, Schiavone DJ. Use of 5-fluorocytosine in patients with impaired renal function. *Br Med J* 1973;4(889):382–384.

88. Block ER, Bennett JE. Pharmacological studies with 5-fluorocytosine. *Antimicrob Agents Chemother* 1972;1(6):476–482.

89. Harper KJ, Sawyer WT. Malabsorption of flucytosine in a pediatric patient with Shwachman syndrome. *DICP* 1989;23(10):782–783.

90. Brouwer AE, van Kan HJ, Johnson E, et al. Oral versus intravenous flucytosine in patients with human immunodeficiency virus-associated cryptococcal meningitis. *Antimicrob Agents Chemother* 2007;51(3):1038–1042.

91. Eisenberg ES. Intraperitoneal flucytosine in the management of fungal peritonitis in patients on continuous ambulatory peritoneal dialysis. *Am J Kidney Dis* 1988;11(6):465–467.

92. Holdsworth SR, Atkins RC, Scott DF, Jackson R. Management of *Candida* peritonitis by prolonged peritoneal lavage containing 5-fluorocytosine. *Clin Nephrol* 1975;4(4):157–159.

93. van der Voort PH, Boerma EC, Yska JP. Serum and intraperitoneal levels of amphotericin B and flucytosine during intravenous treatment of critically ill patients with *Candida* peritonitis. *J Antimicrob Chemother* 2007;59(5):952–956.

94. Daneshmend TK, Warnock DW. Clinical pharmacokinetics of systemic antifungal drugs. *Clin Pharmacokinet* 1983;8(1):17–42.

95. Ittel TH, Legler UF, Polak A, Glockner WM, Sieberth HG. 5-Fluorocytosine kinetics in patients with acute renal failure undergoing continuous hemofiltration. *Chemotherapy* 1987;33(2):77–84.

96. Fuzibet JG, Squara P, Verdier JM, et al. Candida albicans spondylitis. Review of the literature apropos of a case with study of bone penetration of 5-fluorocytosine. *Ann Med Interne (Paris)* 1982;133(6):410–415.

97. Levinson DJ, Silcox DC, Rippon JW, Thomsen S. Septic arthritis due to nonencapsulated *Cryptococcus neoformans* with coexisting sarcoidosis. *Arthritis Rheum* 1974;17(6):1037–1047.

98. Weisse ME, Person DA, Berkenbaugh JT, Jr. Treatment of Candida arthritis with flucytosine and amphotericin. *J Perinatol* 1993;13(5):402–404.

99. O'Day DM. Studies in experimental keratomycosis. *Curr Eye Res* 1985;4(3):243–252.

100. Walsh A, Haft DA, Miller MH, Loran MR, Friedman AH. Ocular penetration of 5-fluorocytosine. *Invest Ophthalmol Vis Sci* 1978;17(7):691–694.

101. Polak A. Pharmacokinetics of amphotericin B and flucytosine. *Postgrad Med J* 1979;55(647):667–670.

102. Smego RA, Jr., Devoe PW, Sampson HA, et al. *Candida* meningitis in two children with severe combined immunodeficiency. *J Pediatr* 1984;104(6):902–904.

103. Muther RS, Bennett WM. Peritoneal clearance of amphotericin B and 5-fluorocytosine. *West J Med* 1980;133(2):157–160.

104. Brasseur P, Bonmarchand G, Caron F, Lecomte F, Leroy J, Humbert G. Diffusion of 5-fluorocytosine in bronchial secretions in patients with respiratory insufficiency. *Ann Biol Clin (Paris)* 1987;45(6):685–688.

105. Hayashi Y, Asano T, Ito G, Yamada Y. Study of serial bronchoalveolar lavage in patients with aspergilloma: Cell reaction at the affected sites and penetration of miconazole and flucytosine into the lesion. *Kansenshogaku Zasshi* 1995;69(5):517–523.

106. Stafford CR, Fisher JF, Fadel HE, Espinel-Ingroff AV, Shadomy S, Hamby M. Cryptococcal meningitis in pregnancy. *Obstet Gynecol* 1983;62(suppl 3):35s–37s.

107. Vialaneix JP, Malet-Martino MC, Hoffmann JS, Pris J, Martino R. Direct detection of new flucytosine metabolites in human biofluids by 19F nuclear magnetic resonance. *Drug Metab Dispos* 1987;15(5):718–724.

108. Harris BE, Manning BW, Federle TW, Diasio RB. Conversion of 5-fluorocytosine to 5-fluorouracil by human intestinal microflora. *Antimicrob Agents Chemother* 1986;29(1):44–48.

109. Malet-Martino MC, Martino R, de Forni M, Andremont A, Hartmann O, Armand JP. Flucytosine conversion to fluorouracil in humans: Does a correlation with gut flora status exist? A report of two cases using fluorine-19 magnetic resonance spectroscopy. *Infection* 1991;19(3):178–180.

110. Vermes A, Kuijper EJ, Guchelaar HJ, Dankert J. An *in vitro* study on the active conversion of flucytosine to fluorouracil by microorganisms in the human intestinal microflora. *Chemotherapy* 2003;49(1–2):17–23.

111. Chouinilalanne N, Maletmartino MC, Gilard V, Ader JC, Martino R. Structural determination of a glucuronide conjugate of flucytosine in humans. *Drug Metab Dispos* 1995;23(8):813–817.

112. Williams KM, Duffield AM, Christopher RK, Finlayson PJ. Identification of minor metabolites of 5-fluorocytosine in man by chemical ionization gas chromatography mass spectrometry. *Biomed Mass Spectrom* 1981;8(4):179–182.

113. Cutler RE, Blair AD, Kelly MR. Flucytosine kinetics in subjects with normal and impaired renal function. *Clin Pharmacol Ther* 1978;24(3):333–342.

114. Schonebeck J, Polak A, Fernex M, Scholer HJ. Pharmacokinetic studies on the oral antimycotic agent 5-fluorocytosine in individuals with normal and impaired kidney function. *Chemotherapy* 1973;18(6):321–336.

115. Block ER, Bennett JE, Livoti LG, et al. Flucytosine and amphotericin B: Hemodialysis effects on the plasma concentration and clearance. Studies in man. *Ann Intern Med* 1974;80(5):613–617.

116. Rault RM, Hulme B, Davies RR. 5-Fluorocytosine treatment of candidiasis on a patient receiving regular hemodialysis. *Clin Nephrol* 1975;3(6):225–227.

117. Muther RS, Bennett WM. Clearance of amphotericin B and 5-fluorocytosine by peritoneal dialysis. *Proc Clin Dial Transplant Forum* 1979;9:100–101.

118. Lau AH, Kronfol NO. Elimination of flucytosine by continuous hemofiltration. *Am J Nephrol* 1995;15(4):327–331.

119. Kunka ME, Cady EA, Woo HC, Thompson Bastin ML. Flucytosine pharmacokinetics in a critically ill patient receiving continuous renal replacement therapy. *Case Rep Crit Care* 2015;2015:927496.

120. Baley JE, Meyers C, Kliegman RM, Jacobs MR, Blumer JL. Pharmacokinetics, outcome of treatment, and toxic effects of amphotericin B and 5-fluorocytosine in neonates. *J Pediatr* 1990;116(5):791–797.

121. Soltani M, Tobin CM, Bowker KE, Sunderland J, MacGowan AP, Lovering AM. Evidence of excessive concentrations of 5-flucytosine in children aged below 12 years: A 12-year review

of serum concentrations from a UK clinical assay reference laboratory. *Int J Antimicrob Agents* 2006;28(6):574–577.

122. Stockmann C, Constance JE, Roberts JK, et al. Pharmacokinetics and pharmacodynamics of antifungals in children and their clinical implications. *Clin Pharmacokinet* 2014;53(5):429–454.

123. Gillum JG, Johnson M, Lavoie S, Venitz J. Flucytosine dosing in an obese patient with extrameningeal cryptococcal infection. *Pharmacotherapy* 1995;15(2):251–253.

124. Francis P, Walsh TJ. Evolving role of flucytosine in immunocompromised patients: New insights into safety, pharmacokinetics, and antifungal therapy. *Clin Infect Dis* 1992;15(6):1003–1018.

125. Vermes A, Guchelaar HJ, van Kuilenburg AB, Dankert J. 5-fluorocytosine-related bone-marrow depression and conversion to fluorouracil: A pilot study. *Fundam Clin Pharmacol* 2002;16(1):39–47.

126. Kauffman CA, Frame PT. Bone marrow toxicity associated with 5-fluorocytosine therapy. *Antimicrob Agents Chemother* 1977;11(2):244–247.

127. Stamm AM, Diasio RB, Dismukes WE, et al. Toxicity of amphotericin B plus flucytosine in 194 patients with cryptococcal meningitis. *Am J Med* 1987;83(2):236–242.

128. Vermes A, van Der SH, Guchelaar HJ. Flucytosine: Correlation between toxicity and pharmacokinetic parameters. *Chemotherapy* 2000;46(2):86–94.

129. Day JN, Chau TT, Lalloo DG. Combination antifungal therapy for cryptococcal meningitis. *N Engl J Med* 2013;368(26):2522–2523.

130. Bicanic T, Bottomley C, Loyse A, et al. Toxicity of amphotericin B deoxycholate-based induction therapy in patients with HIV-associated cryptococcal meningitis. *Antimicrob Agents Chemother* 2015;59(12):7224–7231.

131. Bryan CS, McFarland JA. Cryptococcal meningitis. Fatal marrow aplasia from combined therapy. *JAMA* 1978;239(11):1068–1069.

132. Meyer R, Axelrod JL. Fatal aplastic anemia resulting from flucytosine. *JAMA* 1974;228(12):1573–1573.

133. Chuck SL, Sande MA. Infections with *Cryptococcus neoformans* in the acquired immunodeficiency syndrome. *N Engl J Med* 1989;321(12):794–799.

134. Inselmann G, Holzlohner U, Heidemann HT. Effect of 5-fluorocytosine and 5-fluorouracil on human and rat hepatic cytochrome P 450. *Mycoses* 1989;32(12):638–643.

135. Record CO, Skinner JM, Sleight P, Speller DC. *Candida* endocarditis treated with 5-fluorocytosine. *Br Med J* 1971;1(5743):262–264.

136. Folk A, Cotoraci C, Balta C, et al. Evaluation of hepatotoxicity with treatment doses of flucytosine and amphotericin B for invasive fungal infections. *Biomed Res Int* 2016;2016:5398730.

137. Kyriakidis I, Tragiannidis A, Munchen S, Groll AH. Clinical hepatotoxicity associated with antifungal agents. *Expert Opin Drug Saf* 2016.

138. Shelley WB, Sica PA, Jr. Disseminate sporotrichosis of skin and bone cured with 5-fluorocytosine: Photosensitivity as a complication. *J Am Acad Dermatol* 1983;8(2):229–235.

139. Kotani S, Hirose S, Niiya K, Kubonishi I, Miyoshi I. Anaphylaxis to flucytosine in a patient with AIDS [letter]. *JAMA* 1988;260(22):3275–3276.

140. Heidemann HT, Brune KH, Sabra R, Branch RA. Acute and chronic effects of flucytosine on amphotericin B nephrotoxicity in rats. *Antimicrob Agents Chemother* 1992;36(12):2670–2675.

141. Mitchell RT, Marshall LH, Lefkowitz LB, Jr., Stratton CW. Falsely elevated serum creatinine levels secondary to the presence of 5-fluorocytosine. *Am J Clin Pathol* 1985;84(2):251–253.

142. Hospenthal DR, Bennett JE. Flucytosine monotherapy for cryptococcosis. *Clin Infect Dis* 1998;27(2):260–264.

143. Kerkering TM, Duma RJ, Shadomy S. The evolution of pulmonary cryptococcosis: Clinical implications from a study of 41 patients with and without compromising host factors. *Ann Intern Med* 1981;94:611–614.

144. Utz JP, Shadomy S, McGehee KF. Flucytosine: Experience in patients with pulmonary and other forms of cryptococcosis. *Ann Rev Resp Dis* 1969;99:975–979.

145. de Gans J, Portegies P, Tiessens G, et al. Itraconazole compared with amphotericin B plus flucytosine in AIDS patients with cryptococcal meningitis. *AIDS* 1992;6(2):185–190.

146. Loyse A, Wilson D, Meintjes G, et al. Comparison of the early fungicidal activity of high-dose fluconazole, voriconazole, and flucytosine as second-line drugs given in combination with amphotericin B for the treatment of HIV-associated cryptococcal meningitis. *Clin Infect Dis* 2012;54(1):121–128.

147. Brouwer AE, Rajanuwong A, Chierakul W, et al. Combination antifungal therapies for HIV-associated cryptococcal meningitis: A randomised trial. *Lancet* 2004;363(9423):1764–1767.

148. Yao ZW, Lu X, Shen C, Lin DF. Comparison of flucytosine and fluconazole combined with amphotericin B for the treatment of HIV-associated cryptococcal meningitis: A systematic review and meta-analysis. *Eur J Clin Microbiol Infect Dis* 2014;33(8):1339–1344.

149. Chotmongkol V, Jitpimolmard S. Treatment of cryptococcal meningitis with combination itraconazole and flucytosine. *J Med Assoc Thai* 1994;77(5):253–256.

150. Viviani MA. Cryptococcal meningitis: Diagnosis and treatment. *Int J Antimicrob Agents* 1996;6(3):169–173.

151. Witt MD, Lewis RJ, Larsen RA, et al. Identification of patients with acute AIDS-associated cryptococcal meningitis who can be effectively treated with fluconazole: The role of antifungal susceptibility testing. *Clin Infect Dis* 1996;22(2):322–328.

152. Mayanja-Kizza H, Oishi K, Mitarai S, et al. Combination therapy with fluconazole and flucytosine for cryptococcal meningitis in Ugandan patients with AIDS. *Clin Infect Dis* 1998;26(6):1362–1366.

153. Milefchik E, Leal MA, Haubrich R, et al. Fluconazole alone or combined with flucytosine for the treatment of AIDS-associated cryptococcal meningitis. *Med Mycol* 2008;46(4):393–395.

154. Jackson AT, Nussbaum JC, Phulusa J, et al. A phase II randomized controlled trial adding oral flucytosine to high-dose fluconazole, with short-course amphotericin B, for cryptococcal meningitis. *AIDS* 2012;26(11):1363–1370.

155. Nussbaum JC, Jackson A, Namarika D, et al. Combination flucytosine and high-dose fluconazole compared with fluconazole monotherapy for the treatment of cryptococcal meningitis: A randomized trial in Malawi. *Clin Infect Dis* 2010;50(3):338–344.

156. Horowitz BJ. Topical flucytosine therapy for chronic recurrent *Candida tropicalis* infections. *J Reprod Med* 1986;31(9):821–824.

157. Kivinen S, Tarkkila T, Laakso L, Laakso K. Short-term topical treatment of vulvovaginal candidiasis with the combination of 5-fluorocytosine and candicidin. *Curr Med Res Opin* 1979;6(2):88–92.

158. Rubio-Lotvin B, Gonzalez Ansorena R, Bolio Arista R, Ruiz Moreno JA. Treatment of vaginal candidiasis with 5-fluorocytosine. *Ginecol Obstet Mex* 1975;37(219):23–25.

159. Seligman SA. Letter: Treatment of vulval candidiasis with 5-fluorocytosine. *Br Med J* 1974;3(924):173–174.

160. Sobel JD, Chaim W, Nagappan V, Leaman D. Treatment of vaginitis caused by *Candida glabrata*: Use of topical boric acid and flucytosine. *Am J Obstet Gynecol* 2003;189(5):1297–1300.

161. Shann S, Wilson J, Shann S, Wilson J. Treatment of *Candida glabrata* using topical amphotericin B and flucytosine. *Sex Transm Infect* 2003;79(3):265–266.

162. Mendling W, Brasch J. Guideline vulvovaginal candidosis (2010) of the German Society for Gynecology and Obstetrics, the Working Group for Infections and Infectimmunology in Gynecology and Obstetrics, the German Society of Dermatology, the Board of German Dermatologists and the German Speaking Mycological Society. *Mycoses* 2012;55 Suppl 3:1–13.

163. Barbaro G, Barbarini G, Dilorenzo G. Fluconazole vs. flucytosine in the treatment of esophageal candidiasis in AIDS patients: A double-blind, placebo-controlled study. *Endoscopy* 1995;27(5):377–383.

164. Wise GJ, Kozinn PJ, Goldberg P. Flucytosine in the management of genitourinary candidiasis: 5 years of experience. *J Urol* 1980;124(1):70–72.

165. Yasumoto R, Asakawa M, Umeda M, et al. Clinical efficacy of flucytosine on urinary candidiasis. *Hinyokika Kiyo* 1988;34(9):1679–1682.

166. Fisher JF, Sobel JD, Kauffman CA, Newman CA. Candida urinary tract infections Treatment. *Clin Infect Dis* 2011;52 Suppl 6:S457–466.

167. Kauffman CA. Diagnosis and management of fungal urinary tract infection. *Infect Dis Clin North Am* 2014;28(1):61–74.

168. Thomas L, Tracy CR. Treatment of fungal urinary tract infection. *Urol Clin North Am* 2015;42(4):473–483.

169. Tokunaga S, Ohkawa M, Nakashima T, et al. [Clinical evaluation of flucytosine in patients with urinary fungal infections]. [Japanese]. *Jpn J Antibiot* 1992;45(8):1060–1064.

170. Lempert KD, Jones JM. Flucytosine-miconazole treatment of *Candida* peritonitis. Its use during continuous ambulatory peritoneal dialysis. *Arch Intern Med* 1982;142(3):577–578.

171. Struijk DG, Krediet RT, Boeschoten EW, Rietra PJ, Arisz L. Antifungal treatment of *Candida* peritonitis in continuous ambulatory peritoneal dialysis patients. *Am J Kidney Dis* 1987;9(1):66–70.

172. Pomeranz A, Reichenberg Y, Mor J, Drukker A. *Candida* peritonitis-inefficacy of amphotericin-B and 5-fluorocytosine treatment. *Int J Pediatr Nephrol* 1983;4(2):127–128.

173. Dismukes WE. Combination therapy with amphotericin B and flucytosine for selected systemic mycoses. In: Holmberg K, Meyer RD (Eds.). *Diagnosis and Therapy of Systemic Fungal Infections*. New York: Raven Press, 1989:121–132.

174. Walsh TJ, Pizzo PA. Fungal infections in granulocytopenic patients: Current approaches to classification, diagnosis and treatment. In: Holmberg K, Meyer RD (Eds.). *Diagnosis and Therapy of Systemic Fungal Infections*. New York: Raven Press, 1989:47–70.

175. Smego RA, Jr., Perfect JR, Durack DT. Combined therapy with amphotericin B and 5-fluorocytosine for *Candida* meningitis. *Rev Infect Dis* 1984;6(6):791–801.

176. Fennelly AM, Slenker AK, Murphy LC, Moussouttas M, DeSimone JA. Candida cerebral abscesses: A case report and review of the literature. *Med Mycol* 2013;51(7):779–784.

177. Benjamin DK, Jr., Stoll BJ, Fanaroff AA, et al. Neonatal candidiasis among extremely low birth weight infants: Risk factors, mortality rates, and neurodevelopmental outcomes at 18 to 22 months. *Pediatrics* 2006;117(1):84–92.

178. Verweij PE, Donnelly JP, Kullberg BJ, Meis JF, De Pauw BE. Amphotericin B versus amphotericin B plus 5-flucytosine: Poor results in the treatment of proven systemic mycoses in neutropenic patients. *Infection* 1994;22(2):81–85.

179. Horn R, Wong B, Kiehn TE, Armstrong D. Fungemia in a cancer hospital: Changing frequency, earlier onset, and results of therapy. *Rev Infect Dis* 1985;7(5):646–655.

180. Marr B, Gross S, Cunningham C, Weiner L. Candidal sepsis and meningitis in a very-low-birth-weight infant successfully treated with fluconazole and flucytosine. *Clin Infect Dis* 1994;19(4):795–796.

181. Saag MS, Graybill RJ, Larsen RA, et al. Practice guidelines for the management of cryptococcal disease. Infectious Diseases Society of America. *Clin Infect Dis* 2000;30(4):710–718.

182. Dumaine V, Eyrolle L, Baixench MT, et al. Successful treatment of prosthetic knee *Candida glabrata* infection with caspofungin combined with flucytosine. *Int J Antimicrob Agents* 2008;31(4):398–399.

183. Polak A, Scholer HJ, Wall M. Combination therapy of experimental candidiasis, cryptococcosis and aspergillosis in mice. *Chemotherapy* 1982;28(6):461–479.

184. Arroyo J, Medoff G, Kobayashi GS. Therapy of murine aspergillosis with amphotericin B in combination with rifampin of 5-fluorocytosine. *Antimicrob Agents Chemother* 1977;11(1):21–25.

185. Karp JE, Burch PA, Merz WG. An approach to intensive antileukemia therapy in patients with previous invasive aspergillosis. *Am J Med* 1988;85(2):203–206.

186. Walsh TJ, Anaissie EJ, Denning DW, et al. Treatment of aspergillosis: Clinical practice guidelines of the Infectious Diseases Society of America. *Clin Infect Dis* 2008;46(3):327–360.

187. Patterson TF, Thompson GR, 3rd, Denning DW, et al. Practice guidelines for the diagnosis and management of aspergillosis: 2016 update by the Infectious Diseases Society of America. *Clin Infect Dis* 2016;63(4):e1–e60.

188. Verweij PE, Ananda-Rajah M, Andes D, et al. International expert opinion on the management of infection caused by azole-resistant Aspergillus fumigatus. *Drug Resist Updat* 2015;21–22:30–40.

189. Chermsirivathana S, Bunyaratavej K, Pupaibul K. The treatment of chromomycosis with 5-fluorocystine. *Int J Dermatol* 1979;18(5):377–379.

190. Lopes CF, Alvarenga RJ, Cisalpino EO, Resende MA, Oliveira LG. Six years' experience in treatment of chromomycosis with 5-fluorocytosine. *Int J Dermatol* 1978;17(5):414–418.

191. Jacyk WK. Chromomycosis due to *Cladosporium carrionii* treated with 5-fluorocytosine. A case report from northern Nigeria. *Cutis* 1979;23(5):649–650.

192. Uitto J, Santa-Cruz DJ, Eisen AZ, Kobayashi GS. Chromomycosis. Successful treatment with 5-fluorocytosine. *J Cutan Pathol* 1979;6(1):77–84.

193. Gonzaga de Oliveira L, Aparecida de Rezende M, Osorio Cisalpino E, Peixoto de Figueiredo Y, Ferreira Lopes C. *In vitro* sensitivity to 5-fluorocytosine of strains isolated from patients under treatment for chromomycosis. *Int J Dermatol* 1975;14(2):141–143.

194. Murakawa GJ, Mccalmont T, Altman J, Hoffman MD, Kantor GR, Berger TG. Disseminated acanthamebiasis in patients with aids A report of five cases and a review of the literature. *Arch Dermatol* 1995;131(11):1291–1296.

195. Hope WW, Warn PA, Sharp A, et al. Optimization of the dosage of flucytosine in combination with amphotericin B for disseminated candidiasis: A pharmacodynamic rationale for reduced dosing. *Antimicrob Agents Chemother* 2007;51(10):3760–3762.

196. Thomson AH, Shankland G, Clareburt C, Binning S. Flucytosine dose requirements in a patient receiving continuous veno-venous haemofiltration. *Intensive Care Med* 2002;28(7):999.

197. Block ER. Effect of hepatic insufficiency on 5-fluorocytosine concentrations in serum. *Antimicrob Agents Chemother* 1973;3(1):141–142.

198. Panel on Opportunistic Infections in HIV-Infected Adults and Adolescents. Guidelines for the prevention and treatment of opportunistic infections in HIV-infected adults and adolescents: Recommendations from the Centers for Disease Control and Prevention, the National Institutes of Health, and the HIV Medicine Association of the Infectious Diseases Society of America. Available at http://aidsinfo.nih.gov/contentfiles/lvguidelines/adult_oi.pdf (accessed 5/17/17). 2017.

199. Ancobon Product Information. Physicians Desk Reference; 1996.

200. Govender NP, Meintjes G, Banoo S. Access to flucytosine for HIV-infected patients with cryptococcal meningitis: An urgent need. *S Afr Med J* 2014;104(9):594–595.

201. Perfect JR. Editorial commentary: Life-saving antimicrobial drugs: What are we doing to pricing and availability? *Clin Infect Dis* 2016;62(12):1569–1570.

202. Loyse A, Dromer F, Day J, Lortholary O, Harrison TS. Flucytosine and cryptococcosis: Time to urgently address the worldwide accessibility of a 50-year-old antifungal. *J Antimicrob Chemother* 2013;68(11):2435–2444.

203. Kneale M, Bartholomew JS, Davies E, Denning DW. Global access to antifungal therapy and its variable cost. *J Antimicrob Chemother* 2016;71(12):3599–3606.

204. Rajasingham R, Rolfes MA, Birkenkamp KE, Meya DB, Boulware DR. Cryptococcal meningitis treatment strategies in resource-limited settings: A cost-effectiveness analysis. *PLoS Med* 2012;9(9):e1001316.

205. Merry M, Boulware DR. Cryptococcal meningitis treatment strategies affected by the explosive cost of flucytosine in the United States: A cost-effectiveness analysis. *Clin Infect Dis* 2016;62(12):1564–1568.

206. Wintermeyer SM, Nahata MC. Stability of flucytosine in an extemporaneously compounded oral liquid. *Am J Health Syst Pharm* 1996;53(4):407–409.

207. VandenBussche HL, Johnson CE, Yun J, Patel SA. Stability of flucytosine 50 mg/mL in extemporaneous oral liquid formulations. *Am J Health Syst Pharm* 2002;59(19):1853–1855.

208. Chotmongkol V, Siricharoensang S. Cryptococcal meningitis in pregnancy: A case report. *J Med Assoc Thai* 1991;74(9):421–422.

209. Curole DN. Cryptococcal meningitis in pregnancy. *J Reprod Med* 1981;26(6):317–319.

210. Pereira CA, Fischman O, Colombo AL, Moron AF, Pignatari AC. Cryptococcal meningitis in pregnancy. Review of the literature. Report of 2 cases. *Rev Inst Med Trop Sao Paulo* 1993;35(4):367–371.

211. Philpot CR, Lo D. Cryptococcal meningitis in pregnancy. *Med J Aust* 1972;2(18):1005–1007.

212. Schonebeck J, Segerbrand E. *Candida albicans* septicaemia during first half of pregnancy successfully treated with 5-fluorocytosine. *Br Med J* 1973;4(888):337–338.

213. Chen CP, Wang KG. Cryptococcal meningitis in pregnancy. *Am J Perinatol* 1996;13(1):35–36.

214. Goodwin ML, Drew RH. Antifungal serum concentration monitoring: An update. *J Antimicrob Chemother* 2008;61(1):17–25.

215. Petersen D, Demertzis S, Freund M, Schumann G, Oellerich M. Individualization of 5-fluorocytosine therapy. *Chemotherapy* 1994;40(3):149–156.

216. Richardson RA. Rapid fluorimetric determination of 5-fluorocytosine in serum. *Clin Chim Acta* 1975;63(2):109–114.

217. Hulsewede JW. Comparison of high-performance liquid chromatography and bioassay for the determination of 5-fluorocytosine in serum. *Int J Med Microbiol Virol Parasitol Infect Dis* 1994;281(4):513–518.

218. Ng TKC, Chan RCY, Adeyemidoro FAB, Cheung SW, Cheng AFB. Rapid high performance liquid chromatographic assay for antifungal agents in human sera. *J Antimicrob Chemother* 1996;37(3):465–472.

219. St.-Germain G, Lapierre S, Tessier D. Performance characteristics of two bioassays and high-performance liquid chromatography for determination of flucytosine in serum. *Antimicrob Agents Chemother* 1989;33(8):1403–1405.

220. Huang CM, Kroll MH, Ruddel M, Washburn RG, Bennett JE. An enzymatic method for 5-fluorocytosine. *Clin Chem* 1988;34(1):59–62.

221. Shivji A, Bernstein M, Noble MA. Enzyme rate assay for 5-fluorocytosine. *Am J Clin Pathol* 1993;100(3):299–300.

222. Washburn RG, Klym DM, Kroll MH, Bennett JE. Rapid enzymatic method for measurement of serum flucytosine levels. *J Antimicrob Chemother* 1986;17(5):673–677.

223. Wee SH, Anhalt JP. Gas chromatographic determination of 5-fluorocytosine: A modified extraction method. *Antimicrob Agents Chemother* 1977;11(5):914–915.

224. Pasqualotto AC, Howard SJ, Moore CB, Denning DW. Flucytosine therapeutic monitoring: 15 years experience from the UK. *J Antimicrob Chemother* 2007;59(4):791–793.

225. Bennett JE. Antifungal agents. In: Mandell GL, Bennett JE, Dolin R (Eds.). *Principles and Practice of Infectious Diseases.* Vol. 1, 4th ed. New York: Churchill Livingstone Inc, 1995:401–410.

226. Wingfield HJ. Absence of fungistatic antagonism between flucytosine and cytarabine *in vitro* and *in vivo. J Antimicrob Chemother* 1987;20(4):523–527.

12

Pharmacology of azole antifungal agents

ELIZABETH S. DODDS ASHLEY

INTRODUCTION

Azole antifungal drugs are the most widely employed antifungal agents in clinical practice. When first introduced in the late 1970s, these agents greatly changed the way fungal infections were managed by introducing choice for clinicians and presenting oral therapy options for treating systemic fungal diseases. Today, their clinical utility spans every aspect of treating fungal infection from topical therapy for superficial diseases to intravenous preparations for the most severe, life-threatening invasive mycoses.

This class can be divided into two distinct groups, based on the number of nitrogen atoms within the 5-membered azole ring of their chemical structure [1]. The imidazoles (butoconazole, clotrimazole, econazole, ketoconazole, miconazole, oxiconazole, sulconazole, terconazole, and tioconazole) are limited to largely topical use owing to their sub-optimal pharmacokinetics and intolerable safety profiles. Comparatively, the triazoles (fluconazole, itraconazole, isavuconazole, voriconazole, posaconazole) demonstrate a broader spectrum of activity and have become first-line treatment options for many serious infections.

The azoles cannot be thought of as a single class with similar pharmacologic profiles. Instead, each member

must be specifically understood for its unique role in the management of fungal disease. This chapter will focus on the pharmacology of the azole class, primarily the triazole agents currently available for systemic administration. Where possible, similarities and differences will be highlighted.

STRUCTURE AND MECHANISM OF ACTION

The key structural component of all members of the azole class is the 5-membered azole ring (Figure 12.1). The imidazoles contain 2 nitrogen atoms in this ring, while the triazoles incorporate a third nitrogen into this structure. Many triazoles are derived from earlier members of the imidazole class such as itraconazole and posaconazole, which are structurally similar to the long lipophilic molecule—ketoconazole. This is in contrast to fluconazole that is less lipophilic and has a smaller molecular size that is more akin to the structures of clotrimazole and similarly appearing imidazoles. Although more lipophilic than fluconazole, voriconazole most closely resembles the structure of fluconazole [1]. The newest azole antifungal, isavuconazole, is most structurally similar to voriconazole [2].

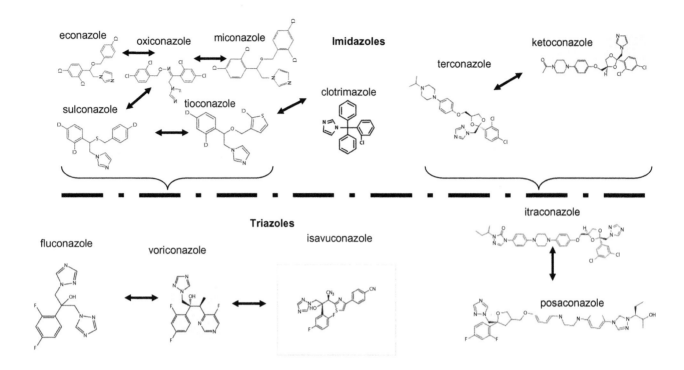

Figure 12.1 Similarities among the structures of the azoles.

All azole antifungal agents share a common, primary mechanism of action, inhibition of the cytochrome P-450 dependent enzyme lanosterol 14-alpha-demethylase [3]. This enzyme is necessary for the conversion of lanosterol to ergosterol, a vital component of the cellular membrane of fungi. Disruptions in the biosynthesis of ergosterol cause significant damage to the cell membrane by increasing its permeability, resulting in cell lysis and death.

SPECTRUM OF ACTIVITY

The agents within this class vary importantly in regards to spectrum of activity.

Fluconazole, the first member of this class, has activity limited to yeasts and some of the endemic fungi. It has excellent activity against most *Candida* species, but has less activity against *C. glabrata* and no activity against *C. krusei*. In a survey of over 200,000 yeast isolates collected from a 7 year period from the 1990s and early 2000s, fluconazole retained activity against most species of *Candida* with resistance found in less than 5% of all isolates tested [4]. This was in contrast to nearly 80% resistance for *C. krusei* and more than 15% for *C. glabrata*.

Updated clinical breakpoints from the Clinical and Laboratory Standards Institute (CLSI), changed minimum inhibitory concentration (MIC) ranges considered susceptible and gave species specific breakpoints for the azole agents [5]. These changes led to an increase in reported resistance. For example, in a survey of more than 1000 *C. albicans* isolates at a reference laboratory, a resistance rate of 5.7% for fluconazole was reported using the updated guidelines compared with 2.1% when previous guidance was applied [6].

Similar results were seen for *C. tropicalis* (9.8% vs. 5.8%) and *C. parapsilosis* (2.2% vs. 0.6%). The breakpoint for fluconazole against *C. glabrata* was not changed, and resistance is reported to be around 7.9% for the more than 800 isolates tested.

The activity of fluconazole against *Cryptococcus* spp. was reported at just above 70%. Overall, fluconazole activity for other yeasts, including *Trichosporon* and *Saccharomyces* spp., was lower than that observed for candidal isolates [4].

Itraconazole offers a broader spectrum of activity than fluconazole, including some mold pathogens, such as *Aspergillus* species and dimorphic fungi. In a sample of nearly 20,000 clinical isolates, itraconazole susceptibilities compared favorably with other azole antifungal agents [7]. The itraconazole MIC50 was ≤1 mcg/mL for all species tested with the exception of *Fusarium* spp., *Scedosporium prolificans*, and many *Zygomycetes* [7].

Voriconazole has a broad spectrum of activity that includes the most frequently isolated yeasts and molds causing opportunistic disease [8,9]. Additionally, this agent has activity against common dermatophytes and the pathogens causing the endemic mycoses [10,11]. *In vitro* data have shown that voriconazole is also effective against emerging fungal pathogens, including *Scedosporium apiospermum*, *Trichosporon* spp., *Acremonium* spp., and *Fusarium* spp. [12–17].

Voriconazole, like fluconazole, has fungistatic activity against *Candida* spp.; however, offers better activity against most isolates than its predecessor and has the added activity against most isolates of *C krusei* [4]. The 2012 CLSI revised breakpoints also resulted in increased reported resistance for voriconazole [5]. For *C. glabrata*, resistance to voriconazole is more than 18% as compared to only 6% using older guidance [6]. Voriconazole also retains activity against some fluconazole-resistant strains of *Candida*. This may represent a therapeutic niche for this agent when results of susceptibility testing are available [18].

Fungicidal activity is seen against filamentous fungi, including *Aspergillus* spp. In a survey of more than 400 clinical isolates, voriconazole was active against more than 95% of *Aspergillus* isolates, compared with only 90% being susceptible to itraconazole [19]. Resistance in *Aspergillus* spp. has been reported for the entire azole class, including high-level voriconazole resistance [20,21]. Although best described in Europe it is important to continue to monitor for spread of resistance. The notable hole in the spectrum of voriconazole is the *Zygomycetes* [12,22,23].

Both posaconazole and isavuconazole provide a similar spectrum of activity to voriconazole with added activity against the *Zygomycetes* [12–17,23–25]. It is important to note that MICs for isavuconazole were comparable but consistently 2- to 4-fold higher than corresponding MICs for posaconazole when tested together [25]. This should be interpreted cautiously, because there are currently no interpretive criteria for these pathogen-drug combinations so the clinical meaning of this difference is unknown. For determining ideal treatment options, relying on clinical data regarding treatment outcomes is best.

PHARMACOKINETICS

The kinetic properties of the azole antifungal agents differ between each member of the class and even among formulations for an individual agent. These distinguishing factors play an important role in drug selection and can affect the ultimate success of the regimen if the agent is administered inappropriately. An understanding of the absorption, distribution, metabolism and elimination of these drugs is the basis for many aspects of these therapies, including use of certain formulations, optimal administration conditions, as well as drug–drug interactions.

Absorption

Currently, all systemic triazole antifungal agents are available as oral formulations and each achieves serum drug concentrations suitable for treating systemic disease. However, several factors are involved in optimal drug absorption.

Fluconazole is very hydrophilic allowing easy intravenous administration. It is almost completely absorbed with a reported oral bioavailability of 85%–90%, when compared with intravenous exposure, among the highest for the class [26]. Unlike many other agents in the class, fluconazole absorption is unaffected by changes in gastric pH or contents.

In contrast, itraconazole has the most unpredictable serum drug concentrations following oral administration. The capsule formulation has a very limited bioavailability, which is completely dependent upon an acidic gastric pH to attain even minimal serum drug concentrations [27].

In order to optimize absorption, this formulation needs to be administered with a full meal and without any acid suppressive therapies, such as proton pump inhibitors or H_2 receptor antagonists [28–31].

A cyclodextrin solution of itraconazole was developed to improve bioavailability. This formulation does result in improved drug exposure, with an increase in area under the curve (AUC) of 30% compared with the capsule [32]. This newer and now preferred formulation is free of effects from acid suppressive therapy, but absorption can be impeded when concomitantly administered with food [33–35]. Consequently, it is important that this formulation be administered on an empty stomach, and patients and caregivers alike need to be educated accordingly.

The cyclodextrin component of the itraconazole oral solution is employed as a solubilizing agent, and this same excipient was used to develop an intravenous formulation of itraconazole initially marketed in the United States (US) in the late 1990s. However, due to limitations of administering cyclodextrin via this route and limited use following the availability of newer antifungal agents, this product has been removed from the US market and sees little use worldwide.

Similarly, voriconazole has limited solubility but readily goes into solution when formulated with cyclodextrin. This has allowed an intravenous preparation of voriconazole that is currently offered in addition to tablets and suspension both for oral administration. When administered orally, voriconazole demonstrates a greater than 90% bioavailbility [36]. This is enhanced by administration on an empty stomach [37]. In similar fashion to its azole predecessor, fluconazole, voriconazole does not otherwise rely on gastric pH for absorption as evidenced by a lack of any effect on absorption with acid suppressive therapies.

Bioavailability of posaconazole is perhaps the most intriguing of the class. Initially available as only an oral suspension, this formulation required administration with a high fat meal and had drug absorption that seemed to maximize at a total daily dosage of 800 mg [34,38,39]. In order to optimize exposure, clinicians had to craft administration regimens to further optimize drug absorption that could be accomplished by administering the drug in small, frequent doses with a high fat meal or nutritional supplement [38,40,41]. These interventions increased serum drug concentrations by 2.5 and 4-fold, respectively [40,42]. Gastric acid can also enhance absorption, and, therefore, acid suppressive therapies should be avoided if at all possible [43].

Subsequent availability of a delayed-release oral tablet and IV formulation have greatly eased issues of serum drug exposure related to this agent, and the suspension is now reserved for patients unable to tolerate another form. The delayed-release oral tables are recommended to be taken with food, but even under fasting conditions, they produce serum drug exposures equivalent to the suspension under ideal administration conditions [44]. The IV formulation contains the cyclodextrin excipient that can limit administration of IV voriconazole; thus, it is recommended that the formulation be avoided in patients with moderate to severe renal impairment [44].

Isavuconazole, the newest member of the class circumvents the need for a cyclodextrin excipient and absorption difficulties through use of a pro-drug for administration [45]. All isovoconazole is actually administered as isovuconazonium sulfate. This is rapidly cleaved to the active compound isovuconazole and an inert product that is eliminated within 30 minutes of IV administration [46]. As a result of the pro-drug, the dose of isavuconazonium administered is actually 372 mg for each 200 mg dose of active drug.

The use of the pro-drug also eases oral administration. Bioavailability is greater than 98% and is not effected by food. Neither the pro-drug nor the cleavage product are detectable systemically after administration [45,46].

Distribution

Drug distribution is an important consideration when treating invasive fungal infections particularly when the infection occurs at a distant site that may not be amenable to drug penetration. In general, all of the triazole antifungal agents are well distributed throughout the body with volumes of distribution ranging from approximately 40 L (volume of total body water) for fluconazole to more than 1500 L for posaconazole [26,47]. While initially appearing to vary largely, these values reflect the volume of distribution for total drug rather than free active drug. This highlights the importance of considering the degree of protein binding for each of these agents, which is the smallest for fluconazole (10%–12%) and highest for itraconazole, posaconazole, and isavuconazole (>98%) [2,26,47,48].

In addition to total body exposure of a drug, certain anatomical sites, including cerebrospinal fluid (CSF), urine, and eyes, are of particular interest regarding drug penetration.

Azole agents are attractive options for treating diseases of the central nervous system (CNS). This is secondary to their oral routes of administration for patients who require long treatment courses as is the case with CNS disease. CSF penetration is the best for fluconazole (>60%) compared to other agents in the class [49,50]. Voriconazole is also detected in the CSF at high concentrations at approximately 50% of those observed in serum [51,52]. CSF concentrations of both itraconazole, isavuconazole, and posaconazole are minimal or not well-described; however, this does not mean that these agents cannot effectively treat diseases of the CNS. For example, the success of posaconazole in treating cryptococcal meningitis, as well as other fungal diseases of the CNS, has been reported and results from a small number of patients suggest adequate penetration across inflamed meninges [53–55]. Similarly, itraconazole has been shown to effectively treat patients with cryptococcal meningitis despite nearly undetectable CSF concentrations although this activity is still inferior to fluconazole [56]. Likewise, isavuconazole has demonstrated brain tissue concentrations almost twice those of serum in a pre-clinical rat model [57].

Fungal infections of the urinary tract remain an area of controversy as positive cultures often represent colonization rather than true infection. This has limited clinical trials to assess the efficacy of antifungal agents in treating fungal infections of the urine. Owing to their routes of elimination, fluconazole is the only azole antifungal with detectable concentrations in the urine that are adequate to treat lower urinary tract disease [36,46,58–60].

Additional data exist regarding penetration of the azole agents into other anatomic sites. Data are most complete for fluconazole, which has demonstrated concentrations in saliva, sputum, vitreous, blister fluid, skin, nails, prostate, liver, spleen, kidney, pericardium, heart tissue, synovial fluid, and vaginal tissues exceeding half of those detected in serum and in many cases at or above serum concentrations [26,61–63] Voriconazole, which is the azole most structurally similar to fluconazole, is detected in saliva, vitreous humor, brain, liver, kidney, heart, lung, epithelial lining fluid, bone, and spleen [51,63–67]. Both itraconazole and posaconazole also have decent vitreal penetration of greater than 10% [68,69]. Itraconazole penetration into sputum is variable, but concentrations within lung tissue appear adequate to treat pulmonary disease [59,70,71]. It also has excellent concentrations in the skin and nails; thus, supporting its use for treating infections due to dermatophytes and onychomycosis [72,73]. Posaconazole achieves excellent concentrations in epithelial lining fluid, at least equal to that of plasma, as well as alveolar cell concentration several fold greater than human serum [74]. It has also demonstrated high concentrations in toenails [75]. Data to date are very limited for the newest agent isavuconazole independent of isolated case reports and pre-clinical animal data [57].

Metabolism and elimination

All of the azole antifungal agents undergo some degree of hepatic metabolism (Table 12.1) [3,26,33,34,36,37,42,46–48,51,52,58,65,66,68,76–78]. For fluconazole, this only contributes minimally to overall elimination with more than 80% excreted unchanged in the urine [58]. Oxidative metabolism is the primary process involved in the metabolism for voriconazole and itraconazole while glucoronide conjugation is more prominent with posaconazole and isavuconazole [36,46,48,79]. Of note, only one antifungal metabolite has clinically meaningful activity; the itraconazole metabolite hydroxyitraconazole [79]. For the inactive metabolites of the remaining azole agents, elimination occurs via a combination of urinary and fecal routes.

The cytochrome P450 enzyme system plays a significant role in the metabolism of voriconazole (2C19, 2C9, and 3A4), isavuconazole (3A4) and to a lesser extent, itraconazole (3A4) [36,46,48,81] (Table 12.2) [81–84]. In the case of voriconazole, this process is saturable and as a result, the drug exhibits non-linear pharmacokinetics [64]. Therefore, clinicians should be cautious when considering dose escalation for this agent. Another variable that influences the kinetics of voriconazole is genetic polymorphisms that

Table 12.1 Properties and pharmacokinetics of the azole antifungals

	Fluconazole	Itraconazole oral solution	Isavuconazole	Voriconazole	Posaconazole
Available formulations	IV/PO	PO	IV/PO	IV/PO	IV/PO
Drug dosing ranges (Adult)	50–800 mg once daily	200–800 mg daily (doses greater than 400 mg/day should be divided)	Load: 200 mg q8h for 48 hours Maintenance: 200 mg q24h	IV: Load: 6 mg/kg q12h × 2 doses Maintenance: 4 mg/kg q12h Oral: Load: 400 mg q12h × 2 doses Maintenance: 200–300 mg q12h	Delayed-release tablets and IV: 300 mg q12h × 2 doses then 300 mg q24h Oral Suspension: 200 mg three times a day (prophylaxis) 200 mg four times a day (treatment)
Oral bioavailability (%)	95	50	98	96	ND
Food effect	No effect	Decreases	No effect	Decreases	Increases—Optimal with high fat meal
Distribution					
Total C_{max} (µg/mL)	0.7	11	4	4.6	7.8
AUC (mg*h/L)	400	29.2	60	20.3	8.9
Volume of distribution (L)	40	796	450	322	1774
Protein binding (%)	10	99.8	>99	58	99
CSF penetration (%)	>60	<10	Low	60	<1–50
Vitreal penetration (%)	28–75	10[a]	Not Reported	38[a]	26
Urine penetration(%)§	90	1–10	<1	<2	<2
Metabolism	Minor hepatic	Hepatic	Hepatic	Hepatic	Hepatic
Elimination	Urine	Hepatic	Feces/Urine	Urine	Feces
Half-life (h)	31	24	80–130	6	25

Source: Rybak, J.M. et al., *Pharmacotherapy*, 35, 1037–1051, 2015; Groll, A.H. et al., *Adv Pharmacol*, 44, 343–500, 1998; Diflucan [package insert], Roerig, New York, 2004; Barone, J.A. et al., *Pharmacotherapy*, 18, 295–301, 1998; Van de Velde, V.J. et al., *Pharmacotherapy*, 16, 424–428, 1996; Petitcollin, A. et al., *Drug Metab Pharmacokinet*, 31, 389–393, 2016; Purkins, L. et al., *Br. J. Clin. Pharmacol.*, 56, 17–23, 2003; Courtney, R. et al., *Br. J. Clin. Pharmacol.*, 57, 218–222, 2004; Noxafil [Package Insert], Merck&Co Inc, Whitehouse Station, 2017; Noxafil [package insert], Schering Plough, Kenilworth, NJ, 2008; Sporanox [package insert], Janssen, Titusville, NY, 2008; Lutsar, I. et al., *Clin. Infect. Dis.*, 37, 728–732, 2003; Mian, U.K. et al., *J. Ocul. Pharmacol. Ther.*, 14, 459–471, 1998; Calcagno, A. et al., *J. Antimicrob. Chemother.*, 66, 224–225, 2011; Ruping, M.J. et al., *J. Antimicrob. Chemother.*, 62, 1468–1470, 2008; Brammer, K.W. et al., *Drug Metab. Dispos.*, 19, 764–767, 1991; Boucher, H.W. et al., *Drugs*, 64, 1997–2020, 2004; Hariprasad, S.M. et al., *Archives Opthalmol.*, 122, 42–47, 2004; Savani, D.V. et al., *Antimicrob. Agent Chemother.*, 31, 6–10, 1987; O'Day, D.M. et al., *Arch Ophthalmol.*, 108, 1006–1008, 1990; Zimmermann, T. et al., *European J. Clin. Pharmacol.*, 46, 147–150, 1994; Zimmermann, T. et al., *Int. J. Clin. Pharmacol. Ther.*, 32, 491–496, 1994; Cornely, O.A. et al., *Antimicrob. Agents Chemother.*, 59, 2078–2085, 2015.

[a] Data reported for oral formulations.

can lead to a complete lack of 2C19 expression in various patient populations. Just over 2% of Caucasians and 15.8% of Asians are poor metabolizers via 2C19 [85]. The influence of this polymorphism on drug exposure has been demonstrated with voriconazole and may be an indication for serum concentration monitoring [86,87]. Although less common, genetic polymorphisms of *Cyp2C9* also occur, although not in Southeast Asians and in only 1% of Caucasians [88]. Limited experience in patients who are poor metabolizers via 2C9 did not result in altered voriconazole kinetics [89].

As previously mentioned, metabolism of posaconazole occurs via a non-cytochrome P450 mediated pathway carried out by UDP-glucuronosyltransferase (UGT) enzymes [90].

Table 12.2 Azole antifungal activity via cytochrome P450 and P-Glycoprotein

	Cyp3A4	Cyp2C9	Cyp2C19	P-glycoprotein
Substrates				
Fluconazole				Yes
Itraconazole	Major			Yes
Isavuconazole	Major			
Posaconazole				Yes
Voriconazole	Minor	Minor	Major	
Inhibitors				
Fluconazole	Moderate (>200 mg)	Moderate	Minor	
Itraconazole	Strong	Weak		Yes
Isavuconazole	Moderate			Weak
Posaconazole	Moderate			Yes
Voriconazole	Moderate	Moderate	Moderate	

Source: US Food and Drug Administration. Isavuconazonium—Invasive aspergillosis and invasive mucormycosis. Advisory Committee Briefing Document 2015. (Accessed November 25, 2017, www. FDA.gov/downloads/advisorycommittees/committeesmeetingmaterials/drugs/anti-infectivedrugsadvisorycommittee/ucm430748.pdf.); Hyland, R. et al., *Drug Metab. Dispos.,* 31, 540–547, 2003; Thummel, K.E. and Wilkinson, G.R., *Ann. Rev. Pharmacol. Toxicol.,* 38, 389–430, 1998; Isoherranen, N. et al., *Drug Metab. Dispos.,* 32, 1121–1131, 2004; Wang, E. et al., *Antimicrob. Agent Chemother.,* 46, 160–165, 2002.

The two glucoronide metabolites are excreted in the urine with the majority of drug being eliminated unchanged in the stool [60].

Isavuconazole is a substrate of *Cyp3A4.* The inactive metabolite is eliminated primarily through the urine and any unchanged drug is eliminated in the stool [46]. It has been noted that patients of Chinese origin have a more than 50% increased exposure to isavuconazole, as compared with Caucasian patients [46]. This is interesting; however, as the drug is not metabolized by 2C19 and further explanation of this difference is not yet available.

Special populations

ORGAN DYSFUNCTION

The effect of organ dysfunction on drug elimination has been studied with each of the azole agents. Renal dysfunction is a concern for patients receiving fluconazole. In patients with renal dysfunction, it is advised to decrease the total daily dose of fluconazole by 50% [26]. Studies have also been conducted in patients requiring renal replacement therapy with either hemodialysis or continuous hemofiltration. For a traditional hemodialysis session, 25%–40% of fluconazole is removed depending on the duration of the session [91,92]. Therefore, supplementation is suggested following each dialysis session [26]. Continuous hemofiltration increased clearance of fluconazole ranging from 20 to 400 times baseline elimination in patients with acute renal failure suggesting that daily dosing should be continued in this population [93].

While one would expect that the other triazole agents are free from kinetic changes due to renal dysfunction, this is actually not the case. The solubilizing agent cyclodextrin that is used in the intravenous formulation of voriconazole can accumulate in patients with renal disease. While the exact effects of this are largely unknown, prescribing information cautions against use of this preparation in patients with decreased renal function (defined as creatinine clearance <50 mL/min) [36]. While the same agent is employed in the oral solution formulation of itraconazole, it is not absorbed from the gastrointestinal tract and, therefore, similar concerns do not exist. Studies of itraconazole in patients with renal disease, including those requiring dialysis, did not suggest that any dose modifications are required [94]. Posaconazole is also free from significant kinetic changes in patients with varying degrees of renal dysfunction [95].

Hepatic dysfunction is a concern with itraconazole, voriconazole and posaconazole therapy as each of these agents relies heavily on the liver for metabolism. Unfortunately no firm guidelines exist for any of these agents in regards to specific dosing guidance for patients with hepatic dysfunction. The most precise recommendation is available for voriconazole that suggests considering a dose modification in patients with mild to moderate cirrhosis [36]. Data from the manufacturer indicate that in patients with moderate hepatic insufficiency defined as Child-Pugh class B, the mean C_{max} for voriconazole increased by 20% compared with subjects receiving traditional doses and that dose reductions should be considered in these patients accordingly [36,96]. In patients with chronic liver disease, maximum serum concentrations of posaconazole were decreased while half-life and time to maximum serum concentration were prolonged; however, data were inconclusive to recommend dose modifications [97]. Therefore, current recommendations for both itraconazole and posaconazole are to carefully monitor patients when administering them to patients with liver disease [47,48].

PEDIATRIC PATIENTS

The azole antifungal agents have all been used in pediatric patient populations. The kinetic properties for each drug are altered in this population leading to different dosing strategies depending on patient age.

Fluconazole clearance in pediatric patients is accelerated when compared with adults as evidenced by a shorter half-life (20 vs. 30 hours, respectively) [98]. Some advocate addressing this by doubling the daily dose of fluconazole in children who are more than 3 months old [99]. The FDA-approved prescribing information for fluconazole also offers guidance depending on the adult target dose [26] (Table 12.3).

Experience with the cyclodextrin solution of itraconazole in children has resulted in much lower concentrations than those seen in adults, particularly when a once daily dosing regimen is used [105]. In order to obtain equivalent exposure to once daily doses of itraconazole in adults, a comparable total daily dose needs to be divided into a q12h regimen [101].

Voriconazole, which demonstrates non-linear pharmacokinetics in adult patients, has linear elimination in children [100]. As a result, children are able to eliminate more voriconazole per kg of total body weight than their adult counterparts and higher daily doses may be needed in this population. This appears to remain true through the age of 15 and for patients <50 kg. Dosing guidance varies by age and indication for use and the following outlines dosing recommendations for treatment of presumed or confirmed fungal disease. In children less than 2 years, current dosing recommendations are based on data from fewer than 20 patients. An initial dose 9 mg/kg given every 12 hours coupled with prompt initiation of pharmacokinetic monitoring is recommended [106,107]. The ultimate total daily dose requirements may lower or far exceed this initial starting point. The same starting dose of 9 mg/kg q12h is recommended for the first two doses of a regimen for children aged 2–12. This is followed by a maintenance dose of 8 mg/kg q12h monitored to maintain serum concentrations above targets of 2 mcg/mL for treatment.

The role of genetic polymorphisms in *Cyp2C19* expression as previously discussed also contribute to interpatient variability in serum exposures to voriconazole. There are currently guidelines, specifically addressing *Cyp2C19* polymorphisms, including recommending appropriate scenarios where alternative antifungal agents should be used [108].

Table 12.3 Equivalent pediatric dosing

	Pediatric patient age	Pediatric dose	Equivalent adult dose
Fluconazole	>3 months	3 mg/kg	100 mg q24h
		6 mg/kg	200 mg q24h
		12 mg/kg	400 mg q24h
		(not to exceed 600 mg/day)	
Itraconazole	>5 years	2.5 mg/kg q12h	200 mg q24h
Isavuconazole	Currently under study		
Posaconazole	Prophylaxis		
	8 months to 12 years	4 mg/kg/dose tid of suspension	600 mg/day
	>12 years	Use adult dosing with delayed release tablets	
	Treatment		
	8–18 years	800 mg per day (suspension)	800 mg/day
	All ages	20 mg/kg/day (suspension) with close monitoring	800 mg/day
Voriconazole	Infants to 12 years (up to 50 kg)	IV: 9 mg/kg IV q12 × 2 doses load then 8 mg/kg q12h	3–4 mg/kg q12h
		Oral suspension: 9 mg/kg po q12h	

Source: Diflucan [package insert], Roerig, New York, 2004; Walsh, T.J. et al., *Antimicrob. Agents Chemother.*, 48, 2166–2172, 2004; Groll, A.H. et al., *Antimicrob. Agents Chemother.*, 46, 2554–2563, 2002; Groll, A.H. et al., *CurrFungal Infect Rep.*, 2, 49–56, 2008; Krishna, G. et al., *Antimicrob. Agents Chemother.*, 51, 812–818, 2007; A Study of Intravenous Isavuconozonium Sulfate in Pediatric Patients (Accessed November 25, 2017 at: https://clinicaltrials.gov/ct2/show/NCT03241550), 2017; Gerin, M. et al., *Ther. Drug Monit.*, 33, 464–466, 2011; Bartelink, I.H. et al., *Antimicrob. Agents Chemother.*, 57, 235–240, 2013; Bernardo, V.A. et al., *Ann. Pharmacother.*, 47, 976–983, 2013; Doring, M. et al. *BMC Infect. Dis.*, 12:263, 2012; Andes, D. et al., *Antimicrob. Agent Chemother.*, 53, 24–34, 2009; Ashbee, H.R. et al., *J. Antimicrob. Chemother.*, 69, 1162–1176, 2014; Desai, A.V. et al. *Antimicrob Agents Chemother.* 2017;61:e01034.

Note: Please note, at the time up this update, several ongoing pharmacokinetic studies of pediatric dosing for the newer azole antifungals were underway and as always, current recommended doses should be verified in these patient populations.

Additionally, equivalency between the various oral formulations of voriconzole have not been established. Therefore, current data for treatment of pediatric patients is based on use of the oral suspension formulation, which is the preferred product for this population [109].

Data for use of posaconazole in pediatric patients suggest that dosing of each formulation mimics that of adult patients for patients aged 13 years or greater [103]. Children 12 years old and younger should receive weight based dosing [110]. At present, the recommendation is to administer 12 mg/kg/day in four divided doses using the oral suspension formulation [111]. This has been studied as part of a prophylactic regimen in children.

The newest azole antifungal agent, isavuconazole is currently under study for use in pediatric patients. Data are insufficient at this time to recommend routine doses for this agent in the pediatric population [112].

ADVERSE EFFECTS

As a class, the azoles are generally well tolerated. Gastrointestinal symptoms are most frequently reported, including nausea, abdominal pain, vomiting, and diarrhea [26,36,47,48]. The latter is most notable with the itraconazole oral solution and is caused by the cyclodextrin vehicle that enhances its solubility [113].

The other most common class-wide adverse effect is hepatic dysfunction. These reactions range from mild elevations in transaminases occurring in 1%–20% of patients to severe hepatic reactions including hepatitis, cholestasis, and fulminant hepatic failure resulting in transplantation or death [114–122]. In the case of voriconazole, this reaction appears to be concentration related [123,124].

Careful monitoring of liver function is recommended for all patients receiving systemic azole therapy as this adverse effect does not appear to be associated with duration of antifungal therapy. Current recommendations are to monitor patients at baseline and routinely throughout the entire course of treatment for development of elevations in hepatic enzymes [26,36,47,48]. Interestingly, hepatotoxicity to one azole agent does not predict reactions to other members of the class [125].

Another serious effect common to the whole azole class is prolongation of the QT interval and although rare, is associated with cases of torsade de pointes [126–132]. Many of these cases are associated with drug–drug interaction between the azoles and other agents also associated with QTc prolongation or additive QTc prolongation with agents, such as the anthracycline antineoplastic agents. It is important to consider this effect when adding azoles to complicated medication regimens and monitor accordingly [26,36,47,48,133]. Interestingly, the newest member of this class, isavuconazole actually results in shortened QTc and should be avoided in patients with familial short QTc syndrome [122,134].

Adrenal insufficiency is also common to all of the azole antifungal agents [26,36,47,48]. This is most often associated with high-drug doses and may go undetected or underreported especially in the critically ill [135–139]. The mechanism for this effect is inhibition of cytochrome P450 enzymes, and, therefore, it is considered to be a class-wide side effect although it has been best described with flucaonzole and ketoconazole.

Fluconazole should be avoided in pregnant women because of well-documented cases of fetal abnormalities [140,141]. Although recent experiences suggest that short courses as low doses may be tolerated and no studies have been performed with the other triazoles in pregnant women, the class as a whole should be routinely avoided in this patient population [36,47,48,142].

In addition to the class effects already discussed, each of the triazole agents also carry a unique side effect profile that are discussed below.

Fluconazole

Fluconazole is associated with minimal side effects with safety data in millions of patients; however, there are two distinct reactions worth noting. Alopecia has been reported following long courses of high-dose fluconazole [143]. This condition is reversible after discontinuation of the agent. Another, more serious condition associated with fluconazole is the development of Stevens-Johnson syndrome following administration [144].

Itraconazole

High doses of itraconazole (600 mg/day) have been associated with an aldosterone-like effect, with manifestations including hypertension, hypokalemia, and, less often, peripheral edema [139]. Peripheral edema can also be seen with lower doses of itraconazole. Cases of heart failure have been described [145]. The manufacturer recommends reconsideration of the use of the drug in patients with a history of heart failure and to avoid use of the agent altogether for treatment of onychomycosis in patients with evidence of ventricular dysfunction [48,146].

Voriconazole

Voriconazole is associated with two distinct adverse reactions compared with the other triazoles: abnormal vision and rash. Abnormal vision (photophobia, color changes, or blurred vision) is reported in up to 20% of patients who receive this triazole [36]. This transient effect is temporally associated with drug dosing, occurring within 30 minutes of oral administration. Symptoms usually last for approximately 30–60 minutes. Photopsia (flashes of light) and visual hallucinations have also been reported [124,147,148]. Ocular toxicity has been linked to elevated serum concentrations of voriconazole [124,149,150].

Rash associated with voriconazole therapy is reported in approximately 10% of patients [36]. This photosensitivity reaction is not prevented by administration of sunscreens.

Therefore, avoidance of sun exposure is required to prevent this condition. Although the rash is usually mild and will abate with withdrawal of therapy, it has precipitated discontinuation of voriconazole, particularly in pediatric patients and caused more significant reactions in isolated patients [124,151–157]. As more experience has been gained with this agent, it is clear that there may be more permanent damage associated with this phototoxicity reaction. Voriconazole has been identified as an independent risk factor for developing cutaneous malignancy, particularly in immunocompromised patients [158].

Another rare complication of voriconazole therapy is pancreatitis and resultant hypoglycemia [159,160]. This can be difficult to predict in patients, particularly in the complex scenarios that are often associated with invasive fungal disease, but withdrawal of this agent should be considered in patients who develop pancreatitis while on treatment.

Posaconazole and isavuconazole

In general, posaconazole isavuconazole did not result in a significant increase in adverse events compared with other azole agents in randomized clinical trials [161–163]. In general use, no specific adverse events have emerged beyond those seen for the class as a whole [122,164].

DRUG–DRUG INTERACTIONS

Drug–drug interactions involving the azole antifungal agents pose some of the most difficult challenges in administering these therapies to patients. Their occurrence is common with more than 70% of patients on azole treatment concurrently receiving another agent with the potential for interaction [146]. The importance of understanding these complicated relationships cannot be understated. In addition to those involving altered azole absorption already discussed, there are numerous interactions involving drug metabolism. The complexity of drug–drug interactions arises from the similarities between the mechanism of action for the azole antifungals and the physiologic effects of the cytochrome P450 enzyme system and p-glycoprotein transport proteins. In addition, select azole antifungals are themselves substrates of p-glycoprotein and the cytochrome P450 enzymes resulting in multi-directional interactions that can be more difficult to predict.

Cytochrome P450 mediated interactions

Cyp3A4

All azole antifungals and some of their metabolites inhibit cytochrome P450 3A4 to a degree [81–83,165,166]. These agents vary in their affinity for the 3A4 isoenzyme leading to different degrees of inhibition. Of the available agents, itraconazole and voriconazole are the most potent inhibitors of 3A4 followed by fluconazole [81,83,167]. Head-to-head comparative studies have not yet been conducted with posaconazole; however, its structural similarity to itraconazole and relative equivalent requirement in dose modifications

for immunosuppressive agents when compared with voriconazole imply that it is also a potent inhibitor of Cyp3A4 [36,47,166]. It also appears that the posaconazole inhibition of Cyp3A4 may be concentration dependent given case reports of significantly elevated concentrations of 3A4 substrates, such as posacoazole, when the tablet formulation is used resulting in higher serum drug exposures than seen with the suspension [36]. Isavuconazole is also a moderate inhibitor of Cyp3A4 [168].

Interestingly, the weakest of the inhibitors, fluconazole appears to exhibit dose-dependent inhibition of Cyp3A4 that is only seen at doses exceeding 200 mg/day [169,170]. There have been reports of interactions with fluconazole occurring at daily doses less than 200 mg per day. However, one must carefully consider renal function in these cases as systemic drug exposure may be similar in the setting of decreased renal elimination despite a smaller amount of administered drug [171,172].

Interactions involving Cyp3A4 are particularly problematic. This isoenzyme is prevalent in the liver and gastrointestinal tract and accounts for the majority of cytochrome P450 enzymes present in humans [173]. It is also involved in the metabolism of numerous medications. Therefore, inhibition can significantly affect the metabolism of these agents and lead to negative consequences, such as added physiologic effect or toxicities of target medications.

Perhaps the most prominent of these are the immunosuppressants cyclosporine, tacrolimus and sirolimus [174–176]. Significant toxicities have occurred with each of these agents and concomitant triazole therapy [174]. Empiric dose reductions are required when an azole agent is added to a regimen containing any of these drugs [26,36,47,48]. Failure to recognize the impact of this interaction and appropriately increase immunosuppressant doses when terminating azole therapy has resulted in negative consequences including loss of the graft and death [177–179]. In some cases, azole agents have been proposed as a method to decrease the required daily dose of immunosuppressant, a practice more commonly employed with calcium channel blockers [180–182]. However, given the rising incidence of azole resistance and toxicities of these agents, azoles should not be used for the sole purpose of decreasing daily requirements of immunosuppressive agents.

Many clinicians do not realize that glucocorticoid metabolism is also completed in part by intestinal and hepatic cytochrome P450 3A4 leading to potential interactions with the triazole class [174,175]. This is best described with itraconazole, but it is a theoretical concern with each of the other triazoles as well [183–185]. While there are no empiric dose modifications suggested, it should be considered in patients demonstrating symptoms of excess glucocorticoid therapy or rapid steroid withdrawal in the setting of azole initiation or discontinuation, respectively.

Several antineoplastic agents also rely on Cyp3A4 for metabolism or activation. Inhibition of the clearance of vincristine by itraconazole has been noted to result in added neurotoxicity of vincristine and other vinca alkaloids [186,187].

Prescribing information for itraconazole, posaconazole and voriconazole caution against use of these drugs in combination with any vinca alkaloid [36,47,48]. Cyclophosphamide metabolism is also affected by azole antifungals [188]. Inhibition of *Cyp3A4* leads to preferential production of the more toxic metabolite of cyclophosphamide. Interestingly, inhibition of 2C9 as is seen with fluconazole and voriconazole may be protective against this effect. Busulfan kinetics are known to be affected by itraconazole therapy, an effect that has been attributed to its elimination via cytochrome P450 [189]. As a result, conventional wisdom is to try and avoid this agent with any of the azoles, if possible.

Several cardiac medications including members of the dihydropyridine calcium channel blockers and the statin class of lipid lowering agents are also metabolized via the cytochrome P450 3A4 [174,175,190–192]. Management of these interactions ranges from close monitoring for signs and symptoms of excess drug concentrations (calcium channel blockers) or use of an agent from the class less prone to interactions, such as pravastatin for the HMG CoA reductase inhibitors [191].

Several additional classes of medications are also known substrates of *Cyp450* 3A4 leading to potential interactions with the azole antifungals. These include benzodiazepines, macrolide antimicrobials, protease inhibitors, and the antiarrhythmic agent quinidine [174,175]. Given the complexity of drug interactions involving the azole antifungal agents, it is always prudent to consult current prescribing information and other drug information resources to determine the most appropriate course of action for managing the azole as well as the other medication therapies. Several Internet-based sources maintain current information regarding drug–drug interactions such as Indiana University, which provides an excellent resource at the following website: www.medicine. iupui.edu/flockhart/table.htm [193].

In addition to drug–drug interactions occurring as a result of triazole inhibition via 3A4, four members of this class—voriconazole, fluconazole, itraconazole, and isavuconazole—are also substrates of this isoenzyme [36,48,81,168]. As a result, inducers of 3A4, including phenytoin, carbamazepine, phenobarbital, and the rifamycins (rifampin and rifabutin), can result in decreased concentrations of these azole antifungal agents [36,194–200]. Great caution should be exercised if azoles are to be administered with any of these agents.

Cyp2C9

Voriconazole and fluconazole are both moderate inhibitors of *Cyp2C9* [176,201]. Fortunately, fewer drugs are metabolized via this route than 3A4; however, there are some notable interactions worthy of discussion. Most significant on this list are the sulfonylurea hypoglycemic agents and the active enantiomer of warfarin (S-warfarin) [174,175,202–204]. The magnitude of these interactions can be significant. For example, when voriconazole was added to a stable warfarin regimen, the average increase in prothrombin time was 17 seconds in one trial [202]. Careful monitoring is essential when either voriconazole or fluconazole are added to a regimen containing any of these agents.

Cyp2C19

Fluconazole and voriconazole are also the only azole agents known to inhibit *Cyp2C19* [176,201]. The most clinically significant interaction that has been identified via this mechanism occurs with voriconazole and omeprazole. Voriconazole can lead to elevated omeprazole concentrations if daily doses of the proton pump inhibitor exceed 40 mg daily [205]. As a result, prescribing information for voriconazole recommends halving the daily omeprazole dose for patients receiving more than 40 mg daily when voriconazole is initiated [36].

UGT mediated interactions

The majority of drug-interactions involving posaconazole stem from its inhibition of cytochrome P450 3A4 [176]. Given the unique elimination route of this agent compared with other triazoles, posaconazole itself is relatively free of drug–drug interactions unrelated to absorption. However, some agents are able to induce the UGT enzymes responsible for posaconazole metabolism and decrease concentrations of the drug. These include the rifamycins and phenytoin, which should be used cautiously with posaconazole [47,206,207].

P-glycoprotein mediated interactions

P-glycoprotein is an ATP dependent transport protein that is found throughout the human body and is involved in the transport of many drugs. There are significant similarities in the list of agents that are substrates and inhibitors between cytochrome P450 3A4 and p-glycoprotein [84]. As a result, the azole antifungals can also inhibit p-glycoprotein and many, with the exception of voriconazole and posaconazole are also substrates [176,208]. Often it is difficult to differentiate the role of p-glycoprotein in azole-induced drug–drug interactions from that of *Cyp3A4*.

The best described pure interaction involving an azole agent and p-glycoprotein is that of itraconazole and digoxin [209,210]. Itraconazole is known to increase digoxin concentrations. This is surprising given that digoxin is not a substrate for any of the cytochrome P450 enzymes [211–213]. The mechanism of this interaction is p-glycoprotein inhibition by itraconazole. This is further supported by the lack of an interaction between digoxin and voriconazole, which is not a p-glycoprotein inhibitor, and digoxin and also only weak modification of digoxin by isavuconazole a known weak inhibitor of p-glycoprotein [208,214].

THERAPEUTIC DRUG MONITORING

Assays to determine azole drug concentrations are available for each member of the class [215]. The role of drug concentration monitoring in antifungal therapy continues

Table 12.4 Recommendations for therapeutic drug monitoring of triazole antifungal agents

	Indication	Minimal time to first measurement after initiation of therapy (days)	Target trough concentration for efficacy (mcg/mL)	Target trough concentration for safety (mcg/mL)
Itraconazole	Routine during first week of therapy, lacking response, gastrointestinal dysfunction, drug–drug interactions	4–7	Prophylaxis: >0.5 Treatment: >0.5–2	NA
Isavuconazole	Not currently recommended			
Posaconazole	Lacking response, gastrointestinal dysfunction, therapy with proton pump inhibitors, drug–drug interactions, questionable compliance	2–7	Prophylaxis: >0.7 Treatment: >1–1.5	NA
Voriconazole	Lacking response, gastrointestinal dysfunction, within 7 days of initiating treatment for documented IFI or prophylaxis, drug–drug interactions, children, intravenous to oral switch, severe hepatopathy, unexplained neurologic symptoms	4–7	Prophylaxis: >1 Treatment: >1 to 2	<6

Source: Andes, D. et al., *Antimicrob. Agent Chemother.*, 53, 24–34, 2009; Ashbee, H.R. et al., *J. Antimicrob. Chemother.*, 69, 1162–1176, 2014; Desai, A.V. et al. *Antimicrob. Agents Chemother.*, 61, e01034, 2017.

to evolve, and available data for each of the agents has established a framework for where this practice may be most useful (Table 12.4). In 2014, the British Society for Medical Mycology issues guidelines for therapeutic drug monitoring of all antifungal agents to help guide the practice [216].

Fluconazole

Of all the azole antifungals, fluconazole achieves relatively consistent drug exposures when administered via the oral route. In addition, available susceptibility breakpoints are based in part on efficacy data from clinical trials [217]. Together these two factors have largely obviated the need for routine therapeutic drug monitoring of this agent.

Itraconazole

Serum drug concentration monitoring for itraconazole has become an established practice and is recommended in treatment guidelines for many fungal infections when itraconazole is used [218–220]. The erratic absorption associated with each of its oral formulations underlies this practice [32,59]. Initially, these concentrations were obtained solely to confirm oral absorption of the drug. However, data from studies linking success of therapy with drug concentration have been conducted and support thresholds for efficacy with many indications [217,221–226] (Table 12.4).

When obtaining serum drug concentrations with itraconazole, the effect of the active metabolite, hydroxyitraconazole also needs to be considered [80]. If monitoring is performed via bioassay, this activity is accounted for in the result. High performance liquid chromatography (HPLC) measures itraconazole and hydroxyitraconazole separately, sometimes leaving the impression that HPLC results can be 2–10 fold lower than those obtained by bioassay [227]. However, the true activity of the drug can be obtained by adding the results for hydroxyitraconazole to those for itraconazole.

Voriconazole

Voriconazole has several qualities that make it an attractive candidate for therapeutic drug monitoring. These include its oral bioavailability that is dependent on optimal gastric conditions [37], significant inter-patient variability in pharmacokinetics [64], and subject to cytochrome P450 mediated metabolism and drug–drug interactions that can decrease its systemic exposure [36,48,81]. Several toxicities of voriconazole have also been linked to serum drug concentrations [147,149,150,159,228].

Voriconazole concentration monitoring data are available beginning with the earliest clinical trials for this agent [124]. Clinical failures of voriconazole in patients with invasive fungal disease are often linked to low or undetectable serum drug concentrations [124,229,230]. Low drug exposures can also be associated with breakthrough fungal infections in patients receiving prophylactic voriconazole [231,232].

Posaconazole

Posaconazole is also an attractive candidate for routine drug concentration monitoring as it is only available orally and is relied upon to prevent or treat severe, life-threatening infections. Other reasons to promote monitoring include variable drug exposure as a result of changes in gastric pH, fat content of food, and frequent use in patients with altered gastrointestinal integrity [42,43,162]. Although limited, data are available that support a positive linear relationship between success and drug exposure in patients with aspergillosis [233]. A similar experience has been noted for antifungal prophylaxis [162].

Isavuconazole

The newest triazole antifungal agent has excellent oral bioavailability as it is administered as a water soluble pro-drug. This eliminates many of the exposure concerns that support routine concentration monitoring for other oral azole formulations. Serum drug exposures and response, as well as toxicity attributed to isavuconazole, was assessed in the comparative study of isavuconazole compared with voriconazole in the treatment of invasive aspergillosis [234]. Based on these results, there was no clear evidence to support routine monitoring for either efficacy or toxicity for patients receiving isavuconaozle.

SUMMARY

The triazole antifungal agents are the most widely used antifungal drugs today. Their development has revolutionized the treatment of many invasive fungal diseases. Part of their attractiveness is a perception that this drug class is relatively easy to administer and is less toxic than systemic alternatives. However, each member of this drug class has unique properties that need to be understood and considered when these therapies are being administered. Based on available data regarding the kinetics, drug–drug interactions, toxicities, and appropriate monitoring of these agents, clinicians can now further optimize therapy in complex patient populations.

REFERENCES

1. Como JA, Dismukes WE. Oral azole drugs as systemic antifungal therapy. N Engl J Med 1994;330:263–272.
2. Rybak JM, Marx KR, Nishimoto AT, Rogers PD. Isavuconazole: Pharmacology, pharmacodynamics, and current clinical experience with a new triazole antifungal agent. Pharmacotherapy 2015;35:1037–1051.
3. Groll AH, Piscitelli SC, Walsh TJ. Clinical pharmacology of systemic antifungal agents: A comprehensive review of agents in clinical use, current investigational compounds, and putative targets for antifungal drug development. Adv Pharmacol 1998;44:343–500.
4. Pfaller MA, Diekema DJ, Gibbs DL, et al. Results from the ARTEMIS DISK Global Antifungal Surveillance study, 1997 to 2005: An 8.5-year analysis of susceptibilities of Candida species and other yeast species to fluconazole and voriconazole determined by CLSI standardized disk diffusion testing. J Clin Microbiol 2007;45:1735–1745.
5. CLSI. Reference Method for Broth Dilution Antifungal Susceptibility Testing of Yeasts; 4th Informational Supplement. CLSI document M27-S4. Wayne, PA: Clinical and Laboratory Standards Institute, 2012.
6. Fothergill AW, Sutton DA, McCarthy DI, Wiederhold NP. Impact of new antifungal breakpoints on antifungal resistance in Candida species. J Clin Microbiol 2014;52:994–997.
7. Sabatelli F, Patel R, Mann PA, et al. In vitro activities of posaconazole, fluconazole, itraconazole, voriconazole, and amphotericin B against a large collection of clinically important molds and yeasts. Antimicrob Agent Chemother 2006;50:2009–2015.
8. Pfaller MA, Diekema DJ, Messer SA, Boyken L, Hollis RJ, Jones RN. In vitro activities of voriconazole, posaconazole, and four licensed systemic antifungal agents against Candida species infrequently isolated from blood. J Clin Microbiol 2003;41:78–83.
9. Pfaller MA, Messer SA, Hollis RJ, Jones RN. Antifungal activities of posaconazole, ravuconazole, and voriconazole compared to those of itraconazole and amphotericin B against 239 clinical isolates of Aspergillus spp., and other filamentous fungi: Report from SENTRY Antimicrobial Surveillance Program. Antimicrob Agents Chemother 2002;21:1032–1037.
10. Perea S, Fothergill AW, Sutton DA, Rinaldi MG. Comparison of in vitro activities of voriconazole and five established antifungal agents against different species of dermatophytes using a broth macrodilution method. J Clin Microbiol 2001;39:385–388.
11. Li RK, Ciblak MA, Nordoff N, Pasarell L, Warnock DW, McGinnis MR. In vitro activities of voriconazole, itraconazole, and amphotericin B against Blastomyces dermatitidis, Coccidioides immitis, and Histoplasma capsulatum. Antimicrob Agents Chemother; 2000;44:1734–1736.
12. Espinel-Ingroff A, Boyle K, Sheehan DJ. In vitro antifungal activities of voriconazole and reference agents as determined by NCCLS methods: Review of the literature. Mycopathologia 2001;150:101–115.
13. Carrillo AJ, Guarro J. In vitro activities of four novel triazoles against Scedosporium spp. Antimicrob Agent Chemother 2001;41:2151–2153.
14. Cuenca-Estrella M, Ruiz-Diez B, Martinez-Suarez JV, Monzon A, Rodriguez-Tudela JL. Comparative in-vitro activity of voriconazole (UK-109,496) and six

other antifungal agents against clinical isolates of *Scedosporium prolificans* and *Scedosporium apiospermum*. *J Antimicrob Chemother* 1999;43:149–151.

15. Meletiadis J, Meis J, Mouton JW, Rodriquez-Tudela JL, Donnelly JP, Verweij PE. In vitro activities of new and conventional antifungal agents against clinical *Scedosporium* isolates. *Antimicrob Agent Chemother* 2002;46:62–68.

16. Paphitou NI, Ostrosky-Zeichner L, Paetznick VL, Rodriguez JR, Chen E, Rex JH. In vitro activities of investigational triazoles against *Fusarium* species: Effects of inoculum size and incubation time on broth microdilution susceptibility test results. *Antimicrob Agent Chemother* 2002;46:3298–3300.

17. Paphitou NI, Ostrosky-Zeichner L, Paetznick VL, Rodriguez JR, Chen E, Rex JH. In vitro antifungal susceptibilities of *Trichosporon* species. *Antimicrob Agent Chemother* 2002;46:1144–1146.

18. Ruhnke M, Schmidt-Westhausen A, Trautmann M. In vitro activities of voriconazole (UK-109,496) against fluconazole-susceptible and-resistant *Candida albicans* isolates from oral cavities of patients with human immunodeficiency virus infection. *Antimicrob Agent Chemother* 1997;41:575–577.

19. Diekema DJ, Messer SA, Hollis RJ, Jones RN, Pfaller MA. Activities of caspofungin, itraconazole, posaconazole, ravuconazole, voriconazole, and amphotericin B against 448 recent clinical isolates of filamentous fungi. *JClin Microbiol* 2003;41:3623–3626.

20. Verweij PE, Chowdhary A, Melchers WJ, Meis JF. Azole resistance in *Aspergillus fumigatus*: Can we retain the clinical use of mold-active antifungal azoles? *Clin Infect Dis* 2016;62:362–368.

21. Fuhren J, Voskuil WS, Boel CH, et al. High prevalence of azole resistance in *Aspergillus fumigatus* isolates from high-risk patients. *J Antimicrob Chemother* 2015;70:2894–2898.

22. Dannaoui E, Meletiadis J, Mouton JW, Meis J, Verweij PE. In vitro susceptibilities of zygomycetes to conventional and new antifungals. *Br Soc Antimicrob Chemo;* 2003;51:45–52.

23. Sun QN, Fothergill AW, McCarthy DI, Rinaldi MG, Graybill JR. In vitro activities of posaconazole, itraconazole, voriconazole, amphotericin B, and fluconazole against 37 clinical isolates of zygomycetes. *Antimicrob Agent Chemother;* 2002;46:1581–1582.

24. Pfaller MA, Messer SA, Hollis RJ, Jones RN. Antifungal activities of posaconazole, ravuconazole, and voriconazole compared to those of itraconazole and amphotericin B against 239 clinical isolates of *Aspergillus* spp. and other filamentous fungi: Report from SENTRY Antimicrobial Surveillance Program, 2000. *Antimicrob Agents Chemother* 2002;46:1032–1037.

25. Thompson GR, 3rd, Wiederhold NP. Isavuconazole: A comprehensive review of spectrum of activity of a new triazole. *Mycopathologia* 2010;170:291–313.

26. Diflucan [package insert]. New York, NY: Roerig, 2004.

27. Lim SG, Sawyerr AM, Hudson M, Sercombe J, Pounder RE. Short report: The absorption of fluconazole and itraconazole under conditions of low intragastric acidity. *Aliment Pharmacol Ther* 1993;7:317–321.

28. Jaruratanasirikul S, Sriwiriyajan S. Effect of omeprazole on the pharmacokinetics of itraconazole. *E J Clin Pharmacol* 1998;54:159–161.

29. Lange D, Pavao JH, Wu J, Klausner M. Effect of a cola beverage on the bioavailability of itraconazole in the presence of H2 blockers. *J Clin Pharmacol* 1997;37:535–540.

30. Van Peer A, Woestenborghs R, Heykants J, Gasparini R, Gauwenbergh G. The effects of food and dose on the oral systemic availability of itraconazole in healthy subjects. *E J Clin Pharmacol* 1989;36:423–426.

31. Kanda Y, Kami M, Matsuyama T, et al. Plasma concentration of itraconazole in patients receiving chemotherapy for hematological malignancies: The effect of famotidine on the absorption of itraconazole. *Hematol Oncol* 1998;16:33–37.

32. Barone JA, Moskovitz BL, Guarnieri J, et al. Enhanced bioavailability of itraconazole in hydroxypropylß-cyclodextrin solution versus capsules in healthy volunteers. *Antimicrob Agent Chemother* 1998;42:1862–1865.

33. Barone JA, Moskovitz BL, Guarnieri J, et al. Food interaction and steady-state pharmacokinetics of itraconazole oral solution in healthy volunteers. *Pharmacotherapy* 1998;18:295–301.

34. Van de Velde VJ, Van Peer AP, Heykants JJ, et al. Effect of food on the pharmacokinetics of a new hydroxypropyl-beta-cyclodextrin formulation of itraconazole. *Pharmacotherapy* 1996;16:424–428.

35. Johnson MD, Hamilton CD, Drew RH, Sanders LL, Pennick GJ, Perfect JR. A randomized comparative study to determine the effect of omeprazole on the peak serum concentration of itraconazole oral solution. *Br Soc Antimicrob Chemo;* 2003;51:453–457.

36. Petitcollin A, Crochette R, Tron C, et al. Increased inhibition of cytochrome P450 3A4 with the tablet formulation of posaconazole. *Drug Metab Pharmacokinet* 2016;31:389–393.

37. Purkins L, Wood N, Kleinermans D, Greenhalgh K, Nichols D. Effect of food on the pharmacokinetics of multiple-dose oral voriconazole. *Br J Clin Pharmacol* 2003;56:17–23.

38. Courtney R, Pai S, Laughlin M, Lim J, Batra V. Pharmacokinetics, safety, and tolerability of oral posaconazole administered in single and multiple doses in healthy adults. *Antimicrob Agent Chemother* 2003;47:2788–2795.

39. Ezzet F, Wexler D, Courtney R, Krishna G, Lim J, Laughlin M. Oral bioavailability of posaconazole in fasted healthy subjects: Comparison between three regimens and basis for clinical dosage recommendations. *Clin Pharmacokinet* 2005;44:211–220.

40. Courtney R, Radwanski E, Lim J, Laughlin M. Pharmacokinetics of posaconazole coadministered with antacid in fasting or nonfasting healthy men. *Antimicrob Agents Chemother* 2004;48:804–808.

41. Sansone-Parsons A, Krishna G, Calzetta A, et al. Effect of a nutritional supplement on posaconazole pharmacokinetics following oral administration to healthy volunteers. *Antimicrob Agent Chemother* 2006;50:1881–1883.

42. Courtney R, Wexler D, Radwanski E, Lim J, Laughlin M. Effect of food on the relative bioavailability of two oral formulations of posaconazole in healthy adults. *BrJ Clin Pharmacol* 2004;57:218–222.

43. Krishna G, Moton A, Ma L, Medlock MM, McLeod J. The pharmacokinetics and absorption of posaconazole oral suspension under various gastric conditions in healthy volunteers. *Antimicrob Agent Chemother* 2008;53:958–966.

44. Noxafil [Package Insert]. Whitehouse Station, NJ: Merck&Co Inc., 2017.

45. Ohwada J, Tsukazaki M, Hayase T, et al. Design, synthesis and antifungal activity of a novel water soluble prodrug of antifungal triazole. *Bioorg Med Chem Lett* 2003;13:191–196.

46. US Food and Drug Administration. Isavuconazonium—invasive aspergillosis and invasive mucormycosis. Advisory Committee Briefing Document 2015. (Accessed November 25, 2017, www. FDA.gov/downloads/advisorycommittees/ committeesmeetingmaterials/drugs/anti-infective-drugsadvisorycommittee/ucm430748.pdf.)

47. Noxafil [package insert]. Kenilworth, NJ: Schering Plough, 2008.

48. Sporanox [package insert]. Titusville, NY:Janssen 2008.

49. Arndt CAS, Walsh TJ, McCully CL, Balis FM, Pizzo PA, Poplack DG. Fluconazole penetration into cerebrospinal fluid: Implications for treating fungal infections of the central nervous system. *J Infect Dis* 1988;157:178–180.

50. Foulds G, Brennan DR, Wajszczuk C, et al. Fluconazole penetration into cerebrospinal fluid in humans. *J Clin Pharmacol* 1988;28:363–366.

51. Lutsar I, Roffey S, Troke P. Voriconazole concentrations in the cerebrospinal fluid and brain tissue of guinea pigs and immunocompromised patients. *Clin Infect Dis* 2003;37:728–732.

52. Mian UK, Mayers M, Garg Y, et al. Comparison of fluconazole pharmacokinetics in serum, aqueous humor, vitreous humor, and cerebrospinal fluid following a single dose and at steady state. *J Ocul Pharmacol Ther* 1998;14:459–471.

53. Pitisuttithum P, Negroni R, Graybill JR, et al. Activity of posaconazole in the treatment of central nervous system fungal infections. *J Antimicrob Chemother* 2005;56:745–755.

54. Calcagno A, Baietto L, De Rosa FG, et al. Posaconazole cerebrospinal concentrations in an HIV-infected patient with brain mucormycosis. *J Antimicrob Chemother* 2011;66:224–225.

55. Ruping MJ, Albermann N, Ebinger F, et al. Posaconazole concentrations in the central nervous system. *J Antimicrob Chemother* 2008;62:1468–1470.

56. van der Horst CM, Saag MS, Cloud GA, et al. Treatment of cryptococcal meningitis associated with the acquired immunodeficiency syndrome. *N Engl J Med* 1997;337:15–21.

57. Schmitt-Hoffmann AH, Kato K, Townsend R, et al. Tissue distribution and elimination of isavuconazole following single and repeat oral-dose administration of isavuconazonium sulfate to rats. *Antimicrob Agents Chemother* 2017;61:e01292–17.

58. Brammer KW, Coakley AJ, Jezequel SG, Tarbit MH. The disposition and metabolism of [14C] fluconazole in humans. *Drug Metab Dispos* 1991;19:764–767.

59. Hardin TC, Graybill JR, Fetchick R, Woestenborghs R, Rinaldi MG, Kuhn JG. Pharmacokinetics of itraconazole following oral administration to normal volunteers. *Antimicrob Agent Chemother* 1988;32:1310–1313.

60. Krieter P, Flannery B, Musick T, Gohdes M, Martinho M, Courtney R. Disposition of posaconazole following single-dose oral administration in healthy subjects. *Antimicrob Agent Chemother* 2004;48:3543–3551.

61. Finley RW, Cleary JD, Goolsby J, Chapman SW. Fluconazole penetration into the human prostate. *Antimicrob Agent Chemother* 1995;39:553–555.

62. Fischman AJ, Alpert NM, Livni E, et al. Pharmacokinetics of 18F-labeled fluconazole in healthy human subjects by positron emission tomography. *Antimicrob Agent Chemother* 1993;37:1270–1277.

63. Felton T, Troke PF, Hope WW. Tissue penetration of antifungal agents. *Clin Microbiol Rev* 2014;27:68–88.

64. Purkins L, Wood N, Ghahramani P, Greenhalgh K, Allen MJ, Kleinermans D. Pharmacokinetics and safety of voriconazole following intravenous-to oral-dose escalation regimens. *Antimicrob Agent Chemother* 2002;46:2546–2553.

65. Boucher HW, Groll AH, Chiou CC, Walsh TJ. Newer systemic antifungal agents: Pharmacokinetics, safety and efficacy. *Drugs* 2004;64:1997–2020.

66. Hariprasad SM, Mieler WF, Holz ER, et al. Determination of vitreous, aqueous, and plasma concentration of orally administered voriconazole in humans. *Archives Opthalmol;* 2004;122:42–47.

67. Capitano B, Potoski BA, Husain S, et al. Intrapulmonary penetration of voriconazole in patients receiving an oral prophylactic regimen. *Antimicrobial Agents and Chemotherapy* 2006;50:1878–1880.

68. Savani DV, Perfect JR, Cobo LM, Durack DT. Penetration of new azole compounds into the eye and efficacy in experimental *Candida* endophthalmitis. *Antimicrob Agent Chemother* 1987;31:6–10.

69. Sponsel WE, Graybill JR, Nevarez HL, Dang D. Ocular and systemic posaconazole (SCH-56592) treatment of invasive *Fusarium solani* keratitis and endophthalmitis. *Br J Opthalmol* 2002;86:829–830.

70. Sermet-Gaudelus I, Lesne-Hulin A, Lenoir G, Singlas E, Berche P, Hennequin C. Sputum itraconazole concentrations in cystic fibrosis patients. *Antimicrob Agent Chemother* 2001;45:1937–1938.

71. Coronel B, Levron JC, Van Devenne D, Archimbaud E, Mercatello A. Itraconazole lung concentrations in haematological patients. *Mycoses* 2000;43:125–127.

72. Matthieu L, Doncker P, Cauwenbergh G, et al. Itraconazole penetrates the nail via the nail matrix and the nail bed-an investigation in onychomycosis. *Clin Exp Dermatol* 1991;16:374–376.

73. Seishima M, Oyama Z, Oda M, Ishigo S. Distribution of an antifungal drug, itraconazole, in pathological and non-pathological tissues. *Eur J Dermatol* 2004;14:24–27.

74. Conte JE, Jr., Golden JA, Krishna G, McIver M, Little E, Zurlinden E. Intrapulmonary pharmacokinetics and pharmacodynamics of posaconazole at steady state in healthy subjects. *Antimicrob Agents Chemother* 2009;53:703–707.

75. Krishna G, Ma L, Martinho M, Prasad P, Wahl J, Tavakkol A. Determination of posaconazole levels in toenails of adults with onychomycosis following oral treatment with four regimens of posaconazole for 12 or 24 weeks. *Antimicrob Agents Chemother* 2011;55:4424–4426.

76. O'Day DM, Foulds G, Williams TE, Robinson RD, Allen RH, Head WS. Ocular uptake of fluconazole following oral administration. *Arch Ophthalmol* 1990;108:1006–1008.

77. Zimmermann T, Yeates RA, Laufen H, Pfaff G, Wildfeuer A. Influence of concomitant food intake on the oral absorption of two triazole antifungal agents, itraconazole and fluconazole. *European J Clin Pharmacol* 1994;46:147–150.

78. Zimmermann T, Yeates RA, Riedel KD, Lach P, Laufen H. The influence of gastric pH on the pharmacokinetics of fluconazole: The effect of omeprazole. *Int J Clin Pharmacol Ther* 1994;32:491–496.

79. Odds FC, Bossche HV. Antifungal activity of itraconazole compared with hydroxy-itraconazole in vitro. *Br Soc Antimicrob Chemo*; 2000;45:371–373.

80. Cornely OA, Bohme A, Schmitt-Hoffmann A, Ullmann AJ. Safety and pharmacokinetics of isavuconazole as antifungal prophylaxis in acute myeloid leukemia patients with neutropenia: Results of a phase 2, dose escalation study. *Antimicrob Agents Chemother* 2015;59:2078–2085.

81. Hyland R, Jones BC, Smith DA. Identification of the cytochrome P450 enzymes involved in the N-oxidation of voriconazole. *Drug Metab Dispos* 2003;31:540–547.

82. Thummel KE, Wilkinson GR. In vitro and in vivo drug interactions involving human CYP3A. *Ann Rev Pharmacol Toxicol* 1998;38:389–430.

83. Isoherranen N, Kunze KL, Allen KE, Nelson WL, Thummel KE. Role of itraconazole metabolites in CYP3A4 inhibition. *Drug Metab Dispos* 2004;32:1121–1131.

84. Wang E, Lew K, Casciano CN, Clement RP, Johnson WW. Interaction of common azole antifungals with P glycoprotein. *Antimicrob Agent Chemother* 2002;46:160–165.

85. Shimizu T, Ochiai H, ÅSell F, et al. Bioinformatics research on inter-racial difference in drug metabolism I. Analysis on frequencies of mutant alleles and poor metabolizers on CYP2D6 and CYP2C19. *Drug Metab Pharmacokinet* 2003;18:48–70.

86. Mikus G, Schöwel V, Drzewinska M, et al. Potent CYP2C19 genotype related interaction between voriconazole and the CYP3A4 inhibitor ritonavir. *Clin Pharmacol Ther* 2006;80:126–135.

87. Rengelshausen J, Banfield M, Riedel KD, et al. Opposite effects of short-term and long-term StJohn's wort intake on voriconazole pharmacokinetics. *Clin Pharmacol Ther* 2005;78:25–33.

88. Wilkinson GR. Drug metabolism and variability among patients in drug response. *N Engl J Med* 2005;352:2211–2221.

89. Geist MJP, Egerer G, Burhenne J, Mikus G. Safety of voriconazole in a patient with CYP2C9 * 2/CYP2C9 * 2 Genotype. *Antimicrob Agent Chemother* 2006;50:3227–3228.

90. Ghosal A, Hapangama N, Yuan Y, et al. Identification of human udp-glucuronosyltransferase enzyme(s) responsible for the glucuronidation of posaconazole (Noxafil). *Drug Metab Dispos* 2004;32:267–271.

91. Toon S, Ross CE, Gokal R, Rowland M. An assessment of the effects of impaired renal function and hemodialysis on the pharmacokinetics of fluconazole. Antifungal agents 75 76 L. Silvestri, D. Mur Laffon, A. Gullo 49858 (fluconazole). *Am Rev Respir Dis* 1990;134:768–770.

92. Oono S, Tabei K, Tetsuka T, Asano Y. The pharmacokinetics of fluconazole during haemodialysis in uraemic patients. *EJ Clin Pharamcol* 1992;42:667–669.

93. Valtonen M. Effect of continuous venovenous haemofiltration and haemodiafiltration on the elimination of fluconazole in patients with acute renal failure. *J Antimicrob Chemother*; 1997;40:695–700.

94. Boelaert J, Schurgers M, Matthys E, et al. Itraconazole pharmacokinetics in patients with renal dysfunction. *Antimicrob Agent Chemother* 1988;32:1595–1597.

95. Courtney R, Sansone A, Smith W, et al. Posaconazole pharmacokinetics, safety, and tolerability in subjects with varying degrees of chronic renal disease. *J Clin Pharmacol* 2005;45:185–192.

96. Child CG, Turcotte JG. Surgery and portal hypertension. In: *The Liver and Portal Hypertension*. Philadelphia, PA: Saunders, 1964.

97. Courtney R, Laughlin M, Gontz H. Single-dose pharmacokinetics of posaconazole in subjects with various degrees of chronic liver disease. *J Clin Pharmacol* 2005;45:185–192.

98. Brammer KW, Coates PE. Pharmacokinetics of fluconazole in pediatric patients. *Eur J Clin Microbiol Infect Dis* 1994;13:325–329.

99. Zaoutis TE, Benjamin DK, Steinbach WJ. Antifungal treatment in pediatric patients. *Drug Resistance Updates* 2005;8:235–245.

100. Walsh TJ, Karlsson MO, Driscoll T, et al. Pharmacokinetics and safety of intravenous voriconazole in children after single-or multiple-dose administration. *Antimicrob Agents Chemother* 2004;48:2166–2172.

101. Groll AH, Wood L, Roden M, et al. Safety, pharmacokinetics, and pharmacodynamics of cyclodextrin itraconazole in pediatric patients with oropharyngeal candidiasis. *Antimicrob Agents Chemother* 2002;46:2554–2563.

102. Groll AH, Roilides E, Walsh TJ. Pediatric pharmacology of antifungal agents. *CurrFungal Infect Rep* 2008;2:49–56.

103. Krishna G, Sansone-Parsons A, Martinho M, Kantesaria B, Pedicone L. Posaconazole plasma concentrations in juvenile patients with invasive fungal infection? *Antimicrob Agents Chemother* 2007;51:812–818.

104. A Study of Intravenous Isavuconozonium Sulfate in Pediatric Patients. 2017. (Accessed November 25, 2017 at: https://clinicaltrials.gov/ct2/show/NCT03241550).

105. de Repentigny L, Ratelle J, Leclerc JM, et al. Repeated-dose pharmacokinetics of an oral solution of itraconazole in infants and children. *Antimicrob Agents Chemother* 1998;42:404–408.

106. Gerin M, Mahlaoui N, Elie C, et al. Therapeutic drug monitoring of voriconazole after intravenous administration in infants and children with primary immunodeficiency. *Ther Drug Monit* 2011;33:464–466.

107. Bartelink IH, Wolfs T, Jonker M, et al. Highly variable plasma concentrations of voriconazole in pediatric hematopoietic stem cell transplantation patients. *Antimicrob Agents Chemother* 2013;57:235–240.

108. Moriyama B, Obeng AO, Barbarino J, et al. Clinical Pharmacogenetics Implementation Consortium (CPIC) guidelines for CYP2C19 and voriconazole therapy. *Clin Pharmacol Ther* 2017;102:45–51.

109. Voriconazole Accord. 2017. (Accessed January 5, 2018., 2018, at http://www.ema.europa.eu/docs/en_GB/document_library/EPAR_-_Product_Information/human/000387/WC500049756.pdf.)

110. Bernardo VA, Cross SJ, Crews KR, et al. Posaconazole therapeutic drug monitoring in pediatric patients and young adults with cancer. *Ann Pharmacother* 2013;47:976–983.

111. Doring M, Muller C, Johann PD, et al. Analysis of posaconazole as oral antifungal prophylaxis in pediatric patients under 12 years of age following allogeneic stem cell transplantation. *BMC Infect Dis* 2012;12:263.

112. A Study of Intravenous Isavuconazonium Sulfate in Pediatric Patients. (Accessed January 5, 2018. at https://clinicaltrials.gov/ct2/show/NCT03241550.)

113. Vandewoude K, Vogelaers D, Decruyenaere J, et al. Concentrations in plasma and safety of 7 days of intravenous itraconazole followed by 2 weeks of oral itraconazole solution in patients in intensive care units. *Antimicrob Agents Chemother* 1997;41:2714–2718.

114. Gearhart MO. Worsening of liver function with fluconazole and review of azole antifungal hepatotoxicity. *Ann Pharmacother* 1994;28:1177–1181.

115. Crerar-Gilbert A, Boots R, Fraenkel D, Macdonald GA. Survival following fulminant hepatic failure from fluconazole induced hepatitis. *Anaesth Intensive Care* 1999;27:650–652.

116. Bronstein JA, Gros P, Hernandez E, Larroque P, Molinie C. Fatal acute hepatic necrosis due to dose-dependent fluconazole hepatotoxicity. *Clin Infect Dis* 1997;25:1266–1267.

117. Munoz P, Moreno S, Berenguer J, Bernaldo QJC, Bouza E. Fluconazole-related hepatotoxicity in patients with acquired immunodeficiency syndrome. *Arch Intern Med* 1991;151:1020–1021.

118. Adriaenssens B, Roskams T, Steger P, Van Steenbergen W. Hepatotoxicity related to itraconazole: Report of three cases. *Acta Clinica Belgica* 2001;56:364–369.

119. Gallardo-Quesada S, Luelmo-Aguilar J, Guanyabens-Calvet C. Hepatotoxicity associated with itraconazole. *Int J Dermatol* 1995;34:589.

120. Talwalkar JA, Soetikno RE, Carr-Locke DL, Berg CL. Severe cholestasis related to itraconazole for the treatment of onychomycosis. *Am J gastroenterol* 1999;94:3632–3633.

121. Srebrnik A, Levtov S, Ben-Ami R, Brenner S. Liver failure and transplantation after itraconazole treatment for toenail onychomycosis. *J Eur Acad Dermatol Vemereal* 2005;19:205–207.

122. Miceli MH, Kauffman CA. Isavuconazole: A new broad-spectrum triazole antifungal agent. *Clin Infect Dis* 2015;61:1558–1565.

123. Potoski BA, Brown J. The safety of voriconazole. *Clin Infect Dis* 2002;35:1273–1275.

124. Denning DW, Ribaud P, Milpied N, et al. Efficacy and safety of voriconazole in the treatment of acute invasive aspergillosis. *Clin Infect Dis* 2002;34:563–571.

125. Spellberg B, Rieg G, Bayer A, Edwards JJE. Lack of cross-hepatotoxicity between fluconazole and voriconazole. *Clin Infect Dis* 2003;36:1091–1093.

126. Alkan Y, Haefeli WE, Burhenne J, Stein J, Yaniv I, Shalit I. Voriconazole-induced QT interval prolongation and ventricular tachycardia: A non-concentration-dependent adverse effect. *Clin Infect Dis* 2004;39:884,e49–e52.

127. Dorsey ST, Biblo LA. Prolonged QT interval and torsades de pointes caused by the combination of fluconazole and amitriptyline. *A J Emerg Med* 2000;18:227–229.

128. Hoover CA, Carmichael JK, Nolan Jr PE, Marcus FI. Cardiac arrest associated with combination cisapride and itraconazole therapy. *J Cardiovasc Pharmacol Ther* 1996;1:255–258.

129. Khazan M, Mathis AS. Probable case of torsades de pointes induced by fluconazole. *Pharmacotherapy* 2002;22:1632–1637.

130. Pohjola-Sintonen S, Viitasalo M, Toivonen L, Neuvonen P. Itraconazole prevents terfenadine metabolism and increases risk of torsades de pointes ventricular tachycardia. *Eur J Clin Pharmacol* 1993;45:191–193.

131. Tholakanahalli VN. Fluconazole-induced torsade de pointes. *Ann Pharmacother* 2001;35:432–434.

132. Wassmann S, Nickenig G, Bohm M. Long QT syndrome and torsade de pointes in a patient receiving fluconazole. *Am Coll Physicians* 1999;10:797.

133. Owens Jr RC, Nolin TD. Antimicrobial-associated QT interval prolongation: Pointes of interest. *Clin Infect Dis* 2006;43:1603–1611.

134. Mellinghoff SC, Bassetti M, Dorfel D, et al. Isavuconazole shortens the QTc interval. *Mycoses* 2017 (epub ahead of print).

135. Albert SG, DeLeon MJ, Silverberg AB. Possible association between high-dose fluconazole and adrenal insufficiency in critically ill patients. *Crit Care Med* 2001;29:668–670.

136. Shibata S, Kami M, Kanda Y, et al. Acute adrenal failure associated with fluconazole after administration of high-dose cyclophosphamide. *Am J Hematol* 2001;66:303–305.

137. Gradon JD, Sepkowitz DV. Fluconazole-associated acute adrenal insufficiency. *Postgrad Med J* 1991;67:1084–1085.

138. Michaelis G, Zeiler D, Biscoping J, Fussle R, Hempelmann G. Function of the adrenal cortex during therapy with fluconazole in intensive care patients. *Mycoses* 1993;36:117–123.

139. Sharkey PK, Rinaldi MG, Dunn JF, Hardin TC, Fetchick RJ, Graybill JR. High-dose itraconazole in the treatment of severe mycoses. *Antimicrob Agent Chemother* 1991;35:707–713.

140. Pursley TJ, Blomquist IK, Abraham J, Andersen HF, Bartley JA. Fluconazole-induced congenital anomalies in three infants. *Clin Infect Dis* 1996;22:336–340.

141. Esther Lee B, Feinberg M, Abraham JJ, Murthy ARK. Congenital malformation in an infant born to a woman treated with fluconazole. *Pediatr Infect Dis J* 1992;11:1062–1064.

142. Norgaard M, Pedersen L, Gislum M, et al. Maternal use of fluconazole and risk of congenital malformations: A Danish population-based cohort study. *J Antimicrob Chemother* 2008;62:172–176.

143. Pappas PG, Kauffman CA, Perfect J, et al. Alopecia associated with fluconazole therapy. *Am Coll Physicians*; 1995;123:354–357.

144. Gussenhoven MJ, Haak A, Peereboom-Wynia JD, van't Wout JW. Stevens-Johnson syndrome after fluconazole. *Lancet* 1991;338:120.

145. Ahmad SR, Singer SJ, Leissa BG. Congestive heart failure associated with itraconazole. *Lancet* 2001;357:1766–1767.

146. Yu DT, Peterson JF, Rph DLS, Mba WCG, Bates DW. Frequency of potential azole drug–drug interactions and consequences of potential fluconazole drug interactions. *Pharmacoepidemiol Drug Saf* 2005;14:755–767.

147. Herbrecht R, Denning DW, Patterson TF, et al. Voriconazole versus amphotericin B for primary therapy of invasive aspergillosis. *N Engl J Med* 2002;347:408–415.

148. Zonios DI, Gea-Banacloche J, Childs R, Bennett JE. Hallucinations during voriconazole therapy. *Clin Infect Dis* 2008;47:e7–e10.

149. Tan K, Brayshaw N, Tomaszewski K, Troke P, Wood N. Investigation of the potential relationships between plasma voriconazole concentrations and visual adverse events or liver function test abnormalities. *J Clin Pharmacol* 2006;46:235–243.

150. Imhof A, Schaer DJ, Schwarz U, Schanz U. Neurological adverse events to voriconazole: Evidence for therapeutic drug monitoring. *Swiss Med Wkly* 2006;136:739–742.

151. Swift AC, Denning DW. Skull base osteitis following fungal sinusitis. *J Laryngol Otol* 2007;112:92–97.

152. Curigliano G, Formica V, De Pas T, et al. Life-threatening toxic epidermal necrolysis during voriconazole therapy for invasive aspergillosis after chemotherapy. *Ann Oncol* 2006;17:1174–1175.

153. Racette AJ, Roenigk HH, Hansen R, Mendelson D, Park A. Photoaging and phototoxicity from long-term voriconazole treatment in a 15-year-old girl. *Journal of the Am Acad Dermatol* 2005;52:81–85.

154. Vandecasteele S, Wijngaerden E, Peetermans W. Two cases of severe phototoxic reactions related to long-term outpatient treatment with voriconazole. *Eur J Clin Microbiol Infect Dis* 2004;23:656–657.

155. McCarthy KL, Playford EG, Looke DF, Whitby M. Severe photosensitivity causing multifocal squamous cell carcinomas secondary to prolonged voriconazole therapy. *Clin Infect Dis* 2007;44:e55–e56.

156. Anonymous. Voriconazole: Phototoxicity and squamous cell cancer: Case report. *Reactions Weekly* 2008;1200:30.

157. Brunel AS, Fraisse T, Lechiche C, Pinzani V, Mauboussin JM, Sotto A. Multifocal squamous cell carcinomas in an HIV-infected patient with a long-term voriconazole therapy. *AIDS* 2008;22:905–906.

158. Williams K, Mansh M, Chin-Hong P, Singer J, Arron ST. Voriconazole-associated cutaneous malignancy: A literature review on photocarcinogenesis in organ transplant recipients. *Clin Infect Dis* 2014;58:997–1002.

159. Boyd AE, Modi S, Howard SJ, Moore CB, Keevil BG, Denning DW. Adverse reactions to voriconazole. *Clin Infect Dis* 2004;39:1241–1244.

160. Robatel C, Rusca M, Padoin C, Marchetti O, Liaudet L, Buclin T. Disposition of voriconazole during continuous veno-venous haemodiafiltration (CVVHDF) in a single patient. *J Antmicrob Chemother* 2004;54:269–270.

161. Cornely OA, Maertens J, Winston DJ, et al. Posaconazole vs. fluconazole or itraconazole prophylaxis in patients with neutropenia. *N Engl J Med* 2007;356:348–359.

162. Ullmann AJ, Lipton JH, Vesole DH, et al. Posaconazole or fluconazole for prophylaxis in severe graft-versus-host disease. *N Engl J Med* 2007;356:335–347.

163. Maertens JA, Raad, II, Marr KA, et al. Isavuconazole versus voriconazole for primary treatment of invasive mould disease caused by Aspergillus and other filamentous fungi (SECURE): A phase 3, randomised-controlled, non-inferiority trial. *Lancet* 2016;387:760–769.

164. Raad II, Graybill JR, Bustamante AB, et al. Safety of long-term oral posaconazole use in the treatment of refractory invasive fungal infections. *Clin Infect Dis* 2006;42:1726–1734.

165. Niwa T, Shiraga T, Takagi A. Effect of antifungal drugs on cytochrome P450 (CYP) 2C9, CYP2C19, and CYP3A4 activities in human liver microsomes. *Biol Pharm Bull* 2005;28:1805–1808.

166. Wexler D, Courtney R, Richards W, Banfield C, Lim J, Laughlin M. Effect of posaconazole on cytochrome P450 enzymes: A randomized, open-label, two-way crossover study. *EurJ Pharm Sci* 2004;21:645–653.

167. Omar G, Whiting PH, Hawksworth GM, Humphrey MJ, Burke MD. Ketoconazole and fluconazole inhibition of the metabolism of cyclosporin A by human liver in vitro. *Ther Drug Monit* 1997;19:436–445.

168. Townsend R, Dietz A, Hale C, et al. Pharmacokinetic evaluation of CYP3A4-mediated drug-drug interactions of isavuconazole with rifampin, ketoconazole, midazolam, and ethinyl estradiol/norethindrone in healthy adults. *Clin Pharmacol Drug Dev* 2017;6:44–53.

169. Lopez-Gil JA. Fluconazole-cyclosporine interaction: A dose-dependent effect? *Ann Pharmacother* 1993;27:427–430.

170. Venkatakrishnan K, von Moltke LL, Greenblatt DJ. Effects of the antifungal agents on oxidative drug metabolism: Clinical relevance. *Clin Pharmacokinet* 2000;38:111.

171. Toda F, Tanabe K, Ito S, et al. Tacrolimus trough level adjustment after administration of fluconazole to kidney recipients. *Transplant Proc* 2002;34:1733–1735.

172. Sugar AM, Saunders C, Idelson BA, Bernard DB. Interaction of fluconazole and cyclosporine. *Ann Intern Med* 1989;110:844.

173. Slaughter RL. Recent advances: The cytochrome P450 enzymes. *Ann Pharmacother* 1995;29:619–624.

174. Lomaestro BM. Update on drug interactions with azole antifungal agents. *Ann Pharmacother* 1998;32:915–928.

175. Gubbins PO, Amsden JR. Drug-drug interactions of antifungal agents and implications for patient care. *Expert Opin Pharmacother* 2005;6:2231–2243.

176. Nivoix Y, Levêque D, Herbrecht R, Koffel JC, Beretz L, Ubeaud-Sequier G. The enzymatic basis of drug-drug interactions with systemic triazole antifungals. *Clin Pharmacokinet* 2008;47:779–792.

177. Hairhara Y, Makuuchi M, Kawarasaki H, et al. Effect of fluconazole on blood levels of tacrolimus. Transplant Proc 1999;31:2767.

178. Shitrit D, Ollech JE, Ollech A, et al. Itraconazole prophylaxis in lung transplant recipients receiving tacrolimus (FK 506): Efficacy and drug interaction. *J Heart Lung Transplant* 2005;24:2148–2152.

179. Groll AH, Kolve H, Ehlert K, Paulussen M, Vormoor J. Pharmacokinetic interaction between voriconazole and ciclosporin A following allogeneic bone marrow transplantation. *J Antimicrob Chemother;* 2004;53:113–114.

180. Florea NR, Capitano B, Nightingale CH, Hull D, Leitz GJ, Nicolau DP. Beneficial pharmacokinetic interaction between cyclosporine and itraconazole in renal transplant recipients. *Transplant Proc* 2003;35:2873–2877.

181. Dhawan A, Mowat AP, Tredger JM, Gonde CE, North-Lewis PJ, Heaton NJ. Tacrolimus (FK506) malabsorption: Management with fluconazole coadministration. *Transpl Int* 1997;10:331–334.

182. Martin JE, Daoud AJ, Schroeder TJ, Royfirst M. The clinical and economic potential of cyclosporin drug interactions. *PharmacoEconomics* 1999;15:317–337.

183. Varis T, Kivistö KT, Backman JT, Neuvonen PJ. The cytochrome P450 3A4 inhibitor itraconazole markedly increases the plasma concentrations of dexamethasone and enhances its adrenal-suppressant effect. *Clin Pharmacol Toxicol* 2000;68:487–494.

184. Varis T, Kivisto KT, Backman JT, Neuvonen PJ. Itraconazole decreases the clearance and enhances the effects of intravenously administered methylprednisolone in healthy volunteers. *Pharmacol Toxicol* 1999;85:29.

185. Lebrun-Vignes B, Archer VC, Diquet B, et al. Effect of itraconazole on the pharmacokinetics of prednisolone and methylprednisolone and cortisol secretion in healthy subjects. *Br J Clin Pharmacol* 2001;51:443–450.

186. Böhme A, Ganser A, Hoelzer D. Aggravation of vincristine-induced neurotoxicity by itraconazole in the treatment of adult ALL. *Ann Hematol* 1995;71:311–312.

187. Gillies J, Hung KA, Fitzsimons E, Soutar R. Severe vincristine toxicity in combination with itraconazole. *Clin Lab Haematol* 1998;20:123–124.

188. Marr KA, Leisenring W, Crippa F, et al. Cyclophosphamide metabolism is affected by azole antifungals. *Blood* 2004;103:1557–1559.

189. Buggia I, Zecca M, Alessandrino EP, et al. Itraconazole can increase systemic exposure to busulfan in patients given bone marrow transplantation. GITMO (Gruppo Italiano Trapianto di Midollo Osseo). *Anticancer Res* 1996;16:2083–2088.

190. Kantola T, Kivistö KT, Neuvonen PJ. Effect of itraconazole on the pharmacokinetics of atorvastatin. *Clin Pharmacol Ther* 1998;64:58–65.

191. Igel M, Sudhop T, von Bergmann K. Metabolism and drug interactions of 3-hydroxy-3-methylglutaryl coenzyme A-reductase inhibitors (statins). *Eur J Clin Pharamcol* 2001;57:357–364.

192. Guengerich FP, Brian WR, Iwasaki M, Sari MA, Baeaernhielm C, Berntsson P. Oxidation of dihydropyridine calcium channel blockers and analogs by human liver cytochrome P-450 IIIA4. *J Med Chem* 1991;34:1838–1844.

193. Indiana University Department of Medicine. Cytochrome P450 Drug Interaction Table. (Accessed January 10, 2018, at www.medicine.iupui.edu/flockhart/table.htm.)

194. Geist MJP, Egerer G, Burhenne J, Riedel KD, Mikus G. Induction of Voriconazole Metabolism by Rifampin in a Patient with Acute Myeloid Leukemia: Importance of Interdisciplinary Communication To Prevent Treatment Errors with Complex Medications? *Antimicrobial Agent and Chemother* 2007;51:3455–3456.

195. Todd JR, Arigala MR, Penn RL, King JW. Possible clinically significant interaction of itraconazole plus rifampin. *AIDS patient care STDs* 2001;15:505–510.

196. Jaruratanasirikul S, Sriwiriyajan S. Effect of rifampicin on the pharmacokinetics of itraconazole in normal volunteers and AIDS patients. *Eur J Clin Pharmacol* 1998;54:155–158.

197. Drayton J, Dickinson G, Rinaldi MG. Coadministration of rifampin and itraconazole leads to undetectable levelsof serum itraconazole. *Clin Infect Dis* 1994;18:266.

198. Purkins L, Wood N, Ghahramani P, Love ER, Eve MD, Fielding A. Coadministration of voriconazole and phenytoin: Pharmacokinetic interaction, safety, and toleration. *Br J Clin Pharmacol* 2003;56:37–44.

199. Ducharme MP, Slaughter RL, Warbasse LH, et al. Itraconazole and hydroxyitraconazole serum concentrations are reduced more than tenfold by phenytoin. *Clin Pharmacol Ther* 1995;58:617–624.

200. Bonay M, Jonville-Bera AP, Diot P, Lemarie E, Lavandier M, Autret E. Possible interaction between phenobarbital, carbamazepine and itraconazole. *Drug Saf* 1993;9:309–311.

201. Jeong S, Nguyen PD, Desta Z. Comprehensive in vitro inhibition analysis of 8 cytochrome P450 (CYP) enzymes by voriconazole: Major effect on CYPs 2B6, 2C9, 2C19 and 3A. *Antimicrob Agent Chemother* 2009;53:541–551.

202. Purkins L, Wood N, Kleinermans D, Nichols D. Voriconazole potentiates warfarin-induced prothrombin time prolongation. *Br J Clin Pharmacol* 2003;56:24–29.

203. Hervé EA, Tillement JP. Systemic antifungal agents: Drug interactions of clinical significance. *Drug Saf* 1998;18:83–97.

204. Kunze KL, Wienkers LC, Thummel KE, Trager WF. Warfarin-fluconazole. I. Inhibition of the human cytochrome P450-dependent metabolism of warfarin by fluconazole: In vitro studies. *Drug Metab Dispos* 1996;24:414–421.

205. Wood N, Tan K, Purkins L, et al. Effect of omeprazole on the steady-state pharmacokinetics of voriconazole. *Br J Clin Pharmacol* 2003;56:56–61.

206. Krishna G, Sansone-Parsons A, Kantesaria B. Drug interaction assessment following concomitant administration of posaconazole and phenytoin in healthy men. *Curr Med Res Opin* 2007;23:1415–1422.

207. Krishna G, Parsons A, Kantesaria B, Mant T. Evaluation of the pharmacokinetics of posaconazole and rifabutin following co-administration to healthy men. *Curr Med Res Opin* 2007;23:545–552.

208. Yamazaki T, Desai A, Goldwater R, et al. Pharmacokinetic interactions between isavuconazole and the drug transporter substrates atorvastatin, digoxin, metformin, and methotrexate in healthy subjects. *Clin Pharmacol Drug Dev* 2017;6:66–75.

209. Sachs MK, Blanchard LM, Green PJ. Interaction of itraconazole and digoxin. *Clin Infect Dis* 1993;16:400–403.

210. Partanen J, Jalava KM, Neuvonen PJ. Itraconazole increases serum digoxin concentration. *Pharmacol Toxicol* 1996;79:274–276.

211. Jalava KM, Partanen J, Neuvonen PJ. Itraconazole decreases renal clearance of digoxin. *Ther Drug Monit* 1997;19:609–613.

212. Alderman CP. Digoxin-itraconazole interaction: Possible mechanisms. *Ann Pharmacother* 1997;31:438–440.

213. Angirasa AK, Koch AZ. P-glycoprotein as the mediator of itraconazole-digoxin interaction. *Am Podiatric Med Assoc;* 2002;92:471–472.

214. Purkins L, Wood N, Kleinermans D, Nichols D. Voriconazole does not affect the steady-state pharmacokinetics of digoxin. *Br J Clin Pharmacol* 2003;56:45–50.

215. Andes D, Pascual A, Marchetti O. Antifungal therapeutic drug monitoring: established and emerging indications? *Antimicrob Agent Chemother* 2009;53:24–34.

216. Ashbee HR, Barnes RA, Johnson EM, Richardson MD, Gorton R, Hope WW. Therapeutic drug monitoring (TDM) of antifungal agents: Guidelines from the British Society for Medical Mycology. *J Antimicrob Chemother* 2014;69:1162–1176.

217. Rex JH, Pfaller MA, Galgiani JN, et al. Development of interpretive breakpoints for antifungal susceptibility testing: Conceptual framework and analysis of in vitro-in vivo correlation data for fluconazole, itraconazole, and *Candida* infections. Subcommittee on Antifungal Susceptibility Testing of the National Committee for Clinical Laboratory Standards. *Clin Infect Dis* 1997;24:235–247.

218. Patterson TF, Thompson GR3rd, Denning DW, et al. Practice guidelines for the diagnosis and management of aspergillosis: 2016 update by the Infectious Diseases Society of America. *Clin Infect Dis* 2016;15:e1–e60.

219. Wheat J, Freifeld AG, Kleiman MB, et al. Clincial practice guidelines for the management of patients with histoplasmosis: 2007 update by the Infectious Diseases Society of America. *Clin Infect Dis* 2007;45:807–825.

220. Chapman SW, DIsmukes WE, Proia LA. Practice guidelines for the management of patients with blastomycosis. *Clin Infect Dis* 2008;63:112–146.

221. Cartledge JD. Itraconazole solution: Higher serum drug concentrations and better clinical response rates than the capsule formulation in acquired immunodeficiency syndrome patients with candidosis. *J Clin Pathol* 1997;50:477–480.

222. Denning DW, Tucker RM, Hanson LH. Treatment of invasive aspergillosis with itraconazole. *Am J Med* 1989;86:791–800.

223. Denning DW, Tucker RM, Hanson LH, Hamilton JR, Stevens DA. Itraconazole therapy for cryptococcal meningitis and cryptococcosis. *Arch Intern Med* 1989;149:2301–2308.

224. Poirier M, Cheymol G. Optimisation of itraconazole therapy using target drug concentrations. *Clinical Pharmacokinet* 1998;35:461–473.

225. Glasmacher A, Hahn C, Molitor E, Marklein G, Sauerbruch T, Schmidt-Wolf IGH. Itraconazole trough concentrations in antifungal prophylaxis with six different dosing regimens using hydroxypropyl-ß-cyclodextrin oral solution or coated-pellet capsules. *Mycoses* 1999;42:591–600.

226. Glasmacher A, Hahn C, Leutner C, et al. Breakthrough invasive fungal infections in neutropenic patients after prophylaxis with itraconazole. *Mycoses* 1999;42:443–451.

227. Hostetler JS, Heykants J, Clemons KV, Woestenborghs R, Hanson LH, Stevens DA. Discrepancies in bioassay and chromatography determinations explained by metabolism of itraconazole to hydroxyitraconazole: Studies of interpatient variations in concentrations. *Antimicrob Agent Chemother* 1993;37:2224–2227.

228. Lutsar I, Hodges MR, Tomaszewski K, Troke PF, Wood ND. Safety of voriconazole and dose individualization. *Clin Infect Dis* 2003;36:1087–1088.

229. Smith J, Safdar N, Knasinski V, et al. Voriconazole therapeutic drug monitoring. *Antimicrob Agent Chemother* 2006;50:1570–1572.

230. Pascual A, Calandra T, Bolay S, Buclin T, Bille J, Marchetti O. Voriconazole therapeutic drug monitoring in patients with invasive mycoses improves efficacy and safety outcomes. *Clin Infect Dis* 2008;46:201–211.

231. Trifilio S, Ortiz R, Pennick G, et al. Voriconazole therapeutic drug monitoring in allogeneic hematopoietic stem cell transplant recipients. *Bone Marrow Transplant* 2005;35:509–513.

232. Trifilio S, Pennick G, Pi J, et al. Monitoring plasma voriconazole levels may be necessary to avoid subtherapeutic levels in hematopoietic stem cell transplant recipients. *Cancer* 2007;109:1532–1535.

233. Walsh TJ, Raad I, Patterson TF, et al. Treatment of invasive aspergillosis with posaconazole in patients who are refractory to or intolerant of conventional therapy: An externally controlled trial. *Clin Infect Dis* 2007;44:2–12.

234. Desai AV, Kovanda LL, Hope WW, et al. Exposure-response relationships for isavuconazole in patients with invasive aspergillosis and other filamentous fungi. *Antimicrob Agents Chemother* 2017;61:e01034.

13

Echinocandins for prevention and treatment of invasive fungal infections

MELISSA D. JOHNSON, JOHN MOHR, AND AHMAD MOURAD

INTRODUCTION

Echinocandins are the most recent addition to the antifungal armamentarium, with a unique mechanism of action. There are currently three echinocandin antifungal agents in clinical use: caspofungin, micafungin, and anidulafungin. These agents block fungal cell wall synthesis through inhibition of (1,3)-beta-D-glucan synthase, resulting in fungicidal effects against *Candida* spp. and fungistatic effects against *Aspergillus* spp. Echinocandins have also been shown to have some activity, alone or in combination with other agents, against a variety of other fungal pathogens. Several clinical trials have evaluated performance of echinocandins in the setting of oropharyngeal/esophageal candidiasis and invasive candidiasis. Others have reported experience with echinocandins as salvage therapy for invasive aspergillosis, and case reports describe efficacy of these agents in the treatment of a variety of other fungal infections. In general, echinocandins have become preferred agents in the hospital setting for invasive candidiasis because of broad activity against non-albicans *Candida* as well as *Candida albicans* infections, while having an excellent safety profile and relative lack of drug interactions. Since they are available only in intravenous form, their use is limited in patients where oral antifungal therapy is preferable.

CHEMICAL STRUCTURE AND FORMULATIONS

Structurally, echinocandins are all large lipoprotein molecules containing an amphiphilic cyclic hexapeptide. All three echinocandins have a unique *N*-linked acyl lipid side chain, which imparts different physicochemical properties to each agent [1,2]. Caspofungin was derived from *Glarea lozoyensis*, while micafungin and anidulafungin are fermentation by-products of the fungi *Coleophoma empetri* F-11899 and *Aspergillus nidulans*, respectively [2–5]. Owing to their lipophilicity and large size, echinocandins have low bioavailability and, therefore, are only available for parenteral (intravenous) delivery. With its fatty acid side chain, caspofungin is soluble in water. Similarly, micafungin is soluble in water due to it complex aromatic side chain. In contrast, anidulafungin is insoluble in water due to its alcoxytriphenyl side chain. Both caspofungin and anidulafungin are somewhat soluble in ethanol, but micafungin is not. Therefore, reconstitution of vials containing echinocandin must be done carefully, according to the manufacturers specific instructions (Table 13.1).

MECHANISM OF ACTION

Echinocandins exert their antifungal effects by inhibiting the synthesis of (1,3)-beta-D-glucan, an integral component of the fungal cell wall [6]. 13-(1,3)-D-Glucan is a major component of the cell wall of many fungi, along with other cell wall components including (1,6)-beta-D-glucan, chitin, galactomannan, and various glycoproteins. The effects of echinocandins result in decreased (1,3)-beta-D-glucan production, loss of cell integrity, and eventually cell lysis [6].

SPECTRUM OF ACTIVITY

Echinocandins have antifungal activity against the most common yeasts and molds, although these agents generally lack activity as single agents against *Cryptococcus neoformans* and *Zygomycetes*. Because of their mechanism of action, beta-glucan content of the specific fungus may affect activity of echinocandins against individual fungal species [7]. Echinocandins have fungicidal activity against *Candida* spp. and fungistatic activity against many invasive molds [8–14] (Tables 13.2 and 13.3). In 2008, the Clinical and Laboratory Standards Institute (CLSI) recommended that *Candida* spp. with minimum inhibitory concentrations (MICs) ≤ 2 μg/mL are considered susceptible to echinocandins [15]. The recommendations were updated in 2012 to include new drug and species-specific clinical breakpoints [16]. Except for *Candida parapsilosis* and *Candida guilliermondii*, the breakpoints

Table 13.1 Dosing, chemical, and pharmacological properties of echinocandin formulations

	Caspofungin	Micafungin	Anidulafungin
Brand Name	Cancidas	Mycamine	Eraxis
Relative Molecular Weight	1213.42	1292.26	1140.3
Origin	*Glarea lozovensis*	*Coleophoma empetri*	*Aspergillus nidulans*
FDA-approved Dose			
Adults			
Candidemia/invasive candidiasis	70 mg IV loading dose followed by 50 mg IV daily	100 mg IV daily	200 mg IV loading dose followed by 100 mg IV daily
Esophageal candidiasis	50 mg IV daily	150 mg IV daily	100 mg IV loading dose followed by 50 mg IV daily
Children			
Age	3 months to 17 years	≥ 4 months	
Candidemia, acute disseminated candidiasis, *Candida peritonitis* and abscesses	70 mg/m² IV loading dose followed by 50 mg/m² IV daily up to 70 mg daily maximum	2 mg/kg IV daily not to exceed 100 mg/day	
Esophageal candidiasis		≤ 30 kg: 3 mg/kg IV daily >30 kg: 2.5 mg/kg IV daily not to exceed 150 mg/day	
Prophylaxis of *Candida* infections in HSCT recipients		1 mg/kg IV daily not to exceed 50 mg/day	

(Continued)

Table 13.1 (*Continued*) Dosing, chemical, and pharmacological properties of echinocandin formulations

	Caspofungin	Micafungin	Anidulafungin
Other FDA-approved Indications	Invasive Aspergillosis (intolerant/refractory to other therapies), and empirical therapy in febrile neutropenics: 70 mg IV loading dose followed by 50 mg IV daily	Prophylaxis in HSCT recipients: 50 mg IV daily	
Reconstitution	Any of the following: 1. 0.9% Sodium chloride injection 2. Sterile water for injection 3. Bacteriostatic water for injection with methylparaben and propylparaben 4. Bacteriostatic water for injection with 0.9% benzyl alcohol	0.9% Sodium chloride injection, USP Alternative: 5% Dextrose injection	Sterile water for Injection only
Dilution	0.9%, 0.45%, or 0.225% Sodium chloride injection or lactated ringers injection	0.9% Sodium chloride injection or 5% dextrose injection	0.9% Sodium chloride injection USP (normal saline) or 5% dextrose injection
Duration of infusion/ Infusion Rate	One hour	One hour	Rate not to exceed 1.1 mg/min

Source: Wagner, C. et al., *Pharmacology*, 78, 161–177, 2006; Astellas Pharma US. *Mycamine (micafungin) [Prescribing Information]*, Astellas Pharma US, Deerfield, IL, 2013; Pfizer & Co. *Eraxis (anidulafungin) [Prescribing Information]*, Pfizer & Co., New York, 2006; Merck & Co. *Cancidas (caspofungin) [Prescribing Information]*, Merck & Co., Whitehouse Station, NJ, 2008.

Table 13.2 MIC_{90} of 1846 invasive *Candida* spp. from global surveillance (2013)

Organism (number of isolates tested)	MIC/MEC$_{90}$ µg/mL		
	Caspofungin	Micafungin	Anidulafungin
C. albicans (712)	0.03	0.03	0.06
C. parapsilosis (215)	0.5	2	2
C. glabrata (251)	0.06	0.03	0.12
C. tropicalis (155)	0.03	0.06	0.03
C. krusei (49)	0.25	0.12	0.06
C. dubliniensis (32)	0.12	0.06	0.06
C. lusitaniae (24)	0.5	0.25	0.5
C. guillermondii (16)	1	1	4
C. orthopsilosis (16)	0.25	1	1

Source: Castanheira, M. et al., *Diagn. Microbiol. Infect. Dis.*, 85, 200–204, 2016.

Table 13.3 Comparative MEC_{90} values for *Aspergillus* spp.

Organism (number of isolates tested)	Median MIC/MEC$_{90}$ µg/mL		
	Caspofungin	Micafungin	Anidulafungin
A. fumigatus (142)	0.03	0.03	0.03
A. section Nigri (23)	0.06	0.03	≤0.008
A. section Flavi (22)	0.03	0.015	≤0.008

Source: Castanheira, M. et al., *Diagn. Microbiol. Infect. Dis.*, 85, 200–204, 2016.

Table 13.4 CLSI Clinical breakpoints for echinocandin resistance

Antifungal	Clinical Breakpoints (µg/ml)				
	C. albicans	C. glabrata	C. tropicalis	C. krusei	C. parapsilosis
Caspofungin					
Previous	≥4	≥4	≥4	≥4	≥4
Revised	>1	>0.5	>1	>1	>8
Micafungin					
Previous	≥4	≥4	≥4	≥4	≥4
Revised	≥1	≥0.25	≥1	≥1	≥8
Anidulafungin					
Previous	≥4	≥4	≥4	≥4	≥4
Revised	≥1	≥0.5	≥1	≥1	≥8

Source: Fothergill, A.W. et al., J. Clin. Microbiol., 52, 994–997, 2014.

were lowered from previous recommendations (Table 13.4). As a result, resistance was seen to increase for most *Candida* spp. isolates, most notably *C. glabrata* [17].

The guidelines also recommend performing the MIC determination for echinocandins after 24 hours of incubation [18]. In an *in vitro* comparison of more than 5000 *Candida* isolates collected from patients with invasive *Candida* infections at 91 medical centers from 2001 to 2006, the majority of *Candida* isolates demonstrated MICs ≤2 µg/mL to all three echinocandins with no change in susceptibility observed over the six-year observation period (Table 13.2) [8]. Six of the isolates tested had MIC >4 µg/mL: *C. guillermondii* (three isolates with caspofungin MIC ≥8 µg/mL), *C. glabrata* (one isolate with caspofungin MIC ≥8 µg/mL), *C. tropicalis* (one isolate with caspofungin MIC ≥8 µg/mL), and *C. rugosa* (one isolate with anidulafungin MIC ≥8 µg/mL).

In many studies, the MIC90 for *C. parapsilosis* for all the echinocandins has been 2 µg/mL, which is at the breakpoint of susceptibility [19,20]. The clinical relevance of this finding among patients with invasive *Candida* spp. infections is not known. A naturally occurring proline-to-alanine substitution in the region of *FKS1p* may explain the higher MICs observed with *C. parapsilosis* and echinocandins [21]. *Candida auris* has recently emerged as a new global nosocomial pathogen with resistance to antifungals, including echinocandins. The number of isolates resistant to echinocandins remains relatively low (~7%) compared to those resistant to some of the azoles (~93%) and amphotericin B (~35%). As such, the first line for therapy remains echinocandins, given a susceptibility panel is performed as soon as possible [22].

The *in vitro* activity of echinocandins against dimorphic fungi, such as *Histoplasma, capsulatum, Blastomyces dermatitidis,* and *C. occidiodes immitis/posadasii,* has been variable and it is not clear if this translates to clinical efficacy. Caspofungin MICs of 0.5–8 µg/mL for *B. dermatitidis* and 0.5–4 µg/mL for *H. capsulatum* have been reported [23]. Anidulafungin MICs of 2–8 µg/mL have been reported for *B. dermatitidis* and 2–4 µg/mL for *H. capsulatum*, respectively [23]. The wide range and variability of the MICs could be attributed to the

different fungal forms. The antifungal effect of echinocandins on yeast forms of fungal species, such as histoplasma, can differ greatly from its effects on hyphal forms [24]. Recent studies exploring the use of echinocandins against *Coccidioides* spp. have shown that they do have variable activity with MIC90 at 8, 0.25, and 0.125 µg/mL for caspofungin, anidulafungin and micafungin respectively [25].

Activity of echinocandins against *Trichosporon* spp. has not been investigated extensively but may be insufficient; cases of breakthrough infections with this species have been reported [23,26–28]. Activity of echinocandins against mold species has been described in several *in vitro* studies [12,29,30]. Minimum effective concentration (MEC) is the lowest concentration of drug that produces growth of small, rounded, compact hyphal forms of the organism and has shown to have better reproducibility than MIC testing for echinocandins against molds [31]. MECs have not been correlated with clinical outcome in studies to date, and breakpoints for susceptibility or resistance have not been approved by CLSI for *in vitro* testing of mold species. MECs for most echinocandins against *Aspergillus* spp. are generally ≤1 µg/mL. In one study, *A. versicolor* was found to have slightly higher MICs to caspofungin (MIC90 = 0.12 µg/mL, range: 0.015–4 µg/mL) and approximately 90% of strains were inhibited at an MEC of ≤1 µg/mL [12]. In other studies, anidulafungin and micafungin have been found to have similar *in vitro* activity against *Aspergillus* spp. with MIC90s of <0.03 µg/mL [29,30]. Other molds including *Scedosporium apiospermum, Lomentospora prolificans, Exophiala jeanselmei,* and *Fonsecaea pedrosoi* may be inhibited by echinocandins, but extensive incubation periods have sometimes been used to demonstrate this activity [32]. Appreciable *in vitro* activity of echinocandins against *Cryptococcus neoformans, Fusarium* spp., *Rhizopus* spp., or *Mucor* spp. as single agents has not been demonstrated [33].

There has been some animal data suggesting that echinocandins have antifungal activity against *Pneumocystis* pneumonia (PCP), specifically the cyst forms. Rodent models have shown that therapeutic and prophylactic echinocandins significantly reduced the cyst forms of PCP but spared the trophic forms [34]. There has also been a case report of combining caspofungin with clindamycin for the successful treatment of a patient with PCP who was intolerant to TMP/SMX [35]. New drugs in development, such as rezafungin (CD-101), may provide this extended spectrum of activity to be used against PCP in the future [36]. More studies are needed to make substantial conclusions about the use of echinocandins for PCP.

MECHANISM OF RESISTANCE

Recent reports have documented isolates with higher MICs to echinocandins, and mechanisms by which these isolates may be echinocandin resistant. Generally, *Candida* isolates with higher MICs in patients failing caspofungin, micafungin, or anidulafungin therapy have had mutations in the *FKS1* and *FKS2* genes [37–43]. A recent investigation also highlighted apparent differences in susceptibility between echinocandins among *C. parapsilosis* in an outbreak situation in a burn unit [44]. However, these differences in susceptibility were not due to differences in *FKS1* gene mutations. In another study, isolates from other patients failing caspofungin with MICs of 0.5–1 μg/mL were found to have upregulation of cell wall integrity pathway genes and increases in the minimum fungicidal activity without changes in FKS genes [45]. A study evaluating echinocandin resistance in *Candida glabrata* found that the proportion of resistant isolates increased between 2001 and 2010. Eighty percent of patients with an FKS mutant isolate that had intermediate or resistant MICs to echinocandins failed to respond to therapy or had recurrence [46]. Prior echinocandin therapy was shown to be a predictor of having an FKS mutant isolate [46]. There are other reports of clinical failures due to isolates with reduced susceptibility to echinocandins, suggesting that other unknown mechanisms may also contribute to echinocandin resistance [47]. The mechanisms of *Candida auris* resistance are still unclear but whole genome sequencing has revealed single copies of *FKS1, 2* and *3* [48].

A paradoxical effect of fungal organisms with regrowth at high echinocandin concentrations has been reported in several *in vitro* investigations, and further complicates the study of echinocandin resistance [49]. In the presence of high concentrations of echinocandin, it has been suggested that resistance mechanisms among *Candida* and *Aspergillus* spp. are derepressed. The majority of reports have occurred with caspofungin, but one recent paper also observed these effects with micafungin and anidulafungin against certain isolates [49–54]. These concentrations are much higher than those typically achieved with human doses, and notably these *in vitro* findings have not been consistently replicated in animal models [55]. This effect was also not apparent in clinical studies of invasive candidiasis [52,56–58]. One study suggests that high concentrations of echinocandins restore the enzyme β-1,3-glucan synthase, possibly by recruiting chaperone proteins [59]. Based on these data, additional studies are needed to further elucidate the clinical and microbiologic significance of the paradoxical effect reported with echinocandins.

PHARMACOKINETICS

The pharmacokinetics of echinocandins have been described in both animal models and humans. All present echinocandins have limited oral bioavailability. Thus, they are only available as a therapeutic solution for parenteral administration.

Caspofungin

Caspofungin is extensively bound to albumin in serum (approximately 97%), with rapid distribution into tissues after intravenous dosing in humans [5,60,61]. It has a relatively low volume of distribution (9.67 L after a single 70 mg dose in healthy adults) [61]. Caspofungin exhibits triphasic elimination from plasma, with a short a-phase following infusion ($t_{1/2}$ 1–2 hours), and then a beta-phase 6–48 hours post-dose ($t_{1/2}$ 9–11 hours) that accounts for most of the plasma clearance. The third or gamma phase has a half-life of 40–50 hours [61]. Administration of a 70-mg loading dose followed by 50 mg intravenously, typically, results in serum concentrations exceeding 1 μg/mL. Caspofungin is metabolized to inactive metabolites by hydrolysis and N-acetylation [62]. It is also spontaneously degraded to a ring-opened peptide compound called L-747969 [5]. Inactive caspofungin metabolites are then excreted in urine (41%) and feces (35%) [62,63]. However, a very small amount of active, unchanged drug is excreted in bile (<1%) or urine (1.4%). It is important to note that urine caspofungin concentrations are minimal, and since it lacks active metabolites its clinical utility in treating urinary infections with *Candida* spp. might be compromised. However, it has been effective in isolated cases of candiduria [64].

Results of four different pharmacokinetic studies using various doses of caspofungin on a single- and multiple-dose basis were published in one paper [61]. In one study, pharmacokinetics of caspofungin was compared for healthy men receiving 50 mg IV daily or a loading dose of 70 mg IV followed by 50 mg daily IV for 14 days total. Serum concentrations at the end of a 1-hour infusion and at 24 hours were higher for the loading dose group on day 1 (trough concentration 1 hour postdosing [C_{1h}] 7.64 and 12.09 μg/mL, trough concentration 24 hours postdosing [C_{24h}] 0.76 and 1.41 μg/mL), and this finding indicated that a loading dose is necessary to achieve an inhibitory target concentration over 24 hours of 1 μg/mL, which is predicted to be effective against most *Candida* species. After 14 days of dosing, the differences between those who had received a loading dose and the nonloading dose group were less pronounced, with C_{1h} approximately 9 μg/mL and C_{24h} approximately 1.7 μg/mL. Caspofungin doses of 70 mg daily for 14 or 21 days resulted in higher serum concentrations at the end of infusion (approximately 15 μg/mL) and higher concentrations 24 hours after the dose (approximately 2.5 μg/mL) [61]. Day 21 to Day 14 ratios for $AUC_{0–24h}$ (area under the time-concentration profile), C_{1h}, and C_{24h} indicated that there was also accumulation of serum concentrations between 14 and 21 days of dosing. This suggests that steady-state was not reached by day 14, but subjects were approaching steady-state by the third week of dosing [61].

Micafungin

Like other echinocandins, micafungin is extensively bound to proteins in serum, primarily albumin and to a lesser extent alpha acid glycoprotein. In animals, micafungin has also been shown to bind high-density lipoprotein (HDL) and gamma globulin [65]. Following doses of 50–150 mg/day, micafungin exhibits linear pharmacokinetics with dose-proportional increases in serum concentrations. Single doses of 100 or 150 mg result in trough concentrations of 2 and 2.5 µg/mL, respectively. Steady-state concentrations typically are achieved after 4 days of intravenous dosing. Micafungin undergoes ring opening and liver metabolism to three metabolites: M1, M2, and M5. M1 undergoes arylsulfatase transformation to a catechol form, which is then transformed by catechol-o-methyltransferase to a methoxy form (M2). M5 is a minor metabolite and is the result of $Cyp450$ hydroxylation of micafungin's side chain. Like other echinocandins, <1% of unchanged drug is excreted in urine. Fecal excretion is the primary route of elimination, with 71% of the dose eliminated as parent drug and metabolites 28 days after dosing.

A population pharmacokinetic analysis based on a range of doses from 12.5 to 200 mg micafungin daily in adult hematopoietic stem cell transplant recipients (HSCT) suggested that body weight significantly impacted micafungin AUC [66]. The investigators estimated that patients weighing ≥66.3 or <66.3 kg would have AUC_{0-24h} of 81 or 121 mg·h/L, respectively. Doses of 150 mg daily would be necessary in those weighing ≥66.3 kg to achieve exposures similar to that observed after 100 mg doses among lower-weight adults. One study suggests that when weight increases to above 66 kg, the systemic clearance of micafungin increases by a measurable factor and continues to increase with weight with no observable plateau This suggests that obese patients may require adjusted dosing [67].

Anidulafungin

Anidulafungin is highly protein bound (>99%) and has a larger apparent volume of distribution (30–50 L) and somewhat longer half-life (26–40 hours) than the other echinocandins (Table 13.5). This echinocandin is also unique in that it is not metabolized in the liver, but rather undergoes chemical degradation to inactive open-ring products. Less than 10% of the drug is excreted unchanged in feces [68].

Doses of 100 mg once daily, following a loading dose of 200 mg intravenously result in trough concentrations of 2.5 µg/mL on day 1. Population pharmacokinetics have been determined for anidulafungin on the basis of combined data from four Phase II/III clinical trials receiving 50–100 mg of anidulafungin daily [69,70].

Overall, pharmacokinetic parameters in infected patients were similar to that previously reported among healthy volunteers. Drug clearance was faster among males and those with increased body weight, but only explained a small proportion (20%) of intersubject variability observed with anidulafungin. In addition, both males and females with invasive candidiasis appeared to have approximately 30% faster clearance than subjects with oropharyngeal/esophageal candidiasis or invasive aspergillosis. Body weight also explained a small amount of variability in volume of distribution observed among study subjects, but overall body weight is not currently recommended as a consideration when dosing anidulafungin in adults.

Tissue concentrations

Substantial data describing tissue concentrations of echinocandins have emerged from both animal models and human investigations (Table 13.6). In animal models, echinocandins

Table 13.5 Comparative pharmacokinetics of echinocandins in adults

	Caspofungin	Micafungin	Anidulafungin
Steady state C_{max} (range) (µg/mL)	12 (11–13)	10 (SD ± 4.4)	9 (% CV 16)
Steady state AUC_{0-24} (µg · h/mL)	101 (range 88–115)	97 (SD ± 29)	112 (% CV 24.9)
$t_{1/2}$ 13 (h)	11 (SD ± 1.1)	11–17	36(69)–52 (% CV 12)
Clearance (mL/min)	10–13	11	0.94–0.99 L/h (SD ± 0.1)
Vd (L/kg)	0.15	0.2	0.5
Half-life in hepatic impairment (h ± SD)	Prolonged	14 (± 0.8)	Mild: 34 (± 2.5) Moderate: 42 (± 8.6) Severe: 35 (± 7)
Half-life in severe renal impairment (h ± SD)	NA	14 (± 1.5)	33–39 (± 5–7)
Protein binding (%)	96	99.8	>99
Urine concentration (% of plasma)	1.4	<1	<1
CSF concentration	Low	Low	Low

Source: Azuma, J. et al., *Jap. J. Chemother.*, 50, 148–154, 2002; Mochizuki, N. et al., *Transplant Proc.*, 38, 3649–3650, 2006; Azuma, J. et al., Phase 1 study of FK463, a new antifungal agent, in healthy adult male volunteers, *38th International Conference on Antimicrobial Agents and Chemotherapy*, American Society of Microbiology, Washington, DC, 1998; Mukai, T. et al., Pharmacokinetics of FK463, a novel echinocandin analogue, in elderly and non-elderly subjects, *41st International Conference on Antimicrobial Agents and Chemotherapy*, American Society of Microbiology, Washington, DC, 2001; Hiemenz, J. et al., *Antimicrob. Agents Chemother.*, 49, 1331–1336, 2005; Chandrasekar, P.H. and Sobel, J.D., *Clin. Infect. Dis.*, 42, 1171–1178, 2006.

Table 13.6 Concentration of echinocandins in tissues and body fluids relative to plasma concentration

| | Eye | | | Skin | Heart | | | | Bone | Brain | | Lung | | | | |
	Aqueous	Vitreous	Cornea	Tissue	Tissue	Liver	Pancreas	Kidney	Tissue	Tissue	CSF	Tissue	Alveolar cells	Epithelial lining fluid	Spleen	Muscle
Anidulafungin	-[a]	-[a]		+[a]	+[a]	+[a]		+[a]	+[a]	-[a]	+[a]	+[a]/++[a]	++[b]	-[b]	-[a]/++[a]	
Caspofungin	-[b]/+[a]	-[b]	++[a]		++[a]	++[a]		++[a]		-[a]	-[b]	-[a]	++[b]		-[a]	-[a]
Micafungin	-[a]	-[a]	-[b]			-[a]/+[a]	-[b]	-[a]/+[a]		-[b]	-[b]/+[b]	-[a]/+[a]	+[b]	-[b]	-[a]	-[a]

Source: Felton, T. et al., Clin. Microbiol. Rev., 27, 68–88, 2014.

-; Below level of detection to ≤0.5 times the plasma concentration of the echinocandin

+; >0.5 to ≤5 times the plasma concentration of the echinocandin

++; >5 times the plasma concentration of the echinocandin

blank; no data

[a] Data based on animal studies

[b] Data based on human studies

-/-; variable data

had the highest ratio of tissue-to-plasma concentrations in the liver, lungs, and kidneys. After intraperitoneal administration in murine models (60), caspofungin had the highest ratio of tissue-to-plasma concentrations in the liver (16), followed by kidneys (2.9), large intestine (2), small intestine (1.3), lungs (1.1), and spleen (1). In this model, caspofungin had little penetration into heart (0.3), thigh (0.2), and brain (0.1) tissue. In rats, micafungin had the highest concentrations in lung, kidney, and liver with tissue:plasma ratios of 3.6, 3.2, and 7.8, respectively, after 1 mg/kg of nonradiolabeled drug [71]. Micafungin was shown to achieve concentrations in the retina-choroid similar to plasma in rabbits, but the drug could not be detected in vitreous humor [72]. In a rabbit model of *C. albicans* hematogenous meningoencephalitis, micafungin was found in highest concentrations in the meninges and choroid but had low and variable concentrations in the cerebrospinal fluid (CSF) [73]. This suggested that high doses may be necessary to achieve therapeutic concentrations in the central nervous symptoms (CNS) [73]. CSF concentrations of micafungin were measured clinically in a patient receiving treatment for CNS aspergillosis. CSF:plasma concentration ratio was 0.2%–0.05%, despite a dose of 300 mg daily. The patient responded clinically; however, suggesting that tissue concentrations rather than CSF may be an important factor in treating these infections.

Administration of a single intravenous dose of 5 mg/kg of radiolabeled anidulafungin in rats resulted in the highest tissue-to-plasma concentrations in liver [12.4], lung [10.4], kidney [10.7], and spleen [9.2] [74]. Anidulafungin had little to no measurable concentrations in CSF, brain tissue, or the eye.

Although human studies and case reports are scarce some have shown the extent of tissue penetration of the echinocandins. Anidulafungin in the lungs of healthy adults predominantly concentrated in the alveolar macrophages but did remain above MIC90 for *Aspergillus* species for up to 24 hours after administration in the epithelial lining fluid (ELF) and alveolar macrophages at a dose of 200 mg on day 1 followed by 100 mg a day for 3 days, in combination with voriconazole [75]. However, in a patient with *Candida empyema*, the AUC_{0-T} ratio of anidulafungin in concentration in the pleural fluid to serum concentration was only 12.5% [76].

Caspofungin ocular penetration is poor with case reports describing undetectable to very low intraocular levels (6% of plasma concentration) in patients with fungal endophthalmitis [77,78]. Furthermore, a report of caspofungin used to treat fungal meningitis described poor CSF penetration with undetectable levels after 22 days of therapy [79]. However, caspofungin has excellent lung penetration with high levels (more than five times the plasma concentration) being reported in the alveolar cells of a lung transplant patient receiving therapy for suspected pulmonary aspergillosis [80].

Micafungin has excellent penetration into the cellular components of the lung with more than 100% of plasma concentration depositing in alveolar macrophages of healthy volunteers. However, only 5% of plasma concentration was detected in the ELF [81]. In adult lung transplant patients, a single 150 mg dose of micafungin was enough to achieve levels above MIC_{90} of *Aspergillus fumigatus* in alveolar macrophages and ELF for 24 hours [82]. Reports suggest that micafungin has poor penetration into the CNS, with tissue concentrations at the lower limit of detection (0.05 μg/ml) and CSF concentrations ranging from 0.05% to 0.2% of plasma concentration [83,84].

PHARMACOKINETICS IN SPECIAL POPULATIONS

The pharmacokinetics of echinocandins have also been reported among special populations including elderly patients [85,86], women [87], adults with renal or hepatic insufficiency, intensive care unit (ICU) patients, and children [88].

Elderly

Pharmacokinetics of caspofungin and micafungin has been studied in elderly subjects, and were similar to nonelderly adults [85,86]. With caspofungin dosing, six elderly men and six elderly women (67–77 years of age) with creatinine clearances ≥60 mL/min had slightly higher serum concentrations of caspofungin at 1 hour and 24 hours after infusion compared to young men (aged 24–44 years) [86]. Mean AUC_{0-24h} was higher among elderly men (28% greater) and women (18% greater), but these differences were not statistically significant. With micafungin, pharmacokinetics among 10 elderly (66–78 years of age) volunteers was similar to 10 young men (20–24 years of age) receiving single intravenous doses of micafungin 50 mg [85]. Pharmacokinetics of anidulafungin has not been specifically reported in elderly patients.

Women

Serum concentrations among women receiving echinocandins may be relatively higher than that among men, but no dosage adjustments are currently recommended on the basis of gender [3–5]. Mean AUC_{0-24h} at day 14 was increased a mean of 22% among healthy women when compared to healthy men receiving caspofungin (70 mg IV loading dose, followed by 50 mg IV daily for a total of 14 days) [87]. AUC was increased by 23% in women compared to men after 14 days of 150 mg micafungin daily, but this difference in serum concentrations was attributed to lower body weight among women [3]. In a population pharmacokinetic model based on serum concentrations obtained from participants in Phase II/III studies with anidulafungin, gender impacted clearance of anidulafungin but in concert with body weight and a diagnosis of invasive candidiasis, it explained the less than 20% of inter-subject pharmacokinetic variability [4].

Renal insufficiency

Dosage adjustment of echinocandins is not recommended for those with renal insufficiency or those requiring hemodialysis [5]. Plasma concentrations of caspofungin among patients with mild- to end-stage renal disease receiving 50 mg daily for treatment of invasive aspergillosis or candidiasis were similar to that among patients with no renal impairment [5]. In a single dose study of 70 mg, caspofungin serum concentrations were moderately higher (AUC 30%–49% increased) among those with moderate, advanced, or end-stage renal insufficiency. However, dosage adjustments are not recommended for those with renal insufficiency receiving caspofungin. Hemodialysis does not remove caspofungin, so dose supplementation is not necessary in patients requiring dialysis. There are clinical data but no published pharmacokinetic data from patients requiring peritoneal dialysis; however, continuous ambulatory peritoneal is not likely to affect plasma concentrations of caspofungin. Renal impairment (CrCl <30 mL/min) also did not affect the pharmacokinetics of micafungin after single 100 mg doses [89]. Continuous hemodiafiltration does not increase the elimination of micafungin [90]. Anidulafungin pharmacokinetics among 26 subjects with renal impairment or end-stage renal disease were similar to eight subjects with normal renal function following single intravenous doses of 50 mg anidulafungin [91]. Pharmacokinetics of anidulafungin was not affected in those undergoing hemodialysis, whether anidulafungin was given before or after a dialysis session [91].

Hepatic insufficiency

Hepatic insufficiency appears to reduce elimination of caspofungin and micafungin, while plasma concentrations of anidulafungin are decreased in those with severe hepatic impairment receiving anidulafungin [5,92]. Dose reduction should be considered when administering caspofungin to patients with moderate hepatic insufficiency [5]. In a single dose study of 70 mg, those with Child Pugh scores of 5–6 experienced an increase in AUC of 55% compared to historical healthy controls, while those with Child Pugh scores of 7–9 experienced a mean AUC increase of 76% [63]. These differences were not as pronounced with daily caspofungin doses of 50 mg, where subjects with mild hepatic insufficiency experienced increases in AUC of approximately 19%–25% compared to healthy controls. In this study, subjects with moderate hepatic impairment received 35 mg daily, following the 70 mg loading dose. Patients with severe liver dysfunction (Child Pugh score >9) were excluded from clinical trials with caspofungin, so there is limited clinical experience with the drug in this severely ill patient population.

Single 100 mg doses of micafungin have been administered to subjects with Child Pugh scores of 7–9, who experienced 22% lower values for C_{max} and AUC compared to age-, gender-, and weight-matched individuals with no hepatic impairment [89]. Pharmacokinetics of micafungin in those with severe hepatic impairment was described among nine liver transplant recipients. A graft recipient with small-for-size graft had substantially higher AUC and elimination half-life after micafungin doses of 100 mg, and the authors suggest that lower doses of 50 mg daily may be appropriate for such patients [93].

Pharmacokinetics of anidulafungin among subjects with mild-to-moderate hepatic dysfunction was similar to healthy controls receiving single 50 mg doses of anidulafungin. Peak serum concentration and AUC were 36% and 33% lower, respectively, in those with severe hepatic impairment (Child Pugh score 10–15) compared to healthy controls. Clearance was increased by 57% in those with severe hepatic impairment, with 78% increase in volume of distribution that could be potentially attributed to ascites and edema. Since concentrations remained above the MIC for most relevant organisms, the authors suggest that these differences in pharmacokinetic parameters among subjects with severe hepatic failure are probably not clinically relevant.

Burn patients

The use of caspofungin to treat candidemia in burn patients was investigated in a case report of two patients. Although one patient had PK parameters similar to those of healthy individuals, the other patient had significantly lower therapeutic exposure. One explanation is the hypoalbuminemia seen in burn patients, since caspofungin is nearly 97% bound to albumin. However, a larger sample size is required to investigate this variability among burn patients. It may be necessary to monitor therapeutic drug levels in burn patients receiving echinocandins to optimize dosing [94].

Critically ill patients in the intensive care unit

In a study of 40 Surgical Intensive Care Unit patients, caspofungin doses of 50 mg daily were associated with higher concentrations at 24 hours post-dose than that previously reported among healthy volunteers (mean C_{24h} 2.16 vs. 1.41 µg/mL, respectively) [95]. Serum concentrations were reduced with increasing body weight (>75 kg), but were increased among those with albumin concentrations >23.6 g/L. Of the subjects studied, 75% were within the target concentration range of 1–3 µg/mL for the duration of treatment. Of those with subtherapeutic concentrations, 10 of 17 weighed more than 75 kg, suggesting that weight may be an important covariate in caspofungin serum concentrations among critically ill adults. A recent large multicenter European study of critically ill patients receiving antifungal therapy showed that there was a significant degree of individual variability of drug concentrations, measured as AUC_{0-24h}, C_{max} and C_{min}, of caspofungin and anidulafungin among patients [96].

Pharmacokinetics of micafungin was determined in nine Japanese ICU patients receiving doses of 150–300 mg daily [90]. In this study, clearance of micafungin appeared to be greater than that previously reported among healthy volunteers (1.4 vs. 0.7 L/hr, respectively). The investigators suggest that this increased clearance observed in the ICU setting may be attributed to decreased albumin and total protein concentrations in serum of these critically ill patients, which may lead to increases in free drug available for clearance. Thus, individualized optimization of dosing may be required to maintain therapeutic echinocandin levels in critically ill patients.

Extracorporeal membrane oxygenation (ECMO)

Invasive candidiasis and candidemia are common occurrences in patients during ECMO. The nature of the ECMO circuit is such that drug may be extracted from the blood during recirculation resulting in subtherapeutic blood levels. An *ex-vivo* study has shown that recovery of micafungin from recirculated blood can be as low as 26% after 24 hours [97]. However, blood levels of caspofungin and anidulafungin were not significantly affected during ECMO [98,99]. These findings suggest that micafungin might require adjusted dosing during ECMO support, while caspofungin and anidulafungin do not.

Older children

Children have been the focus of several recent investigations of echinocandin pharmacokinetics (Table 13.7). In general, clearance of echinocandins is increased in children relative to adults. In a small study of caspofungin prophylaxis in children and adolescents with fever and neutropenia, AUC_{0-24h} among children receiving 1 mg/kg daily doses was 46% lower than that of adults receiving 50 mg daily [88]. The beta-phase elimination half-life was similarly reduced by approximately 32%–43% in these children compared to adults. These effects appeared to be more pronounced among younger, smaller subjects than older, larger

subjects, so increases in dosage may be especially important for younger children. On the basis of these data, the authors suggest that a dose of 50 mg/m² in children and adolescents 2–17 years of age may more closely approximate pharmacokinetic parameters achieved in adults. Micafungin clearance was also increased in children relative to adults [100]. Studies are limited in children under 4 months of age, but for children 4 months or older dosing is recommended once a day based on a weight and indication. Patients with candidemia, acute disseminated candidiasis, *Candida peritonitis* or abscesses are dosed at 2 mg/kg with a maximum daily dose of 100 mg. Patients being treated for esophageal candidiasis are dosed at 3 or 2.5 mg/kg if they weigh 30 kg or less or more than 30 kg, respectively with a maximum daily dose of 150 mg. HSCT recipients are dosed at 1 mg/kg with a maximum daily dose of 50 mg [3].

Anidulafungin pharmacokinetics was found to be similar among older children (2–17 years of age) receiving maintenance doses of 0.75 or 1.5 mg/kg/day in the setting of neutropenia. Concentrations achieved at these dosages approximated that of adults receiving 50 or 100 mg of anidulafungin daily [101]. Body weight, but not age, was associated with variability in clearance and volume of distribution in this patient population.

Neonates

Among the echinocandins, micafungin has been studied most extensively in preterm infants. Clearance of micafungin among neonates appears to be substantially greater than that in older children and adults [73,102,103]. Doses of 9 mg/kg in neonates have been estimated to yield exposures similar to 150 mg daily in adults and 2 mg/kg in older children [73]. Doses of 15 mg/kg/day in preterm infants (median 27 weeks of age, 775 grams at birth) yielded concentrations similar to 5 mg/kg/day in adults [103]. A more recent study of neonates and young infants with disseminated candidiasis showed that dosing at 10 mg/kg/day resulted in ~83% of patients with AUCs associated with significant decline in fungal burden [104]. A small multicenter study reported pharmacokinetics following caspofungin doses of 25 mg/m² among 18 infants less than 3 months

Table 13.7 Comparative pharmacokinetics of echinocandins in children (single dose administration)

	Caspofungin	Micafungin	Anidulafungin
Age range (years)	2–17	≥4 months	2–17
Dose[a]	50 mg/m²/day	1–3 mg/kg/day	0.75 or 1.5 mg/kg/day
C_{max} (µg/mL)	13	15	4
AUC_{0-24h} (µg · h/mL)	96	83	48
$t_{1/2}$ (h)	8.2–16.5	12.2–17.3	18.9–26.0
Plasma clearance (mL/h/kg)	5.2–8.6 mL/min/m²	14.2–24.3	13.3–21.7
Vd_{ss} (L/kg)	N/A	0.24–0.42	0.42–0.58

Source: Groll, A.H. et al., *Curr. Fungal Infect. Rep.*, 2, 49–56, 2008; VandenBussche, H.L. and Van Loo, D.A., *Ann. Pharmacother.*, 44, 166–177, 2010; Chiou, C.C. et al., *Expert. Opin. Pharmacother.*, 8, 2465–2489, 2007.

[a] not loading doses

of age with documented or suspected invasive candidiasis [105]. Pharmacokinetics in neonates receiving this dose was similar to adults receiving 50 mg caspofungin daily for invasive candidiasis.

PHARMACODYNAMICS

The pharmacodynamics of echinocandins has been extensively evaluated in *in vitro* studies and animal models of infection. As mentioned previously, a paradoxical effect has been reported *in vitro* with some isolates, but this phenomenon has not been validated in the clinical setting. Post-antifungal effects have been reported for echinocandins against *Candida* infections, but not against *Aspergillus* [106,107]. In animal models of invasive candidiasis, C_{max}:MIC and the AUC_{0-24h}:MIC ratios were most predictive of echinocandin activity [108–111]. In these studies, C_{max}:MIC ratio >10 or AUC_{0-24h}:MIC >250 has been suggestive of efficacy. Likewise, in animal models of invasive pulmonary aspergillosis, the C_{max}/MIC ratio for caspofungin or C_{max}:MEC ratio for micafungin was best correlated with efficacy [111,112]. More recently, clinical experience has been published, and supports the hypotheses generated in laboratory investigations that the echinocandins exhibit concentration-dependent killing. A study in Japanese patients with candidiasis or aspergillosis has suggested that a $C_{max} > 5$ μg/mL after doses of 50 mg or more of micafungin was associated with efficacy [113]. A later study suggested that higher concentrations ($C_{min} > 5$ μg/mL) were necessary for optimal outcome in managing invasive aspergillosis [114]. For anidulafungin, based upon data from Phase II and Phase III studies, a steady-state AUC of more than 35 mg·hr/L, a steady-state serum concentration of more than 1.5 mg/L, and trough concentration >1 mg/L have been suggestive of efficacy in oropharyngeal/esophageal candidiasis [115]. These concentrations are readily achievable following daily doses of 50 mg.

SAFETY

Overall, echinocandins have been well tolerated with few serious side effects. In a summary evaluation of several caspofungin clinical trials, the most commonly reported drug-related adverse events were fever (12%–26%) and infusion-related phlebitis (12%–18%) [116]. The most common laboratory abnormalities reported were increased liver transaminases, alkaline phosphatase, and decreased hemoglobin and hematocrit concentrations, although these rates were similar to those among comparators. There have been isolated reports of histamine-related symptoms with caspofungin; however, these reports are rare [117,118]. In addition, there have been rare reports of hepatotoxicity in patients receiving caspofungin and cyclosporine concomitantly, but the contribution of caspofungin was uncertain [119]. However, the benefit of the caspofungin therapy should be carefully weighed against the risks in those receiving cyclosporine, and liver function tests should be monitored [5].

Micafungin has been approved for use in Japan for years and has a large body of evidence in Japanese literature. In a dose escalation study of 74 patients receiving doses of micafungin up to 200 mg/day, who were undergoing peripheral blood or stem cell transplantation, the most common adverse events were rash, headache, arthralgia, and hypophosphatemia [120]. In clinical trials with micafungin, the most common adverse events were nausea (2.8%), vomiting (2.4%), increased AST (2.7%), increased ALT (2.6%), and increased alkaline phosphatase (2.0%) [3]. In clinical trials of patients receiving anidulafungin for the treatment of candidemia, the most frequent adverse events were diarrhea (3.1%), hypokalemia (3.1%), and increased ALT (2.3%), which were not different than that seen with the comparator group [121]. A large multicenter study of adult and pediatric patients receiving micafungin and other parenteral antifungal agents showed that there was no significant difference in rates of liver injury between micafungin and other parenteral antifungals (13 vs. 12 events per 100 patients). Micafungin was shown to have lower rates of renal injury; however, the measurable effect may not be clinically significant [122]. In terms of long term risks of receiving echinocandin therapy, some animal studies have found liver tumors in animals receiving very high doses of micafungin [123]. However, these findings have not been replicated in humans or even repeated with other echinocandins. There have been several reports of infusion-related toxicities, including hypotension and flushing with anidulafungin [4,124]. However, the overall incidence of infusion-related reactions can be minimized by infusing anidulafungin at a rate not to exceed 1.1 mg/min [4].

DOSING AND ADMINISTRATION

Dosing of the echinocandins differs among the agents and according to indication for use [3–5]. FDA-approved recommended doses for each agent are summarized in Table 13.1. In addition to these doses, the prescribing information for some countries recommend doses of caspofungin of 70 mg IV daily throughout the course of therapy for adult patients weighing more than 80 kg [125]. A recent study in adults with candidemia/invasive candidiasis also investigated higher doses of caspofungin (150 mg daily) and found no differences in safety compared to standard dosages [56]. Dosages of caspofungin may need to be increased to 70 mg daily (or 70 mg/m² in older children) in the setting of invasive aspergillosis when patients have not responded to 50 mg (or 50 mg/m²) daily, or in those receiving inducers of drug clearance such as rifampin, nevirapine, efavirenz, carbamazepine, dexamethasone, or phenytoin (see drug interactions below). Dose reductions of caspofungin to 35 mg daily are recommended for adults with moderate hepatic insufficiency (Child Pugh score 7–9). Based on pharmacokinetic data, caspofungin doses of 25 mg/m² for children less than 3 months of age can be considered but are not FDA approved for this use. Among HSCT recipients, doses as high as 8 mg/kg/day (maximum 896 mg) of micafungin have been tolerated [120]. However, micafungin is typically administered in doses of 50–150 mg daily for adults based on clinical indication (Table 13.1). In clinical studies of the pediatric population, dosages of 2.1 (mean, ± 1.25) mg/kg/day and 2 mg/kg/day have been administered for treatment of invasive aspergillosis and candidiasis, respectively [126,127]. In one study, dose escalation was permitted and as much as 325 mg daily (8.6 mg/kg/day) was administered to a child less than 16 years of age [127]. Current recommendations for dosing micafungin in pediatric patients ≥4 months of age range between 1 and 3 mg/kg/day [3]. Dose optimization is still being determined for neonates, but up to 15 mg/kg/day has been given safely for up to 5 days in neonates >48 hours of life and infants less than 3 months of age [103]. Micafungin dosages do not need to be adjusted for drug interactions (see Drug Interactions below).

Anidulafungin is typically given as a 100 or 200 mg loading dose, followed by 50 or 100 mg daily for esophagitis or candidemia/invasive candidiasis, respectively [4]. In clinical trials, a dose as high as 400 mg was administered on one occasion without adverse event in one patient, and, in healthy subjects, doses of 130 mg daily following a 260 mg loading dose were well tolerated [4]. Among children, a dose of 1.5 mg/kg/day of anidulafungin can be considered on the basis of pharmacokinetics studies, but anidulafungin is not FDA approved for this use.

DRUG INTERACTIONS

Drug interactions with all three echinocandins are fairly limited. Caspofungin is not an inhibitor, inducer, or substrate for any of the cytochrome P450 isoenzymes, nor a substrate for P-glycoprotein. However, when caspofungin is coadministered with cyclosporine, a 35% increase in the AUC of caspofungin, without a concomitant increase in the AUC of cyclosporine has been observed [5]. In addition, the AUC and C_{max} of tacrolimus is reduced by 20% and 16% respectively when coadministered with caspofungin [5]. However, in patients receiving caspofungin concomitantly with cyclosporine and/or tacrolimus in the clinical setting, the need for dose adjustments of immunosuppressants is not common [5,128]. Coadministration of caspofungin with rifampin also results in a 30% decrease in the caspofungin trough concentrations and an increase in caspofungin dose to 70 mg/day is recommended [5]. The mechanism of the drug–drug interactions is unclear; however, this may be due to an overexpression of organic anion transporter proteins (OATP) that are responsible for hepatic uptake [129].

Although micafungin is a substrate for *Cyp*3A4, this is a minor pathway of metabolism and inhibitors and inducers of this isoenzyme system do not affect the pharmacokinetics of either drug. However, sirolimus coadministration with micafungin resulted in a 21% increase in the AUC of sirolimus and nifedipine AUC was increased by 18% with an increase of 42% of the C_{max} with coadministration of micafungin [3]. Thus, it is recommended to monitor for nifedipine and sirolimus toxicity if coadministration is necessary.

Anidulafungin has been evaluated in several drug interaction studies to evaluate the effects of *Cyp*450 isoenzymes inducers. Anidulafungin is not an inducer, inhibitor, or substrate for any of the common isoenzymes, and clinically relevant drug–drug interactions were not present between anidulafungin and cyclosporine, tacrolimus, liposomal amphotericin B, voriconazole, or rifampin [4].

CLINICAL EFFICACY

Clinical efficacy of all three echinocandins has been well established in clinical trials for oropharyngeal/esophageal candidiasis and treatment of candidemia/invasive candidiasis [20,58,121]. In a review of randomized trials evaluating patients with candidemia and invasive candidiasis, treatment with an echinocandin versus other antifungal agents resulted in improved survival (OR = 0.65, 95% CI = 0.45 to 0.94, p = 0.02) [130]. All of these clinical trials excluded subjects with meningitis, endocarditis, endophthalmitis, and osteomyelitis. Sufficient penetration of echinocandins into these spaces at concentrations required for clinical efficacy has been questioned. Some success has been reported with echinocandins for these indications (alone or in combination), but clinical failures have also been observed [131–135]. There are four sites of the body where reduced penetration of echinocandins into the site of infection makes efficacy questionable. These sites include eye, CNS, pleural space, and bladder. None of the echinocandins has received FDA approval for such deeply invasive *Candida* spp. infections. In addition to efficacy in management of invasive candidiasis, the individual agents have demonstrated activity as salvage therapy for invasive aspergillosis (caspofungin), as empirical therapy in those with neutropenic fever (caspofungin), and prophylaxis in HSCT recipients (micafungin). Additional experience is evolving with micafungin for invasive aspergillosis [127,136], and for all candins as combination agents in the management of invasive fungal infections.

CASPOFUNGIN

Oropharyngeal/esophageal candidiasis

Efficacy of caspofungin has been demonstrated in the management of esophageal candidiasis in several clinical trials that involved primarily HIV-infected patients. In all of these trials, *C. albicans* was the most common pathogen isolated. Favorable responses in subjects with esophageal candidiasis at the end of IV therapy (14 days) with 50 or 70 mg of caspofungin daily were 85% and 96%, respectively. For the 70 mg caspofungin group, this response rate was significantly greater at 2 weeks after therapy than the comparison group receiving intravenous amphotericin B 0.5 mg/kg daily [89% vs. 63%, mean difference 26% (95% CI = 4%–50%)] [137]. In a dose ranging study, favorable responses 3 to 4 days after 7–14 days of 35, 50, or 70 mg of caspofungin were observed in more than 70% of patients with oropharyngeal/esophageal candidiasis. Favorable responses were observed in 63% of subjects randomized to 0.5 mg/kg/day of amphotericin B, but these differences were not statistically significant [138]. In both these studies, fewer subjects receiving caspofungin experienced drug-related adverse events than those receiving amphotericin B. Caspofungin (50 mg daily) was also compared to fluconazole (200 mg daily) in HIV patients with esophageal candidiasis [139]. The overall clinical response was 90% for the caspofungin-treated patients and 89% for the fluconazole-treated patients, with a median time to symptom resolution of 4–5 days in both groups. However, relapse rates 4 weeks after treatment were numerically higher in caspofungin-treated patients than in those who had received fluconazole, but this was not statistically significant (28% vs. 17%, respectively; difference = 12%; 95% CI = −5%–29%, p = 0.19).

In a pooled analysis of data from four phase II/III clinical trials including 115 evaluable patients who received caspofungin for esophagitis, relapse was experienced by 17% of patients [140]. In a multivariate analysis, only severe symptoms and extensive esophageal disease by endoscopic assessment at baseline were predictive of relapse at 14 days after the end of therapy. Duration of antifungal therapy (range 7–21 days) with caspofungin was not predictive of relapse.

Candidemia/invasive candidiasis

Caspofungin's efficacy in the management of candidemia/invasive candidiasis has been demonstrated in a large randomized, double-blind clinical trial of 239 patients [20]. Caspofungin (50 mg daily following a 70 mg loading dose) or AmBd (0.6–0.7 mg/kg) were administered for at least 10 days, followed by oral fluconazole (400 mg daily), for a total of 14 days after the last positive culture for *Candida* spp. In the intent to treat population, the overall response rate was 73.4% versus 61.7% (difference = 12.7%, 95.6% CI = −0.7%–26%, p = 0.09) for caspofungin-versus amphotericin B–treated patients, respectively. The difference in the treatment groups increased to 15.4% (95.6% CI = 1.1–29.7, p = 0.03) among clinically evaluable patients. Caspofungin (50 mg daily, following a 70 mg loading dose) was also compared to two different doses of micafungin (100 and 150 mg) for candidemia/invasive candidiasis in a double-blind, controlled clinical trial of 595 subjects [58]. Treatment success at the end of IV therapy was experienced by 72.3% of subjects receiving caspofungin, which was similar to the success rates among those receiving micafungin 100 or 150 mg (76.4% and 71.4%, respectively) (see Micafungin efficacy). Relapse, mortality, and treatment-related adverse rates were similar between the treatment groups. Treatment-related adverse events were experienced by approximately 23% of patients in the study, and most commonly included liver transaminase elevations, gastrointestinal disturbances, hypokalemia, and rash. Another study investigated the safety and efficacy of high-dose (150 mg daily) caspofungin compared to standard caspofungin dosages (50 mg

daily after a 70 mg loading dose) in adults with candidemia/invasive candidiasis [56]. This study was designed primarily to assess safety, but efficacy was a secondary objective. At the end of caspofungin therapy, favorable overall response was experienced by 71.6% and 77.9% of patients, who received standard- and high-dose caspofungin, respectively. This difference was not statistically significant (6.3%; 95% CI = −5.9%–18.4%). Numerical trends for fewer relapses in the high-dose arm were apparent at 2 and 8 weeks after treatment discontinuation, but the numbers of cases were small, and these differences were not statistically significant. Rates of significant or serious drug-related adverse events (2%–3%) were similar between treatment groups, and overall adverse event rates were similar to rates from other published studies with caspofungin at approximately 20%.

Aspergillosis

Caspofungin has been investigated as a single agent and as part of combination antifungal therapy for invasive aspergillosis. In a multicenter, open label, noncomparative clinical trial, caspofungin (50 mg daily following a 70 mg loading dose) was administered to 48 patients with proven or probable aspergillosis [141]. Most patients (75%) had pulmonary infections refractory (90%) or intolerant (10.4%) to initial therapy. Among those with pulmonary disease, response was experienced by 53%. Among those with extra-pulmonary disease, there was only an 18% response, which probably reflects the challenge of treating disseminated aspergillosis. Caspofungin has also been studied in combination with other antifungal agents in the management of invasive aspergillosis [142,143]. In a small, single-center open label study, patients with pulmonary aspergillosis who were failing therapy with amphotericin B received either voriconazole (n = 31) or voriconazole in combination with caspofungin (n = 16) [143].

Combination therapy was associated with improved survival relative to a historical cohort of patients who received voriconazole alone (HR = 0.28, 95% CI = 0.28–0.92, p = 0.01). In another study, the combination of caspofungin and voriconazole was used as initial therapy for invasive aspergillosis in a prospective, multicenter cohort of solid-organ transplant recipients (n = 40) and compared to a historical cohort of patients (n = 47), who had received a lipid formulation of amphotericin B (LFAB) as primary therapy. Pulmonary infection was most common among both cases and controls (92.5% and 87.2%, respectively). Treatment success was 70% among those receiving the combination of caspofungin plus voriconazole compared to 51% among those who received LFAB, but this difference was not statistically significant (p = 0.08). Other smaller studies have been performed and suggest that this echinocandin combination may be promising, but conclusive evidence of synergistic effects in combination with other agents for invasive aspergillosis remains to be shown [144–146].

Empiric treatment of IFI in febrile neutropenia

Caspofungin has also demonstrated efficacy as empirical antifungal therapy in patients with neutropenia and persistent fever despite ≥96 hours of broad-spectrum antibacterials. In a double-blind randomized trial, 1123 subjects received either caspofungin (70 mg loading dose, followed by 50 mg/day) or liposomal amphotericin B (L-AmB, 3 mg/kg daily). Overall, clinical response based on a composite endpoint (successful treatment of any baseline fungal infection, absence of breakthrough fungal infection, survival for at least 7 days after the end of therapy, no discontinuation of drug due to treatment-related adverse event or lack of efficacy, and resolution of fever <38°C for ≥48 hours) was similar between treatment groups: 33.9% and 33.7% of the caspofungin- and liposomal amphotericin B–treated patients, respectively (difference 0.2%, 95.2% CI = −5.6%–6%). Caspofungin was associated with a higher rate of treatment success among those with baseline fungal infections (51.9% vs. 25.9%, difference 25.9%, 95.2% CI = 0.9%–51%). In addition, the proportion of patients surviving to seven days was greater among those receiving caspofungin, compared to L-AmB (p = 0.04). Nephrotoxicity, infusion-related adverse events, and treatment discontinuation due to adverse events were significantly less common among patients receiving caspofungin. Thus, as empirical therapy in patients with fever and neutropenia, caspofungin was as effective and better tolerated than liposomal amphotericin B.

Prophylaxis in patients with hematologic malignancies

The use of caspofungin (70 and 50 mg/day) for IFI prophylaxis in acute leukemia patients undergoing induction therapy was compared to other antifungal regimens. Over a two-year period, 175 patients were randomized to receive caspofungin prophylaxis or other antifungal regimens. The overall incidence of breakthrough IFIs was ~18% with no significant difference between the groups, suggesting caspofungin can be used for prophylaxis [147].

Efficacy in pediatric patients

Efficacy of caspofungin in children with invasive fungal infections has been demonstrated in an open-label, noncomparative study [148]. Forty-nine children 3 months to 17 years of age received caspofungin 70 mg/m² as a loading dose, followed by 50 mg/m² daily as primary or salvage therapy for invasive candidiasis (n = 37), esophageal candidiasis (n = 1), or invasive aspergillosis (n = 10). Among those with invasive candidiasis, 92% had candidemia and 82% received caspofungin as primary therapy. All 10 patients with invasive aspergillosis were refractory to prior antifungal therapies, and 80% had pulmonary involvement. Overall, success

at the end of caspofungin therapy was experienced by 81% of patients with invasive candidiasis and 50% of those with invasive aspergillosis. Treatment was also successful in one child with esophageal candidiasis. Doses were increased up to 70 mg/m² in four patients with candidiasis and one with aspergillosis. Of these, three patients with candidiasis responded favorably, while one patient each with candidiasis and aspergillosis had unfavorable responses and discontinued caspofungin therapy after 1 and 3 days, respectively. Caspofungin was generally well tolerated, with 27% of patients having at least one clinical adverse event and 35% having at least one laboratory adverse event that was possibly related to caspofungin. These rates are similar to those reported in other similar studies in adults.

Comparing caspofungin to L-AmB for the treatment of invasive candidiasis in newborn infants showed more favorable response with caspofungin. Thirty-two patients were randomized to caspofungin (15 patients) at a maintenance dose of 50 mg/m² daily with a maximum daily dose of 70 mg or amphotericin (17 patients) at a dose of 3 mg/kg daily. Approximately 87% of patients on caspofungin had favorable response whereas only 42% had favorable response with L-AmB (p = 0.04) [149]. These results suggest that caspofungin should be used as primary therapy for management of invasive candidiasis in infants.

Caspofungin has also been compared to L-AmB in a double-blind randomized trial as empirical antifungal therapy in children with persistent fever and neutropenia in children 2–17 years of age [150]. Eighty-two children were randomized in a 2:1 fashion to receive caspofungin 70 mg/m² loading dose, followed by 50 mg/m² daily or L-AmB 3 mg/kg/day. Efficacy was assessed using the same composite endpoint used in the adult studies mentioned previously [151]. Twenty-seven percent of patients in both treatment groups were considered high-risk (allogeneic HSCT recipients or had relapsed acute leukemia). Prior antifungal prophylaxis had been used in 51% of the 81 patients evaluable for efficacy. Success rates were 46% for caspofungin- and 32% for L-AmB–treated patients [5]. Among high-risk patients, success was higher among those receiving caspofungin (9 of 15 patients, 60%) compared to L-AmB (0 of 7 patients, 0%). Among low-risk patients, success rates were similar between treatment groups: 17 of 41 children (41.5%) receiving caspofungin and 8 of 18 (44.4%) children receiving L-AmB had favorable responses. Overall rates of clinical and laboratory treatment-related adverse events were similar between groups [150]. This information suggests that caspofungin is safe and effective as empirical therapy in febrile neutropenic children.

Based on these studies, the FDA has approved caspofungin for use in children 3 months and older as treatment for candidemia and intraabdominal abscesses, peritonitis, and pleural space infections caused by Candida spp., esophageal candidiasis, invasive aspergillosis that is refractory to other therapies, and as empirical therapy for presumed fungal infections in febrile neutropenic patients.

MICAFUNGIN

Oropharyngeal/esophageal candidiasis

Micafungin has demonstrated efficacy in the treatment of oropharyngeal/esophageal candidiasis in several clinical trials. In a multicenter, randomized, double-blind study, micafungin (50, 100, or 150 mg) was compared to fluconazole (200 mg/day) in the treatment of esophageal candidiasis with or without oropharyngeal candidiasis in 245 HIV-infected adults [152]. A dose- response was demonstrated with micafungin, based on end-of-treatment endoscopic cure rates of 68.8%, 77.4%, and 89.8% for micafungin dosages of 50, 100, and 150 mg daily, respectively. Fluconazole response rates were 86.7% overall. Micafungin response rates were comparable to fluconazole at micafungin doses of 100 or 150 mg daily, but inferior at micafungin 50 mg daily doses. As in trials with caspofungin, relapse occurred more frequently with the echinocandin compared to the azole in the post-treatment phase period (9 vs. 0 patients).

A multicenter, randomized, double-blind study compared micafungin 150 mg to fluconazole 200 mg per day for 14 days in the treatment of esophageal candidiasis [153]. Ninety-four percent of study subjects were HIV-infected, although antiretroviral therapy was only used in 10% of the study subjects. Treatment success, as determined by endoscopy at the end of antifungal therapy, was similar between the two treatment groups: 87.7% for micafungin and 88.0% for fluconazole-treated patients. Relapse rates at week 2, week 4, and through week 4 were also similar between groups. Relapse through the week 4 visit was 15.2% for micafungin versus 11.3% for fluconazole (p = 0.257). No differences in overall adverse event rates were observed between treatment groups (27.7% micafungin vs. 21.3% fluconazole, p = NS).

Another multinational, double-blind randomized trial compared micafungin to caspofungin for oropharyngeal/esophageal candidiasis, but these results have not been published in a peer-reviewed journal [154]. In this study, 454 subjects were randomized to receive micafungin 150 mg daily, micafungin 300 mg every other day, or caspofungin 50 mg daily. Approximately 90% of subjects had both oropharyngeal and esophageal candidiasis. There were no differences found between treatment groups in endoscopic cure rate, clinical response rate, or overall therapeutic response at the end of antifungal therapy. Incidence of relapse was numerically lower in the two micafungin treatment groups than in the caspofungin treatment group at the two-week follow-up visit and through four weeks of follow up. In particular, relapse rates were approximately 7% lower with micafungin 300 mg QOD than caspofungin 50 mg daily.

Together, these studies demonstrate that micafungin is safe and effective for management of oropharyngeal/esophageal candidiasis.

Candidemia/invasive candidiasis

Experience with micafungin for management of candidemia and invasive candidiasis has been published from both open-label noncomparative studies [155] and randomized clinical trials [58,156]. One hundred twenty-six adults and children with newly diagnosed (n = 72) or refractory candidemia (n = 54) received micafungin in a multicenter, open-label, noncomparative study [155]. Patients with infections due to C. albicans were initially administered 50 mg daily, while those with infections caused by other species of Candida initially received 100 mg daily (or 1–2 mg/kg/day if <40 kg). Incremental dose escalation in 50 mg increments was permitted up to 200 mg daily after at least 5 days of dosing for those with stable or progressive disease. Combination antifungal therapy was allowed in those with refractory Candida spp. infections. Approximately 80% of the patients received ≤100 mg of micafungin daily. Of the patients receiving micafungin as initial therapy for candidemia, 87.5% experienced a complete or partial response at end of therapy. Among patients who had failed prior antifungal therapy, 76% responded to micafungin alone while 79.3% responded to micafungin in combination with another agent. These data provided preliminary evidence of the efficacy of micafungin as both primary and salvage therapy for candidemia.

Micafungin has been compared to other antifungals in two multicenter, randomized, double-blind controlled trials in patients with invasive candidiasis or candidemia [58,156]. Micafungin 100 mg daily was compared to L-AmB 3 mg/kg/day in 531 patients ≥16 years of age [156]. A large proportion of the patients were in the ICU (51%), and/or receiving mechanical ventilation (35%). Most infections were caused by non-C. albicans species and approximately 16% had sites of infection outside the bloodstream. Overall clinical and mycological response at the end of IV therapy in the per-protocol population was 89.6% for micafungin versus 89.5% for L-AmB. In the modified intention-to-treat analysis, overall success was lower but still similar between treatment groups (74.1% micafungin, 69.6% L-AmB, difference when stratified by neutropenic status: 4.9% [95% CI = −3%–12.8%]). No differences in treatment efficacy between the two groups were observed on the basis of infecting pathogen. There were more infusion-related reactions (28.8% vs. 17%) and increases in serum creatinine from baseline to above upper level of normal (29.9% vs. 10.3%) in the L-AmB group compared to the micafungin group. Micafungin doses of 100 and 150 mg/day were compared to caspofungin (50 mg daily following a 70 mg loading dose) in a phase III, double-blind, multicenter study in 595 patients with invasive candidiasis or candidemia [58]. Approximately 85% of the patients were candidemic, and 55% of the infections were due to non-C. albicans spp. Overall, success at the end of IV therapy was experienced in 73.9%, 70.3%, and 71.4% of patients treated with micafungin 100 mg, micafungin 150 mg, and caspofungin 50 mg, respectively (p = NS). Of the study participants, 29.6% died but there were no statistical differences in survival between the treatment groups. Rates of treatment-related adverse events were similar between treatment groups (range 22%–23.8%), and rates of discontinuation due to treatment-related adverse events were quite low overall (3%). Based on the data in these studies, 100 mg has become the standard daily dose for micafungin in the treatment of adults with invasive candidiasis or candidemia [3].

Aspergillosis

No randomized comparative trials have been performed with micafungin as primary treatment for invasive aspergillosis, but experience from several open-label studies for this indication has been published [127,136,157].

In a small open label, multicenter Japanese study, experience with micafungin doses of 25–150 mg/day with 46 pulmonary aspergillosis patients was described [157]. Among 42 patients evaluable for efficacy at the end of antifungal therapy, 57% of patients experienced complete or partial improvement. Response rates were similar for the range of aspergillosis diagnoses included in this study: 60% (6/10) in those with invasive pulmonary aspergillosis, 55% (12/22) in those with pulmonary aspergilloma, and 67% (6/9) in those with chronic necrotizing pulmonary aspergillosis.

Micafungin was also investigated as a single agent or in combination antifungal therapy in some recent studies [127,136,158]. The first study describes 225 evaluable adults and children who received micafungin for proven or probable invasive aspergillosis refractory or intolerant to initial antifungal therapy [127]. Eighty-five percent of these patients added micafungin to a failing antifungal regimen. Complete/partial responses were experienced by 35.6% (8% complete, 27.6% partial) of patients at the end of antifungal therapy, while 53.5% of patients experienced progression of infection. This study showed no advantage of a combination antifungal therapy compared to micafungin alone as either primary (29.4% vs. 50%) or salvage (34.5% vs. 40.9%) therapy; however, the overall number of patients included in these groups was small, so it was underpowered to detect such differences. In a second, multicenter, open-label study, 98 adult and pediatric HSCT recipients with invasive aspergillosis received micafungin as a single agent (8%) or in combination with other antifungals (92%) as primary (15%) or salvage (85%) therapy [136]. Most of the patients (83%) had invasive pulmonary aspergillosis. Amphotericin B or its lipid formulations were most commonly used in conjunction with micafungin. Treatment success was experienced by 26% of patients, who had either complete (5%) or partial (20%) responses. Success rates were similar among those receiving micafungin as primary therapy (22%) and as salvage therapy (24%). Success was 24% among those receiving micafungin in combination with other antifungals, and 38% among the eight patients receiving micafungin alone. Thus, micafungin demonstrated some success in treating invasive aspergillosis in this very challenging patient population. Another randomized trial evaluating the use of micafungin as salvage therapy in patients with invasive aspergillosis, who were intolerant or refractory to other systemic antifungals, showed 25% of patients on 300 mg/day of micafungin monotherapy and 60% of patients in the control arm achieved treatment success. However, the study was concluded early due to the common use of combination antifungals for salvage therapy at the time, and no clear conclusion could be made about the use of micafungin monotherapy for salvage therapy [158].

Together, these data demonstrate that micafungin may be an effective treatment option for patients with pulmonary aspergillosis and further blinded, comparative clinical trials are needed.

Empiric treatment of IFI in febrile neutropenia

A study comparing micafungin to voriconazole for empriric therapy of patients with febrile neutropenia did not yield any differences in efficacy in terms of successfully-treated patients, absence of breakthrough infections (96% vs. 87%), survival 7 days after completion of therapy (98% vs. 100%), and resolution of fever during neutropenia (65% vs. 62%). However, significantly fewer patients had adverse events requiring withdrawal of treatment due to adverse events on micafungin compared to voriconazole (10% vs. 36%) [159]. Comparing micafungin to another azole, itraconazole, for empiric therapy of febrile neutropenic patients with hematological malignancies yielded non-inferior results. Overall, success was not significantly different between micafungin and itraconazole (64% vs. 57%). Duration of fever and length of hospital stay were shorter with micafungin (6 vs. seven days and 22 vs. 27 days, respectively) and grade 3 adverse events were fewer with micafungin compared to itraconazole (10% vs. 19%) [160].

Prophylaxis in patients undergoing hematopoietic stem cell transplant

The role of micafungin as antifungal prophylaxis has been established through a randomized, double-blind trial in 882 patients undergoing autologous (46%) or allogeneic (54%) HSCT [161]. Micafungin 50 mg IV daily or fluconazole 400 mg IV daily was started within 48 hours of initiating pre-transplant conditioning and continued up to a maximum of 42 days and discontinued when the patient's ANC was >500 cells/mm^3. Treatment success (absence of systemic IFI) was higher among those receiving micafungin compared to fluconazole (80% vs. 73.5%, difference 6.5%, 95% CI = 0.9%–12%). Accordingly, breakthrough infections were more common with fluconazole therapy. These breakthrough infections included two candidemia and seven aspergillosis (four proven and three probable) cases in patients who received fluconazole. Four cases of candidemia and one probable aspergillosis case were reported among those who received micafungin. Overall mortality was similar between treatment groups (4.2% micafungin vs. 5.7% fluconazole, p = NS). Discontinuations due to treatment-related adverse events were low in both treatment groups (4.2% micafungin vs. 7.2% fluconazole, p = NS). In summary, this study demonstrated that micafungin was superior in efficacy and as safe as fluconazole for antifungal prophylaxis in HSCT recipients.

A study comparing 50 mg/day of micafungin to 5 mg/kg/day of itraconazole for IFI prophylaxis in HSCT recipients showed non-inferiority of micafungin in preventing fungal infections. Approximately 93% versus 95% of patients had treatment success with micafungin compared to itraconazole, with no significant difference between the groups. Furthermore, patients receiving micafungin experienced significantly fewer drug-related adverse events compared to those on itraconazole (8% vs. 26.5%), as well as a lower incidence of treatment withdrawal due to adverse events (4.4% vs. 21.1%) [162].

Prophylaxis of IFI in high-risk liver transplant recipients

An assessment of the use of micafungin compared to other center-specific regimens for prophylaxis in liver transplant patients demonstrated non-inferiority of micafungin when compared to standard prophylaxis; clinical success with micafungin was 96.5% versus 93.6% for standard prophylaxis. Furthermore, adverse event rates did not differ significantly at 11.6% versus 16.3%, but kidney function was better overall in patients receiving micafungin [163].

Efficacy in pediatric patients

Several studies investigating micafungin efficacy have included children as well as adults [126,127,136,155,161]. Not all of these have reported outcomes separately for children. A multicenter, noncomparative study of micafungin for management of candidemia included 20 patients less than 16 years of age [155]. Micafungin was given as a single agent for primary therapy (n = 6) or as salvage therapy (n = 6), or in combination with other antifungals as salvage therapy (n = 8). Eleven neonates were included, and all but one of these received micafungin as salvage therapy. Treatment success was experienced by 15 of the 20 children (75%, 95% CI = 51%–91%). This was similar to the rate among adults (84.9%, 95% CI = 77%–91%). Eight of the eleven neonates (72%) had a complete response while three failed the therapy. In a larger substudy of a double-blind, randomized multicenter trial, micafungin (2 mg/kg/day) was compared to L-AmB (3 mg/kg/day) as primary therapy for candidemia/invasive candidiasis [126]. Ninety-eight children under 16 years of age with confirmed candidiasis were included. 57 patients were less than 2 years of age, and 19 of these were premature infants. Approximately 18% of the children were neutropenic. Overall clinical and microbiologic success at

the end of therapy was 73% versus 76% (difference −2.4%, 95% CI = −20.1%–15.3%) for the children who had received micafungin versus L-AmB, respectively. Seven patients in each treatment group had persistently positive cultures at the end of antifungal therapy. Mortality and overall adverse event rates were also similar between treatment groups. During the post treatment follow-up, three patients who had received micafungin and no patients who had received L-AmB experienced recurrent infection. Two cases involved recurrences of candidemia, and one additional recurrence involved Candida meningitis in a four-week-old infant who initially presented with disseminated candidiasis. Higher dosages of micafungin are subsequently being investigated in neonates to achieve greater CNS penetration, but efficacy of these dosages needs to be established in a clinical trial.

Children were included in two open-label studies of micafungin as primary or salvage therapy for invasive aspergillosis [127,136]. The first study included 58 children, and 27 of these were less than 10 years of age [127]. Premature neonates were excluded from the study, and the youngest child was 3 months of age. Micafungin was initially administered as 1.5 mg/kg/day for children weighing ≤40 kg, but dose escalation was allowed after 7 days of dosing in 1.5 mg/kg/day increments. The mean dose administered to patients less than 16 years of age was 2.1 ± 1.25 mg/kg/day and mean maximum daily dose was 2.8 ± 1.7 mg/kg/day. Twelve children received 4 mg/kg/day or more, with daily doses of more than 200 mg in five children and as high as 325 mg (8.6 mg/kg) in one child. Overall treatment success (complete and partial response) in children was 45%, with a similar rate among children less than 10 years of age. These rates are comparable to the success rate of the overall study (36%). Treatment was discontinued due to adverse events in 24% of children, but this rate was similar to that in the overall study (26%). In the second study, HSCT recipients received micafungin (1.5 mg/kg/day) alone or as part of combination antifungal therapy for primary or salvage treatment of invasive aspergillosis. Twenty-seven children less than or equal to 16 years of age were included in the study. Treatment success was experienced by 19% (5/27) of these children, while success was experienced by 28% (20/71) among adult study participants. No additional information is provided about the outcomes among children in the study, but these rates of success are not surprising given the challenge of managing invasive aspergillosis in HSCT recipients.

Finally, 84 children (6 months to 16 years of age) were included in a large randomized, double-blind clinical trial of antifungal prophylaxis in HSCT recipients [161]. Patients were randomized to micafungin (1 mg/kg/day in those <50 kg, n = 39) or fluconazole (8 mg/kg/day in those <50 kg, n = 45). Treatment success was experienced by 61% of children overall, which is somewhat lower than the success rates among adults 16–64 years of age (78%) and >64 years of age (86%). Of the children receiving micafungin, 69.2% had treatment success while only 53% of those receiving fluconazole were successfully prophylaxed (difference 15.9%). Statistical comparisons were not presented for children, probably reflecting the small sample size. However, the authors state that there were no differences between children and adults in frequency of treatment-related adverse events. In summary, micafungin has demonstrated that it is at least as effective as fluconazole as antifungal prophylaxis in children undergoing HSCT.

ANIDULAFUNGIN

Oropharyngeal/esophageal candidiasis

Efficacy of anidulafungin in managing oropharyngeal/esophageal candidiasis has been investigated in one small open-label study and one large clinical trial [124,164]. In a noncomparative, open-label Phase II study, anidulafungin (50 mg daily following a 100 mg loading dose) was administered for up to 21 days to 19 adults with azole-refractory oropharyngeal/esophageal candidiasis [164]. Eighty-nine percent of patients were HIV-infected, with a median CD4+ cell count of 9 cells/mm^3. Study subjects had a median of 5.5 prior episodes of mucosal candidiasis. Endoscopic success was achieved in 92% of study subjects with esophageal candidiasis at the end of therapy, with 75% experiencing cure and 17% experiencing improvement of lesions. Among those with oropharyngeal candidiasis, the success rate was similar (94%), with 61% cured and 33% improved at the end of therapy. Clinical success was not universally sustained through the post treatment period 10–14 days after the end of therapy. Success was 47% at this visit, with 8/18 (44%) of patients with oropharyngeal candidiasis and 6/12 (50%) of patients with esophageal candidiasis experiencing success. Four patients were successfully re-treated with anidulafungin. Use of antiretroviral therapy was not described in this study, but 76% of patients had CD4 cell count ≤50 cells/mm^3, which could have impacted ability to sustain a clinical response after antifungal therapy was discontinued. Anidulafungin (50 mg daily, following a 100 mg loading dose) was compared to fluconazole (100 mg daily, following a 200 mg loading dose) in a randomized, double-blind clinical trial in 601 predominantly HIV-infected adults with esophageal candidiasis [124]. Endoscopic resolution of lesions after 14–21 days of treatment was graded as either cured (complete resolution of lesions) or improved. In addition, clinical response, defined as an absence or improvement in symptoms compared to baseline was determined. At the end of treatment, success based on endoscopic assessment and clinical response was similar between anidulafungin and fluconazole. Endoscopic cure or improvement was present in 97.2% and 98.8% of anidulafungin- and fluconazole-treated patients, respectively. Clinical response was 98.8% with anidulafungin, versus 99.6% for fluconazole. However, at the two-week follow up, only 64.4% of the anidulafungin-treated patients had a sustained endoscopic success compared to 89.5% of the fluconazole-treated patients (p < 0.001). The lack of sustained response in the anidulafungin compared to the fluconazole-treated patients was complicated by higher use of antiretroviral therapy among patients receiving fluconazole. It has also been suggested that salivary enzymes or pharmaceutical replacement enzymes could digest anidulafungin through ring digestion, and this could contribute to the lack of a sustained response when treating esophageal candidiasis with anidulafungin [165].

Candidemia

Anidulafungin has been investigated in at least two prospective studies of invasive candidiasis [121,166]. In a Phase II open-label, noncomparative study, 123 patients were randomized to 50, 75, or 100 mg of anidulafungin daily [166]. Overall clinical success rate at the end of treatment was 84%, 90%, and 89% with 50, 75, and 100 mg daily, respectively. In a phase III, randomized, double-blind study of candidemia and invasive candidiasis, anidulafungin (100 mg daily, after a 200 mg loading dose) was compared to fluconazole (400 mg daily, after an 800 mg loading dose] [121]. Treatment was continued for at least 14 days from the last positive blood culture. Patients included in this study were predominantly non-neutropenic (97%) with APACHE II (Acute Physiology and Chronic Health) scores less than 20 (80%). The majority of infections were due to *C. albicans* (62%) and involved candidemia (89%). At the end of intravenous therapy, there was a 75.6% overall clinical response with anidulafungin compared to 60.2% response with fluconazole (difference = 15.4%, 95% CI = 3.9%–27%, p = 0.01). This improvement in efficacy with anidulafungin was maintained at 2 weeks after the end of therapy. There was no apparent association between fluconazole MICs of the organisms and eradication rates observed in this study, but few isolates (*n* = 5) had fluconazole MICs ≥16 μg/mL. Microbiologic and overall treatment success among patients with *C. parapsilosis* infections were numerically higher with fluconazole, but these differences were not statistically significant. Overall mortality among study subjects was lower among patients receiving anidulafungin (33%) compared to fluconazole (23%), but these differences were not statistically significant in a survival analysis. Fewer patients receiving anidulafungin had adverse events leading to discontinuation of study treatment (11.5% anidulafungin group vs. 21.6% fluconazole group, p = 0.02), but overall rates of treatment-related adverse events were similar between groups (24.4% anidulafungin vs. 26.4% fluconazole). In summary, anidulafungin had superior efficacy and was similarly safe as fluconazole in treating adults with candidemia/invasive candidiasis. Additional studies are needed to confirm these findings that echinocandins may be more efficacious than azoles for *Candida* spp. infections.

Aspergillosis

A randomized, double-blind, placebo controlled multicenter trial evaluated 277 patients with confirmed invasive aspergillosis who received either a combination of anidulafungin and voriconazole or voriconazole monotherapy. Six-week mortality was significantly lower with combination therapy at ~16% versus ~27% with monotherapy. However, the low power of the study limited any conclusions about superiority of combination therapy versus monotherapy [167].

Prophylaxis of IFI in high-risk liver transplant recipients

A randomized, double-blind trial of 200 patients comparing the use of anidulafungin to fluconazole for prophylaxis of IFI in liver transplant recipients showed no significant difference between incidence of IFI (approximately 5% vs. 8% respectively). Patients receiving anidulafungin did show lower rates of *Aspergillus* colonization or infection and lower rates of breakthrough infection compared to those who had received pretransplant fluconazole. However, the results were not significant [168]. More data are needed to make an accurate conclusion for the use of anidulafungin in this important patient population.

New echinocandins

Preclinical studies with rezafungin (CD-101), a new echinocandin in development (NCT02734862, NCT02733432), suggest that it has an improved safety profile than other echinocandins. This, in part, is due to its structural stability, infrequent *Cyp*450 enzyme interactions, as well as not forming reactive intermediates like the other echinocandins [169]. A phase I clinical trial has shown doses of rezafungin (CD-101) of 400 mg once weekly for up to 3 weeks to be very well tolerated with no incidents of serious or severe adverse events and none requiring discontinuation of therapy. It's long half-life and linear pharmacokinetics suggest it may require less frequent dosing for therapeutic success [170].

SUMMARY OF EFFICACY AND RECOMMENDATIONS

Given their excellent activity against *Candida* spp. and their safety profile, echinocandins are recognized as primary therapy for candidemia/invasive candidiasis and also have demonstrated efficacy in esophageal/oropharyngeal candidiasis. The Infectious Diseases Society of America (IDSA) currently recommends echinocandins as initial therapy for candidemia in neutropenic and non-neutropenic patients as well as for treatment of chronic disseminated candidiasis. The IDSA also recommends use of an echinocandin as initial empiric therapy for suspected candidiasis in non-neutropenic patients in the ICU [171].

In addition, caspofungin is an option as prophylaxis among patients receiving induction chemotherapy for the duration of neutropenia, and micafungin is an option as prophylaxis in neutropenic HSCT recipients. The IDSA suggests echinocandins should be reserved as alternatives to fluconazole or amphotericin B in neonates and is generally reserved for salvage therapy or intolerance to other antifungal agents [171].

Experience with echinocandins in treatment of invasive aspergillosis is evolving, although these agents are largely employed as salvage or when other first-line options for primary treatment of invasive aspergillosis cannot be used. Caspofungin has an FDA indication for treatment of invasive aspergillosis in patients who are refractory or intolerant to other therapies. Micafungin has generally been employed as part of combination antifungal therapy as salvage for invasive aspergillosis [127,136,141,143]. Anidulafungin was paired with voriconazole in the only randomized double-blind placebo-controlled trial to evaluate combination therapy for invasive aspergillosis [167]. While IDSA does not recommend echinocandins for primary treatment of invasive aspergillosis except in cases where a patient cannot tolerate azoles or polyenes, echinocandins may be combined with voriconazole in select patients with documented invasive pulmonary aspergillosis [172]. Echincandins may also be considered as part of salvage therapy, as recommended by IDSA.

REFERENCES

1. Kurtz MB, Rex JH. Glucan synthase inhibitors as antifungal agents. *Adv Protein Chem* 2001;56:423–475.
2. Wagner C, Graninger W, Presterl E, Joukhadar C. The echinocandins: Comparison of their pharmacokinetics, pharmacodynamics and clinical applications. *Pharmacology* 2006;78(4):161–177.
3. Astellas Pharma US. *Mycamine (micafungin) [Prescribing Information].* Deerfield, IL: Astellas Pharma US.; Revised 2013.
4. Pfizer & Co. *Eraxis (anidulafungin) [Prescribing Information].* New York: Pfizer & Co.; 2006.
5. Merck & Co. *Cancidas (caspofungin) [Prescribing Information].* Whitehouse Station, NJ: Merck & Co.; 2008.
6. Douglas CM, D'Ippolito JA, Shei GJ, et al. Identification of the *FKS1* gene of *Candida albicans* as the essential target of 1,3-beta-D-glucan synthase inhibitors. *Antimicrob Agents Chemother* 1997;41(11):2471–2479.
7. Odabasi Z, Paetznick VL, Rodriguez JR, Chen E, McGinnis MR, Ostrosky-Zeichner L. Differences in beta-glucan levels in culture supernatants of a variety of fungi. *Med Mycol.* 2006;44(3):267–272.
8. Pfaller MA, Boyken L, Hollis RJ, et al. *In vitro* susceptibility of invasive isolates of *Candida* spp. to anidulafungin, caspofungin, and micafungin: Six years of global surveillance. *J Clin Microbiol* 2008;46(1):150–156.
9. Rautemaa R, Richardson M, Pfaller MA, Perheentupa J, Saxen H. Activity of amphotericin B, anidulafungin, caspofungin, micafungin, posaconazole, and voriconazole against *Candida albicans* with decreased susceptibility to fluconazole from APECED

patients on long-term azole treatment of chronic mucocutaneous candidiasis. *Diagn Microbiol Infect Dis* 2008;62(2):182–185.

10. Pfaller MA, Diekema DJ, Messer SA, Hollis RJ, Jones RN. *In vitro* activities of caspofungin compared with those of fluconazole and itraconazole against 3,959 clinical isolates of *Candida* spp., including 157 fluconazole-resistant isolates. *Antimicrob Agents Chemother* 2003;47(3):1068–1071.

11. Marco F, Pfaller MA, Messer SA, Jones RN. Activity of MK-0991 (L-743,872), a new echinocandin, compared with those of LY303366 and four other antifungal agents tested against blood stream isolates of *Candida* spp. *Diagn Microbiol Infect Dis* 1998;32(1):33–37.

12. Diekema DJ, Messer SA, Hollis RJ, Jones RN, Pfaller MA. Activities of caspofungin, itraconazole, posaconazole, ravuconazole, voriconazole, and amphotericin B against 448 recent clinical isolates of filamentous fungi. *J Clin Microbiol* 2003;41(8):3623–3626.

13. Bowman JC, Abruzzo GK, Flattery AM, et al. Efficacy of caspofungin against *Aspergillus flavus*, *Aspergillus terreus*, and *Aspergillus nidulans*. *Antimicrob Agents Chemother* 2006;50(12):4202–4205.

14. Bowman JC, Abruzzo GK, Anderson JW, et al. Quantitative PCR assay to measure *Aspergillus fumigatus* burden in a murine model of disseminated aspergillosis: Demonstration of efficacy of caspofungin acetate. *Antimicrob Agents Chemother* 2001;45(12):3474–3481.

15. Pfaller MA, Diekema DJ, Ostrosky-Zeichner L, et al. Correlation of MIC with outcome for *Candida* species tested against caspofungin, anidulafungin, and micafungin: Analysis and proposal for interpretive MIC breakpoints. *J Clin Microbiol* 2008;46(8):2620–2629.

16. Institute CaLS. *Reference Method for Broth Dilution Antifungal Susceptibility Testing of Yeasts*. Wayne, PA: Institute CaLS, 2012.

17. Fothergill AW, Sutton DA, McCarthy DI, Wiederhold NP. Impact of new antifungal breakpoints on antifungal resistance in *Candida* species. *J Clin Microbiol* 2014;52(3):994–997.

18. Institute CaLS. *Reference Method for Broth Dilution Antifungal Susceptibility Testing of Yeasts*. Wayne, PA: Institute CaLS, 2008.

19. Colombo AL, Perfect J, DiNubile M, et al. Global distribution and outcomes for *Candida* species causing invasive candidiasis: Results from an international randomized double-blind study of caspofungin versus amphotericin B for the treatment of invasive candidiasis. *Eur J Clin Microbiol Infect Dis* 2003;22(8):470–474.

20. Mora-Duarte J, Betts R, Rotstein C, et al. Comparison of caspofungin and amphotericin B for invasive candidiasis. *N Engl J Med* 2002;347(25):2020–2029.

21. Garcia-Effron G, Katiyar SK, Park S, Edlind TD, Perlin DS. A naturally occurring proline-to-alanine amino acid change in Fks1p in *Candida*

parapsilosis, *Candida orthopsilosis*, and *Candida metapsilosis* accounts for reduced echinocandin susceptibility. *Antimicrob Agents Chemother* 2008;52(7):2305–2312.

22. Chowdhary A, Sharma C, Meis JF. *Candida auris*: A rapidly emerging cause of hospital-acquired multidrug-resistant fungal infections globally. *PLoS Pathog* 2017;13(5):e1006290.

23. Espinel-Ingroff A. Comparison of *In vitro* activities of the new triazole SCH56592 and the echinocandins MK-0991 (L-743,872) and LY303366 against opportunistic filamentous and dimorphic fungi and yeasts. *J Clin Microbiol* 1998;36(10):2950–2956.

24. Goughenour KD, Rappleye CA. Antifungal therapeutics for dimorphic fungal pathogens. *Virulence* 2017;8(2):211–221.

25. Thompson GR, 3rd, Barker BM, Wiederhold NP. Large-scale evaluation of *in vitro* amphotericin B, triazole, and echinocandin activity against coccidioides species from U.S. institutions. *Antimicrob Agents Chemother* 2017;61(4):e02634-16.

26. Akagi T, Yamaguti K, Kawamura T, Nakumura T, Kubo K, Takemori H. Breakthrough trichosporonosis in patients with acute myeloid leukemia receiving micafungin. *Leuk Lymphoma* 2006;47(6):1182–1183.

27. Matsue K, Uryu H, Koseki M, Asada N, Takeuchi M. Breakthrough trichosporonosis in patients with hematologic malignancies receiving micafungin. *Clin Infect Dis* 2006;42(6):753–757.

28. Goodman D, Pamer E, Jakubowski A, Morris C, Sepkowitz K. Breakthrough trichosporonosis in a bone marrow transplant recipient receiving caspofungin acetate. *Clin Infect Dis* 2002;35(3):E35–E36.

29. Serrano Mdel C, Valverde-Conde A, Chavez MM, et al. *In vitro* activity of voriconazole, itraconazole, caspofungin, anidulafungin (VER002, LY303366) and amphotericin B against *Aspergillus* spp. *Diagn Microbiol Infect Dis* 2003;45(2):131–135.

30. Nakai T, Uno J, Otomo K, et al. *In vitro* activity of FK463, a novel lipopeptide antifungal agent, against a variety of clinically important molds. *Chemotherapy* 2002;48(2):78–81.

31. Institute CaLS. *Reference Method for Broth Dilution Antifungal Susceptibility Testing of Filamentous Fungi*. Wayne, PA: Institute CaLS, 2008.

32. Del Poeta M, Schell WA, Perfect JR. *In vitro* antifungal activity of pneumocandin L-743,872 against a variety of clinically important molds. *Antimicrob Agents Chemother* 1997;41(8):1835–1836.

33. Espinel-Ingroff A. *In vitro* antifungal activities of anidulafungin and micafungin, licensed agents and the investigational triazole posaconazole as determined by NCCLS methods for 12,052 fungal isolates: Review of the literature. *Rev Iberoam Micol* 2003;20(4):121–136.

34. Cushion MT, Linke MJ, Ashbaugh A, et al. Echinocandin treatment of pneumocystis pneumonia in rodent models depletes cysts leaving trophic burdens that cannot transmit the infection. *PLoS One* 2010;5(1):e8524.

35. Li H, Huang H, He H. Successful treatment of severe Pneumocystis pneumonia in an immunosuppressed patient using caspofungin combined with clindamycin: A case report and literature review. *BMC Pulm Med* 2016;16(1):144.

36. Cushion M, Ashbaugh A, Lynch K, Linke MJ, Bartizal K. Efficacy of CD101, a novel echinocandin, in prevention of pneumocystis pneumonia (PCP): Thwarting the biphasic life cycle of pneumocystis. *Blood* 2016;128(22):3396.

37. Laverdiere M, Lalonde RG, Baril JG, Sheppard DC, Park S, Perlin DS. Progressive loss of echinocandin activity following prolonged use for treatment of *Candida albicans* oesophagitis. *J Antimicrob Chemother* 2006;57(4):705–708.

38. Baixench MT, Aoun N, Desnos-Ollivier M, et al. Acquired resistance to echinocandins in *Candida albicans*: Case report and review. *J Antimicrob Chemother* 2007;59(6):1076–1083.

39. Desnos-Ollivier M, Bretagne S, Raoux D, et al. Mutations in the fks1 gene in *Candida albicans*, C. tropicalis, and C. krusei correlate with elevated caspofungin MICs uncovered in AM3 medium using the method of the European committee on antibiotic susceptibility testing. *Antimicrob Agents Chemother* 2008;52(9):3092–3098.

40. Cleary JD, Garcia-Effron G, Chapman SW, Perlin DS. Reduced *Candida glabrata* susceptibility secondary to an FKS1 mutation developed during candidemia treatment. *Antimicrob Agents Chemother* 2008;52(6):2263–2265.

41. Thompson GR, 3rd, Wiederhold NP, Vallor AC, Villareal NC, Lewis JS, 2nd, Patterson TF. Development of caspofungin resistance following prolonged therapy for invasive candidiasis secondary to *Candida glabrata* infection. *Antimicrob Agents Chemother* 2008;52(10):3783–3785.

42. Pasquale T, Tomada JR, Ghannoun M, Dipersio J, Bonilla H. Emergence of *Candida tropicalis* resistant to caspofungin. *J Antimicrob Chemother* 2008;61(1):219.

43. Garcia-Effron G, Kontoyiannis DP, Lewis RE, Perlin DS. Caspofungin-resistant *Candida tropicalis* strains causing breakthrough fungemia in patients at high risk for hematologic malignancies. *Antimicrob Agents Chemother* 2008;52(11):4181–4183.

44. Ghannoum MA, Chen A, Buhari M, et al. Differential *in vitro* activity of anidulafungin, caspofungin and micafungin against *Candida parapsilosis* isolates recovered from a burn unit. *Clin Microbiol Infect* 2009;15(3):274–279.

45. Mohr JF, Wanger, A, Rogers, PD, et al. Phenotypic and molecular characteristics of relapsing *Candida glabrata* bloodstrem infection during caspofungin treatment. *46th International Conference on Antimicrobial Agents and Chemotherapy*. Washington, DC: American Society of Microbiology; 2006.

46. Alexander BD, Johnson MD, Pfeiffer CD, et al. Increasing echinocandin resistance in *Candida glabrata*: Clinical failure correlates with presence of FKS mutations and elevated minimum inhibitory concentrations. *Clin Infect Dis* 2013;56(12):1724–1732.

47. Hakki M, Staab JF, Marr KA. Emergence of a *Candida krusei* isolate with reduced susceptibility to caspofungin during therapy. *Antimicrob Agents Chemother* 2006;50(7):2522–2524.

48. Sharma C, Kumar N, Pandey R, Meis JF, Chowdhary A. Whole genome sequencing of emerging multidrug resistant *Candida auris* isolates in India demonstrates low genetic variation. *New Microbes New Infect* 2016;13:77–82.

49. Stevens DA, Espiritu M, Parmar R. Paradoxical effect of caspofungin: Reduced activity against *Candida albicans* at high drug concentrations. *Antimicrob Agents Chemother* 2004;48(9):3407–3411.

50. Wiederhold NP, Kontoyiannis DP, Prince RA, Lewis RE. Attenuation of the activity of caspofungin at high concentrations against Candida albicans: Possible role of cell wall integrity and calcineurin pathways. *Antimicrob Agents Chemother* 2005;49(12):5146–5148.

51. Stevens DA, Ichinomiya M, Koshi Y, Horiuchi H. Escape of *Candida* from *caspofungin* inhibition at concentrations above the MIC (paradoxical effect) accomplished by increased cell wall chitin; evidence for beta-1,6-glucan synthesis inhibition by caspofungin. *Antimicrob Agents Chemother* 2006;50(9):3160–3161.

52. Chamilos G, Lewis RE, Albert N, Kontoyiannis DP. Paradoxical effect of Echinocandins across *Candida species in vitro*: Evidence for echinocandin-specific and *Candida* species-related differences. *Antimicrob Agents Chemother* 2007;51(6):2257–2259.

53. Clemons KV, Espiritu M, Parmar R, Stevens DA. Assessment of the paradoxical effect of caspofungin in therapy of candidiasis. *Antimicrob Agents Chemother* 2006;50(4):1293–1297.

54. Antachopoulos C, Meletiadis J, Sein T, Roilides E, Walsh TJ. Comparative *in vitro* pharmacodynamics of caspofungin, micafungin, and anidulafungin against germinated and nongerminated *Aspergillus conidia*. *Antimicrob Agents Chemother* 2008;52(1):321–328.

55. Lewis RE, Albert ND, Kontoyiannis DP. Comparison of the dose-dependent activity and paradoxical effect of caspofungin and micafungin in a neutropenic murine model of invasive pulmonary aspergillosis. *J Antimicrob Chemother* 2008;61(5):1140–1144.

56. Betts RF, Nucci M, Talwar D, et al. A Multicenter, double-blind trial of a high-dose caspofungin treatment regimen versus a standard caspofungin treatment regimen for adult patients with invasive candidiasis. *Clin Infect Dis* 2009;48(12):1676–1684.

57. Kartsonis N, Killar J, Mixson L, et al. Caspofungin susceptibility testing of isolates from patients with esophageal candidiasis or invasive candidiasis: Relationship of MIC to treatment outcome. *Antimicrob Agents Chemother* 2005;49(9):3616–3623.

58. Pappas PG, Rotstein CM, Betts RF, et al. Micafungin versus caspofungin for treatment of candidemia and other forms of invasive candidiasis. *Clin Infect Dis* 2007;45(7):883–893.

59. Loiko V, Wagener J. The paradoxical effect of echinocandins in *Aspergillus fumigatus* relies on recovery of the beta-1,3-Glucan Synthase Fks1. *Antimicrob Agents Chemother* 2017;61(2):e01690-16.

60. Hajdu R, Thompson R, Sundelof JG, et al. Preliminary animal pharmacokinetics of the parenteral antifungal agent MK-0991 (L-743,872). *Antimicrob Agents Chemother* 1997;41(11):2339–2344.

61. Stone JA, Holland SD, Wickersham PJ, et al. Single- and multiple-dose pharmacokinetics of caspofungin in healthy men. *Antimicrob Agents Chemother* 2002;46(3):739–745.

62. Balani SK, Xu X, Arison BH, et al. Metabolites of caspofungin acetate, a potent antifungal agent, in human plasma and urine. *Drug Metab Dispos* 2000;28(11):1274–1278.

63. Mistry GC, Migoya E, Deutsch PJ, et al. Single- and multiple-dose administration of caspofungin in patients with hepatic insufficiency: Implications for safety and dosing recommendations. *J Clin Pharmacol* 2007;47(8):951–961.

64. Sobel JD, Bradshaw SK, Lipka CJ, Kartsonis NA. Caspofungin in the treatment of symptomatic candiduria. *Clin Infect Dis* 2007;44(5):e46–e49.

65. Abe F, Ueyama J, Kawasumi N, et al. Role of plasma proteins in pharmacokinetics of micafungin, an antifungal antibiotic, in analbuminemic rats. *Antimicrob Agents Chemother* 2008;52(9):3454–3456.

66. Gumbo T, Hiemenz J, Ma L, Keirns JJ, Buell DN, Drusano GL. Population pharmacokinetics of micafungin in adult patients. *Diagn Microbiol Infect Dis* 2008;60(3):329–331.

67. Hall RG, Swancutt MA, Gumbo T. Fractal geometry and the pharmacometrics of micafungin in overweight, obese, and extremely obese people. *Antimicrob Agents Chemother* 2011;55(11):5107–5112.

68. Brown GL, White, RJ., Taubel, J. Phase 1 dose optimization study for V-echinocandin. *40th International Conference on Antimicrobial Agents and Chemotherapy*. Washington, DC: American Society of Microbiology, 2000.

69. Thye D, Shepherd, B, White, RJ, et al. Anidulafungin: A phase 1 study to identify the maximum tolerated dose in healthy volunteers. *41st International Conference on Antimicrobial Agents and Chemotherapy*. Washington, DC: American Society of Microbiology, 2001.

70. Dowell JA, Knebel W, Ludden T, Stogniew M, Krause D, Henkel T. Population pharmacokinetic analysis of anidulafungin, an echinocandin antifungal. *J Clin Pharmacol* 2004;44(6):590–598.

71. Niwa T, Yokota Y, Tokunaga A, et al. Tissue distribution after intravenous dosing of micafungin, an antifungal drug, to rats. *Biol Pharm Bull* 2004;27(7):1154–1156.

72. Suzuki T, Uno T, Chen G, Ohashi Y. Ocular distribution of intravenously administered micafungin in rabbits. *J Infect Chemother* 2008;14(3):204–207.

73. Hope WW, Mickiene D, Petraitis V, et al. The pharmacokinetics and pharmacodynamics of micafungin in experimental hematogenous *Candida meningoencephalitis*: Implications for echinocandin therapy in neonates. *J Infect Dis* 2008;197(1):163–171.

74. Damle B, Stogniew M, Dowell J. Pharmacokinetics and tissue distribution of anidulafungin in rats. *Antimicrob Agents Chemother* 2008;52(7):2673–2676.

75. Crandon JL, Banevicius MA, Fang AF, et al. Bronchopulmonary disposition of intravenous voriconazole and anidulafungin given in combination to healthy adults. *Antimicrob Agents Chemother* 2009;53(12):5102–5107.

76. Moriyama B, Ditullio M, Wilson E, et al. Pharmacokinetics of anidulafungin in pleural fluid during the treatment of a patient with *Candida empyema*. *Antimicrob Agents Chemother* 2011;55(5):2478–2480.

77. Gauthier GM, Nork TM, Prince R, Andes D. Subtherapeutic ocular penetration of caspofungin and associated treatment failure in *Candida albicans* endophthalmitis. *Clin Infect Dis* 2005;41(3):e27–e28.

78. Spriet I, Delaere L, Lagrou K, Peetermans WE, Maertens J, Willems L. Intraocular penetration of voriconazole and caspofungin in a patient with fungal endophthalmitis. *J Antimicrob Chemother* 2009;64(4):877–878.

79. Hsue G, Napier JT, Prince RA, Chi J, Hospenthal DR. Treatment of meningeal coccidioidomycosis with caspofungin. *J Antimicrob Chemother* 2004;54(1):292–294.

80. Burkhardt O, Ellis S, Burhenne H, et al. High caspofungin levels in alveolar cells of a lung transplant patient with suspected pulmonary aspergillosis. *Int J Antimicrob Agents* 2009;34(5):491–492.

81. Nicasio AM, Tessier PR, Nicolau DP, et al. Bronchopulmonary disposition of micafungin in healthy adult volunteers. *Antimicrob Agents Chemother* 2009;53(3):1218–1220.

82. Walsh TJ, Goutelle S, Jelliffe RW, et al. Intrapulmonary pharmacokinetics and pharmacodynamics of micafungin in adult lung transplant patients. *Antimicrob Agents Chemother* 2010;54(8):3451–3459.

83. Okugawa S, Ota Y, Tatsuno K, Tsukada K, Kishino S, Koike K. A case of invasive central nervous system aspergillosis treated with micafungin with monitoring of micafungin concentrations in the cerebrospinal fluid. *Scand J Infect Dis* 2007;39(4):344–346.

84. Lat A, Thompson GR, 3rd, Rinaldi MG, Dorsey SA, Pennick G, Lewis JS, 2nd. Micafungin concentrations from brain tissue and pancreatic pseudocyst fluid. *Antimicrob Agents Chemother* 2010;54(2):943–944.

85. Azuma J, Nakahara, K., Kagayama, A., et al. Pharmacokinetic study of micafungin in elderly subjects. *Jap J Chemother* 2002;50(Supplement 1):148–154.

86. Stone JA, Ballow, CH, Holland, SD, et al. Single dose caspofungin pharmacokinetics in healthy elderly subjects. *40th International Conference on Antimicrobial Agents and Chemotherapy.* Washington, DC: American Society of Microbiology, 2000.

87. Stone JA, McCrea, JB., Wickersham, PJ, et al. A phase 1 study of caspofungin evaluating the potential for drug interactions with itraconazole, the effect of gender and the use of a loading dose regimen. *40th International Conference on Antimicrobial Agents and Chemotherapy.* Washington, DC: American Society of Microbiology, 2000.

88. Walsh TJ, Adamson PC, Seibel NL, et al. Pharmacokinetics, safety, and tolerability of caspofungin in children and adolescents. *Antimicrob Agents Chemother* 2005;49(11):4536–4545.

89. Hebert MF, Smith HE, Marbury TC, et al. Pharmacokinetics of micafungin in healthy volunteers, volunteers with moderate liver disease, and volunteers with renal dysfunction. *J Clin Pharmacol* 2005;45(10):1145–1152.

90. Hirata K, Aoyama T, Matsumoto Y, et al. Pharmacokinetics of antifungal agent micafungin in critically ill patients receiving continuous hemodialysis filtration. *Yakugaku Zasshi* 2007;127(5):897–901.

91. Dowell JA, Stogniew M, Krause D, Damle B. Anidulafungin does not require dosage adjustment in subjects with varying degrees of hepatic or renal impairment. *J Clin Pharmacol* 2007;47(4):461–470.

92. Thye D, Kilfoil, T, Kilfoil, G, et al. Anidulafungin: Pharmacokinetics in subjects with severe hepatic impairment. *42nd International Conference on Antimicrobial Agents and Chemotherapy.* Washington, DC: American Society of Microbiology, 2002.

93. Mochizuki N, Matsumoto K, Ohno K, et al. Effects of hepatic CYP3A4 activity on disposition of micafungin in liver transplant recipients with markedly small-for-size grafts. *Transplant Proc* 2006;38(10):3649–3650.

94. Jullien V, Blanchet B, Benyamina M, Tod M, Vinsonneau C. Pharmacokinetics of caspofungin in two patients with burn injuries. *Antimicrob Agents Chemother* 2012;56(8):4550–4551.

95. Nguyen TH, Hoppe-Tichy T, Geiss HK, et al. Factors influencing caspofungin plasma concentrations in patients of a surgical intensive care unit. *J Antimicrob Chemother* 2007;60(1):100–106.

96. Sinnollareddy MG, Roberts JA, Lipman J, et al. Pharmacokinetic variability and exposures of fluconazole, anidulafungin, and caspofungin in intensive care unit patients: Data from multinational defining antibiotic levels in intensive care unit (DALI) patients study. *Crit Care* 2015;19:33.

97. Watt KM, Cohen-Wolkowiez M, Williams DC, et al. Antifungal extraction by the extracorporeal membrane oxygenation circuit. *J Extra Corpor Technol* 2017;49(3):150–159.

98. Aguilar G, Ferriols R, Carbonell JA, et al. Pharmacokinetics of anidulafungin during venovenous extracorporeal membrane oxygenation. *Crit Care* 2016;20(1):325.

99. Hahn J, Choi JH, Chang MJ. Pharmacokinetic changes of antibiotic, antiviral, antituberculosis and antifungal agents during extracorporeal membrane oxygenation in critically ill adult patients. *J Clin Pharm Ther* 2017; 42(6):661–671.

100. Seibel NL, Schwartz C, Arrieta A, et al. Safety, tolerability, and pharmacokinetics of Micafungin (FK463) in febrile neutropenic pediatric patients. *Antimicrob Agents Chemother* 2005;49(8):3317–3324.

101. Benjamin DK, Jr., Driscoll T, Seibel NL, et al. Safety and pharmacokinetics of intravenous anidulafungin in children with neutropenia at high risk for invasive fungal infections. *Antimicrob Agents Chemother* 2006;50(2):632–638.

102. Heresi GP, Gerstmann DR, Reed MD, et al. The pharmacokinetics and safety of micafungin, a novel echinocandin, in premature infants. *Pediatr Infect Dis J* 2006;25(12):1110–1115.

103. Smith PB, Walsh TJ, Hope W, et al. Pharmacokinetics of an elevated dosage of micafungin in premature neonates. *Pediatr Infect Dis J* 2009;28(5):412–415.

104. Hope WW, Smith PB, Arrieta A, et al. Population pharmacokinetics of micafungin in neonates and young infants. *Antimicrob Agents Chemother* 2010;54(6):2633–2637.

105. Saez-Llorens X, Macias M, Maiya P, et al. Pharmacokinetics and safety of caspofungin in neonates and infants less than 3 months of age. *Antimicrob Agents Chemother* 2009;53(3):869–875.

106. Groll AH, Roilides E, Walsh TJ. Pediatric pharmacology of antifungal agents. *Curr Fungal Infect Rep* 2008;2(1):49–56.

107. Andes D. *In vivo* pharmacodynamics of antifungal drugs in treatment of candidiasis. *Antimicrob Agents Chemother* 2003;47(4):1179–1186.

108. Louie A, Deziel M, Liu W, Drusano MF, Gumbo T, Drusano GL. Pharmacodynamics of caspofungin in a murine model of systemic candidiasis:

Importance of persistence of caspofungin in tissues to understanding drug activity. *Antimicrob Agents Chemother* 2005;49(12):5058–5068.

109. Andes DR, Diekema DJ, Pfaller MA, Marchillo K, Bohrmueller J. In vivo pharmacodynamic target investigation for micafungin against *Candida albicans* and C. glabrata in a neutropenic murine candidiasis model. *Antimicrob Agents Chemother* 2008;52(10):3497–3503.

110. Andes D, Diekema DJ, Pfaller MA, et al. In vivo pharmacodynamic characterization of anidulafungin in a neutropenic murine candidiasis model. *Antimicrob Agents Chemother* 2008;52(2):539–550.

111. Petraitis V, Petraitiene R, Groll AH, et al. Comparative antifungal activities and plasma pharmacokinetics of micafungin (FK463) against disseminated candidiasis and invasive pulmonary aspergillosis in persistently neutropenic rabbits. *Antimicrob Agents Chemother* 2002;46(6):1857–1869.

112. Wiederhold NP, Kontoyiannis DP, Chi J, Prince RA, Tam VH, Lewis RE. Pharmacodynamics of caspofungin in a murine model of invasive pulmonary aspergillosis: Evidence of concentration-dependent activity. *J Infect Dis* 2004;190(8):1464–1471.

113. Tabata K, Katashima M, Kawamura A, Kaibara A, Tanigawara Y. Population pharmacokinetic analysis of micafungin in Japanese patients with fungal infections. *Drug Metab Pharmacokinet* 2006;21(4):324–331.

114. Shimoeda S, Ohta S, Kobayashi H, Yamato S, Sasaki M, Kawano K. Effective blood concentration of micafungin for pulmonary aspergillosis. *Biol Pharm Bull* 2006;29(9):1886–1891.

115. Dowell J, Stogniew, M, Krause, D, et al. Anidulafungin pharmacokinetic/pharmacodynamic correlation: Treatment of esophageal candidiases. *43rd International Conference on Antimicrobial Agents and Chemotherapy*. Washington, DC: American Society of Microbiology, 2003.

116. Sable CA, Nguyen BY, Chodakewitz JA, DiNubile MJ. Safety and tolerability of caspofungin acetate in the treatment of fungal infections. *Transpl Infect Dis* 2002;4(1):25–30.

117. Cleary JD, Schwartz M, Rogers PD, de Mestral J, Chapman SW. Effects of amphotericin B and caspofungin on histamine expression. *Pharmacotherapy* 2003;23(8):966–973.

118. Kartsonis NA, Nielsen J, Douglas CM. Caspofungin: The first in a new class of antifungal agents. *Drug Resist Updat* 2003;6(4):197–218.

119. Marr KA, Hachem R, Papanicolaou G, et al. Retrospective study of the hepatic safety profile of patients concomitantly treated with caspofungin and cyclosporin A. *Transpl Infect Dis* 2004;6(3):110–116.

120. Sirohi B, Powles RL, Chopra R, et al. A study to determine the safety profile and maximum tolerated dose of micafungin (FK463) in patients undergoing haematopoietic stem cell transplantation. *Bone Marrow Transplant* 2006;38(1):47–51.

121. Reboli AC, Rotstein C, Pappas PG, et al. Anidulafungin versus fluconazole for invasive candidiasis. *N Engl J Med* 2007;356(24):2472–2482.

122. Schneeweiss S, Carver PL, Datta K, et al. Short-term risk of liver and renal injury in hospitalized patients using micafungin: A multicentre cohort study. *J Antimicrob Chemother* 2016;71(10):2938–2944.

123. Kofla G, Ruhnke M. Pharmacology and metabolism of anidulafungin, caspofungin and micafungin in the treatment of invasive candidosis: Review of the literature. *Eur J Med Res* 2011;16(4):159–166.

124. Krause DS, Simjee AE, van Rensburg C, et al. A randomized, double-blind trial of anidulafungin versus fluconazole for the treatment of esophageal candidiasis. *Clin Infect Dis* 2004;39(6):770–775.

125. Bellmann R. Clinical pharmacokinetics of systemically administered antimycotics. *Curr Clin Pharmacol* 2007;2(1):37–58.

126. Queiroz-Telles F, Berezin E, Leverger G, et al. Micafungin versus liposomal amphotericin B for pediatric patients with invasive candidiasis: Substudy of a randomized double-blind trial. *Pediatr Infect Dis J* 2008;27(9):820–826.

127. Denning DW, Marr KA, Lau WM, et al. Micafungin (FK463), alone or in combination with other systemic antifungal agents, for the treatment of acute invasive aspergillosis. *J Infect* 2006;53(5):337–349.

128. Sanz-Rodriguez C, Arranz R, Cisneros JM, et al. Absence of clinically relevant effect of caspofungin on cyclosporin pharmacokinetics. *Swiss Med Wkly* 2005;135(43–44):658–659.

129. Sandhu P, Lee W, Xu X, et al. Hepatic uptake of the novel antifungal agent caspofungin. *Drug Metab Dispos* 2005;33(5):676–682.

130. Andes DR, Safdar N, Baddley JW, et al. Impact of treatment strategy on outcomes in patients with candidemia and other forms of invasive candidiasis: A patient-level quantitative review of randomized trials. *Clin Infect Dis* 2012;54(8):1110–1122.

131. Prabhu RM, Orenstein R. Failure of caspofungin to treat brain abscesses secondary to *Candida albicans* prosthetic valve endocarditis. *Clin Infect Dis* 2004;39(8):1253–1254.

132. Liu KH, Wu CJ, Chou CH, et al. Refractory candidal meningitis in an immunocompromised patient cured by caspofungin. *J Clin Microbiol* 2004;42(12):5950–5953.

133. Rajendram R, Alp NJ, Mitchell AR, Bowler IC, Forfar JC. *Candida* prosthetic valve endocarditis cured by caspofungin therapy without valve replacement. *Clin Infect Dis* 2005;40(9):e72–e74.

134. Bacak V, Biocina B, Starcevic B, Gertler S, Begovac J. *Candida albicans* endocarditis treatment with caspofungin in an HIV-infected patient--case report and review of literature. *J Infect* 2006;53(1):e11–e14.

135. Cornely OA, Lasso M, Betts R, et al. Caspofungin for the treatment of less common forms of invasive candidiasis. *J Antimicrob Chemother* 2007;60(2):363–369.

136. Kontoyiannis DP, Ratanatharathorn V, Young JA, et al. Micafungin alone or in combination with other systemic antifungal therapies in hematopoietic stem cell transplant recipients with invasive aspergillosis. *Transpl Infect Dis* 2009;11(1):89–93.

137. Villanueva A, Arathoon EG, Gotuzzo E, Berman RS, DiNubile MJ, Sable CA. A randomized double-blind study of caspofungin versus amphotericin for the treatment of candidal esophagitis. *Clin Infect Dis* 2001;33(9):1529–1535.

138. Arathoon EG, Gotuzzo E, Noriega LM, Berman RS, DiNubile MJ, Sable CA. Randomized, double-blind, multicenter study of caspofungin versus amphotericin B for treatment of oropharyngeal and esophageal candidiases. *Antimicrob Agents Chemother* 2002;46(2):451–457.

139. Villanueva A, Gotuzzo E, Arathoon EG, et al. A randomized double-blind study of caspofungin versus fluconazole for the treatment of esophageal candidiasis. *Am J Med* 2002;113(4):294–299.

140. Dinubile MJ, Lupinacci RJ, Berman RS, Sable CA. Response and relapse rates of candidal esophagitis in HIV-infected patients treated with caspofungin. *AIDS Res Hum Retroviruses* 2002;18(13):903–908.

141. Kartsonis NA, Saah AJ, Joy Lipka C, Taylor AF, Sable CA. Salvage therapy with caspofungin for invasive aspergillosis: Results from the caspofungin compassionate use study. *J Infect* 2005;50(3):196–205.

142. Singh N, Limaye AP, Forrest G, et al. Combination of voriconazole and caspofungin as primary therapy for invasive aspergillosis in solid organ transplant recipients: A prospective, multicenter, observational study. *Transplantation.* 2006;81(3):320–326.

143. Marr KA, Boeckh M, Carter RA, Kim HW, Corey L. Combination antifungal therapy for invasive aspergillosis. *Clin Infect Dis* 2004;39(6):797–802.

144. Maertens J, Glasmacher A, Herbrecht R, et al. Multicenter, noncomparative study of caspofungin in combination with other antifungals as salvage therapy in adults with invasive aspergillosis. *Cancer* 2006;107(12):2888–2897.

145. Caillot D, Thiebaut A, Herbrecht R, et al. Liposomal amphotericin B in combination with caspofungin for invasive aspergillosis in patients with hematologic malignancies: A randomized pilot study (Combistrat trial). *Cancer* 2007;110(12):2740–2746.

146. Nivoix Y, Zamfir A, Lutun P, et al. Combination of caspofungin and an azole or an amphotericin B formulation in invasive fungal infections. *J Infect* 2006;52(1):67–74.

147. Cattaneo C, Monte S, Algarotti A, et al. A randomized comparison of caspofungin versus antifungal prophylaxis according to investigator policy in acute leukaemia patients undergoing induction chemotherapy (PROFIL-C study). *J Antimicrob Chemother* 2011;66(9):2140–2145.

148. Zaoutis TE, Jafri HS, Huang LM, et al. A prospective, multicenter study of caspofungin for the treatment of documented *Candida* or *Aspergillus* infections in pediatric patients. *Pediatrics* 2009;123(3):877–884.

149. Mohamed WA, Ismail M. A randomized, double-blind, prospective study of caspofungin vs. amphotericin B for the treatment of invasive candidiasis in newborn infants. *J Trop Pediatr* 2012;58(1):25–30.

150. Maertens JA, Madero L, Reilly AF, et al. A randomized, double-blind, multicenter study of caspofungin versus liposomal amphotericin B for empiric antifungal therapy in pediatric patients with persistent fever and neutropenia. *Pediatr Infect Dis J* 2010;29(5):415–420.

151. Walsh TJ, Teppler H, Donowitz GR, et al. *Caspofungin versus* liposomal amphotericin B for empirical antifungal therapy in patients with persistent fever and neutropenia. *N Engl J Med* 2004;351(14):1391–1402.

152. de Wet N, Llanos-Cuentas A, Suleiman J, et al. A randomized, double-blind, parallel-group, dose-response study of micafungin compared with fluconazole for the treatment of esophageal candidiasis in HIV-positive patients. *Clin Infect Dis* 2004;39(6):842–849.

153. de Wet NT, Bester AJ, Viljoen JJ, et al. A randomized, double blind, comparative trial of micafungin (FK463) vs. fluconazole for the treatment of oesophageal candidiasis. *Aliment Pharmacol Ther* 2005;21(7):899–907.

154. Astellas Pharma I. Trial of Two Dosing Regimens of Micafungin Versus Caspofungin for the Treatment of Esophageal Candidiasis, 2008. [online.] 08/20/2014. https://clinicaltrials.gov/show/NCT00665639.

155. Ostrosky-Zeichner L, Kontoyiannis D, Raffalli J, et al. International, open-label, noncomparative, clinical trial of micafungin alone and in combination for treatment of newly diagnosed and refractory candidemia. *Eur J Clin Microbiol Infect Dis* 2005;24(10):654–661.

156. Kuse ER, Chetchotisakd P, da Cunha CA, et al. Micafungin versus liposomal amphotericin B for candidaemia and invasive candidosis: A phase III randomised double-blind trial. *Lancet* 2007;369(9572):1519–1527.

157. Kohno S, Masaoka T, Yamaguchi H, et al. A multicenter, open-label clinical study of micafungin (FK463) in the treatment of deep-seated mycosis in Japan. *Scand J Infect Dis* 2004;36(5):372–379.

158. Cornely OA, Meems L, Herbrecht R, Viscoli C, van Amsterdam RG, Ruhnke M. Randomised, multicentre trial of micafungin vs. an institutional standard regimen for salvage treatment of invasive aspergillosis. *Mycoses* 2015;58(1):58–64.

159. Oyake T, Kowata S, Murai K, et al. Comparison of micafungin and voriconazole as empirical antifungal therapies in febrile neutropenic

patients with hematological disorders: A randomized controlled trial. *Eur J Haematol* 2016;96(6):602–609.

160. Jeong SH, Kim DY, Jang JH, et al. Efficacy and safety of micafungin versus intravenous itraconazole as empirical antifungal therapy for febrile neutropenic patients with hematological malignancies: A randomized, controlled, prospective, multicenter study. *Ann Hematol* 2016;95(2):337–344.

161. van Burik JA, Ratanatharathorn V, Stepan DE, et al. Micafungin versus fluconazole for prophylaxis against invasive fungal infections during neutropenia in patients undergoing hematopoietic stem cell transplantation. *Clin Infect Dis* 2004;39(10):1407–1416.

162. Huang X, Chen H, Han M, et al. Multicenter, randomized, open-label study comparing the efficacy and safety of micafungin versus itraconazole for prophylaxis of invasive fungal infections in patients undergoing hematopoietic stem cell transplant. *Biol Blood Marrow Transplant* 2012;18(10):1509–1516.

163. Saliba F, Pascher A, Cointault O, et al. Randomized trial of micafungin for the prevention of invasive fungal infection in high-risk liver transplant recipients. *Clin Infect Dis* 2015;60(7):997–1006.

164. Vazquez JA, Schranz JA, Clark K, Goldstein BP, Reboli A, Fichtenbaum C. A phase 2, open-label study of the safety and efficacy of intravenous anidulafungin as a treatment for azole-refractory mucosal candidiasis. *J Acquir Immune Defic Syndr* 2008;48(3):304–309.

165. Kelly K, Chapman, S., Cleary, J.D. Digestion of echinocandins. *46th International Conference on Antimicrobial Agents and Chemotherapy.* Washington, DC: American Society of Microbiology, 2006.

166. Krause DS, Reinhardt J, Vazquez JA, et al. Phase 2, randomized, dose-ranging study evaluating the safety and efficacy of anidulafungin in invasive candidiasis and candidemia. *Antimicrob Agents Chemother* 2004;48(6):2021–2024.

167. Marr KA, Schlamm HT, Herbrecht R, et al. Combination antifungal therapy for invasive aspergillosis: A randomized trial. *Ann Intern Med* 2015;162(2):81–89.

168. Winston DJ, Limaye AP, Pelletier S, et al. Randomized, double-blind trial of anidulafungin versus fluconazole for prophylaxis of invasive fungal infections in high-risk liver transplant recipients. *Am J Transplant* 2014;14(12):2758–2764.

169. Ong V, Hough G, Schlosser M, et al. Preclinical evaluation of the stability, safety, and efficacy of CD101, a novel echinocandin. *Antimicrob Agents Chemother* 2016;60(11):6872–6879.

170. Sandison T, Ong V, Lee J, Thye D. Safety and pharmacokinetics of CD101 IV, a novel echinocandin, in healthy adults. *Antimicrob Agents Chemother* 2017;61(2):e01627-16.

171. Pappas PG, Kauffman CA, Andes DR, et al. Clinical practice guideline for the management of candidiasis: 2016 update by the infectious diseases society of America. *Clin Infect Dis* 2016;62(4):e1–e50.

172. Patterson TF, Thompson GR, 3rd, Denning DW, et al. Practice guidelines for the diagnosis and management of aspergillosis: 2016 update by the infectious diseases society of America. *Clin Infect Dis* 2016;63(4):e1–e60.

173. Castanheira M, Messer SA, Rhomberg PR, Pfaller MA. Antifungal susceptibility patterns of a global collection of fungal isolates: Results of the SENTRY antifungal surveillance program (2013). *Diagn Microbiol Infect Dis* 2016;85(2):200–204.

174. Azuma J, Yamamoto Y., Ogura M, et al. Phase 1 study of FK463, a new antifungal agent, in healthy adult male volunteers. *38th International Conference on Antimicrobial Agents and Chemotherapy.* Washington, DC: American Society of Microbiology, 1998.

175. Mukai T, Ohkuma T, Nakahara K, et al. Pharmacokinetics of FK463, a novel echinocandin analogue, in elderly and non-elderly subjects. *41st International Conference on Antimicrobial Agents and Chemotherapy.* Washington, DC: American Society of Microbiology, 2001.

176. Hiemenz J, Cagnoni P, Simpson D, et al. Pharmacokinetic and maximum tolerated dose study of micafungin in combination with fluconazole versus fluconazole alone for prophylaxis of fungal infections in adult patients undergoing a bone marrow or peripheral stem cell transplant. *Antimicrob Agents Chemother* 2005;49(4):1331–1336.

177. Chandrasekar PH, Sobel JD. Micafungin: A new echinocandin. *Clin Infect Dis* 2006;42(8):1171–1178.

178. Felton T, Troke PF, Hope WW. Tissue penetration of antifungal agents. *Clin Microbiol Rev* 2014;27(1):68–88.

179. VandenBussche HL, Van Loo DA. A clinical review of echinocandins in pediatric patients. *Ann Pharmacother* 2010;44(1):166–177.

180. Chiou CC, Walsh TJ, Groll AH. Clinical pharmacology of antifungal agents in pediatric patients. *Expert Opin Pharmacother* 2007;8(15):2465–2489.

14

Novel methods of antifungal administration

RICHARD H. DREW

INTRODUCTION

Despite the availability of systemic antifungal agents with potent activity *in vitro* against a wide variety of fungal pathogens, treatment outcomes for many invasive fungal infections (IFIs) (especially in immunocompromised hosts) remain poor. Numerous strategies have been employed in an attempt to optimize therapy, including use of prophylaxis in high-risk patient populations, early diagnosis, pre-emptive antifungal therapy, pharmacodynamic-based dosing of antifungals, antifungal serum concentration monitoring, and the introduction of newer therapies. In an effort to optimize antifungal concentration at the infection site while minimizing the consequences of systemic administration (including adverse reactions and drug interactions), antifungals tested and approved for systemic therapy (i.e., oral and parenteral administration) have been administered in a variety of novel (i.e., unconventional and/or unapproved) methods [1]. While most of the older reports involve administration of the polyene amphotericin B, other antifungal classes (notably select azoles and echinocandins) have also been administered in novel methods, including (but not limited to) aerosols, irrigations, topical administration, and direct (local) administration (via injection or the use of antifungal-impregnated beads or orthopedic cement).

Novel methods to administer antifungals have been reviewed previously, including detailed descriptions of the administered preparations (when available) [1]. With the exception of select trials evaluating the impact of aerosols and urinary irrigants, much of the published data are restricted to uncontrolled case reports and case series of small numbers of patients. Most cases involve treatment in patients who are refractory to conventional therapy and/or have or are receiving systemic therapy concomitantly. Adequate descriptions of the agent's preparation and stability are lacking in most reports. In many cases, safety and tolerability information is either scarce or omitted. Finally, it is likely that significant publication bias exists in reporting interventions with positive outcomes in patients who are often refractory to conventional therapies. Thus, it is often difficult to determine the contribution of the novel antifungal in the treatment outcome.

It is the intent of this chapter to provide an overview regarding the potential role of novel antifungal administration in the current treatment of a variety of IFIs. With one exception (specifically the administration of polyhexamethylene biguanide [PHMB]), the descriptions in this chapter utilize FDA-approved drugs for unapproved indications and/or unapproved routes of administration to humans. Inclusion of information in this chapter should *not* be considered an endorsement of such use, and clinicians should refer to the original publications and current treatment guidelines for details and verification regarding dose and frequency, formulation, administration methods, and adverse effects.

AEROSOLS AND ENDOBRONCHIAL ADMINISTRATION

Aerosols

Numerous case reports and limited clinical trials have been published evaluating the use of aerosolized antifungals in the prevention and adjunctive therapy of IFIs in select populations [2–5]. Although early reports described the use of nystatin [6–8], more recent investigations in both animals and humans describe various formulations of amphotericin B (usually amphotericin B deoxycholate [AmBd] or a lipid-based formulation of amphotericin B [LFAmB]) [2]. The focus of recent human investigations has been in the prevention and adjunctive treatment of invasive aspergillosis in high-risk patients [2]. Since disease occurs after inhalation and deposition of the fungal propagule into the lungs, aerosolized formulations of amphotericin B may provide high antifungal concentrations at the site of initial infection while minimizing its potential for systemic side effects [2,9–12].

Aerosolized amphotericin B deoxycholate (aAmBd) has been studied for the prophylaxis of fungal infections in several patient populations, including neutropenic patients receiving chemotherapy [13–15], bone marrow transplant recipients [16,17], and solid organ transplant recipients, most notably heart or lung transplant recipients [18–21]. Doses vary between trials, ranging from 5 to 20 mg once daily to three times daily with and without additional systemic prophylaxis. The trials utilize a variety of nebulizers and durations of drug exposure. More recently, aerosolized amphotericin B lipid complex (aABLC) [21–23] and aerosolized liposomal amphotericin B (aLAmB) [24–26] have been investigated for their potential roles in the prevention of IFIs in both solid organ recipients, hematopoietic stem cell transplants, and high-risk hematology-oncology patients. In one such study, a randomized, placebo-controlled trial was conducted in 271 patients with prolonged neutropenia [24]. Patients were randomized to receive either aLAmB or placebo twice weekly. A total of 18/132 in the placebo group and 6/139 patients in the aLAmB developed invasive pulmonary aspergillosis (odds ratio, 0.26; 95% confidence interval, 0.09–0.72; p = 0.005) and significantly favored the use of aLAmB in preventing pulmonary aspergillosis.

The potential role of aerosolized formulations of amphotericin B as adjuncts to systemic therapy for the treatment of IFIs has been studied in the animal model [27]. However, reports in humans are generally restricted to the use of case reports or case series in patients receiving concomitant systemic therapy [6,28–34], which make definitive statements regarding efficacy impossible.

Adverse events associated with the administration of aerosolized amphotericin B formulations include nausea, bad taste, cough, dizziness, chest tightness, mild bronchospasm, and sputum production [13–20,24,34]. The incidence of such reactions varies between preparations and patient populations. When compared to aAmBd, aABLC has demonstrated improved tolerability in lung transplant recipients [21]. Concerns have been raised with the isolation of fungal pathogens with reduced susceptibility to amphotericin B that may be a consequence of widespread aerosolized prophylaxis [26].

The current role of aerosolized amphotericin B formulations in the prevention and treatment of IFIs (most notably invasive pulmonary aspergillosis) in high-risk patients is still evolving. Numerous questions still need to be addressed, including cost, optimal preparation, dose, delivery system, need for concomitant systemic antifungals, timing, and duration of therapy [3,4,35,36]. In addition, the safety of healthcare practitioners who administer this (and any other) aerosol must be considered [37]. Recent guidelines for the management of aspergillosis recognize the potential role of aerosolized formulations of amphotericin B for the prevention of infection in patients at highest risk of invasive aspergillosis (notably in patients with prolonged neutropenia and lung transplant recipients), and as adjunctive therapy in those with tracheobronchial aspergillosis [38]. In contrast to the 2017 prevention and treatment guidelines for hematology-oncology patients published by the National Comprehensive Cancer Center [39] where alternate antifungal strategies are preferred, published guidelines by the German Society for Haematology and Oncology [40] recommend aLAmB 12.5 mg twice weekly or aAmBd 20 mg daily (in conjunction with systemic fluconazole) for fungal prevention in patients with prolonged neutropenia.

In contrast to the use of amphotericin B formulations, data on the use of aerosolized echinocandins or azoles in humans is limited. The characteristics of aerosolized micafungin utilizing the Pari LC Star, Hudson Updraft (Small Volume) nebulizer, and Aeroclipse II nebulizer were studied in one report [41], while nebulized voriconazole (40 mg once daily) was used adjunctively in an adolescent with cystic fibrosis for treatment of a severe *Scedosporium apiospermum* pulmonary infection [42]. However, the method of delivery was not described in this report.

Endobronchial instillations

Reports on endobronchial instillations of antifungals are generally restricted to treatment of pulmonary aspergillosis [43–48]. Less frequently, these involve administration of intracavitary ketoconazole [48] or fluconazole [46]. Most of this endobronchial experience is from case reports involving the administration of amphotericin B deoxycholate [43–46] or amphotericin B lipid complex [49] in the treatment of aspergillomas. In patients who received amphotericin B deoxycholate, doses ranged from 5 to 50 mg administered between every other day and four times daily [43,44,46]. Complete remission occurred in 2/7 patients [43,44]. Four out of five patients not achieving complete remission demonstrated improvement [43,45,46]. Adverse effects were cough and fever [46]. More recent are reports of the use of lipid-based formulations of amphotericin (notably amphotericin B lipid complex) in combination with both oral voriconazole and inhaled amphotericin B lipid complex [49]. A patient who underwent a bilateral lung transplant and placement of a double endobronchial prosthesis with depots adherent to the prosthetic material had *Aspergillus fumigatus*, *Scedosporium prolificans*, and *C. glabrata* isolated from a bronchial aspirate. A solution of amphotericin B lipid complex 25 mg instilled weekly for 5 weeks, before and after bronchoscopy, was well-tolerated and resulted in negative cultures for the follow-up period of 2 years. More recently, the use of weekly endobronchial instillation of liposomal amphotericin B (25 mg diluted in 20 cc of saline and administered under visualization over the left lower lobe endobronchial growth) was reported in a patient with endobronchial mucormycosis without apparent adverse effect [50].

Given the availability of newer treatment options for the treatment of pulmonary aspergillosis (such as echinocandins and extended-spectrum triazoles) and the lack of sufficient efficacy and safety data to support its use, endobronchial instillations of antifungal agents should not be routinely used for the treatment of pulmonary aspergillosis [38].

NASAL IRRIGATIONS

Initial interest in the intranasal administration of antifungal-containing solutions was for the prevention of IFIs (primarily aspergillosis) in high-risk patients. The vast majority of reports involve amphotericin B [51–55]. Use of intranasal amphotericin B-containing solutions (2 mL of a 5 mg/mL solution [10 mg total] administered three times daily) was first described in 1984 as a potential method to prevent pulmonary aspergillosis infections in neutropenic patients [51]. Subsequent reports of nasal use describe a variety of doses, formulations, and durations of therapy [52–58]. In general, clinical trials evaluating the potential role of antifungal-containing nasal irrigants and sprays for the prevention of IFIs are significantly limited by the use of historical controls and/or the co-administration of systemic prophylaxis. However, the administrations were generally well-tolerated, with mild rhinorrhagia the most frequent adverse event reported. Currently, antifungal-containing nasal irrigations are not recommended for the prevention of invasive fungal infections. Such use has largely been replaced by use of either aerosolized or systemic therapies in most high-risk patient populations.

Fungal colonization has been implicated as a precipitating factor in select patients with chronic rhinosinusitis. However, the role of amphotericin B-containing nasal solutions in the treatment of patients with chronic rhinosinusitis (with or without polyps) continues to be poorly-defined [57,59–64]. Some investigators have proposed that nasal polyps represent an allergic reaction to fungal colonization of the nares [62]. Conflicting information exists regarding the effect of amphotericin B on inflammatory markers [63,65,66]. A recent randomized, double-blind placebo-controlled trial in patients with chronic sinusitis without nasal polyps demonstrated improved symptoms and endoscopic findings in patients receiving intranasal amphotericin B [57]. However, overall treatment outcomes did not improve. In addition, existing studies to date do not justify their routine use in patients with rhinosinusitis [38,58,67].

While isolated reports have described the nasal use of alternative agents, such as fluconazole (100 mg in 500 mL of normal saline solution administered as 5–0.5 mL sprays twice daily) [68] and liposomal amphotericin B [69], adjunctive use of nasal irrigations containing amphotericin B have been reported for the treatment of various forms of fungal sinusitis. Again, lack of adequately-controlled clinical trials makes it difficult to determine its efficacy in these medical settings. However, surgery and (in select cases) systemic antifungal therapy are likely to be mainstays of therapy for most forms of fungal sinusitis.

URINARY TRACT IRRIGANTS

Prior to the availability of fluconazole, options for the treatment of fungal urinary tract infections (most commonly due to *Candida* spp.) were limited. Rare case reports describe the use of bladder irrigations containing miconazole [70], nystatin [71] or methylene blue [72]. However, the overwhelming majority of clinical experience with antifungal urinary irrigations is with amphotericin B deoxycholate bladder irrigations. Amphotericin B bladder irrigations were first reported in two 59-year old male patients with complaints of frequent urination, dysuria, and nocturia [73]. Since that report, attempts have been made to determine the optimal dose, method of administration, duration of therapy, and comparative efficacy with alternate therapies.

Early experience with amphotericin B bladder irrigations was reported from an open-labeled, noncomparative study in 40 patients with noninvasive candiduria receiving amphotericin B 50 mg/L of sterile water (administered through a 3-way catheter or an indwelling urethral catheter or suprapubic tube at a rate of 40 mL/hour until urine became clear of *Candida*) [74]. *Candida* was eliminated from the urine in 92.5% of cases. Eight of the fourteen patients with follow-up cultures were also negative, while two patients experienced recurrence. Subsequently, a report of similar doses in 65 nursing home residents with candiduria determined a response rate of 72% after 2 days of therapy [75].

The use of a single amphotericin B bladder irrigation (30 mg in 100 mL of sterile water infused through a 3-way catheter clamped for 2 hours) as a diagnostic strategy to distinguish between upper and lower urinary tract infections has been reported [76]. Forty-four out of 62 (71%) single bladder irrigations caused clearance of *Candida* from the urine, with 12 of these experiencing recurrence 1–3 weeks after treatment. Persistence of positive cultures occurred in 18, of which 10 lacked evidence of upper tract infection or invasive candidiasis. Therefore, the use of the irrigation as a diagnostic tool is questionable or (at best) has limited applicability.

Continuous versus intermittent administrations of amphotericin B bladder irrigation were compared in a randomized, prospective study [77]. Ten men were randomized to either continuous infusion (50 mg/L sterile water per day through a 3-way catheter for 48 hours) or intermittent (10 mg/100 mL through a catheter that was clamped for 30 minutes and released 3 times). Eight out of 10 patients in the continuous infusion group had clearance of fungus from the urine at 72 hours versus only 3 out of 10 patients in the intermittent treatment group (p = 0.035). Reinfection at day 7 was seen in 2 patients and 1 patient, respectively. These findings do suggest the method of administration may be important.

Amphotericin B bladder irrigations have been compared to oral fluconazole therapy [78–81]. In the first of these trials in patients with noninvasive candiduria, no difference in efficacy could be detected in patients receiving either fluconazole 200 mg daily for 7 days, continuous amphotericin B bladder irrigations 50 mg/L for 1 day, or continuous amphotericin B bladder irrigations at 50 mg/L for 7 days [78]. A randomized, placebo-controlled trial comparing oral fluconazole (200 mg × 1, then 100 mg/d × 4), a single 15 mg dose of amphotericin B IV, and three concentrations of amphotericin B bladder washes (5 mcg/mL, 100 mcg/mL or 200 mcg/mL three times daily for 3 days) for treatment of fungal urinary tract infections in 180 adults failed to demonstrate differences between the three active treatment strategy groups [79]. However, when oral fluconazole (200 mg on day 1 followed by 100 mg daily for 4 days) was compared with amphotericin B bladder irrigations (25 mg in 500 mL of D5W continuous infusion for 5 days) in elderly patients, with microbiologic response rates of 73% (33/45) and 96% (49/51), respectively (p < 0.05) [80]. Finally, an observational trial in 530 patients with funguria reported resolution in 75.5% of untreated patients, 45.5% of patients treated with fluconazole alone, and 54.4% of patients treated with amphotericin B bladder irrigations alone [81].

The optimal concentration of amphotericin B to use as a bladder irrigation remains controversial. Recommendations generally range between 5 and 50 mg/L [75,82,83]. In one randomized study of 28 patients with funguria, patients received either 10 or 50 mg of amphotericin B per liter of sterile water as a continuous irrigation for 72 hours [84]. All treatment failures (33%) occurred in the 10 mg/L group. Current guidelines recommend a concentration of 50 mg/L for a period of 5 days [85]. Amphotericin B bladder irrigation solutions must be protected from light and heat, and are usually added to sterile water for irrigation, since amphotericin B will precipitate in normal saline [70,74,78,86,87].

Adverse effects associated with the use of amphotericin B bladder washes appear to be infrequent, but may include hematuria, cramping, bladder discomfort, dysuria, and burning during irrigation [83].

In the majority of patients with uncomplicated candiduria, no treatment is needed [85]. Given the availability of alternative oral treatment options for fungal infections, the current role of amphotericin B bladder irrigations for the treatment of Candida cystitis is for the treatment of fluconazole-resistant isolates [85]. Prior to use of amphotericin B irrigations, it is important to define desired goals (such as diagnosis of upper tract disease, relief of symptoms associated with symptomatic cystitis, or eradication of yeast in the urine in a patient undergoing urinary catheterization). Use of amphotericin B bladder irrigation does not treat upper urinary tract disease, while lower tract disease remains difficult to define. Use of amphotericin B bladder irrigations is not needed in most patients with candiduria [85].

In addition to bladder irrigations, the use of antifungals as irrigants for nephrostomy tubes has also been reported. The majority of the published experience with amphotericin B in this role is in pediatric patients [88–93]. Less experience is published in adult patients [94,95]. Due to the lack of controlled trials, it is unclear whether or not the efficacy in case reports is due to surgical intervention, the process of irrigation (independent of antifungal), amphotericin B, or a combination of these factors. Currently, amphotericin B deoxycholate (25–50 mg in 200–500 mL sterile water) is recommended for Candida urinary tract infection associated with fungus balls if nephrostomy tubes are present [85]. The optimal method (continuous vs. intermittent, volumes, and frequency) are not well-defined.

Fluconazole [96–99] and caspofungin irrigation [100] have also been described in literature as an irrigation for nephrostomy tubes to treat upper urinary tract fungal infections. Concentrations of fluconazole in these reports ranged from 10–1000 mg/L administered once-six times daily [96–99]. For caspofungin, a continuous irrigation of caspofungin 50 mg in 100 mL 0.9% sodium chloride was utilized [100]. As with many of the previous reports, most patients received concomitant systemic antifungal therapy, making the efficacy of the irrigant difficult to determine.

PERITONEAL LAVAGE

Administration of intraperitoneal antifungals in patients with fungal peritonitis secondary to peritoneal lavage is generally considered as adjunctive to catheter management and administration of systemic antifungals [101]. Direct instillation of antifungals (specifically amphotericin B) directly into the peritoneal fluid in patient undergoing peritoneal dialysis with fungal peritonitis (most often due to Candida spp) was first described in the early 1970s [102–105]. Amphotericin B concentrations in dialysate varied from 1–4 µg/mL [102,105]. Concomitant use of IV therapy with amphotericin B was common in these reports. Adverse effects have included mild/moderate abdominal discomfort [103,106] and hypokalemia [105]. Intraperitoneal amphotericin B has also been associated with chemical peritonitis and pain [101].

Administration of peritoneal lavage containing flucytosine has also been reported [106,107]. In one report, peritoneal lavage containing flucytosine 50 mg/L was administered at a rate of 1.2 L/hour for 5 days for the treatment of fungal peritonitis [107]. Peritoneal lavage with flucytosine has also been reported in pediatric patients [106].

Intraperitoneal administration of azoles has been reported for both fluconazole [108] and voriconazole [109]. Current guidelines for the treatment of fungal peritonitis identify either continuous amphotericin B (1.5 mg/L dialysate) or either fluconazole 200 mg or voriconazole 2.5 mg/kg intraperitoneally in one exchange per day, every 24–48 hours (depending upon the pathogen) [101]. Of particular note was the detection of serum concentrations of voriconazole (>1 mcg/mL) after 48 hours of intraperitoneal administration [109]. While the role of intraperitoneal irrigation of antifungals may be limited in the treatment of peritonitis caused by *Candida* spp. [85], amphotericin B-containing lavage solutions (in addition to systemic administration and catheter removal) may play more of a role in the treatment of peritonitis caused by *Aspergillus* spp. [38].

PERCUTANEOUS DELIVERY

Percutaneous administration of antifungals has been reported in a variety of dosage forms, including injections of antifungal medications, infusions, pastes, and gelatins [1]. Reports in the literature are generally restricted to use in patients with pulmonary aspergilloma, often accompanied by hemoptysis [45,110–122].

English language reports of delivery of antifungals via percutaneous catheter generally involve amphotericin B [112,113,117–122]. Most reports have utilized amphotericin B 50 mg in 20 mL of D5W [116–118,121,122]. Total doses generally have ranged between 500 mg [121,122] and 3 g via catheter [119]. Reported toxicities of the instillations vary with the side of administration, and include coughing [118,120–122], fever [117,121,122], headaches [122], and vomiting [122]. Reports of fluconazole via percutaneous catheter instillation are rare [113].

The percutaneous administration of pastes and gelatins containing either amphotericin B or nystatin has been described in the treatment of patients with aspergilloma [110,114]. Final concentrations of amphotericin B and nystatin in one of these reports were 5 mg/mL and 45,000 units/mL, respectively [114]. Five mL (25 mg of amphotericin B and 225,000 units of nystatin) were injected at one time into patients, usually every 5–7 days [114]. In other reports, 10 mL of amphotericin B per dose were administered every 1–3 weeks [110]. One published report to date described percutaneous injection of amphotericin B in a gelatin solution [111].

Based on the availability of alternative treatment options and the lack of adequate efficacy, safety and stability data, percutaneous delivery of antifungals is not routinely recommended for the treatment of *Aspergillus* infections [38].

INTRATHECAL ADMINISTRATION

Low penetration of intravenously-administered amphotericin B into cerebrospinal fluid [123–125], combined with poor treatment outcomes for amphotericin B monotherapy for central nervous system (CNS) fungal infections, stimulated

reports regarding the potential role of direct drug administration to the CNS. While intrathecal (IT) administration was first investigated for amphotericin B as adjunctive treatment for cryptococcal meningitis [126–132], it was soon investigated as adjunctive therapy for other systemic fungal infections involving spread to the CNS, such as cococciodidal [133–140], candidal [85,141], histoplasmosis [142,143], mucormycosis [144], and blastomycosis [145,146]. With the incurable nature of coccidioidal meningitis, this condition is the most likely infection being treated with intrathecal amphotericin B deoxycholate [139,140]. A detailed description of its preparation, storage, dose (0.1 mg IT AmBd 3 times a week gradually increased by 0.1 mg per week as tolerated), administration (lumbar, ventricular, cisternal), tolerability, and monitoring for this infection has recently been published [139].

Numerous and frequent adverse effects secondary to intrathecal administration of amphotericin B have been reported, including (but not limited) to paraplegia [130,142,145,147], pain in the back and legs [130], nausea and vomiting [130], loss of bowel and bladder control [145,147], headache [130,131], chemical meningitis [139], and arachnoiditis [139] Amphotericin B deoxycholate may be co-administered with intrathecal corticosteroids (such as preservative-free methylprednisolone) in attempt to reduce the potential side effects resulting from IT administration [139]. Of note is the concern for the potential for drug-drug interactions between amphotericin B and hydrocortisone [139,148].

Methods of administering antifungals directly into the CNS have been investigated in attempts to address the serious adverse effects associated with intrathecal administration via lumbar injection of amphotericin B. Cisternal administration of amphotericin B has been reported for the treatment of coccidioidal meningitis [149] and cryptococcal infections [150,151]. Severe adverse effects have also been reported with cisternal administration, including a report of subarachnoid hemorrhage, brain stem decompensation, and subsequent death [152]. Intrathecal administration of amphotericin B using ventricular reservoirs (such as the Ommaya reservoir [153–159] and Rickham reservoir [160,161]) have been used for the treatment of cryptococcal meningitis, coccidioidal meningitis, mucormycotic brain abscess, and other unidentified invasive mold infection of the CNS. Amphotericin B doses ranged from 0.05 mg [159] to 1 mg [154], most commonly 1–3 times per week [153,157,158]. Less frequently, the Ommaya reservoir administration of amphotericin B was used for the treatment of mucormycotic brain abscesses [157,159] and *Aspergillus* [155]. Chemically-induced arachnoiditis and bacterial colonization of the reservoir have been reported to be complications of such administration [156].

Relative to administration of amphotericin B, direct administration of other antifungals into the CNS is infrequently reported. Miconazole has been administered intrathecally in the treatment of various CNS infections, to include coccidioidal meningitis, cryptococcal meningitis, histoplasmosis meningitis, and *Candida albicans* infections [162–167]. Doses in adults ranged from 1 to 30 mg [162–167], with lower doses of 3–5 mg in children [166,167]. Adverse effects of intrathecal miconazole may include arachnoiditis [124,164], cisternal hemorrhage [124,147,164], ventricle hemorrhage [162], transient numbness [162], and bacterial infections when administered via Ommaya reservoir [166].

Because of the complications associated with intrathecal or intracisternal administration of amphotericin B, most treatment guidelines for the management of IFIs involving the CNS do not recommend the routine use of such administration [38,85,132,143,146]. However, in desperate situations (notably in the treatment of coccidioidal meningitis), intrathecal amphotericin B is still recommended by some experts [139,140].

INTRA-ARTICULAR INJECTIONS

Direct intra-articular injection of amphotericin B was first described in the literature in the late 1960s [168]. Subsequent reports for the management of fungal synovitis and arthritis utilized doses ranging between 0.05 and 20 mg (most commonly 2–5 mg) [168–177]. However, such administration is rarely employed today in the treatment of IFIs, since many of the systemic treatment options achieve high concentrations in joint fluid and intra-articular administrations of amphotericin B may cause significant pain and irritation.

ORTHOPEDIC APPLICATIONS

Use of fluconazole- [178] and amphotericin B- [179,180] containing irrigants has been described as adjuncts to surgical intervention and systemic antifungal therapy in the treatment of select fungal bone and joint infections. One description included local therapy with amphotericin B (10 mg in 10 mL normal saline) during surgical debridement for the treatment of mucormycosis [179]. However, in select settings (such as mediastinitis due to *Candida*), use of amphotericin B-containing lavage solutions should be discouraged due to the potential for chemical mediastinitis to occur [181].

Treatment of fungal osteomyelitis due to pathogens resistant to most antifungals is especially problematic. Polyhexamethylene biguanide (PHMB) is a chemical most commonly used for cleaning pools. Use of adjunctive administration of a PHMB 0.2% solution as irritation for fungal osteomyelitis (one due to *Fusarium* and the other was polymicrobial, including *Aspergillus fumigatus*, a *Fusarium* species, *Scedosporium prolificans*, and *Trichoderma* species) has been reported [182,183]. In another report, a case of *Scedosporium prolificans* osteomyelitis in an immunocompetent child was treated adjunctively with locally-applied PHMB [183].

High concentrations of amphotericin B incorporated into cement beads may elude in high enough concentrations to serve as adjunctive therapy for the treatment of periprosthetic infections [184]. Limited published information is available to describe the use of antifungals incorporated into bone cement for the treatment of fungal osteomyelitis and/or prosthetic joint infections [185–188]. Successful use of an amphotericin B-containing bone cement was reported in a patient developing a knee infection due to *Candida glabrata* [185]. In addition to systemic therapy and local irrigations containing amphotericin B, bone cement saturated amphotericin B was inserted into the knee. Amphotericin B has also been incorporated into spacers [189,190] and use of fluconazole-impregnated beads was reported for adjunctive treatment for a prosthetic joint infection [191]. While controlled clinical data are lacking, the incorporation of amphotericin B appears to be a safe adjunct for the treatment of osteomyelitis caused by *Candida* spp. [181].

OPHTHALMIC ADMINISTRATION

The limited commercial therapeutic options, combined with poor treatment outcomes with systemic therapies, has stimulated interest and experience in the novel of administration of antifungals for the treatment of invasive fungal infections involving the eye.

Topical

At present, natamycin (a polyene antifungal) is the only topical agent commercially available and FDA-approved for the treatment of ocular fungal infections [192–194]. In one study, natamycin 5% eye drops was compared with itraconazole 1% eye drops in 100 patients with fungal keratitis due to a variety of pathogens, including *Fusarium*, *Aspergillus*, and *Curvularia* [192]. Overall, favorable response rates were seen in 72% and 60% of natamycin and itraconazole-treated patients, respectively. In the subset of patients with fungal keratitis due to *Fusarium* spp, 19/24 (79%) and 8/18 (44%) demonstrated a favorable response, respectively (p < 0.02). Natamycin has become a treatment option primarily for the treatment of keratitis due to filamentous fungi [195]. Natamycin 5% ophthalmic suspension is approved for use in the US for the treatment of fungal blepharitis, conjunctivitis, and keratitis. Topical administration of other polyene antifungals has also been described. Amphotericin B eye drops have been used in the treatment of a variety of fungal pathogens such as *Aspergillus*, *Candida*, *Curvalaria lunata*, *Phialophora*, *Gibberella*, *Alternaria*, *Scopularisopsis brevicaulis*, *Rhinosporidiosis*, *Macrophoma*, and *Fusarium* [196–201]. Solutions containing 0.5–1.5 mg/mL of amphotericin B were administered every 30 minutes to 1 hour [196–201].

There are case reports of the use of topical azole antifungals [202–214] and flucytosine [215] for the treatment of ophthalmic fungal infections. Flucytosine 1% eye drops given every hour were used in conjunction with oral flucytosine therapy for the treatment of corneal ulcers in two patients caused by *Candida* [215]. Miconazole 10 mg/mL solution has also been administered (in combination with subconjunctival miconazole) for the treatment of keratomycosis caused by *Candida* [216], while miconazole 2%

ointment has been utilized in the treatment of a patient with *Aspergillus conicus* endophthalmitis following a cataract extraction [217]. Case reports also describe the use of both amphotericin B and miconazole administered as a topical ointment for corneal ulcers and endophthalmitis caused by *Aspergillus* and *Fusarium* [217,218]. In general, the application of topical fluconazole is limited because of high concentration following oral administration. Successful use of topical posaconazole (using the suspension containing 10 mg/0.1 mL) administered every hour (in conjunction with oral posaconazole) was reported for keratitis caused by *Fusarium solani* [212]. More recently, topical voriconazole (in combination with systemic administration) has also been reported [202,205,206,211,213,214], likely due to its activity against mold infections combined with significant intra- and interpatient kinetic variability following systemic administration.

Topical ophthalmic administration of echinocandins (alone or in combination with other antifungals) has also been reported, and most frequently involves caspofungin [219–225]. Use of caspofungin 0.5% (in combination with intrastromal voriconazole) was reported in the treatment of *Alternaria* keratitis [226,227]. Caspofungin 1% solution has also been used in the setting of *C. albicans* infections refractory to topical and oral voriconazole [219] and as a lacrimal sac irrigant for recurrent *C. parapsilosis* keratitis [228]. The successful use of topical administration of micafungin 0.1% has been reported in the treatment of keratitis due to both *Candida* [229] and *Wickerhamomyces* [230].

Subconjunctival, intracameral, and intravitreal injections

Because of the limited penetration of most agents when applied topically, antifungals (most commonly amphotericin B) have been administered via subconjunctival, intracameral and intravitreal injections. Subconjunctival administration of antifungals has been reported in combination with other local therapies [216,231–233]. While both amphotericin B [231–233] and miconazole [216,234] have been used in this manner, subconjunctival amphotericin B is likely to be limited due to poor aqueous penetration when given in this manner [231]. Subconjunctival miconazole (in combination with amphotericin B IV) was used in the treatment of blastomycosis [234], keratomycosis [216] and in one patient for the treatment of blastomycosis [234].

Various case reports describe intracameral injection of amphotericin B in the treatment of keratomycosis caused by *Aspergillus* and other molds, like *Colletotrichum*, and in endophthalmitis caused by molds such as *Paecilomyces* [232,233,235–237]. Six of 7 patients treated with intracameral injections achieved resolution or significant improvement of this infection [236]. The only reported adverse effect in these reports is uveitis. Anterior chamber injections have been described for amphotericin B in the treatment of endophthalmitis in doses ranging from 5 mcg to 50 mcg for

the treatment of endophthalmitis caused by *Paecilomyces* [238,239], *Coccidioides* [240], *Cylindrocarpon* [238], and *Acremonium* [238]. Intravitreous injections of amphotericin B (concurrent with surgery [i.e., vitrectomy], systemic, and other local antifungal therapies) have also been utilized in the treatment of ophthalmic fungal infections in an attempt to compensate for its poor penetration into vitreal fluid. Endophthalmitis due to *Fusarium* [238,241], *Acremonium* [238,241–243], *Aspergillus* [238], and *Candida* [238,243–249] has been treated with intravitreal doses of amphotericin ranging from 5 to 10 mcg, and many reports have used multiple intravitreous injections per infection. Fibrinous iritis has been reported with intravitreal injections of amphotericin B at doses of 10 mcg, but not after dosage reduction to 5 mcg [246]. Retinal or pigment epithelial toxicity secondary to such use has also been described [238]. Loss of retinal ganglion cells, vitreous inflammation, corneal edema, neovascularization, and inflammation have also been reported as consequences of such administration [225].

Numerous reports describe the use of voriconazole administered via intravitreal, intracameral or intrastromal administration for the treatment of refractory and/or resistant fungal endophthalmitis as an adjunct to systemic antifungal therapy [204,250–263]. Intracameral doses range from 2.5 mcg/0.1 mL [253] to 100 mcg/0.1 mL [204,254]. The concentration utilized for intravitreal administration was 25 mcg in 0.1 mL in one report [250].

ANTIBIOTIC LOCK ADMINISTRATION

The instillation and retention of high concentrations of antibiotics within the lumen of a catheter with the intent to sterilize *in situ* has been described in the medical literature in situations where catheter-related infections occur and that catheter removal (generally considered essential to treatment success) is impractical. While most frequently reported in the treatment of catheter-related bacteremias, antibiotic lock therapy for fungemia has also been reported [264–278]. Most of these reports utilize amphotericin B [264–267,274–277]. The first case report of antibiotic lock use in fungemia was for the treatment of *Malassezia furfur*, for which 2 mL of amphotericin B 2.5 mg/mL solution in normal saline was utilized [265]. A second report examined the use of amphotericin B deoxycholate 2.5 mg/mL solution daily instilled into catheters to remain for 8–12 hours in 2 patients with *Candida* catheter-related infections (in addition to systemic therapy) [264]. However, relapse was reported in both patients. In general, reports of the use of amphotercin B deoxycholate as a lock solution generally utilize concentrations ranging from 0.33–2.5 mg/mL for 6–24 hours/day for 14–21 days [265,274–277].

Animal models have suggested a potential role for the use of lipid-based formulations of amphotericin B (specifically liposomal amphotericin B) [278], amphotericin B lipid complex [279], caspofungin [270,272,280] micafungin [281,282] and anidulafungin [268] in catheter-related infections, due to their increased activity (relative to AmBd) against organisms producing biofilms. Reports of the use of lipid-based formulations of amphotericin B as an antibiotic lock solution are infrequent. In one such report, liposomal amphotericin B was successful in 4/4 in fungal eradication despite continued catheter use [283]. In another, liposomal amphotericin B 8 mg/3 mL was used successfully [271]. More recently, a pilot study in children (primarily with infected catheters due to *Candida* spp) examined the use of liposomal amphotericin B 2 mg/mL (as an adjunct to systemic therapy) [269]. Liposomal amphotericin B 2mg/mL was allowed to dwell for 8–12 hours before its removal for a minimum of 14 days. Lines were cleared of infection in 9/12 subjects without apparent adverse effect.

Despite the potential application of echinocandins for use a lock solution for the treatment of catheter-related fungal infections, clinical reports of their use are sparse. One report described the adjunctive use of caspofungin (10 mg/3 mL in 5% dextrose allowed to dwell for 12 hour) for the treatment of *Candida lipolytica* line-related fungaemia in a 9-year-old boy [284].

SUMMARY

The novel administration of antifungals most frequently involves the delivery of amphotericin B in a variety of manners, other than intravenous administration. Adequately controlled clinical studies to support the use of novel methods of antifungal drug administration for the adjunctive treatment of IFIs (generally in combination with systemic antifungal therapy) are lacking for most indications.

Data are emerging for the use of aerosolized formulations of amphotericin B in the prevention of invasive aspergillosis in high-risk patients (most notably hematology-oncology patients with prolonged neutropenia and in lung transplant recipients). Use of antifungal-containing irrigating solutions (usually amphotericin B) most frequently involves their use as bladder irrigations (for the treatment of funguria), peritoneal lavage fluid (for management of fungal peritonitis), and nasal solutions (for the treatment of fungal sinusitis). Among these indications, amphotericin B bladder irrigations and nasal solutions are perhaps the best-studied. However, the role of such therapies (in the setting of adequate systemic antifungal therapy) is often questionable. In contrast, despite lack of controlled clinical studies, novel administrations of amphotericin B (such as in the use for the treatment of candidal osteomyelitis, or endophthalmitis due to *Candida* or *Aspergillus* spp) has been identified by treatment guidelines as adjunctive therapy for these infections.

REFERENCES

1. Arthur RR, Drew RH, Perfect JR. Novel modes of antifungal drug administration. *Expert Opin Investig Drugs* 2004;13:903–932.
2. Drew R. Potential role of aerosolized amphotericin B formulations in the prevention and adjunctive treatment of invasive fungal infections. *Int J Antimicrob Agents* 2006;27 Suppl 1:36–44.
3. Le J, Schiller DS. Aerosolized delivery of antifungal agents. *Curr Fungal Infect Rep* 2010;4:96–102.
4. Le J, Ashley ED, Neuhauser MM, et al. Consensus summary of aerosolized antimicrobial agents: Application of guideline criteria. Insights from the Society of Infectious Diseases Pharmacists. *Pharmacotherapy* 2010;30:562–584.
5. Xia D, Sun WK, Tan MM, et al. Aerosolized amphotericin B as prophylaxis for invasive pulmonary aspergillosis: A meta-analysis. *Int J Infect Dis* 2015;30:78–84.
6. Oehling A, Giron M, Subira M. Aerosol chemotherapy in bronchopulmonary candidiasis. *Respiration* 1975;32:179–184.
7. McKendrick GM, Medlock JM. Pulmonary moniliasis treated with nystatin aerosol. *Lancet* 1958;1:621–622.
8. Gero S, Szekely J. Pulmonary moniliasis treated with nystatin aerosol. *Lancet* 1958;1:1229–1230.
9. Klepser M. Amphotericin B in lung transplant recipients. *Ann Pharmacother* 2002;36:167–169.
10. Husain S, Capitano B, Corcoran T, et al. Intrapulmonary disposition of amphotericin B after aerosolized delivery of amphotericin B lipid complex (Abelcet; ABLC) in lung transplant recipients. *Transplantation* 2010;90:1215–1219.
11. Monforte V, Ussetti P, Gavalda J, et al. Feasibility, tolerability, and outcomes of nebulized liposomal amphotericin B for *Aspergillus* infection prevention in lung transplantation. *J Heart Lung Transplant* 2010;29:523–530.
12. Rodvold KA, Yoo L, George JM. Penetration of anti-infective agents into pulmonary epithelial lining fluid: Focus on antifungal, antitubercular and miscellaneous anti-infective agents. *Clin Pharmacokinet* 2011;50:689–704.
13. Behre G, Schwartz S, Lenz K, et al. Aerosol amphotericin B inhalations for prevention of invasive pulmonary aspergillosis in neutropenic cancer patients. *Ann Hematol* 1995;71:287–291.
14. Schwartz S, Behre G, Heinemann V, et al. Aerosolized amphotericin B inhalations as prophylaxis of invasive *Aspergillus* infections during prolonged neutropenia: Results of a prospective randomized multicenter trial. *Blood* 1999;93:3654–3661.
15. De Laurenzi A, Matteocci A, Lanti A, Pescador L, Blandino F, Papetti C. Amphotericin B prophylaxis against invasive fungal infections in neutropenic patients: A single center experience from 1980 to 1995. *Infection* 1996;24:361–366.
16. Conneally E, Cafferkey M, Daly P, Keane C, McCann S. Nebulized amphotericin B as prophylaxis against invasive aspergillosis in granulocytopenic patients. *Bone Marrow Transplant* 1990;5:403–406.

17. Hertenstein B, Kern W, Schmeiser T, et al. Low incidence of invasive fungal infections after bone marrow transplantation in patients receiving amphotericin B inhalations during neutropenia. *Ann Hematol* 1994;68:21–26.

18. Reichenspurner H, Gamberg P, Nitschke M, et al. Significant reduction in the number of fungal infections after lung-, heart-lung, and heart transplantation using aerosolized amphotericin B prophylaxis. *Transplant Proc* 1997;29:627–628.

19. Calvo V, Borro J, Morales P, et al. Antifungal prophylaxis during the early postoperative period of lung transplantation. Valencia Lung Transplant Group. *Chest* 1999;115:1301–1304.

20. Monforte V, Roman A, Gavalda J, et al. Nebulized amphotericin B prophylaxis for *Aspergillus* infection in lung transplantation: Study of risk factors. *J Heart Lung Transplant* 2001;20:1274–1281.

21. Drew RH, Dodds AE, Benjamin DK, Jr., Duane DR, Palmer SM, Perfect JR. Comparative safety of amphotericin B lipid complex and amphotericin B deoxycholate as aerosolized antifungal prophylaxis in lung-transplant recipients. *Transplantation* 2004;77:232–237.

22. Palmer S, Drew R, Whitehouse J, et al. Safety of aerosolized amphotericin B lipid complex in lung transplant recipients. *Transplantation* 2001;72:545–548.

23. Alexander BD, Dodds Ashley ES, Addison RM, Alspaugh JA, Chao NJ, Perfect JR. Non-comparative evaluation of the safety of aerosolized amphotericin B lipid complex in patients undergoing allogeneic hematopoietic stem cell transplantation. *Transplant Infect Dis* 2006;8:13–20.

24. Rijnders BJ, Cornelissen JJ, Slobbe L, et al. Aerosolized liposomal amphotericin B for the prevention of invasive pulmonary aspergillosis during prolonged neutropenia: A randomized, placebo-controlled trial. *Clin Infect Dis* 2008;46:1401–1408.

25. Hullard-Pulstinger A, Holler E, Hahn J, Andreesen R, Krause SW. Prophylactic application of nebulized liposomal amphotericin B in hematologic patients with neutropenia. *Onkologie* 2011;34:254–258.

26. Peghin M, Monforte V, Martin-Gomez MT, et al. 10 years of prophylaxis with nebulized liposomal amphotericin B and the changing epidemiology of *Aspergillus* spp. infection in lung transplantation. *Transpl Int* 2016;29:51–62.

27. Ruijgrok EJ, Fens MH, Bakker-Woudenberg IA, Van Etten EW, Vulto AG. Nebulized amphotericin B combined with intravenous amphotericin B in rats with severe invasive pulmonary aspergillosis. *Antimicrob Agents Chemother* 2006;50:1852–1854.

28. Dalconte I, Riva G, Obert R, et al. Tracheobronchial aspergillosis in a patient with AIDS treated with aerosolized amphotericin B combined with itraconazole. *Mycoses* 1996;39:371–374.

29. Palmer S, Perfect J, Howell D, et al. Candidal anastomotic infection in lung transplant recipients: Successful treatment with a combination of systemic and inhaled antifungal agents. *J Heart Lung Transplant* 1998;17:1029–1033.

30. Kanj S, Welty-Wolf K, Madden J, et al. Fungal infections in lung and heart-lung transplant recipients. Report of 9 cases and review of the literature. *Medicine (Baltimore)* 1996;75:142–156.

31. Birsan T, Taghavi S, Klepetko W. Treatment of *Aspergillus*-related ulcerative tracheobronchitis in lung transplant recipients. *J Heart Lung Transplant* 1998;17:437–438.

32. Casey P, Garrett J, Eaton T. Allergic bronchopulmonary aspergillosis in a lung transplant patient successfully treated with nebulized amphotericin. *J Heart Lung Transplant* 2002;21:1237–1241.

33. Suzuki K, Iwata S, Iwata H. Allergic bronchopulmonary aspergillosis in a 9-year-old boy. *Eur J Pediatr* 2002;161:408–409.

34. Kilburn K. The innocuousness and possible therapeutic use of aerosol amphotericin B. *Am Rev Respir Dis* 1959;80:441–442.

35. Perfect JR. Use of newer antifungal therapies in clinical practice: What do the data tell us? *Oncology (Huntington)* 2004;18:15–23.

36. Chong GL, Broekman F, Polinder S, et al. Aerosolised liposomal amphotericin B to prevent aspergillosis in acute myeloid leukaemia: Efficacy and cost effectiveness in real-life. *Int J Antimicrob Agents* 2015;46:82–87.

37. Tsai RJ, Boiano JM, Steege AL, Sweeney MH. Precautionary practices of respiratory therapists and other healthcare practitioners who administer aerosolized medications. *Respir Care* 2015;60:1409–1417.

38. Patterson TF, Thompson GR, 3rd, Denning DW, et al. Practice guidelines for the diagnosis and management of aspergillosis: 2016 update by the Infectious Diseases Society of America. *Clin Infect Dis* 2016;63:e1–e60.

39. Network NCC. *Prevention and Treatment of Cancer-Related Infections (version 2.2017)*. Available at https://www.nccn.org/professionals/physician_gls/pdf/infections.pdf. (accessed May 19, 2017).

40. Tacke D, Buchheidt D, Karthaus M, et al. Primary prophylaxis of invasive fungal infections in patients with haematologic malignancies. 2014 update of the recommendations of the Infectious Diseases Working Party of the German Society for Haematology and Oncology. *Ann Hematol* 2014;93:1449–1456.

41. Alexander BD, Winkler TP, Shi S, Ashley ES, Hickey AJ. Nebulizer delivery of micafungin aerosols. *Pharmacotherapy* 2011;31:52–57.

42. Holle J, Leichsenring M, Meissner PE. Nebulized voriconazole in infections with *Scedosporium apiospermum*—Case report and review of the literature. *J Cyst Fibros* 2014;13:400–402.

43. Ramirez RJ. Pulmonary aspergilloma: Endobronchial treatment. *N Engl J Med* 1964;271:1281–1285.

44. Bennett M, Weinbaum D, Fiehler P. Chronic necrotizing pulmonary aspergillosis treated by endobronchial amphotericin B. *South Med J* 1990;83:829–832.

45. Ikemoto H. Medical treatment of pulmonary aspergilloma. *Intern Med* 2000;39:191–192.

46. Yamada H, Kohno S, Koga H, Maesak iS, Kaku M. Topical treatment of pulmonary aspergilloma by antifungals: Relationship between duration of the disease and efficacy of treatment. *Chest* 1993;103:1421–1425.

47. Hamamoto T, Watanabe K, Ikemoto H. Endobronchial miconazole for pulmonary aspergilloma. *Ann Intern Med* 1983;98:1030.

48. Guleria R, Gupta D, Jindal S. Treatment of pulmonary aspergilloma by endoscopic intracavitary instillation of ketoconazole. *Chest* 1993;103:1301–1302.

49. Morales P, Galan G, Sanmartin E, Monte E, Tarrazona V, Santos M. Intrabronchial instillation of amphotericin B lipid complex: A case report. *Transplant Proc* 2009;41:2223–2224.

50. Nattusamy L, Kalai U, Hadda V, Mohan A, Guleria R, Madan K. Bronchoscopic instillation of liposomal amphotericin B in management of nonresponding endobronchial mucormycosis. *Lung India* 2017;34:208–209.

51. Meunier-Carpentier F, Snoeck R, Gerain J, Muller C, Klastersky J. Amphotericin B nasal spray as prophylaxis against aspergillosis in patients with neutropenia. *N Engl J Med* 1984;311:1056.

52. Jorgensen C, Dr, fus F, et al. Failure of amphotericin B spray to prevent aspergillosis in granulocytopenic patients. *Nouv Rev Fr Hematol* 1989;31:327–328.

53. Jeffery G, Beard M, Ikram R, et al. Intranasal amphotericin B reduces the frequency of invasive aspergillosis in neutropenic patients. *Am J Med* 1991;90:685–692.

54. Todeschini G, Murari C, Bonesi R, et al. Oral itraconazole plus nasal amphotericin B for prophylaxis of invasive aspergillosis in patients with hematological malignancies. *Eur J Clin Microbiol* 1993;12:614–618.

55. Trifilio SM, Heraty R, Zomas A, et al. Amphotericin B deoxycholate nasal spray administered to hematopoietic stem cell recipients with prior fungal colonization of the upper airway passages is associated with low rates of invasive fungal infection. *Transpl Infect Dis* 2015;17:1–6.

56. Ebbens FA, Georgalas C, Luiten S, et al. The effect of topical amphotericin B on inflammatory markers in patients with chronic rhinosinusitis: A multicenter randomized controlled study. *Laryngoscope* 2009;119:401–408.

57. Liang KL, Su MC, Shiao JY, et al. Amphotericin B irrigation for the treatment of chronic rhinosinusitis without nasal polyps: A randomized, placebo-controlled, double-blind study. *Am J Rhinol* 2008;22:52–58.

58. Wang T, Su J, Feng Y. The effectiveness topical amphotericin B in the management of chronic rhinosinusitis: A meta-analysis. *Eur Arch Otorhinolaryngol* 2015;272:1923–1929.

59. Stankiewicz JA, Musgrave BK, Scianna JM. Nasal amphotericin irrigation in chronic rhinosinusitis. *Curr Opin Otolaryngol Head Neck Surg* 2008;16:44–46.

60. Shirazi MA, Stankiewicz JA, Kammeyer P. Activity of nasal amphotericin B irrigation against fungal organisms *in vitro. Am J Rhinol* 2007;21:145–148.

61. Ebbens FA, Scadding GK, Badia L, et al. Amphotericin B nasal lavages: Not a solution for patients with chronic rhinosinusitis. *J Allergy Clin Immunol* 2006;118:1149–1156.

62. Ricchetti A, Landis B, Maffioli A, Giger R, Zeng C, Lacroix J. Effect of anti-fungal nasal lavage with amphotericin B on nasal polyposis. *J Laryngol Otol* 2002;116:261–263.

63. Ponikau JU, Sherris DA, Weaver A, Kita H. Treatment of chronic rhinosinusitis with intranasal amphotericin B: A randomized, placebo-controlled, double-blind pilot trial. *J Allergy Clin Immunol* 2005;115:125–131.

64. Weschta M, Rimek D, Formanek M, Polzehl D, Podbielski A, Riechelmann H. Topical antifungal treatment of chronic rhinosinusitis with nasal polyps: A randomized, double-blind clinical trial. *J Allergy Clin Immunol* 2004;113:1122–1128.

65. Helbling A, Baumann A, Hanni C, et al. Amphotericin B nasal spray has no effect on nasal polyps. *J Laryngol Otol* 2006;120:1023–1025.

66. Weschta M, Rimek D, Formanek M, et al. Effect of nasal antifungal therapy on nasal cell activation markers in chronic rhinosinusitis. *Arch Otolaryngol Head Neck Surg* 2006;132:743–747.

67. Hashemian F, Hashemian F, Molaali N, Rouini M, Roohi E, Torabian S. Clinical effects of topical antifungal therapy in chronic rhinosinusitis: A randomized, double-blind, placebo-controlled trial of intranasal fluconazole. *Excli J* 2016;15:95–102.

68. Jen A, Kacker A, Huang C, Anand V. Fluconazole nasal spray in the treatment of allergic fungal sinusitis: A pilot study. *Ear Nose Throat J* 2004;83:692–695.

69. Piccaluga PP, Ricci P, Martinelli G, et al. Prompt resolution of nasal aspergillosis with intranasal instillation of liposomal amphotericin-B (AmBisome) and granulocyte transfusions. *Leuk Lymphoma* 2004;45:637–638.

70. Wise G, Goldman W, Goldberg P, Rothenberg R. Miconazole: A cost-effective antifungal genitourinary irrigant. *J Urol* 1987;138:1413–1415.

71. Kennelly B. *Candida albicans* cystitis cured by nystatin bladder instillations. *S Afr Med J* 1965:414–417.

72. Aktug T, Olguner M, Akgur F, Aldirmaz C, Hosgor M, Yulug N. A new ancient irrigation therapy for childhood renal candidiasis. *Int Urol Nephrol* 1998;30:127–132.

73. Goldman H, Littman M, Oppenheimer G, Glickman S. Monilial cystitis—Effective treatment with instillations of amphotericin B. *JAMA* 1960;174:359–362.

74. Wise G, Kozinn P, Goldberg P. Amphotericin B as a urologic irrigant in the management of noninvasive candiduria. *J Urol* 1982;128:82–84.

75. Hsu C, Ukleja B. Clearance of *Candida* colonizing the urinary bladder by a two-day amphotericin B irrigation. *Infection* 1990;18:280–282.

76. Fong I. The value of a single amphotericin B bladder washout in candiduria. *J Antimicrob Chemother* 1995;36:1067–1071.

77. Trinh T, Simonian J, Vigil S, Chin D, Bidair M. Continuous versus intermittent bladder irrigation of amphotericin B for the treatment of candiduria. *J Urol* 1995;154:2032–2034.

78. Fan-Havard P, O'Donovan C, Smith S, Oh J, Bamberger M, Eng R. Oral fluconazole versus amphotericin B bladder irrigation for treatment of candidal funguria. *Clin Infect Dis* 1995;21:960–965.

79. Leu H, Huang C. Clearance of funguria with short-course antifungal regimens: A prospective, randomized, controlled study. *Clin Infect Dis* 1995;20:1152–1157.

80. Jacobs LG, Skidmore EA, Freeman K, Lipschultz D, Fox N. Oral fluconazole compared with bladder irrigation with amphotericin B for treatment of fungal urinary tract infections in elderly patients. *Clin Infect Dis* 1996;22:30–35.

81. Kauffman CA, Vazquez JA, Sobel JD, et al. Prospective multicenter surveillance study of funguria in hospitalized patients. The National Institute for Allergy and Infectious Diseases (NIAID) Mycoses Study Group. *Clin Infect Dis* 2000;30:14–18.

82. Gnau T. Amphotericin B dosage for bladder irrigation. *Am J Hosp Pharm* 1992;49:2705–2706.

83. Drew RH, Arthur RR, Perfect JR. Is it time to abandon the use of amphotericin B bladder irrigation? *Clin Infect Dis* 2005;40:1465–1470.

84. Nesbit SA, Katz LE, McClain BW, Murphy DP. Comparison of two concentrations of amphotericin B bladder irrigation in the treatment of funguria in patients with indwelling urinary catheters. *Am J Health Syst Pharm* 1999;56:872–875.

85. Pappas PG, Kauffman CA, Andes DR, et al. Clinical practice guideline for the management of Candidiasis: 2016 Update by the Infectious Diseases Society of America. *Clin Infect Dis* 2016;62:e1–e50.

86. Cuetara M, Mallo N, Dalet F. Amphotericin B lavage in the treatment of candidial cystitis. *Br J Urol* 1972;44:475–480.

87. Wise G, Wainstein S, Goldberg P, Kozinn P. Candidal cystitis. Management by continuous bladder irrigation with amphotericin B. *JAMA* 1973;224:1636–1637.

88. Fisher JF, Sobel JD, Kauffman CA, Newman CA. *Candida* urinary tract infections—Treatment. *Clin Infect Dis* 2011;52 Suppl 6:S457–S466.

89. Hill J. Candidiasis of the urinary tract. *Proc R Soc Med* 1974;67:1155–1156.

90. Keller M, Sellers B, Jr, Melish M, Kaplan G, Miller K, Mendoza S. Systemic candidiasis in infants: A case presentation and literature review. *Am J Dis Child* 1977;131:1260–1263.

91. Schmitt G, Hsu A. Renal fungus balls: Diagnosis by ultrasound and percutaneous antegrade pyelography and brush biopsy in a premature infant. *J Ultrasound Med* 1985;4:155–156.

92. Aragona F, Passerini G, Pavanello L, Perale R, Rizzoni G, Pagano F. Upper urinary tract obstruction in children caused by *Candida* fungus balls. *Eur Urol* 1985;11:188–191.

93. Bartone F, Hurwitz R, Rojas E, Steinberg E, Franceschini R. The role of percutaneous nephrostomy in the management of obstructing candidiasis of the urinary tract in infants. *J Urol* 1988;140:338–341.

94. Mazer J, Bartone F. Percutaneous antegrade diagnosis and management of candidiasis of the upper urinary tract. *Urol Clin North Am* 1982;9:157–164.

95. Walzer Y, Bear R. Ureteral obstruction of renal transplant due to ureteral candidiasis. *Urology* 1983;21:295–297.

96. Oliver S, Walker R, Woods D. Fluconazole infused via a nephrostomy tube: A novel and effective route of delivery. *J Clin Pharm Ther* 1995;20:317–318.

97. Clark M, Gaunt T, Czachor J. The use of fluconazole as a local irrigant for nephrostomy tubes. *Mil Med* 1999;164:239–241.

98. Chung B, Chang S, Kim S, Choi H. Successfully treated renal fungal ball with continuous irrigation of fluconazole. *J Urol* 2001;166:1835–1836.

99. Simsek U, Akinci H, Oktay B, Kavrama I, Ozyurt M. Treatment of catheter-associated Candiduria with fluconazole irrigation. *Br J Urol* 1995;75:75–77.

100. Garcia H, Guitard J, Peltier J, et al. Caspofungin irrigation through percutaneous calicostomy catheter combined with oral flucytosine to treat fluconazole-resistant symptomatic candiduria. *J Mycol Med* 2015;25:87–90.

101. Li PK, Szeto CC, Piraino B, et al. ISPD peritonitis recommendations: 2016 Update on prevention and treatment. *Perit Dial Int* 2016;36:481–508.
102. Bayer A, Blumenkrantz M, Montgomerie J, Galpin J, Coburn J, Guze L. *Candida* peritonitis. Report of 22 cases and review of the English language. *Am J Med* 1976;61:832–840.
103. Arfania D, Everett E, Nolph K, Rubin J. Uncommon causes of peritonitis in patients undergoing peritoneal dialysis. *Arch Intern Med* 1981;141:61–64.
104. Brewer T, Caldwell F, Patterson R, Flanigan W. Indwelling peritoneal (tenckhoff) dialysis catheter. Experience with 24 patients. *JAMA* 1972;219:1011–1015.
105. Bortolussi R, MacDonald M, Bannatyne R, Arbus G. Treatment of *Candida* peritonitis by peritoneal lavage with Amphotericin B. *J Pediatr* 1975;87:987–988.
106. Raaijmakers R, Schroder C, Monnens L, Cornelissen E, Warris A. Fungal peritonitis in children on peritoneal dialysis. *Pediatr Nephrol* 2007;22:288–293.
107. Holdsworth S, Atkins R, Scott D, Jackson R. Management of *Candida* peritonitis by prolonged peritoneal lavage containing 5-Fluorocytosine. *Clin Nephrol* 1975;4:157–159.
108. Kameoka H, Kumakawa K, Matuoka T, Nakano M, Shiraiwa Y, Yamaguchi O. Intraperitoneal fluconazole for fungal peritonitis in CAPD: Report of two cases. *Perit Dial Int* 1999;19:481–483.
109. Roberts DM, Kauter G, Ray JE, Gillin AG. Intraperitoneal voriconazole in a patient with *Aspergillus* peritoneal dialysis peritonitis. *Perit Dial Int* 2013;33:92–93.
110. Giron J, Poey C, Fajadet P, et al. Inoperable pulmonary aspergilloma: Percutaneous CT-guided injection with glycerin and amphotericin B paste in 15 cases. *Radiology* 1993;188:825–827.
111. Munk P, Vellet A, Rankin R, Muller N, Ahmad D. Intracavitary aspergilloma: Transthoracic percutaneous injection of amphotericin gelatin solution. *Radiology* 1993;188:821–823.
112. Aslam P, Larkin J, Eastridge C, Hughes F. Endocavitary infusion through percutaneous endobronchial catheter. *Chest* 1970;57:94–96.
113. Tsushima K, Fujimoto K, Kubo K, Sekiguchi M. Successful treatment of fungus ball in a patient with allergic bronchopulmonary aspergillosis: Continuous percutaneous instillation of antifungal agents into the cavity. *Intern Med* 1996;35:736–741.
114. Krakowka P, Traczyk K, Walczak J, Halweg H, Elsner Z, Pawlicka L. Local treatment of aspergilloma of the lung with a paste containing nystatin or amphotericin B. *Tubercle, Lond* 1970;51:184–191.
115. Veltri A, Anselmetti G, Bartoli G, et al. Percutaneous treatment with amphotericin B of mycotic lung lesions from invasive aspergillosis: Results in 10 immunocompromised patients. *Eur Radiol* 2000;10:1939–1044.
116. Cochrane L, Morano J, Norman J, Mansel J. Use of intracavitary amphotericin B in a patient with aspergilloma and recurrent hemoptysis. *Am J Med* 1991;90:654–656.
117. Lee K, Kim Y, Bae W. Percutaneous intracavitary treatment of a giant aspergilloma. *AJR Am J Roentgenol* 1990;154:1346.
118. Lee H, Kim H, Kim Y, Choe K. Treatment of hemoptysis in patients with cavitary aspergilloma of the lung: Value of percutaneous instillation of amphotericin B. *AJR Am J Roentgenol* 1993;161:727–731.
119. Jackson M, Flower C, Shneerson J. Treatment of symptomatic pulmonary aspergillomas with intracavitary instillation of amphotericin B through an indwelling catheter. *Thorax* 1993;48:928–930.
120. Klein J, Fang K, Chang M. Percutaneous transcatheter treatment of an intracavitary aspergilloma. *Cardiovasc Intervent Radiol* 1993;16:321–324.
121. Shapiro M, Albelda S, Mayock R, McLean G. Severe hemoptysis associated with pulmonary aspergilloma: Percutaneous intracavitary treatment. *Chest* 1988;94:1225–1231.
122. Hargis J, Bone R, Stewar J, Rector N, Hiller F. Intracavitary amphotericin B in the treatment of symptomatic pulmonary aspergillomas. *Am J Med* 1980;68:389–394.
123. Drutz D, Catanzaro A. Coccidioidomycosis, part II. *Am Rev Respir Dis* 1978;117:727–768.
124. Stevens DA, Shatsky SA. Intrathecal amphotericin in the management of coccidioidal meningitis. *Semin Respir Infect* 2001;16:263–269.
125. Bennett J. Amphotericin B toxicity: Review of selected aspects of pharmacology. *Ann Intern Med* 1964;61:335–339.
126. Butler W, Alling D, Spickard A, Utz J. Diagnostic and prognostic value of clinical and laboratory findings in cryptococcal meningitis. *N Engl J Med* 1964;270:59–66.
127. Halkin H, Ravid M, Zulman J, Reichert N. Cryptococcal meningitis treated with 5-fluorocytosine and amphotericin B. *Isr J Med Sci* 1974;10:1148–1152.
128. Littman M. Cryptococcosis (Torulosis): Current concepts and therapy. *Am J Med* 1959;27:976–998.
129. Seabury J, Dascomb H. Experience with amphotericin B. *Ann N York Acad Sci* 1960;89:202–220.
130. Spickard A, Butler W, Andriole V, Utz J. The improved prognosis of cryptococcal meningitis with amphotericin B therapy. *Ann Intern Med* 1963;58:66–83.

131. Mishima T, Kobayashi Y, Ohkubo M, Marumo F, Yoshimura H. A case of renal transplant recipient complicated with cryptococcosis and amphotericin B induced acute tubular necrosis. *Jpn Circ J* 1977;41:1009–1013.

132. Perfect JR, Dismukes WE, Dromer F, et al. Clinical practice guidelines for the management of cryptococcal disease: 2010 update by the Infectious Diseases Society of America. *Clin Infect Dis* 2010;50:291–322.

133. Caudill R, Smith C, Reinarz J. Coccidioidal meningitis: A diagnostic challenge. *Am J Med* 1970;49:360–365.

134. Bouza E, Dreyer J, Hewitt W, Meyer R. Coccidioidal meningitis: An analysis of thirty-one cases and review of the literature. *Medicine (Baltimore)* 1981;60:139–171.

135. Labadie E, Hamilton R. Survival improvement in coccidioidal meningitis by high-dose intrathecal amphotericin B. *Arch Intern Med* 1986;146:2013–2018.

136. Glynn K, Alazraki N, Waltz T. Coccidioidal meningitis. Intrathecal treatment with hyperbaric amphotericin B. *Calif Med* 1973;119:6–9.

137. LeClerc M, Giammona S. Coccidioidal meningitis the use of amphotericin B intravenously and intrathecally by repeated lumbar punctures. *West J Med* 1975;122:251–254.

138. Peterson C, Johnson S, Kelly J, Kelly P. Coccidioidal meningitis and pregnancy: A case report. *Obstet Gynecol* 1989;73:835–836.

139. Goldstein EJC, Ho J, Fowler P, Heidari A, Johnson RH. Intrathecal amphotericin B: A 60-year experience in treating coccidioidal meningitis. *Clin Infect Dis* 2017;64:519–524.

140. Galgiani JN, Ampel NM, Blair JE, et al. 2016 Infectious Diseases Society of America (IDSA) Clinical Practice Guideline for the Treatment of Coccidioidomycosis. *Clin Infect Dis* 2016;63:e112–e146.

141. Rao H, Myers G. *Candida* meningitis in the newborn. *South Med J* 1979;72:1468–1471.

142. Snyder C, White R. Successful treatment of histoplasma meningitis with amphotericin B. *J Pediatr* 1961;58:554–558.

143. Wheat LJ, Freifeld AG, Kleiman MB, et al. Clinical practice guidelines for the management of patients with histoplasmosis: 2007 update by the Infectious Diseases Society of America. *Clin Infect Dis* 2007;45:807–825.

144. Grannan BL, Yanamadala V, Venteicher AS, Walcott BP, Barr JC. Use of external ventriculostomy and intrathecal anti-fungal treatment in cerebral mucormycotic abscess. *J Clin Neurosci* 2014;21:1819–1821.

145. Loudon R, Lawson R. Systemic blastomycosis: Recurrent neurological relapse in a case treated with amphotericin B. *Ann Intern Med* 1961;55:139–147.

146. Chapman SW, Dismukes WE, Proia LA, et al. Clinical practice guidelines for the management of blastomycosis: 2008 update by the Infectious Diseases Society of America. *Clin Infect Dis* 2008;46:1801–1812.

147. Carnevale N, Galgiani J, Stevens D, Herrick M, Langston J. Amphotericin B-induced myelopathy. *Arch Intern Med* 1980;140:1189–1192.

148. Hodge G, Cohen SH, Thompson GR, 3rd. *In vitro* interactions between amphotericin B and hydrocortisone: Potential implications for intrathecal therapy. *Med Mycol* 2015;53:749–753.

149. WA W. The treatment of coccidioidal meningitis—The use of amphotericin B in a group of 25 patients. *Calif Med* 1964;101:78–89.

150. McIntyre H. Cryptococcal meningitis. A case successfully treated by cisternal administration of amphotericin B with a review of recent literature. *Bull Los Angeles Neurol Soc* 1967;32:213–219.

151. van Dellen J, Buchanan N. Intrathecal cryptococcal lesion of the cauda equina successfully treated with intrathecal amphotericin B: A case report. *S Afr Med J* 1980;58:137–138.

152. Keane J. Cisternal puncture complications. Treatment of coccidioidal meningitis with amphotericin B. *Calif Med* 1973;119:10–15.

153. Witorsch P, Williams T, Jr, Ommaya A, Utz J. Intraventricular administration of amphotericin B. Use of subcutaneous reservoir in four patients with mycotic meningitis. *JAMA* 1965;194:699–702.

154. LePage E. Using a ventricular reservoir to instill amphotericin B. *J Neurosci Nurs* 1993;25:212–217.

155. Buxhofer V, Ruckser R, Kier P, et al. Successful treatment of invasive mould infection affecting lung and brain in an adult suffering from acute leukaemia. *Eur J Haematol* 2001;67:128–132.

156. Graybill J, Ellenbogen C. Complications with the Ommaya reservoir in patients with granulomatous meningitis. *J Neurosurg* 1973;38:477–480.

157. Hamill R, Oney L, Crane L. Successful therapy for rhinocerebral mucormycosis with associated bilateral brain abscesses. *Arch Intern Med* 1983;143:581–583.

158. Craven P, Graybill J, Jorgensen J, Dismukes W, Levine B. High-dose ketoconazole for treatment of fungal infections of the central nervous system. *Ann Intern Med* 1983;98:160–167.

159. Fong K, Seneviratne E, McCormack J. Mucor cerebral abscess associated with intravenous drug abuse. *Aust N Z J Med* 1990;20:74–77.

160. Davis S, Donovan W. Combined intravenous miconazole and intrathecal amphotericin B for treatment of disseminated coccidioidomycosis. *Chest* 1979;76:235–236.

161. Schonheyder H, Thestrup-Pedersen K, Esmann V, Stenderup A. Cryptococcal meningitis: Complications due to intrathecal treatment. *Scand J Infect Dis* 1980;12:155–157.

162. Deresinski S, Lilly R, Levine H, Galgiani J, Stevens D. Treatment of fungal meningitis with miconazole. *Arch Intern Med* 1977;137:1180–1185.

163. Sung J, Grendahl J, Levine H. Intravenous and intrathecal miconazole therapy for systemic mycoses. *West J Med* 1977;126:5–13.

164. Sung J, Campbell G, Grendahl J. Miconazole therapy for fungal meningitis. *Arch Neurol* 1978;35:443–447.

165. Morison A, Erasmus D, Bowie M. Treatment of *Candida albicans* meningitis with intravenous and intrathecal miconazole. A case report. *S Afr Med J* 1988;74:235–236.

166. Shehab Z, Britton H, Dunn J. Imidazole therapy of coccidioidal meningitis in children. *Pediatr Infect Dis J* 1988;7:40–44.

167. Harrison H, Galgiani J, Reynolds A, Jr, Sprunger L, Friedman A. Amphotericin B and imidazole therapy for coccidioidal meningitis in children. *Pediatr Infect Dis* 1983;2:216–221.

168. Aidem H. Intra-articular amphotericin B in the treatment of coccidioidal synovitis of the knee. Case report. *J Bone Joint Surg Am* 1968;50:1663–1638.

169. Klein J, Yamauchi T, Horlick S. Neonatal candidiasis, meningitis, and arthritis: Observations and a review of the literature. *J Pediatr* 1972;81:31–34.

170. Greenman R, Becker J, Campbell G, Remington J. Coccidioidal synovitis of the knee. *Arch Intern Med* 1975;135:526–530.

171. Winter WJ, Larson R, Honeggar M, Jacobsen D, Pappagianis D, Huntington RJ. Coccidioidal arthritis and its treatment. *J Bone Joint Surg Am* 1975;57:1152–1157.

172. Bayer A, Guze L. Fungal arthritis. II. Coccidioidal synovitis: Clinical, diagnostic, therapeutic, and prognostic considerations. *Semin Arthritis Rheum* 1979;8:200–211.

173. Pruitt A, Achord J, Fales F, Patterson J. Glucose-galactose malabsorption complicated by monilial arthritis. *Pediatrics* 1969;43:106–110.

174. Gullberg R, Quintanilla A, Levin M, Williams J, Phair J. *Sporotrichosis*: Recurrent cutaneous, articular, and central nervous system infection in a renal transplant recipient. *Rev Infect Dis* 1987;9:369–375.

175. Lachman R, Yamauchi T, Klein J. Neonatal systemic candidiasis and arthritis. *Radiology* 1972;105:631–632.

176. Poplack D, Jacobs S. *Candida* arthritis treated with amphotericin B. *J Pediatr* 1975;87:989–990.

177. Cooper LG, Heydemann J, Misenhimer G, Antony SJ. Use of intra-articular amphotericin B in the treatment of *Candida parasilosis* and *albicans* in prosthetic joint infections (PJI): A novel approach to this difficult problem. *Infect Disord Drug Targets* 2017;17:36–42.

178. Wada M, Baba H, Imura S. Prosthetic knee *Candidaparapsilosis* infection. *J Arthroplasty* 1998;13:479–482.

179. Chen F, Lu G, Kang Y, et al. Mucormycosis spondylodiscitis after lumbar disc puncture. *Eur Spine J* 2006;15:370–376.

180. Miller AO, Gamaletsou MN, Henry MW, et al. Successful treatment of *Candida* osteoarticular infections with limited duration of antifungal therapy and orthopedic surgical intervention. *Infect Dis (Lond)* 2015;47:144–149.

181. Pappas PG, Rex JH, Sobel JD, et al. Guidelines for treatment of candidiasis. *Clin Infect Dis* 2004;38:161–189.

182. Walls G, Noonan L, Wilson E, Holland D, Briggs S. Successful use of locally applied polyhexamethylene biguanide as an adjunct to the treatment of fungal osteomyelitis. *Can J Infect Dis Med Microbiol* 2013;24:109–112.

183. Steinbach WJ, Schell WA, Miller JL, Perfect JR. Scedosporium prolificans osteomyelitis in an immunocompetent child treated with voriconazole and caspofungin, as well as locally applied polyhexamethylene biguanide. *J Clin Microbiol* 2003;41:3981–3985.

184. Houdek MT, Greenwood-Quaintance KE, Morrey ME, Patel R, Hanssen AD. Elution of high dose amphotericin B deoxycholate from polymethylmethacrylate. *J Arthroplasty* 2015;30:2308–2310.

185. Selmon G, Slater R, Shepperd J, Wright E. Successful 1-stage exchange total knee arthroplasty for fungal infection. *J Arthroplasty* 1998;13:114–115.

186. Marra F, Robbins GM, Masri BA, et al. Amphotericin B-loaded bone cement to treat osteomyelitis caused by *Candida albicans*. *Can J Surg* 2001;44:383–386.

187. Deelstra JJ, Neut D, Jutte PC. Successful treatment of *Candida albicans*-infected total hip prosthesis with staged procedure using an antifungal-loaded cement spacer. *J Arthroplasty* 2013;28:374.e5–e8.

188. Zhu ES, Thompson GR, Kreulen C, Giza E. Amphotericin B-impregnated bone cement to treat refractory coccidioidal osteomyelitis. *Antimicrob Agents Chemother* 2013;57:6341–6343.

189. Gaston G, Ogden J. *Candida glabrata* periprosthetic infection: A case report and literature review. *J Arthroplasty* 2004;19:927–930.

190. Wu MH, Hsu KY. Candidal arthritis in revision knee arthroplasty successfully treated with sequential parenteral-oral fluconazole and amphotericin B-loaded cement spacer. *Knee Surg Sports Traumatol Arthrosc* 2011;19:273–276.

191. Bruce AS, Kerry RM, Norman P, Stockley I. Fluconazole-impregnated beads in the management of fungal infection of prosthetic joints. *J Bone Joint Surg Br* 2001;83:183–184.

192. Kalavathy CM, Parmar P, Kaliamurthy J, et al. Comparison of topical itraconazole 1% with topical natamycin 5% for the treatment of filamentous fungal keratitis. *Cornea* 2005;24:449–452.

193. Prajna NV, Nirmalan PK, Mahalakshmi R, Lalitha P, Srinivasan M. Concurrent use of 5% natamycin and 2% econazole for the management of fungal keratitis. *Cornea* 2004;23:793–796.

194. Prajna NV, John RK, Nirmalan PK, Lalitha P, Srinivasan M. A randomised clinical trial comparing 2% econazole and 5% natamycin for the treatment of fungal keratitis. *Br J Ophthalmol* 2003;87:1235–1237.

195. Thomas PA. Current perspectives on ophthalmic mycoses. *Clin Microbiol Rev* 2003;16:730–797.

196. Bhomaj S, Das J, Chaudhuri Z, Bansal R, Sharma P. Rhinosporidiosis and peripheral keratitis. *Ophthalmic Surg Lasers* 2001;32:338–340.

197. Lotery A, Kerr J, Page B. Fungal keratitis caused by *Scopulariopsis brevicaulis*: Successful treatment with topical amphotericin B and chloramphenicol without the need for surgical debridement. *Br J Ophthalmol* 1994;78:730.

198. Wood T, Williford W. Treatment of keratomycosis with amphotericin B 0.15%. *Am J Ophthalmol* 1976;81:847–849.

199. Wood T, Tuberville A. Keratomycosis and amphotericin B. *Trans Am Ophth Soc* 1985;83:397–409.

200. Jones D, Sexton R, Rebell G. Mycotic keratitis in south Florida: A review of thirty-nine cases. *Trans Ophth Soc UK* 1969;89:781–797.

201. Anderson B, Chick E. Mycokeratitis: Treatment of fungal corneal ulcers with amphotericin B and mechanical debridement. *South Med J* 1963;56:270–274.

202. Amoros-Reboredo P, Bastida-Fernandez C, Guerrero-Molina L, Soy-Muner D, Lopez-Cabezas C. Stability of frozen 1% voriconazole ophthalmic solution. *Am J Health Syst Pharm* 2015;72:479–482.

203. Bui DK, Carvounis PE. Favorable outcomes of filamentous fungal endophthalmitis following aggressive management. *J Ocul Pharmacol Ther* 2016;32:623–630.

204. Chang YF, Yang CS, Lee FL, Lee SM. Voriconazole for Candida endophthalmitis. *Ophthalmology* 2012;119:2414–2415.

205. Malhotra S, Khare A, Grover K, Singh I, Pawar P. Design and evaluation of voriconazole eye drops for the treatment of fungal keratitis. *J Pharm (Cairo)* 2014;2014:490595.

206. Neoh CF, Leung L, Chan E, et al. The absorption and clearance of voriconazole 1% eye drops—An open label study. *Antimicrob Agents Chemother* 2016.

207. Parchand S, Gupta A, Ram J, Gupta N, Chakrabarty A. Voriconazole for fungal corneal ulcers. *Ophthalmology* 2012;119:1083.

208. Qiu S, Zhao GQ, Lin J, et al. Natamycin in the treatment of fungal keratitis: A systematic review and Meta-analysis. *Int J Ophthalmol* 2015;8:597–602.

209. Rose-Nussbaumer J, Prajna NV, Krishnan T, et al. Risk factors for low vision related functioning in the Mycotic Ulcer Treatment Trial: A randomised trial comparing natamycin with voriconazole. *Br J Ophthalmol* 2016;100:929-932.

210. Servais AC, Moldovan R, Farcas E, Crommen J, Roland I, Fillet M. Development and validation of a liquid chromatographic method for the stability study of a pharmaceutical formulation containing voriconazole using cellulose tris(4-chloro-3-methylphenylcarbamate) as chiral selector and polar organic mobile phases. *J Chromatogr A* 2014;1363:178–182.

211. Sharma S, Das S, Virdi A, et al. Re-appraisal of topical 1% voriconazole and 5% natamycin in the treatment of fungal keratitis in a randomised trial. *Br J Ophthalmol* 2015;99:1190–1195.

212. Sponsel W, Graybill J, Nevarez H, Dang D. Ocular and systemic posaconazole(SCH-56592) treatment of invasive *Fusarium solani* keratitis and endophthalmitis. *Br J Ophthalmol* 2002;86:829–830.

213. Jhanji V, Sharma N, Mannan R, Titiyal JS, Vajpayee RB. Management of tunnel fungal infection with voriconazole. *J Cataract Refract Surg* 2007;33:915–917.

214. Ozbek Z, Kang S, Sivalingam J, Rapuano CJ, Cohen EJ, Hammersmith KM. Voriconazole in the management of *Alternaria* keratitis. *Cornea* 2006;25:242–244.

215. Jones B. Jackson memorial lecture. *Am J Ophthalmol* 1975;79:719–751.

216. Foster C. Miconazole therapy for keratomycosis. *Am J Ophthalmol* 1981;91:622–629.

217. Jones D. Therapy of postsurgical fungal endophthalmitis. *Ophthalmology* 1978;85:357–373.

218. Hirose H, Terasaki H, Awaya S, Yasuma T. Treatment of fungal corneal ulcers with amphotericin B ointment. *Am J Ophthalmol* 1997;124:836–838.

219. Hurtado-Sarrio M, Duch-Samper A, Cisneros-Lanuza A, Diaz-Llopis M, Peman-Garciia J, Vazquez-Polo A. Successful topical application of caspofungin in the treatment of fungal keratitis refractory to voriconazole. *Arch Ophthalmol* 2010;128:941–942.

220. Kernt M, Kampik A. Intraocular caspofungin: *In vitro* safety profile for human ocular cells. *Mycoses* 2011;54:e110–e121.

221. Livermore JL, Felton TW, Abbott J, et al. Pharmacokinetics and pharmacodynamics of anidulafungin for experimental *Candida* endophthalmitis: Insights into the utility of echinocandins for treatment of a potentially sight-threatening infection. *Antimicrob Agents Chemother* 2013;57:281–288.

222. Neoh CF, Daniell M, Chen SC, Stewart K, Kong DC. Clinical utility of caspofungin eye drops in fungal keratitis. *Int J Antimicrob Agents* 2014;44:96–104.

223. Neoh CF, Leung L, Misra A, et al. Penetration of topically administered 0.5-percent caspofungin eye drops into human aqueous humor. *Antimicrob Agents Chemother* 2011;55:1761–1763.

224. Shen YC, Liang CY, Wang CY, et al. Pharmacokinetics and safety of intravitreal caspofungin. *Antimicrob Agents Chemother* 2014;58:7234–7239.

225. Patil A, Majumdar S. Echinocandins in ocular therapeutics. *J Ocul Pharmacol Ther* 2017.

226. Tu EY. Alternaria keratitis: Clinical presentation and resolution with topical fluconazole or intrastromal voriconazole and topical caspofungin. *Cornea* 2009;28:116–119.

227. Neoh CF, Leung L, Vajpayee RB, Stewart K, Kong DC. Treatment of *Alternaria* keratitis with intrastromal and topical caspofungin in combination with intrastromal, topical, and oral voriconazole. *Ann Pharmacother* 2011;45:e24.

228. Gregory ME, Macdonald EC, Lockington D, Ramaesh K. Recurrent fungal keratitis following penetrating keratoplasty: An unusual source of infection. *Arch Ophthalmol* 2010;128:1490–1491.

229. Matsumoto Y, Murat D, Kojima T, Shimazaki J, Tsubota K. The comparison of solitary topical micafungin or fluconazole application in the treatment of *Candida* fungal keratitis. *Br J Ophthalmol* 2011;95:1406–1409.

230. Kamoshita M, Matsumoto Y, Nishimura K, et al. Wickerhamomyces anomalus fungal keratitis responds to topical treatment with antifungal micafungin. *J Infect Chemother* 2015;21:141–143.

231. Green W, Bennett J, Goos R. Ocular penetration of amphotericin B. *Arch Ophthalmol* 1965;73:769–775.

232. Kermani N, Aggarwal S. Isolated post-operative *Aspergillus niger* endophthalmitis. *Eye* 2000;14:114–116.

233. Pettit T, Olsen R, Foos R, Martin W. Fungal endophthalmitis following intraocular lens implantation: A surgical epidemic. *Arch Ophthalmol* 1980;98:1025–1039.

234. Mason J, III, Parker J. Subconjunctival miconazole and anterior segment blastomycosis. *Am J Ophthalmol* 1993;116:506–507.

235. Ritterband DC, Shah M, Seedor JA. *Colletotrichum graninicola*: A new corneal pathogen. *Cornea* 1997;16:362–364.

236. Kuriakose T, Kothari M, Paul P, Jacob P, Thomas R. Intracameral amphotericin B injection in the management of deep keratomycosis. *Cornea* 2002;21:653–656.

237. Kaushik S, Ram J, Brar G, Jain A, Chakraborti A, Gupta A. Intracameral amphotericin B: Initial experience in severe keratomycosis. *Cornea* 2001;20:715–719.

238. Pflugfelder S, Flynn H, Jr, Zwickey T, et al. Exogenous fungal endophthalmitis. *Ophthalmology* 1988;95:19–30.

239. Scott I, Flynn H, Jr, Miller D, Speights J, Snip R, Brod R. Exogenous endophthalmitis caused by amphotericin B-resistant *Paecilomyces lilacinus*: Treatment options and visual outcomes. *Arch Ophthalmol* 2001;119:916–919.

240. Cutler JE, Binder PS, Paul TO, Beamis JF. Metastatic coccidioidal endophthalmitis. *Arch Ophthalmol* 1978;96:689–691.

241. Weissgold D, Orlin S, Sulewski M, Frayer W, Eagle R, Jr. Delayed-onset fungal keratitis after endophthalmitis. *Ophthalmology* 1998;105:258–262.

242. Weissgold DJ, Maguire AM, Brucker AJ. Management of postoperative *Acremonium* endophthalmitis. *Ophthalmology* 1996;103:749–756.

243. Brod RD, Flynn HW, Clarkson JG, Pflugfelder SC, Culbertson WW, Miller D. Endogenous *Candida* endophthalmitis. *Ophthalmology* 1990;97:666–674.

244. Borne M, Elliott J, O'Day D. Ocular fluconazole treatment of *Candida parapsilosis* endophthalmitis after failed intravitreal amphotericin B. *Arch Ophthalmol* 1993;111:1326–1327.

245. Goodman D, Stern W. Oral ketoconazole and intraocular amphotericin B for treatment of postoperative *Candida parapsilosis* endophthalmitis. *Arch Ophthalmol* 1987;105:172–173.

246. Stern W, Tamura E, Jacobs R, et al. Epidemic postsurgical *Candida parapsilosis* endophthalmitis. Clinical findings and management of 15 consecutive cases. *Ophthalmology* 1985;92:1701–1709.

247. Gilbert CM, Novak MA. Successful treatment of postoperative *Candida* endophthalmitis in an eye with an intraocular lens implant. *Am J Ophthalmol* 1984;97:593–595.

248. Hogeweg M, De Jong PTVM. *Candida* endophthalmitis in heroin addicts. *Doc Ophthalmol* 1983;55:63–71.

249. Stransky TJ. Postoperative endophthalmitis secondary to *Candida parapsilosis*. *Retina* 1981;1:179–183.

250. Lin RC, Sanduja N, Hariprasad SM. Successful treatment of postoperative fungal endophthalmitis using intravitreal and intracameral voriconazole. *J Ocul Pharmacol Ther* 2008;24:245–248.

251. Amiel H, Chohan AB, Snibson GR, Vajpayee R. Atypical fungal sclerokeratitis. *Cornea* 2008;27:382–383.

252. Shen YC, Wang MY, Wang CY, et al. Clearance of intravitreal voriconazole. *Invest Ophthalmol Vis Sci* 2007;48:2238–2241.

253. Alves da Costa Pertuiset PA, Logrono JF. *Fusarium* endophthalmitis following cataract surgery: Successful treatment with intravitreal and systemic voriconazole. *Case Rep Ophthalmol Med* 2016;2016:4593042.

254. Funakoshi Y, Yakushijin K, Matsuoka H, Minami H. Fungal endophthalmitis successfully treated with intravitreal voriconazole injection. *Intern Med* 2011;50:941.

255. Goyal J, Fernandes M, Shah SG. Intracameral voriconazole injection in the treatment of fungal endophthalmitis resulting from keratitis. *Am J Ophthalmol* 2010;150:939; author reply -40.

256. Haddad RS, El-Mollayess GM. Combination of intracameral and intrastromal voriconazole in the treatment of recalcitrant Acremonium fungal keratitis. *Middle East Afr J Ophthalmol* 2012;19:265–268.

257. Kim EL, Patel SR, George MS, Ameri H. *Ochroconis gallopava* endophthalmitis successfully treated with intravitreal voriconazole and amphotericin b. *Retin Cases Brief Rep* 2016.

258. Lekhanont K, Nonpassopon M, Nimvorapun N, Santanirand P. Treatment with intrastromal and intracameral voriconazole in 2 eyes with Lasiodiplodia theobromae keratitis: Case reports. *Medicine (Baltimore)* 2015;94:e541.

259. Mithal K, Pathengay A, Bawdekar A, et al. Filamentous fungal endophthalmitis: Results of combination therapy with intravitreal amphotericin B and voriconazole. *Clin Ophthalmol* 2015;9:649–655.

260. Mittal V, Mittal R. Intracameral and topical voriconazole for fungal corneal endoexudates. *Cornea* 2012;31:366–370.

261. Niki M, Eguchi H, Hayashi Y, Miyamoto T, Hotta F, Mitamura Y. Ineffectiveness of intrastromal voriconazole for filamentous fungal keratitis. *Clin Ophthalmol* 2014;8:1075–1079.

262. Shen YC, Wang CY, Tsai HY, Lee HN. Intracameral voriconazole injection in the treatment of fungal endophthalmitis resulting from keratitis. *Am J Ophthalmol* 2010;149:916–921.

263. Vila Arteaga J, Suriano MM, Stirbu O. Intravitreal voriconazole for the treatment of *Aspergillus chorioretinitis*. *Int Ophthalmol* 2011;31:341–344.

264. Benoit J, Carandang G, Sitrin M, Arnow P. Intraluminal antibiotic treatment of central venous catheter infections in patients receiving parenteral nutrition at home. *Clin Infect Dis* 1995;21:1286–1288.

265. Arnow P, Kushner R. *Malassezia furfur* catheter infection cured with antibiotic lock therapy. *Am J Med* 1991;90:128–130.

266. Bestul MB, Vandenbussche HL. Antibiotic lock technique: Review of the literature. *Pharmacotherapy* 2005;25:211–227.

267. Segarra-Newnham M, Martin-Cooper EM. Antibiotic lock technique: A review of the literature. *Ann Pharmacother* 2005;39:311–318.

268. Basas J, Morer A, Ratia C, et al. Efficacy of anidulafungin in the treatment of experimental *Candida parapsilosis* catheter infection using an antifungal-lock technique. *J Antimicrob Chemother* 2016;71:2895–2901.

269. McGhee W, Michaels MG, Martin JM, Mazariegos GV, Green M. Antifungal lock therapy with liposomal amphotericin B: A prospective trial. *J Pediatr Infect Dis Soc* 2016;5:80–84.

270. Oncu S. *In vitro* effectiveness of antifungal lock solutions on catheters infected with *Candida* species. *J Infect Chemother* 2011;17:634–639.

271. DiMondi VP, Townsend ML, Johnson M, Durkin M. Antifungal catheter lock therapy for the management of a persistent *Candida albicans* bloodstream infection in an adult receiving hemodialysis. *Pharmacotherapy* 2014;34:e120–e127.

272. Simitsopoulou M, Kyrpitzi D, Velegraki A, Walsh TJ, Roilides E. Caspofungin at catheter lock concentrations eradicates mature biofilms of *Candida lusitaniae* and *Candida guilliermondii*. *Antimicrob Agents Chemother* 2014;58:4953–4956.

273. Walraven CJ, Lee SA. Antifungal lock therapy. *Antimicrob Agents Chemother* 2013;57:1–8.

274. Benoit JL, Carandang G, Sitrin M, Arnow P. Intraluminal antibiotic treatment of central venous catheter infections in patients receiving parenteral nutrition at home. *Clin Infect Dis* 1997;24:743–744.

275. Johnson DC, Johnson FL, Goldman S. Preliminary results treating persistent central venous catheter infections with the antibiotic lock technique in pediatric patients. *Pediatr Infect Dis J* 1994;13:930–931.

276. Krzywda EA, Andris DA, Edmiston CE, Jr., Quebbeman EJ. Treatment of Hickman catheter sepsis using antibiotic lock technique. *Infect Control Hosp Epidemiol* 1995;16:596–598.

277. Wu CY, Lee PI. Antibiotic-lock therapy and erythromycin for treatment of catheter-related *Candida parapsilosis* and *Staphylococcus aureus* infections. *J Antimicrob Chemother* 2007;60:706–707.

278. Schinabeck MK, Long LA, Hossain MA, et al. Rabbit model of *Candida albicans* biofilm infection: Liposomal amphotericin B antifungal lock therapy. *Antimicrob Agents Chemother* 2004;48:1727–1732.

279. Kuhn DM, George T, Chandra J, et al. Antifungal susceptibility of *Candida* biofilms: Unique efficacy of amphotericin B lipid formulations and echinocandins. *Antimicrob Agents Chemother* 2002;46:1773–1780.

280. Shuford JA, Rouse MS, Piper KE, Steckelberg JM, Patel R. Evaluation of caspofungin and amphotericin B deoxycholate against *Candida albicans* biofilms in an experimental intravascular catheter infection model. *J Infect Dis* 2006;194:710–713.

281. Lown L, Peters BM, Walraven CJ, Noverr MC, Lee SA. An optimized lock solution containing micafungin, ethanol and doxycycline inhibits *Candida albicans* and mixed *C. albicans*—*Staphyloccoccus aureus* biofilms. *PLoS One* 2016;11:e0159225.

282. Marcos-Zambrano LJ, Escribano P, Gonzalez del Vecchio M, Bouza E, Guinea J. Micafungin is more active against *Candida albicans* biofilms with high metabolic activity. *J Antimicrob Chemother* 2014;69:2984–2987.

283. Buckler BS, Sams RN, Goei VL, et al. Treatment of central venous catheter fungal infection using liposomal amphotericin-B lock therapy. *Pediatr Infect Dis J* 2008;27:762–764.

284. Ozdemir H, Karbuz A, Ciftci E, et al. Successful treatment of central venous catheter infection due to *Candida lipolytica* by caspofungin-lock therapy. *Mycoses* 2011;54:e647–e649.

15

Dermatophytosis

MAHMOUD A. GHANNOUM, IMAN SALEM, AND NANCY ISHAM

DERMATOPHYTOSIS

Cutaneous fungal infections are a worldwide health concern. While the majority of dermatophyte infections are benign when affecting otherwise healthy individuals, infections in elderly or immunocompromised patients may be accompanied by significant morbidity or mortality. Some forms of dermatomycosis are increasing in incidence, whereas others remain rare [1]. Although newer oral antifungal agents for the treatment of invasive and superficial infections have significantly improved the efficacy of treatment for many fungal infections, side effects, drug interactions, and resistant organisms have created a challenge to find safer and more effective treatments. This chapter blends current clinical knowledge of superficial and cutaneous fungal infections with recent advances in management.

Introduction

Dermatophytes are fungi causing localized infection of the stratum corneum, hair, and nails that may infect up to 20% of the population at any given time [2]. Three genera of dermatophytes account for the majority of infections: *Epidermophyton*, *Trichophyton*, and *Microsporum*. In the United States, *Trichophyton* species account for the majority of dermatophytoses [3,4]. Clinical infections are commonly named based on the region of the body affected. For instance, *tinea pedis* refers to a dermatophyte infection of the foot. Likewise, *tinea manuum, tinea corporis, tinea cruris, tinea facei, tinea capitis, tinea barbae, and tinea unguium* refer to dermatophyte infections of the hand, body, genitalia, face, scalp, beard, and nails, respectively.

History

Charif and Elewski highlight the history and epidemiology of dermatophytoses in Europe and the United States [5]. *Trichophyton rubrum* originated in West Africa, Southeast Asia, Northern Australia, and Indonesia mostly in the form of *tinea corporis*. *Tinea pedis* was not reported in Europe until 1908 (Great Britain). Until then, *tinea pedis* was considered a rare, sporadic, nonrecurring phenomenon, likely due to the limited use of footwear. Increased population mobility through migration, recreational travel, as well as World War I allowed *T. rubrum* to translocate to the Americas, with the first case in the United States being reported shortly after World War I [5]. Thereafter, the incidence of *tinea pedis* and onychomycosis increased as a result of future wars, frequent use of health clubs, occlusive footwear, and greater ease of travel. Although the incidence of *tinea capitis* initially remained relatively low due to rigorous screening of immigrants, *tinea pedis* flourished unchecked [5].

Epidemiology

Trichophyton rubrum is the most prevalent pathogen and most common etiologic agent in the United States for most dermatophytic infections except tinea capitis and fingernail onychomycosis. A recent epidemiological study in the United States from 1999 to 2002 reported increasing incidence of *T. rubrum* in onychomycosis, *tinea corporis*, *tinea cruris*, *tinea manuum*, and *tinea pedis* [6]. *Trichophyton tonsurans* and *Candida albicans*, on the other hand, were the predominant species for tinea capitis and fingernail onychomycosis, respectively. The primary etiologic agents for the various dermatophytic infections are listed in Table 15.1.

Pathogenesis

Dermatophytes use keratin as a nutrient source. Unlike most other fungi, dermatophytes produce keratinases allowing invasion into and subsequent colonization of the keratinized stratum corneum. They generally do not invade viable tissue and rarely extend below the epidermis. Involvement of underlying and surrounding tissues usually results from allergic or inflammatory host responses to the presence of the fungi. The circular morphology results from the inflammatory reaction forcing dermatophytes outward to inflammation-free areas. Outward migration continues as long as the infection persists [7].

In dermatophyte species infecting the hair (tinea capitis and tinea barbae), infection may occur in one of the two ways: (*i*) in ectothrix invasion (i.e., *M. canis*, *M. gypseum*, *T. equinum*, and *T. verrucosum*), the arthroconidia form on the outside of the hair shaft and destroy the cuticle; (*ii*) in endothrix infections (i.e., *T. tonsurans* and *T. violaceum*), the arthroconidia form within the hair shaft leaving the cuticle intact.

Transmission of dermatophytes to humans is classified into one of three categories: geophilic, zoophilic, and anthropophilic. Geophilic transmission involves transfer of fungal spores, or hyphae, from the soil to either a human or animal host, whereas zoophilic and anthropophilic

Table 15.1 Etiologic organisms in cutaneous mycotic infections

Condition	Dermatophyte	Non-dermatophyte	Yeast
Tinea capitis	*T. tonsurans*		
	T. verrucosum		
	T. violaceum		
	T. schoenleinii		
	M. canis		
	M. gypseum		
	M. audouinii		
Tinea corporis	*T. rubrum*		
	T. tonsurans		
	T. verrucosum		
	Microsporum canis		
Tinea cruris	*T. rubrum*		
	E. floccosum		
	T. mentagrophytes var. interdigitale		
Tinea pedis	*Trichophyton rubrum*	*Scytalidium hyalinum*	*Candida albicans*
	Epidermophyton floccosum		
	T. mentagrophytes		
Tinea unguium (onychomycosis)	*T. rubrum*	*Acremonium spp.*	*C. albicans*
	T. mentagrophytes	*Aspergillus terreus*	
	E. floccosum	*Fusarium spp.*	
		Neoscytalidium dimidiatum	
		Onychocola canadensis	
		Scopulariopsis spp.	
		Scytalidium hyalinum	

Source: Melody, R.V.S. et al., *Infect. Dis. Clin. North Am.*, 17, 87–112, 2003.

transmission involves transfer of fungal spores and hyphae from animals to humans or humans to humans, respectively. Geophilic species survive by decomposing keratinaceous debris. Dermatophytes are often transmitted by either direct contact with infected humans or animals or indirectly by human contact with desquamated skin harboring the fungi (which can persist for months to years without an animal host). Human carriers occur when dermatophytes cause clinical or subclinical infections of the hair, skin, or nails. Subclinical infections usually occur within interdigital spaces or on the scalp and not only create a public health hazard but also act as reservoirs for autoinoculation, making eradication of dermatophytoses difficult.

Dermatophytes thrive in warm moist conditions. Conditions predisposing to fungal infections include immobility from increased age or medical comorbidities, immunosuppression, warm climates, poor hygiene, disruption of the skin barrier or skin maceration, and contact with infected individuals or surfaces (Figure 15.1). Immunosuppression not only increases the risk for fungal infections but also may lead to more severe disease with increased rates of recurrence and possible direct deep dermal invasion [8].

Clinical features

TINEA PEDIS

Tinea pedis is the most common dermatophytosis with a lifetime incidence of up to 70% [4]. The incidence of *tinea pedis* has been estimated at 3% in the United States but may be up to 5% in the elderly and in excess of 20% in populations who use communal showers or locker rooms [9]. *T. rubrum* causes the majority of infections. Risk factors for infection or conversion to symptomatic carriage include hyperhydrosis secondary to warm humid climates or occlusive footwear and walking barefoot on surfaces at risk for contamination, such as communal locker rooms and shower stalls.

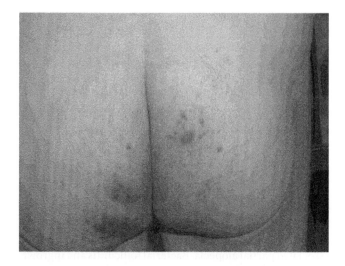

Figure 15.1 *Tinea cruris* in a transplant patient.

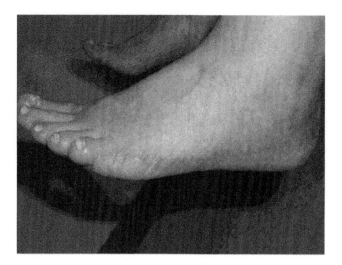

Figure 15.2 *Tinea pedis*.

Three clinical forms of tinea pedis predominate: (*i*) interdigital, (*ii*) moccasin, and (*iii*) vesiculobullous [1]. Interdigital infection involves the web spaces, most commonly between the fourth and fifth toes. It is often malodorous because of bacterial superinfection and pruritic. The infection can be dry and scaly, resembling psoriasis, or moist and macerated (Figure 15.2). Unlike interdigital infection, moccasin-type infections involve the heel, plantar, lateral, and medial aspects of the foot. It may present as mild asymptomatic scale or as silvery-white scale on a red, thickened base, resembling psoriasis or contact dermatitis. Moccasin-type *tinea pedis* infections can be recalcitrant to treatment and may be complicated by onychomycosis, *tinea manuum, tinea cruris,* or *tinea corporis* [10]. Vesiculobullous *tinea pedis* usually occurs on the sole but may also be on the side of the foot. Vesicles or pustules are present, and the area may become macerated and secondarily infected with bacteria. This form may be misdiagnosed as dyshidrotic eczema, contact dermatitis, nummular eczema, or pustular psoriasis. Other conditions that may resemble tinea pedis include candidiasis, erythrasma, pyoderma, secondary syphilis, and pitted keratolysis.

TINEA MANUUM

Tinea manuum is a much less prevalent infection than *tinea pedis* and involves the palmar, dorsal, or interdigital surface of the hands and fingernails. It may appear diffusely dry and hyperkeratotic or resemble *tinea corporis* (Figure 15.3). Only one hand is usually involved; however, both may be affected. Bilateral *tinea pedis* is also frequently an accompanying feature. Differential diagnosis includes psoriasis, eczema, dyshidrotic eczema, callous formation, secondary syphilis, contact dermatitis, and infection with nondermatophytic fungi.

TINEA CORPORIS

Tinea corporis, or "ringworm," is an infection of the glabrous skin, usually on the trunk and extremities. The predominant pathogens are *T. rubrum* and to a lesser extent *T. tonsurans*.

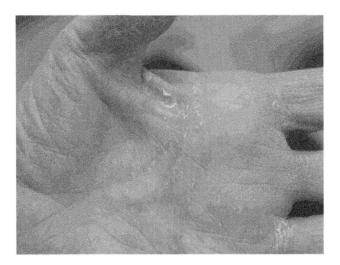

Figure 15.3 *Tinea manuum.*

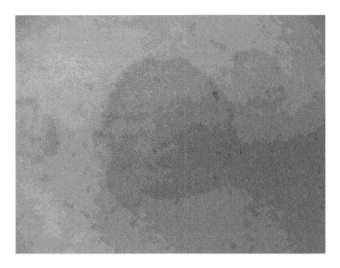

Figure 15.5 *Tinea incognito.*

Infection in wrestlers is referred to as tinea corporis gladiatorum and is most often caused by *T. tonsurans*. In teams without known epidemics, prevalence rates ranged from 20% to 44% [11]. Majocchi's granuloma, tinea imbricata, and tinea incognito are three variants of tinea corporis. Deep-seated tinea corporis, referred to as Majocchi's granuloma, is most often due to *T. rubrum* or *T. mentagrophytes*. It occurs most frequently in women and is typically located on the lower extremities [4] (Figure 15.4). Tinea imbricata is caused by *T. concentricum* and is limited geographically to southwest Polynesia, Melanesia, Southeast Asia, India, and Central America. Lastly, tinea incognito is a term applied to atypical clinical lesions of tinea that have been treated with topical corticosteroids (Figure 15.5).

Tinea corporis is characterized by an erythematous, round, annular plaque with central pallor and scaly, raised advancing border that may contain papules or pustules (Figure 15.6). These infections are sometimes pruritic and can resemble nummular eczema, plaque psoriasis, granuloma annulare, erythema nodosum, contact dermatitis,

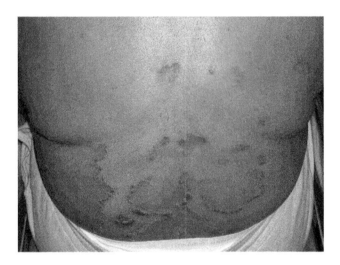

Figure 15.6 *Tinea corporis.*

cutaneous lupus erythematosus, drug eruptions, and erythema multiforme.

TINEA FACIEI

Tinea faciei affects the nonbearded areas of the face. It may present as itchy, red poorly demarcated patches or may resemble tinea corporis with scaly, red annular plaques (Figure 15.7). It should be considered in all erythematous eruptions on the face [1]. The differential diagnosis includes rosacea, contact dermatitis, seborrheic dermatitis, lymphocytic infiltration, and discoid lupus erythematosus.

TINEA BARBAE

Tinea barbae is a rare infection of the beard area. It most often occurs in men who are in close contact with farm animals [4]. The fungi infect the hair shaft, forming either nodular, boggy, exudative lesions, or crusted patches with associated partial alopecia. Bacterial folliculitis and ingrown hairs may complicate the condition. Tinea barbae may be confused with folliculitis, sporotrichosis, candidiasis,

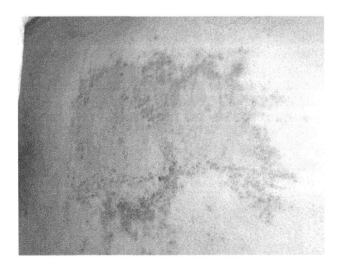

Figure 15.4 Majocchi's granuloma.

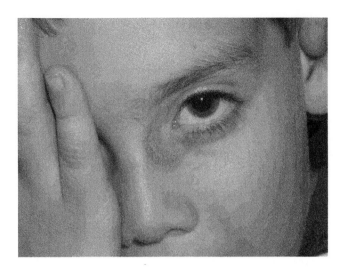

Figure 15.7 *Tinea faciei.*

pseudofolliculitis barbae, contact dermatitis, herpes labialis, acne, syphilis, and even malignant lymphoma.

TINEA CRURIS

Tinea cruris, or "jock itch," is an invasion of the hair follicles that can easily be confused with cutaneous candidal infection. It is most commonly caused by *T. rubrum* and often occurs during the summer, in young men, and in persons with tight-fitting clothing. Tinea cruris forms an erythematous, pruritic patch on the intertriginous inguinal folds and medial thighs with characteristic sparing of the scrotum and penis (Figure 15.8). The patch spreads peripherally with partial central clearing and may have small follicular papules, pustules, or vesicles along the advancing border. Infections with *Candida* species may closely resemble tinea cruris; however, it may be distinguished by their moist appearance, presence of satellite lesions, and possible scrotal involvement. Mechanical intertrigo, or "chafing," may also be misdiagnosed as tinea cruris; however, it is usually sharply demarcated, tender, and lacking scale. Erythrasma can be distinguished by Wood's lamp examination, under which it fluoresces coral red. Lastly, inverse psoriasis and

seborrheic dermatitis may be difficult to distinguish from tinea cruris without biopsy if other lesions outside the genital region are absent. Concurrent *tinea pedis* infection or onychomycosis can predispose to recurrence, suggesting possible transfer of organisms [4].

TINEA CAPITIS

Tinea capitis primarily affects preadolescent children, although adult carrier states have been reported [12]. It can be transmitted via direct contact with infected persons and select animal vectors or indirectly through use of contaminated clothing, combs, and furniture. Prevalence in the United States is generally estimated to be between 3% and 8% of the pediatric population, with carriers occurring in as many as 34% of household contacts [13]. Over the past 50 years, the primary etiologic agent of tinea capitis has changed from *Microsporum audouinii* to *T. tonsurans*. Recent studies report *T. tonsurans* as the predominant dermatophyte isolated in the United States, frequently achieving near exclusionary proportions [14–16]. In contrast, *M. canis* is the most commonly isolated pathogen in Europe [8], and *T. violaceum* is the main infecting agent in children in India with tinea capitis [15].

The presentation of tinea capitis is highly variable. The primary lesions may be papules, pustules, plaques, or nodules on the scalp (Figure 15.9). Inflammation and secondary infection lead to secondary processes, such as scaling, alopecia, erythema, exudate, and edema. The initial presentation may be subtle and asymptomatic. As the inflammatory response increases, inflammatory alopecia occurs with scaling and black dot alopecia due to breakage of weakened hairs at the scalp's surface (Figure 15.10). A kerion may develop as a result of an intense cell-mediated immune response and is characterized by an inflamed, exudative, nodular, boggy swelling with associated hair loss and cervical lymphadenopathy (Figure 15.11). An unusual scaling reaction, known as favus, confers a doughy or waxy appearance to the scalp by way of a saucer-shaped, yellow crust over hair follicles (called a scutula) with resultant scarring alopecia (Figure 15.12). *T. schoenleinii* is responsible for this appearance [1,9].

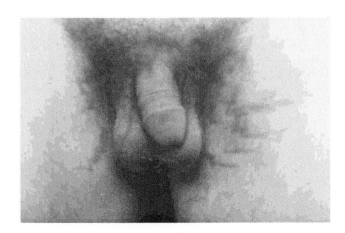

Figure 15.8 *Tinea cruris.*

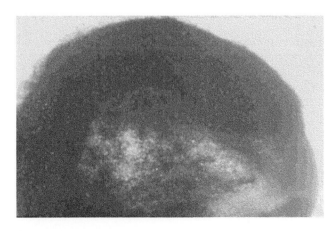

Figure 15.9 *Tinea capitis.*

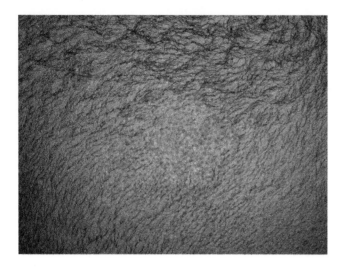

Figure 15.10 *Tinea capitis* with black dot alopecia.

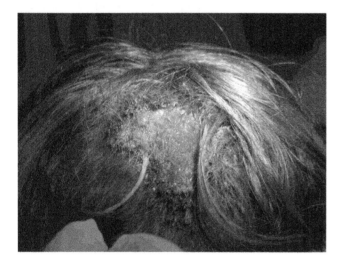

Figure 15.11 Kerion.

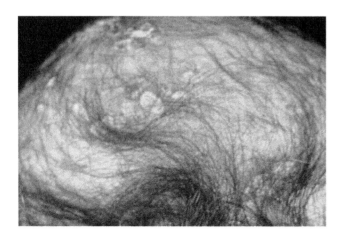

Figure 15.12 Flavus.

Laboratory diagnosis

Microscopic examination is the most efficient and cost-effective laboratory technique to diagnose dermatophyte infections. Diagnosis of *tinea pedis, tinea corporis, tinea cruris, tinea faciei, tinea barbae,* and *tinea manuum* can usually be made with 10%–20% potassium hydroxide (KOH) preparation of scale scraped from the leading edge of the lesion. In vesicular or pustular lesions, the roof and contents of the vesicle or pustule should be examined. *Tinea capitis* can also be diagnosed by KOH via examination of extracted hairs. To speed the clearing of keratin, the slide is heated or dimethyl sulfoxide (DMSO) is added. Calcofluor is a stain specific for chitin, a fungal cell wall component that may enhance the visualization of fungal elements. Under fluorescent microscopy, fungal elements fluoresce apple-green.

Fungal culture is used to confirm a diagnosis, especially in long-standing or recalcitrant disease, or when species identification is desired. Sabouraud dextrose agar with chloramphenicol and cycloheximide allows growth of dermatophytes while suppressing nondermatophytes and bacterial contaminants. The specimen (scale or extracted hair) is placed on the media and cultured at 26°C–28°C for up to 4 weeks [9]. In tinea capitis, cultures must involve extracted hairs, not simply scale, to provide accurate results. Any growth of dermatophytes is considered significant. Molecular sequencing is a more rapid alternative for species identification; however, its availability is limited. Lastly, a Wood's lamp can be used to diagnosis certain tinea capitis infections. Hair infected by ectothrix organisms, except for *T. verrucosum*, fluoresce bright green or yellow-green, while endothrix organisms, such as *T. tonsurans*, do not fluoresce (Figure 15.13).

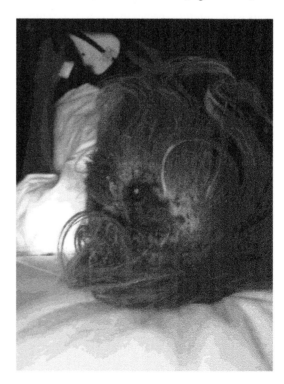

Figure 15.13 Kerion fluorescence due to ectothrix infection.

Treatment and prevention

TINEA PEDIS

Tinea pedis usually responds to topical antifungal agents, many of which are available over the counter in a variety of formulations (creams, gels, powders, and aerosols). Antifungal powders (clotrimazole, miconazole, and tolnaftate) or gel formulations (naftifine, ciclopirox, and terbinafine) can be helpful, especially when there is appreciable moisture. Duration of topical treatment varies based on the antifungal agent and ranges from a single application with the new terbinafine film-forming solution to multiple applications daily for up to 4 weeks. While the various topical antifungal agents and formulations have variable dosing regimens, their clinical and mycologic cure rates appear comparable [18]. Recurrence is common, especially if there is concomitant untreated onychomycosis. Furthermore, topical antifungal treatments have been reported to fail in up to 33% of patients with *tinea pedis* [19]. Oral therapy can be considered for extensive, severe, or recalcitrant disease. Some of the more common and effective oral treatments include terbinafine, itraconazole, and fluconazole. Considering relative cost-effectiveness, griseofulvin is also an option; however, current data suggests it may be significantly less effective than terbinafine [20]. The recommended doses for the oral antifungal agents are as follows: Griseofulvin 500 mg twice daily for 4–8 weeks with higher doses used for relapse, itraconazole 400 mg daily for 1 week or 200 mg daily for 2 weeks, fluconazole 150–300 mg once weekly for 4–6 weeks, and terbinafine 250 mg daily for 2–6 weeks [21,22]. Table 15.2 summarizes the dosing regimens for *tinea pedis* for the oral antifungal agents. The addition of products containing glycolic or lactic acids or urea may decrease the amount of hyperkeratosis.

Table 15.2 Treatment of cutaneous mycotic infections

Condition	Medication	Dose and regimen	Comments
Tinea barbae			
Oral	Fluconazole		Combine with regular shaving and cleansing with antibacterial soaps
	Griseofulvin	0.5–1 g/day × 2–4 weeks	
	Itraconazole		
	Terbinafine		
Tinea capitis			
Topical	Ketoconazole cream	Daily	Adjunct only;
	Ketoconazole shampoo	Daily	reduce fungal shedding
Oral	Griseofulvin	20–25 mg/kg/day × 8 weeks or 10–15 mg/kg/day (ultra microsize)	Continue 2 weeks beyond cure
	Fluconazole	3–6 mg/kg/day × 6 weeks (oral solution)	
	Itraconazole	5 mg/kg/day × 4–6 weeks	Avoid oral solution
	Ketoconazole	200 mg daily × 4 weeks	
	Terbinafine	125 mg/day (<25 kg) 187.5 mg/day (25–35 kg) 250 mg/day (>35 kg)	
Tinea corporis			
Topical	Clotrimazole cream	BID	Continue topicals for 7–14 days beyond symptom resolution
	Econazole cream	BID	
	Ketoconazole cream	BID	
	Miconazole cream	BID	
	Terbinafine cream	BID × 1 weeks	
Oral	Fluconazole	150–300 mg once weekly × 4–6 weeks	
	Griseofulvin	500 mg BID × 4–8 weeks	
	Itraconazole	200–400 mg daily × 1 weeks	
	Terbinafine	250 mg qd × 10 days	

(Continued)

Table 15.2 (*Continued*) Treatment of cutaneous mycotic infections

Condition	Medication	Dose and regimen	Comments
Tinea cruris			
Topical	Ciclopirox cream	BID × 2–3 weeks	Continue topicals for 7–14 days beyond symptom resolution. May help to add antifungal powders.
	Econazole cream	BID × 2–3 weeks	
	Ketoconazole cream	BID × 2–3 weeks	
	Miconazole cream	BID × 2–3 weeks	
	Terbinafine cream	BID × 2–3 weeks	
Oral	Fluconazole	150–300 mg once weekly × 2 weeks	
	Griseofulvin	500 mg BID × 2–4 weeks	
	Itraconazole	200–400 mg daily × 1 weeks	
	Terbinafine	250 mg daily × 10 days	
Tinea faiei			
Topical	Econazole cream	Daily × 2 weeks	
	Ketoconazole cream	Daily × 2 weeks	
	Miconazole cream	Daily × 2 weeks	
Tinea manuum			
Topical	Lac-Hydrin 12% lotion	BID	
Oral	Fluconazole	150–300 mg once weekly × 4–6 weeks	
	Griseofulvin	500 mg BID × 4–8 weeks	
	Itraconazole	400 mg daily × 1 weeks or 200 mg daily × 2 weeks	
	Terbinafine	250 mg daily × 2–6 weeks	
Tinea pedis			
Topical	Ciclopirox cream	Daily to BID 1–4 weeks	Antifungal powders or gel formulations of ciclopirox
	Econazole nitrate cream	Daily to BID 1–4 weeks	or naftifine for moist web spaces
	Ketoconazole cream	Daily to BID 1–4 weeks	
	Terbinafine hydrochloride cream	Daily to BID 1–4 weeks	
	Terbinafine film-forming solution	Single use	
Oral	Fluconazole	150–300 mg once weekly × 4–6 weeks	
	Griseofulvin	500 mg BID × 4–8 weeks	Higher doses for relapse
	Itraconazole	400 mg daily × 1 weeks or 200 mg daily × 2 weeks	
	Terbinafine	250 mg daily × 2–6 weeks	
Tinea unguium			
Topical	Ciclopirox 8% nail lacquer	Daily, 8 hours before showering Remove weekly with alcohol	
	Efinaconazole	Apply twice daily × 48 weeks	
	Tavaborole	Apply twice daily × 48 weeks	

(*Continued*)

Table 15.2 (*Continued*) Treatment of cutaneous mycotic infections

Condition	Medication	Dose and regimen	Comments
Oral	Fluconazole	100–300 mg once weekly	3–6 months for fingernails, 6–12 months for toenails
	Itraconazole	200 mg BID for 1 weeks/month	Pulse dosing × 2 months (fingernails) × 3 months (toenails)
		200 mg once daily	Continuous dosing × 6 weeks (fingernails) × 12 weeks (toenails)
	Terbinafine	250 mg once daily	
			× 6 weeks (fingernails) × 12 weeks (toenails)

Source: Melody, R.V.S. et al., *Infect. Dis. Clin. North Am.*, 17, 87–112, 2003.

TINEA MANUUM

Tinea manuum, like *tinea pedis*, can usually be treated effectively with topical antifungal agents and keratolytics. Infections may recur if untreated *tinea pedis* or onychomycosis is present [1]. Oral antifungal agents may be used for refractory disease and are dosed similarly to tinea pedis [17,23].

TINEA CORPORIS, TINEA FACIEI, AND TINEA CRURIS

Tinea corporis, tinea faciei, and *tinea cruris* usually respond well to topical antifungal creams or powders. Treatment should be continued 7–14 days beyond symptom resolution to minimize recurrence. Similar to *tinea pedis* and *tinea manuum*, oral medications are reserved for extensive or recalcitrant disease. Commonly prescribed doses of oral antifungals are listed in Table 15.2 and include itraconazole, 200–400 mg daily for 1 week; fluconazole, 150–300 mg once weekly for 2 weeks (*tinea cruris*) or 4–6 weeks (*tinea corporis*); terbinafine, 250 mg daily for 10 days; and griseofulvin, 500 mg daily for 2–4 weeks [24].

TINEA CAPITIS

Oral antifungals are currently the mainstay of treatment for *tinea capitis*. Griseofulvin has long been the standard of care for the treatment of *tinea capitis* and, until recently, had been the only FDA-approved medication for *tinea capitis* in children. Griseofulvin continues to be widely used among pediatricians and dermatologists. Griseofulvin comes in both oral suspension and crushable tablet formulations. As it is poorly water soluble, absorption can be enhanced if taken with a fatty meal. Over the past few decades, higher doses have been required to eradicate infection. The current recommended dose is 20–25 mg/kg/day of the microsize formulation or 10–15 mg/kg/day of the ultramicrosize formulation for 6–8 weeks, or 2 weeks beyond clinical cure [14]. In 2007, terbinafine was approved by the FDA for treatment of *tinea capitis* in children older than 4 years of age. Results of a meta-analysis by Fleece et al. indicated that terbinafine is as effective as or more effective than griseofulvin for the treatment of *tinea capitis*

caused by *T. tonsurans*, with equivalent side-effect profiles [25]. Terbinafine is available in easy to use granules that can be sprinkled on nonacidic food. The approved pediatric dose is based on weight according to the following guidelines: 125 mg/day for children less than 25 kg, 187.5 mg/day for children weighing between 25 and 35 kg, and 250 mg/day for children over 35 kg. Therapy should be given once daily for 6 weeks. Serum transaminases are advised prior to treatment. While currently not FDA approved for *tinea capitis*, studies suggest that itraconazole and fluconazole may be effective alternative treatments [25,26]. Additional studies are required to determine appropriate dosing of the azole antifungal agents, including pulse versus continuous scheduling, and to evaluate their safety in children. Currently available off label, itraconazole's oral suspension is not recommended due to concerns of potential carcinogenicity of its vehicle, hydroxypropyl-B-cyclodextrin.

Optimal treatment of asymptomatic carriers remains to be established. Topical therapy with antifungal shampoos, such as ketoconazole or selenium sulfide, may help to reduce shedding of viable spores. Combs, hats, pillows should also be frequently disinfected to prevent transmission of conidia to household contacts.

TINEA BARBAE

Oral antifungal agents are also considered the first-line treatment for *tinea barbae*. Oral griseofulvin is conventionally used at a dose of 0.5 to 1 g/day for 2–4 weeks. Itraconazole, terbinafine, and fluconazole may also be used for difficult-to-treat cases. Regular shaving and cleansing with antibacterial soaps also aid in treatment.

ONYCHOMYCOSIS

Onychomycosis, or *tinea unguium*, is an infection of the nail plate or nail bed that interferes with normal nail function (Figure 15.14). Eighty to ninety percent of infections are caused by dermatophytes, such as *T. rubrum* and *T. mentagrophytes var interdigitale*. The remainder of infections is caused by a combination of nondermatophytic filamentous fungi (3%–5%),

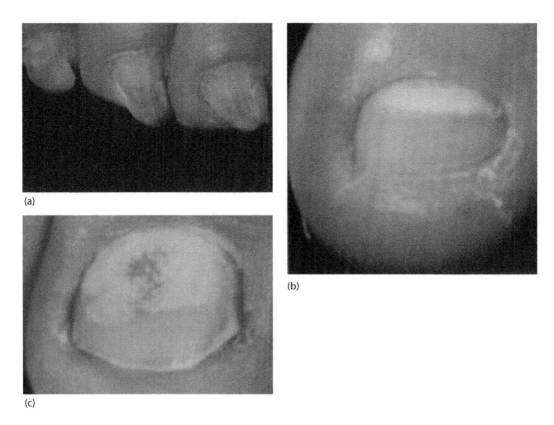

Figure 15.14 **(a)** Distal subungual, **(b)** proximal white subungual, and **(c)** white superficial.

molds, and yeasts (1%–2%) [3,23,24]. Patients with onychomycosis may experience pain, difficulty performing daily activities, and embarrassment over their condition due to associated nail disfigurement and limitation of mobility. Factors predisposing to onychomycosis infections include immunosuppression, diabetes, hemodialysis, concurrent dermatophyte infections at other locations, age greater than 60 years, obesity, male gender, poor peripheral circulation, smoking, genetic pre-disposition, and history of nail trauma [1,3,21,27,28]. Conflicting data exists as to whether psoriasis, a condition that can be associated with nail deformity, is also a predisposing factor to onychomycosis [29]. A recent prospective study of 2761 patients in Poland found 42.8% of patients with toenail onychomycosis had a concurrent second dermatophyte infection with *tinea pedis* being the most common concurrent fungal infection occurring in 33.8% of patients. Less common infections included fingernail onychomycosis (7.4%), *tinea cruris* (4.2%), *tinea corporis* (2.1%), *tinea manuum* (1.6%), and *tinea capitis* (0.5%) [30].

Epidemiology

Onychomycosis accounts for up to 50% of all nail disorders. The incidence of onychomycosis is increasing worldwide as a result of an aging population, occlusive footwear, and increasing numbers of immunocompromised patients [1]. The prevalence of dermatophyte nail infections was found to be 8.7% in a 1997 cross-sectional survey conducted in a dermatology clinic waiting room in Cleveland. Prevalence ranged from 1.1% in children less than 18 years of age to as high as 28.1% in adults over the age of 60 with an average prevalence of 6.5% in women and 13.3% in men [31]. A more comprehensive multicenter study of 1832 patients reported a prevalence of 13.8% by microscopic examination with KOH and 7.2% by culture confirmation [3]. The association of onychomycosis infection and increasing age may partially be attributed to an age-related decrease in immune function, lower vascular efficiency, and less efficient T cells and phagocytes.

Up to a third of diabetic patients may develop onychomycosis [32]. Diabetic patients tend to have higher rates of complication including rapid spread to unaffected nails or the development of osteomyelitis and cellulitis, which may progress to necrosis and amputation if not aggressively treated [21,32]. Patients with HIV are also at increased risk for complications including more clinically aggressive disease, higher incidence of atypical presentations, resistance to conventional therapy, and higher rates of recurrence. As many as 11%–67% of patients with AIDS suffer from onychomycosis, with infection more likely when CD4 cell count is less than 450 cells/mm^3 [33].

Clinical features

Onychomycosis may be divided into four clinical types: (*i*) proximal subungual, (*ii*) distal subungual, (*iii*) white superficial, and (*iv*) mucocutaneous candidiasis. Each type differs in clinical presentation and causative etiologic agents.

Dermatophytes are the principal causative agent for distal subungual, proximal subungual, and white superficial onychomycosis with *Candida* present in less than 1% of cases [1].

Proximal subungual onychomycosis is most commonly caused by *T. rubrum* but may also be caused by *T. megnini, T. tonsurans,* and *T. mentagrophytes* [34]. Toenails are affected more often than fingernails. It is the least common clinical presentation among healthy individuals and may be an early indicator of HIV infection. Infection enters the cuticle and involves the proximal nail bed. If left untreated, infection spreads distally eventually involving the entire nail plate. The nail plate is usually white in color with associated subungual hyperkeratosis and proximal onycholysis [1].

Distal subungual onychomycosis, in contrast, is the most common clinical presentation comprising more than 90% of all nail infections [1]. Its most frequent etiologic agent is *T. rubrum,* but is also caused by *T. tonsurans, T. mentagrophytes,* and *E. floccosum.* It also preferentially affects the toenails. Fungal hyphae enter distally under the nail plate and spread proximally digesting the stratum corneum of the nail bed and nail plate. As the infection spreads, subungual hyper- keratosis, paronychia, and onycholysis can occur. Splinter hemorrhages can be seen secondary to mild inflammation compressing small vessels, and discoloration of the nail plate may occur as a result of secondary infection with mold or bacteria.

White superficial onychomycosis occurs in only 10% of cases. It is most commonly caused by *T. mentagrophytes* but may also be caused by nondermatophyte molds, such as *Aspergillus terreus, Fusarium oxysporum, Acremonium potonii,* and *A. roseogrisum.* The dorsal surface of the nail plate is attacked. Minimal inflammation occurs as viable tissue is typically not involved. Clinically, the nail becomes crumbly and soft with a white discoloration and rough texture. If unchecked, the infection may spread through the nail plate to the cornified layer of the nail bed [1].

Candidal onychomycosis is usually found in patients with chronic mucocutaneous candidiasis. The typical pathogen is *Candida albicans,* though *C. tropicalis, C. krusei, C. guilliermondii,* and *C. parapsilosis* may also be found (*C. parapsilosis* is thought to be part of the normal skin flora) [3]. *Candida* may cause a direct infection of the nail bed or plate, or it may indirectly involve the nail through infection of the nail folds, nail bed, or hyponychium after trauma or exposure to excessive moisture or irritants. Furthermore, other body sites may be involved including the face and arms. Candidal organisms causing onychomycosis have shown some resistance to oral antifungal agents [35].

Onychomycosis may resemble other disorders that involve the nails such as psoriasis, lichen planus, distal onycholysis, subungual tumor, verruca vulgaris, Reiter's syndrome, Hallopeau's acrodermatitis, yellow nail syndrome, paronychia congenita, contact dermatitis, traumatic onychodystrophies, and bacterial superinfection [1,3]. Psoriasis can occasionally be clinically differentiated from onychomycosis by the presence of skin lesions and its symmetrical distribution compared to the frequently unilateral distribution of onychomycosis [36]. Fungal culture is necessary in questionable cases, although the two conditions may coexist. Notably, treatment for psoriasis may worsen onychomycosis; conversely, the presence of a fungal nail infection may inhibit response to psoriasis treatment. Approximately 10% of patients with lichen planus develop nail abnormalities that may also be difficult to differentiate from onychomycosis. These abnormalities usually consist of onychorrhexis, longitudinal ridging of the nail plate, and "angel-wing" deformity. Additional findings of lichen planus—including violaceous polygonal papules on the extremities and mucous membranes, Wickham's striae, and pterygium—may help to differentiate the nail findings of lichen planus from onychomycosis [1,3]. A culture may be required to distinguish these conditions. Lastly, distal onycholysis caused by formaldehyde in nail products, repetitive nail trauma, and contact dermatitis may cause hyperkeratosis of the nail bed with resultant onycholysis. History, culture, or patch testing may distinguish these conditions from onychomycosis.

Laboratory diagnosis

Culture is the definitive diagnostic tool for onychomycosis [1]. Microscopic preparation of debris underneath the nail plate in 10%–15% KOH with calcofluor and gentle heating may aid in diagnosis, with sensitivity of 92% and specificity of 95% [37]. Culture is considered the mainstay of diagnosis because it not only isolates the organism but also allows for identification of the etiologic agent allowing treatment to be tailored appropriately. Other diagnostic tests include nail unit biopsy, immunochemistry, polymerase chain reaction, restriction enzyme analysis, and flow cytometry. Most of these tests are more difficult or more expensive (although probably faster) than culture and are currently only available as research tools.

Treatment and prevention

Systemic therapy is the mainstay of treatment for onychomycosis as less than 20% of cases respond to topical treatment alone due to poor penetration of the nail bed [1]. Terbinafine, itraconazole, and fluconazole (not FDA approved) are the most frequently used oral antifungal agents for onychomycosis. Oral griseofulvin may also be effective for infections caused solely by dermatophytes. Dose and length of treatment differ for toenail and fingernail involvement. The recommended dose of terbinafine is 250 mg daily for 6 weeks (fingernails) or 12 weeks (toenails) [1,31,38]. Itraconazole and fluconazole may be given in a pulsed dosing regimen. Itraconazole (pulsed dose) is given at 400 mg daily (or 200 mg twice a day) for 7 days repeating in 1 month for fingernails and continuing 3–4 months in toenail infections [27,31,38,39]. Itraconazole (continuous dosing) may also be given at 200 mg daily for 2 months (fingernails) or 3 months (toenails) [40]. Fluconazole (pulsed dosing) is usually effective at 150–300 mg once weekly for 3–6 months (fingernails) or 6–12 months (toenails). Several recent studies suggest an added benefit of adjuvant topical therapy with ciclopirox nail lacquer to systemic antifungal treatment [27,40]. When treating onychomycosis, it is important to realize that visible clearance of infection occurs after the process of nail-plate turnover is complete, which typically takes 12–18 months for toenails and 4–6 months for fingernails. Some investigators recommend continuation of treatment until the diseased nail is replaced by normal growth; however, this issue remains controversial [41].

Topical treatment with ciclopirox 8% nail lacquer may be effective in mild-to-moderate (early) *T. rubrum* onychomycosis infections without lunula involvement when used every day, 8 hours before washing hands, with removal once a week with alcohol. Treatment may take 6 months to 1 year to be effective with a clinical cure rate of 5%–8% and a mycological cure rate of 29%–36% [42]. Two new topical agents have been approved by the FDA for the treatment of onychomycosis. Efinaconazole 10% solution achieved a complete cure rate (defined as KOH and culture negative and normal nail appearance) of 15%–18% in pivotal randomized clinical trials [43]. Tavaborole 5% solution, a novel, boron-based antifungal with low molecular weight, which allows a high amount of penetration through the human nail plate, achieved a complete cure rate of 6.5%–9.1% [44]. Both of these new topical agents are applied once daily for 48 weeks.

Despite treatment, recurrence of onychomycosis is not uncommon, with reported rates ranging from 10% to 53% of cases [45].

TINEA VERSICOLOR

Tinea versicolor, otherwise known as *pityriasis versicolor*, is a common superficial mycotic infection of otherwise healthy young and middle-aged adults caused by lipophilic yeast of the *Malassezia* genus. Recent evidence has suggested *Malassezia* species are not only the causative agent of *tinea versicolor* but also seborrheic dermatitis and possibly atopic dermatitis [46].

Epidemiology

Malassezia species are found worldwide. Affected individuals are typically young adults; how- ever, people of all ages may develop the disease. Use of new molecular techniques recently allowed for better classification of the *Malassezia* genus including the identification of seven species: *M. furfur*, *M. pachydermatitis*, *M. sympodialis*, *M. globosa*, *M. slooffiae*, *M. restricta*, and *M. obtuse* with possibly five additional species awaiting validation. While *tinea versicolor* had long been attributed to *M. furfur*, the aid of newer molecular techniques recently uncovered *M. globosa* as the predominant species of *tinea versicolor* reaching incidences of up to 90% [47].

Pathogenesis and host defense

Malassezia species may be part of the normal human flora. *Tinea versicolor* occurs when the yeast form transforms into the mycelial form. This transformation has been reported to occur in the presence of high temperature or high humidity, oily skin, excessive sweating, immunodeficiency, malnutrition, pregnancy, and hereditary predisposition. The change from the saprophytic to mycelial phase; however, is not completely understood. *Malassezia* species have an oil requirement for growth likely accounting for the increased incidence of disease in adolescents and preference for sebum-rich areas of the skin. The yeast does not cause an inflammatory response in the host but may lead to decreased pigmentation. The reduction in pigmentation has been hypothesized to result from inhibitory effects of dicarboxylic acids and lipoperoxidases produced by the metabolism of surface lipids by yeast on melanocytes [47]. Overall, the condition causes minimal morbidity with most patients seeking treatment for cosmetic reasons.

Clinical features

Tinea versicolor causes erythematous, hypopigmented, or hyperpigmented macules or patches, which may or may not be pruritic (Figure 15.15). Fine scaling may be elicited with scratching of the skin surface. Sebum-rich areas, in particular the upper chest, upper back, and shoulders, are frequent sites of involvement. In temperate climates, facial involvement occurs primarily in children, whereas in tropical and subtropical regions, it is common in both adults and children [47]. *Tinea versicolor* may be confused with *tinea corporis*, vitiligo, pityriasis rosea, pityriasis alba, and secondary syphilis, among others [17].

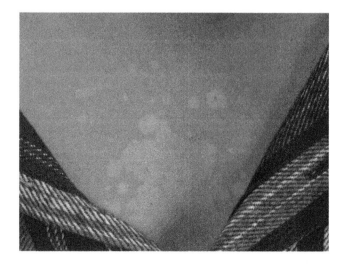

Figure 15.15 Tinea versicolor.

Laboratory diagnosis

Clinical diagnosis of *tinea versicolor* is easily confirmed with direct microscopic examination. Microscopic examination with KOH demonstrates characteristic short, angular hyphae and budding yeast commonly referred to as "spaghetti and meatballs" appearance. Wood's lamp can also be used to diagnose *tinea versicolor*; however, the yellow fluorescence is only elicited in cases caused by *M. furfur*, as it is the only *Malassezia* species that produces fluorochromes. As a result, fluorescence is not appreciated in up to two-thirds of cases. Culture is usually not necessary for diagnosis but can be used for species identification. Special media (mDixon or Leeming-Notman) with an exogenous lipid source is needed as only *M. pachydermatis* grows in routine mycologic media such as Sabouraud dextrose agar. In addition, as several species are inhibited above 37°C, cultures should be incubated between 30°C and 35°C [47].

Treatment and prevention

Tinea versicolor does not clear spontaneously and alterations in pigment may take years to normalize despite treatment. Due to the organism's lipophilic nature, patients are instructed to avoid oils applied to the skin or bath. For eradication of the *Malassezia*, both topical and oral medications have been found to be effective. Topical treatments include azole antifungal agents, terbinafine, and selenium sulfide preparations. Various dosing regimens have been suggested. Possible regimens include azole creams daily for 1–2 weeks, ketoconazole 2% shampoo daily for one week, or selenium sulfide 2.5% shampoo daily (left on the skin for 3–5 minutes and then rinsed off) for 7 days. Oral therapy may be preferred in patients with extensive skin involvement or frequent recurrences. Ketoconazole, itraconazole, and fluconazole are the three main oral therapies used. Recommended dosing regimens include ketoconazole 400 mg once, itraconazole 200 mg daily for 5–7 days, or fluconazole 400 mg once or 300 mg weekly for 2 weeks [47]. Oral terbinafine and griseofulvin are ineffective in the treatment of *tinea versicolor*. Periodic retreatment or prophylactic treatment; for example, ketoconazole shampoo or selenium sulfide 2.5% shampoo once weekly, may be needed due to *tinea versicolor's* high recurrence rate reaching up to 80% after 2 years [45].

SIDE EFFECTS OF ORAL ANTIFUNGALS

Newer, oral antifungal agents have greatly improved the management of dermatomycoses but not without consequence. Some are quite expensive (although this is changing with some of the oral agents becoming generic), have side effects and organ toxicity that may or may not be tolerable, or have significant drug interactions [23,48–50]. As a result, treatment selection should be based on a patient's likelihood of compliance, age, concomitant medical conditions, and potential drug interactions.

Griseofulvin is an effective inexpensive treatment option for dermatophyte infections; however, it is ineffective against yeast and nondermatophyte organisms. Hepatotoxicity is a concern especially with long-term use, as in the treatment of onychomycosis. Other less severe but more common side effects include rash, headache, photosensitivity, nausea, and vomiting. Less commonly, arthralgia, peripheral neuritis, memory lapse, confusion, and insomnia have been reported [1,4,51]. Griseofulvin has interactions with barbiturates, alcohol, cyclosporine, oral contraceptives, aspirin, and warfarin [49,50].

Hepatotoxicity is also a concern with ketoconazole occurring in one out of 10,000 to 15,000 people. Other side effects include nausea, vomiting, abdominal pain, diarrhea, headache, pruritus, insomnia, leukopenia, hemolytic anemia, decreased libido, and impotence [1,4,51]. A key concern with the use of ketoconazole and the other azole antifungal agents are their numerous drug–drug interactions. Use of H1 blockers (astemizole, terfenadine), as well as cisapride and triazolam, are absolute contraindication for use of ketoconazole. A complete list of interactions can be found in a review on drug interactions by Brodell and Elewski [49].

Similar to ketoconazole, itraconazole is associated with numerous medication interactions. Use of itraconazole is contraindicated in patients taking terfenadine, astemizole, diazepam, oral triazolam, oral midazolam, cisapride, and HMG-CoA reductase inhibitors (lovastatin, simvastatin). Numerous additional interactions exist [1,49]. Absorption is optimized with an acidic environment, so it should also be taken 1 hour before or 2 hours after antacid use. Similarly, ingestion of a cola beverage can improve absorption in patients with achlorhydria. Absorption is also improved if taken with food [11]. Side effects of itraconazole include diarrhea, headache, rhinitis, dyspepsia, nausea, dry skin, rash, weakness, pruritus, dizziness, hypertension, and loss of libido. Hepatotoxicity has only rarely been reported [1,4,51].

Similar to ketoconazole and itraconazole, fluconazole is associated with numerous medication interactions. Significant reactions have been associated with terfenadine, tacrolimus, astemizole, rifabutin, oral hypoglycemics, coumarin derivatives, phenytoin sodium, cyclosporine, theophylline, cisapride, and rifampin [1,4,49]. Side effects occur with fluconazole, more often in HIV-positive patients [4] and include nausea, vomiting, headache, rash, diarrhea, dizziness, abdominal pain, dyspepsia, and taste perversion. Rare cases of hepatotoxicity, anaphylaxis, and exfoliative skin disorders have been reported [1,4,49].

Terbinafine has been associated with diarrhea, pruritus, dyspepsia, rash, taste disturbance, urticaria, abdominal pain, headache, visual disturbance, and neutropenia. Rare cases of cholestatic hepatitis and fulminant hepatic failure have been reported [52–54]. Terbinafine should be avoided in patients with renal impairment or hepatic cirrhosis, as terbinafine clearance is reduced by 50%. In addition, terbinafine levels are potentiated by cimetidine and antagonized by rifampin. Cyclosporine levels should be monitored if taken concurrently with terbinafine [1,4,51].

Laboratory monitoring is recommended during treatment with the oral antifungal medications especially for prolonged therapy. Baseline liver function tests should be obtained for terbinafine and itraconazole. When itraconazole is prescribed to patients on concurrent cyclosporine, cyclosporine levels should be closely monitored in addition to serum creatinine concentration. Similarly, in patients on oral hypoglycemic agents, blood glucose levels should be closely monitored if concurrent fluconazole is prescribed. Renal, hepatic, and hematopoietic functions should be obtained for patients on prolonged griseofulvin therapy. Lastly, ketoconazole should be avoided for durations greater than 7 to 10 days. With this duration, monitoring is not needed. It is generally agreed that treatment with oral antifungals should be avoided during pregnancy as the risk of use does not outweigh the benefits.

SUMMARY

Cutaneous fungal infections cause significant morbidity for healthy and ill patients. The incidence of some dermatomycoses is increasing despite availability of newer and better topical and systemic treatments. Fungal remnants last months to years under ideal conditions allowing continued spread of infection. Mycoses treated in one area may recur because of organism travel from concomitant areas of infection. Failure of patients and physicians to recognize a fungal etiology early may lead to more extensive, severe, or difficult-to-treat infections. Finally, a patient's concurrent illnesses may play a part in susceptibility and ability to manage fungal infections. For these reasons, scientists have studied and developed newer antifungal agents with better efficacy and great convenience in dosing. These drugs, however, still have side effects and drug–drug interactions that may limit their use in some patients. Better efforts to educate patients and physicians alike may aid in faster recognition, diagnosis, and treatment of dermatophytoses. More research is needed to continue to develop drugs suitable for use in a broader range of patients and diagnostic tests that may be quicker or more specific than conventional ones.

COMMON CLINICAL QUESTIONS

1. It is important to perform a culture to diagnose *tinea capitis* because:
   a. There are no clear clinical signs or symptoms of fungal infection of the scalp.
   b. Different fungal species that cause *tinea capitis* are treated by different antifungal drugs.
   c. Identification of certain species will require treatment of household pets to remove the dermatophyte reservoir.
   d. Most insurance companies will not cover the cost of prescription drugs without a laboratory diagnosis.

   Correct answer: c, *Microsporum canis is commonly spread by dogs living in the household.*

2. Which of these statements about *tinea pedis* is false?
   a. *Tinea pedis* is always caused by a fungus.
   b. *Tinea pedis* is self-containing and will not spread.
   c. *Tinea pedis* is the most common superficial fungal infection.
   d. *Tinea pedis* can present with a secondary bacterial infection.

   Correct answer: b, *Tinea pedis, if left untreated, can spread to the toenails and result in onychomycosis infection.*

3. Which conditions can be confused with onychomycosis?
   a. Lichen planus
   b. Secondary syphilis
   c. Mineral deficiencies
   d. Both a and c

   Correct answer: a, *Lichen planus causes similar nail abnormalities as fungal infection, but the presence of violaceous polygonal papules on the extremities and mucous membranes, wickham's striae, and pterygium—may help to differentiate the nail findings of lichen planus from onychomycosis.*

4. Which of the following statements about the newer topical treatments for onychomycosis are true?
   a. They are more effective than oral medications because they come into direct contact with the infecting fungus.
   b. They can to be administered for a shorter period of time than oral drugs.
   c. They can be used to treat moderate-to-severe cases if the laboratory diagnosis confirms the presence of a dermatophyte.
   d. None of the above.

   Correct answer: d, *None of the above. Topical agents have limited ability to penetrate the nail plate to reach the nail bed where the fungus resides, they must be used for long periods of time, and are usually successful only against mild-to-moderate infections.*

REFERENCES

1. Zuber T, Baddam K. Superficial fungal infection of the skin: Where and how it appears help determine therapy. *Postgrad Med* 2001;109:117–132.

2. Drake LA, Dinehart SM, Farmer ER, et al. Guidelines of care for superficial mycotic infections of the skin: *Tinea corporis, tinea cruris, tinea faciei, tinea manuum,* and *tinea pedis. J Am Acad Dermatol* 1996;34(2 pt 1):282–286.

3. Ghannoum M, Hajjeh R, Scher R, et al. A large-scale North American study of fungal isolates from nails: The frequency of onychomycosis, fungal distribution, and antifungal susceptibility patterns. *J Am Acad Dermatol* 2000;43:641–648.

4. Goldstein A, Smith K, Ives T, et al. Mycotic infections: Effective management of conditions involving the skin, hair, and nails. *Geriatrics* 2000;55:40–52.

5. Charif M, Elewski B. A historical perspective on onychomycosis. *Dermatol Ther* 1997;3:43–45.

6. Foster KW, Ghannoum MA, Elewski BE. Epidemiologic surveillance of cutaneous fungal infection in the United States from 1999 to 2002. *JAAD* 2004;50(5):748–752.

7. Hossain M, Ghannoum M. New developments in chemotherapy for non-invasive fungal infections. *Expert Opin Investig Drugs* 2001;10:1–11.

8. Smith KJ, Welsh M, Skelton H. *Trichophyton rubrum* showing deep dermal invasion directly from the epidermis in immunosuppressed patients. *Br J Dermatol* 2001;145(20):344–348.

9. www.mycology.adelaide.edu.au. Accessed September 2001.

10. Svejgaard E. Recalcitrant dermatophyte infection. *Dermatol Ther* 1997;3:75–78.

11. Adams BB. Tinea corporis gladiatorum. *J Am Acad Dermatol* 2002;47:286–290.

12. Gupta A, DeDoncker P, Degreef H. Tinea manus treated with 1-week itraconazole vs. terbinafine. *Int J Dermatol* 2000;39:521–538.

13. Babel DE, Baughman SA. Evaluation of the adult carrier state in juvenile tinea capitis caused by *Trichophyton tonsurans. J Am Acad Dermatol* 1989;21(6):1209–1212.

14. Elewski B. Tinea capitis: A current perspective. *J Am Acad Dermatol* 2000;42(1 pt 1):1–20.

15. Roberts BJ, Friedlander SF. Tinea capitis: A treatment update. *Pediatr Ann* 2005;34(3):191–200.

16. Ghannoum M, Isham N, Sheehan D. Voriconazole susceptibility of dermatophyte isolates obtained from a large worldwide tinea capitis clinical trial. *J Clin Microbiol* 2006;44(7):2579–2580.

17. Ghannoum M, Isham N, Hajjeh R, et al. Tinea capitis in Cleveland: Survey of elementary school students. *J Am Acad Dermatol* 2003;48(2):189–193.

18. Korting HC, Kiencke P, Nelles S, et al. Comparable efficacy and safety of various topical formulations of terbinafine in *tinea pedis* irrespective of the treatment regimen: Results of a meta-analysis. *Am J Clin Dermatol* 2007;8(6):357–364.

19. Hart R, Bell-Syer SE, Crawford F, et al. Systematic review of topical treatments for fungal infections of the skin and nails of the feet. *BMJ* 1999;319(7202):79–82.

20. Bell-Syer SE, Hart R, Crawford F, et al. Oral treatments for fungal infections of the skin of the foot. *Cochrane Database Syst Rev* 2002;2:CD003584.

21. Del Rosso J. Current management of onychomycosis and dermatomycoses. *Curr Infect Dis Rep* 2000;2:438–445.

22. McClellan K, Wiseman L, Markham A. Terbinafine: An update of its use in superficial mycoses. *Drugs* 1999;58:179–202.

23. Hall M, Monka C, Krupp P, et al. Safety of oral terbinafine: Results of a postmarketing surveillance study in 25,884 patients. *Arch Dermatol* 1997;133:1213–1219.

24. Stary A, Sarnow E. Fluconazole in the treatment of tinea corporis and tinea cruris. *Dermatology* 1998;196:237–241.

25. Fleece D, Gaughan JP, Aronoff SC. Griseofulvin versus terbinafine in the treatment of tinea capitis: A meta-analysis of randomized, clinical trials. *Pediatrics* 2004;114(5):1312–1315.

26. De Rosso J, Gupta A. Oral itraconazole therapy for superficial, subcutaneous, and systemic infections: A panoramic view. *Postgrad Med* 1999;Spec No:46–52.

27. Gupta AK, Cooper EA, Ryder JE, et al. Optimal management of fungal infections of the skin, hair, and nails. *Am J Clin Dermatol* 2004;5(4):225–237.

28. Kuvandik G, Cetin M, Genctoy G, et al. The prevalence, epidemiology and risk factors for onychomy-cosis in hemodialysis patients. *BMC Infect Dis* 2007;7:102.

29. Szepietowski JC, Salomon J. Do fungi play a role in psoriatic nails? *Mycoses* 2007;50:437–442.

30. Szepietowski JC, Reich A, Garlowska E, et al. Factors influencing coexistence of toenail onychomycosis with *tinea pedis* and other dermatophycoses. *Arch Dermatol* 2006;142:1279–1284.

31. Elewski B. Prevalence of onychomycosis in patients attending a dermatology clinic in northeastern Ohio for other conditions. *Arch Dermatol* 1999;133:1172–1173.

32. Albreski D, Gupta A, Gross E. Onychomycosis in diabetes; management considerations. *Postgrad Med* 1999;Spec No:26–30.

33. Durden F, Elewski B. Fungal infections in HIV-infected patients. *Semin Cutan Med Surg* 1997;16:200–212.

34. Faergemann J, Baran R. Epidemiology, clinical presentation and diagnosis of onychomycosis. *Br J Dermatol* 2003;149(65):1–4.

35. Evans E. Resistance of *Candida* species to antifungal agents used in the treatment of onychomycosis: A review of current problems. *Br J Dermatol* 1999;141(suppl 56):33–35.

36. Amadio P. Fungal infections of the hand. *Hand Clin* 1998;14:605–612.

37. Haldane DJM, Robert E. A comparison of calcofluor white, potassium hydroxide and culture for the laboratory diagnosis of superficial fungal infection. *Diagn Microbiol Infect Dis* 1990;13:337–339.

38. Evans E, Sigurgeirsson B. Double-blind, randomised study of continuous terbinafine compared with intermittent itraconazole in treatment of toenail onychomycosis. *BMJ* 1999;318:1031–1035.

39. Havu V, Brandt H, Heikkila H, et al. Continuous and intermittent itraconazole dosing schedules for the treatment of onychomycosis: A pharmacokinetic comparison. *Br J Dermatol* 1999;140:96–101.

40. Avner S, Nir N, Henri T. Combination of oral terbinafine and topical ciclopirox compared to oral terbinafine for the treatment of onychomycosis. *J Dermatolog Treat* 2005;16(5–6):327–330.

41. Zaias N. Onychomycosis treated until the nail is replaced by normal growth or there is failure. *Arch Dermatol* 2000;136:940.

42. Gupta AK, Fleckman P, Baron R. Ciclopirox nail lacquer topical solution 8% in the treatment of toenail onychomycosis. *J Am Acad Dermatol* 2000; 43(4 suppl):S70–S80.

43. Del Rosso J. Onychomycosis of toenails and *post-hoc* analyses with efinaconazole 10% solution once-daily treatment. *J Clin Aesthet Dermatol* 2016;9(2):42–47.

44. Sharma N, Sharma D. An upcoming drug for onychomycosis: Tavaborole. *J Pharmacol Pharmacother* 2015;6(4):236–239.

45. Scher RK, Tavakkol A, Sigurgeirsson B. Onychomycosis: Diagnosis and definition of cure. *JAAD* 2007;56(6):939–944.

46. Ashbee HR. Update on the genus *Malassezia*. *Med Mycol* 2007;45(4):287–303.

47. Crespo-Erchiga V, Florencio VD. *Malassezia* yeasts and pityriasis versicolor. *Curr Opin Infect Dis* 2006;19(2):139–147.

48. Amichai B, Grunwald M. Adverse drug reactions of the new oral antifungal agents terbinafine, flu-conazole, and itraconazole. *Int J Dermatol* 1998;37:410–415.

49. Brodell R, Elewski B. Antifungal drug interactions: Avoidance requires more than memorization. *Postgrad Med* 2000;107:41–43.

50. Katz H. Possible drug interactions in oral treatment of onychomycosis. *J Am Podiatr Med Assoc* 1997;87:571–574.

51. Moossavi M, Bagheri B, Scher R. Systemic antifungal therapy. *Dermatol Clin* 2001;19:35–52.

52. Agarwal K, Manas DM, Hudson M. Terbinafine and fulminant hepatic failure. *N Engl J med* 1999;340:1292–1293.

53. Perveze Z, Johnson MW, Rublin RA, et al. Terbinafine-induced hepatic failure requiring liver transplantation. *Liver Transpl* 2007;13(1):162–164.

54. Lazaros GA, Papatheodoridis GV, Delladetsima JK, et al. Terbinafine-induced cholestatic liver disease. *J Hepatol* 1996;24(6):753–756.

16

Invasive candidiasis

RICHARD R. WATKINS AND TRACY LEMONOVICH

INTRODUCTION

The term "invasive candidiasis" (IC) encompasses both candidemia and deep organ involvement; it excludes more superficial and less severe diseases, such as oropharyngeal and esophageal candidiasis. Emerging trends in IC are notable for a dramatic increase in infections due to non-*albicans Candida* spp [1]. The common use of prophylactic antifungal agents, mainly fluconazole, the widespread use of broad-spectrum antibacterial agents, more aggressive management of patient with leukemia and malignancy, the frequency of organ transplantation, and, importantly, the extensive use of invasive medical devices (e.g., chronic indwelling intravascular catheters) have contributed toward the changing epidemiology of IC. *Candida* spp. represents the fourth leading cause of hospital-acquired bloodstream infection (BSI) in the United States, accounting for 8%–10% of all BSIs [2]. One of the major concerns with IC is an associated excess attributable mortality rate of up to 72% [3–7] and an excess length of hospital stay of 3–30 days [8,9]. Furthermore, the estimated additional cost for each episode of IC in adults is approximately $40,000 [5]. Similar impacts of IC have been seen in the pediatric population [10].

This chapter addresses the epidemiology and risk factors associated with IC, with particular emphasis on common clinical presentations, diagnostic testing, and the new treatment guidelines.

EPIDEMIOLOGY AND RISK FACTORS

Most IC infections are caused by one of five *Candida* spp. (*albicans, parapsilosis, tropicalis, glabrata,* and *krusei*), with *C. albicans* accounting for approximately 38%–70% of infections based on geographic area [11]. However, recent reports have noted an increasing trend in the isolation of non-*albicans* spp. in some clinical settings [1,12–14]. Furthermore, each of the non-*albicans Candida* spp. has been associated with a specific patient population and risk factors (Table 16.1). *Candida auris* is an emerging strain associated with high mortality and is often multidrug-resistant. Transmission of *C. auris* has likely occurred in health care facilities in the United Sates (US), highlighting the need for infection control measures to contain this pathogen [15].

Candida glabrata ranks second to *C. albicans* as a cause of BSI in the United States, accounting for 12%–24% of all *Candida* BSIs [11]. Among *Candida* spp., *C. glabrata* alone has increased as a cause of BSI in US intensive care units (ICUs) since 1993 [16]. On a global scale, the frequency of *C. glabrata* as a cause of BSI varies 4%–12% in Latin America [17,18], 9.8% in Europe [19], and 13.6% in the Asia–Pacific region [20]. The prevalence of this species is related to different factors, including geographic characteristics [17,18,20], patient age [21,22], characteristics of the patient population studied [23–24], and the frequent use of fluconazole [23–25]. Numerous studies have demonstrated that both colonization and infection with *C. glabrata* are rare among infants and children and increase significantly with increasing patient age [26–29]. Notably, obese children seem to have less diversity in their fungal gut microbiome (including *C. glabrata*) compared to normal weight controls [30]. More than one-third of *Candida*-associated BSIs among patients >60 years of age are due to *C. glabrata* [21,22,31]. In addition to age, the use of broad-spectrum antibiotics, particularly piperacillin/tazobactam and vancomycin, the frequent use of central

Table 16.1 Risk factors associated with candidemia by species

Candida species	Risk factors
C. glabrata	Age, azole exposure, HIV/AIDS, surgery, urinary, and vascular catheter
C. guilliermondii	Polyene use
C. krusei	Azole exposure, bone marrow transplant, neutropenia
C. lusitaniae	Polyene use
C. parapsilosis	Central venous catheter, neonates, parenteral nutrition, hematologic malignancy
C. tropicalis	Neutropenia, hematologic malignancy, bone marrow transplantation

Source: Arendrup, M.C., *Curr. Opin. Crit. Care*, 16, 445–452, 2010; Hachem, R. et al., *Cancer* 112, 2493–2499, 2008; Huang, Y.C. et al., *Infection*, 27, 97–102, 1999; Kontoyiannis, D.P. et al., *Clin. Infect. Dis.*, 33, 1676–1681, 2001.

venous catheters, the receipt of parenteral nutrition, and a prolonged stay in ICU have all been associated with an increased risk of *C. glabrata* BSI [22]. Also, renal failure requiring hemodialysis in patients with *C. glabrata* BSI is a risk factor associated with higher mortality [32]. The widespread use of fluconazole has contributed to the emergence of resistant non-*albicans* spp., including *C. glabrata* [23,33]. In one study investigating the impact of fluconazole prophylaxis on *Candida* spp. in the pre- and post-fluconazole era, the incidence of infections caused by *C. albicans* isolates decreased by 50% (decreasing from 2.1% to 1.6%), with a corresponding significant increase in infections caused by *C. glabrata* spp. [34].

In contrast to the US, *C. parapsilosis* is the most common non-*albicans* spp. of *Candida* recovered from blood cultures in other parts of the world [11]. *C. parapsilosis* is an important species to consider in hospitalized patients with vascular catheters. In the neonatal population, *C. parapsilosis* accounts for more than 30% of all *Candida* bloodstream isolates, compared with only 10%–15% of *Candida* bloodstream isolates in adults [2,6,35,36]. With the exception of prematurity and congenital abnormalities, risk factors for the development of IC in infants and children are similar to those in adults. *C. parapsilosis* infections are especially associated with hyperalimentation solutions (TPN), prosthetic devices, and indwelling catheters. Moreover, *C. parapsilosis* is the most common species found on the hands of healthcare workers, which has been associated with nosocomial infections [37]. A number of nosocomial outbreaks of catheter-associated candidemia due to *C. parapsilosis* have been reported, highlighting the importance of hand hygiene and proper catheter care in hospital settings [35,38–40].

C. tropicalis is the fourth most frequent cause of candidemia in the US [11]. *C. tropicalis* ranks second in Latin America and is more common than *C. glabrata* in the Asia-Pacific region [17,20]. *C. tropicalis* is an important fungal pathogen in patients with chemotherapy-induced neutropenia and those with hematologic malignancies, especially leukemia, and in bone marrow transplant recipients [23,24,41–43]. Among patients with neutropenia who are found to be colonized with *C. tropicalis*, 60%–80% develop invasive infection [44–46]. *C. tropicalis* has remained highly susceptible to fluconazole and this drug is frequently given to neutropenic patients for prophylaxis [24].

C. krusei causes 2%–4% of all *Candida*-associated BSIs [17,26,29] and is best known for its propensity to emerge in the setting of fluconazole prophylaxis due to its innate resistance to this azole. Colonization and infection with *C. krusei* were noticeable in certain medical centers among stem cell transplant recipients and patients who had leukemia and received fluconazole as part the prophylaxis regimen [41,43,47–49]. *C. krusei* organisms are inherently resistant to fluconazole [25,26,28]. This has a considerable impact on patient outcomes, as BSIs due to *C. krusei* were reported to be associated with a high mortality rate (59%–80% crude mortality and 40% attributable mortality), primarily related to its poor response to standard antifungal therapy [26,50].

Other important risk factors for IC among adults are listed in Table 16.2 and include the development of acute kidney injury, hemodialysis (acute or chronic), severe pancreatitis, diabetes mellitus, immunosuppressive therapy, and any surgery that requires general anesthesia (especially upper gastrointestinal tract surgeries).

Table 16.2 Risk factors associated with invasive candidiasis

Prolonged length of stay in an ICU
High acute physiology and chronic health evaluation (APACHE) II score
Central venous catheter
Parenteral nutrition
Broad spectrum antibiotics
Prolonged antibiotic use
Malignancy
Neutropenia
Bone marrow transplant recipients
Solid organ transplant recipient
HIV/AIDS
Diabetes mellitus
Liver disease
Hemodialysis within 3 months
Kidney disease
Autoimmune disease
Immunosuppressive therapy
Surgery in the last 90 days
Candida colonization at multiple sites
Very low birth weight neonate
Extensive burns
Malnutrition
Severe pancreatitis

Source: Diekema, D. et al., *Diagn. Microbiol. Infect. Dis.*, 73, 45–48, 2012; Kauffman, C.A., *Clin. Infect. Dis.*, 33, 550–555, 2001; Husain, S. et al., *Transplantation*, 75, 2023–2029, 2003.

CLINICAL MANIFESTATIONS OF INVASIVE CANDIDIASIS

Candidemia

The isolation of *Candida* spp. in one or more blood cultures is the most commonly recognized manifestation of IC, and occurs in approximately 50% of patients with this disorder. A positive blood culture for *Candida* spp. should never be regarded as a contaminant, and should trigger immediate intervention with effective antifungal therapy and appropriate management strategies.

A wide spectrum of clinical manifestations has been described for IC, ranging from "transient" or self-limited candidemia to sepsis, multiorgan failure, and death. Also, the clinical presentation of candidemia varies in different patient populations. Respiratory distress and apnea are the prominent clinical signs of candidemia in neonates. Spread to multiple organs including the skin (66%), the central nervous system (64%), and the retina (54%) has been commonly reported [52]. Fever is the most common presentation of candidemia in adults [53].

Acute disseminated candidiasis is usually seen in patients who are neutropenic as a result of cytotoxic chemotherapy for an underlying hematologic malignancy. Discrete erythematous or hemorrhagic palpable rash, which is consistent with small vessel vasculitis, is a major clinical manifestation of this form of IC and has been described in neutropenic hosts (Figure 16.1) [54]. A prompt recognition and management of candidemia is crucial, as the overall mortality rate is high.

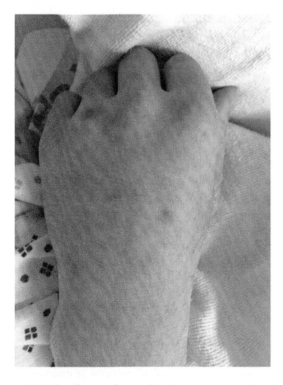

Figure 16.1 Small vessel vasculitis in a neutropenic patient with invasive candidiasis.

Candida endophthalmitis

Candida chorioretinitis with or without macular involvement and with or without vitreitis is a serious complication of untreated candidemia, underscoring the ability of *Candida* spp. to attach to and invade endothelial cells [55]. Ocular presentations may be the first clinical manifestation of hematogenous spread and can develop after the diagnosis of candidemia, leading to permanent blindness if not identified and treated adequately [56,57]. *Candida* endophthalmitis begins as a choroidal lesion that progresses to an area of retinal necrosis, followed by vitreitis and endophthalmitis (Figure 16.2). The most frequent initial symptoms are eye redness, pain, and diminished or blurry vision. Unilateral involvement is most common, although bilateral endophthalmitis can occur. Recent guidelines recommend all patients with candidemia should have a dilated retinal exam, preferably by an ophthalmologist, within the first week of therapy in nonneutropenic patients to determine if endophthalmitis is present [58]. This exam should be delayed in neutropenic patients until neutrophil recovery.

Candida spp. may also cause endocarditis, meningitis, septic arthritis, tenosynovitis, isolated involvement of the kidney, and pneumonia, which are less common manifestations of IC and are not discussed in detail in this chapter.

Chronic disseminated candidiasis (hepatosplenic candidiasis)

Chronic disseminated candidiasis (CDC, formerly hepatosplenic candidiasis) is almost exclusively described in patients who have undergone myeloablative chemotherapy [59]. CDC is usually associated with recovery from neutropenia, and may occur after the treatment of an episode

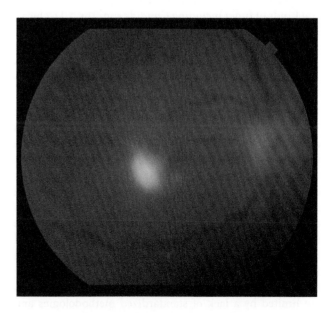

Figure 16.2 *Candida albicans* endophthalmitis.

of candidemia. Clinical signs and symptoms include fever unresponsive to antibiotics, abdominal pain, and hepatosplenomegaly. Laboratory studies may reveal negative blood cultures and elevated transaminases and alkaline phosphatase. Imaging studies often show multiple focal lesions in the liver and spleen although such lesions may be absent early in the course of disease. In the absence of candidemia to guide the diagnosis, a liver biopsy is often recommended. Fortunately, the frequency of CDC has been decreasing due to the widespread use of antifungal prophylaxis [59].

DIAGNOSTIC ASSAYS

Recovery of *Candida* spp. from blood is commonly achieved by using standard bacterial blood culture media in automated blood culture systems [60,61]. Generally, blood cultures are positive in one to two days for *C. albicans*, *C. parapsilosis*, and *C. tropicalis*, whereas *C. glabrata* and *C. krusei* may require longer incubation times [62]. One of the major drawbacks of blood cultures is that they give false-negative data in nearly 50% of cultures in spite of biopsy-proven infection.

Once isolated, *C. albicans* can be presumptively identified in 90 minutes by germ tube formation [63]. Other species may require 72 hours to be identified by morphology and carbo- hydrate metabolism determined by many available commercial kits (e.g., API 20 C BioMerieux, Durham, NC). Several agar-based systems are available to more rapidly differentiate *Candida* spp. [64]. Peptide nucleic acid fluorescence *in situ* hybridization (PNA FISH) targets rRNA of *Candida* and can provide clinicians with rapid (in 2.5 hours) species identification [65,66]. One of the major advantages of PNA FISH is its ability to be performed directly using aliquots from positive blood culture bottles.

Aside from culture, nonculture methods have been developed to assist clinicians with an early diagnosis of IC. β-D-glucan is a component of the fungal cell wall of several kinds of fungi including *Candida* spp. The β-D-glucan assay can identify invasive candidiasis days to weeks before positive blood cultures [67]. Furthermore, decreasing levels of β-D-glucan may correspond with the response to antifungal therapy and can be used to guide treatment [68]. Meta-analyses of β-D-glucan studies showed the sensitivity and specificity of the assay for diagnosing IC were 76% and 85%, respectively [69,70]. False positive results can occur, especially in hemodialysis patients and those with bacteremia.

An assay to detect *Candida* spp. antigenemia has been described but is not commercially available [71]. Polymerase chain reaction (PCR) assays have potential advantages over the β-D-glucan assay and antigen detection methods including the capacity to provide species identification and to detect markers of drug resistance [58]. A meta-analysis of PCR for IC determined the pooled sensitivity and specificity to be 95% and 92%, respectively [72]. However, PCR assays are limited by a lack of standardized methodologies and multicenter validation of assay performance [58]. Recently, a miniaturized, magnetic resonance-based diagnostic approach has been described that allows for sensitive and specific detection of *Candida* pathogens directly in whole blood without the need for culture or a nucleic acid extraction step [73].

PREDICTION RULES

Several investigators have tried to identify independent factors that are predictive of IC, and to use these factors to design clinically relevant scores to help clinicians to identify, implement, and adapt an optimal therapeutic approach [74,75]. In this regard, Ostrosky-Zeichner et al. attempted to identify patients at high risk for IC in the ICU. The best performing rule in this case was ≥1 day of systemic antibiotic therapy or presence of a central venous catheter, and at least two of the following: total parenteral nutrition, any form of dialysis, any major surgery, pancreatitis, any use of steroids, or use of an immunosuppressive agent. The rate of IC among patients meeting the rule was 9.9%, capturing 34% of cases of IC, with the following performance: relative risk 4.36, sensitivity 0.34, specificity 0.90, positive predictive value 0.01, and negative predictive value 0.97 [76]. A more recent study reported that administration of total parenteral nutrition, prior antibiotic exposure, transfer from an outside hospital or admission from a nursing home, mechanical ventilation and presence of a central vein catheter were independent predictors of candidemia in patients with sepsis and septic shock, while a pulmonary source for infection was protective [77].

ANTIFUNGAL SUSCEPTIBILITY TESTING

The role of antifungal susceptibility testing (AST) is to aid in selecting the best agent for the treatment of fungal infections. Routine use of AST is generally uncommon. Expert opinion suggests that laboratories perform routine AST against fluconazole for *C. glabrata* isolates from blood and sterile sites, for other *Candida* spp. that have failed to respond to antifungal therapy or where azole resistance is strongly suspected [58,78,79]. Also, testing for echinocandin susceptibility should be considered in patients with prior treatment with an echinocandin and in those with infections from *C. glabrata* or *C. parapsilosis* [58]. Minimum inhibitory concentration (MIC) breakpoints have been established for *Candida* spp. against fluconazole, itraconazole, voriconazole, and flucytosine, enabling selection of a suitable therapeutic agent [80]. Interpretive MIC breakpoints for echinocandins (anidulafungin, caspofungin, and micafungin) were recently added [81] (Table 16.3).

Among the five most common *Candida* spp., *C. albicans*, *C. parapsilosis* and *C. tropicalis* are usually susceptible to azoles, polyenes, flucytosine, and the echinocandins [80], while *C. parapsilosis* exhibits higher MICs than other species of *Candida* for the echinocandins. The correlation of this *in vitro* finding to clinical outcome is uncertain, since this species generally responds well clinically to echinocandin therapy (Table 16.4).

Table 16.3 Minimum Inhibitory Concentration (MIC) breakpoints of approved antifungal agents against *Candida* spp.

Antifungal agent	Susceptible (S)	Susceptible-dose dependent (S-DD)	Intermediate (I)	Resistant (R)	Nonsusceptible
Anidulafungin	≤2	–	–	–	≥2
Caspofungin	≤2	–	–	–	≥2
Fluconazole	≤8	16–32	–	≥64	
Flucytosine	≤4	–	8–16	≥32	
Itraconazole	≤0.125	0.25–0.5	–	≥1	
Micafungin	≤2		–		≥2
Voriconazole	≤1	2	–	≥4	

Source: Clinical and Laboratory Standards Institute, *Reference Method for Broth Dilution Antifungal Susceptibility Testing of Yeasts*, 3rd ed., Approved standard M27-A3, Clinical and Laboratory Standards Institute, Wayne, PA, 2008; Pfaller, M.A. et al., *J. Clin. Microbiol.*, 46, 2620–2629, 2008.

Table 16.4 Antifungal susceptibility of *Candida* spp. to approved antifungal agents

Species	Amphotericin B	5-FC	Fluconazole and itraconazole	Voriconazole	Echinocandins
C. albicans	S	S	S	S	S
C. glabrata	S tol	S	S-DD toR	S to S-DD	S
C. krusei	S tol	I toR	R	S to S-DD	S
C. lusitaniae	S to R	S	S	S	S
C. parapsilosis	S	S	S	S	S to I
C. tropicalis	S	S	S	S	S

Abbreviations: S, Susceptible; I, Intermediate; R, Resistant; S-DD, Susceptible dose dependent.
Source: Pappas, P.G. et al., *Clin. Infect. Dis.*, 62, e1–e50, 2016.

C. glabrata is inherently less susceptible to fluconazole than are most other species of *Candida*. Voriconazole, posaconazole and isavuconazole are often more active against *C. glabrata* isolates than fluconazole [82]. Although cross-resistance within the azole class is documented for this species, certain strains remain susceptible to voriconazole (therefore, it is recommended that prior to using voriconazole, *C. glabrata* AST should be performed). *C. glabrata* is usually susceptible to the echinocandins, although investigators recently reported that 3.95% of bloodstream isolates were resistant to anidulafungin [83,84]. This has important clinical implications and highlights the necessity of knowing local epidemiology and resistance patterns.

In addition to its intrinsic resistance to fluconazole, *C. krusei* shows decreased susceptibility to both amphotericin B and flucytosine. In contrast, this species is very susceptible to both the extended-spectrum triazoles (posaconazole, voriconazole, and isavuconazole) and the echinocandin antifungal agents [83,85].

TREATMENT

The armamentarium of anticandidal agents has expanded during the past decade to include the new echinocandins (anidulafungin, caspofungin, and micafungin), voriconazole, posaconazole, and isavuconazole. The Infectious

Diseases Society of America (IDSA) has recently updated the guidelines for the treatment of candidemia and IC [58]. As a general rule, the treatment for IC should take into account any history of recent antifungal exposure, the dominant *Candida* species and current susceptibility in a specific clinical unit, severity of illness, relevant co-morbidities, and evidence for central nervous system or cardiac involvement [58] (Table 16.5).

Fluconazole remains the standard therapy in selected patients who do not have a previous history of azoles exposure, have mild-to-moderate illness, and are not at high risk for *C. glabrata* (see above) [58,86,87]. However, a recent study found that initial fluconazole treatment was not associated with a poorer outcome than that obtained with echinocandins/liposomal amphotericin B (AmB) regimens in patients with *C. glabrata* BSI [88]. Although itraconazole has a spectrum of antifungal activity comparable to fluconazole, it has a limited role in the treatment of IC because of its pharmacokinetics properties. Fluconazole is not advisable as primary therapy for proven or suspected IC in patients with neutropenia, severe illness (e.g., Acute Physiology and Chronic Health Evaluation [APACHE] >20), and in special clinical scenarios when involvement of cardiac valves, myocardium, or the central nervous system is suspected. Fluconazole is a reasonable "step-down therapy" for patients who are improving on more aggressive initial antifungal

Table 16.5 Treatment recommendations for candidemia and other forms of invasive candidiasis therapy

Condition	Primary	Alternative	Duration	Comments
Nonneutropenic adults	An echinocandin[a]	Fluconazole 800 mg (12 mg/kg) loading dose, then 400 mg (6 mg/kg) daily; or LFAmB 3–5 mg/kg daily; or AmB 0.5–1 mg/kg daily; or voriconazole 400 mg (6 mg/kg) bid for 2 doses, then 200 mg (3 mg/kg) bid	14 days after last positive blood culture and resolution of signs and symptoms	Ophthalmological examination is recommended in all patients with candidemia. Remove all intravascular catheters, if possible.
Neutropenic Patients	An echinocandin[a]	LFAmB 3–5 mg/kg daily; or Fluconazole 800 mg (12 mg/kg) loading dose, then 400 mg (6 mg/kg) daily; or voriconazole 400 mg (6 mg/kg) bid for 2 doses, then 200 mg (3 mg/kg) bid	14 days after last positive blood culture and resolution of signs, symptoms and neutropenia	Ophthalmological exam should be performed within first week of recovery from neutropenia. Source of candidemia often GI tract. Catheter removal should be considered. G-CSF should be considered in cases of persistent candidemia.
Empiric treatment for suspected IC in nonneutropenic patients in the ICU	An echinocandin[a]	Fluconazole 800 mg (12 mg/kg) loading dose, then 400 mg (6 mg/kg) daily; or LFAmB 3–5 mg/kg daily	14 days	Stop antifungal therapy if no clinical response after 4–5 days or have a negative non-culture-based diagnostic test.
Chronic disseminated candidiasis	LFAmB 3–5 mg/kg daily; or an echinocandin[a] for several weeks, followed by oral fluconazole 400 mg (6 mg/kg) daily for patients unlikely to have a fluconazole-resistant isolate		Until lesions resolve on repeat imaging, usually in several months	Short term (1–2 weeks) treatment with nonsteroidal anti-inflammatory drugs or corticosteroids can be considered for patients with persistent debilitating fevers.
Prophylaxis to prevent IC in the ICU	Fluconazole 800 mg (12 mg/kg) loading dose, then 400 mg (6 mg/kg) daily in high-risk patients	An echinocandin[a]		Daily chlorhexidine bathing has been shown to decrease incidence of IC.
CNS candidiasis	LFAmB 3–5 mg/kg with or without 5-FC 25 mg/kg qid for several weeks, followed by fluconazole 400–800 mg (6–12 mg/kg) daily		Until all signs and symptoms resolve including CSF and radiological abnormalities	
Candida endophthalmitis	LFAmB 3–5 mg/kg with or without oral flucytosine 25 mg/kg qid	Fluconazole 800 mg (12 mg/kg) loading dose, then 400 mg (6 mg/kg) daily; or voriconazole 400 mg (6 mg/kg) bid for 2 doses, then 200 mg (3 mg/kg) bid	4–6 weeks depending on resolution of lesions	With macular involvement add intravitreal injection of either AmB 5–10 µg/0.1 mL sterile water; or voriconazole 100 µg/0.1 mL sterile water or normal saline.

(Continued)

Table 16.5 (*Continued*) Treatment recommendations for candidemia and other forms of invasive candidiasis therapy

Condition	Primary	Alternative	Duration	Comments
Symptomatic *Candida* cystitis	Fluconazole 200 mg (3 mg/kg) daily; For *C. glabrata* AmB 0.3–0.6 mg/kg daily or flucytosine 25 mg/kg qid; for *C. krusei* AmB 0.3–0.6 mg/kg daily	AmB bladder irrigation 50 mg/L sterile water daily for 5 days to treat fluconazole-resistant strains	14 days for fluconazole-susceptible strains; 7 days for AmB or flucytosine	Removal of indwelling catheter is strongly recommended.
Candida endocarditis	LFAmB 3–5 mg/kg with or without 5-FC 25 mg/kg qid; or high dose echinocandin (caspofungin 150 mg daily, micafungin 150 mg daily, or anidulafungin 200 mg daily)[b] for initial therapy followed by step down therapy to fluconazole 400–800 mg (6–12 mg/kg) daily	Oral voriconazole 200–300 mg (3–4 mg/kg) bid or posaconazole 300 mg daily can be used for step down therapy instead of fluconazole for susceptible isolates	6 weeks after surgery and longer for patients with perivalvular abscesses and other complications; fluconazole 400–800 mg (6–12 mg/kg daily) for patients who cannot undergo valve replacement if isolate is susceptible	Valve replacement is recommended. Give fluconazole lifelong for prosthetic valve endocarditis.
Candida septic arthritis	Fluconazole 400 mg (6 mg/kg) daily for 6 weeks; or an echinocandin[a] for 2 weeks followed by fluconazole 400 mg (6 mg/kg) daily for at least 4 weeks	LFAmB 3–5 mg/kg daily for 2 weeks followed by fluconazole 400 mg (6 mg/kg) daily for at least 4 weeks	At least 6 weeks	Surgical drainage in all cases, device removal when a prosthetic joint is in place. If device cannot be removed then chronic suppression with fluconazole 400 mg (6 mg/kg) daily if susceptible.
Neonatal candidiasis	AmB 1 mg/kg daily	Fluconazole 12 mg/kg daily in patents who have not been on fluconazole prophylaxis; or LFAmB 3–5 mg/kg daily; or echinocandins when resistance or toxicity preclude use of other agents	14 days after clearance of *Candida* from bloodstream and resolution of signs and symptoms	A lumbar puncture and ophthalmological exam are recommended when blood and/or urine cultures are positive for *Candida*.

Abbreviations: G-CSF: Granulocyte stimulating factor; AmB: Amphotericin B deoxycholate; LFAmB: Lipid formulation amphotericin B.

Source: Pappas, P.G. et al., *Clin. Infect. Dis.*, 62, e1–e50, 2016.

a Echinocandin dosing in adults is as follows: anidulafungin, 200 mg loading dose, then 100 mg/day; caspofungin, 70-mg loading dose, then 50 mg/day; and micafungin, 100 mg/day.

b For patients with other cardiovascular infections e.g. pericarditis, myocarditis, suppurative thrombophlebitis, infected pacemaker, ICD, or VAD, higher daily doses of an echinocandin may be appropriate (e.g., caspofungin 50–150 mg/day, micafungin 100–150 mg/day, or anidulafungin 100–200 mg/day).

therapy (e.g., echinocandin or AmB), who are infected with a susceptible organism, and who are ready for transition to oral therapy [58].

Although voriconazole has broad activity against most *Candida* spp. especially *C. krusei* and most *C. glabrata* isolates, it is not indicated as primary therapy in IC. Voriconazole is considered an excellent oral alternative to intravenous AmB or an echinocandin in clinically stable patients with *Candida* isolates resistant to fluconazole and are ready for transition to oral therapy [89]. Significant underlying liver disease is a contraindication for voriconazole therapy. A number of points should be considered when prescribing voriconazole: its unpredictable pharmacokinetics, drug–drug interactions, and toxicities including visual disturbances [90]. Periostitis with elevated blood fluoride levels can be a complication of long-term use [91].

Despite excellent *in vitro* activity against most *Candida* spp., posaconazole and isavuconazole have limited roles in the treatment of candidemia except for selected patients for whom transition to an expanded-spectrum oral azole is an acceptable option [92].

The echinocandins have become the agents of choice for primary therapy of IC because of their ease of administration, safety profile, few drug–drug interactions, and, in general, broad fungicidal activity against most *Candida* spp. Echinocandins are indicated as first-line therapy in patients who have a recent history of exposure to azoles, ongoing neutropenia, are hemodynamically unstable, have a history of allergy or intolerance to azoles or amphotericin B, or at high risk for infection with *C. krusei* or *C. glabrata*. However, echinocandins should not be used to treat central nervous system (CNS) infections because of their poor CNS penetration. The safety, tolerability, and efficacy of these compounds in the treatment of candidemia and other forms of IC have been well studied in large, controlled, randomized phase III clinical trials [93,94]. All echinocandins demonstrate diminished *in vitro* activity, expressed by a higher MIC, against *C. parapsilosis*. There is a difference in activity among echinocandins against certain *C. parapsilosis* isolates, in that susceptibility was observed to anidulafungin but not to caspofungin or micafungin [95]. Thus, it is recommended that fluconazole remain the preferred agent over the echinocandins for treatment of IC due to *C. parapsilosis*.

With the availability of alternatives and less toxic antifungal agents, AmB deoxycholate or lipid formulation AmB are only recommended for the treatment of IC as initial therapy in special circumstances: when alternative therapy is unavailable or unaffordable, when there is a history of intolerance to echinocandins or azoles, when the infection is refractory to other therapy, when the organism is resistant to other agents, or when there is a suspicion of infection due to non-*Candida* yeast, such as *Cryptococcus neoformans* [94,96,97]. *C. lusitaniae* is frequently resistant to AmB and should be treated with fluconazole or one of the echinocandins.

Up to 20% of patients with candidemia will have some manifestation of ocular involvement, with *C. albicans* being a greater risk factor compared to other *Candida* species (p = 0.021) [98]. Therefore, a dilated funduscopic examination (preferably by an ophthalmologist) along with blood cultures is strongly recommended for all patients with candidemia within the first week after initiation of therapy. Such strategy has an influence on the duration of treatment. For instance, if there are no metastatic complications, such as endophthalmitis, meningitis, or endocarditis, the duration of antifungal therapy is 14 days after resolution of signs and symptoms attributable to infection and clearance of *Candida* spp. from the bloodstream [58] (Table 16.5).

PROPHYLAXIS

Antifungal prophylaxis has led to a significant decrease in mortality related to fungal infections in critically ill and in cancer patients [99,100]. Several antifungal agents have proved to reduce the rate of IC in clinical trials in populations at high risk to develop IC. A dramatic reduction in the rates of invasive fungal infection was observed when fluconazole or liposomal AmB was used as a prophylactic regimen in liver transplant recipients [101,102]. Prophylactic fluconazole therapy after liver transplantation prevented invasive fungal infections caused by most *Candida* spp., except *C. glabrata* [101].

Other at risk populations who benefit from fluconazole prophylaxis include pancreas and small bowel transplant recipients [103,104]. The risk of IC after transplantation of other solid organs, such as kidney and heart, is too low to warrant routine prophylaxis [105].

A meta-analysis found that prophylactic antifungal agents reduced the number of superficial and invasive fungal infections in patients with chemotherapy-induced neutropenia [100]. In patients undergoing chemotherapy for acute myelogenous leukemia or the myelodysplastic syndrome, posaconazole prevented invasive fungal infections more effectively than fluconazole or itraconazole and improved overall survival [106]. Although another meta-analysis showed that itraconazole administered orally and/or intravenously as antifungal prophylaxis is effective in reducing the rate of fungal infection in neutropenic patients with hematologic malignancies, itraconazole has little advantage over more tolerable antifungal agents [107]. Recently, isavuconazole has been shown to be effective in preventing IC for acute myeloid leukemia patients with neutropenia [108].

Micafungin administered at 50 mg daily before engraftment was effective in reducing the rate of candidiasis in stem cell transplant recipients, compared with fluconazole administered at a dosage of 400 mg daily [109]. Because of its broad spectrum of activity, posaconazole was shown to be more effective than fluconazole in preventing invasive fungal infections in stem cell transplant recipients who had severe graft-versus-host disease [110]. The optimal duration of prophylaxis is not known but should usually include the period of neutropenia risk.

Patients in ICU settings are among the population at high risk for IC. For those ICUs that have a very high risk of IC (>5%), antifungal prophylaxis may be warranted for those patients with the highest risk [111]. Two meta-analyses showed that fluconazole prophylaxis was associated with a reduction in IC and reduced candidemia [112,113]. An alternative to fluconazole is prophylaxis with an echinocandin [57]. Skin decolonization with antiseptic agents is another emerging strategy to prevent IC. One randomized clinical trial found a significant reduction in catheter-associated *Candida* spp. BSIs [114]. Although more robust data are needed, there is likely little downside in using daily chlorhexidine baths in ICU patients for BSI prevention.

ACKNOWLEDGMENTS

We would like to thank Dr. Misha Rosenbach from the University of Pennsylvania Perelman School of Medicine for kindly providing Figure 16.1 and Dr. Marlene Durand from Harvard Medical School for kindly providing Figure 16.2.

COMMON CLINICAL QUESTIONS

1. Which of the following is the second most common cause of candidemia in the US?
   A. *C. parapsilosis*
   B. *C. albicans*
   C. *C. glabrata*
   D. *C. krusei*
2. What is the most common clinical manifestation of candidemia?
   A. Hypotension
   B. Fever
   C. Endophthalmitis
   D. Nausea
3. Which of the following statements about invasive candidiasis is true?
   A. The risk of invasive candidiasis is high after kidney transplantation
   B. The frequency of chronic disseminated candidiasis has been increasing in recent years
   C. Amphotericin B is the recommended as the empiric drug of choice in most cases
   D. *C. krusei* has intrinsic resistance to fluconazole
4. A 75-year-old man is diagnosed with multiple myeloma and started on chemotherapy. Two days later he develops a fever of 39.2° and blood cultures subsequently grow *C. albicans*. Which of the following statements is correct?
   A. An ophthalmologist should be consulted for a dilated retinal examination
   B. The *C. albicans* is likely a contaminant and not a true pathogen
   C. The central intravenous catheter is unlikely to be the source of the bloodstream infection and does not need to be removed
   D. Due to his immunocompromised status, he should be treated with amphotericin B

ANSWERS TO CLINICAL QUESTIONS

1. C. *C. glabrata* is the second most common cause of candidemia behind *C. albicans* accounting for 12%–24% of *Candida* BSIs. This species is associated with increasing age, use of broad spectrum antibiotics, azole exposure, use of central venous catheters, parenteral nutrition, and ICU stay.
2. B. Fever is the most common clinical manifestation of candidemia in adults. The clinical presentation may vary based on the patient population. In neonates, respiratory distress and apnea are the most prominent clinical signs of candidemia.
3. D. *C. krusei* has intrinsic resistance to fluconazole, but is very susceptible to both the extended-spectrum triazoles (posaconazole, voriconazole, and isavuconazole) and echinocandins. Given the availability of effective and less toxic alternatives, amphotericin B is rarely the recommended first-line empiric antifungal therapy for invasive candidiasis.
4. A. A dilated funduscopic exam, preferably by an ophthalmologist, is recommended for all patients with candidemia within the first week after diagnosis, given that up to 20% of patients with candidemia will manifest ocular involvement. Central venous catheters are common causes of candidemia, and removal of the catheter is indicated in the setting of catheter-associated candidemia.

REFERENCES

1. Horn DL, Neofytos D, Anaissie EJ, et al. Epidemiology and outcomes of candidemia in 2019 patients: Data from the prospective antifungal therapy alliance registry. *Clin Infect Dis* 2009;48(12):1695–1703.
2. Wisplinghoff H, Bischoff T, Tallent SM, et al. Nosocomial bloodstream infections in US hospitals: Analysis of 24,179 cases from a prospective nationwide surveillance study. *Clin Infect Dis* 2004;39(3):309–317.
3. Gudlaugsson O, Gillespie S, Lee K, et al. Attributable mortality of nosocomial candidemia, revisited. *Clin Infect Dis* 2003;37(9):1172–1177.
4. Wenzel RP. Nosocomial candidemia: Risk factors and attributable mortality. *Clin Infect Dis* 1995;20(6):1531–1534.
5. Morgan J, Meltzer MI, Plikaytis BD, et al. Excess mortality, hospital stay, and cost due to candidemia: A case-control study using data from population-based candidemia surveillance. *Infect Control Hosp Epidemiol* 2005;26(6):540–547.
6. Pappas PG, Rex JH, Lee J, et al. A prospective observational study of candidemia: Epidemiology, therapy, and influences on mortality in hospitalized adult and pediatric patients. *Clin Infect Dis* 2003;37(5):634–643.

7. Kawano Y, Togawa A, Nakamura Y, et al. Prognostic factors for candidaemia in intensive care unit patients: A retrospective analysis. *Singapore Med J* 2017;58(4):196–200.

8. Wey SB, Mori M, Pfaller MA, et al. Hospital-acquired candidemia. The attributable mortality and excess length of stay. *Arch Intern Med* 1988;148(12):2642–2645.

9. Haltmeier T, Inaba K, Effron Z, et al. *Candida* score as a predictor of worse outcomes and mortality in severely injured trauma patients with positive *Candida* cultures. *Am Surg* 2015;81(10):1067–1073.

10. Benjamin DK, DeLong E, Cotten CM, et al. Mortality following blood culture in premature infants: Increased with Gram-negative bacteremia and candidemia, but not Gram-positive bacteremia. *J Perinatol* 2004;24(3):175–180.

11. Guinea J. Global trends in the distribution of *Candida* species causing candidemia. *Clin Microbiol Infect* 2014;20 Suppl 6:5–10.

12. Diekema D, Arbefeville S, Boyken L, et al. The changing epidemiology of healthcare-associated candidemia over three decades. *Diagn Microbiol Infect Dis* 2012;73(1):45–48.

13. Arendrup MC. Epidemiology of invasive candidiasis. *Curr Opin Crit Care* 2010;16(5):445–452.

14. Hachem R, Hanna H, Kontoyiannis D, et al. The changing epidemiology of invasive candidiasis: *Candida glabrata* and *Candida krusei* as the leading causes of candidemia in hematologic malignancy. *Cancer* 2008;112(11):2493–2499.

15. Vallabhaneni S, Kallen A, Tsay S, et al. Investigation of the first seven reported cases of *Candida auris*, a globally emerging invasive, multidrug-resistant fungus—United States, May 2013–August 2016. *MMWR Morb Mortal Wkly Rep* 2016;65 (44):1234-1237.

16. Trick WE, Fridkin SK, Edwards JR, et al. Secular trend of hospital-acquired candidemia among intensive care unit patients in the United States during 1989–1999. *Clin Infect Dis* 2002;35(5):627–630.

17. Pfaller MA, Diekema DJ. Twelve years of fluconazole in clinical practice: Global trends in species distribution and flin clinic susceptibility of bloodstream isolates of *Candida*. *Clin Microbiol Infect* 2004;10(Suppl 1):11–23.

18. Doi AM, Pignatari AC, Edmond MB, et al. Epidemiology and microbiologic characterization of nosocomial candidemia from a Brazilian National Surveillance Program. *PLoS One* 2016;11(1):e0146909.

19. Tadec L, Talarmin JP, Gastinne T, et al. Epidemiology, risk factor, species distribution, antifungal resistance and outcome of candidemia at a single French hospital: A 7-year study. *Mycoses* 2016;59(5):296–303.

20. Tan TY, Hsu LY, Alejandria MM, et al. Antifungal susceptibility of invasive *Candida* bloodstream isolates from the Asia-Pacific region. *Med Mycol* 2016;54(5):471–477.

21. Diekema DJ, Messer SA, Brueggemann AB, et al. Epidemiology of candidemia: 3-Year results from the emerging infections and the epidemiology of Iowa organisms study. *J Clin Microbiol* 2002;40(4):1298–1302.

22. Malani A, Hmoud J, Chiu L, et al. *Candida glabrata* fungemia: Experience in a tertiary care center. *Clin Infect Dis* 2005;41(7):975–981.

23. Abi-Said D, Anaissie E, Uzun O, et al. The epidemiology of hematogenous candidiasis caused by different *Candida* species. *Clin Infect Dis* 1997;24(6):1122–1128.

24. Marr KA, Seidel K, White TC, et al. Candidemia in allogeneic blood and marrow transplant recipients: Evolution of risk factors after the adoption of prophylactic fluconazole. *J Infect Dis* 2000;181(1):309– 316.

25. Antoniadou A, Torres HA, Lewis RE, et al. Candidemia in a tertiary care cancer center: *In vitro* susceptibility and its association with outcome of initial antifungal therapy. *Medicine (Baltimore)* 2003;82(5):309–321.

26. Pfaller MA, Diekema DJ. Rare and emerging opportunistic fungal pathogens: Concern for resistance beyond *Candida albicans* and *Aspergillus fumigatus*. *J Clin Microbiol* 2004;42(10):4419–4431.

27. Kauffman CA. Fungal infections in older adults. *Clin Infect Dis* 2001;33(4):550–555.

28. Hajjeh RA, Sofair AN, Harrison LH, et al. Incidence of bloodstream infections due to *Candida* species and *in vitro* susceptibilities of isolates collected from 1998 to 2000 in a population-based active surveillance program. *J Clin Microbiol* 2004;42(4):1519–1527.

29. Vermitsky JP, Self MJ, Chadwick SG, et al. Survey of vaginal-flora *Candida* species isolates from women of different age groups by use of species-specific PCR detection. *J Clin Microbiol* 2008;46(4):1501–1503.

30. Borgo F, Verduci E, Riva A, et al. Relative abundance in bacterial and fungal gut microbes in obese children: A case control study. *Child Obes* 2017;13(1)78–84.

31. Kao AS, Brandt ME, Pruitt WR, et al. The epidemiology of candidemia in two United States cities: Results of a population-based active surveillance. *Clin Infect Dis* 1999;29(5):1164–1170.

32. Gupta A, Gupta A, Varma A. *Candida glabrata* candidemia: An emerging threat in critically ill patients. *Indian J Crit Care Med* 2015;19(3):151–154.

33. Nguyen MH, Peacock JE Jr, Morris AJ, et al. The changing face of candidemia: Emergence of non-*Candida albicans* species and antifungal resistance. *Am J Med* 1996;100(6):617–623.

34. Swoboda SM, Merz WG, Lipsetta PA. Candidemia: The impact of antifungal prophylaxis in a surgical intensive care unit. *Surg Infect (Larchmt)* 2003;4(4):345–354.

35. Saxen H, Virtanen M, Carlson P, et al. Neonatal *Candida parapsilosis* outbreak with a high case fatality rate. *Pediatr Infect Dis J* 1995;14(9):776–781.

36. Saiman L, Ludington E, Pfaller M, et al. Risk factors for candidemia in neonatal intensive care unit patients. The National Epidemiology of Mycosis Survey study group. *Pediatr Infect Dis J* 2000;19(4):319–324.

37. Delfino D, Scordino F, Pernice I, et al. Potential association of specific *Candida parapsilosis* genotypes, bloodstream infections and colonization of health workers' hands. *Clin Microbiol Infect* 2014;20(11):O946–O951.

38. Reissa E, Lasker BA, Iqbal NJ, et al. Molecular epidemiology of *Candida parapsilosis* sepsis from outbreak investigations in neonatal intensive care units. *Infect Genet Evol* 2008;8(2):103–109.

39. Kappstein I, Krause G, Hauer T, et al. Pseudo-outbreak of candidaemia with *Candida parapsilosis*. *J Hosp Infect* 1998;40(2):164–165.

40. Huang YC, Lin TY, Leu HS, et al. Outbreak of *Candida parapsilosis* fungemia in neonatal intensive care units: Clinical implications and genotyping analysis. *Infection* 1999;27(2):97–102.

41. Baran J Jr, Muckatira B, Khatib R. Candidemia before and during the fluconazole era: Prevalence, type of species and approach to treatment in a tertiary care community hospital. *Scand J Infect Dis* 2001;33(2):137–139.

42. Kontoyiannis DP, Vaziri I, Hanna HA, et al. Risk factors for *Candida tropicalis* fungemia in patients with cancer. *Clin Infect Dis* 2001;33(10):1676–1681.

43. Wingard JR. Importance of *Candida* species other than *C. albicans* as pathogens in oncology patients. *Clin Infect Dis* 1995;20(1):115–125.

44. Pfaller M, Cabezudo I, Koontz F, et al. Predictive value of surveillance cultures for systemic infection due to *Candida* species. *Eur J Clin Microbiol* 1987;6(6):628–633.

45. Sandford GR, Merz WG, Wingard JR, et al. The value of fungal surveillance cultures as predictors of systemic fungal infections. *J Infect Dis* 1980;142(4):503–509.

46. Walsh TJ, Merz WG. Pathologic features in the human alimentary tract associated with invasiveness of *Candida tropicalis*. *Am J Clin Pathol* 1986;85(4):498–502.

47. Iwen PC, Kelly DM, Reed EC, et al. Invasive infection due to *Candida krusei* in immunocompromised patients not treated with fluconazole. *Clin Infect Dis* 1995;20(2):342–347.

48. Merz WG, Karp JE, Schron D, et al. Increased incidence of fungemia caused by *Candida krusei*. *J Clin Microbiol* 1986;24(4):581–584.

49. Rodríguez D, Almirante B, Cuenca-Estrella M, et al. Predictors of candidaemia caused by non-albicans *Candida* species: Results of a population-based surveillance in Barcelona, Spain. *Clin Microbiol Infect* 2010;16(11):1676–1682.

50. Viudes A, Peman J, Canton E, et al. Candidemia at a tertiary-care hospital: Epidemiology, treatment, clinical outcome and risk factors for death. *Eur J Clin Microbiol Infect Dis* 2002;21(11):767–774.

51. Husain S, Tollemar J, Dominguez EA, et al. Changes in the spectrum and risk factors for invasive candidiasis in liver transplant recipients: Prospective, multicenter, case-controlled study. *Transplantation* 2003;75(12):2023–2029.

52. Faix RG, Kovarik SM, Shaw TR, et al. Mucocutaneous and invasive candidiasis among very low birth weight (less than 1,500 grams) infants in intensive care nurseries: A prospective study. *Pediatrics* 1989;83(1):101–107.

53. Sims CR, Ostrosky-Zeichner L, Rex JH. Invasive candidiasis in immunocompromised hospitalized patients. *Arch Med Res* 2005;36(6):660–671.

54. Anaissie EJ, Rex JH, Uzun O, et al. Predictors of adverse outcome in cancer patients with candidemia. *Am J Med* 1998;104(3):238–245.

55. Tanaka H, Ishida K, Yamada W, et al. Study of ocular candidiasis during nine-year period. *J Infect Chemother* 2016;22(3):149–156.

56. Rodriguez-Adrian LJ, King RT, Tamayo-Derat LG, et al. Retinal lesions as clues to disseminated bacterial and candidal infections: Frequency, natural history, and etiology. *Medicine (Baltimore)* 2003;82(3):187–202.

57. Krishna R, Amuh D, Lowder CY, et al. Should all patients with candidaemia have an ophthalmic examination to rule out ocular candidiasis? *Eye* 2000;14(Pt 1):30–34.

58. Pappas PG, Kauffman CA, Andes DR, et al. Clinical practice guideline for the management of candidiasis: 2016 update by the Infectious Diseases Society of America. *Clin Infect Dis* 2016;62(4):e1–e50.

59. Kontoyiannis DP, Luna MA, Samuels BI, et al. Hepatosplenic candidiasis. A manifestation of chronic disseminated candidiasis. *Infect Dis Clin North Am* 2000;14(3):721–739.

60. Horvath LL, George BJ, Murray CK, et al. Direct comparison of the BACTEC 9240 and BacT/ALERT 3D automated blood culture systems for *Candida* growth detection. *J Clin Microbiol* 2004;42(1):115–118.

61. Horvath LL, George BJ, Hospenthal DR. Detection of fifteen species of *Candida* in an automated blood culture system. *J Clin Microbiol* 2007;45(9):3062–3064.

62. Fernandez J, Erstad BL, Petty W, et al. Time to positive culture and identification for *Candida* blood stream infections. *Diagn Microbiol Infect Dis* 2009;64(4):402–407.

63. Terlecka JA, du Cros PA, Orla Morrissey C, et al. Rapid differentiation of *Candida albicans* from non-albicans species by germ tube test directly from BacTAlert blood culture bottles. *Mycoses* 2007;50(1):48–51.

64. Freydiere AM, Buchaille L, Gille Y. Comparison of three commercial media for direct identification and discrimination of *Candida* species in clinical specimens. *Eur J Clin Microbiol Infect Dis* 1997;16(6):464–467.

65. Gherna M, Merz WG. Identification of *Candida albicans* and *Candida glabrata* within 1.5 hours directly from positive blood culture bottles with a shortened peptide nucleic acid flurs direct *in situ* hybridization protocol. *J Clin Microbiol* 2009;47(1):247–248.

66. Radic M, Goic-Barisic I, Novak A, et al. Evaluation of PNA FISH® Yeast Traffic Light in identification of *Candida* species from blood and non-blood culture specimens. *Med Mycol* 2016;54(6):654–658.

67. Tissot F, Lamoth F, Hauser PM, et al. Beta-glucan antigenemia anticipates diagnosis of blood culture-negative intraabdominal candidiasis. *Am J Respir Crit Care Med* 2013;188(9):1100–1109.

68. Jaijakul S, Vazquez JA, Swanson RN, Ostrosky-Zeichner L. (1,3)-Beta-D-glucan as a prognostic marker of treatment response in invasive candidiasis. *Clin Infect Dis* 2012;55(4):521–526.

69. Lu Y, Chen YQ, Guo YL, et al. Diagnosis of invasive fungal disease using serum (1–>3)-beta-D-glucan: A bivariate meta-analysis. *Intern Med* 2011;50(22):2783–2791.

70. Karageorgopoulos DE, Vouloumanou EK, Ntziora F, et al. Beta-D-glucan assay for the diagnosis of invasive fungal infections: A meta-analysis. *Clin Infect Dis* 2011;52(6):750–770.

71. Berzaghi R, Colombo AL, Machado AM, et al. New approach for diagnosis of candidemia based on detection of a 65-kilodalton antigen. *Clin Vaccine Immunol* 2009;16(11):1538–1545.

72. Avni T, Leibovici L, Paul M. PCR diagnosis of invasive candidiasis: Systematic review and meta-analysis. *J Clin Microbiol* 2011;49(2):665–670.

73. Pfaller MA, Wolk DM, Lowery TJ. T2MR and T2Candida: Novel technology for the rapid diagnosis of candidemia and invasive candidiasis. *Future Microbiol* 2016;11(1):103–117.

74. Michalopoulos AS, Geroulanos S, Mentzelopoulos SD. Determinants of candidemia and candidemia-related death in cardiothoracic ICU patients. *Chest* 2003;124(6):2244–2255.

75. Leon C, Ruiz-Santana S, Saavedra P, et al. A bedside scoring system ("*Candida* score") for early antifungal treatment in nonneutropenic critically ill patients with *Candida* colonization. *Crit Care Med* 2006;34(3):730–737.

76. Ostrosky-Zeichner L, Sable C, Sobel J, et al. Multicenter retrospective development and validation of a clinical prediction rule for nosocomial invasive candidiasis in the intensive care setting. *Eur J Clin Microbiol Infect Dis* 2007;26(4):271–276.

77. Guillamet CV, Vazquez R, Micek ST, et al. Development and validation of a clinical prediction rule for candidemia in hospitalized patients with severe sepsis and septic shock. *J Crit Care* 2015;30(4):715–720.

78. Baddley JW, Patel M, Jones M, et al. Utility of real-time antifungal susceptibility testing for fluconazole in the treatment of candidemia. *Diagn Microbiol Infect Dis* 2004;50(2):119–124.

79. Hospenthal DR, Murray CK, Rinaldi MG. The role of antifungal susceptibility testing in the therapy of candidiasis. *Diagn Microbiol Infect Dis* 2004;48(3):153–160.

80. Clinical and Laboratory Standards Institute. 2008. *Reference Method for Broth Dilution Antifungal Susceptibility Testing of Yeasts*, 3rd ed. Approved standard M27-A3. Wayne, PA: Clinical and Laboratory Standards Institute.

81. Pfaller MA, Diekema DJ, Ostrosky-Zeichner L, et al. Correlation of MIC with outcome for *Candida* species tested against caspofungin, anidulafungin, and micafungin: Analysis and proposal for interpretive MIC breakpoints. *J Clin Microbiol* 2008;46(8):2620–2629.

82. Pfaller MA, Messer SA, Rhomberg PR, et al. *In vitro* activities of isavuconazole and comparator antifungal agents tested against a global collection of opportunistic yeasts and molds. *J Clin Microbiol* 2013;51(8):2608–2611.

83. Pfaller MA, Diekema DJ, Gibbs DL, et al. Results from the ARTEMIS DISK Global Antifungal Surveillance study, 1997 to 2005: An 8.5-year analysis of susceptibilities of *Candida* species and other yeast species to fluconazole and voriconazole determined by CLSI standardized disk diffusion testing. *J Clin Microbiol* 2007;45(6):1735–1745.

84. Rajendran R, Sherry L, Deshpande A, et al. A prospective surveillance study of candidaemia: Epidemiology, risk factors, antifungal treatment and outcome in hospitalized patients. *Front Microbiol* 2016;7:915.

85. Espinel-Ingroff A, Alvarez-Fernandez M, Cantón E, et al. Multicenter study of epidemiological cutoff values and detection of resistance in *Candida* spp. to anidulafungin, caspofungin, and micafungin using the Sensititre YeastOne colorimetric method. *Antimicrob Agents Chemother* 2015;59(11):6725–6732.

86. Rex JH, Bennett JE, Sugar AM, et al. A randomized trial comparing fl randomiz with amphotericin B for the treatment of candidemia in patients without neutropenia. Candidemia Study Group and the National Institute. *N Engl J Med* 1994;331(20):1325–1330.

87. Rex JH, Pappas PG, Karchmer AW, et al. A randomized and blinded multicenter trial of high-dose fluconazole plus placebo versus fluconazole plus amphotericin B as therapy for candidemia and its consequences in nonneutropenic subjects. *Clin Infect Dis* 2003;36(10):1221–1228.

88. Puig-Asensio M, Fernández-Ruiz M, Aguado JM, et al. Propensity score analysis of the role of initial antifungal therapy in the outcome of *Candida glabrata* bloodstream infections. *Antimicrob Agents Chemother* 2016;60(6):3291–3300.

89. Pfaller MA, Messer SA, Hollis RJ, et al. Antifungal activities of posaconazole, ravuconazole, and voriconazole compared to those of itraconazole and amphotericin B against 239 clinical isolates of *Aspergillus* spp. and other filamentous fungi: Report from SENTRY Antimicrobial Surveillance Program, 2000. *Antimicrob Agents Chemother* 2002;46(4):1032–1037.

90. Johnson LB, Kauffman CA. Voriconazole: A new triazole antifungal agent. *Clin Infect Dis* 2003;36(5):630–637.

91. Moon WJ, Scheller EL, Suneja A, et al. Plasma fluoride level as a predictor of voriconazole-induced periostitis in patients with skeletal pain. *Clin Infect Dis* 2014;59(9):1237–1245.

92. Rybak JM, Marx KR, Nishimoto AT, et al. Isavuconazole: Pharmacology, pharmacodynamics, and current clinical experience with a new triazole antifungal agent. *Pharmacotherapy* 2015;35(11):1037–1051.

93. Reboli AC, Rotstein C, Pappas PG, et al. Anidulafungin versus fluconazole for invasive candidiasis. *N Engl J Med* 2007;356(24):2472–2482.

94. Kuse ER, Chetchotisakd P, da Cunha CA, et al. Micafungin versus liposomal amphotericin B for candidaemia and invasive candidosis: A phase III randomised double-blind trial. *Lancet* 2007;369(9572):1519–1527.

95. Ghannoum MA, Chen A, Buhari M, et al. Differential *in vitro* activity of anidulafungin, caspofungin and micafungin against *Candida parapsilosis* isolates recovered from a burn unit. *Clin Microbiol Infect* 2009;15(3):274–279.

96. Mora-Duarte J, Betts R, Rotstein C, et al. Comparison of caspofungin and amphotericin B for invasive candidiasis. *N Engl J Med* 2002;347(25):2020–2029.

97. Phillips P, Shafran S, Garber G, et al. Multicenter randomized trial of fluconazole versus amphotericin B for treatment of candidemia in non-neutropenic patients. Canadian Candidemia Study Group. *Eur J Clin Microbiol Infect Dis* 1997;16(5):337–345.

98. Blennow O, Tallstedt L, Hedquist B, et al. Duration of treatment for candidemia and risk for late-onset ocular candidiasis. *Infection* 2013;41(1):129–134.

99. Rex JH, Sobel JD. Prophylactic antifungal therapy in the intensive care unit. *Clin Infect Dis* 2001;32(8):1191–1200.

100. Bow EJ, Laverdiere M, Lussier N, et al. Antifungal prophylaxis for severely neutropenic chemotherapy recipients: A meta analysis of randomized-controlled clinical trials. *Cancer* 2002;94(12):3230–3246.

101. Winston DJ, Pakrasi A, Busuttil RW. Prophylactic fluconazole in liver transplant recipients. A randomized, double-blind, placebo-controlled trial. *Ann Intern Med* 1999;131(10):729–737.

102. Hadley S, Huckabee C, Pappas PG, et al. Outcomes of antifungal prophylaxis in high-risk liver transplant recipients. *Transpl Infect Dis* 2009;11(1):40–48.

103. Benedetti E, Gruessner AC, Troppmann C, et al. Intra-abdominal fungal infections after pancreatic transplantation: Incidence, treatment, and outcome. *J Am Coll Surg* 1996;183(4):307–316.

104. Guaraldi G, Cocchi S, Codeluppi M, et al. Outcome, incidence, and timing of infectious complications in small bowel and multivisceral organ transplantation patients. *Transplantation* 2005;80(12):1742–1748.

105. Grossi P, Farina C, Fiocchi R, et al. Prevalence and outcome of invasive fungal infections in 1,963 thoracic organ transplant recipients: A multicenter retrospective study. Italian Study Group of Fungal Infections in Thoracic Organ Transplant Recipients. *Transplantation* 2000;70(1):112–116.

106. Cornely OA, Maertens J, Winston DJ, et al. Posaconazole vs. fluconazole or itraconazole prophylaxis in patients with neutropenia. *N Engl J Med* 2007;356(4):348–359.

107. Glasmacher A, Prentice A, Gorschluter M, et al. Itraconazole prevents invasive fungal infections in neutropenic patients treated for hematologic malignancies: Evidence from a meta-analysis of 3,597 patients. *J Clin Oncol* 2003;21(24):4615–4626.

108. Cornely OA, Böhme A, Schmitt-Hoffmann A, et al. Safety and pharmacokinetics of isavuconazole as antifungal prophylaxis in acute myeloid leukemia patients with neutropenia: Results of a phase 2, dose escalation study. *Antimicrob Agents Chemother* 2015;59(4):2078–2085.

109. van Burik JA, Ratanatharathorn V, Stepan DE, et al. Micafungin versus fluconazole for prophylaxis against invasive fungal infections during neutropenia in patients undergoing hematopoietic stem cell transplantation. *Clin Infect Dis* 2004;39(10):1407–1416.

110. Ullmann AJ, Lipton JH, Vesole DH, et al. Posaconazole or fluconazole for prophylaxis in severe graft-versus-host disease. *N Engl J Med* 2007;356(4):335–347.

111. Ostrosky-Zeichner L. Prophylaxis or preemptive therapy of invasive candidiasis in the intensive care unit? *Crit Care Med* 2004;32(12):2552–2553.

112. Vardakas KZ, Samonis G, Michalopoulos A, Soteriades ES, Falagas ME. Antifungal prophylaxis with azoles in high-risk, surgical intensive care unit patients: A meta-analysis of randomized, placebo-controlled trials. *Crit Care Med* 2006;34(4):1216–1224.

113. Cruciani M, de Lalla F, Mengoli C. Prophylaxis of *Candida* infections in adult trauma and surgical intensive care patients: A systematic review and meta-analysis. *Intensive Care Med* 2005;31(11):1479–1487.

114. O'Horo JC, Silva GL, Munoz-Price LS, Safdar N. The efficacy of daily bathing with chlorhexidine for reducing healthcare-associated bloodstream infections: A meta-analysis. *Infect Control Hosp Epidemiol* 2012;33(3):257–267.

17

Invasive aspergillosis

FRANK ESPER

INTRODUCTION

Invasive aspergillosis (IA) continues to be a leading cause of death in severely immunocompromised patients, particularly patients with malignancy and recipients of solid or hematopoietic stem cell transplant (HSCT) [1,2]. The incidence has significantly increased due to the development of new intensive chemotherapy regimens, increased use of high-dose corticosteroids, worldwide increase in solid organ and bone marrow transplantation, and increased use of chronic immunosuppressive regimens for autoimmune diseases [3,4]. Recent reports demonstrate that *Aspergillus* species are the second leading cause of invasive fungal illness overall behind *Candida* [5]. Despite a high incidence, a significant decrease in mortality in patients with a diagnosis of IA was noticed in recent years coinciding with multiple changes in transplantation practices, including the use of nonmyeloablative conditioning regimens, receipt of peripheral blood stem cells, earlier and improved surveillance and diagnosis, employing antifungal prophylaxis in at risk populations, and the use of voriconazole as the primary antifungal agent [6]. This chapter addresses the risk factors associated with IA, the common clinical presentation, novel approaches for early detection of subclinical infection and diagnosis modalities, and updated treatment strategies.

EPIDEMIOLOGY AND RISK FACTORS

Invasive aspergillosis in Hematopoietic Stem Cell Transplant (HSCT)

Invasive aspergillosis is most often caused by *A. fumigatus* and to a lesser extent by *A. flavus*, *A. niger*, and *A. terreus* [5]. Transplant recipients and those with acute myeloid leukemia are among the most significant groups at risk for IA. The cumulative incidence of IA has been reported from several multicenter study in the United States [5,7]. In the HSCT population, *Aspergillus* now exceeds *Candida* as the most common invasive fungal pathogen. The cumulative incidence is higher at 12 months in patients with allogeneic unrelated donors (3.9%) than in those with allogeneic human leukocyte antigen (HLA)-mismatched (3.2%), HLA-matched (2.3%), and autologous (0.5%) donors [7]. The rates were similar for myeloablative and nonmyeloablative conditioning regimen before allogeneic HSCT (3.1% vs. 3.3%). Risk factors for IA in the HSCT population include prolonged and profound neutropenia resulting from antineoplastic chemotherapy and secondary neutropenia associated with failure of hematopoietic stem cell engraftment [8,9]. Typically, IA occurs in the preengraftment period where neutropenia is the predominant immune defect associated with early IA. In the nonneutropenic host, however, IA occurs as a late infection (typically more than three months after engraftment) when recipients are receiving immunosuppressive drugs (especially high doses of corticosteroids) for the treatment of graft-versus-host disease (GvHD) [2,8,10]. In addition to neutropenia, other risk factors for IA in HSCT include acute and chronic GvHD, a prior history of fungal infection, corticosteroids therapy for GvHD, HLA mismatch, unrelated donor, receipt of T-cell depleted or CD34 selected transplant, and higher age of the recipients [11,12]. Cytomegalovirus (CMV) and respiratory virus infection, lymphopenia, the use of ganciclovir and alemtuzumab therapy, and increased bone marrow iron stores secondary to repeated transfusion have been identified in various studies as potential risk factors for IA [2,8,9,13].

Invasive aspergillosis in Solid Organ Transplant (SOT)

Although the net state of immunosuppression and intensity of the immunosuppressive regimen is a major determinant for the development of IA in SOT recipients, the incidence of IA and risk factors varies by the type of SOT. The rates of IA are low among all solid organ transplant recipients with the exception of lung transplant recipients. Lung transplant recipients have a reported cumulative incidence of IA up to 2.4% at 12 months following transplantation. Whereas, the cumulative incidence of IA is 0.8% after heart transplantation, 0.3% after liver transplantation, and 0.1% after kidney transplantation [7].

INVASIVE ASPERGILLOSIS IN LUNG TRANSPLANT RECIPIENT

Lung transplant recipients have a unique predisposition and clinical manifestation for *Aspergillus* infection. Impairment of local host defenses (e.g., mucociliary clearance and cough reflex), ischemic airway injury, altered alveolar phagocytic function, direct communication of the transplanted organ with the environment and an overall higher intensity of immunosuppression, render these patients uniquely susceptible to airway colonization with *Aspergillus* and invasive disease [14]. In addition, Anastomotic complication and airways or graft ischemia, during the surgery, predispose lung transplant recipients to IA. In the posttransplant period, *Aspergillus* infection has been reported in patients with reperfusion injury and poor allograft function. CMV infection and requirement of a higher degree of immunosuppressive therapy for rejection or bronchiolitis are also described to be a risk factor for IA following lung transplant [15,16]. In one large retrospective review of 362 lung transplant recipients, over 30% had evidence of *Aspergillus* infection. This investigation demonstrated that 25% of lung transplant patients develop colonization and 6% develop invasive pulmonary or disseminated aspergillosis [17]. The majority of infections occurring in the first few months following transplantation [7,17]. Interestingly, a higher incidence of invasive pulmonary aspergillosis occurs in recipients with single lung transplant than in those with

bilateral lung transplant [18] and the native lung if affected more frequently than the transplanted lung [19]. The mortality rate of IA in lung transplant recipients varies between 20% and 83% depending on the study [7,17,20].

INVASIVE ASPERGILLOSIS IN HEART TRANSPLANT RECIPIENT

Heart transplantation has been reported as the only type of solid organ transplantation in which fungal infection is caused predominantly (i.e., in 68% of cases) by *Aspergillus* spp. [21]. The of occurrence IA has been studied by several groups with an incidence between 0.8% and 14% [7,22]. A large single-center study found the incidence of invasive aspergillosis in 6.5% of 479 consecutive heart transplant recipients over a 24-year period [22]. Independent risk factors for IA following heart transplantation includes reoperation (RR:5.8; 95% CI = 1.8–18; p = 0.002), CMV disease (RR:5.2; 95% CI = 2–13.9; p = 0.001), requirement of hemodialysis posttransplant (RR:4.9; 95% CI = 1.2–18; p = 0.02), and the existence of an episode of IA in the institutional transplant program 2 months before or after the date of transplantation (RR:4.6; 95% CI = 0.3–0.8; p = 0.007) [22–24]. Early disease is commonly confined to the lung, but late disease (>3 months from transplant) has a higher proportion of disseminated involvement [22]. Historically, the mortality rate of IA following heart transplant was between 66% and 78% [7,14]. However, owing to numerous improvements, including usage of improved antifungal prophylaxis, earlier diagnosis, targeted immunosuppressive therapies, and better support and management of critical patients, mortality has decreased to as low as 36% [22].

INVASIVE ASPERGILLOSIS IN LIVER TRANSPLANT RECIPIENT

A number of well-characterized risk factors have been shown to carry a high risk of IA after liver transplantation. Retransplantation and renal failure are among the most significant risk factors for IA in these patient populations [25,26]. Other factors associated with IA in liver transplant recipients include transplantation for fulminant liver failure, steroid resistant rejection, CMV infection, use of broad spectrum antibiotics, and prolonged intensive care stay [25,27–29]. The median time of onset of IA after renal replacement therapy and retransplantation was 13 and 28 days, respectively, in one study [30]. Hepatitis C and CMV are independent risk factors for late onset IA (>3 months) in liver transplant recipients. There is a poor prognosis in liver transplant patients who develop IA, with a 1 year survival of 35% in one large study [25].

INVASIVE ASPERGILLOSIS IN KIDNEY TRANSPLANT RECIPIENT

Renal transplant recipients are at lower risk for IA than other transplant recipients. The incidence of IA following kidney transplantation ranges from 0.1% to 2.2% [7,31–33]. High dose and prolonged duration of corticosteroids, graft failure requiring hemodialysis, and potent immunosuppressive therapy have been associated with increased risk of IA [14,34,35]. Despite a low incidence compared to other solid transplant recipients, IA in kidney transplant recipients carry a high mortality rate ranging from 67% to 75% [14,20].

Invasive aspergillosis in hematologic malignancy

Patients with hematologic malignancies are at an increased risk for developing IA. Acute myeloid leukemia is the most frequent underlying condition [5,36], but in recent years, IA has been increasingly diagnosed in patients with multiple myeloma. In a study of HSCT recipients, the risk of IA was 4.5 times greater in patients with multiple myeloma, compared with the risk for patients with chronic myeloid leukemia [2].

Corticosteroid therapy

The risk of IA is a function of the dose and duration of steroid therapy [2,12,37]. Corticosteroids affect the host immune response to *Aspergillus* by preventing killing of phagocytosed *A. fumigatus* conidia by alveolar macrophages [38] and by blunting alveolar macrophage production of proinflammatory cytokines (IL-1a and TNF-a) and chemokines (macrophage inhibitory factor-1a) that are pivotal for recruiting neutrophils and monocytes [39]. Corticosteroids also affect the type of T helper cell response to IA. Corticosteroids therapy is associated with induction of TH2 cell responses and poor outcome [40]. It was shown that hydrocortisone enhances the doubling time and the hyphal extension rate of *A. fumigatus* grown *in vitro* [41]. Such characteristics have a clinical impact on patients receiving corticosteroids therapy for various indications. From a clinical perspective, the administration of 0.5 mg/kg of body weight/day for a period of more than 30 days or >1 mg/kg for a period of more than 21 days has been associated with an increased risk of IA, which starts within two weeks of steroid administration (>1 mg/kg/day of prednisone or equivalent) and has a dose response extending to more than six weeks [1,42,43]. Even lower doses (0.25–1 mg/kg/day) for 2 to 10 weeks have shown to increase the risk of IA [9].

Other risk factors

Other at-risk groups for IA include critically ill patients without traditional risk factors, those who have poorly controlled diabetes mellitus or AIDS, and those with primary immunodeficiency (e.g., chronic granulomatous disease) [44–47]. Immunomodulatory antibodies have revolutionized the treatment of patients with a variety of malignancies and inflammatory conditions [48]. TNF-α inhibitors are widely employed but have been associated with very few cases of IA [49]. Conversely, infliximab and alemtuzumab are associated with high risks of IA [50,51].

CLINICAL MANIFESTATIONS OF INVASIVE DISEASE

Invasive pulmonary aspergillosis

Aspergillus is ubiquitous in the outdoor environment and their spores are easily aerosolized and inhaled. As such, Invasive pulmonary aspergillosis (IPA) is the most common form of invasive *Aspergillus* disease. Clinical presentation is highly dependent on the host immune status and the risk factors for disease development. Patients usually present with nonspecific respiratory symptoms that are consistent with bronchopneumonia including fever, cough, and dyspnea [52]. Two concerning symptoms that raise the possibility of IPA are pleuritic chest pain and mild to severe hemoptysis. These symptoms develop due to vascular invasion leading to pulmonary infarctions, thrombosis, and necrosis [53]. IPA is one of the most common causes of hemoptysis in neutropenic patients and has been reported to be associated with cavitation that occurs with neutrophil recovery [54]. Pulmonary immune reconstitution inflammatory syndrome has been described in patients with pulmonary aspergillosis, who present with a worsening of respiratory clinical features and imaging changes in the absence of dissemination to other organs [55]. This clinical picture was observed after neutrophil recovery and coincided with microbiological and clinical response in 84% of the subjects [56]. The clinical presentation in other hosts, such as SOT recipients and patients on high dose corticosteroids, tend to be less fulminant than that seen in HSCT recipients or patients with hematologic malignancies [17,57]. Other pulmonary manifestations of IA include isolated tracheobronchitis with severe inflammation of the airways that is associated with ulcerations and plaque formation leading to airway obstruction and secondary atelectasis. This form of IPA has been most commonly reported in patients with AIDS and in lung transplant recipients [58,59].

Cerebral aspergillosis

With the predilection of *Aspergillus* to invade blood vessels, IPA commonly leads to hematogenous spread and dissemination to other organs, most commonly the brain and less commonly the skin, kidneys, pleura, heart, esophagus, and liver [60]. Cerebral aspergillosis may also arise by continuous invasion from adjacent anatomical sites, such as the paranasal sinuses, as well as following neurosurgical procedure or vascular intervention or in association with endocarditis [61–65]. It should be noted that this form of IA almost exclusively occurs in severely immunocompromised patients and carries a particularly poor prognosis and high mortality rate approaching 100% [66,67]. While cerebral aspergillosis is rarely found in patients with mild immunosuppression (e.g., diabetes and short course of corticosteroids) [68,69], it is concerning in patients with inherited defects of phagocytes [70].

Clinical symptoms in cerebral aspergillosis are variable and nonspecific. Altered mental status, focal neurologic deficits, and seizures are the most common symptoms reported. Meningeal signs are uncommon [10]. Following hematogenous spread, *Aspergillus* hyphae lodge and obstruct cerebral vessels, often large and intermediate-sized vessels, causing arterial thrombosis and infarction, typically hemorrhagic [71]. Head imaging including CT and MRI with contrast are essential in establishing the diagnosis of cerebral aspergillosis. Although angioinvasion is a common finding in IA, true mycotic aneurysms due to *Aspergillus* species are infrequently observed, often fatal, and most commonly involve the proximal part of large vessels at the base of the brain [72,73]. Abscess formation is the most common finding in a patient with cerebral aspergillosis [74]. Screening asymptomatic patients with IPA for CNS involvement remains controversial [10].

Invasive *Aspergillus sinusitis*

ACUTE

Aspergillus species are the most frequently identified fungal pathogens in patients with sinusitis [75] with *A. flavus* being the most common isolated organism [76]. Similar to pulmonary disease, Aspergillosis of the paranasal sinus is virtually always acquired by inhalation of aerosolized conidia. The disease occurs almost exclusively in immunocompromised hosts, including patients with prolonged neutropenia, AIDS patients, and after HSCT [77,78]. Acute invasive *Aspergillus* sinusitis is less common than invasive pulmonary aspergillosis with a frequency of sinus infections of only 5% among immunocompromised patients [79,80]. Acute IA sinusitis is characterized by an abrupt onset with rapid progression and a tendency of destructive invasion into neighboring structures resulting in orbital cellulitis, retinitis, palate destruction, or brain abscess formation. Patient at risk usually present with fever, facial pain, nasal discharge or congestion, epistaxis, and periorbital swelling [78,81,82]. Over 90% of disease occurs in the maxillary sinuses. However, involvement of the ethmoid sinus carries a particularly high risk of extension to the cavernous sinus and potentially the internal carotid artery [10]. Early signs of ophthalmoplegia may precede radiologic evidence of cavernous sinus thrombosis. Systemic or local antifungals have a limited role in therapy. Surgical excision is paramount for successful treatment in the severely immunocompromised [10].

CHRONIC

Unlike acute invasive *Aspergillus* sinusitis, the chronic form of the disease tends to occur in patients carrying a lesser degree of immunosuppression, such as patients with poorly controlled diabetes mellitus and patients on chronic steroids therapy [83]. Patients usually present with the orbital apex syndrome are characterized by decreasing vision and ocular immobility resulting from orbital mass. Chronic invasive sinus aspergillosis carries a poor prognosis and should be managed similar to acute invasive disease.

DIAGNOSIS

A high index of clinical suspicion is required especially in the setting of severe immunosuppression given the nonspecific presentation and high mortality associated with invasive disease. Early identification of patients at risk who require antifungal therapy is an important goal, as a prompt diagnosis and institution of the right antifungal agent has been associated with improved patient outcome and increased survival [6,84]. The diagnosis of invasive aspergillosis relies on a combination of clinical suspicion along with microbiologic and/ or histological findings [85]. While diagnostic sensitivity of histopathology is poor, histopathologic evidence is crucial in determining the significance of culture growth [10].

When a pulmonary IA is suspected, a high-resolution computed tomography (CT) scan is recommended [10,86,87]. Pulmonary nodules are the most common findings in early IPA in neutropenic patients and HSCT recipients and can be easily missed by a regular chest radiograph [86,88]. The "halo sign," a haziness surrounding a nodule or infiltrate, is a characteristic chest CT feature of angioinvasive organisms and is highly suggestive of IPA in patients with prolonged neutropenia. Other findings on chest CTs may include consolidative lesions, wedge shaped infarcts, cavitation, and pleural effusions. Analysis of the high-resolution CT images of patients with probable and proven IPA showed that those with a halo sign at initiation of antifungal therapy had a significantly better response and greater survival than those presenting with other CT images [86]. In patients with cerebral or sinus IA, magnetic resonance imaging (MRI) is the preferred modality and allows early detection of inflammatory soft tissue edema, bone destruction, or invasion into adjacent structures and guides the subsequent diagnostic approach and surgical management [10,89,90].

Although radiological features may be characteristic, they are not diagnostic of IA. For instance, infections due to other angioinvasive filamentous fungi, such as Zygomycetes, *Fusarium* spp., and *Scedosporium* spp., as well as due to *Pseudomonas aeruginosa* and *Nocardia* spp., may cause a halo sign and other radiologic patterns of IPA. Therefore, culture and histopathology confirmation is important to differentiate *Aspergillus disease* from other filamentous fungal infections or simple colonization. Recovery of *Aspergillus* spp. from nonsterile sites is suggestive of infection, but is not diagnostic. Host immune status is critical in culture interpretation. The positive predictive value of finding *Aspergillus* spp. in immunocompromised host with neutropenia was 64% in one study compared to 1% in patients with cystic fibrosis [91]. Definitive diagnosis often requires an invasive procedure with tissue biopsy (e.g., thoracoscopic biopsy, endoscopy for sinusitis). Fluid and tissue specimens from these procedures may reveal characteristic angular dichotomously branching septate hyphae on direct microscopic examination and/or *Aspergillus* spp. on culture. However, lack of positive culture or direct smear results do not rule out the diagnosis of IA. Moreover, clinical conditions in severely immunocompromised patients, such as thrombocytopenia, often preclude invasive procedure for tissue diagnosis. Thus, other markers are often used in the assessment of IA.

There is a growing number of publications detailing the use of nucleic acid tests for the detection of *Aspergillus* from clinical specimens. Detection of *Aspergillus* DNA has been performed on numerous patient samples including whole blood, respiratory fluids, cerebral spinal fluid, and tissues including skin, lung, and bone. The sensitivity and specificity vary with the tissue type: Whole blood PCR was found to have a sensitivity and specificity of 84% and 76%, respectively, in one study [92]. Whereas the sensitivity of *Aspergillus* DNA detection in BAL fluid were 77% and 94% [93]. However, PCR diagnosis for IA is not recommended for routine use at this time [10].

LABORATORY MARKERS

Laboratory markers that detect *Aspergillus* antigen can be used as a diagnostic adjunct, as a surveillance tool in high-risk patients (e.g., allogeneic HSCT recipients) to detect subclinical infection, and as a monitoring response to antifungal therapy. A serum test for detection of galactomannan (a fungal cell wall constituent of *Aspergillus*) was approved in the United States as an adjunct tool for the diagnosis of IA [94,95]. The combination of the host factors predisposition to IA (e.g., prolonged neutropenia), a compatible clinical and radiologic finding (e.g., pulmonary nodule), and two consecutive positive serum galactomannan assays is equated with "probable invasive aspergillosis." This could avoid the need for an invasive procedure and tissue biopsy when the clinical status of the patient precludes invasive intervention [96]. The use of galactomannan has also decreased the use of empiric antifungal agents [97]. Galactomannan antigen has been detected in the cerebral spinal fluid of patients with CNS aspergillosis and the bronchoalveolar lavage fluid specimens of patients with IPA [98,99].

It should be noted that the sensitivity and the specificity of the assay is affected by host factors and medications [100,101]. Most notably, the sensitivity of the assay is reduced by concomitant use of antifungal agents with activity against molds [101]. False-positive galactomannan results testing have been reported in several contexts, including in patients who had received certain antibiotics (piperacillin/tazobactam and amoxicillin/clavulanate), in cases of neonatal colonization with bifidobacterium, and in patients with other invasive mycoses (*Penicillium*, histoplasmosis, and blastomycosis) [102–104]. The sensitivity of galactomannan is also reduced in non-neutropenic patients, CGD, and those who received solid organ transplants [105–107].

The value of surveillance serum galactomannan monitoring is still unclear. Overall the sensitivity of galactomannan is 70% in hematologic malignancy and stem cell transplant recipients [10]. It appears best in allogeneic HSCT recipients where positive and negative predictive values are 94.4% and 98.8%, respectively, and antigenemia preceded radiographic findings by more than a week in 80% of cases of IA [108]. In malignancies, the sensitivity was only 64.5% in cases of definite IA [79]. As such, the current recommendations suggest use of serum galactomannan in these specific populations of hematological malignancies and HSCT recipients but not in SOT recipients, CGD, or those on broad anti-mold therapy as a marker for IA [10].

Detection of serum β-glucan, a fungal cell wall constituent, received Food and Drug Administration approval for the diagnosis of invasive mycosis, including aspergillosis [109,110]. Elevated levels of this marker is suggestive of invasive fungal infection but is not specific for invasive *Aspergillus* disease. In patients with acute myeloid leukemia and myelodysplastic syndrome, the assay was highly sensitive and specific in detecting early invasive fungal infections, including candidiasis, fusariosis, trichosporonosis, and aspergillosis [96]. Our understanding of this assay in other at-risk populations is limited. More research is required to define the utility of this assay in nonneutropenic patients at high risk for invasive mold infections, most notably, in allogeneic HSCT recipients with GvHD. Also there is controversy as to which biomarker (β-glucan vs. galactomannan) is superior for the detection of IA [111,112].

PHARMACOLOGIC TREATMENT OF INVASIVE ASPERGILLOSIS

The Infectious Disease Society of America (IDSA) has recently updated the guidelines for the treatment of various forms of aspergillosis, including IA, chronic (and saprophytic) forms of aspergillosis, and allergic forms of aspergillosis [10]. This chapter focuses on the different strategic treatments for invasive aspergillosis, summarized in Table 17.1. Pharmacologic description of each antifungal agent is beyond the scope of this chapter and can be found elsewhere [10].

Voriconazole is now the preferred antifungal compound in the United States for primary treatment of all forms of IA. Because of its excellent bioavailability and excellent CNS penetration, voriconazole in conjunction with a surgical intervention is recommended for patients with CNS and invasive sinus aspergillosis [72,102,103]. Deoxycholate amphotericin B (D-AMB) along with its lipid formulations (AMB lipid complex, liposomal-AMB, and AMB colloidal dispersion) may be used as an initial therapy when voriconazole is unavailable or due to patient intolerance [10,113]. In a randomized trial, isavuconazole was found to be noninferior to voriconazole in the treatment of IPA and is now approved as an alternative primary therapy against IPA [114].

There are few randomized trials on the treatment of IA. The largest landmark randomized, controlled trial demonstrates that voriconazole is superior to D-AMB as a primary treatment for IA [115]. In this study, a total of 277 patients with definite or probable aspergillosis were randomized to receive voriconazole or D-AMB for 12 weeks. In most

Table 17.1 Recommendations for the treatment of aspergillosis (See IDSA Guidelines for Specific Parameters) [10]

Presentation	Primary therapy	Alternative	Salvage therapy
Invasive pulmonary Invasive sinus Tracheobronchial CNS	Voriconazole	L-AMB Isavuconazole	Caspofungin Micafungin Posaconazole Itraconazole Surgical debridement when feasible
Chronic cavitary pulmonary	Voriconazole Itraconazole	L-AMB Isavuconazole	Caspofungin Micafungin Posaconazole Itraconazole Anecdotal response to IFN-γ
Endocarditis Pericarditis Myocarditis Osteomyelitis Septic arthritis	Voriconazole	L-AMB Isavuconazole	Caspofungin Micafungin Posaconazole Itraconazole Surgical debridement is required with endocardial lesions or devitalized bone

Endophthalmitis
Keratitis
	Voriconazole plus
	  intravitreal AmB
	
	Voriconazole with
	  partial vitrectomy
	
	Close consultation
	  with ophthalmology
		L-AMB
		Isavuconazole
			Caspofungin
			Micafungin
			Posaconazole
			Itraconazole
			
			Topical therapy for keratitis is indicated

Cutaneous	Voriconazole	L-AMB Isavuconazole	Caspofungin Micafungin Posaconazole Itraconazole Surgical debridement when feasible
Peritonitis	Voriconazole Removal of dialysis catheters	L-AMB Isavuconazole	Caspofungin Micafungin Posaconazole Itraconazole

Aspergilloma	No therapy or Surgical
	  resection
		Voriconazole
		Itraconazole
			Utility of medical therapy in the
			  treatment of aspergilloma is unclear

Allergic bronchopulmonary	Itraconazole Corticosteroids	Voriconazole Posaconazole	
Invasive pulmonary prophylaxis	Posaconazole	Voriconazole Itraconazole Micafungin	

Source: Patterson, T.F. et al., Clin. Infect. Dis., 63, e1–e60, 2016.

of the patients, the underlying condition was allogeneic hematopoietic-cell transplantation or hematologic malignancies, and the majority of IA disease was IPA. Partial (significant clinical improvement and at least 50% decrease in size of radiological lesions) or complete responses were considered a successful outcome. Patients given voriconazole had higher successful outcome rates with a 53% response (complete 21%, partial 32%) compared to 32% response rate in those given amphotericin B (complete 17%, partial 15%). Furthermore, the survival rate at 12 weeks was 70.8% in the voriconazole group compared to only 57.9% in the amphotericin B group (hazard ratio, 0.59; 95% CI = 0.40–0.88). Because of better survival and improved responses of initial therapy with voriconazole, primary therapy with D-AMB is no longer recommended for the treatment of IA [10].

Itraconazole and posaconazole, in addition to isavuconazole, are approved for salvage therapy of IA. Posaconazole is licensed for prophylaxis of IA in neutropenic patients with leukemia and myelodysplasia and in allogeneic HSCT recipients with GvHD for its expanded coverage against other mold species [116]. Posaconazole also was approved in the European Union for treatment of IA that is refractory to an AMB formulation or to itraconazole. Posaconazole is not recommended for a primary therapy of IA. Measurement of serum levels for all anti-*Aspergillus* azoles are recommended when the oral form is used because of their erratic bioavailability, which may affect therapeutic efficacy [10].

Micafungin and anidulafungin are members of the class of echinocandins, have *in vitro*, *in vivo*, and clinical activity against aspergillosis. Echinocandins are considered effective as salvage therapy in patients with IA. A favorable response was seen in 37 (45%) of the 83 patients refractory to or intolerant to conventional therapy [117]. They are not used as a monotherapy for primary treatment against AI. Echinocandins have been studied in combination therapy with polyenes and azoles against IA in order to maximize antimicrobial targeting against the invasive fungus. The rationale is that echinocandins target the 13-glucan constituents of the fungal cell wall, a site distinct from the fungal cell membrane targeted by polyenes and azoles. Synergistic effects of combination therapy have been seen in human and animal studies [118–120] but not in all studies [121–123]. Combination therapy is currently only considered as salvage in refractory disease

IMMUNE AUGMENTATION STRATEGIES

Methods for immune reconstitution are often employed in addition to antifungal agents for patients with IA. These strategies often include reestablishing immune function or reduction in immune suppression vital to effective fungal clearance.

Augmentation of neutrophil number colony-stimulating factors

Colony-stimulating factors (CSFs) are used to accelerate neutrophil count recovery in neutropenic patients. Macrophage CSF increases phagocytosis, chemotaxis, and secondary cytokine production in monocytes and macrophages [124]. Granulocyte macrophage CSF (GM-CSF) stimulates various neutrophil effectors functions and prolongs neutrophil survival *in vitro*, accelerates the proliferation of the monocyte–macrophage system, and is a potent activator of monocytes and macrophages [124].

A meta-analysis of prophylactic G-CSF showed a reduction in neutropenic fever and deaths, as well as decreased mortality due to infections [125,126]. However, our understanding on CSFs as adjunctive therapy for fungal infections is unclear, and clinical trials have led to conflicting results. Multiple randomized clinical trials of prophylactic recombinant G-CSF and GM-CSF have shown the benefit of CSF in reducing the time to neutrophil recovery and the duration of fever and hospitalization in patients with acute myelogenous leukemia [126,127]. In one randomized study in patients receiving chemotherapy for AML, prophylaxis with GM-CSF led to a lower frequency of fungal infections

and overall mortality compared to placebo [126,128]. The American Society of Clinical Oncology has established authoritative guidelines related to the use of prophylactic CSF in standards practice [129].

Granulocyte transfusions

Granulocyte transfusions provide supportive therapy for patients with neutropenia with a life-threatening infection by augmenting the number of circulating neutrophils until neutrophil recovery occurs. This strategy is recommended for patients with prolonged neutropenia and life-threatening infections refractory to conventional therapy when granulocyte recovery is predicted [10,130]. A randomized study of adjunctive granulocyte transfusions among neutropenic patients with severe bacterial and fungal infections was performed, but there was no overall effect of granulocyte transfusion. This study did not meet recruitment goals so the power to detect an effect was limited [131].

Recombinant interferon-γ

Studies *in vitro*, from animal models, and limited patient data provide a rational for adjunctive IFN-γ for the treatment of IA [132]. IFN-γ confers protection against a variety of experimental fungal infections in animals. Recombinant IFN-γ augments the human neutrophil oxidative response and killing of *A. fumigatus* hyphae *in vitro* and acted additively with G-CSF [133]. It also prevents corticosteroid-mediated suppression of neutrophil killing of hyphae and enhances killing of *A. fumigatus* by human monocytes [134,135]. Recombinant IFN-γ is licensed as a prophylactic agent in patients with congenital granulomatous disease [136]. Supporting the recommendation of its use in IA originate mainly from small uncontrolled series [137]. Recombinant IFN-γ is currently reserved for patients with life-threatening mold infection refractory to standard antifungal therapy.

PROPHYLAXIS AGAINST INVASIVE ASPERGILLOSIS

Antifungal prophylaxis with the aim to prevent IA is recommended in patients at high risk to develop IA, including patients with prolonged neutropenia and severe GvHD, lung transplant recipients, patients receiving long-term, high-dose corticosteroid therapy, some liver transplant recipients, and those with certain inherited immunodeficiency disorders (e.g., CGD) [10,116]. Preferred prophylactic regimens to prevent IA include the use of posaconazole, voriconazole, or an echinocandin (micafungin) during episodes of prolonged neutropenia. Posaconazole is recommended for patients with GvHD following HSCT. Itraconazole, while effective, is often limited by poor absorption and issues with tolerance. Prophylaxis is continued for the duration of substantial immune suppression [10].

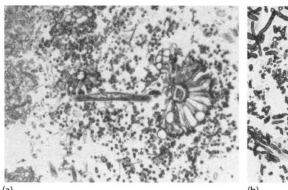 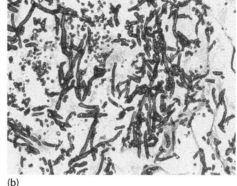

(a)　　　　　　　　　　　　　　(b)

Figure 17.1 Paranasal sinus biopsy showing **(a)** the *Aspergillus* fruiting head (GMS stain) and **(b)** branching septate hyphae (H&E stain). (Courtesy of Dr. Michael Jacobs, University Hospitals Cleveland Medical Center, Cleveland, OH.)

Patients with a previous history of IA are at high risk for recurrence during subsequent immunosuppression [138,139]. Therefore, an antifungal therapy with a mold activity is a reasonable approach during the entire period of immunosuppression as secondary prophylaxis against IA [116,138]. Several studies indicate that secondary prophylaxis against IA can be successful when an anti-*Aspergillus* azole (voriconazole, posaconazole, or itraconazole) or lipid formulation of amphotericin B is given to patients receiving ongoing immunosuppressive therapy following treatment of a documented episode of IA [139,140] (Figure 17.1).

REFERENCES

1. Baddley JW. Clinical risk factors for invasive aspergillosis. *Med Mycol* 2011;49 Suppl 1:S7–S12.
2. Marr KA. Invasive aspergillosis in allogeneic stem cell transplant recipients: Changes in epidemiology and risk factors. *Blood* 2002;100(13):4358–4366.
3. Martino R, Subira M. Invasive fungal infections in hematology: New trends. *Ann Hematol* 2002;81(5):233–243.
4. Warris A, Bjorneklett A, Gaustad P. Invasive pulmonary aspergillosis associated with infliximab therapy. *N Engl J Med* 2001;344(14):1099–1100.
5. Azie N, Neofytos D, Pfaller M, Meier-Kriesche HU, Quan SP, Horn D. The PATH (Prospective Antifungal Therapy) Alliance(R) registry and invasive fungal infections: Update 2012. *Diagn Microbiol Infect Dis* 2012;73(4):293–300.
6. Upton A, Kirby KA, Carpenter P, Boeckh M, Marr KA. Invasive aspergillosis following hematopoietic cell transplantation: Outcomes and prognostic factors associated with mortality. *Clin Infect Dis* 2007;44(4):531–540.
7. Morgan J, Wannemuehler KA, Marr KA, Hadley S, Kontoyiannis DP, Walsh TJ, et al. Incidence of invasive aspergillosis following hematopoietic stem cell and solid organ transplantation: Interim results of a prospective multicenter surveillance program. *Med Mycol* 2005;43(s1):49–58.
8. Mihu CN, King E, Yossepovitch O, Taur Y, Jakubowski A, Pamer E, et al. Risk factors and attributable mortality of late aspergillosis after T-cell depleted hematopoietic stem cell transplantation. *Transpl Infect Dis* 2008;10(3):162–167.
9. Thursky K, Byrnes G, Grigg A, Szer J, Slavin M. Risk factors for post-engraftment invasive aspergillosis in allogeneic stem cell transplantation. *Bone Marrow Transplant* 2004;34(2):115–121.
10. Patterson TF, Thompson GR, 3rd, Denning DW, Fishman JA, Hadley S, Herbrecht R, et al. Practice guidelines for the diagnosis and management of aspergillosis: 2016 Update by the Infectious Diseases Society of America. *Clin Infect Dis* 2016;63(4):e1–e60.
11. Jantunen E, Nihtinen A, Anttila VJ. Changing landscape of invasive aspergillosis in allogeneic stem cell transplant recipients. *Transpl Infect Dis* 2008;10(3):156–161.
12. Wald A, Leisenring W, van Burik JA, Bowden RA. Epidemiology of *Aspergillus* infections in a large cohort of patients undergoing bone marrow transplantation. *J Infect Dis* 1997;175(6):1459–1466.
13. Kontoyiannis DP, Chamilos G, Lewis RE, Giralt S, Cortes J, Raad II, et al. Increased bone marrow iron stores is an independent risk factor for invasive aspergillosis in patients with high-risk hematologic malignancies and recipients of allogeneic hematopoietic stem cell transplantation. *Cancer* 2007;110(6):1303–1306.
14. Paterson DL, Singh N. Invasive aspergillosis in transplant recipients. *Medicine* 1999;78(2):123–133.
15. Dauber JH, Paradis IL, Dummer JS. Infectious complications in pulmonary allograft recipients. *Clin Chest Med* 1990;11(2):291–308.
16. Husni RN, Gordon SM, Longworth DL, Arroliga A, Stillwell PC, Avery RK, et al. Cytomegalovirus infection is a risk factor for invasive aspergillosis in lung transplant recipients. *Clin Infect Dis* 1998;26(3):753–755.

17. Iversen M, Burton CM, Vand S, Skovfoged L, Carlsen J, Milman N, et al. *Aspergillus* infection in lung transplant patients: Incidence and prognosis. *Eur J Clin Microbiol Infect Dis* 2007;26(12):879–886.

18. Singh N, Husain S. *Aspergillus* infections after lung transplantation: Clinical differences in type of transplant and implications for management. *J Heart Lung Transplant* 2003;22(3):258–266.

19. Sandur S, Gordon SM, Mehta AC, Maurer JR. Native lung pneumonectomy for invasive pulmonary aspergillosis following lung transplantation: A case report. *J Heart Lung Transplant* 1999;18(8):810–813.

20. Gavalda J, Len O, San Juan R, Aguado JM, Fortun J, Lumbreras C, et al. Risk factors for invasive aspergillosis in solid-organ transplant recipients: A case–control study. *Clin Infect Dis* 2005;41(1):52–59.

21. Grossi P, Farina C, Fiocchi R, Dalla Gasperina D. Prevalence and outcome of invasive fungal infections in 1,963 thoracic organ transplant recipients: A multicenter retrospective study. Italian Study Group of Fungal Infections in Thoracic Organ Transplant Recipients. *Transplantation* 2000;70(1):112–116.

22. Munoz P, Ceron I, Valerio M, Palomo J, Villa A, Eworo A, et al. Invasive aspergillosis among heart transplant recipients: A 24-year perspective. *J Heart Lung Transplant* 2014;33(3):278–288.

23. Munoz P, Alcala L, Sanchez Conde M, Palomo J, Yanez J, Pelaez T, et al. The isolation of *Aspergillus fumigatus* from respiratory tract specimens in heart transplant recipients is highly predictive of invasive aspergillosis. *Transplantation* 2003;75(3):326–329.

24. Munoz P, Guinea J, Pelaez T, Duran C, Blanco JL, Bouza E. Nosocomial invasive aspergillosis in a heart transplant patient acquired during a break in the HEPA air filtration system. *Transpl Infect Dis* 2004;6(1):50–54.

25. Barchiesi F, Mazzocato S, Mazzanti S, Gesuita R, Skrami E, Fiorentini A, et al. Invasive aspergillosis in liver transplant recipients: Epidemiology, clinical characteristics, treatment, and outcomes in 116 cases. *Liver Transpl* 2015;21(2):204–212.

26. Fortún J, Martín-Dávila P, Moreno S, de Vicente E, Nuño J, Candelas A, et al. Risk factors for invasive aspergillosis in liver transplant recipients. *Liver Transpl* 2002;8(11):1065–1070.

27. Collins LA, Samore MH, Roberts MS, Luzzati R, Jenkins RL, David Lewis W, et al. Risk factors for invasive fungal infections complicating orthotopic liver transplantation. *J Infect Dis* 1994;170(3):644–652.

28. George MJ, Snydman DR, Werner BG, Griffith J, Falagas ME, Dougherty NN, et al. The independent role of cytomegalovirus as a risk factor for invasive fungal disease in orthotopic liver transplant recipients. *Am J Med* 1997;103(2):106–113.

29. Osawa M, Ito Y, Hirai T, Isozumi R, Takakura S, Fujimoto Y, et al. Risk factors for invasive aspergillosis in living donor liver transplant recipients. *Liver Transpl* 2007;13(4):566–570.

30. Singh N, Gayowski T, Wagener MM. Posttransplantation dialysis-associated infections: Morbidity and impact on outcome in liver transplant recipients. *Liver Transpl* 2001;7(2):100–105.

31. Alangaden GJ, Thyagarajan R, Gruber SA, Morawski K, Garnick J, El-Amm JM, et al. Infectious complications after kidney transplantation: Current epidemiology and associated risk factors. *Clin Transplant* 2006;20(4):401–409.

32. Ergin F, Arslan H, Azap A, Demirhan B, Karakayali H, Haberal M. Invasive aspergillosis in solid-organ transplantation: Report of eight cases and review of the literature. *Transpl Int* 2003;16(4):280–286.

33. Pappas PG, Alexander BD, Andes DR, Hadley S, Kauffman CA, Freifeld A, et al. Invasive fungal infections among organ transplant recipients: Results of the Transplant-Associated Infection Surveillance Network (TRANSNET). *Clin Infect Dis* 2010;50(8):1101–1111.

34. Gustafson TL, Schaffner W, Lavely GB, Stratton CW, Johnson HK, Hutcheson RH. Invasive aspergillosis in renal transplant recipients: Correlation with corticosteroid therapy. *J Infect Dis* 1983;148(2):230–238.

35. Panackal AA, Dahlman A, Keil KT, Peterson CL, Mascola L, Mirza S, et al. Outbreak of invasive aspergillosis among renal transplant recipients. *Transplantation* 2003:1050–1053.

36. Cornet M, Fleury L, Maslo C, Bernard JF, Brücker G. Epidemiology of invasive aspergillosis in France: A six-year multicentric survey in the Greater Paris area. *J Hosp Infect* 2002;51(4):288–296.

37. Fukuda T. Risks and outcomes of invasive fungal infections in recipients of allogeneic hematopoietic stem cell transplants after nonmyeloablative conditioning. *Blood* 2003;102(3):827–833.

38. Philippe B, Ibrahim-Granet O, Prevost MC, Gougerot-Pocidalo MA, Sanchez Perez M, Van der Meeren A, et al. Killing of *Aspergillus fumigatus* by alveolar macrophages is mediated by reactive oxidant intermediates. *Infect Immun* 2003;71(6):3034–3042.

39. Brummer E, Kamberi M, Stevens David A. Regulation by granulocyte-macrophage colony-stimulating factor and/or steroids given *in vivo* of proinflammatory cytokine and chemokine production by bronchoalveolar macrophages in response to *Aspergillus* conidia. *J Infect Dis* 2003;187(4):705–709.

40. Hebart H. Analysis of T-cell responses to *Aspergillus fumigatus* antigens in healthy individuals and patients with hematologic malignancies. *Blood* 2002;100(13):4521–4528.

41. Ng TTC, Robson GD, Denning DW. Hydrocortisone-enhanced growth of *Aspergillus* spp.: Implications for pathogenesis. *Microbiology* 1994;140(9):2475–2479.

42. Cordonnier C, Ribaud P, Herbrecht R, Milpied N, Valteau-Couanet D, Morgan C, et al. Prognostic factors for death due to invasive aspergillosis after hematopoietic stem cell transplantation: A 1-year retrospective study of consecutive patients at French transplantation centers. *Clin Infect Dis* 2006;42(7):955–963.

43. Grow WB, Moreb JS, Roque D, Manion K, Leather H, Reddy V, et al. Late onset of invasive *Aspergillus* infection in bone marrow transplant patients at a university hospital. *Bone Marrow Transplant* 2002;29(1):15–19.

44. Almyroudis NG, Holland SM, Segal BH. Invasive aspergillosis in primary immunodeficiencies. *Med Mycol* 2005;43(s1):247–259.

45. Groll A, Shah P, Mentzel C, Schneider M, Justnuebling G, Huebner K. Trends in the postmortem epidemiology of invasive fungal infections at a University Hospital. *J Infect* 1996;33(1):23–32.

46. Vandewoude KH, Blot SI, Depuydt P, Benoit D, Temmerman W, Colardyn F, et al. Clinical relevance of *Aspergillus* isolation from respiratory tract samples in critically ill patients. *Crit Care* 2006;10(1):R31.

47. Meersseman W, Van Wijngaerden E. Invasive aspergillosis in the ICU: An emerging disease. *Intensive Care Med* 2007;33(10):1679–1681.

48. Kyi C, Hellmann MD, Wolchok JD, Chapman PB, Postow MA. Opportunistic infections in patients treated with immunotherapy for cancer. *J Immunother Cancer* 2014;2:19.

49. Baddley JW, Winthrop KL, Chen L, Liu L, Grijalva CG, Delzell E, et al. Non-viral opportunistic infections in new users of tumour necrosis factor inhibitor therapy: Results of the SAfety Assessment of Biologic ThERapy (SABER) study. *Ann Rheum Dis* 2014;73(11):1942–1948.

50. Gallamini A, Zaja F, Patti C, Billio A, Specchia MR, Tucci A, et al. Alemtuzumab (Campath-1H) and CHOP chemotherapy as first-line treatment of peripheral T-cell lymphoma: Results of a GITIL (Gruppo Italiano Terapie Innovative nei Linfomi) prospective multicenter trial. *Blood* 2007;110(7):2316–2323.

51. Marty FM, Lee SJ, Fahey MM, Alyea EP, Soiffer RJ, Antin JH, et al. Infliximab use in patients with severe graft-versus-host disease and other emerging risk factors of non-*Candida* invasive fungal infections in allogeneic hematopoietic stem cell transplant recipients: A cohort study. *Blood* 2003;102(8):2768–2776.

52. Sherif R, Segal BH. Pulmonary aspergillosis: Clinical presentation, diagnostic tests, management and complications. *Curr Opin Pulm Med* 2010;16(3):242–250.

53. Naaraayan A, Kavian R, Lederman J, Basak P, Jesmajian S. Invasive pulmonary aspergillosis—Case report and review of literature. *J Community Hosp Intern Med Perspect* 2015;5(1):26322.

54. Albelda SM, Talbot GH, Gerson SL, Miller WT, Cassileth PA. Pulmonary cavitation and massive hemoptysis in invasive pulmonary aspergillosis. Influence of bone marrow recovery in patients with acute leukemia. *Am Rev Respir Dis* 1985;131(1):115–120.

55. Miceli MH, Maertens J, Buvé K, Grazziutti M, Woods G, Rahman M, et al. Immune reconstitution inflammatory syndrome in cancer patients with pulmonary aspergillosis recovering from neutropenia: Proof of principle, description, and clinical and research implications. *Cancer* 2007;110(1):112–120.

56. Todeschini G, Murari C, Bonesi R, Pizzolo G, Verlato G, Tecchio C, et al. Invasive aspergillosis in neutropenic patients: Rapid neutrophil recovery is a risk factor for severe pulmonary complications. *Eur J Clin Invest* 1999;29(5):453–457.

57. Davies S, Guidry C, Politano A, Rosenberger L, McLeod M, Hranjec T, et al. *Aspergillus* infections in transplant and non-transplant surgical patients. *Surg Infect (Larchmt)* 2014;15(3):207–212.

58. Judson MA, Sahn SA. Endobronchial lesions in HIV-infected individuals. *Chest* 1994;105(5):1314–1323.

59. Nathan SD, Shorr AF, Schmidt ME, Burton NA. *Aspergillus* and endobronchial abnormalities in lung transplant recipients. *Chest* 2000;118(2):403–407.

60. Boes B, Bashir R, Boes C, Hahn F, McConnell JR, McComb R. Central nervous system aspergillosis. Analysis of 26 patients. *J Neuroimaging* 1994;4(3):123–129.

61. Darras-Joly C, Veber B, Bedos J-P, Gachot B, Regnier B, Wolff M. Nosocomial cerebral aspergillosis: A report of 3 cases. *Scand J Infect Dis* 1996;28(3):317–319.

62. Kim DG, Hong SC, Kim HJ, Chi JG, Hee Han M, Choi KS, et al. Cerebral aspergillosis in immunologically competent patients. *Surg Neurol* 1993;40(4):326–331.

63. Saah D, Braverman I, Drakos PE, Or R, Elidan J, Nagler A. Rhinocerebral aspergillosis in patients undergoing bone marrow transplantation. *Ann Otol Rhinol Laryngol* 1994;103(4):306–310.

64. Scherer M, Fieguth H-G, Aybek T, Ujvari Z, Moritz A, Wimmer-Greinecker G. Disseminated *Aspergillus fumigatus* infection with consecutive mitral valve endocarditis in a lung transplant recipient. *J Heart Lung Transplant* 2005;24(12):2297–2300.

65. van de Beek D, Patel R, Campeau NG, Badley A, Parisi JE, Rabinstein AA, et al. Insidious sinusitis leading to catastrophic cerebral aspergillosis in transplant recipients. *Neurology* 2008;70(Issue 24, Part 2):2411–2413.

66. Baddley JW, Salzman D, Pappas PG. Fungal brain abscess in transplant recipients: Epidemiologic, microbiologic, and clinical features. *Clin Transplant* 2002;16(6):419–424.

67. Lin SJ, Schranz J, Teutsch SM. Aspergillosis case-fatality rate: Systematic review of the literature. *Clin Infect Dis* 2001;32(3):358–366.

68. Apostolidis J. Short-course corticosteroid-induced pulmonary and apparent cerebral aspergillosis in a patient with idiopathic thrombocytopenic purpura. *Blood* 2001;98(9):2875–2877.

69. Leroy P, Smismans A, Seute T. Invasive pulmonary and central nervous system aspergillosis after near-drowning of a child: Case report and review of the literature. *Pediatrics* 2006;118(2):e509–e513.

70. Alsultan A, Williams MS, Lubner S, Goldman FD. Chronic granulomatous disease presenting with disseminated intracranial aspergillosis. *Pediatr Blood Cancer* 2006;47(1):107–110.

71. Erdogan E, Beyzadeoglu M, Arpaci F, Celasun B. Cerebellar aspergillosis: Case report and literature review. *Neurosurgery* 2002;50(4):874–877.

72. Ho CL, Deruytter MJ. CNS aspergillosis with mycotic aneurysm, cerebral granuloma and infarction. *Acta Neurochir* 2004;146(8):851–856.

73. Sundaram C, Goel D, Uppin SG, Seethajayalakshmi S, Borgohain R. Intracranial mycotic aneurysm due to *Aspergillus* species. *J Clin Neurosci* 2007;14(9):882–886.

74. Pagano L, Ricci P, Montillo M, Cenacchi A, Nosari A, Tonso A, et al. Localization of aspergillosis to the central nervous system among patients with acute leukemia: Report of 14 cases. *Clin Infect Dis* 1996;23(3):628–630.

75. Parikh SL, Venkatraman G, DelGaudio JM. Invasive fungal sinusitis: A 15-year review from a single institution. *Am J Rhinol* 2004;18(2):75–81.

76. Kennedy C, Adams G, Neglia J, Giebink G. Impact of surgical treatment on paranasal fungal infections in bone marrow transplant patients. *Otolaryngol Head Neck Surg* 1997;116(6):610–616.

77. Mylonakis E, Rich J, Skolnik PR, De Orchis DF, Flanigan T. Invasive *Aspergillus* sinusitis in patients with human immunodeficiency virus infection: Report of 2 cases and review. *Medicine* 1997;76(4):249–255.

78. Schwartz S, Thiel E. Palate destruction by *Aspergillus*. *N Engl J Med* 1997;337(4):241.

79. Herbrecht R, Letscher-Bru V, Oprea C, Lioure B, Waller J, Campos F, et al. *Aspergillus* galactomannan detection in the diagnosis of invasive aspergillosis in cancer patients. *Am J Clin Oncol* 2002;20(7):1898–1906.

80. Patterson TF, Kirkpatrick WR, White M, Hiemenz JW, Wingard JR, Dupont B, et al. Invasive aspergillosis. Disease spectrum, treatment practices, and outcomes. *Medicine* 2000;79(4):250–260.

81. Gillespie MB, O'Malley BW, Francis HW. An approach to fulminant invasive fungal rhinosinusitis in the immunocompromised host. *Arch Otolaryngol Head Neck Surg* 1998;124(5):520.

82. Iwen PC, Rupp ME, Hinrichs SH. Invasive mold sinusitis: 17 Cases in immunocompromised patients and review of the literature. *Clin Infect Dis* 1997;24(6):1178–1184.

83. deShazo RD, Chapin K, Swain RE. Fungal sinusitis. *N Engl J Med* 1997;337(4):254–259.

84. von Eiff M, Roos N, Schulten R, Hesse M, Zühlsdorf M, van de Loo J. Pulmonary aspergillosis: Early diagnosis improves survival. *Respiration* 2009;62(6):341–347.

85. De Pauw B, Walsh TJ, Donnelly JP, Stevens DA, Edwards JE, Calandra T, et al. Revised definitions of invasive fungal disease from the European Organization for Research and Treatment of Cancer/Invasive Fungal Infections Cooperative Group and the National Institute of Allergy and Infectious Diseases Mycoses Study Group (EORTC/MSG) Consensus Group. *Clin Infect Dis* 2008;46(12):1813–1821.

86. Greene RE, Schlamm HT, Oestmann JW, Stark P, Durand C, Lortholary O, et al. Imaging findings in acute invasive pulmonary aspergillosis: Clinical significance of the halo sign. *Clin Infect Dis* 2007;44(3):373–379.

87. Kuhlman JE, Fishman EK, Burch PA, Karp JE, Zerhouni EA, Siegelman SS. Invasive pulmonary aspergillosis in acute leukemia. *Chest* 1987;92(1):95–99.

88. Hauggaard A, Ellis M, Ekelund L. Early chest radiography and CT in the diagnosis, management and outcome of invasive pulmonary aspergillosis. *Acta Radiol* 2002;43(3):292–298.

89. Aribandi M, McCoy VA, Bazan C. Imaging features of invasive and noninvasive fungal sinusitis: A review. *Radiographics* 2007;27(5):1283–1296.

90. Siddiqui AA, Bashir SH, Ali Shah A, Sajjad Z, Ahmed N, Jooma R, et al. Diagnostic MR imaging features of craniocerebral aspergillosis of sino-nasal origin in immunocompetent patients. *Acta Neurochir (Wien)* 2006;148(2):155–166; discussion 66.

91. Perfect JR, Cox GM, Lee JY, Kauffman CA, de Repentigny L, Chapman SW, et al. The impact of culture isolation of *Aspergillus* species: A hospital-based survey of aspergillosis. *Clin Infect Dis* 2001;33(11):1824–1833.

92. Arvanitis M, Ziakas PD, Zacharioudakis IM, Zervou FN, Caliendo AM, Mylonakis E. PCR in diagnosis of invasive aspergillosis: A meta-analysis of diagnostic performance. *J Clin Microbiol* 2014;52(10):3731–3742.

93. Avni T, Levy I, Sprecher H, Yahav D, Leibovici L, Paul M. Diagnostic accuracy of PCR alone compared to galactomannan in bronchoalveolar lavage fluid for diagnosis of invasive pulmonary aspergillosis: A systematic review. *J Clin Microbiol* 2012;50(11):3652–3658.

94. Maertens J, Buve K, Theunissen K, Meersseman W, Verbeken E, Verhoef G, et al. Galactomannan serves as a surrogate endpoint for outcome of pulmonary invasive aspergillosis in neutropenic hematology patients. *Cancer* 2009;115(2):355–362.

95. Mennink-Kersten MASH, Donnelly JP, Verweij PE. Detection of circulating galactomannan for the diagnosis and management of invasive aspergillosis. *Lancet Infect Dis* 2004;4(6):349–357.

96. Ascioglu S, Rex JH, de Pauw B, Bennett JE, Bille J, Crokaert F, et al. Defining opportunistic invasive fungal infections in immunocompromised patients with cancer and hematopoietic stem cell transplants: An international consensus. *Clin Infect Dis* 2002;34(1):7–14.

97. Maertens J, Theunissen K, Verhoef G, Verschakelen J, Lagrou K, Verbeken E, et al. Galactomannan and computed tomography-based preemptive antifungal therapy in neutropenic patients at high risk for invasive fungal infection: A prospective feasibility study. *Clin Infect Dis* 2005;41(9):1242–1250.

98. Verweij PE, Brinkman K, Kremer HP, Kullberg BJ, Meis JF. *Aspergillus* meningitis: Diagnosis by non-culture-based microbiological methods and management. *J Clin Microbiol* 1999;37(4):1186–1189.

99. Viscoli C, Machetti M, Gazzola P, De Maria A, Paola D, Van Lint MT, et al. *Aspergillus* galactomannan antigen in the cerebrospinal fluid of bone marrow transplant recipients with probable cerebral aspergillosis. *J Clin Microbiol* 2002;40(4):1496–1499.

100. Maertens JA, Klont R, Masson C, Theunissen K, Meersseman W, Lagrou K, et al. Optimization of the cutoff value for the *Aspergillus* double-sandwich enzyme immunoassay. *Clin Infect Dis* 2007;44(10):1329–1336.

101. Marr KA, Laverdiere M, Gugel A, Leisenring W. Antifungal therapy decreases sensitivity of the *Aspergillus* galactomannan enzyme immunoassay. *Clin Infect Dis* 2005;40(12):1762–1769.

102. Mennink-Kersten MASH, Klont RR, Warris A, Op den Camp HJM, Verweij PE. Bifidobacterium lipoteichoic acid and false ELISA reactivity in *Aspergillus* antigen detection. *Lancet* 2004;363(9405):325–327.

103. Singh N, Obman A, Husain S, Aspinall S, Mietzner S, Stout JE. Reactivity of Platelia *Aspergillus* galactomannan antigen with piperacillin-tazobactam: Clinical implications based on achievable concentrations in serum. *Antimicrob Agents Chemother* 2004;48(6):1989–1992.

104. Sulahian A, Touratier S, Ribaud P. False positive test for *Aspergillus* antigenemia related to concomitant administration of piperacillin and tazobactam. *N Engl J Med* 2003;349(24):2366–2367.

105. Fortun J, Martin-Davila P, Alvarez ME, Norman F, Sanchez-Sousa A, Gajate L, et al. False-positive results of *Aspergillus* galactomannan antigenemia in liver transplant recipients. *Transplantation* 2009;87(2):256–260.

106. Ku NS, Han SH, Choi JY, Kim SB, Kim HW, Jeong SJ, et al. Diagnostic value of the serum galactomannan assay for invasive aspergillosis: It is less useful in non-haematological patients. *Scand J Infect Dis* 2012;44(8):600–604.

107. Verweij PE, Weemaes CM, Curfs JH, Bretagne S, Meis JF. Failure to detect circulating *Aspergillus* markers in a patient with chronic granulomatous disease and invasive aspergillosis. *J Clin Microbiol* 2000;38(10):3900–3901.

108. Maertens J, Van Eldere J, Verhaegen J, Verbeken E, Verschakelen J, Boogaerts M. Use of circulating galactomannan screening for early diagnosis of invasive aspergillosis in allogeneic stem cell transplant recipients. *J Infect Dis* 2002;186(9):1297–1306.

109. Odabasi Z, Mattiuzzi G, Estey E, Kantarjian H, Saeki F, Ridge RJ, et al. Beta-D-glucan as a diagnostic adjunct for invasive fungal infections: validation, cutoff development, and performance in patients with acute myelogenous leukemia and myelodysplastic syndrome. *Clin Infect Dis* 2004;39(2):199–205.

110. Ostrosky-Zeichner L, Alexander BD, Kett DH, Vazquez J, Pappas PG, Saeki F, et al. Multicenter clinical evaluation of the (1->3)-D-glucan assay as an aid to diagnosis of fungal infections in humans. *Clin Infect Dis* 2005;41(5):654–659.

111. Badiee P, Alborzi A, Karimi M, Pourabbas B, Haddadi P, Mardaneh J, et al. Diagnostic potential of nested PCR, galactomannan EIA, and beta-D-glucan for invasive aspergillosis in pediatric patients. *J Infect Dev Ctries* 2012;6(4):352–357.

112. Sulahian A, Porcher R, Bergeron A, Touratier S, Raffoux E, Menotti J, et al. Use and limits of (1–3)-beta-d-glucan assay (Fungitell), compared to galactomannan determination (Platelia *Aspergillus*), for diagnosis of invasive aspergillosis. *J Clin Microbiol* 2014;52(7):2328–2333.

113. Cornely OA, Maertens J, Bresnik M, Ebrahimi R, Ullmann AJ, Bouza E, et al. Liposomal amphotericin B as initial therapy for invasive mold infection: A randomized trial comparing a high-loading dose regimen with standard dosing (AmBiLoad trial). *Clin Infect Dis.* 2007;44(10):1289–1297.

114. Maertens JA, Raad II, Marr KA, Patterson TF, Kontoyiannis DP, Cornely OA, et al. Isavuconazole versus voriconazole for primary treatment of

invasive mould disease caused by *Aspergillus* and other filamentous fungi (SECURE): A phase 3, randomised-controlled, non-inferiority trial. *Lancet* 2016;387(10020):760–769.

115. Herbrecht R, Denning DW, Patterson TF, Bennett JE, Greene RE, Oestmann JW, et al. Voriconazole versus amphotericin B for primary therapy of invasive aspergillosis. *N Engl J Med* 2002;347(6):408–415.

116. Tomblyn M, Chiller T, Einsele H, Gress R, Sepkowitz K, Storek J, et al. Guidelines for preventing infectious complications among hematopoietic cell transplant recipients: A global perspective. Preface. *Bone Marrow Transplant* 2009;44(8):453–455.

117. Maertens J, Raad I, Petrikkos G, Boogaerts M, Selleslag D, Petersen Finn B, et al. Efficacy and safety of caspofungin for treatment of invasive aspergillosis in patients refractory to or intolerant of conventional antifungal therapy. *Clin Infect Dis* 2004;39(11):1563–1571.

118. Mukherjee PK, Sheehan DJ, Hitchcock CA, Ghannoum MA. Combination treatment of invasive fungal infections. *Clin Microbiol Rev* 2005;18(1):163–194.

119. Wirk B, Wingard JR. Combination antifungal therapy: From bench to bedside. *Curr Infect Dis Rep* 2008;10(6):466–472.

120. Zhang M, Sun WK, Wu T, Chen F, Xu XY, Su X, et al. Efficacy of combination therapy of triazole and echinocandin in treatment of invasive aspergillosis: A systematic review of animal and human studies. *J Thorac Dis* 2014;6(2):99–108.

121. Chandrasekar PH, Cutright JL, Manavathu EK. Efficacy of voriconazole plus amphotericin B or micafungin in a guinea-pig model of invasive pulmonary aspergillosis. *Clin Microbiol Infect* 2004;10(10):925–928.

122. Graybill JR. Combination antifungal therapy of murine aspergillosis: Liposomal amphotericin B and micafungin. *J Antimicrob Chemother* 2003;52(4):656–662.

123. Sivak O, Bartlett K, Risovic V, Choo E, Marra F, Scotty Batty D, et al. Assessing the antifungal activity and toxicity profile of amphotericin B lipid complex (ABLC; Abelcet®) in combination with caspofungin in experimental systemic aspergillosis. *J Pharm Sci* 2004;93(6):1382–1389.

124. Nemunaitis J. Use of macrophage colony-stimulating factor in the treatment of fungal infections. *Clin Infect Dis* 1998;26(6):1279–1281.

125. Kuderer NM, Dale DC, Crawford J, Lyman GH. Impact of primary prophylaxis with granulocyte colony-stimulating factor on febrile neutropenia and mortality in adult cancer patients receiving chemotherapy: A systematic review. *J Clin Oncol* 2007;25(21):3158–3167.

126. Lyman GH, Dale DC, Wolff DA, Culakova E, Poniewierski MS, Kuderer NM, et al. Acute myeloid leukemia or myelodysplastic syndrome in randomized controlled clinical trials of cancer chemotherapy with granulocyte colony-stimulating factor: A systematic review. *J Clin Oncol* 2010;28(17):2914–2924.

127. Rowe JM. Treatment of acute myeloid leukemia with cytokines: Effect on duration of neutropenia and response to infections. *Clin Infect Dis* 1998;26(6):1290–1294.

128. Rowe JM, Andersen JW, Mazza JJ, Bennett JM, Paietta E, Hayes FA, et al. A randomized placebo-controlled phase III study of granulocyte-macrophage colony-stimulating factor in adult patients (>55 to 70 years of age) with acute myelogenous leukemia: A study of the Eastern Cooperative Oncology Group (E1490). *Blood* 1995;86(2):457–462.

129. Smith TJ, Bohlke K, Lyman GH, Carson KR, Crawford J, Cross SJ, et al. Recommendations for the use of WBC growth factors: American Society of Clinical Oncology clinical practice guideline update. *J Clin Oncol* 2015;33(28):3199–3212.

130. Segal BH, Walsh TJ. Current approaches to diagnosis and treatment of invasive aspergillosis. *Am J Respir Crit Care Med* 2006;173(7):707–717.

131. Price TH, Boeckh M, Harrison RW, McCullough J, Ness PM, Strauss RG, et al. Efficacy of transfusion with granulocytes from G-CSF/dexamethasone-treated donors in neutropenic patients with infection. *Blood* 2015;126(18):2153–2161.

132. Nagai H, Guo J, Choi H, Kurup V. Interferon- and tumor necrosis factor-protect mice from invasive aspergillosis. *J Infect Dis* 1995;172(6):1554–1560.

133. Roilides E, Uhlig K, Venzon D, Pizzo PA, Walsh TJ. Enhancement of oxidative response and damage caused by human neutrophils to *Aspergillus fumigatus* hyphae by granulocyte colony-stimulating factor and gamma interferon. *Infect Immun* 1993;61(4):1185–1193.

134. Roilides E, Holmes A, Blake C, Venzon D, Pizzo PA, Walsh TJ. Antifungal activity of elutriated human monocytes against *Aspergillus fumigatus* hyphae: Enhancement by granulocyte-macrophage colonystimulating factor and Interferon-Y. *J Infect Dis* 1994;170(4):894–899.

135. Roilides E, Uhlig K, Venzon D, Pizzo PA, Walsh TJ. Prevention of corticosteroid-induced suppression of human polymorphonuclear leukocyte-induced damage of *Aspergillus fumigatus* hyphae by granulocyte colony-stimulating factor and gamma interferon. *Infect Immun* 1993;61(11):4870–4877.

136. A controlled trial of interferon gamma to prevent infection in chronic granulomatous disease. *N Engl J Med* 1991;324(8):509–516.

137. Safdar A, Rodriguez G, Ohmagari N, Kontoyiannis DP, Rolston KV, Raad II, et al. The safety of interferon-gamma-1b therapy for invasive fungal infections after hematopoietic stem cell transplantation. *Cancer* 2005;103(4):731–739.

138. Fukuda T, Boeckh M, Guthrie KA, Mattson DK, Owens S, Wald A, et al. Invasive aspergillosis before allogeneic hematopoietic stem cell transplantation: 10-Year experience at a single transplant center. *Biol Blood Marrow Transplant* 2004;10(7):494–503.

139. Offner F, Cordonnier C, Ljungman P, Prentice HG, Engelhard D, De Bacquer D, et al. Impact of previous aspergillosis on the outcome of bone marrow transplantation. *Clin Infect Dis* 1998;26(5):1098–1103.

140. Martino R, Lopez R, Sureda A, Brunet S, Domingo-Albos A. Risk of reactivation of a recent invasive fungal infection in patients with hematological malignancies undergoing further intensive chemo-radiotherapy. A single-center experience and review of the literature. *Haematologica* 1997;82(3):297–304.

18

Management of cryptococcosis

JOHN R. PERFECT AND AHMAD MOURAD

INTRODUCTION

Cryptococcosis is a global invasive mycosis with significant morbidity and mortality [1]. HIV significantly increased the burden of cryptococcal disease with several studies showing that the incidence of cryptococcal disease increased by up to 5-fold with the emergence of the HIV pandemic in developed countries and this was reversed after access to highly active antiretroviral therapy (HAART) [2]. Although the widespread use of HAART has lowered the incidence of cases in medically developed countries [3], the incidence of this infection is extremely high in areas where large numbers of HIV disease still persist and there is limited access to HAART and/or health care. It has been estimated at the peak of the pandemic and before use of HAART that the global burden of HIV-associated cryptococcosis approached a million cases per year with over 700,000 deaths [4]. A recent assessment has lowered the yearly rate to approximately 200,000 cases per year with over 1,200,000 deaths [5]. However, despite widespread availability of HAART in some countries, the rate of cryptococcosis has leveled off at a continued high rate [6,7]. Clearly, cryptococcosis will remain a major invasive fungal infection at present and into the immediate future. Even in medically-developed countries, this infection continues to find new risk groups such as those receiving high doses of corticosteroids, monoclonal antibodies (such as alemtuzumab and infliximab), ibrutinib (tyrosine kinase inhibitor) for cancer therapy, or other immunosuppressive agents used with transplantation [8–10]. Therefore, modern medicine from the severely immunosuppressed patients with HIV infection or organ transplantation to the apparently normal host must deal with the management of this encapsulated yeast with a propensity to invade the central nervous system.

Antifungal drug regimens for the management of cryptococcosis represent some of the best characterized for invasive fungal diseases [1,11,12]. However, there remain many strategy gaps and no new classes of anticryptococcal agent(s) have been developed for use in over 25 years. Furthermore, despite access to advanced medical care with availability to HAART, the 3-month mortality rate during management of acute cryptococcal meningoencephalitis still approximates 20%–30% with less-resourced health care systems reporting approximately 50%, and, without HAART treatment or antifungal agents, certain HIV-infected populations have reported mortality rates of 100% within 2 weeks of presentation to health care facilities [13–15]. It is apparent that there is a wide spectrum of needs for successful management of this life-threatening infection. They revolve around access to antifungal drugs, diagnostic strategies, and adjunctive medical care. However, there are also complex clinical scenarios in which correcting host immunodeficiency and immune reconstitution can be extremely difficult and requires careful clinical strategies one patient at a time.

This chapter attempts to provide information and insights into the management of this infection. The 2000 and updated 2010 IDSA guidelines for management of cryptococcosis have been previously published and form the foundation for this chapter, but there has been an attempt to update clinical practices and principles [16,17].

CRYPTOCOCCAL MENINGOENCEPHALITIS

The treatment strategies for the patient with cryptococcal meningoencephalitis will be divided up into three risk groups (HIV-infected, transplant recipient, and non-HIV, nontransplant host). Although the principles are similar, some risk groups have different demands on management. However, several important issues carry across all patient groups. First, the treatment goal is to rapidly and consistently reduce the burden of yeasts in the host and particularly the central nervous system (CNS). This goal was validated by the landmark clinical trial of Day et al. in which effective fungicidal activity (EFA) was correlated with improved mortality [18]. This therapeutic goal is primarily achieved with a polyene-driven induction regimen and then patients are placed on consolidation/maintenance regimens. Second, there are a series of complications and confounders that need to be addressed in many patients from increased intracranial pressure to immune reconstitution inflammatory syndrome (IRIS). Third, control of the underlying disease will be essential to improve final outcome. For instance, patients with an underlying disease of HIV infection or transplant recipients with cryptococcosis have a better prognosis than disseminated cryptococcosis in a patient with severe liver disease because of our limited abilities to manages the end-stage liver disease [19,20].

HIV-infection with cryptococcal meningoencephalitis

Treatment of cryptococcal meningoencephalitis in an HIV-infected individual is based on the principles of a high burden of cerebrospinal fluid (CSF) yeasts and a severely depressed immune system (profound CD4 lymphocytopenia). In medically-advanced countries, the treatment strategy has been formalized into the concept of induction, consolidation (clearance), and maintenance (suppression) phases. Table 18.1 gives the details and is adapted from the (2010) IDSA Guidelines. It places an emphasis on combination therapy with amphotericin B and flucytosine, which has been shown to be the most fungicidal regimen for cryptococcal meningitis [11,21–23]. It is also noted that with the Van der Horst et al. study, the use of a higher amphotericin B dose (0.7 mg/kg/day) and lower flucytosine dose (100 mg/kg/day) provided the best regimen to reliably sterilize the CSF, and most but not all patients receiving this regimen will be CSF culture negative after 2 weeks of induction therapy [24]. Newer studies have evaluated the use of even higher doses of amphotericin B (1 mg/kg/day) with flucytosine and found that fungicidal activity improved (vs. 0.7 mg/kg/day). However, there was an increase in serious adverse events related to the higher dose [25]. Nonetheless, this substantial rapid reduction in the burden of yeasts is a much better position clinically to start fluconazole treatment in

Table 18.1 Treatment recommendations for cryptococcal meningoencephalitis in HIV-infected individuals

Initial antifungal regimen (induction and consolidation)	Duration
Liposomal AmB 3–4 mg/kg/day or ABLC 5 mg/kg/day[a]	2 weeks
Then fluconazole 400 mg/day	8 weeks
AmBd ≥0.7–1.0 mg/kg/day + 5FC 100 mg/kg/day	2 weeks
Then fluconazole 400 mg/day	8 weeks
AmBd 0.7–1.0 mg/kg/day or liposomal AmB 3–6 mg/kg/day or ABLC 5 mg/kg/day (5FC intolerant)	4–6 weeks
Then fluconazole 400 mg/day	8 weeks
[b]*Alternatives:* AmBd + fluconazole, fluconazole + 5FC, fluconazole, itraconazole	
Maintenance	
Fluconazole 200 mg/day[a]	≥1 year[d]
Alternatives: Itraconazole 400 mg/day[c]	≥1 year[d]
AmBd 1 mg/kg × week[c]	

Source: Perfect, J.R. et al., *Clin. Infect. Dis.*, 50, 291–322, 2010.
Abbreviations: AmBd, amphotericin B deoxycholate; 5FC, flucytosine.
[a] Begin HAART 2–10 weeks after start of initial antifungal treatment.
[b] Alternatives: Because of unique clinical situations, primary recommendations are not available, then consideration of alternative regimens may be made but not encouraged as substitutes.
[c] Inferior to primary recommendation.
[d] With successful introduction of HAART: CD4 count > 100 cells/μL and negative viral load for >3 months with minimum of 1 year of antifungal therapy.

the consolidation and maintenance phases of treatment. It has been shown in multiple studies that fluconazole acts in a fungistatic manner in cryptococcal meningitis and for a significant impact with this azole there needs to be either a small burden of yeasts at the site of infection or very high doses of fluconazole must be administered [26–30]. Therefore, a polyene-based regimen when available is the first-line induction therapy and not an azole alone. In fact, polyene exposure and combination therapy in induction therapy is so critical that when flucytosine is not available in many countries, experts will recommend amphotericin B and fluconazole together. Furthermore, there are now studies demonstrating in resource-limited settings that short course polyene therapy with an azole base can be successful [31]. Thus, the polyene treatment toxicity and interruption of the induction therapy schedule has been found to impact the therapeutic outcome, so that the lipid formulations of amphotericin B have become the primary polyenes of choice in healthcare-resourced countries. This change has occurred despite no formal comparative studies with lipid formulations of amphotericin B and flucytosine together but importantly, it allows a more smooth, consistent induction regimen without drug interruptions. In the general guidelines, it is recommended that induction therapy last at least 2 weeks, but for very high burden CSF yeast infections and those anticipated to have prolonged positive fungal CSF cultures, a longer induction may be necessary, and this is a bedside decision. A complete uninterrupted induction period is so critical to a consistently successful outcome. In patients with developing renal dysfunction, the substitution of lipid formulations of amphotericin B for amphotericin B is appropriate at the doses recommended in Table 18.1 [32–36]. There is now substantial clinical experience that robustly support this strategy but, in fact, the vast majority of treatment strategies today start with the lipid formulations of amphotericin B. There are a series of other alternative induction regimens that might be necessary to consider for a variety of reasons [37–40]. One retrospective meta-analysis did reveal that combining amphotericin B with flucytosine for induction did not improve outcome compared to amphotericin B alone [41] but the vast majority of evidence supports this combination for primary induction therapy. Therefore, not using the standard induction regimen will need to be defended with clinical and economic considerations. Unfortunately, flucytosine is still not available in many areas of the world with high rates of cryptococcal meningoencephalitis and in some areas of the world high prices of flucytosine can challenge the system's ability to pay for it [42]. The consolidation phase allows fluconazole exposure in relatively high doses for approximately 8 weeks and this azole was found to be superior to itraconazole [43]. If the patient continues to be stable, then the patient is placed on maintenance (suppressive) therapy with fluconazole.

Prior to HAART, the relapse rate after initial therapy for cryptococcal meningoencephalitis was high (15%),

and, therefore, several studies validated that fluconazole dramatically reduced relapses and was actually superior to itraconazole and weekly intravenous amphotericin B (1 mg/kg) for this suppression strategy [43–45]. The fluconazole suppressive or maintenance regimen has become an entrenched standard policy in HIV-infected patients and has been frequently continued for at least 1 year. With the immune reconstitution associated with HAART, several studies have now supported discontinuing suppressive therapy with fluconazole when CD4 cell count returns above 100 cell/μL and an undetectable HIV RNA level is sustained for ≥3 months [46–50]. Therefore, clinicians may consider stopping suppressive therapy when the previous conditions of immune reconstitution are met, and the patient has received at least a minimum of 12 months of therapy. If successful with this three-part strategy, the patient can then be followed closely for symptoms and periodic serum cryptococcal antigen tests.

There are several distinct clinical issues related to cryptococcal meningoencephalitis and coinfection with HIV infection.

1. In resource-limited environments, intravenous amphotericin B deoxycholate may not be available or combination therapy with flucytosine nonexistent. High dose amphotericin B deoxycholate (1 mg/kg/day) should be encouraged for ideally 2 weeks, but at least 1 week, of combination therapy during induction period. Studies with even less exposure to a lipid amphotericin B formulation seem to be successful and more formal studies are presently attempting to validate these polyene short courses with daily fluconazole [51]. The polyene-based combination regimen with fluconazole provides induction therapy advantages in its fungicidal activity. If fluconazole is the only drug available for treatment in some countries or certain geographical areas then doses of ≥1200 mg per day of fluconazole are recommended.

2. When does a clinician start HAART during management of meningoencephalitis? There have been suggestions that early HAART administration can be both helpful and deleterious [52]. It can help immune reconstitution but could add to IRIS or drug–drug interaction toxicities so timing of HARRT is critical. A recent landmark study has suggested that delaying HAART for 5 weeks after diagnosis and start of anticryptococcal therapy, improved survival compared to starting HAART within 1 to 2 weeks after diagnosis and start of antifungal treatment [53]. The critical message is that very early HAART is not recommended during cryptococcal meningoencephalitis treatment and the 2010 IDSA Guidelines remain liberal in a 2–10-week window for starting HAART. For countries with less- resourced health care earlier HAART (4–5 weeks) to control the underlying disease may be necessary within this window.

3. Asymptomatic cryptococcal antigenemia (CRAG) can occur in HIV-infected individuals [54–58]. If it is detected, generally clinicians will use this biomarker as a strategy for preemptive therapy. It is recommended that blood and CSF cultures are obtained to rule out proven disease but if cultures are negative most clinicians still would consider fluconazole therapy until immune reconstitution occurs with HAART in asymptomatic cryptococcal antigenemia patients. For example, a positive CRAG in a HIV-infected individual with low CD4 count does identify a patient who is higher risk of dying in the next 1–3 years [59]. There have now been policies to integrate a cheap accurate lateral flow assay (LFA) testing during HAART assessment in areas with a 2%–3% general prevalence of CRAG positivity. To further bolster its impact, there is recent data suggesting high serum CRAG titers (≥1:160) in an asymptomatic patient should signal an initiation of a lumbar puncture for detection of CNS disease and potentially more aggressive preemptive therapies.

4. Primary antifungal prophylaxis for cryptococcosis. A retrospective meta-analysis has shown that primary prophylaxis reduced the incidence of cryptococcal meningoencephalitis but did not decrease overall mortality. However, there was some benefit in resource-limited settings [60]. Therefore, although it is not routinely recommended in HIV-infected patients in developed countries, in areas with limited HAART availability, high antiretroviral drug resistance, and high burden of cryptococcal disease, consideration of prophylaxis or a preemptive strategy using the serum CRAG might be advisable [61,62]. Because of costs and potential development of drug resistance, most high incidence areas have generally followed the pathway of preemptive therapy based on CRAG testing.

Organ transplant recipients

Cryptococcosis has been found in approximately 2%–3% of solid organ transplant recipients and the majority of disease will occur after the first 1–2 years posttransplant and most individuals have disseminated disease on presentation [63–66]. Cases occur due to reactivation of prior infections, acquisition of a new infection from the environment or even acquired through the transplanted organ [67]. In many respects, the strategies for treatment in the highly immunosuppressed transplant recipients are similar to HIV-infected patients (Table 18.2). However, an important emphasis is that these patients have potentially compromised renal functions or are receiving nephrotoxic agents, such as calcineurin inhibitors, and, therefore, lipid formulations of amphotericin B are particularly preferred polyenes for induction therapy in these particular patients [68]. Also, there needs to be a concerted effort to carefully adjust the immunosuppressive drugs used in this risk group. Following the recommendations in Table 18.2, there is a good chance for treatment success

Table 18.2 Treatment recommendations for cryptococcal meningoencephalitis in transplant recipients

Initial antifungal regimen[a] (induction and consolidation)	Duration
Liposomal AmB 3–4 mg/kg/day or ABLC 5 mg/kg/day + 5FC 100 mg/kg/day	2 weeks
Then fluconazole 400–800 mg/day	8 weeks
Alternative: Liposomal AmB 6 mg/kg/day or ABLC 5 mg/kg/day	4–6 weeks
Then fluconazole 400–800 mg/day	8 weeks
AmB use (must weigh risk of renal dysfunction)[b]	(see lipid products of AmB)
Maintenance	
Fluconazole 200 mg/day	6 months–1 year

Source: Perfect, J.R. et al., *Clin. Infect. Dis.*, 50, 291–322, 2010.
Abbreviations: AmBd, amphotericin B deoxycholate; 5FC, flucytosine; ABLC, amphotericin B lipid complex.
[a] Immunosuppressive management may require sequential or step-wise reductions.
[b] Many transplant recipients have been successfully managed with AmBd; however, issues of renal dysfunction with calcineurin inhibitors are important.

but there are several issues with transplant recipients and their cryptococcal disease management:

First, transplant recipients with disseminated disease are generally treated for a total of at least 1 year. Second, immunosuppressive management should include an individualized sequential or step-wise reduction of immunosuppressants with corticosteroids being considered the first adjusted immunosuppressive, since calcineurin inhibitors may have some direct anticryptococcal activity and even synergize the antifungal activity of the azole treatments [69]. Third, it is important to recognize IRIS in these patients since its appearance may be diagnosed as failure and/or associated with organ rejection. Fourth, if a patient received 1 year of antifungal treatment and is off an antifungal drug for another year with normal CSF, consideration for transplantation or re-transplantation could be re-initiated (e.g., renal transplants). Finally, transplanted organs may contain Cryptococcus at the time of transplantation. If this is detected, it will require that the recipient be aggressively treated because the risk of disseminated yeast disease from the transplanted organ is substantial in these cases.

Non-HIV, non-transplant hosts

This is a heterogeneous group of patients from liver to connective tissue diseases to sarcoidosis and many of these disease processes are linked to the use of corticosteroids [70,71]. There is also the "presumably immunocompetent hosts" in which it is difficult to define their immune state. Recently, some in this group have been found to possess autoantibodies to GM-CSF [72,73]. However, it is clear that those with apparently much less severe or variable immune defects, compared with HIV infection or transplant recipients, can present significant therapeutic challenges [74]. There have been few studies in this group since the classical comparative studies of Bennett and Dismukes in the 1970s and 1980s [75,76]. In these studies, the combination of amphotericin B and fl in these was validated as an effective regimen, and the length of induction therapy for 6 weeks appeared better than 4 weeks [76]. However, despite the guidance of these studies, the use of higher doses of the polyene today and the integration of fluconazole in the therapeutic strategy has transformed the proposed management of cryptococcal meningoencephalitis in this risk group without robust studies for the present recommendations. In Table 18.3, there is a set of guidelines for the treatment of cryptococcal meningoencephalitis in this group and they represent reasonable starting points for management, but future studies are needed to precisely determine best strategies and as can be observed these guidelines have been co-opted from the severely immunosuppressed populations. Relapse of cryptococcal meningoencephalitis in the non-HIV-infected patient ranged from 15% to 25% prior to the AIDS epidemic and integration of fluconazole use and thus there has been a focus to treat (suppress) patients for at least a year with fluconazole after induction and consolidation phases of treatment

Table 18.3 Treatment recommendations for cryptococcal meningoencephalitis in non-HIV-infected and nontransplant individuals

Initial antifungal regimen	Duration
AmBd ≥0.7–1.0 mg/kg/day + 5FC 100 mg/kg/day	≥4 weeks[a,b]
AmBd ≥0.7–1.0 mg/kg/day (5FC intolerant)	≥6 weeks[a,b]
Liposomal AmB 3–4 mg/kg/day or ABLC 5 mg/kg/day combined with 5FC when possible (AmBd intolerant)	≥4 weeks[a,b]
AmBd 0.7 mg/kg/day + 5FC 100 mg/kg/day (low-risk patients for therapeutic failure)[c]	2 weeks
Consolidation	
Fluconazole 400 mg/day	8 weeks
Maintenance	
Fluconazole 200 mg/day[b]	6–12 months

Source: Perfect, J.R. et al., Clin. Infect. Dis., 50, 291–322, 2010.
Abbreviations: AmBd, amphotericin B; 5FC, flucytosine.
[a] Four weeks are reserved for patients with meningitis without neurological complications; no significant underlying diseases or immunosuppression and with end of two weeks treatment CSF sample without viable yeasts on culture; second two weeks may substitute LF AmB for AmBd.
[b] Fluconazole at 200 mg daily to prevent relapse following induction and consolidation therapy is recommended.
[c] Low risk = early diagnosis by history, no uncontrolled underlying or immunocompromised state, excellent response to initial two weeks combination course.

and this strategy likely reduces true relapses. Actually, the recommendations of 4–6 weeks induction therapy in this group reflects both the worse prognosis of this group and the lack of recent randomized studies. However, many clinicians still will use a 2-week induction therapy with the combination of polyene and flucytosine similar to HIV and transplant recipients. The value of the extending the induction therapy period will depend on overall prognosis status and initial clinical response of the patient.

ISSUES WITH MANAGEMENT OF CRYPTOCOCCAL MENINGOENCEPHALITIS

There are a series of complications that may occur during management of cryptococcal meningoencephalitis, and the following issues are specifically examined: (i) persistence/relapse, (ii) increased intracranial pressure, (iii) immune reconstitution inflammatory syndrome (IRIS), and (iv) cryptococcomas.

Persistence/relapse

The definition of persistent infection is arbitrary but a reasonable starting point is persistently positive CSF cultures after 4 weeks of proven antifungal therapy at a proper dose as suggested by 2010 IDSA Guidelines. Relapse has three features: recovery of viable yeasts from CSF, previous cultures at the site are negative, and recrudescence of signs and symptoms. It is important to note that positive India ink exams, changing antigen titers, and abnormal cellular reactions or chemistries are insufficient to alter direct antifungal treatment strategies [77]. Most cases of relapse are due to inadequate primary induction therapy or failure of compliance with outpatient regimens. In these cases, it is important to check initial and relapse isolates for direct in vitro drug resistance since there are a few direct drug resistance strains [78–80]. Although there are no formal in vitro susceptibility breakpoints established for Cryptococcus, a MICs ≥16 μg/mL for fluconazole may be associated with treatment failure [81–83]. It may be best to compare the two isolates and an increase of 3 dilutions or greater in the relapse isolate over the initial isolate may support the yeast strain acquiring direct antifungal resistance. Furthermore, most primary isolates of C. neoformans and C. gattii do not have high MICs by direct in vitro susceptibility testing [78]. In most cases of true relapse there will be a need to reintroduce an induction regimen with at least a polyene for a longer period of re-introduction time and then ensure compliance. In some cases, voriconazole or posaconazole might be considered for the suppressive phase of treatment but in most cases these agents will not likely improve outcome over readministration of high doses of fluconazole [84,85]. One randomized controlled trial has shown that adjunctive interferon gamma increases the rate of yeast clearance within CSF with no reported significant adverse events and although its use has not been formalized in initial therapies, it might be tried in difficult relapse cases with other antifungal therapies [86]. However, there may not be enough data to make confident conclusions regarding its routine use and its administration must be assessed on an individual basis [86]. There have also been well-established reports of anti-GM-CSF antibodies being produced in immunocompetent patients with cryptococcal meningoencephalitis and prompting the suggestion that administering GM-CSF to these specific patients could be of utility [72,73]. However, GM-CSF has rarely been used in cryptococcosis, and there is too little data to make any specific comment on its usefulness in cryptococcosis [87].

Elevated cerebrospinal fluid (CSF)/pressure

One of the most critical acute determinants of cryptococcal meningoencephalitis outcome is control of CSF pressure [88,89]. Approximately half the HIV-infected patients with cryptococcal CNS disease have elevated baseline intracranial pressures (>25 cm of CSF) and this CSF pressure can rise further as treatment is started with a subsequent increased morbidity and mortality [88]. Most patients in resource-available health care systems will receive CT/MRI scan on their initial evaluation and any patients without mass lesions but with persistent symptoms and increased intracranial pressure should have repeated daily lumbar punctures. If symptoms persist after several days of CSF withdrawal strategy, then lumbar drains can be considered [90]. Ventriculo-peritoneal (VP) shunts are a more permanent solution and are used in subacute/chronic conditions of hydrocephalus [91]. Generally, these VP shunts can be placed during active infection if appropriate antifungals agents have been started [92,93]. Increased intracranial pressure in cryptococcosis is not helped by medical treatments like acetazolamide, corticosteroids, and mannitol [89,94]. If there is a careful effort to control intracranial pressure, outcomes of these CNS infections appear to be improved and unfortunately, at this point only retrospective data have favored the use of repeated lumbar punctures [95].

Immune reconstitution inflammatory syndrome (IRIS)

In cryptococcosis, IRIS can occur in two forms: (i) unmasking IRIS when cryptococcal symptoms first appear after the start of HAART or (ii) paradoxical IRIS during the treatment of cryptococcosis and administration of HAART [96–100]. It is important to emphasize that Cryptococcus-associated IRIS has also been reported as a complication in both solid organ transplant recipients and normal hosts as well as HIV-infected individuals [74,101]. Cryptococcosis lives within the classic Goldilocks' immunity paradigm of "not too much or not too little immunity but need to get it just right" [102]. Many times, cryptococcosis occurs when immunity is depressed and during treatment the goal is to improve immunity but subsequently the host overshoots its immune attack. In many cases, IRIS just needs to be

identified and observed but in the CNS the excess inflammation can cause new, prolonged and even life-threatening symptoms. With major complications such as CNS inflammation with an associated increased CSF intracranial pressure, consideration of corticosteroid therapy may be necessary for IRIS management [103].

For instance, in a cohort of patients with cryptococcal spinal arachnoiditis, it was shown that excess inflammatory and neuronal damage markers at the site of infection prolonged symptoms, but they improved with corticosteroid therapy [104]. It is clear that routine use of dexamethasone in treatment of cryptococcal meningitis may be harmful with prolonged killing of yeasts and increased morbidity during steroid therapy; however, its specific use during IRIS can be life-saving [15]. Based mainly on expert opinion, generally, a taper of corticosteroids is considered over 2–6 weeks or even the tapered dexamethasone regimen used in tuberculosis might be beneficial [105]. There have also been salvage/refractory reports of anti-TNF-α and thalidomide use for treatment of IRIS but no robust recommendations for management with these agents [106,107]. It is important to realize that IRIS may present early in the management of meningitis or after several months of treatment. There are a series of criteria reported to diagnose IRIS but in sum, it is increased inflammation with all biomarkers or cultures for yeasts either reducing or negative. A recent small study, which needs confirmation, suggests that a positive Biofire® PCR test can distinguish fungal infection relapse from IRIS [108]. IRIS must be considered in all patients when new symptoms and radiographic findings occur suggesting failure while receiving appropriate antifungal therapy [109]. In transplant patients, IRIS can actually lead to graft loss [101].

Cerebral cryptococcomas

Cerebral cryptococcomas can cause significant short- and long-term sequela. They are more commonly observed in *C. gattii* infections but may also be detected in *C. neoformans* infections. It is essential in severely immunosuppressed patients with a nonresponding parenchymal brain mass(s) that the mass may also be considered as caused by a second pathogen, and a brain biopsy or aspirate will be necessary. However, most of these lesions in the presence of known cryptococcal meningoencephalitis are cryptococcal parenchymal lesions, which change their sizes slowly with host immune recovery and antifungal therapies. Brain lesions detected by CT scan are seen in apparently normal hosts (14%), AIDS patients (4%–5%), or those with other risk factors (10%). Although there are no definitive studies for CNS cryptococcoma management, recommendations are based on case reports, retrospective and prospective observational studies, and expert opinions. In general, an induction regimen with amphotericin B and flucytosine is prolonged and the suppressive phase with fluconazole is also extended from 1–2 years. Of course, these guidelines can be adjusted depending on the patient's response and other underlying conditions. However, radiographically it may take a long time for these lesions to completely disappear [110]. The successful use of anti-TNF-α monoclonal antibody to reduce inflammation has been reported in a cerebral cryptococcoma management in the setting of IRIS [111]. In very large cryptococcomas (>3 cm) there have been successful cases managed in which surgically the parenchymal lesion was debulked. However, surgery should probably be reserved for persistently symptomatic individuals.

CRYPTOCOCCAL MENINGOENCEPHALITIS TREATMENT IN SPECIAL CLINICAL SITUATIONS

1. *Pregnancy [112–115]*
   The goal is to use a polyene regimen and avoid fluconazole, especially early in pregnancy (first trimester) [116]. The use of flucytosine must be a bedside decision. It is important to watch for IRIS during the postpartum period [117].
2. *Children [118–123]*
   Cryptococcal disease occurs less frequently in children than in adults. There are some unique childhood conditions, such as Hyper IgM Syndrome, Severe Combined Immunodeficiency Syndrome, Acute Lymphoblastic Leukemia, and Sarcoma, associated with pediatric cryptococcosis. In general, pediatric meningoencephalitis is treated like it is with an adult except higher doses of amphotericin B and lipid formulations can be used, and, similarly, fluconazole dosing is increased to approximate a child's metabolism and clearance [124,125].

CRYPTOCOCCOSIS IN A RESOURCE-LIMITED HEALTH ENVIRONMENT

Sub-Saharan Africa is a common area for cryptococcal disease and it is primarily related to HIV infection. Details of treatment issues have been addressed by multiple studies, but, specifically, more aggressive induction therapy is needed with either short courses of high doses of intravenous amphotericin B (1 mg/kg/day for 1–2 weeks) or lipid formulations of amphotericin B and/or high doses of fluconazole (≥1200 mg/day) [25,126–129].

CRYPTOCOCCUS GATTII INFECTIONS

Infections caused by this species predominantly occur in apparently normal hosts or those with cancer although occasionally there are HIV-infected and transplant recipient cases [130,131]. Despite some very difficult cases because of IRIS and variable drug susceptibility, at present most clinicians still treat *C. gattii* infections similar to *C. neoformans* infections [132,133]. In fact, recent data suggest that mortality from *C. gattii* infections is less than *C. neoformans* infections [134].

Table 18.4 Recommendations for nonmeningeal cryptococcosis

Initial antifungal regimen	Duration
Immunosuppressed and immunocompetent patient with pulmonary cryptococcosis (mild-to-moderate), fluconazole 400 mg/day	6–12 months
Immunosuppressed[a] and immunocompetent patients with pulmonary cryptococcosis (severe), same as CNS disease	12 months
Nonmeningeal, nonpulmonary cryptococcosis	
1. Cryptococcemia, same as CNS disease	12 months
2. CNS disease ruled out and no fungemia, single site, and no immunosuppressive risk factor, fluconazole 400 mg/day	6–12 months

Source: Perfect, J.R. et al., *Clin. Infect. Dis.*, 50, 291–322, 2010.
[a] Must directly rule out CNS disease with lumbar puncture.

The appropriate treatment strategies for patients with nonmeningeal cryptococcosis have been much less studied, and only pulmonary cryptococcosis has enough cases reported to make robust recommendations (Table 18.4).

PULMONARY CRYPTOCOCCOSIS

Pulmonary cryptococcosis includes clinical presentations ranging from asymptomatic colonization to pneumonia to severe acute respiratory distress syndrome [135–139]. Once Cryptococcus is isolated from the lung or airway of the host, there is an assessment of whether the patient is immunosuppressed or not. An immunosuppressed patient needs consideration of a lumbar puncture to rule out CNS disease even in a patient who is asymptomatic. In the immunocompetent patient who has no CNS symptoms or signs, it is less critical to determine whether CNS involvement has occurred since it is very unlikely to present in the CNS in this group without symptoms [140,141]. Of course, it is important to identify CNS cryptococcosis since it has a different induction therapeutic regimen and prognosis. Pneumonia associated with CNS or documented dissemination and/or severe pneumonia (ARDS) should be treated like CNS disease as outlined in the prior sections. However, for those with mild-to-moderate symptoms or simply positive cultures or histopathology from a pulmonary lesion, fluconazole 400 mg/day for 6–12 month is a reasonable starting strategy [141–143]. It can be adapted depending on patient's response, condition, and the impact of other therapies like starting HAART or stopping monoclonal antibodies like anti-TNF-α or anti-CD52. Although some clinicians do not treat what is diagnosed as asymptomatic airway colonization or lung nodule(s) in a normal host, others recommend treating all patients with viable Cryptococcus isolated from the airways. Since there are no randomized, prospective drug studies, the dose and duration of fluconazole is not precise and represents clinical experience and opinions more than robust evidence-based studies.

The nonmeningeal, nonpulmonary cryptococcosis is not common [144–148]. There are occasional cases of primary (inoculation) skin infection, but most skin infections are primarily the consequence of dissemination even if only a single site is identified. In these cases, one should check HIV test and work-up symptoms/signs and body sites, such as CSF and blood. If cryptococcemia or high-level dissemination (at least two noncontiguous sites) is involved or if there is evidence of high fungal burden based on cryptococcal antigen ≥1:512, then treat as CNS disease. If CNS disease is ruled out such as no fungemia, single site, and no major immunosuppressive risk factor(s), then consider fluconazole 400 mg/day for 6–12 months for mild, non-CNS disease.

Cryptococcal infection can involve any body site or structure such as liver, bone, lymph nodes, peritoneum, kidney, adrenal, or eyes. In the ocular infections, there will be a need for individualized strategy depending on the extent of ocular involvement. Consulting an ophthalmologist will be necessary since antifungal drugs like fluconazole and flinfeosine penetrate eye tissue well, but the patient may also need intravitreal amphotericin B.

CRAG SCREENING OF HIGH-RISK INDIVIDUALS

Cryptococcal antigen (CRAG) is a polysaccharide antigen that can be detected in serum more than 3 weeks before onset of symptoms of cryptococcal meningoencephalitis. The percentage of patients with HIV who test positive for CRAG is measurable, and CRAG positivity has been significantly correlated with decreased survival [149]. This brings to question whether CRAG testing should be routinely performed on HIV patients with low CD4 counts in areas of known endemicity for CRAG positivity in HIV-infected patients (≥2%–3% prevalence of CRAG positivity). In 2011, the World Health Organization (WHO) recommended that HIV patients with CD4 ≤100 cells/μL be tested for cryptococcal infection [150]. Once positivity is established, initiation of preemptive antifungal therapy with fluconazole has been shown to decrease incidence of cryptococcal disease and improve survival [151,152]. This strategy has been proven to be cost-effective in resource-limited settings [151]. With the development of cheap, accurate lateral flow assays using serum or CSF, CRAG can be detected with a sensitivity and specificity approaching 100% [153] and potentially improving costs. The utility of this preemptive strategy must also be assessed thoroughly in developed countries as it may have the potential to improve outcomes significantly. A recent issue has been an attempt to make the CRAG test

more effective in screening. It appears that titers of 1:160 or greater predict disseminated disease and require more aggressive diagnostics and drug treatments [154].

REFERENCES

1. Chayakulkeeree M, Perfect JR. Cryptococcosis. *Infect Dis Clin North Am* 2006;20(3):507–544, v–vi.
2. Sloan DJ, Parris V. Cryptococcal meningitis: Epidemiology and therapeutic options. *Clin Epidemiol* 2014;6:169–182.
3. van Elden LJ, Walenkamp AM, Lipovsky MM, Reiss P, Meis JF, de Marie S, et al. Declining number of patients with cryptococcosis in the Netherlands in the era of highly active antiretroviral therapy. *AIDS* 2000;14(17):2787–2788.
4. Park BJ, Wannemuehler KA, Marston BJ, Govender N, Pappas PG, Chiller TM. Estimation of the current global burden of cryptococcal meningitis among persons living with HIV/AIDS. *AIDS* 2009;23(4):525–530.
5. Rajasingham R, Smith RM, Park BJ, et al. Global burden of disease of HIV-associated cryptococcal meningitis: An updated analysis. *Lancet Infect Dis* 2017;17:873–881.
6. Tenforde MW, Mokomane M, Leeme T, et al. Advance HIV disease in Botswana following successful antiretroviral therapy rollout: Incidence of and temporal trends in cryptococcal meningitis. *Clin Infect Dis* 2017;65:779–786.
7. Scriven JE, Lalloo DG, Meintjes G. Changing epidemiology of HIV-associated cryptococcosis in sub-Saharan Africa. *Lancet Infect Dis* 2016;16(8):891–892.
8. Messina JA, Maziarz EK, Spec A, Kontoyiannis DP, Perfect JR. Disseminated cryptococcosis with brain involvement in patients with chronic lymphoid malignancies on ibrutinib. *Open Forum Infect Dis* 2017;4(1):ofw261.
9. Nath DS, Kandaswamy R, Gruessner R, Sutherland DE, Dunn DL, Humar A. Fungal infections in transplant recipients receiving alemtuzumab. *Transplant Proc* 2005;37(2):934–936.
10. Hage CA, Wood KL, Winer-Muram HT, Wilson SJ, Sarosi G, Knox KS. Pulmonary cryptococcosis after initiation of anti-tumor necrosis factor-alpha therapy. *Chest* 2003;124(6):2395–2397.
11. Dromer F, Bernede-Bauduin C, Guillemot D, Lortholary O, French Cryptococcosis Study Group. Major role for amphotericin B-flucytosine combination in severe cryptococcosis. *PLoS One* 2008;3(8):e2870.
12. Dromer F, Mathoulin-Pelissier S, Launay O, Lortholary O, French Cryptococcosis Study Group. Determinants of disease presentation and outcome during cryptococcosis: The CryptoA/D study. *PLoS Med* 2007;4(2):e21.

13. Hakim JG, Gangaidzo IT, Heyderman RS, Mielke J, Mushangi E, Taziwa A, et al. Impact of HIV infection on meningitis in Harare, Zimbabwe: A prospective study of 406 predominantly adult patients. *AIDS* 2000;14(10):1401–1407.

14. Bratton EW, El Husseini N, Chastain CA, Lee MS, Poole C, Sturmer T, et al. Comparison and temporal trends of three groups with cryptococcosis: HIV-infected, solid organ transplant, and HIV-negative/non-transplant. *PLoS One* 2012;7(8):e43582.

15. Beardsley J, Wolbers M, Kibengo FM, Ggayi AB, Kamali A, Cuc NT, et al. Adjunctive dexamethasone in HIV-associated cryptococcal meningitis. *N Engl J Med* 2016;374(6):542–554.

16. Saag MS, Graybill RJ, Larsen RA, Pappas PG, Perfect JR, Powderly WG, et al. Practice guidelines for the management of cryptococcal disease. Infectious Diseases Society of America. *Clin Infect Dis* 2000;30(4):710–718.

17. Perfect JR, Dismukes WE, Dromer F, Goldman DL, Graybill JR, Hamill RJ, et al. Clinical practice guidelines for the management of cryptococcal disease: 2010 update by the Infectious Diseases Society of America. *Clin Infect Dis* 2010;50(3):291–322.

18. Day JN, Chau TT, Wolbers M, Mai PP, Dung NT, Mai NH, et al. Combination antifungal therapy for cryptococcal meningitis. *N Engl J Med* 2013;368(14):1291–1302.

19. Bratton EW, El Husseini N, Chastain CA, Lee MS, Poole C, Sturmer T, et al. Approaches to antifungal therapies and their effectiveness among patients with cryptococcosis. *Antimicrob Agents Chemother* 2013;57(6):2485–2495.

20. Spec A, Raval K, Powderly WG. End-stage liver disease is a strong predictor of early mortality in cryptococcosis. *Open Forum Infect Dis* 2016;3(1):ofv197.

21. Brouwer AE, Rajanuwong A, Chierakul W, Griffin GE, Larsen RA, White NJ, et al. Combination antifungal therapies for HIV-associated cryptococcal meningitis: A randomised trial. *Lancet* 2004;363(9423):1764–1767.

22. Larsen RA, Leal MA, Chan LS. Fluconazole compared with amphotericin B plus flucytosine for cryptococcal meningitis in AIDS. A randomized trial. *Ann Intern Med* 1990;113(3):183–187.

23. de Gans J, Portegies P, Tiessens G, Eeftinck Schattenkerk JK, van Boxtel CJ, van Ketel RJ, et al. Itraconazole compared with amphotericin B plus flucytosine in AIDS patients with cryptococcal meningitis. *AIDS* 1992;6(2):185–190.

24. van der Horst CM, Saag MS, Cloud GA, Hamill RJ, Graybill JR, Sobel JD, et al. Treatment of cryptococcal meningitis associated with the acquired immunodeficiency syndrome. National Institute of Allergy and Infectious Diseases Mycoses Study Group and AIDS Clinical Trials Group. *N Engl J Med* 1997;337(1):15–21.

25. Bicanic T, Wood R, Meintjes G, Rebe K, Brouwer A, Loyse A, et al. High-dose amphotericin B with flucytosine for the treatment of cryptococcal meningitis in HIV-infected patients: A randomized trial. *Clin Infect Dis* 2008;47(1):123–130.

26. Bicanic T, Meintjes G, Wood R, Hayes M, Rebe K, Bekker LG, et al. Fungal burden, early fungicidal activity, and outcome in cryptococcal meningitis in antiretroviral-naive or antiretroviral-experienced patients treated with amphotericin B or fluconazole. *Clin Infect Dis* 2007;45(1):76–80.

27. Robinson PA, Bauer M, Leal MA, Evans SG, Holtom PD, Diamond DA, et al. Early mycological treatment failure in AIDS-associated cryptococcal meningitis. *Clin Infect Dis* 1999;28(1):82–92.

28. Saag MS, Powderly WG, Cloud GA, Robinson P, Grieco MH, Sharkey PK, et al. Comparison of amphotericin B with fluconazole in the treatment of acute AIDS-associated cryptococcal meningitis. The NIAID Mycoses Study Group and the AIDS Clinical Trials Group. *N Engl J Med* 1992;326(2):83–89.

29. Menichetti F, Fiorio M, Tosti A, Gatti G, Bruna Pasticci M, Miletich F, et al. High-dose fluconazole therapy for cryptococcal meningitis in patients with AIDS. *Clin Infect Dis* 1996;22(5):838–840.

30. Haubrich RH, Haghighat D, Bozzette SA, Tilles J, McCutchan JA. High-dose fluconazole for treatment of cryptococcal disease in patients with human immunodeficiency virus infection. The California Collaborative Treatment Group. *J Infect Dis* 1994;170(1):238–242.

31. Bicanic T, Bottomley C, Loyse A, Brouwer AE, Muzoora C, Taseera K, et al. Toxicity of amphotericin B deoxycholate-based induction therapy in patients with HIV-associated cryptococcal meningitis. *Antimicrob Agents Chemother* 2015;59(12):7224–7231.

32. Leenders AC, Reiss P, Portegies P, Clezy K, Hop WC, Hoy J, et al. Liposomal amphotericin B (AmBisome) compared with amphotericin B both followed by oral fluconazole in the treatment of AIDS-associated cryptococcal meningitis. *AIDS* 1997;11(12):1463–1471.

33. Sharkey PK, Graybill JR, Johnson ES, Hausrath SG, Pollard RB, Kolokathis A, et al. Amphotericin B lipid complex compared with amphotericin B in the treatment of cryptococcal meningitis in patients with AIDS. *Clin Infect Dis* 1996;22(2):315–321.

34. Baddour LM, Perfect JR, Ostrosky-Zeichner L. Successful use of amphotericin B lipid complex in the treatment of cryptococcosis. *Clin Infect Dis* 2005;40 Suppl 6:S409–S413.

35. Coker RJ, Viviani M, Gazzard BG, Du Pont B, Pohle HD, Murphy SM, et al. Treatment of cryptococcosis with liposomal amphotericin B (AmBisome) in 23 patients with AIDS. *AIDS* 1993;7(6):829–835.

36. Hamill RJ, Sobel JD, El-Sadr W, Johnson PC, Graybill JR, Javaly K, et al. Comparison of 2 doses of liposomal amphotericin B and conventional amphotericin B deoxycholate for treatment of AIDS-associated acute cryptococcal meningitis: A randomized, double-blind clinical trial of efficacy and safety. *Clin Infect Dis* 2010;51(2):225–232.

37. Larsen RA, Bozzette SA, Jones BE, Haghighat D, Leal MA, Forthal D, et al. Fluconazole combined with flucytosine for treatment of cryptococcal meningitis in patients with AIDS. *Clin Infect Dis* 1994;19(4):741–745.

38. Mayanja-Kizza H, Oishi K, Mitarai S, Yamashita H, Nalongo K, Watanabe K, et al. Combination therapy with fluconazole and flucytosine for cryptococcal meningitis in Ugandan patients with AIDS. *Clin Infect Dis* 1998;26(6):1362–1366.

39. Milefchik E, Leal MA, Haubrich R, Bozzette SA, Tilles JG, Leedom JM, et al. Fluconazole alone or combined with flucytosine for the treatment of AIDS-associated cryptococcal meningitis. *Med Mycol* 2008;46(4):393–395.

40. Pappas PG, Chetchotisakd P, Larsen RA, Manosuthi W, Morris MI, Anekthananon T, et al. A phase II randomized trial of amphotericin B alone or combined with fluconazole in the treatment of HIV-associated cryptococcal meningitis. *Clin Infect Dis* 2009;48(12):1775–1783.

41. Campbell JI, Kanters S, Bennett JE, Thorlund K, Tsai AC, Mills EJ, et al. Comparative effectiveness of induction therapy for human immunodeficiency virus-associated cryptococcal meningitis: A network meta-analysis. *Open Forum Infect Dis* 2015;2(1):ofv010.

42. Perfect JR. Editorial Commentary: Life-saving antimicrobial drugs: What are we doing to pricing and availability? *Clin Infect Dis* 2016;62(12):1569–1570.

43. Saag MS, Cloud GA, Graybill JR, Sobel JD, Tuazon CU, Johnson PC, et al. A comparison of itraconazole versus fluconazole as maintenance therapy for AIDS-associated cryptococcal meningitis. National Institute of Allergy and Infectious Diseases Mycoses Study Group. *Clin Infect Dis* 1999;28(2):291–296.

44. Bozzette SA, Larsen RA, Chiu J, Leal MA, Jacobsen J, Rothman P, et al. A placebo-controlled trial of maintenance therapy with fluconazole after treatment of cryptococcal meningitis in the acquired immunodeficiency syndrome. California Collaborative Treatment Group. *N Engl J Med* 1991;324(9):580–584.

45. Powderly WG, Saag MS, Cloud GA, Robinson P, Meyer RD, Jacobson JM, et al. A controlled trial of fluconazole or amphotericin B to prevent relapse of cryptococcal meningitis in patients with the acquired immunodeficiency syndrome. The NIAID AIDS Clinical Trials Group and Mycoses Study Group. *N Engl J Med* 1992;326(12):793–798.

46. Mussini C, Pezzotti P, Miro JM, Martinez E, de Quiros JC, Cinque P, et al. Discontinuation of maintenance therapy for cryptococcal meningitis in patients with AIDS treated with highly active antiretroviral therapy: An international observational study. *Clin Infect Dis* 2004;38(4):565–571.

47. Vibhagool A, Sungkanuparph S, Mootsikapun P, Chetchotisakd P, Tansuphaswaswadikul S, Bowonwatanuwong C, et al. Discontinuation of secondary prophylaxis for cryptococcal meningitis in human immunodeficiency virus-infected patients treated with highly active antiretroviral therapy: A prospective, multicenter, randomized study. *Clin Infect Dis* 2003;36(10):1329–1331.

48. Aberg JA, Price RW, Heeren DM, Bredt B. A pilot study of the discontinuation of antifungal therapy for disseminated cryptococcal disease in patients with acquired immunodeficiency syndrome, following immunologic response to antiretroviral therapy. *J Infect Dis* 2002;185(8):1179–1182.

49. Martinez E, Garcia-Viejo MA, Marcos MA, Perez-Cuevas JB, Blanco JL, Mallolas J, et al. Discontinuation of secondary prophylaxis for cryptococcal meningitis in HIV-infected patients responding to highly active antiretroviral therapy. *AIDS* 2000;14(16):2615–2617.

50. Rollot F, Bossi P, Tubiana R, Caumes E, Zeller V, Katlama C, et al. Discontinuation of secondary prophylaxis against cryptococcosis in patients with AIDS receiving highly active antiretroviral therapy. *AIDS* 2001;15(11):1448–1449.

51. Molefi M, Chofle AA, Molloy SF, Kalluvya S, Changalucha JM, Cainelli F, et al. AMBITION-cm: Intermittent high dose AmBisome on a high dose fluconazole backbone for cryptococcal meningitis induction therapy in sub-Saharan Africa: Study protocol for a randomized controlled trial. *Trials* 2015;16:276.

52. Zolopa A, Andersen J, Powderly W, Sanchez A, Sanne I, Suckow C, et al. Early antiretroviral therapy reduces AIDS progression/death in individuals with acute opportunistic infections: A multicenter randomized strategy trial. *PLoS One* 2009;4(5):e5575.

53. Boulware DR, Meya DB, Muzoora C, Rolfes MA, Huppler Hullsiek K, Musubire A, et al. Timing of antiretroviral therapy after diagnosis of cryptococcal meningitis. *N Engl J Med* 2014;370(26):2487–2498.

54. Tassie JM, Pepper L, Fogg C, Biraro S, Mayanja B, Andia I, et al. Systematic screening of cryptococcal antigenemia in HIV-positive adults in Uganda. *J Acquir Immune Defic Syndr* 2003;33(3):411–412.

55. Nelson MR, Bower M, Smith D, Reed C, Shanson D, Gazzard B. The value of serum cryptococcal antigen in the diagnosis of cryptococcal infection in patients infected with the human immunodeficiency virus. *J Infect* 1990;21(2):175–181.

56. Desmet P, Kayembe KD, De Vroey C. The value of cryptococcal serum antigen screening among HIV-positive/AIDS patients in Kinshasa, Zaire. *AIDS* 1989;3(2):77–78.

57. Liechty CA, Solberg P, Were W, Ekwaru JP, Ransom RL, Weidle PJ, et al. Asymptomatic serum cryptococcal antigenemia and early mortality during antiretroviral therapy in rural Uganda. *Trop Med Int Health* 2007;12(8):929–935.

58. Micol R, Lortholary O, Sar B, Laureillard D, Ngeth C, Dousset JP, et al. Prevalence, determinants of positivity, and clinical utility of cryptococcal antigenemia in Cambodian HIV-infected patients. *J Acquir Immune Defic Syndr* 2007;45(5):555–559.

59. Jarvis JN, Lawn SD, Vogt M, Bangani N, Wood R, Harrison TS. Screening for cryptococcal antigenemia in patients accessing an antiretroviral treatment program in South Africa. *Clin Infect Dis* 2009;48(7):856–862.

60. Ssekitoleko R, Kamya MR, Reingold AL. Primary prophylaxis for cryptococcal meningitis and impact on mortality in HIV: A systematic review and meta-analysis. *Future Virol* 2013;8(9).

61. Powderly WG, Finkelstein D, Feinberg J, Frame P, He W, van der Horst C, et al. A randomized trial comparing fluconazole with clotrimazole troches for the prevention of fungal infections in patients with advanced human immunodeficiency virus infection. NIAID AIDS Clinical Trials Group. *N Engl J Med* 1995;332(11):700–705.

62. McKinsey DS, Wheat LJ, Cloud GA, Pierce M, Black JR, Bamberger DM, et al. Itraconazole prophylaxis for fungal infections in patients with advanced human immunodeficiency virus infection: Randomized, placebo-controlled, double-blind study. National Institute of Allergy and Infectious Diseases Mycoses Study Group. *Clin Infect Dis* 1999;28(5):1049–1056.

63. Husain S, Wagener MM, Singh N. *Cryptococcus neoformans* infection in organ transplant recipients: Variables influencing clinical characteristics and outcome. *Emerg Infect Dis* 2001;7(3):375–381.

64. Vilchez RA, Fung J, Kusne S. Cryptococcosis in organ transplant recipients: An overview. *Am J Transplant* 2002;2(7):575–580.

65. Singh N, Alexander BD, Lortholary O, Dromer F, Gupta KL, John GT, et al. *Cryptococcus neoformans* in organ transplant recipients: Impact of calcineurin-inhibitor agents on mortality. *J Infect Dis* 2007;195(5):756–764.

66. Shaariah W, Morad Z, Suleiman AB. Cryptococcosis in renal transplant recipients. *Transplant Proc* 1992;24(5):1898–1899.

67. Singh N, Dromer F, Perfect JR, Lortholary O. Cryptococcosis in solid organ transplant recipients: Current state of the science. *Clin Infect Dis* 2008;47:1321–1327.

68. Singh N, Lortholary O, Alexander BD, Gupta KL, John GT, Pursell KJ, et al. Antifungal management practices and evolution of infection in organ transplant recipients with *Cryptococcus neoformans* infection. *Transplantation* 2005;80(8):1033–1039.

69. Kontoyiannis DP, Lewis RE, Alexander BD, Lortholary O, Dromer F, Gupta KL, et al. Calcineurin inhibitor agents interact synergistically with antifungal agents *in vitro* against *Cryptococcus neoformans* isolates: Correlation with outcome in solid organ transplant recipients with cryptococcosis. *Antimicrob Agents Chemother* 2008;52(2):735–738.

70. Dromer F, Mathoulin S, Dupont B, Brugiere O, Letenneur L. Comparison of the efficacy of amphotericin B and fluconazole in the treatment of cryptococcosis in human immunodeficiency virus-negative patients: Retrospective analysis of 83 cases. French Cryptococcosis Study Group. *Clin Infect Dis* 1996;22 Suppl 2:S154–S160.

71. Pappas PG, Perfect JR, Cloud GA, Larsen RA, Pankey GA, Lancaster DJ, et al. Cryptococcosis in human immunodeficiency virus-negative patients in the era of effective azole therapy. *Clin Infect Dis* 2001;33(5):690–699.

72. Saijo T, Chen J, Chen SC, Rosen LB, Yi J, Sorrell TC, et al. Anti-granulocyte-macrophage colony-stimulating factor autoantibodies are a risk factor for central nervous system infection by *Cryptococcus gattii* in otherwise immunocompetent patients. *MBio* 2014;5(2):e00912–e00914.

73. Rosen LB, Freeman AF, Yang LM, Jutivorakool K, Olivier KN, Angkasekwinai N, et al. Anti-GM-CSF autoantibodies in patients with cryptococcal meningitis. *J Immunol* 2013;190(8):3959–3966.

74. Ecevit IZ, Clancy CJ, Schmalfuss IM, Nguyen MH. The poor prognosis of central nervous system cryptococcosis among nonimmunosuppressed

patients: A call for better disease recognition and evaluation of adjuncts to antifungal therapy. *Clin Infect Dis* 2006;42(10):1443–1447.

75. Bennett JE, Dismukes WE, Duma RJ, Medoff G, Sande MA, Gallis H, et al. A comparison of amphotericin B alone and combined with flucytosine in the treatment of cryptoccal meningitis. *N Engl J Med* 1979;301(3):126–131.

76. Dismukes WE, Cloud G, Gallis HA, Kerkering TM, Medoff G, Craven PC, et al. Treatment of cryptococcal meningitis with combination amphotericin B and flucytosine for four as compared with six weeks. *N Engl J Med* 1987;317(6):334–341.

77. Powderly WG, Cloud GA, Dismukes WE, Saag MS. Measurement of cryptococcal antigen in serum and cerebrospinal fluid: Value in the management of AIDS-associated cryptococcal meningitis. *Clin Infect Dis* 1994;18(5):789–792.

78. Cuenca-Estrella M, Diaz-Guerra TM, Mellado E, Rodriguez-Tudela JL. Flucytosine primary resistance in *Candida* species and *Cryptococcus neoformans*. *Eur J Clin Microbiol Infect Dis* 2001;20(4):276–279.

79. Schwarz P, Dromer F, Lortholary O, Dannaoui E. Efficacy of amphotericin B in combination with flucytosine against flucytosine-susceptible or flucytosine-resistant isolates of *Cryptococcus neoformans* during disseminated murine cryptococcosis. *Antimicrob Agents Chemother* 2006;50(1):113–120.

80. Schwarz P, Janbon G, Dromer F, Lortholary O, Dannaoui E. Combination of amphotericin B with flucytosine is active *in vitro* against flucytosine-resistant isolates of *Cryptococcus neoformans*. *Antimicrob Agents Chemother* 2007;51(1):383–385.

81. Aller AI, Martin-Mazuelos E, Lozano F, Gomez-Mateos J, Steele-Moore L, Holloway WJ, et al. Correlation of fluconazole MICs with clinical outcome in cryptococcal infection. *Antimicrob Agents Chemother* 2000;44(6):1544–1548.

82. Witt MD, Lewis RJ, Larsen RA, Milefchik EN, Leal MA, Haubrich RH, et al. Identification of patients with acute AIDS-associated cryptococcal meningitis who can be effectively treated with fluconazole: The role of antifungal susceptibility testing. *Clin Infect Dis* 1996;22(2):322–328.

83. Bicanic T, Harrison T, Niepieklo A, Dyakopu N, Meintjes G. Symptomatic relapse of HIV-associated cryptococcal meningitis after initial fluconazole monotherapy: The role of fluconazole resistance and immune reconstitution. *Clin Infect Dis* 2006;43(8):1069–1073.

84. Pitisuttithum P, Negroni R, Graybill JR, Bustamante B, Pappas P, Chapman S, et al. Activity of posaconazole in the treatment of central nervous system fungal infections. *J Antimicrob Chemother* 2005;56(4):745–755.

85. Perfect JR, Marr KA, Walsh TJ, Greenberg RN, DuPont B, de la Torre-Cisneros J, et al. Voriconazole treatment for less-common, emerging, or refractory fungal infections. *Clin Infect Dis* 2003;36(9):1122–1131.

86. Jarvis JN, Meintjes G, Rebe K, Williams GN, Bicanic T, Williams A, et al. Adjunctive interferon-gamma immunotherapy for the treatment of HIV-associated cryptococcal meningitis: A randomized controlled trial. *AIDS* 2012;26(9):1105–1113.

87. Manfredi R, Coronado OV, Mastroianni A, Chiodo F. Liposomal amphotericin B and recombinant human granulocyte-macrophage colony-stimulating factor (rHuGM-CSF) in the treatment of paediatric AIDS-related cryptococcosis. *Int J STD AIDS* 1997;8(6):406–408.

88. Pappas PG. Managing cryptococcal meningitis is about handling the pressure. *Clin Infect Dis* 2005;40(3):480–482.

89. Graybill JR, Sobel J, Saag M, van Der Horst C, Powderly W, Cloud G, et al. Diagnosis and management of increased intracranial pressure in patients with AIDS and cryptococcal meningitis. The NIAID Mycoses Study Group and AIDS Cooperative Treatment Groups. *Clin Infect Dis* 2000;30(1):47–54.

90. Macsween KF, Bicanic T, Brouwer AE, Marsh H, Macallan DC, Harrison TS. Lumbar drainage for control of raised cerebrospinal fluid pressure in cryptococcal meningitis: Case report and review. *J Infect* 2005;51(4):e221–e224.

91. Woodworth GF, McGirt MJ, Williams MA, Rigamonti D. The use of ventriculoperitoneal shunts for uncontrollable intracranial hypertension without ventriculomegally secondary to HIV-associated cryptococcal meningitis. *Surg Neurol* 2005;63(6):529–531; discussion 31-2.

92. Park MK, Hospenthal DR, Bennett JE. Treatment of hydrocephalus secondary to cryptococcal meningitis by use of shunting. *Clin Infect Dis* 1999;28(3):629–633.

93. Sun HY, Hung CC, Chang SC. Management of cryptococcal meningitis with extremely high intracranial pressure in HIV-infected patients. *Clin Infect Dis* 2004;38(12):1790–1792.

94. Newton PN, Thai le H, Tip NQ, Short JM, Chierakul W, Rajanuwong A, et al. A randomized, double-blind, placebo-controlled trial of acetazolamide for the treatment of elevated intracranial pressure in cryptococcal meningitis. *Clin Infect Dis* 2002;35(6):769–772.

95. Shoham S, Cover C, Donegan N, Fulnecky E, Kumar P. *Cryptococcus neoformans* meningitis at 2 hospitals in Washington, D.C.: Adherence of health care providers to published practice guidelines for the management of cryptococcal disease. *Clin Infect Dis* 2005;40(3):477–479.

96. Shelburne SA, Visnegarwala F, Darcourt J, Graviss EA, Giordano TP, White AC, Jr., et al. Incidence and risk factors for immune reconstitution inflammatory syndrome during highly active antiretroviral therapy. *AIDS* 2005;19(4):399–406.

97. Jenny-Avital ER, Abadi M. Immune reconstitution cryptococcosis after initiation of successful highly active antiretroviral therapy. *Clin Infect Dis* 2002;35(12):e128–e133.

98. Skiest DJ, Hester LJ, Hardy RD. Cryptococcal immune reconstitution inflammatory syndrome: Report of four cases in three patients and review of the literature. *J Infect* 2005;51(5):e289–e297.

99. Lortholary O, Fontanet A, Memain N, Martin A, Sitbon K, Dromer F, et al. Incidence and risk factors of immune reconstitution inflammatory syndrome complicating HIV-associated cryptococcosis in France. *AIDS* 2005;19(10):1043–1049.

100. Shelburne SA, 3rd, Darcourt J, White AC, Jr., Greenberg SB, Hamill RJ, Atmar RL, et al. The role of immune reconstitution inflammatory syndrome in AIDS-related *Cryptococcus neoformans* disease in the era of highly active antiretroviral therapy. *Clin Infect Dis* 2005;40(7):1049–1052.

101. Singh N, Lortholary O, Alexander BD, Gupta KL, John GT, Pursell K, et al. An immune reconstitution syndrome-like illness associated with *Cryptococcus neoformans* infection in organ transplant recipients. *Clin Infect Dis* 2005;40(12):1756–1761.

102. Singh N, Perfect JR. Immune reconstitution syndrome associated with opportunistic mycoses. *Lancet Infect Dis* 2007;7(6):395–401.

103. Lesho E. Evidence base for using corticosteroids to treat HIV-associated immune reconstitution syndrome. *Expert Rev Anti Infect Ther* 2006;4(3):469–478.

104. Panackal AA, Komori M, Kosa P, Khan O, Hammoud DA, Rosen LB, et al. Spinal arachnoiditis as a complication of Cryptococcal meningoencephalitis in non-HIV previously healthy adults. *Clin Infect Dis* 2017;64(3):275–283.

105. Thwaites GE, Nguyen DB, Nguyen HD, Hoang TQ, Do TT, Nguyen TC, et al. Dexamethasone for the treatment of tuberculous meningitis in adolescents and adults. *N Engl J Med* 2004;351(17):1741–1751.

106. Scemla A, Gerber S, Duquesne A, Parize P, Martinez F, Anglicheau D, et al. Dramatic improvement of severe cryptococcosis-induced immune reconstitution syndrome with adalimumab in a renal transplant recipient. *Am J Transplant* 2015;15(2):560–564.

107. Somerville LK, Henderson AP, Chen SC, Kok J. Successful treatment of *Cryptococcus neoformans* immune reconstitution inflammatory syndrome in an immunocompetent host using thalidomide. *Med Mycol Case Rep* 2015;7:12–14.

108. Rhein J, Bahr NC, Hemmert AC, Cloud JL, Bellamkonda S, Oswald C, et al. Diagnostic performance of a multiplex PCR assay for meningitis in an HIV-infected population in Uganda. *Diagn Microbiol Infect Dis* 2016;84(3):268–273.

109. Maziarz EK, Perfect JR. Cryptococcosis. *Infect Dis Clin North Am* 2016;30(1):179–206.

110. Hospenthal DR, Bennett JE. Persistence of cryptococcomas on neuroimaging. *Clin Infect Dis* 2000;31(5):1303–1306.

111. Sitapati AM, Kao CL, Cachay ER, Masoumi H, Wallis RS, Mathews WC. Treatment of HIV-related inflammatory cerebral cryptococcoma with adalimumab. *Clin Infect Dis* 2010;50(2):e7–e10.

112. Ely EW, Peacock JE, Jr., Haponik EF, Washburn RG. Cryptococcal pneumonia complicating pregnancy. *Medicine (Baltimore)* 1998;77(3):153–167.

113. Philpot CR, Lo D. Cryptococcal meningitis in pregnancy. *Med J Aust* 1972;2(18):1005–1007.

114. Dean JL, Wolf JE, Ranzini AC, Laughlin MA. Use of amphotericin B during pregnancy: Case report and review. *Clin Infect Dis* 1994;18(3):364–368.

115. King CT, Rogers PD, Cleary JD, Chapman SW. Antifungal therapy during pregnancy. *Clin Infect Dis* 1998;27(5):1151–1160.

116. Pursley TJ, Blomquist IK, Abraham J, Andersen HF, Bartley JA. Fluconazole-induced congenital anomalies in three infants. *Clin Infect Dis* 1996;22(2):336–340.

117. Singh N, Perfect JR. Immune reconstitution syndrome and exacerbation of infections after pregnancy. *Clin Infect Dis* 2007;45(9):1192–1199.

118. Abadi J, Nachman S, Kressel AB, Pirofski L. Cryptococcosis in children with AIDS. *Clin Infect Dis* 1999;28(2):309–313.

119. Gonzalez CE, Shetty D, Lewis LL, Mueller BU, Pizzo PA, Walsh TJ. Cryptococcosis in human immunodeficiency virus-infected children. *Pediatr Infect Dis J* 1996;15(9):796–800.

120. McCarthy KM, Morgan J, Wannemuehler KA, Mirza SA, Gould SM, Mhlongo N, et al. Population-based surveillance for cryptococcosis in an antiretroviral-naive South African province with a high HIV seroprevalence. *AIDS* 2006;20(17):2199–2206.

121. Likasitwattanakul S, Poneprasert B, Sirisanthana V. Cryptococcosis in HIV-infected children. *Southeast Asian J Trop Med Public Health* 2004;35(4):935–939.

122. Sirinavin S, Intusoma U, Tuntirungsee S. Mother-to-child transmission of *Cryptococcus neoformans*. *Pediatr Infect Dis J* 2004;23(3):278–279.

123. Kaur R, Mittal N, Rawat D, Mathur MD. Cryptococcal meningitis in a neonate. *Scand J Infect Dis* 2002;34(7):542–543.

124. Wiley JM, Seibel NL, Walsh TJ. Efficacy and safety of amphotericin B lipid complex in 548 children and adolescents with invasive fungal infections. *Pediatr Infect Dis J* 2005;24(2):167–174.

125. Seay RE, Larson TA, Toscano JP, Bostrom BC, O'Leary MC, Uden DL. Pharmacokinetics of fluconazole in immune-compromised children with leukemia or other hematologic diseases. *Pharmacotherapy* 1995;15(1):52–58.

126. de Lalla F, Pellizzer G, Vaglia A, Manfrin V, Franzetti M, Fabris P, et al. Amphotericin B as primary therapy for cryptococcosis in patients with AIDS: Reliability of relatively high doses administered over a relatively short period. *Clin Infect Dis* 1995;20(2):263–266.

127. Pitisuttithum P, Tansuphasawadikul S, Simpson AJ, Howe PA, White NJ. A prospective study of AIDS-associated cryptococcal meningitis in Thailand treated with high-dose amphotericin B. *J Infect* 2001;43(4):226–233.

128. Tansuphaswadikul S, Maek-a-Nantawat W, Phonrat B, Boonpokbn L, Mctm AG, Pitisuttithum P. Comparison of one week with two week regimens of amphotericin B both followed by fluconazole in the treatment of cryptococcal meningitis among AIDS patients. *J Med Assoc Thai* 2006;89(10):1677–1685.

129. Longley N, Muzoora C, Taseera K, Mwesigye J, Rwebembera J, Chakera A, et al. Dose response effect of high-dose fluconazole for HIV-associated cryptococcal meningitis in southwestern Uganda. *Clin Infect Dis* 2008;47(12):1556–1561.

130. Speed B, Dunt D. Clinical and host differences between infections with the two varieties of *Cryptococcus neoformans*. *Clin Infect Dis* 1995;21(1):28–34; discussion 5-6.

131. Mitchell DH, Sorrell TC, Allworth AM, Heath CH, McGregor AR, Papanaoum K, et al. Cryptococcal disease of the CNS in immunocompetent hosts: Influence of cryptococcal variety on clinical manifestations and outcome. *Clin Infect Dis* 1995;20(3):611–616.

132. Thompson GR, 3rd, Wiederhold NP, Fothergill AW, Vallor AC, Wickes BL, Patterson TF. Antifungal susceptibilities among different serotypes of *Cryptococcus gattii* and *Cryptococcus neoformans*. *Antimicrob Agents Chemother* 2009;53(1):309–311.

133. Chen S, Sorrell T, Nimmo G, Speed B, Currie B, Ellis D, et al. Epidemiology and host- and variety-dependent characteristics of infection due to *Cryptococcus neoformans* in Australia and New Zealand. Australasian Cryptococcal Study Group. *Clin Infect Dis* 2000;31(2):499–508.

134. Chen SC, Slavin MA, Heath CH, et al. Clinical manifestations of Cryptococcus gattii infection: Determinants of neurological sequelae and death. *Clin Infect Dis* 2012;55:789–798.

135. Vilchez RA, Linden P, Lacomis J, Costello P, Fung J, Kusne S. Acute respiratory failure associated with pulmonary cryptococcosis in non-aids patients. *Chest* 2001;119(6):1865–1869.

136. Visnegarwala F, Graviss EA, Lacke CE, Dural AT, Johnson PC, Atmar RL, et al. Acute respiratory failure associated with cryptococcosis in patients with AIDS: Analysis of predictive factors. *Clin Infect Dis* 1998;27(5):1231–1237.

137. Meyohas MC, Roux P, Bollens D, Chouaid C, Rozenbaum W, Meynard JL, et al. Pulmonary cryptococcosis: Localized and disseminated infections in 27 patients with AIDS. *Clin Infect Dis* 1995;21(3):628–633.

138. Kerkering TM, Duma RJ, Shadomy S. The evolution of pulmonary cryptococcosis: Clinical implications from a study of 41 patients with and without compromising host factors. *Ann Intern Med* 1981;94(5):611–616.

139. Nadrous HF, Antonios VS, Terrell CL, Ryu JH. Pulmonary cryptococcosis in nonimmunocompromised patients. *Chest* 2003;124(6):2143–2147.

140. Aberg JA, Mundy LM, Powderly WG. Pulmonary cryptococcosis in patients without HIV infection. *Chest* 1999;115(3):734–740.

141. Baddley JW, Perfect JR, Oster RA, Larsen RA, Pankey GA, Henderson H, et al. Pulmonary cryptococcosis in patients without HIV infection: Factors associated with disseminated disease. *Eur J Clin Microbiol Infect Dis* 2008;27(10):937–943.

142. Singh N, Alexander BD, Lortholary O, Dromer F, Gupta KL, John GT, et al. Pulmonary cryptococcosis in solid organ transplant recipients: Clinical relevance of serum cryptococcal antigen. *Clin Infect Dis* 2008;46(2):e12–e18.

143. Nunez M, Peacock JE, Jr., Chin R, Jr. Pulmonary cryptococcosis in the immunocompetent host. Therapy with oral fluconazole: A report of four cases and a review of the literature. *Chest* 2000;118(2):527–534.

144. Mitchell TG, Perfect JR. Cryptococcosis in the era of AIDS--100 years after the discovery of *Cryptococcus neoformans*. *Clin Microbiol Rev* 1995;8(4):515–548.

145. Neuville S, Dromer F, Morin O, Dupont B, Ronin O, Lortholary O, et al. Primary cutaneous cryptococcosis: A distinct clinical entity. *Clin Infect Dis* 2003;36(3):337–347.

146. Behrman RE, Masci JR, Nicholas P. Cryptococcal skeletal infections: Case report and review. *Rev Infect Dis* 1990;12(2):181–190.

147. Larsen RA, Bozzette S, McCutchan JA, Chiu J, Leal MA, Richman DD. Persistent *Cryptococcus neoformans* infection of the prostate after successful treatment of meningitis. California Collaborative Treatment Group. *Ann Intern Med* 1989;111(2):125–128.

148. Blackie JD, Danta G, Sorrell T, Collignon P. Ophthalmological complications of cryptococcal meningitis. *Clin Exp Neurol* 1985;21:263–270.

149. McKenney J, Bauman S, Neary B, Detels R, French A, Margolick J, et al. Prevalence, correlates, and outcomes of cryptococcal antigen positivity among patients with AIDS, United States, 1986–2012. *Clin Infect Dis* 2015;60(6):959–965.

150. Organization WH. Rapid Advice: Diagnosis, Prevention and Management of Cryptococcal Disease in HIV-Infected Adults, Adolescents and Children. Geneva, Switzerland 2011.

151. Meya DB, Manabe YC, Castelnuovo B, Cook BA, Elbireer AM, Kambugu A, et al. Cost-effectiveness of serum cryptococcal antigen screening to prevent deaths among HIV-infected persons with a CD4+ cell count < or = 100 cells/microL who start HIV therapy in resource-limited settings. *Clin Infect Dis* 2010;51(4):448–455.

152. Kaplan JE, Vallabhaneni S, Smith RM, Chideya-Chihota S, Chehab J, Park B. Cryptococcal antigen screening and early antifungal treatment to prevent cryptococcal meningitis: A review of the literature. *J Acquir Immune Defic Syndr* 2015;68 Suppl 3:S331–S339.

153. Vijayan T, Chiller T, Klausner JD. Sensitivity and specificity of a new cryptococcal antigen lateral flow assay in serum and cerebrospinal fluid. *MLO Med Lab Obs* 2013;45(3):16–20.

154. Longley N, Jarvis JN, Meintjes G, Boulle A, Cross A, Kelly N, et al. Cryptococcal antigen screening in patients initiating ART in South Africa: A prospective cohort study. *Clin Infect Dis* 2016;62(5):581–587.

19

Management of endemic mycoses

JOHN R. PERFECT AND AHMAD MOURAD

INTRODUCTION

The endemic mycoses are the classical invasive fungal pathogens that have restricted geographical barriers and generally a dimorphic fungal life-cycle. From serological and skin test studies, it is clear that the spectrum of illnesses ranges from subclinical infection to acute or chronic pneumonia, and, in certain hosts, the disease can disseminate to other organs in the body, such as the central nervous system (CNS). Whenever you have this breadth of clinical presentations, it is clear that the individual host responses are critical to the final outcome of the infection. These endemic mycoses have developed the ability to infect human hosts and produce disease. Although, there are described hypervirulent, or hypovirulent strains or mutants, in most cases after exposure, which is primarily by inhalation of spores or direct traumatic implantation into the skin, the individual immune response determines the disease presentation. The management of each of these endemic mycoses is discussed separately, but the principles for management with HIV coinfection are similar. For instance, patients who received induction and then suppressive antifungal therapy should continue treatments until immune reconstitution has occurred with highly active antiretroviral therapy (HAART). It is also important to note that randomized studies in this group were primarily performed with itraconazole, but the extended-spectrum azoles, like voriconazole, posaconazole, and isauvconazole, possess excellent MIC values and, in case reports and open trials, appear to have success in treatment [1].

HISTOPLASMOSIS

Primary lung infection and severity of illness for *Histoplasma capsulatum* depends on the intensity of inhalation exposure to conidia as well as the immune status of the host and the underlying lung architecture [2].

Acute pulmonary disease

In a healthy host, asymptomatic infection or mild pulmonary disease from low aerosol exposure typically requires no therapy. Since it will clear without specific antifungal treatments. However, if the patient remains symptomatic for more than 4 weeks, some clinicians might treat this acute infection with itraconazole (200 mg orally three times daily for 3 days and then 200 mg orally per day or two times daily for 6–12 weeks) [2]. If there is a large inoculum exposure, this may cause severe pulmonary infection with mediastinitis, hypoxia, and respiratory failure. In this setting of severe disease, lipid formulation of amphotericin B (5.0 mg/kg daily intravenously for 2 weeks) or deoxycholate formulation of amphotericin B (0.7–1.0 mg/kg daily intravenously) would be considered a primary therapy until the patient clinically improves, and then followed by itraconazole (200 mg orally tid for 3 days and then 200 mg orally bid for a total of 12 weeks). For patients with severe infection who develop hypoxia or severe respiratory distress, the use of methylprednisolone (0.5–1.0 mg/kg daily intravenously) during the first 1–2 weeks of antifungal therapy is recommended and may help control a brisk inflammatory reaction [2].

Pulmonary nodules

Asymptomatic pulmonary nodules detected by radiographic studies and due to recent or previous infection can be confused with malignancy and sometimes they will show calcifications within them. Therefore, lesions are biopsied or excised and the tissue stains positive for Histoplasma. If the cultures from these lesions are negative, then generally no treatment is given These are generally small 1–2 micron methenamine silver-stained yeasts, which may be intracellular [2]. On the other hand, symptomatic pulmonary nodules with positive cultures and associated mediastinal adenopathy may be considered a recent infection and itraconazole therapy may be considered.

Broncholithiasis and fibrosing mediastinitis

When calcified lymph nodes erode into the airway producing respiratory symptoms or hemoptysis, patients may cough up broncholiths and conservative measures are appropriate. However, for difficult cases these broncholiths may need to be removed during bronchoscopic evaluation [3,4] or even require surgery but antifungal drugs are not necessary for further treatment. Fibrosing mediastinitis can be fatal and is another complication of chronic Histoplasma infection. Although there has been no robust evidence that antifungal treatment makes any impact on the outcome of fibrosing mediastinitis [5], some clinical experts would consider itraconazole therapy for 3 months. The use of adjuvant therapies, like corticosteroids and antifibrotics (such as tamoxifen) [6], are not certain to be of benefit. The use of stenting for mediastinal vessels will require consultation with surgeons specializing in mediastinal disease but may be necessary for the compressive disease of the airways and vascular structures, which can occur with this disease process [7,8].

Chronic histoplasmosis

In patients with mucous membrane involvement (ulcers) or cavitary lung disease, itraconazole (200 mg orally tid for 3 days and then 200 mg orally per day or bid for at least 12 months) is the standard therapy [2]. Chronic histoplasma cavitary lung disease [9], which is generally seen in those with underlying lung disease, can at times be refractory to initial treatment and, therefore, recommendations for itraconazole therapy may be extended for longer periods (18–24 months) [2] or even changed to other antifungal agents.

Disseminated histoplasmosis

For patients with disseminated disease, which primarily occurs in immunocompromised hosts, the treatment strategy will primarily depend on severity of the illness but generally most clinicians will start initial therapy with a polyene regimen. For patients with mild-to-moderate disease, itraconazole (200 mg orally tid for 3 days and then bid for at least 12 months) is recommended. For patients with moderately severe to severe disease, lipid formulations of amphotericin B (5.0 mg/kg daily) or deoxycholate amphotericin B (0.7–1.0 mg/kg daily) is recommended for 4–6 weeks, followed by itraconazole (200 mg orally tid for 3 days and then bid for a total of at least 12 months) is recommended [2]. In fact, one randomized clinical study has even supported the use of liposomal amphotericin B (5 mg/kg/day) being superior over amphotericin B deoxycholate in a group of seriously ill patients with AIDS and disseminated histoplasmosis [10]. After induction therapy for 4–6 weeks, patients may receive itraconazole for 6 months to 1 year [11,12]. In AIDS patients, itraconazole therapy is prolonged for at least a year, and maintenance therapy can be stopped when effective immune reconstitution occurs during HAART (CD4 count > 200/μL and low or undetectable viral load) [13]. Rarely, immunocompromised patients may require lifelong suppressive therapy with itraconazole (200 mg orally per day) if their immunosuppression cannot be reversed [2]. Immunosuppressed patients with disseminated disease may have detection of urine and/or serum histoplasma polysaccharide antigen. For this serology, which can help in diagnosis, change in antigen measurements may also help judge effectiveness of treatment and serial measurements are encouraged. With effective treatment, antigen levels are reduced and/or eliminated. The Histoplasma antigen levels both for diagnosis and treatment may also be helpful in Histoplasma meningitis. For patients with confirmed meningitis/CNS disease, liposomal amphotericin B (5.0 mg/kg daily for 4–6 weeks) is followed by itraconazole (200 mg orally bid or tid) for at least 12 months until resolution of CSF abnormalities, including undetected antigen levels, is recommended [2].

Although previous studies have shown that fluconazole and ketoconazole can be used to treat chronic and acute histoplasmosis, they are currently not recommended as standard therapy and should only be considered [2]. In fact, more effective alternative azoles to itraconazole, when it is not tolerated or has poor absorption, would likely be voriconazole, posaconazole, or isavuconazole. These azoles have excellent *in vitro* activity against Histoplasma and in animal models [14,15] with some occasional successful experience in humans. Their use at present has primarily been in salvage or open-labeled protocols [1,16–18] but successes have been high for these drugs in histoplasmosis. Caspofungin and presumably the other echinocandins have not been found to be effective treatment for Histoplasma infections [19].

Prophylaxis in HIV patients

In HIV-infected patients, prophylaxis with itraconazole (200 mg orally per day) when CD4 cell counts ≤150 cells/

mm³ in endemic areas with an incidence of histoplasmosis of 110 cases per 100 patient-years has been recommended [2]. However, most clinicians have used a more pre-emptive therapeutic approach with antigen testing, radiographs, histopathology, and cultures even in high prevalent areas. The cost of prophylactic azoles is substantial both in acquisition, drug–drug interactions and drug resistance.

General issues in histoplasmosis treatment

There are several issues with Histoplasma infection management. First, if itraconazole is used it should probably have a serum drug level measured at steady state with a goal of ≥0.5 µg/mL, and this is particularly important in patients with serious infections. The capsule formulation can be used but, if absorption problems occur or are anticipated, the suspension formulation might be more appropriate with its better absorption profile. However, it has higher gastrointestinal intolerability. Second, the use of corticosteroids for severe hypoxemia and diffuse pulmonary infiltrates and the development of acute respiratory distress syndrome becomes a bedside decision but should be considered. Third, another area of risk has been the introduction of anti-TNF-α agents for treatment of certain underlying diseases in areas with histoplasmosis [20]. Clinicians should be aware of the association between the use of these agents and Histoplasma disease. At present, there are no formal recommendations for screening, prophylaxis, or management of patients after treatment for Histoplasma infection in regard to restarting the anti-TNF-α agents; however, they are generally discontinued during the initial Histoplasma treatment course. It is assumed that *Histoplasma dubosii* will respond to similar management as *Histoplasma capsulatum*.

SPOROTHRICOSIS

Sporothricosis is a disease caused by several *Sporothrix species*. It is found in decaying vegetation, like sphagnum moss, and, generally, is either directly inoculated into the host tissue by thorns or cat claws and possibly, in the minority of cases, spores are inhaled. The primary presentation of this disease is either the lymphocutaneous or ulcerative forms of the disease but with inhalation, pulmonary sporothricosis can occur. Sporothrix can disseminate to other body sites, primarily bone and large joints, or rarely meningitis as specific body sites. The therapeutic use of heat to skin lesions or the oral use of supersaturated potassium iodide has generally been replaced by itraconazole. Itraconazole is the drug of choice for most forms of sporothricosis and the general dose is 200 mg orally bid. Amphotericin B or its lipid formulations is used for meningeal disease and may need to be used for difficult-to-treat cases of pulmonary and osteoarticular disease. Voriconazole is currently not recommended for use in treatment of sporotrichosis and there have not been enough studies to conclude if posaconazole or isavuconazole have a role [21] but *in vitro* these extended-spectrum azoles have activity and likely would be effective

in treatment of sporothricosis. Terbinafine use has not demonstrated superiority over the azoles and is occasionally added to azoles in patients who do not respond to azole therapy alone [21].

BLASTOMYCOSIS

Blastomyces dermatitidis causes blastomycosis and this fungal infection occurs most often in persons living in the midwestern, south central, or southeastern United States, or Canadian provinces that border the Great Lakes. Blastomycosis generally occurs as localized disease of the lungs but 25%–40% of cases can present as disseminated diseases, such as cutaneous, osteoarticular, genitourinary, or CNS disease. As with most endemic mycoses, disseminated blastomycosis occurs more frequently in immunosuppressed individuals, such as organ transplant recipients and/or those infected with HIV [22].

Pulmonary blastomycosis

Acute (primary) blastomycosis can mimic community-acquired bacterial pneumonia. It is clear from clinical experience that this acute infection in normal hosts can spontaneously clear and, therefore, it is not certain what exactly is the impact of antifungal treatment on the outcome of the primary infection. However, some clinical experts will treat well-documented, symptomatic blastomycete (acute) pneumonia with itraconazole, despite its potential for spontaneous clearing of infection, in an attempt to improve more rapid clearance of symptoms or prevent chronic disease or dissemination. Chronic pulmonary blastomycosis presents as a persistent pneumonia with alveolar infiltrates or masses that appear like lung cancer. Also, there are patients who have diffuse pulmonary infiltrates associated with acute respiratory distress syndrome (ARDS), which is associated with a substantial mortality. Generally, the diagnosis is made with histopathology of tissue or cytology demonstrating wide-based budding yeasts, cultures, or a Blastomyces antigen detection (urine, blood, or other fluids). In patients with mild-to-moderate pulmonary symptoms, itraconazole 200 mg orally tid for 3 days, then 200 mg daily or bid for 6–12 months is the current recommended regimen. Itraconazole has enhanced antifungal activity for this infection compared to ketoconazole or fluconazole [22]. Although there were similar outcomes in 200 mg/day versus 400 mg/day and 400 mg/day versus 800 mg/day fluconazole studies [23,24], the higher dose study (400 mg vs. 800 mg) had higher success rates and, if fluconazole is used, most would recommend starting with higher daily doses. There are simply too few cases treated with the newer triazoles, such as voriconazole, posaconazole, or isavuconazole, to make any robust recommendations, but *in vitro* and animal studies support their activity against Blastomyces [25]. Voriconazole has the most human clinical experience with Blastomyces and with its excellent CNS penetration it has been used to successfully treat CNS blastomycosis [26,27]. In moderate-to-severe pulmonary disease, it is recommended that induction therapy starts with a polyene. It is currently recommended to treat severely ill patients with induction lipid formulation amphotericin B or deoxycholate amphotericin B therapy for 2–4 weeks and then with clinical improvement, patients are switched to finish out 6 months to 1 year with itraconazole [22]. An important area is ARDS in pulmonary blastomycosis. This presentation is a life-threatening event and, although not common, it occasionally occurs, and clinicians need to be prepared for its presentation. In these cases, corticosteroids may be of benefit to help control excess, damaging inflammation in combination with high-dose polyene therapy.

Disseminated disease

For mild-to-moderate disease, such as osteoarticular, skin, and prostate, most patients can be managed with itraconazole [28–30] ensuring that the drug is being absorbed. Patients with osteoarticular disease must be treated for at least 12 months [22]. In patients with severe symptoms or immunosuppression, polyene (either lipid formulation or deoxycholate) should be used for induction therapy for 2–4 weeks and then begin itraconazole. Specifically, for CNS disease, lipid formulations of amphotericin B at ≥5 mg/kg/day for 4–6 weeks should be given, then followed by itraconazole for at least 1 year. No current recommendations can be made for the use of posaconazole, voriconazole, or isavuconazole in treatment of disseminated disease but may be considered in unique clinical circumstances. For certain immunosuppressed patients, length of therapy will depend on how well the immunosuppression is reversed.

Specific issues in blastomycosis treatment

Several issues associated with blastomycosis management need to be emphasized. First, the clinician must ensure that itraconazole levels are adequate. Second, itraconazole treatment is probably better than fluconazole and ketoconazole while voriconazole, isavuconazole, and posaconazole are possible alternative agents. Third, the echinocandins have no clinical activity for treatment of blastomycosis. Fourth, a combination antifungal therapy or immune stimulatory strategies have not been well-established for blastomycosis and are rarely used. Fifth, corticosteroid therapy may be necessary in ARDS. Sixth, polyene induction therapy is used for severe cases of blastomycosis and then, once it is controlled, the patient can be shifted to azole therapy. Seventh, since underlying diseases less often complicate cases of blastomycosis, success rates in management of this infection are relatively high.

COCCIDIOIDOMYCOSIS

Coccidioidomycosis is caused by a soil fungus, which through molecular studies has been divided into two geographically separated species: *Coccidioides immitis* and *Coccidioides posadaii*. From a clinical and treatment standpoint, they are considered together. This fungus has strict geographical boundaries in North America from the arid regions of the southern portion of the San Joaquin Valley of California to south central Arizona and northwestern Mexico. It may also be found in South America. Like many of the inhalational endemic mycoses, there is an acute pulmonary coccidioidomycosis, which presents like a community-acquired pneumonia. It may have some unique features, such as hilar adenopathy, peripheral eosinophilia, and/or appearance of erythema multiforme or erythema nodosum. Diagnosis is made by culture, histopathology that shows spherules, or complement-fixation antibodies in serum or cerebrospinal fluid (CSF) [31].

Acute infection

Primary pulmonary coccidioidomycosis in endemic regions without identified immunosuppressive risk factors is generally considered self-limited and does not require treatment. A retrospective study supports the observation. However, this present strategy continues to suffer from lack of evidence-based prospective, randomized studies and a study is needed to determine outcome of primary antifungal treatment versus placebo for total impact on patients such as time to clearing of symptoms. While nonimmunosuppressed patients with acute pulmonary coccidioidomycosis are not generally treated at present, treatment is given to those with impaired cellular immunity, such as solid organ transplant recipients, HIV-infected patients with low CD4 count, comorbid conditions such as cardiac or pulmonary disease and underlying conditions (i.e., diabetes), and those receiving potent immunosuppressive agents, such as anti-TNF-α therapy [32]. These patients are usually treated with fluconazole, if stable. For more severe disease, treatment is initiated with amphotericin B then de-escalated to fluconazole once stabilized [33]. Chronic pulmonary coccidioidomycosis can be defined as symptoms for more than 3 months and these patients should be treated especially with cavitary lung disease and hemoptysis. The use of surgery in cases with hemoptysis will need expert opinions regarding its need and implementation. All patients should be followed for a year after acute pulmonary coccidioidomycosis for complete resolution since dissemination primarily occurs in this time frame. Clinicians should be able to diagnose disseminated coccidioidomycosis relatively early and particular emphasis needs to be placed on cell-mediated immune defective patients and certain racial types, such as African-American and Filipino males, who have a relatively high rate of disseminated infections. The most common sites for dissemination of infection are skin and soft tissue, bones and joints, and the CNS. Since CNS invasion may occur and be manifested within the first 1–3 months after acute pulmonary infection, if CNS symptoms occur, it will be necessary to rule out coccidioidal meningitis.

Chronic infection

Chronic pulmonary coccidioidomycosis can be defined as symptoms for more than 3 months. Although antifungal treatment for acute pulmonary infection is not used routinely, chronic coccidioidomycosis is treated with antifungal agents for 12 to 18 months and longer courses in immunosuppressed individuals. In CNS involvement with coccidioides infection, treatment is considered for a life time because present antifungal agents cannot reliably cure infection at this site. Available agents for treatment of coccidioidomycosis include azoles and polyenes. In skin and pulmonary infections, outcomes seem similar with fluconazole or itraconazole at a minimum dose of 400 mg/day orally and in bone/joint infections there is one report that suggests itraconazole may be superior to fluconazole [34]. There is a rich history of clinical trials for this chronic infection stage and despite excellent responses there are still a number of patients who relapse after treatment. There are several reports that suggest voriconazole, posaconazole [35,36], and isavuconazole [1] are active in chronic and/or recalcitrant cases, but there remains a need for their performance to be compared to the gold standard—itraconazole. In patients with severe disseminated disease, more consideration should be given to initial induction therapy with polyene (either amphotericin B deoxycholate or lipid formulation of amphotericin B). There are no definitive data suggesting that one polyene preparation is better than another, and the precise length of induction treatment is empirical before switching to azole in the consolidation or suppressive phases of treatment.

Patients with coccidioidal meningitis (cellular reaction in CSF, such as eosinophils and either culture or complement fixation antibody positive with evidence of inflammation) are a special group since the goal appears to be suppression of infection rather than consistent cure. These specific patients with present therapeutic regimens have substantial failure rates if antifungals are stopped [37]. The most common drug for initial treatment of meningitis is fluconazole at ≥800 mg/day orally for non-severely ill patients indefinitely and doses of 800–1200 mg/day are used in severely ill patients [33]. There are reports of successful treatment with voriconazole in patients who failed on fluconazole [38]. In very difficult to control patients, there is still the intermittent use of intrathecal amphotericin B (0.25 mg intrathecal) to control symptoms [39]. However, there are substantial neurological side effects with intrathecal amphotericin B and these may arise and need management.

The use of prophylaxis for high-risk patients in highly endemic areas for coccidioidomycosis is currently not recommended [33]. There has been a substantial history of interest in coccidioidal vaccines, but none have made it into clinical practice.

PENICILLIOSIS

Penicillium (*Takaromyces*) marneffei is a fission yeast in tissue and grows as a red mold on agar plates at room temperature. It has a specific geographical niche and this is primarily present in certain parts of southeast Asia. During the AIDS epidemic, this endemic mycosis rose to prominence as a disseminated opportunistic infection associated with HIV infection. The clinical presentation is similar to histoplasmosis in AIDS patients, but it does have a unique propensity for skin involvement.

Disseminated infection

In the management of disseminated penicilliosis, the primary focus is on both treatment and control of the underlying HIV infection. Both itraconazole and amphotericin B are active against this fungus and have been used in treatment [40]. At present, itraconazole is probably the initial drug of choice but for seriously ill patients, amphotericin B is preferred for best induction therapy before conversion to an azole. In many respects it follows the treatment pattern of histoplasmosis. Studies have also shown that voriconazole can be used as an alternative [41]. Importantly, like all endemic invasive mycoses, in the presence of underlying HIV infection, the use of HAART and documented immune reconstitution will be necessary before antifungal drugs are discontinued, but at a minimum patient should receive 1 year of therapy if available. Finally, there has been a regional disease outbreak caused by the dimorphic genus of Emmonsia in HIV-infected patients [42]. Although precise treatment recommendations cannot be given for Emmonsia infections, it is likely that these infections will respond to treatment with extended-spectrum azoles and/or amphotericin B with HAART immunoreconstitution.

REFERENCES

1. Thompson GR, 3rd, Rendon A, Ribeiro Dos Santos R, Queiroz-Telles F, Ostrosky-Zeichner L, Azie N, et al. Isavuconazole treatment of cryptococcosis and dimorphic mycoses. *Clin Infect Dis* 2016;63(3):356–362.
2. Wheat LJ, Freifeld AG, Kleiman MB, Baddley JW, McKinsey DS, Loyd JE, et al. Clinical practice guidelines for the management of patients with histoplasmosis: 2007 update by the Infectious Diseases Society of America. *Clin Infect Dis* 2007;45(7):807–825.
3. Olson EJ, Utz JP, Prakash UB. Therapeutic bronchoscopy in broncholithiasis. *Am J Respir Crit Care Med* 1999;160(3):766–770.
4. Menivale F, Deslee G, Vallerand H, Toubas O, Delepine G, Guillou PJ, et al. Therapeutic management of broncholithiasis. *Ann Thorac Surg* 2005;79(5):1774–1776.

5. Loyd JE, Tillman BF, Atkinson JB, Des Prez RM. Mediastinal fibrosis complicating histoplasmosis. *Medicine (Baltimore)* 1988;67(5):295–310.

6. Savelli BA, Parshley M, Morganroth ML. Successful treatment of sclerosing cervicitis and fibrosing mediastinitis with tamoxifen. *Chest* 1997;111(4):1137–1140.

7. Doyle TP, Loyd JE, Robbins IM. Percutaneous pulmonary artery and vein stenting: A novel treatment for mediastinal fibrosis. *Am J Respir Crit Care Med* 2001;164(4):657–660.

8. Manali ED, Saad CP, Krizmanich G, Mehta AC. Endobronchial findings of fibrosing mediastinitis. *Respir Care* 2003;48(11):1038–1042.

9. Parker JD, Sarosi GA, Doto IL, Bailey RE, Tosh FE. Treatment of chronic pulmonary histoplasmosis. *N Engl J Med* 1970;283(5):225–229.

10. Johnson PC, Wheat LJ, Cloud GA, Goldman M, Lancaster D, Bamberger DM, et al. Safety and efficacy of liposomal amphotericin B compared with conventional amphotericin B for induction therapy of histoplasmosis in patients with AIDS. *Ann Intern Med* 2002;137(2):105–109.

11. Wheat J, Hafner R, Korzun AH, Limjoco MT, Spencer P, Larsen RA, et al. Itraconazole treatment of disseminated histoplasmosis in patients with the acquired immunodeficiency syndrome. AIDS Clinical Trial Group. *Am J Med* 1995;98(4):336–342.

12. Wheat J, Hafner R, Wulfsohn M, Spencer P, Squires K, Powderly W, et al. Prevention of relapse of histoplasmosis with itraconazole in patients with the acquired immunodeficiency syndrome. *Ann Intern Med* 1993;118(8):610–616.

13. Goldman M, Zackin R, Fichtenbaum CJ, Skiest DJ, Koletar SL, Hafner R, et al. Safety of discontinuation of maintenance therapy for disseminated histoplasmosis after immunologic response to antiretroviral therapy. *Clin Infect Dis* 2004;38(10):1485–1489.

14. Li RK, Ciblak MA, Nordoff N, Pasarell L, Warnock DW, McGinnis MR. *In vitro* activities of voriconazole, itraconazole, and amphotericin B against *Blastomyces dermatitidis*, *Coccidioides immitis*, and *Histoplasma capsulatum*. *Antimicrob Agents Chemother* 2000;44(6):1734–1736.

15. Connolly P, Wheat J, Schnizlein-Bick C, Durkin M, Kohler S, Smedema M, et al. Comparison of a new triazole antifungal agent, Schering 56592, with itraconazole and amphotericin B for treatment of histoplasmosis in immunocompetent mice. *Antimicrob Agents Chemother* 1999;43(2):322–328.

16. Clark B, Foster R, Tunbridge A, Green S. A case of disseminated histoplasmosis successfully treated with the investigational drug posaconazole. *J Infect* 2005;51(3):e177–e180.

17. Perfect JR, Marr KA, Walsh TJ, Greenberg RN, DuPont B, de la Torre-Cisneros J, et al. Voriconazole treatment for less-common, emerging, or refractory fungal infections. *Clin Infect Dis* 2003;36(9):1122–1131.

18. Restrepo A, Tobon A, Clark B, Graham DR, Corcoran G, Bradsher RW, et al. Salvage treatment of histoplasmosis with posaconazole. *J Infect* 2007;54(4):319–327.

19. Kohler S, Wheat LJ, Connolly P, Schnizlein-Bick C, Durkin M, Smedema M, et al. Comparison of the echinocandin caspofungin with amphotericin B for treatment of histoplasmosis following pulmonary challenge in a murine model. *Antimicrob Agents Chemother* 2000;44(7):1850–1854.

20. Wood KL, Hage CA, Knox KS, Kleiman MB, Sannuti A, Day RB, et al. Histoplasmosis after treatment with anti-tumor necrosis factor-alpha therapy. *Am J Respir Crit Care Med* 2003;167(9):1279–1282.

21. Kauffman CA, Bustamante B, Chapman SW, Pappas PG, Infectious Diseases Society of America. Clinical practice guidelines for the management of sporotrichosis: 2007 update by the Infectious Diseases Society of America. *Clin Infect Dis* 2007;45(10):1255–1265.

22. Chapman SW, Dismukes WE, Proia LA, Bradsher RW, Pappas PG, Threlkeld MG, et al. Clinical practice guidelines for the management of blastomycosis: 2008 update by the Infectious Diseases Society of America. *Clin Infect Dis* 2008;46(12):1801–1812.

23. Pappas PG, Bradsher RW, Chapman SW, Kauffman CA, Dine A, Cloud GA, et al. Treatment of blastomycosis with fluconazole: A pilot study. The National Institute of Allergy and Infectious Diseases Mycoses Study Group. *Clin Infect Dis* 1995;20(2):267–271.

24. Pappas PG, Bradsher RW, Kauffman CA, Cloud GA, Thomas CJ, Campbell GD, Jr., et al. Treatment of blastomycosis with higher doses of fluconazole. The National Institute of Allergy and Infectious Diseases Mycoses Study Group. *Clin Infect Dis* 1997;25(2):200–205.

25. Sugar AM, Liu XP. Efficacy of voriconazole in treatment of murine pulmonary blastomycosis. *Antimicrob Agents Chemother* 2001;45(2):601–604.

26. Bakleh M, Aksamit AJ, Tleyjeh IM, Marshall WF. Successful treatment of cerebral blastomycosis with voriconazole. *Clin Infect Dis* 2005;40(9):e69–e71.

27. Borgia SM, Fuller JD, Sarabia A, El-Helou P. Cerebral blastomycosis: A case series incorporating voriconazole in the treatment regimen. *Med Mycol* 2006;44(7):659–664.

28. Saiz P, Gitelis S, Virkus W, Piasecki P, Bengana C, Templeton A. Blastomycosis of long bones. *Clin Orthop Relat Res* 2004(421):255–259.

29. Hadjipavlou AG, Mader JT, Nauta HJ, Necessary JT, Chaljub G, Adesokan A. Blastomycosis of the lumbar spine: Case report and review of the literature, with emphasis on diagnostic laboratory tools and management. *Eur Spine J* 1998;7(5):416–421.

30. Saccente M, Abernathy RS, Pappas PG, Shah HR, Bradsher RW. Vertebral blastomycosis with paravertebral abscess: Report of eight cases and review of the literature. *Clin Infect Dis* 1998;26(2):413–418.

31. Galgiani JN, Ampel NM, Blair JE, Catanzaro A, Johnson RH, Stevens DA, et al. Coccidioidomycosis. *Clin Infect Dis* 2005;41(9):1217–1223.

32. Bergstrom L, Yocum DE, Ampel NM, Villanueva I, Lisse J, Gluck O, et al. Increased risk of coccidioidomycosis in patients treated with tumor necrosis factor alpha antagonists. *Arthritis Rheum* 2004;50(6):1959–1966.

33. Galgiani JN, Ampel NM, Blair JE, Catanzaro A, Geertsma F, Hoover SE, et al. 2016 Infectious Diseases Society of America (IDSA) Clinical Practice Guideline for the Treatment of Coccidioidomycosis. *Clin Infect Dis* 2016;63(6):e112–e146.

34. Galgiani JN, Catanzaro A, Cloud GA, Johnson RH, Williams PL, Mirels LF, et al. Comparison of oral fluconazole and itraconazole for progressive, nonmeningeal coccidioidomycosis. A randomized, double-blind trial. Mycoses Study Group. *Ann Intern Med* 2000;133(9):676–686.

35. Anstead GM, Corcoran G, Lewis J, Berg D, Graybill JR. Refractory coccidioidomycosis treated with posaconazole. *Clin Infect Dis* 2005;40(12):1770–1776.

36. Catanzaro A, Cloud GA, Stevens DA, Levine BE, Williams PL, Johnson RH, et al. Safety, tolerance, and efficacy of posaconazole therapy in patients with nonmeningeal disseminated or chronic pulmonary coccidioidomycosis. *Clin Infect Dis* 2007;45(5):562–568.

37. Dewsnup DH, Galgiani JN, Graybill JR, Diaz M, Rendon A, Cloud GA, et al. Is it ever safe to stop azole therapy for Coccidioides immitis meningitis? *Ann Intern Med* 1996;124(3):305–310.

38. Cortez KJ, Walsh TJ, Bennett JE. Successful treatment of coccidioidal meningitis with voriconazole. *Clin Infect Dis* 2003;36(12):1619–1622.

39. Stevens DA, Shatsky SA. Intrathecal amphotericin in the management of coccidioidal meningitis. *Semin Respir Infect* 2001;16(4):263–269.

40. Al-Abdely HM. Management of rare fungal infections. *Curr Opin Infect Dis* 2004;17(6):527–532.

41. Supparatpinyo K, Schlamm HT. Voriconazole as therapy for systemic *Penicillium marneffei* infections in AIDS patients. *Am J Trop Med Hyg* 2007;77(2):350–353.

42. Kenyon C, Bonorchis K, Corcoran C, Meintjes G, Locketz M, Lehloenya R, et al. A dimorphic fungus causing disseminated infection in South Africa. *N Engl J Med* 2013;369(15):1416–1424.

Human hyalohyphomycoses: A review of human infections due to *Acremonium* spp., *Paecilomyces* spp., *Penicillium* spp., *Talaromyces* spp., and *Scopulariopsis* spp.

NOUR HASAN

Hyalohyphomycosis is the term designated for mycotic infections caused by septate molds with hyaline or light-colored cell walls in tissues. This separates it from phaeo-hyphomycosis where the causative agents are septate molds with dark-colored cell walls [1,2].

Although these filamentous fungi are common environmental saprophytes, they cause a variety of infections mostly thought to be secondary to prior colonization and increased host susceptibility [2].

This chapter will focus on four hyaline molds that cause significant clinical disease. These include *Acremonium* spp., *Paecilomyces* spp., *Penicillium* spp., *Talaromyces* spp., and *Scopulariopsis* spp. *Fusarium*, *Scedosporium*, and *Aspergillus* are covered elsewhere. Within each genus, we will discuss the organisms' mycology, epidemiology, clinical presentation, and treatment.

ACREMONIUM SPECIES

Epidemiology and mycology

The genus *Acremonium*, formerly known as *Cephalosporium*, contains about 100 different species that are ubiquitous in the environment and typically isolated in soil, insects, sewage, plants, and other environmental substrates [3]. The first recorded isolation of this species was *Acremonium cephalosporium* in 1939 [4]. In 1945, *A. cephalosporium* was isolated in the sewage effluent during a search for antibiotic-producing organisms of the coast of Sardinia [4]. By 1953, the active antimicrobial compound cephalosporin C was isolated from *A. cephalosporium* by investigators at Oxford University, United Kingdom, leading to the development of the cephalosporin class of antibiotics [4].

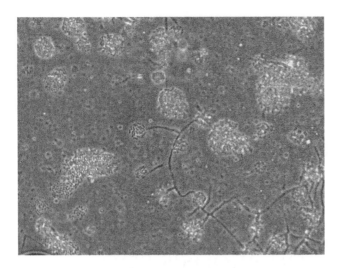

Figure 20.1 *Acremonium* species. Microscopy characterized by narrow hyphae with thin walled, slightly tapered phialides and ellipsoidal conidia forming slimy masses.

Species that have been reported to cause infections in humans are *Acremonium alabamensis, A. sclerotigenum, A. egyptiacum, A. kiliense* (currently *Sarocladium kiliense*), *A. roseogriseum* (currently *Gliomastix roseogrisea*), *A. strictum* (currently *Sarocladium strictum*), *A. potronii*, and *A. recifei* [5,6], with *A. kiliense* being the most common species isolated from clinical samples [7]. *A. falciforme*, on the other hand, is now *Fusarium falciforme*, a member of the *F. solani* species complex [6].

This genus is distinguished by formation of narrow hyphae bearing solitary, slender, unbranched needle-shaped phialides, with some species having shallow collarettes forming conidia in slimy masses (Figure 20.1) [3]. *Acremonium* species grow slowly, forming white, salmon, or pink colonies that are usually velvety, cottony, or fasciculate with flat or slightly raised centers (Figure 20.2) [3].

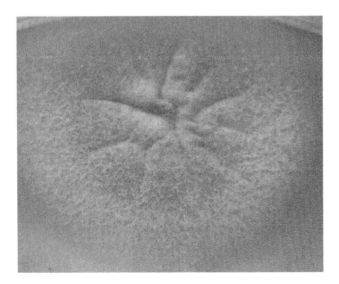

Figure 20.2 Colony of *Acremonium* species. Moderately fast growing with pinkish color, velvety texture, and slightly raised center.

Clinical presentation

Members of this genus are recognized as the etiological agent of many superficial, locally invasive, or disseminated infections. It appears that localized infections account for nearly two-thirds of the *Acremonium* cases reported worldwide in both immunocompetent and immunocompromised individuals; only one-third were reported as disseminated infections, mostly in immunocompromised host [8,9].

Mycetoma [8,10], the most common clinical presentation of *Acremonium* species, usually occur after a traumatic inoculation and are characterized by the clinical triad of swelling, sinus tract formation, and fungal granules. *Acremonium* mycetoma are usually chronic infections of the distal extremities that may lead to underlying bone destruction if left untreated. *Acremonium* species have also been recognized as causative agent in onychomycosis [11].

Ocular infections also represent common infections caused by *Acremonium* species. Multiple cases of keratitis and endophthalmitis [12–14] have been reported in the medical literature. The majority of these infections occur following trauma, surgery, or topical steroid use [9]. The ability of *Acremonium* species to colonize contact lenses has been demonstrated, which may cause ocular infections [9,15].

Several cases of locally invasive *Acremonium* infections have been reported in the literature, including pleuritis [16], lung abscess [17], septic arthritis [18–20], osteomyelitis [21,22], lumbar diskitis [23], and peritonitis secondary to infected peritoneal dialysis [24,25].

Disseminated infections have become more frequent over the past decade, mostly in the immunocompromised population. In one autopsy-proven study of invasive mold infections in cancer patients, 10% of the cases were caused by *Acremonium* spp [26]. These infections include endocarditis [27,28], meningitis [4], pneumonia [29], and diffuse cerebritis [4]. Central line associated blood stream infections have also been reported. These cases have occurred mostly in patients with profound neutropenia and in immunosuppressed patients [30,31]. However, occasional reports of fungemia in patients with subclavian catheters, after mitral valve replacement, or infection of pacemaker pocket, have been reported in patients with no apparent immune depletion [32–34].

The definitive diagnosis requires isolation of *Acremonium* from infected sites, while blood cultures may become positive only after the disease has progressed. *Acremonium* species grow slowly; therefore, culture plates need to be incubated for at least 2 weeks for detection [5].

Treatment

Treatment of *Acremonium* infections presents a challenge to those involved. The optimal therapy for such infections remains unknown, as clinical data are limited to case reports. Clearly, in patients with neutropenia, recovery of the neutrophil count is crucial for clearance of infection. This was well demonstrated in a case report of a woman with line-associated *Acremonium* fungemia that resolved with resolution of neutropenia without antifungal therapy and despite retention of the catheter, only to recur with her next bout of chemotherapy-related neutropenia [35].

In vitro, *Acremonium* isolates demonstrated high minimum inhibitory concentrations (MICs) for the most commonly used antifungal agents, except for terbinafine [7,9]. Perdomo et al. [7] reported MICs of 47 strains obtained from clinical samples testing using the Clinical and Laboratory Standards Institute (CLSI) methodology. Antifungal susceptibility testing of these strains revealed an overall lack of activity for echinocandins and itraconazole. Also, all *Acremonium* isolates were resistant to 5-fluorocytosine and fluconazole, like most other genera of hyaline molds. Amphotericin B had poor activity with elevated MICs. On the other hand, the lowest MICs for all antifungal agents tested against all *Acremonium* species were obtained with terbinafine, followed by posaconazole (MIC range: 0.006–2.0 μg/mL) and voriconazole (MIC range: 0.12–4.0 μg/mL). Guarro et al. also reported antifungal susceptibilities to 33 clinical and environmental isolates [9]. Amphotericin B showed the best results. Nineteen of the strains tested had MICs ≤1.16 mg/mL, while activity of ketoconazole, itraconazole, and miconazole were strain dependent. In another *in vitro* study, posaconazole, voriconazole, itraconazole, and amphotericin B were almost equally effective against the strains tested [36].

Clinical response data are limited to case reports [8,37,38] and, based on the outcomes observed, the executive board of the European Fungal Infection Study Group of the European Society of Clinical Microbiology and Infectious Diseases (ESCMID) and the European Confederation of Medical Mycology (ECMM) recommended treatment with voriconazole, amphotericin B, or posaconazole, guided by susceptibility testing along with surgical debridement and catheter removal [5].

PAECILOMYCES SPECIES

Epidemiology and mycology

Paecilomyces species occur worldwide as saprophytes in soil, decomposing organic matter, and occasionally as insect parasites [1–3]. *Paecilomyces* are rare human pathogens, but some species are implicated in human disease, including *P. variotii* and *P. marquandii*. *P. variotii* is comprised of a complex of five species, of which *P. variotii* and *P. formosus* are the most important clinically [3]. *P. lilacinus* was transferred to the genus *Purpureocillium* and now officially holds the name *Purpureocillium lilacinum* [39–41]. *Paecilomyces* are common contaminants of antiseptic solutions and creams, as they are resistant to most commercially available sterilization techniques [42]. In addition, they may colonize medical foreign bodies, such as catheters and plastic implants [2].

Microscopically *P. variotii* complex form fast-growing yellowish-brown, buff or orange colonies. Conidiophores bear verticillately arranged branches bearing phialides, which are swollen at the base and terminate in long tapering necks. Conidia are single celled and occur in chains. Chlamydospores are usually present [3]. *P. variotii* is thermophilic and can grow well at high temperatures while *P. marquandii* fails to grow at 37°C. On the other hand, *Purpureocillium* exhibits slower growth than *Paecilomyces*. Conidia are lilac colored (Figure 20.3) and chlamydospores are absent [3] (Figure 20.4).

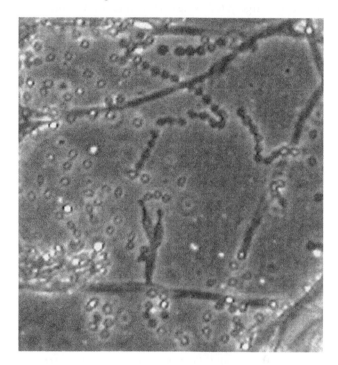

Figure 20.3 *Purpureocillium lilacinum*. Microscopy is notable for phialides that are swollen at the base with long tapered necks and long chains of elliptical conidia.

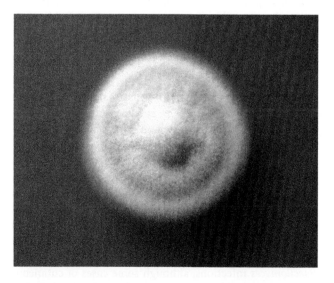

Figure 20.4 Colony of *Purpureocillium lilacinum*. Cottony colonies that gradually become lilac in color.

Clinical presentation

Both *Paecilomyces* spp. and *Purpureocillium lilacinum* are rarely pathogenic in humans, but they are able to infect both immunocompromised and immunocompetent hosts [39,43]. The portal of entry of the fungus usually involves breakdown of the skin barrier, indwelling catheters, or inhalation. On some occasions, infections have been associated with contaminated fluids and solutions [43].

Oculomycosis is the most common clinical presentation [2], usually in the setting of chronic keratopathy, after previous ocular surgery, following corneal trauma, with the use of soft contact lenses, or topical or systemic immunosuppression [44,45]. The most common eye infections include keratitis and endophthalmitis [44]. Cutaneous and subcutaneous infections are the second most common presentations [2], occurring most often in immunocompromised patients but also reported in immunocompetent hosts [43,46]. Recently, invasive infections related to *Paecilomyces* have been increasingly reported [2] with pneumonia being the most common presentation, in addition to pleural effusions and mycetomas [43,47,48]. Other reported clinical presentations include sinusitis [49–51], central line associated fungemia [52–54], disseminated infection in immunocompromised hosts [55], and peritoneal dialysis-associated peritonitis [56]. Less common presentations include infectious endocarditis in patients who have prosthetic valves [57], cerebrospinal fluid shunt infection [58], chronic otitis media [59], pyelonephritis [60], osteomyelitis [61], and synovial infection [62,63].

Treatment

Like other *hyalohyphomycoses*, the optimal treatment for *Paecilomyces* and *Purpureocillium* infections remains uncertain. Differentiation to species level is crucial, as *in vitro* antifungal susceptibility is highly species dependent. In general, *P. lilacinum in vitro* is highly resistant to amphotericin B but susceptible to azoles, while *P. variotii* is usually amphotericin B susceptible [2,5]. In one report [64], *P. lilacinum* strains tested showed high MICs of amphotericin B, itraconazole and echinocandins. In contrast, voriconazole, posaconazole, and terbinafine were active against this species, with posaconazole being the drug with the best *in vitro* activity. By contrast, *P. variotii* showed a different susceptibility pattern and was susceptible to amphotericin B, itraconazole, posaconazole and echinocandins. In addition, 81% of the strains tested showed MICs of ≥2 mg/L for voriconazole. Similar results were reported by Houbraken et al. [65] suggesting that voriconazole is generally not active against members of the *P. variotii* complex. Reported results agreed with previous findings for *P. lilacinum*, except for echinocandins for which contradictory data have been reported. To date, there is no conclusive evidence that echinocandins should be used for treatment of invasive *Paecilomyces* infections, although some cases of cutaneous infection has been successfully treated with echinocandins combined with a topical or systemic triazole [66,67].

For localized infections, especially cutaneous infections, surgical intervention plays a significant role in successful outcomes [43]. For invasive or disseminated infections, removal of infected foci and elimination of indwelling catheters and foreign implants is crucial [43]; species-specific susceptibility data can help to guide antifungal therapy [2]. Reported clinical outcomes of invasive infections attributable to *Paecilomyces* range from 100% recovery to significant rates of morbidity and mortality [2,43]. Several case of successful treatment of *P. lilacinum* invasive infections with triazole therapies [68–70] have been reported, including one successful salvage treatment with posaconazole of a voriconazole-unresponsive *P. lilacinum* lung infection in a bone marrow transplant recipient [69].

PENICILLIUM SPECIES

Epidemiology and mycology

Penicillium is a diverse genus occurring worldwide and its species play important roles as decomposers of organic materials; however, they also cause destructive rots in the food industry. Other species are considered enzyme factories or are common indoor air allergens [71]. However, true *Penicillium* species causing human infections are very rare, and the only pathogenic species previously identified as *Penicillium marneffei* was transferred to the *Talaromyces* genus (the teleomorph stage of *Biverticillium*) and now officially holds the taxonomic name *Talaromyces marneffei*. However, its associated disease is unfortunately still referred to as penicilliosis [72]. This species is dimorphic, growing as a yeast at 37°C in the host and as a filamentous fungus at 25°C in the environment [73]. It is an emerging fungal pathogen causing a fatal mycosis in especially immunocompromised individuals from East Asian countries, such as China, Taiwan, Thailand, and Vietnam [72]. It was initially isolated in 1959 from the bamboo rat *Rhizomys sinensis* in Southeast Asia, but the primary reservoir for this fungus remains unknown [73]. The first reported case of disseminated infection occurred in an American missionary with Hodgkin's disease who had traveled extensively in Southeast Asia [72]. Over the next 10–15 years, a few more sporadic cases were reported. The incidence of *T. marneffei* infection markedly increased after the HIV/AIDS epidemic arrived in Southeast Asia in 1988. *T. marneffei* infection was reported not only among HIV-infected patients residing in endemic areas, but also in HIV-infected patients who had traveled to there [72].

Colonies at 25°C are fast growing, downy, and white with yellowish green conidial heads. Colonies become grayish pink to brown with age and produce a diffusible brown-red pigment (Figure 20.5). Microscopically, the conidiophores bear terminal verticils comprising three to five metulae, each bearing three to seven phialides. Conidia are globose to subglobose, 2–3 μm in diameter, smooth-walled, and are produced in basipetal succession from the phialides producing a typical penicillius, which is a brush-like fruiting structure (Figure 20.6). At 37°C, *T. marneffei*

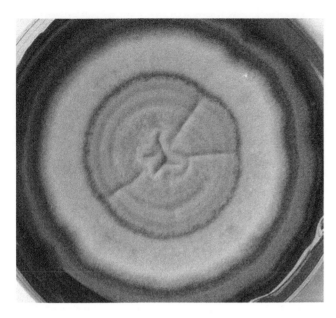

Figure 20.5 White, flat colonies of *Talaromyces marneffei* at 25°C. The colony characteristically exudes red pigment into the media.

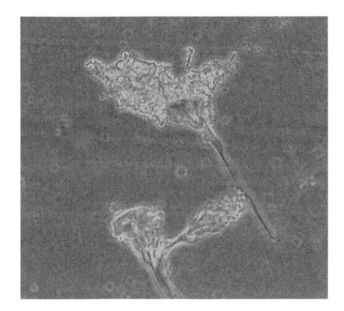

Figure 20.6 *Talaromyces marneffei*. Microscopy reveals three to five metulae on which three to seven pointed phialides rest, each with a chain of one-celled conidia.

converts to yeast-like spherical cells that multiply by fission. Differentiation between *T. marneffei* and *Penicillia* depends on a combination of microscopic evaluation and proof of thermal dimorphism [73].

Clinical presentation

T. marneffei now ranks as the third most common opportunistic infection in HIV/ AIDS patients in endemic regions [73]. Infection has been reported in other immunocompromised patients, including immunodeficiency due to

anti-IFN-γ autoantibodies (an emerging adult-onset immunodeficiency syndrome first described in 2004), solid organ transplantation, hematopoietic stem cell transplantation recipients, and hematological malignancies. *T. marneffei* infection has also been reported in at least 15 patients with various other autoimmune diseases, such as systemic lupus erythematosus, mixed connective tissue disease, Sjögren's syndrome, primary biliary cirrhosis, primary immune thrombocytopenia, and autoimmune hemolytic anemia. *T. marneffei* infection usually occurs when these patients receive high-dose or prolonged treatment with T-lymphocyte-depleting drugs, including corticosteroids, cyclosporine, azathioprine, tacrolimus, and mycophenolate mofetil. The most common manifestations include fever, weight loss, adenopathy, hepatosplenomegaly, pulmonary symptoms, skin lesions, anemia, and leukocytosis or leukopenia [74]. Symptoms may be present for weeks to years prior to diagnosis. In 75% of disseminated infections, umbilicated skin papules, easily confused with molluscum contagiosum, cutaneous cryptococcosis, or histoplasmosis, will be present on the face, trunk, and extremities [74,75]. In addition, bone marrow infection, genital ulcers, osteomyelitis, arthritis, and retropharyngeal abscess have all been reported as complications of disseminated disease [74]. The organism can be isolated from skin lesions, or from blood, bone, or bone marrow. Presumptive diagnosis is made by visualization of yeast-like *T. marneffei* cells in Wright stained smears of skin lesions or biopsy specimens from these sites [73].

Culture remains the gold standard in diagnosis. Culture of the bone marrow is the most sensitive (100%), followed by skin (90%) and blood culture (76%).

T. marneffei infection is associated with a high mortality rate. In one report, 29.7% of non-HIV-infected patients with *T. marneffei* infection died despite most of them having received appropriate antifungal treatment. This rate was higher than that of HIV-infected patients (20%) in the same cohort and might reflect delayed diagnosis of *T. marneffei* infection among non-HIV-infected patients due to the lack of clinical suspicion in the early stage [76].

Treatment

Early treatment of *penicillosis marneffei* is critical to reduce mortality of this infection [73,76] and *in vitro* susceptibility helps to guide therapy. *In vitro*, *T. marneffei* appears to be susceptible to azole compounds, such as ketoconazole, itraconazole, and voriconazole. However, fluconazole appears to be the least active, as 73% of strains were resistant to fluconazole in one report [77]. In the same report, amphotericin B had intermediate activity against the organism, with MIC ranging between 0.25 and 4.0 μg/mL. However, despite the intermediate inhibitory activity of amphotericin B for some strains of *T. marneffei*, patients improved when treated with high doses of the drug administered intravenously. However, clinical response appears to correlate with susceptibility to azoles [77]. In another study from China, voriconazole

MIC against strains of *T. marneffei* ranged from 0.004 to 0.25 mg/L, and it had the lowest MIC in comparison to the other antifungal agents. The MICs of other antifungal agents, in order of lowest to highest, were as follows: itraconazole (0.031–0.5 mg/L), terbinafine (0.031–2.0 mg/L), amphotericin B (0.125–2.0 mg/L), and fluconazole (1.0–16.0 mg/L) [78]. Amphotericin B, voriconazole, and itraconazole are often used to treat penicilliosis [79–84]. In an open-label nonrandomized trial studying the efficacy of 2 weeks of amphotericin B followed by 10 weeks of oral outpatient itraconazole in HIV patients with disseminated *T. marneffei* infection, 72/74 (97.3%) of the patients responded to therapy [80]. Intravenous voriconazole for at least 3 days, followed by transitioning to oral voriconazole for a maximum of 12 weeks, has been used in other studies with good response rate [81]. Oral itraconazole for 8–12 weeks without amphotericin B induction therapy for patients with milder disease has been supported by several reports [82,83]. Alternatively, oral voriconazole for 12 weeks can also be used [81,84]. Following completion of treatment course in HIV positive patients, secondary prophylaxis should be continued until CD4 cell count increases to more than 100 cells/mL^3 for at least 6 months after the patient has been started on HAART [85]. Echinocandins are also active against *T. marneffei in vitro*, but it is more active against the mycelial rather than the yeast form [86]. However, *in vitro* micafungin enhances the efficacy of itraconazole and amphotericin B against *T. marneffei*, so echinocandins may have a potential role in combination therapy in the future [87]. Posaconazole showed potent *in vitro* activity against *T. marneffei* [36] and may be useful clinically but more data are required.

SCOPULARIOPSIS SPECIES

Epidemiology and mycology

Scopulariopsis is a large genus of saprophytic organisms found mostly in soil, but also frequently isolated from wood, paper, decaying organic materials, and animal remains [88]. Within the genus are members of both hyalohyphomycoses and phaeohyphomycoses. Of the hyaline species, *S. brevicaulis* is responsible for causing the majority of human infections. *S. candida* and *S. acremonium* have also been reported to cause disease in humans [3,88]. *S. brumptii* is a dematiaceous *Scopulariopsis* species that has been linked to cases of brain abscess [3].

Hyaline *Scopulariopsis* species grow on Sabouraud dextrose agar at both 28°C and 35°C. Colonies are white, buff, and gray-brown to black (Figure 20.7). Conidiogenous spores are annellides formed on branched condiophores with 1 or 2 levels of branching. Conidia are one celled, globose or ellipsoidal and occur in chains [3]. *S. brevicaulis* has buff or tan granular colonies, with thick-walled, smooth to coarsely roughened conidia that are flattened at the base and rounded or slightly pointed at the tip (Figure 20.8).

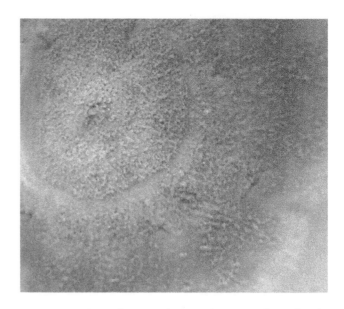

Figure 20.7 *Scopulariopsis brevicaulis*. Expanding whitish, powdery colonies.

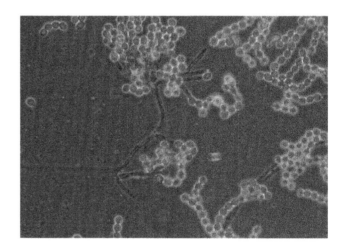

Figure 20.8 *Scopulariopsis brevicaulis*. Microscopy reveals chains of rough-walled conidia on well-developed annellides.

Clinical presentation

Scopulariopsis species are recognized as common causes of non-invasive infections [88] including nondermatophytic onychomycosis [89], keratitis [90,91], and otomycosis [92]. Although uncommon, invasive disease can also occur in both immunocompetent and immunosuppressed patients and include infections such as prosthetic-valve endocarditis [93], sinusitis [94], brain abscess [95], deep cutaneous [96,97], pulmonary [98], and disseminated infection [88].

Treatment

The optimal antifungal treatment has not been established. Invasive infections may require surgical and medical treatment and the mortality rate is very high despite treatment [5].

In vitro, *Scopulariopsis* species are usually quite resistant to most currently available antifungal agents [99–101]. However, susceptibility can vary by isolate, which may be variously susceptible to amphotericin B, miconazole, and ketoconazole [100,101]. In one report [99], antifungal susceptibility was determined for 25 clinical isolates of *S. brevicaulis*. All organisms were highly resistant to amphotericin B, posaconazole, voriconazole, itraconazole, caspofungin, and terbinafine *in vitro*. The activity of combinations of antifungal agents was tested by Cuenca-Estrella et al. [99] and the effect of combinations was not predictable and was dependent on the strain tested. Synergy was observed for some isolates and drug combinations, particularly with posaconazole-terbinafine (68% of strains), amphotericin B-caspofungin (60%), and posaconazole-caspofungin (48%).

There are approximately a dozen published reports of immunocompromised patients with invasive *Scopulariopsis* species infection, and most succumbed to their infection. However, in many patients there was inadequate immune reconstitution, a known essential component to combating an invasive fungal infection [101]. One report identified 12 cases in immunocompromised patients in whom prolonged therapy with amphotericin B with or without surgery was often ineffective [101]. In the same report, combination therapy with voriconazole and caspofungin despite *in vitro* synergy was unsuccessful in treating *S. brevicaulis* invasive infection in a bone marrow transplant recipient. On the other hand, a few cases of *Scopulariopsis* infection in the literature were reportedly successfully treated. Pate et al. reported successful treatment of *S. brumptii* invasive pulmonary infection in a liver transplant recipient with posaconazole and terbinafine combination therapy [102]. Similarly, combined surgery and long-term oral therapy with terbinafine resulted in a favorable outcome in recurrent subcutaneous infection due to *S. brevicaulis* in a liver transplant recipient [96]. Gluck et al. reported a case of *S. brevicaulis* invasive sinonasal infection treated successfully with a combination of wide local excision and antifungal therapy with liposomal amphotericin B [94].

QUESTIONS AND ANSWERS

Q: What is the commonest presentations of infections caused by *Acremonium* species?

A: Mycetomas are the commonest presentations of *Acremonium* species infections, which occur mostly after a traumatic inoculation and are characterized by the clinical triad of swelling, sinus tract formation, and fungal granules.

Q: What is the causative agent of penicilliosis?

A: True *Penicillium* species causing human infections are very rare, and the only pathogenic species previously identified as *Penicillium marneffei* was transferred to the *Talaromyces* genus and now officially holds the name *Talaromyces marneffei*. However, its associated disease is still referred to as penicilliosis

Q: What is the recommended treatment for mild and moderate to severe penicilliosis?

A: For moderate to severe disease, intravenous amphotericin B therapy should be administered for 2 weeks, followed by oral itraconazole for 10 weeks. Patients with mild disease can be initially treated with oral itraconazole for 8–12 weeks without amphotericin B induction therapy.

Q: What is the most common manifestations of *paecilomyces* spp. infection?

A: Oculomycosis and cutaneous infections are the most common clinical presentations of *paecilomyces* spp. infection.

REFERENCES

1. Ajello L. Hyalohyphomycosis and phaeohyphomycosis: Two global disease entities of public health importance. *Eur J Epidemiol* 1986;2(4):243–251.
2. Naggie S, Perfect JR. Molds: Hyalohyphomycosis, phaeohyphomycosis, and zygomycosis. *Clin Chest Med* 2009;30(2):337–353.
3. Zhang SX, O'Donnell K, Sutton DA. *Fusarium* and opportunistic Hyaline fungi: Mycology. In: Jorgensen JH, Pfaller MA, Carroll KC, Funke G, Landry ML, Richter SS, Warnock DW (Eds.). *Manual of Clinical Microbiology*, 11th ed., Vol. 2. Washington, DC: ASM Press, 2015, pp. 2057–2075.
4. Fincher RM, Fisher JF, Lovell RD, Newman CL, Espinel-Ingroff A, Shadomy HJ. Infection due to the fungus *Acremonium* (*cephalosporium*). *Medicine (Baltimore)* 1991;70(6):398–409.
5. Tortorano AM, Richardson M, Roilides E, et al. ESCMID and ECMM joint guidelines on diagnosis and management of hyalohyphomycosis: *Fusarium* spp., *Scedosporium* spp. and others. *Clin Microbiol Infect* 2014;20 Suppl 3:27–46.
6. Summerbell RC, Gueidan C, Schroers HJ, de Hoog GS, Starink M, Arocha Rosete Y. *Acremonium* phylogenetic overveiw and revision of *Gliomastix*, *Scarocladium* and *Trichothecium*. *Persoonia* 2011;68:139–162.
7. Perdomo H, Sutton DA, García D, Fothergill AW, Cano J, Gené J, Summerbell RC, Rinaldi MG, Guarro J. Spectrum of clinically relevant *Acremonium* species in the United States. *J Clin Microbiol* 2011;49(1):243–256.
8. Das S, Saha R, Dar SA, Ramachandran VG. *Acremonium* species: A review of the etiological agents of emerging hyalohyphomycosis. *Mycopathologia* 2010;170:361–375.
9. Guarro J, Gams W, Pujol I, et al. *Acremonium* species: New emerging fungal opportunists—*In vitro* antifungal susceptibilities and review. *Clin Infect Dis* 1997;25(5):1222–1229.
10. Lichon V, Khachemoune A. Mycetoma: A review. *Am J Clin Dermatol* 2006;7(5):315–321.

11. Gupta AK, Summerbell RC. Combined distal and lateral subungual and white superficial onychomycosis in toenails. *J Am Acad Dermatol* 1999;41:938–944.

12. Read RW, Chuck RS, Rao NA, et al. Traumatic *Acremonium atrogriseum* keratitis following laser-assisted in situ keratomileusis. *Arch Ophthalmol* 2000;118(3):418–421.

13. Kennedy SM, Shankland GS, Lee WR, et al. Keratitis due to the fungus *Acremonium* (Cephalosporium). *Eye* 1994;8(pt 6):692–694.

14. Weissgold DJ, Maguire AM, Brucker AJ. Management of postoperative *Acremonium* endophthalmitis. *Ophthalmology* 1996;103(5):749–756.

15. Simmons RB, Buffington JR, Ward M, Wilson LA, Ahearn DG. Ultrastructure of fungi in extended-wear soft contact lenses. *J Clin Microbiol* 1986;24:21–25.

16. Virgilio E, Mercantini P, Abu Samra S, Vitali M, Cavallini M. Pleuritis caused by *Acremoniumstrictum* in a patient with metastatic testicular teratocarcinoma. *Braz J Infect Dis* 2015;19(3):336–337.

17. Qazi MS, Bowalekar SS, Wanjare VS, Shankar A. An unusual case of lung abscess caused by *Acremonium* species treated with itraconazole. *Indian J Med Microbiol* 2015;33(2):307–310.

18. Wu CY, Huang HK, Wu PK, Chen WM, Lai MC, Chung LH. *Acremonium* species combined with *Penicillium* species infection in hip hemiarthroplasty: A case report and literature review. *Hip Int* 2014;24(6):656–659.

19. Beaudreuil S, Buchler M, Al Najjar A, et al. Acute septic arthritis after kidney transplantation due to *Acremonium*. *Nephrol Dial Transplant* 2003;18:850–851.

20. Szombathy SP, Chez MG, Laxer RM. Acute septic arthritis due to *Acremonium*. *J Rheumatol* 1988;15(4):714–715.

21. Brabender W, Ketcherside J, Hodges GR, Rengachary S, Barnes WG. *Acremoniumkiliense* osteomyelitis of the calvarium. *Neurosurgery* 1985;16:554–556.

22. Miyakis S, Velegraki A, Delikou S, Parcharidou A, Papadakis V, Kitra V, Papadatos I, Polychronopoulou S. Invasive *Acremoniumstrictum* infection in a bone marrow transplant recipient. *Pediatr Infect Dis J* 2006;25(3):273–275.

23. Noble RC, Salgado J, Newell SW, et al. Endophthalmitis and lumbar diskitis due to *Acremoniumfalciforme* in a splenectomized patient. *Clin Infect Dis* 1997;24(2):277–278.

24. Manzano-Gayosso P, Hernández-Hernández F, Méndez-Tovar LJ, González-Monroy J, López-Martínez R. Fungal peritonitis in 15 patients on continuous ambulatory peritoneal dialysis (CAPD). *Mycoses* 2003;46(9–10):425–429.

25. Kendirli T, Ciftçi E, Ekim M, Galip N, Düzenli F, Ozçakar ZB, Tapisiz A, Uçar T, Tutar E, Güriz H, Atalay S. Mycoses. *Acremonium* spp. peritonitis in an infant. 2008;51(5):455–457.

26. Krcmery V Jr, Kunova E, Jesenska Z, Trupl J, Spanik S, Mardiak J, Studena M, Kukuckova E. Invasive mold infections in cancer patients: 5 years' experience with *Aspergillus, Mucor, Fusarium* and *Acremonium* infections. *Support Care Cancer* 1996;4(1):39–45.

27. Pânzaru C, Dan M, Balasanian MO, Coadă G, Tinică G, Dabija ER. Subacute fungal endocarditis due to *Acremonium* spp: A case study and review of the literature. *Rev Med Chir Soc Med Nat Iasi* 2014;118(1):182–185.

28. Heitmann L, Cometta A, Hurni M, et al. Right-sided pacemaker-related endocarditis due to *Acremonium* species. *Clin Infect Dis* 1997;25(1):158–160.

29. Fakharian A, Dorudinia A, Alavi Darazam I, Mansouri D, Masjedi MR. *Acremonium* pneumonia: Case report and literature review. *Tanaffos* 2015;14(2):156–160.

30. Rodríguez ZC, Ramos MG. *Acremonium* species associated fungemia: A novel pathogen in the immunosuppressed patient. *Bol Asoc Med P R* 2014;106(3):29–31.

31. Lau YL, Yuen KY, Lee CW, et al. Invasive *Acremoniumfalciforme* infection in a patient with severe combined immunodeficiency. *Clin Infect Dis* 1995;20(1):197–198.

32. Kouvousis N, Lazaros G, Christoforatou E, Deftereos S, Petropoulou MD, Lelekis M. Pacemaker pocket infection due to *Acremonium* species. *Pacing Clin Electrophysiol* 2002;25:378–379.

33. Guarro J, Del Palacio A, Gené J, Cano J, González CG. A case of colonization of a prosthetic mitral valve by *Acremonium strictum*. *Rev Iberoam Micol* 2009;26:146–148.

34. Purnak T, Beyazit Y, Sahin GO, Shorbagi A, Akova M. A novel fungal pathogen under the spotlight—*Acremonium* species associated fungaemia in an immunocompetent host. *Mycoses* 2011;54:78–80.

35. Brown NM, Blundell EL, Chown SR, et al. *Acremonium* infection in a neutropenic patient. *J Infect* 1992;25(1):73–76.

36. Sabatelli F, Patel R, Mann PA, et al. *In vitro* activities of posaconazole, fluconazole, itraconazole, voriconazole, and amphotericin B against a large collection of clinically important molds and yeasts. *Antimicrob Agents Chemother* 2006;50:2009–2015.

37. Herbrecht R, Letscher-Bru V, Fohrer C, et al. *Acremonium strictum* pulmonary infection in a leukemic patient successfully treated with posaconazole after failure of amphotericin B. *Eur J Clin Microbiol Infect Dis* 2002;21:814–817.

38. Mattei D, Mordini N, Lo Nigro C, et al. Successful treatment of *Acremonium* fungemia with voriconazole. *Mycoses* 2003;46:511–514.

39. Luangsa-Ard J, Houbraken J, van Doorn T, et al. *Purpureocillium*, a new genus for the medically important *Paecilomyceslilacinus*. *FEMS Microbiol Lett* 2011;321:141–149.

40. Luangsa-Ard JJ, Hywel-Jones NL, Samson RA. The polyphyletic nature of *Paecilomyces* sensu lato based on 18S-generated rDNA phylogeny. *Mycologia* 2004;96(4):773–780.

41. Sigler L, Gibas CF, Kokotovic B, Bertelsen MF. Disseminated mycosis in veiled chameleons (*Chamaeleo calyptratus*) caused by *Chamaeleomyces granulomatis*, a new fungus related to *Paecilomycesviridis*. *J Clin Microbiol* 2010;48(9):3182–3192.

42. Orth B, Frei R, Itin PH, et al. Outbreak of invasive mycoses caused by *Paecilomyceslilacinus* from a contaminated skin lotion. *Ann Intern Med* 1996;125:799–806.

43. Pastor FJ, and Guarro J. Clinical manifestations, treatment, and outcome of *Paecilomyces lilacinus* infections. *Clin Microbiol Infect* 2006;12:948–960.

44. Yuan X, Wilhelmus KR, Matoba AY, Alexandrakis G, Miller D, Huang AJW. Pathogenesis and outcome of *paecilomyces* keratitis. *Am J Ophthalmol* 2009;147(4):691–696.

45. Turner LD, Conrad D. Retrospective case-series of *Paecilomyces lilacinus* ocular mycoses in Queensland, Australia. *BMC Res Notes* 2015;8:627.

46. Rimawi RH, Carter Y, Ware T, Christie J, Siraj D. Use of voriconazole for the treatment of *Paecilomyces lilacinus* cutaneous infections: Case presentation and review of published literature. *Mycopathologia* 2013;175(3–4):345–349.

47. Steiner B, Aquino VR, Paz AA, Silla LM, Zavascki A, Goldani LZ. *Paecilomyces variotii* as an emergent pathogenic agent of pneumonia. *Case Rep Infect Dis* 2013;2013:273848.

48. Gutiérrez F, Masiá M, Ramos J, Elía M, Mellado E, Cuenca-estrella M. Pulmonary mycetoma caused by an atypical isolate of *Paecilomyces* species in an immunocompetent individual: Case report and literature review of *Paecilomyces* lung infections. *Eur J Clin Microbiol Infect Dis* 2005;24:607–611.

49. Nayak DR, Balakrishnan R, Nainani S, Siddique S. *Paecilomyces* fungus infection of the paranasal sinuses. *Int J Pediatr Otorhinolaryngol* 2000;52(2):183–187.

50. Gucalp R, Carlisle P, Gialanella P, Mitsudo S, McKitrick J, Dutcher J. *Paecilomyces* sinusitis in an immunocompromised adult patient: Case report and review. *Clin Infect Dis* 1996;23:391–393.

51. Swami T, Pannu S, Kumar M, Gupta G. Chronic invasive fungal rhinosinusitis by *Paecilomycesvariotii*: A rare case report. *Indian J Med Microbiol* 2016;34(1):103–106.

52. Ding CH, Tzar MN, Rahman MM, Muttaqillah NA, Redzuan SR, Periyasamy P. *Paecilomyces lilacinus* fungaemia in an AIDS patient: The importance of mycological diagnosis. *Pak J Med Sci* 2014;30(4):914–916.

53. Salle V, Lecuyer E, Chouaki T, Lescure FX, Smail A, Vaidie A, Dayen C, Schmit JL, Ducroix JP, Douadi Y. *Paecilomyces variotii* fungemia in a patient with multiple myeloma: Case report and literature review. *J Infect* 2005;51(3):e93–e95.

54. Labriola L, V B, Ercam, Swinne D, Jadoul M. Successful treatment with voriconazole of prolonged *Paecilomyceslilacinus* fungemia in a chronic hemodialyzed patient. *Clin Nephrol* 2009;71(3):355–358.

55. Chamilos G, Kontoyiannis DP. Voriconazole-resistant disseminated *Paecilomycesvariotii* infection in a neutropenic patient with leukaemia on voriconazole prophylaxis. *J Infect* 2005;51(4):e225–e228.

56. Wright K, Popli S, Gandhi VC, Lentino JR, Reyes CV, Leehey DJ. *Paecilomyces* peritonitis: Case report and review of the literature. *Clin Nephrol* 2003;59(4):305–310.

57. Müller H, Cikirikcioglu M, Lerch R. Subaortic aneurysm caused by *Paecilomyceslilacinus* endocarditis. *Arch Cardiovasc Dis* 2008;101(11–12):803–804.

58. Fagerburg R, Suh B, Buckley HR, Lorber B, Karian J. Cerebrospinal fluid shunt colonization and obstruction by *Paecilomyces variotii*. Case report. *J Neurosurg* 1981;54:257–260.

59. Sherwood JA, Dansky AS. *Paecilomyces* pyelonephritis complicating nephrolithiasis and review of *Paecilomyces* infections. *J Urol* 1983;130:526–528.

60. Dhindsa MK, Naidu J, Singh SM, et al. Chronic suppurative otitis media caused by *Paecilomyces variotii*. *J Med Vet Mycol* 1995;33:59–61.

61. Gompf SG, Paredes A, Quilitz R, Greene JN, Hiemenz JW, Sandin RL. *Paecilomyces lilaceous* osteomyelitis in a bone marrow transplant patient. *Infect Med* 1999;16:766–770.

62. Keshtkar-Jahromi M, McTighe AH, Segalman KA, Fothergill AW, Campbell WN. Unusual case of cutaneous and synovial *Paecilomyces lilacinus* infection of hand successfully treated with voriconazole and review of published literature. *Mycopathologia* 2012;174(3):255–258.

63. Schweitzer KM, Richard MJ, Leversedge FJ, Ruch DS. *Paecilomyces lilacinus* septic olecranon bursitis in an immunocompetent host. *Am J Orthop* 2012;41(5):E74–E75.

64. Castelli MV, Alastruey-Izquierdo A, Cuesta I, et al. Susceptibility testing and molecular classification of *Paecilomyces* spp. *Antimicrobial Agents Chemother* 2008;52:2926–2928.

65. Houbraken J, Verweij PE, Rijs AJ, Borman AM, Samson RA. Identification of *Paecilomyces variotii* in clinical samples and settings. *J Clin Microbiol* 2010;48(8):2754–2761.

66. Kuboi T, Okazaki K, Inotani M, Sugino M, Sadamura T, Nakano A, Kobayashi S, Ota A, Nishimura K, Yaguchi T. A case of cutaneous *Paecilomyces formosus* infection in an extremely premature infant. *J Infect Chemother* 2016;22(5):339–341.

67. Safdar A. Progressive cutaneous hyalohyphomyco-sis due to *Paecilomyces lilacinus*: Rapid response to treatment with caspofungin and itraconazole. *Clin Infect Dis* 2002;34:1415–1417.

68. Martin CA, Roberts S, Greenberg RN. Voriconazole treatment of disseminated *Paecilomyces* infection in a patient with acquired immunodeficiency syndrome. *Clin Infect Dis* 2002;35:e78–e81.

69. Mullane K, Toor AA, Kalnicky C, et al. Posaconazole salvage therapy allows successful allogeneic hema-topoietic stem cell transplantation in patients with refractory invasive mold infections. *Transpl Infect Dis* 2007;9:89–96.

70. Van Schooneveld T, Freifeld A, Lesiak B, et al. *Paecilomyces lilacinus* infection in a liver transplant patient: Case report and review of the literature. *Transpl Infect Dis* 2008;10:117–122.

71. Visagie CM, Houbraken J, Frisvad JC, Hong SB, Klaassen CH, Perrone G, Seifert KA, Varga J, Yaguchi T, Samson RA. Identification and nomenclature of the genus *Penicillium*. *Stud Mycol* 2014;78:343–371.

72. Yilmaz N, Visagie CM, Houbraken J, Frisvad JC, Samson RA. Polyphasic taxonomy of the genus *Talaromyces*. *Stud Mycol* 2014;78:175–341.

73. Chen AC SX, Sorrell TC, Meyer W. *Aspergillus* and *penicillium*: Mycology. In: Jorgensen JH, Pfaller MA, Carroll KC, Funke, Landry ML, Richter SS, Warnock DW (Eds.). *Manual of Clinical Microbiology*, 11th ed., Vol. 2. Washington, DC: ASM Press, 2015:2030–2065.

74. Duong TA. Infection due to *Penicillium marneffei*, an emerging pathogen: Review of 155 reported cases. *Clin Infect Dis* 1996;23(1):125–130.

75. Hilmarsdottir I, Meynard JL, Rogeaux O, et al. Disseminated *Penicillium marneffei* infection associ-ated with human immunodeficiency virus: A report of two cases and a review of 35 published cases. *J Acquir Immune Defic Syndr* 1993;6(5):466–471.

76. Kawila R, Chaiwarith R, Supparatpinyo K. Clinical and laboratory characteristics of *penicilliosis marneffei* among patients with and without HIV infection in Northern Thailand: A retrospective study. *BMC Infect Dis* 2013;13:464.

77. Supparatpinyo K, Nelson KE, Merz WG, et al. Response to antifungal therapy by human immu-nodeficiency virus infected patients with dissemi-nated *Penicillium marneffei* infections and *in vitro* susceptibilities of isolates from clinical specimens. *Antimicrob Agents Chemother* 1993;37:2407–2411.

78. Liu D, Liang L, Chen J. *In vitro* antifungal drug susceptibilities of *Penicillium marneffei* from China. *J Infect Chemother* 2013;19(4):776–778.

79. Sirisanthana T, Supparatpinyo K, Perriens J, et al. Amphotericin B and itraconazole for treatment of disseminated *Penicillium marneffei* infection in human immunodeficiency virus-infected patients. *Clin Infect Dis* 1998;26(5):1107–1110.

80. Supparatpinyo K, Perriens J, Nelson KE, et al. A controlled trial of itraconazole to prevent relapse of *Penicillium marneffei* infection in patients infected with the human immunodeficiency virus. *N Engl J Med* 1998;339(24):1739–1743.

81. Supparatpinyo K, Schlamm HT. Voriconazole as therapy for systemic *Penicillium marneffei* infec-tions in AIDS patients. *Am J Trop Med Hyg* 2007;77(2):350–353.

82. Ranjana KH, Priyokumar K, Singh TJ, Gupta ChC, Sharmila L, Singh PN, Chakrabarti A. Disseminated *Penicillium marneffei* infection among HIV-infected patients in Manipur state, India. *J Infect* 2002;45(4):268.

83. Supparatpinyo K, Chiewchanvit S, Hirunsri P, Baosoung V, Uthammachai C, Chaimongkol B, Sirisanthana T. An efficacy study of itraconazole in the treatment of *Penicillium marneffei* infection. *J Med Assoc Thai* 1992;75(12):688.

84. Perfect JR, Marr KA, Walsh TJ, et al. Voriconazole treatment for less-common, emerging, or refractory fungal infections. *Clin Infect Dis* 2003;36:1122–1131.

85. Kaplan JE, Benson C, Holmes KK, et al. Guidelines for prevention and treatment of opportunistic infections in HIV-infected adults and adolescents: Recommendations from CDC, the National Institutes of Health, and the HIV Medicine Association of the Infectious Diseases Society of America. *MMWR Recomm Rep* 2009;58(RR-4):1–207.

86. Nakai T, Uno J, Ikeda F, Tawara S, Nishimura K, Miyaji M. *In vitro* antifungal activity of Micafungin (FK463) against dimorphic fungi: Comparison of yeast-like and mycelial forms. *Antimicrob Agents Chemother* 2003;47(4):1376–1381.

87. Cao C, Liu W, Li R, Wan Z, Qiao J. *In vitro* interac-tions of micafungin with amphotericin B, itracon-azole or fluconazole against the pathogenic phase of *Penicillium marneffei*. *J Antimicrob Chemother* 2009;63:340–342.

88. Iwen PC, Schutte SD, Florescu DF, Noel-Hurst RK, Sigler L. Invasive *Scopulariopsis brevicaulis* infection in an immunocompromised patient and review of prior cases caused by *Scopulariopsis* and *Microascus* species. *Med Mycol* 2012 Aug;50(6):561–569.

89. Issakainen J, Heikkla H, Vainio E, et al. Occurrence of *Scopulariopsis* and *Scedosporium* in nails and kera-tinous skin. A five-year retrospective multi-center study. *Med Mycol* 2007;45:201–209.

90. Mondal KK, Chattopadhyay C, Ray B, Das D, Biswas S, Banerjee P. Corneal ulcer with *Scopulariopsis brevi-caulis* and *Staphylococcus aureus*—A rare case report. *J Indian Med Assoc* 2012;110(4):253–254.

91. Malecha MA. Fungal keratitis caused by *Scopulariopsis brevicaulis* treated successfully with natamycin. *Cornea* 2004 Mar;23(2):201–203.

92. Besbes M, Makni F, Cheikh-Rouhou F, Sellami H, Kharrat K, Ayadi A. Otomycosis due to *Scopulariopsis brevicaulis*. *Rev Laryngol Otol Rhinol (Bord)* 2002;123(2):77–78.

93. Isidro AM, Amorosa V, Stopyra GA, Rutenberg HL, Pentz WH, Bridges CR. Fungal prosthetic mitral valve endocarditis caused by *Scopulariopsis* species: Case report and review of the literature. *J Thorac Cardiovasc Surg* 2006;131(5):1181–1183.

94. Gluck O, Segal N, Yariv F, Polacheck I, Puterman M, Greenberg D, Daniel B. Pediatric invasive sinonasal *Scopulariopsis brevicaulis*—A case report and literature review. *Int J Pediatr Otorhinolaryngol* 2011;75(7):891–893.

95. Hart AP, Sutton DA, McFeeley PJ, Kornfeld M. Cerebral phaeohyphomycosis caused by a dematiaceous *scopulariopsis* species. *Clin Neuropathol* 2001 Sep–Oct;20(5):224–228.

96. Sellier P, Monsuez JJ, Lacroix C, et al. Recurrent subcutaneous infection due to *Scopulariopsis brevicaulis* in a liver transplant recipient. *Clin Infect Dis* 2000;30:820–823.

97. Wu C, Lee C, HL L, Wu C. Cutaneous granulomatous infection caused by *Scopulariopsis brevicaulis*. *Acta Derm Venereol* 2009;89:103–104.

98. Wheat LJ, Bartlett M, Ciccarelli M, Smith JW. Opportunistic *Scopulariopsis* pneumonia in an immunocompromised host. *South Med J* 1984;77(12):1608–1609.

99. Cuenca-Estrella M1, Gomez-Lopez A, Buitrago MJ, Mellado E, Garcia-Effron G, Rodriguez-Tudela JL. *In vitro* activities of 10 combinations of antifungal agents against the multiresistant pathogen *Scopulariopsis brevicaulis*. *Antimicrob Agents Chemother* 2006;50(6):2248–2250.

100. Cuenca-Estrella M, Gomez-Lopez A, Mellado E, et al. *Scopulariopsis brevicaulis*, a fungal pathogen resistant to broad-spectrum antifungal agents. *Antimicrob Agents Chemother* 2003;47(7):2339–2341.

101. Aguilar C, Pujol I, Guarro J. *In vitro* antifungal susceptibilities of *Scopulariopsis* isolates. *Antimicrob Agents Chemother* 1999;43:1520–1522.

102. Pate MJ, Hemmige V, Woc-Colburn L, Restrepo A. Successful eradication of invasive *Scopulariopsis brumptii* in a liver transplant recipient. *Transpl Infect Dis* 2016;18(2):275–279.

21

Management of phaeohyphomycosis

JOHN R. PERFECT AND AHMAD MOURAD

INTRODUCTION

It is important to emphasize that the term phaeohyphomycosis, which means condition of fungi with dark hyphae, is not based on a single genus or species and, actually, represents many genera and species. Another term, which has been used to describe these fungi, is dematiaceous fungi, but this does not reflect their dark color primarily produced by melanins. However, a unifying theme for these fungi is their ability to produce melanin in their cell walls and form yeasts and/or hyphal-like structures in tissue. It is not surprising that this diversity of fungi is also reflected in their multiple clinical presentations, thus a single management style is not possible. In this chapter, there will be an attempt to incorporate principles that will be helpful once these fungi are properly identified as causing disease.

Although the ability to produce melanin is not unique to this group of mycoses (i.e., *Cryptococcus* and some of the dimorphic fungi can produce melanin), the combination of their ability to produce melanin even during infection and the variety of morphologies of these fungi in tissue have allowed medical mycologists to lump this group of fungi together. In fact, with a broad definition, over 100 dematiaceous molds have been reported to cause medical conditions from simple colonization to invasive disease in the human host and they represent an emerging group of mycoses in the last decade [1]. From solid organ transplant recipients to advanced AIDS patients to cancer victims to iatrogenic outbreaks, multiple risk groups have appeared to be susceptible to phaeohyphomycoses [2–4].

CLINICAL PRESENTATIONS

The "wide net" spread to categorize this group of mycoses allows for a variety of clinical presentations. First, chromoblastomycosis is a chronic disease of the skin and subcutaneous tissue and is classically identified by the appearance of muriform fungal structures (sclerotic bodies) in the tissue. This indolent soft tissue disease is primarily diagnosed in tropical climates. Second, eumycetoma is a chronic deep tissue disease that primarily occurs in lower extremities with the fungi causing sinus tracts and mycotic grains within the subcutaneous and other soft tissues. Third, is the superficial ulceration of the skin and soft tissue or formation of subcutaneous cysts, and these presentations are primarily caused by direct trauma [5]. For example, these lesions may be aided in their appearance by the thinning of the skin with chronic use of corticosteroids therapy. Fourth, foreign body or fomite introduction of these fungi into the body can occur by the contamination of instruments or fluids. Fifth, fungal keratitis is frequently caused by molds, and, along with *Aspergillus* spp., *Fusarium* spp., and *Paecilomyces* spp., the dematiaceous fungi are a major etiological group of fungi for this condition. Sixth, fungal sinusitis is a poorly defined entity, but dematiaceous fungi have frequently been reported to produce allergic fungal sinusitis, fungus ball formation in sinuses, or even invasive disease in which the fungus breaks through sinus tissue planes and invades orbital tissue or the brain. Finally, there is systemic or disseminated phaeohyphomycosis in which several of this group of fungi may spread to multiple organs in severely immunosuppressed individuals or in some individuals with brain abscess(s) since some of these fungi appear to have neurotropic features [6,7].

FUNGAL IDENTIFICATION

Along with a variety of clinical presentations, there are a series of different genera with substantial differences in their ability to produce human disease (Table 21.1) [8–10]. For instance, there are several neurotropic dematiaceous molds, such as the brain abscess-producing fungi (*Cladophialophora bantiana, Dactylaria gallopava, Fonsecaea pedrosoi,* and *Rhinocladiella mackenziei*) [11,12]. In fact, these fungi have enough direct virulence potential that they can produce disease in both immunosuppressed and apparently immunocompetent hosts, and *Scedosporium apiospermum* can uniquely produce meningitis in "near-drowning" freshwater victims [13]. On the other side of the virulence potential scheme are the fungal species that primarily colonize skin and airways, and rarely cause disease. These classic dematiaceous colonizing molds include *Cladosporium* spp., *Aureobadisium* spp., *Hormonema* spp., and certain *Rhinocladiella* spp. With these molds, it is necessary to actually show histopathological evidence or culture from a sterile body site to support their etiologic contribution to disease, since they are rare causes of disease in most host risk groups and frequently colonize skin and/or airways. In the middle of this virulence grouping of the dematiaceous molds are Alternaria, Bipolaris, Exserohilum, Exophiala, Phialophora, and Wangiella species. These fungi have been shown to cause sinusitis, soft tissue disease, keratitis, disseminated disease with or without meningitis, and even endocarditis [14]. Since one can rank the potential virulence of these fungi and most reported disease with these molds occur in small case series, the initial steps in the management of this group of mold infections are to obtain correct

Table 21.1 Dematiaceous fungi and their most common phaeohyphomycosis

Etiologic agent	Clinical presentation	References
Alternaria spp. (*alternata*)	Osteomyelitis, cutaneous, sinusitis	[17–19]
Aureobasidium spp. (*pullulans, mansoni*)	Peritonitis, cutaneous, spleen infection	[18–20]
Bipolaris spp. (*australiensis, hawaiiensis, spicifera*)	Meningitis, sinusitis, keratitis, peritonitis, endocarditis, disseminated infection	[18,19,21–25]
Chaetomium spp. (*atrobrunneum*) *Achaetomium* spp. (*strumarium*)	Fungemia, cutaneous, brain abscess	[19]
Cladophialophora spp. (*carrionii, bantiana*)	Chromoblastomycosis, brain abscess	[11,18,26–29]
Cladosporium spp.	Colonizer, skin, keratitis	[18]
Coniothyrium spp. (*fuckelii*)	Cutaneous, liver infection	[19]
Curvularia spp. (*lunata*)	Sinusitis, keratitis, endocarditis, subcutaneous cyst, pneumonitis	[7,18,30]
Dactylaria spp. (*gallopava*)	Brain abscess, disseminated infection, pneumonitis	[18,31,32]
Exophiala spp. (*jeanselmei*)	Subcutaneous cyst, eumycetoma, keratitis, meningitis/ brain abscess, disseminated infection, mycetoma, peritonitis	[18,33–35]
Exserohilum spp. (*rostratum*)	Sinusitis, cutaneous, subcutaneous cyst, keratitis	[18,22]
Fonsecaea spp. (*pedrosoi*)	Chromoblastomycosis, eumycetoma, pneumonitis	[18,36,37]
Lasiodiplodia spp. (*theobromae*)	Keratitis	[38]
Lecythophora spp. (*hoffmanii*)	Subcutaneous cyst, endocarditis, peritonitis	[38]
Phaeoacremonium spp. (*parasiticum*)	Cutaneous, subcutaneous cyst	[18]
Phaeoannellomyces spp. (*elegans, werneckii*)	Subcutaneous cyst	
Phialemonium spp. (*curvatum, obovatum*)	Subcutaneous cyst, endocarditis, peritonitis	[38]
Phialophora spp. (*verrucosa, richardsiae*)	Chromoblastomycosis, eumycetoma, keratitis, osteomyelitis, endocarditis	[37]
Phoma spp.	Sinusitis, keratitis, subcutaneous cyst	[38]
Ramichloridium spp. (*obovoideum, mackenziei*)	Brain abscess	[12]
Rhinocladiella spp. (*aquaspersa, atrovirens*)	Colonizer; chromoblastomycosis, meningitis	[37–40]
Scedosporium spp. (*apiospermum, prolificans*)	Eumycetoma, meningitis, pneumonitis, fungemia, disseminated infection	[38,41–46]
Scytalidium spp. (*dimidiatum*)	Cutaneous, nail, subcutaneous cyst	[38]
Wangiella spp. (*dermatitidis*)	Cutaneous, subcutaneous cyst, keratitis, brain abscess, arthritis, disseminated infection	[18,47,48]

Source: Schell, W.A., Dematiaceous hyphomycetes, In: Howard, D.H. (Ed.), *Fungi Pathogenic for Humans and Animals*, 2nd ed., Revised and Expanded, Marcel Dekker, New York, pp. 565–636, 2003; Perfect, J.R. et al., Phaeohyphomycosis, *Clinical Mycology*, Oxford Press, New York, pp. 271–282, 2003.

identification of the mold to help predict outcome and plan a therapeutic strategy. Furthermore, during this evaluation of identification, it may also be prudent to obtain *in vitro* susceptibility testing for the strain if it is causing disease and particularly do this testing in difficult cases in which there is a poor clinical track record. It is true that these dematiaceous molds do not have standard "break points" for *in vitro* susceptibility but there is a standard protocol for performing the MICs [15]. In difficult cases, there can be some *in vitro* impression of the antifungal drug activities against the specific dematiaceous mold producing the infection, and, in some cases, MICs are so high that drug resistance can be predicted [16]. In difficult-to-treat cases, this information may be helpful in selection of an antifungal regimen for medical treatment.

TREATMENT MODALITIES

The treatment of phaeohyphomycosis is primarily based on isolated human cases and several small case series [33]. There has been an attempt by the Euopean Society of Microbiology and European Confederation of Medical Mycology to provide some general guidelines for this group of fungi [50]. However, there are no robust randomized, blind studies to provide guidance for the use of any antifungal agents for this group of infections. This deficiency in guidance is a combination of the variety of clinical syndromes produced by this group of fungi, the heterogenous risk groups with underlying diseases, and the number of genus strains that might have varying drug susceptibility. Despite the paucity of robust guidelines with accurate measured outcomes, there are actually several principles that can be followed that will generally provide a positive outcome for phaeohyphomycosis in most patients.

Surgery

The first modality in the management of phaeohyphomycosis is the consideration of surgery. Primary treatment of surgically accessible lesions in selected soft tissue, brain, and sinus locations must be considered. For instance, subcutaneous cysts with dematiaceous fungi can and should be surgically removed as an encapsulated structure(s) since this modality can be curative. It is important that there is no spillage of cyst contents back into the wound during the surgical procedure and a simple aspiration of these cysts alone is probably not optimal. The best results with an ulcerative lesion or without a defined cyst will require very careful debridement and may be even approached with a Moh's like procedure to optimally define the borders of infection for surgical removal [51]. An important principle in the local surgical management of these infections is that these fungi frequently grow with both hyphae and adventitial yeast-like forms in tissue [52]; thus, it is not difficult to surmise that some of these fungal structures may be left or fall back in the wound during surgery to provide a nidus for relapse of infection. Therefore, it is probably wise to carefully lavage residual tissue in the wound after surgery with an antiseptic to help kill or remove these persistent forms. In fact, in many of these local cases, a systemic antifungal agent may also be used after surgery for an empirical period of time to potentially clear any residual fungi from the tissue.

For a single brain abscess, some form of surgical debridement is probably necessary for consistent cure. In this body site, complete surgical removal of a brain abscess that is ideal may not be possible without serious consequences, but even some careful debulking of the lesion may be helpful in reducing the burden of fungi prior to systemic antifungal therapy. Of course, it is possible that surgery might spread the infection to other tissue planes, but it is likely that debulking the mass of fungi far outweighs any concern about infection spread within the brain. Furthermore, all brain abscesses are accompanied by medical treatment with antifungal agents no matter what the extent of surgery. Although occasionally medical therapy alone for brain abscesses has been successful, there are many failures without a combined surgical/medical approach for brain abscesses; therefore, we encourage the combination approach.

Surgery for sinus disease is common. For instance, surgical removal of a fungus ball (eumycetoma) within the sinus may be curative. In some cases of eumycetoma such as Madura foot and chromoblastomycosis, there is chronic scarring, poor lymphatic drainage, many fistulous tracts within the soft tissue, and even underlying bone involvement. These may result in an inability to obtain free margins of disease with surgery, and might create even more destruction of the vascular supply. In these cases, medical therapy alone may be considered the best treatment option. However, even in cases with extensive soft tissue involvement, it is encouraged to have surgical evaluation and follow-up with any initial medical strategy that is planned.

Antifungal drugs

The second component of management of these dematiaceous infections revolves around antifungal drugs. Although there are no robust definitive studies to guide the use of specific antifungal agents in phaeohyphomycosis, there is a rich history of *in vitro* susceptibility testing, animal model results, and reported cases of both failures and successes with antifungal therapy alone. It is impossible to match every phaeohyphomycosis (either genera or individual strains may vary) with a specific antifungal regimen, but it is reasonable to give some general principles that hold for many of these invading pathogens. Potassium iodide has been reported to be successful in cutaneous phaeohyphomycosis, but primarily standard antifungal agents have been used today in the management of phaeohyphomycosis [53]. First, the broad-spectrum polyene class of antifungal agents do possess some *in vitro* activity against these fungi and have been used to treat disseminated phaeohyphomycosis cases successfully. However, for local cases of soft tissue infection, their toxicity profile, need for intravenous administration, occasional resistant strains, and the impreciseness for length of therapy generally do not make this class of agents very attractive for primary use. In most cases, the polyenes are used in cases of disseminated infection and even in these cases are probably most commonly used in combination with other agents rather than as a single agent. Furthermore, it is necessary to identify fungal species and possibly *in vitro* susceptibility before use. Second, flucytosine has excellent *in vitro* activity against many of the genera in this group. It has been used in animal models and patients to successfully treat dematiaceous mold disease [54]. There have always been concerns about the rapid development of direct drug resistance when flucytosine is used alone for antifungal treatment and this concern also includes the management of phaeohyphomycosis. Therefore, flucytosine is generally used in a combination regimen. It is a standard induction therapy regimen with amphotericin B or lipid formulations of amphotericin B for cryptococcal meningitis and is very reasonable to consider it as part of a combination regimen for the treatment of cerebral phaeohyphomycosis. Its different mechanism of action, excellent pharmacokinetics from oral administration, and its high drug levels in the central nervous system make it an antifungal agent that should always be considered in serious, life-threatening phaeohyphomycosis, if the specific infecting fungal strain has basic *in vitro* susceptibility. Third, the newest class of antifungal agents are the echinocandins (caspofungin, micafungin, and anidulafungin) that target the beta-glucan synthase enzyme used for cell wall formation. The echinocandins with their safety, little drug–drug interactions, and antifungal potency for many *Candida* species have become the first line agents in invasive candidiasis and frequently are used in a secondary role for the management of aspergillosis. In fact, these echinocandins do possess *in vitro* activity against some of the genera in the dematiaceous groups [55–57]. Therefore, they may have some role in certain cases of phaeohyphomycosis. Prior to their use in phaeohyphomycosis, it might be wise to determine the direct *in vitro* susceptibility of the strain to be treated in order to understand whether the echinocandin would have any potential to clinically inhibit the fungus in tissue. Furthermore, it is probable that echinocandins will be generally confined to combination therapy, such as in cerebral phaeohyphomycosis that generally uses combination medical therapy. It is still uncertain how effective the echinocandins as a class are in CNS infections with their limited brain penetration. Fourth, terbinafine, the squalene epoxidase inhibitor, which attacks fungal cell membrane formation, has been the pivotal drug in the management of dermatophyte infections. It has not been a linchpin drug for invasive mycoses and its experience in phaeohyphomycosis remains limited. However, it has excellent pharmacokinetics for skin and soft tissue infections; it does possess direct antifungal activity against some of the dematiaceous fungi, and has been successfully used in combination with other antifungal agents [58]. Terbinafine's place in the management of phaeohyphomycosis is probably as a secondary agent that first needs the isolate to be shown to possess some *in vitro* antifungal susceptibility to it [59]. It will primarily be used in combination with another agent, such as an azole, for refractory or relapsed infections. Fifth, the azole drugs have become the most commonly used drugs in the medical management of phaeohyphomycosis. This development as a primary therapeutic choice for this group of fungi was first established by itraconazole and with the report of one series of phaeohyphomycosis successfully treated in over 60% of cases with this antifungal agent [60]. The extended-spectrum oral triazole became established as the drug of choice. Furthermore, the newer extended-spectrum triazoles, such as posaconazole and voriconazole and isavuconazole, also have shown excellent *in vitro* activity against a wide range of dematiaceous fungi, and there have been several case series in which excellent therapeutic outcomes have been demonstrated with these newer azoles [56,61–63]. Importantly, these new azoles have performed very well in CNS phaeohyphomycosis both in animal models and human disease [64–66]. Treatment success has been achieved both in meningitis and brain abscesses with these extended-spectrum azoles [67–69]. There are several advantages of the extended-spectrum azoles (like voriconazole and posaconazole and isavuconazole) in the treatment of phaeohyphomycosis: (i) they can be administered orally, (ii) the pharmacokinetics of these azoles are excellent for both skin/subcutaneous involvement and CNS disease, (iii) the precision of treatment length is still not known for phaeohyphomycosis. However, since these infections are primarily chronic, the length of treatment has also been extended for months of therapy. The azoles allow safe, long-term treatment schedules (iv) through *in vitro* susceptibility testing assessment. The potency and breadth of antifungal activity for these extended-spectrum azoles are broad and potent against many of the dematiaceous molds.

Since there are several classes of antifungal agents with direct antifungal activity against dematiaceous molds, the frequent clinical question in serious and refractory cases is: can combination therapy be of benefit? In fact, drug combinations from *in vitro* susceptibility studies generally show either additive or synergistic activity against many of the dematiaceous fungi [70]. Therefore, there is some clinical support for the use of more than one drug for refractory or serious (life-threatening) disease but within specific isolates or disease locations, the value of using more than one drug remains arbitrary. For disseminated or intracranial disease in which there is a limited surgical option, the use of combinations (polyene, flucytosine, terbinafine, echinocandins, and/or extended-spectrum azoles) is frequently considered. In fact, in most cases in which surgery is performed, antifungal drug treatment is used to insure elimination of any residual infection.

There are specific circumstances that will require creative solutions for treatment of these infections without robust clinical data for guidance.

1. **Fungal keratitis [71,72].** A portion of these infections are caused by dematiaceous molds. Treatment requires careful assessment by an ophthalmologist and generally with initial therapy, ophthalmic drops every one to two hours to control infection. At least one strategy is to alternate antifungal drops with different mechanisms of action, such as amphotericin B, voriconazole, and an antiseptic like polyhexamethylene biquanide. For example, topical natamycin and amphotericin B with or without the combination of a topical azole for a period of 4 weeks to few months is one regimen, but, at times, the natamycin will produce a film over the cornea that may not be helpful for combination therapy and this regimen uses two polyenes with similar mechanism(s) of action [73]. Also, if there is extension deep into cornea or other eye structures in which topical agents may have reduced presence, use of systemic voriconazole may be effective, although topical voriconazole can penetrate through the cornea into the anterior chamber of the eye. Salvage therapy with intrastromal injection of voriconazole has also been reported in patients who did not respond to topical or systemic therapy but its value remains unclear [73].

2. **Allergic fungal sinusitis [74].** As a result of a hypersensitivity reaction to fungal antigens, there has been support for the use of corticosteroids to decrease immune stimulation or immunotherapy to induce tolerance to the fungal antigens in this condition [75]. There are also proponents who would try to reduce antigen loads by prescribing antifungal agents to mimic the strategy that was successful for allergic bronchopulmonary aspergillosis. However, these fungi may be eliminated from sinuses without specific antifungal therapy. Despite these several potential strategies for management, there remain little evidence-based studies to confidently guide antifungal therapies in this condition and this critically needs better studies. Azoles have been suggested for their potential steroid-sparing effect, and oral triazoles have been shown to reduce symptoms in some cases of refractory sinusitis [73]. However, surgery will be required to remove a fungus ball in the sinus cavity [76].

3. **Invasive or disseminated disease in the immunocompromised patient.** It is essential that control of underlying disease is made and maintained. There needs to be an attempt to eliminate or reduce immunosuppressive drugs (i.e., corticosteroids) and correct immunosuppressive conditions, such as neutropenia. Similar to most invasive fungal infections, the use of immune modulators, such as granulocyte-monocyte colony-stimulating factor (GM-CSF), gamma interferon remains a possible option in selecting patients who are refractory to surgery and/or antifungal therapy but their specific use is poorly defined in phaeohyphomycoses. Combination antifungal therapy and adjunctive treatments may have the greatest promise in disseminated disease. For example, some case reports have suggested using a combination of itraconazole or voriconazole and terbinafine for *Scedosporium prolificans*, with improved outcomes [77]. These infections are increasing in our cancer patients and may occur as breakthrough infections during empiric or prophylactic antifungal agents. The mortality rate has reached 33% with *Phaeohyphomycosis* infections. Infections with Scedosporium prolificans, in particular, reach a mortality of 70%–100% [4, 77].

4. **Chronic skin infections.** Chromoblastomycosis and eumycetoma will likely require long-term antifungals (i.e., azoles) with careful surgical intervention when necessary, and control of bacterial superinfections in these chronic conditions that have sinus tracts and at times involvement of the underlying bone. Antifungal therapy also depends on the site and burden of disease. For example, patients with multiple subcutaneous nodules require systemic antifungal therapy with either itraconazole or voriconazole [73]. The length of treatment for all the phaeohyphomycosis is not well defined and will need to be judged individually at the bedside or in the clinic. However, there are situations where these infections will relapse if therapy is stopped early so the majority of infections are treated for months.

5. **Foreign body infections.** The dematiaceous fungi can contaminate catheters, heart valves, and insertion of other foreign bodies (i.e., pacemakers) into sterile sites. For instance, intravenous catheters in cancer patients can act as a source for fungemia with Aureobasidium or patients receiving chronic ambulatory peritoneal dialysis may develop peritonitis with black molds [4,78]. Similar to principles with other infections around foreign bodies, it is prudent to remove the foreign body if possible to guard against antifungal therapy failure related to biofilms and other factors that allow these organisms to persist despite treatment.

6. **Contaminated steroids injections [79–81].** In the United States between 2012 and 2013, there were 749 reported cases of fungal infections spanning over 20 states in patients who received contaminated methylprednisolone acetate injections, purchased from a single pharmacy. Patients had either received epidural or paraspinal steroid injections or peripheral-joint injections, or both. Subsequently, 229 patients developed fungal meningitis with 153 showing laboratory evidence of *Exserohilum rostratum*. Testing of unopened steroid vials from the pharmacy did reveal contamination of the vials with *E. rostratum* and several other non-pathogenic fungi. Prior to this outbreak, *E. rostratum* was not found to be a common pathogenic mold. However, in the setting of direct injection of fungal cells with an immunosuppressive agent (steroid) into human tissue, a host-pathogen interaction did take place. With no previous cases or animal models of *E. rostratum* infection, extrapolating *in vitro* data and clinical experience with antifungal drugs, amphotericin B, and the azoles (voriconazole,

posaconazole, and itraconazole) were recommended to treat infected patients. In patients with CNS disease, a combination of liposomal amphotericin B and voriconazole was recommended due to voriconazole's excellent penetration into the CNS. As of 2013, there were a total of 61 reported deaths with 1–2 still being reported each month. However, this experience has shown that extended-spectrum azoles, like voriconazole, can effectively treat the majority of infections with this black mold in the joints, bone, and meningitis. At times with voriconazole, monotherapy was successful and success occurred in a voriconazole plus polyene combination [82,83]. Additional reports may further identify therapeutic principles, but a reasonable message is that patients responding to antifungal therapy within 6 months of exposure to voriconazole were, generally, cured. The success of extended-spectrum azoles in treatment of serious invasive phaeohyphomycosis was confirmed in this unfortunate outbreak.

REFERENCES

1. Silveira F, Nucci M. Emergence of black moulds in fungal disease: Epidemiology and therapy. *Curr Opin Infect Dis* 2001;14(6):679–684.
2. Singh N, Chang FY, Gayowski T, Marino IR. Infections due to dematiaceous fungi in organ transplant recipients: Case report and review. *Clin Infect Dis* 1997;24(3):369–374.
3. Boggild AK, Poutanen SM, Mohan S, Ostrowski MA. Disseminated phaeohyphomycosis due to *Ochroconis gallopavum* in the setting of advanced HIV infection. *Med Mycol* 2006;44(8):777–782.
4. Ben-Ami R, Lewis RE, Raad, II, Kontoyiannis DP. Phaeohyphomycosis in a tertiary care cancer center. *Clin Infect Dis* 2009;48(8):1033–1041.
5. Ronan SG, Uzoaru I, Nadimpalli V, Guitart J, Manaligod JR. Primary cutaneous phaeohyphomycosis: Report of seven cases. *J Cutan Pathol* 1993;20(3):223–228.
6. Revankar SG, Patterson JE, Sutton DA, Pullen R, Rinaldi MG. Disseminated phaeohyphomycosis: Review of an emerging mycosis. *Clin Infect Dis* 2002;34(4):467–476.
7. Rohwedder JJ, Simmons JL, Colfer H, Gatmaitan B. Disseminated *Curvularia lunata* infection in a football player. *Arch Intern Med* 1979;139(8):940–941.
8. Fader RC, McGinnis MR. Infections caused by dematiaceous fungi: Chromoblastomycosis and phaeohyphomycosis. *Infect Dis Clin North Am* 1988;2(4):925–938.
9. Revankar SG. Phaeohyphomycosis. *Infect Dis Clin North Am* 2006;20(3):609–620.
10. Brandt ME, Warnock DW. Epidemiology, clinical manifestations, and therapy of infections caused by dematiaceous fungi. *J Chemother* 2003;15 Suppl 2:36–47.
11. Dixon DM, Walsh TJ, Merz WG, McGinnis MR. Infections due to *Xylohypha bantiana* (*Cladosporium trichoides*). *Rev Infect Dis* 1989;11(4):515–525.
12. Kanj SS, Amr SS, Roberts GD. *Ramichloridium mackenziei* brain abscess: Report of two cases and review of the literature. *Med Mycol* 2001;39(1):97–102.
13. Neoh CY, Tan SH, Perera P. Cutaneous phaeohyphomycosis due to *Cladophialophora bantiana* in an immunocompetent patient. *Clin Exp Dermatol* 2007;32(5):539–540.
14. Vartian CV, Shlaes DM, Padhye AA, Ajello L. Wangiella dermatitidis endocarditis in an intravenous drug user. *Am J Med* 1985;78(4):703–707.
15. Clinical and Laboratory Standards Institute. *Reference Method for Broth Dilution Anti-Fungal Susceptibility Testing of Conidium-Forming Filamentous Fungi; Proposed Standard.* Wayne, PA: National Committee for Clinical Laboratory Standards (NCCLS), 1998:1–21.
16. Chen YT, Lin HC, Huang CC, Lo YH. Cutaneous phaeohyphomycosis caused by an Itraconazole and Amphoterecin B resistant strain of *Veronaeae botryosa. Int J Dermatol* 2006;45(4):429–432.
17. Viviani MA, Tortorano AM, Laria G, Giannetti A, Bignotti G. Two new cases of cutaneous alternariosis with a review of the literature. *Mycopathologia* 1986;96(1):3–12.
18. Schell WA. Dematiaceous hyphomycetes. In: Howard DH (Ed.). *Fungi Pathogenic for Humans and Animals*, 2nd ed. Revised and Expanded. New York: Marcel Dekker, 2003, pp. 565–636.
19. Schell WA, Pasarell L, Salkin IF. *Bipolaris, Exophiala, Scedosporium, Sporothrix* and other dematiaceous fungi. In: Murray PR, Baron EJ, Pfaller MA (Eds.). *Manual of Clinical Microbiology.* Washington, DC: ASM Press, 2002, pp. 1295–1317.
20. Krcmery V, Jr., Spanik S, Danisovicova A, Jesenska Z, Blahova M. Aureobasidium mansoni meningitis in a leukemia patient successfully treated with amphotericin B. *Chemotherapy* 1994;40(1):70–71.
21. Rolston KV, Hopfer RL, Larson DL. Infections caused by *Drechslera* species: Case report and review of the literature. *Rev Infect Dis* 1985;7(4):525–529.
22. McGinnis MR, Rinaldi MG, Winn RE. Emerging agents of phaeohyphomycosis: Pathogenic species of *Bipolaris* and *Exserohilum. J Clin Microbiol* 1986;24(2):250–259.
23. Karim M, Sheikh H, Alam M, Sheikh Y. Disseminated bipolaris infection in an asthmatic patient: Case report. *Clin Infect Dis* 1993;17(2):248–253.
24. Adam RD, Paquin ML, Petersen EA, Saubolle MA, Rinaldi MG, Corcoran JG, et al. Phaeohyphomycosis caused by the fungal genera *Bipolaris* and *Exserohilum*. A report of 9 cases and review of the literature. *Medicine (Baltimore)* 1986;65(4):203–217.
25. Fuste FJ, Ajello L, Threlkeld R, Henry JE, Jr. Drechslera hawaiiensis: Causative agent of a fatal fungal meningo-encephalitis. *Sabouraudia* 1973;11(1):59–63.

26. Bennett JE, Bonner H, Jennings AE, Lopez RI. Chronic meningitis caused by *Cladosporium trichoides*. *Am J Clin Pathol* 1973;59(3):398–407.

27. Seaworth BJ, Kwon-Chung KJ, Hamilton JD, Perfect JR. Brain abscess caused by a variety of cladosporium trichoides. *Am J Clin Pathol* 1983;79(6):747–752.

28. Palaoglu S, Sav A, Basak T, Yalcinlar Y, Scheithauer BW. Cerebral phaeohyphomycosis. *Neurosurgery* 1993;33(5):894–897.

29. Sekhon AS, Galbraith J, Mielke BW, Garg AK, Sheehan G. Cerebral phaeohyphomycosis caused by *Xylohypha bantiana*, with a review of the literature. *Eur J Epidemiol* 1992;8(3):387–390.

30. de la Monte SM, Hutchins GM. Disseminated *Curvularia* infection. *Arch Pathol Lab Med* 1985;109(9):872–874.

31. Sides EH, 3rd, Benson JD, Padhye AA. Phaeohyphomycotic brain abscess due to *Ochroconis gallopavum* in a patient with malignant lymphoma of a large cell type. *J Med Vet Mycol* 1991;29(5):317–322.

32. Vukmir RB, Kusne S, Linden P, Pasculle W, Fothergill AW, Sheaffer J, et al. Successful therapy for cerebral phaeohyphomycosis due to *Dactylaria gallopava* in a liver transplant recipient. *Clin Infect Dis* 1994;19(4):714–719.

33. Gold WL, Vellend H, Salit IE, Campbell I, Summerbell R, Rinaldi M, et al. Successful treatment of systemic and local infections due to *Exophiala* species. *Clin Infect Dis* 1994;19(2):339–341.

34. Tintelnot K, de Hoog GS, Thomas E, Steudel WI, Huebner K, Seeliger HP. Cerebral phaeohyphomycosis caused by an *Exophiala* species. *Mycoses* 1991;34(5–6):239–244.

35. Sudduth EJ, Crumbley AJ, 3rd, Farrar WE. Phaeohyphomycosis due to *Exophiala* species: Clinical spectrum of disease in humans. *Clin Infect Dis* 1992;15(4):639–644.

36. Morris A, Schell WA, McDonagh D, Chaffee S, Perfect JR. Pneumonia due to Fonsecaea pedrosoi and cerebral abscesses due to *Emericella nidulans* in a bone marrow transplant recipient. *Clin Infect Dis* 1995;21(5):1346–1348.

37. Schell WA. Agents of chromoblastomycosis and sporotrichosis. In: Ajello L, Hay R (Eds.). *Topley & Wilson's Microbiology and Microbial Infections: Mycology*. 4. London, UK: Edward Arnold, 1997:315–336.

38. Sigler L. Miscellaneous opportunistic fungi: Microascaceaea and other ascomycetes, hyphomycetes, coelomyctes and basidiomycetes. In: Howard DH (Ed.). *Fungi Pathogenic for Humans and Animals*, 2nd ed. Revised and Expanded. New York: Marcel Dekker, 2003:637–676.

39. del Palacio-Hernanz A, Moore MK, Campbell CK, del Palacio-Perez-Medel A, del Castillo-Cantero R. Infection of the central nervous system by *Rhinocladiella atrovirens* in a patient with acquired immunodeficiency syndrome. *J Med Vet Mycol* 1989;27(2):127–130.

40. Nucci M, Akiti T, Barreiros G, Silveira F, Revankar SG, Sutton DA, et al. Nosocomial fungemia due to *Exophiala jeanselmei* var. *jeanselmei* and a *Rhinocladiella* species: Newly described causes of bloodstream infection. *J Clin Microbiol* 2001;39(2):514–518.

41. Watanabe S, Hironaga M. An atypical isolate of *Scedosporium apiospermum* from a purulent meningitis in man. *Sabouraudia* 1981;19(3):209–215.

42. Yoo D, Lee WH, Kwon-Chung KJ. Brain abscesses due to *Pseudallescheria boydii* associated with primary non-Hodgkin's lymphoma of the central nervous system: A case report and literature review. *Rev Infect Dis* 1985;7(2):272–277.

43. Dworzack DL, Clark RB, Padgitt PJ. New causes of pneumonia, meningitis, and disseminated infections associated with immersion. *Infect Dis Clin North Am* 1987;1(3):615–633.

44. Berenguer J, Diaz-Mediavilla J, Urra D, Munoz P. Central nervous system infection caused by *Pseudallescheria boydii*: Case report and review. *Rev Infect Dis* 1989;11(6):890–896.

45. Berenguer J, Rodriguez-Tudela JL, Richard C, Alvarez M, Sanz MA, Gaztelurrutia L, et al. Deep infections caused by *Scedosporium prolificans*. A report on 16 cases in Spain and a review of the literature. *Scedosporium Prolificans* Spanish Study Group. *Medicine (Baltimore)* 1997;76(4):256–265.

46. Maertens J, Lagrou K, Deweerdt H, Surmont I, Verhoef GE, Verhaegen J, et al. Disseminated infection by *Scedosporium prolificans*: An emerging fatality among haematology patients. Case report and review. *Ann Hematol* 2000;79(6):340–344.

47. Hiruma M, Kawada A, Ohata H, Ohnishi Y, Takahashi H, Yamazaki M, et al. Systemic phaeohyphomycosis caused by *Exophiala dermatitidis*. *Mycoses* 1993;36(1–2):1–7.

48. Greer KE, Gross GP, Cooper PH, Harding SA. Cystic chromomycosis due to *Wangiella dermatitidis*. *Arch Dermatol* 1979;115(12):1433–1434.

49. Perfect JR, Schell WA, Cox GM. Phaeohyphomycosis. *Clinical Mycology*. New York: Oxford Press, 2003:271–282.

50. Cornely OA, Cuenca-Estrella M, Meis JF, Ullmann AJ. European Society of Clinical Microbiology and Infectious Diseases (ESCMID) Fungal Infection Study Group (EFISG) and European Confederation of Medical Mycology (ECMM) 2013 joint guidelines on diagnosis and management of rare and emerging fungal diseases. *Clin Microbiol Infect* 2014;20 Suppl 3:1–4.

51. Heinz T, Perfect J, Schell W, Ritter E, Ruff G, Serafin D. Soft-tissue fungal infections: Surgical management of 12 immunocompromised patients. *Plast Reconstr Surg* 1996;97(7):1391–1399.

52. Liu K, Howell DN, Perfect JR, Schell WA. Morphologic criteria for the preliminary identification of *Fusarium*, *Paecilomyces*, and *Acremonium* species by histopathology. *Am J Clin Pathol* 1998;109(1):45–54.

53. Gugnani HC, Ramesh V, Sood N, Guarro J, Moin Ul H, Paliwal-Joshi A, et al. Cutaneous phaeohyphomycosis caused by *Caldosporium oxysporum* and its treatment with potassium iodide. *Med Mycol* 2006;44(3):285–288.

54. Polak A. Antimycotic therapy of experimental infections caused by dematiaceous fungi. *Sabouraudia* 1984;22(4):279–289.

55. Del Poeta M, Schell WA, Perfect JR. *In vitro* antifungal activity of pneumocandin L-743,872 against a variety of clinically important molds. *Antimicrob Agents Chemother* 1997;41(8):1835–1836.

56. Espinel-Ingroff A. Comparison of *In vitro* activities of the new triazole SCH56592 and the echinocandins MK-0991 (L-743,872) and LY303366 against opportunistic filamentous and dimorphic fungi and yeasts. *J Clin Microbiol* 1998;36(10):2950–2956.

57. McGinnis MR, Pasarell L, Sutton DA, Fothergill AW, Cooper CR, Jr., Rinaldi MG. *In vitro* evaluation of voriconazole against some clinically important fungi. *Antimicrob Agents Chemother* 1997;41(8):1832–1834.

58. McGinnis MR, Pasarell L. *In vitro* evaluation of terbinafine and itraconazole against dematiaceous fungi. *Med Mycol* 1998;36(4):243–246.

59. Rallis E, Frangoulis E. Successful treatment of subcutaneous phaeohyphomycosis owing to *Exophiala jeanselmei* with oral terbinafine. *Int J Dermatol* 2006;45(11):1369–1370.

60. Santinga JT, Fekety RF, Jr, Bottomley WK, Else B, Willis PW, 3rd. Antibiotic prophylaxis for endocarditis in patients with a prosthetic heart valve. *J Am Dent Assoc* 1976;93(5):1001–1005.

61. Espinel-Ingroff A. *In vitro* activity of the new triazole voriconazole (UK-109,496) against opportunistic filamentous and dimorphic fungi and common and emerging yeast pathogens. *J Clin Microbiol* 1998;36(1):198–202.

62. Proia LA, Trenholme GM. Chronic refractory phaeohyphomycosis: Successful treatment with posaconazole. *Mycoses* 2006;49(6):519–522.

63. Perfect JR, Marr KA, Walsh TJ, Greenberg RN, DuPont B, de la Torre-Cisneros J, et al. Voriconazole treatment for less-common, emerging, or refractory fungal infections. *Clin Infect Dis* 2003;36(9):1122–1131.

64. Al-Abdely HM, Najvar L, Bocanegra R, Fothergill A, Loebenberg D, Rinaldi MG, et al. SCH 56592, amphotericin B, or itraconazole therapy of experimental murine cerebral phaeohyphomycosis due to *Ramichloridium obovoideum* ("*Ramichloridium mackenziei*"). *Antimicrob Agents Chemother* 2000;44(5):1159–1162.

65. Centers for Disease Control and Prevention. Exophiala infection from contaminated injectable steroids prepared by a compounding pharmacy—United States, July-November 2002. *MMWR Morb Mortal Wkly Rep* 2002;51:1109–1112.

66. Li DM, de Hoog GS. Cerebral phaeohyphomycosis—A cure at what lengths? *Lancet Infect Dis* 2009;9(6):376–383.

67. Walsh TJ, Lutsar I, Driscoll T, Dupont B, Roden M, Ghahramani P, et al. Voriconazole in the treatment of aspergillosis, scedosporiosis and other invasive fungal infections in children. *Pediatr Infect Dis J* 2002;21(3):240–248.

68. Revankar SG, Sutton DA, Rinaldi MG. Primary central nervous system phaeohyphomycosis: A review of 101 cases. *Clin Infect Dis* 2004;38(2):206–216.

69. Leechawengwongs M, Milindankura S, Liengudom A, Chanakul K, Viranuvatti K, Clongsusuek P. Multiple *Scedosporium apiospermum* brain abscesses after near-drowning successfully treated with surgery and long-term voriconazole: A case report. *Mycoses* 2007;50(6):512–516.

70. Clancy CJ, Wingard JR, Hong Nguyen M. Subcutaneous phaeohyphomycosis in transplant recipients: Review of the literature and demonstration of in vitro synergy between antifungal agents. *Med Mycol* 2000;38(2):169–175.

71. Forster RK, Rebell G, Wilson LA. Dematiaceous fungal keratitis. Clinical isolates and management. *Br J Ophthalmol* 1975;59(7):372–376.

72. Schell WA. Oculomycosis caused by dematiaceous fungi. In: *Proceedings of the VI International Conference on the Mycoses*. 879. Washington, DC: Pan American Health Organization, 1986:105–109.

73. Chowdhary A, Meis JF, Guarro J, de Hoog GS, Kathuria S, Arendrup MC, et al. ESCMID and ECMM joint clinical guidelines for the diagnosis and management of systemic phaeohyphomycosis: Diseases caused by black fungi. *Clin Microbiol Infect* 2014;20 Suppl 3:47–75.

74. Corey JP, Delsupehe KG, Ferguson BJ. Allergic fungal sinusitis: Allergic, infectious, or both? *Otolaryngol Head Neck Surg* 1995;113(1):110–119.

75. Ferguson BJ. What role do systemic corticosteroids, immunotherapy, and antifungal drugs play in the therapy of allergic fungal rhinosinusitis? *Arch Otolaryngol Head Neck Surg* 1998;124(10):1174–1178.

76. Ferguson BJ. Fungus balls of the paranasal sinuses. *Otolaryngol Clin North Am* 2000;33(2):389–98.

77. Wong EH, Revankar SG. Dematiaceous molds. *Infect Dis Clin North Am* 2016;30(1):165–178.

78. Kerr CM, Perfect JR, Craven PC, Jorgensen JH, Drutz DJ, Shelburne JD, et al. Fungal peritonitis in patients on continuous ambulatory peritoneal dialysis. *Ann Intern Med* 1983;99(3):334–336.

79. Smith RM, Schaefer MK, Kainer MA, Wise M, Finks J, Duwve J, et al. Fungal infections associated with contaminated methylprednisolone injections. *N Engl J Med* 2013;369(17):1598–1609.

80. Casadevall A, Pirofski LA. Exserohilum rostratum fungal meningitis associated with methylprednisolone injections. *Future Microbiol* 2013;8(2):135–137.

81. Pappas PG, Kontoyiannis DP, Perfect JR, Chiller TM. Real-time treatment guidelines: Considerations during the *Exserohilum rostratum* outbreak in the United States. *Antimicrob Agents Chemother* 2013;57(4):1573–1576.

82. Kerkering TM, Grifasi ML, Baffoe-Bonnie AW, Bansal E, Garner DC, Smith JA, et al. Early clinical observations in prospectively followed patients with fungal meningitis related to contaminated epidural steroid injections. *Ann Intern Med* 2013;158(3):154–161.

83. Kauffman CA, Malani AN. Fungal infections associated with contaminated steroid injections. *Microbiol Spectr* 2016;4(2).

22

Pneumocystis

KIM SWINDELL

In 1909, the parasitic fungal genus *Pneumocystis* was discovered by Chagas in the lungs of trypanosome-experimentally infected Guinea pigs [1]. He described the genus as *Scizotrypanum* and thought it to represent a life cycle variant of *Trypanasoma cruzi* [2]. In 1910, Antonio Carinii also identified and mistook similar organisms in rat lungs as a novel trypanosome. In 1912 the Delanoës correctly identified the organism, which was subsequently renamed *Pneumocystis carinii*, in honor of Dr. Carinii [3].

In early twentieth century Europe, Ammich [4] and Benecke [5] described cases of a novel type of pneumonitis associated with mortality rates of 30%–40% [6,7] affecting premature infants and immunocompromised adults and characterized by respiratory distress, cyanosis, and radiographically indicative lung infiltrates. In 1952, Vaněk and Jírovec isolated *Pneumocystis* from the alveolar lumina of immunocompromised adults who had succumbed to interstitial pneumonia [8].

In the 1980s, as the incidence of pneumocystosis rose dramatically coincidently with the advent of human immunodeficiency virus (HIV), keen interest in *Pneumocystis* as a significant pathogen in immunocompromised hosts resumed.

In 1988, analysis of the *Pneumocystis* rRNA gene, along with characterization of cell wall composition and structures of key enzymes, allowed resolution of the genus taxonomy from protozoa to fungi [9].

Of the four identified *Pneumocystis* species, only *Pneumocystis jirovecii*, thusly named in 2001 in honor of Czech parasitologist Otto Jírovec (one of the first researchers to describe *Pneumocystis* infection in humans) causes exclusively human disease [10].

Although the inability of *Pneumocystis* to be propagated in culture continues to complicate genetic manipulation by transformation and complete genomic sequencing, Ma *et al*, have generated near-complete high-quality genome assemblies for three *Pneumocystis* species, including *P. jirovecii* [11].

ORGANISM

Life cycle and genome

The genus *Pneumocystis* comprises a group of ascomycetous single-cell fungi belonging to the class Pneumocystidomycetes, order Pneumocystaidales, and family Pneumocystidaceae. Unique among fungal species, *Pneumocystis* have adapted to and co-evolved with individual mammalian host species such that each *Pneumocystis* species can infect only a single host species; the basis for this specificity is currently unknown.

During its known life cycle, *P. jirovecii* can be found as *trophic* and *cystic* forms (Figure 22.1) [12]. Although the life cycle remains undefined, it has been hypothesized that extra-cystic thin-walled trophic forms (2–6 μm in diameter) can undergo binary fission or, alternatively, conjugate and undergo meiosis, leading to the development of spherical thick-walled cysts (6–8 μm in diameter) containing up to eight intracystic bodies, which can subsequently be released as new trophic forms [13]. Animal studies suggest that the cyst form is responsible for transmission between hosts [14]. During infection, trophic forms (most of which are haploid) predominate over cyst forms [13].

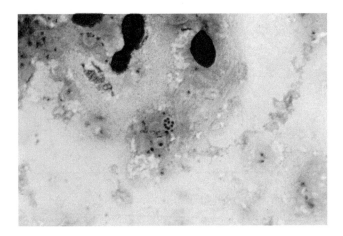

Figure 22.1 *Pneumocystis jirovecii* fungi. Note the round cyst (in the middle of image) containing eight immature haploid nuclei, as well as several freed trophozoites. (Wright-Giemsa, 1000x).

The *P. jirovecii* genome comprises approximately eight million base pairs of DNA divided among 15 linear chromosomes that range in size from 300 to 700 kB [15]. Ma *et al*, have generated near-complete high-quality genome assemblies for three *Pneumocystis* species including *P. jirovecii* [11].

Cell wall and surface antigens

The cell wall of *P. jirovecii* contains chitin. The cyst form also contains β-1,3-glucan, which may help elicit an inflammatory response from the host and may contribute to damage of host alveolar epithelium, within its cell wall. *P. jirovecii* uses mannose carbohydrates to adhere to the host [13]. Cell walls of cysts and trophic forms also contain a number of unique immunogenic mannose-, glucose-, galactose-, and N-acetylglucosamine-containing glycoproteins [16].

One distinguishing characteristic of *Pneumocystis* is the lack of ergosterol in the plasma membrane, a fact that renders the organism resistant to antifungal drugs that target ergosterol synthesis. Instead of ergosterol, the major plasma membrane sterol in *P. jirovecii* is cholesterol, which is postulated to be scavenged from the host lung [17]. Other cell membrane lipids include Δ^7C-24 alkylated sterol and *cis*-9,10-epoystearic acid, both of which are potential drug targets. The major ubiquinone synthesized by *Pneumocystis*, coenzyme Q10, provides a drug target for ubiquinone analogs, such as atovaquone [18].

Pneumocystis contains a family of proteins referred to collectively as the major surface glycoprotein (MSG), an immunogenic protein exhibiting shared and species-specific antigenic determinants [19–24]. Rearrangement of the upstream conserved sequence (UCS) of MSG by recombination and gene conversion results in antigenic variation, which may allow *Pneumocystis* to evade the host immune response [19]. MSG also facilitates interaction with host cell extracellular matrix proteins, such as fibronectin, vitronectin, laminin, surfactant proteins A and D, and the mannose receptor [13,25–29].

EPIDEMIOLOGY

P. jirovecii is an opportunistic pathogen, found worldwide, with humans being the main reservoir. The organism is spread from human to human via the inhalation of airborne particles [30,31]. Exposure to the organism is common, with more than 80% of children having developed antibodies against it by 4 years of age [32]. The organism is typically eradicated by host innate cell-mediated immunity; however, immunocompromised hosts with CD4+ lymphocyte counts <200 cells/μL [33] have increased susceptibility [32,34], in which case the host may develop pneumonia, commonly referred to as *Pneumocystis carinii* pneumonia (PCP), a potentially life-threatening infection.

The prevalence of PCP increased dramatically with the emergence of the HIV epidemic in the 1980s. Coinciding with improvements in viral suppression and immune status of patients receiving increasingly potent and tolerable newer antiretroviral therapy (ART) regimens, persistent reductions in the incidence of PCP pneumonitis was observed in a large longitudinal multi-cohort study of HIV-infected patients in United States and Canada conducted from 2000 to 2010 [35]. However, *Pneumocystis* remains a significant cause of pneumonia in patients with other types of immunodeficiencies, such as transplant recipients, patients with malignancies, and patients who are treated with immunomodulatory drugs [36]. In patients without HIV infection, glucocorticoid use and defects in cell-mediated immunity are the most significant risk factors for PCP [37–40]. Other specific risk factors include other immunosuppressive medications, cancer (particularly hematologic malignancy), hematopoietic cell or solid organ transplantation, treatment for certain inflammatory autoimmune diseases, primary immunodeficiencies, and severe malnutrition.

Evidence exists to suggest that pneumocystosis results from active acquisition from other persons, rather than latent reactivation within the immunocompromised host. For example, in AIDS patients, recurrent episodes of pneumocystosis were found to be caused by differing *Pneumocystis* genotypes [41]. Furthermore, *Pneumocystis* genotypes recovered from patients in different US cities reflected the geographic region of diagnosis rather than the patients' places of birth [42].

PATHOLOGY AND PATHOGENESIS

Pathology

The hallmark histological finding in pneumocystosis is formation of a foamy, eosinophilic exudate within the lung alveoli (Figure 22.2). Microscopically, alveolar-capillary leakage and type 1 pneumocyte destruction have been noted, along with intra-alveolar transudate containing macrophages and a very few neutrophilic granulocytes, dilated capillary tubes, edema, and thickened alveolar septae [43–45].

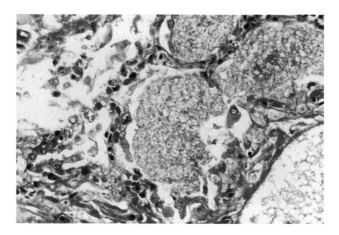

Figure 22.2 Eosinophilic infiltrate in *Pneumocystis* pneumonia within lung alveoli. (H&E stain).

Pathogenesis

Pneumocystis is presumably inhaled into the alveolar space and in the immunocompromised host, adheres [19] to type I alveolar cells and initiates infection resulting in mononuclear cell response, diffuse alveolitis, and impaired oxygenation; physiologic changes similar to that seen in adult respiratory distress syndrome (ARDS) [44–47].

Pneumocystis mitogen-activated protein kinase (MAPK) signal transduction genes, cell wall genes, *Cdc2, Cdc13,* and *Cdc25* have been implicated in organism replication [48–52]. *Pneumocystis* may also scavenge essential nutrients from the host tissue [43].

In HIV-infected persons depletion of CD4+ T lymphocytes strongly correlates with the likelihood of developing PCP. For example, about 95% of PCP cases occurred in HIV-infected patients with CD4+ T lymphocyte counts under 200 cells/µL [53]. In immunocompromised but non-HIV infected persons, CD4+ T lymphocyte counts correlate to a lesser extent [54].

Impaired host humoral immunity may also play a role in the unregulated replication of *Pneumocystis* during PCP. PCP has been recognized in patients with B cell defects, severe combined immunodeficiency disease (SCID), premature infants, organ transplant patients, and oncology patients receiving immunosuppressive drugs [38,55–60]. Outbreaks of PCP have been reported in SCID mice suggesting that impaired cellular immunity contributes to development of the disease [61]. Monoclonal antibodies to MSG and other *Pneumocystis* antigens exert a therapeutic effect in experimental animal models of pneumocystosis [62].

CLINICAL FEATURES

Common symptoms of PCP are dyspnea with exertion, nonproductive cough, and fever. Occasionally, sputum production, hemoptysis, or chest pain is present [63]. In HIV-infected patients, the initial presentation of PCP is

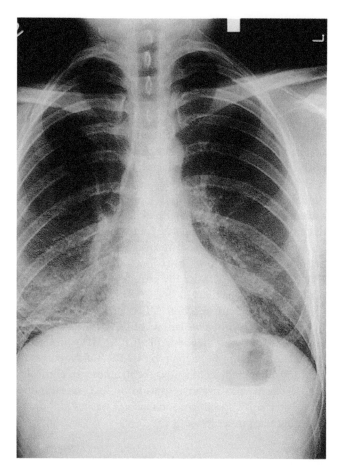

Figure 22.3 Anteroposterior chest radiograph revealing pulmonary pneumocystosis in the form of bilateral pulmonary interstitial infiltrates.

often indolent; although the organism burden in the lung alveoli is higher, the lung damage is less severe [64,65]. Contrastingly, in patients without HIV, PCP typically presents as fulminant respiratory failure associated with fever and dry cough [65]. Acutely ill patients may manifest tachycardia, tachypnea, respiratory distress, and cyanosis.

Lung auscultation is often underwhelming [66]. Characteristic radiographic findings of PCP include bilateral diffuse infiltrates extending from the perihilar region [67] (Figure 22.3). Uncommon radiographic patterns include lobar infiltrates, solitary or multiple nodules, pneumatoceles, and pneumothorax. Upper lobe infiltrates may be seen in patients receiving aerosolized pentamidine due to reduced deposition of pentamidine in the upper lobes. High-resolution computed tomography scanning may demonstrate extensive ground glass opacities or cystic lesions [68–72].

DIAGNOSIS

Given the expansive differential diagnosis of the immunocompromised patient with abnormal respiratory findings, prompt evaluation is warranted. A definitive diagnosis of PCP requires visualization of the cystic or trophic forms in respiratory secretions. Diagnosis is most commonly achieved by microscopy with staining of the organism from sputum or bronchoalveolar lavage (BAL) fluid, as *Pneumocystis* cannot be cultured. *Pneumocystis* can be identified using methenamine silver, toluidine blue O, cresyl echt violet, Wright-Giemsa, or Calcofluor white stains. Direct fluorescent antibody staining using a fluorescein-conjugated monoclonal antibody can visualize both trophic forms and cysts and is the most commonly used technique. The diagnostic yield of microscopy with staining of induced sputum is 50%–90% in patients with HIV infection and PCP but is thought to be lower in those HIV-uninfected patients due to a decreased organism burden [73–77]. If PCP is not able to be diagnosed by analysis of induced sputum, BAL is warranted. The diagnostic yield is of BAL over 90% in HIV-infected patients but may be lower in HIV-uninfected patients [76]. Diagnosis of PCP occasionally requires open-lung biopsy, which carries a sensitivity of 95%–100% [78].

Polymerase chain reaction (PCR) of respiratory fluid, in particular bronchoalveolar lavage (BAL), is increasingly used to support the diagnosis of PCP in HIV-uninfected patients who are immunocompromised [79]. Advantages to PCR testing include confirming the diagnosis in clinically suspect cases with negative sputum or BAL smears, and using alternative specimens such as oral washes and naso-pharyngeal aspirates [80–81].

TREATMENT

Treatment of PCP requires antimicrobial therapy directed against *Pneumocystis jirovecii*. Moreover, some patients may require adjuvant treatment with corticosteroids. Empiric therapy should be initiated promptly when there is a high clinical index of suspicion for PCP, and in HIV-infected patients especially so if the CD4+ T cell count is <200 cells/μL. The recommended duration of therapy for PCP is 21 days [65]. The probability and rate of response to therapy depend on the agent used, number of previous PCP episodes, severity of pulmonary illness, degree of immunodeficiency, timing of initiation of therapy and comorbidities.

Careful monitoring during anti-PCP therapy is important to evaluate response to treatment and to detect toxicity as soon as possible. Follow-up after therapy includes assessment for early relapse, especially when therapy has been with an agent other than TMP-SMX or was shortened for toxicity. PCP prophylaxis should be initiated immediately upon completion of therapy and maintained until the CD4+ T cell count is >200 cells/μL for at least three months [78].

Clinical failure is defined as a lack of improvement or worsening of arterial blood gases (ABGs) after at least 4–8 days of anti-PCP treatment. Treatment failure rates attributed to lack of drug efficacy are estimated to be approximately 10%. Waiting four to eight days prior to changing therapy due to lack of clinical improvement is recommended [78].

Trimethoprim-Sulfamethoxazole (TMP-SMX) TMP-SMX, dosed at 15–20 mg/kg/day (based on the TMP component) in divided doses, is the preferred therapeutic agent for all patients with PCP [82–84]. Multiple randomized clinical trials indicate that TMP-SMX is as effective as parenteral pentamidine and more effective than other regimens. Oral outpatient therapy with TMP-SMX is highly effective in patients with mild-to moderate disease [83]. Patients who have PCP despite TMP-SMX prophylaxis usually can be treated effectively with standard doses of TMP-SMX [78].

Adjunctive corticosteroids

Patients with documented or suspected PCP and moderate-to-severe disease, defined by room air pO2 < 70 mm Hg or Alveolar-arterial O2 gradient ≥35 mm Hg, should receive adjunctive corticosteroids as early as possible and certainly within 72 hours after starting specific PCP therapy [85–90].

Alternative therapies

Alternative therapeutic regimens for mild-to-moderate PCP include: dapsone and TMP [83,91]; primaquine plus clindamycin [92–94]; and atovaquone suspension [82,95–97]. Alternative therapeutic regimens for patients with moderate-to-severe PCP include clindamycin-primaquine or intravenous pentamidine [94,98–99]. Aerosolized pentamidine should be used to treat PCP, because its efficacy is limited and it is associated with more frequent relapse [98,100,101].

PREVENTION

Primary prevention

TMP-SMX is the recommended agent for chemoprophylaxis in patients at significant risk of developing PCP [102–105].

HIV-infected adults and adolescents should receive chemoprophylaxis against PCP if they have CD4+ T cell count of <200 cell/μL or a history of oropharyngeal candidiasis. Patients who have a CD4+ T cell percentage of <14% or a history of an AIDS-defining illness, but who do not otherwise qualify, should be considered for prophylaxis [106–108].

For patients receiving hematopoietic stem cell transplants, guidelines recommend PCP prophylaxis from engraftment through at least 6 months subsequent to transplantation [109]. Patients receiving solid organ transplantation are recommended to receive PCP prophylaxis for at least 6–12 months post-transplant [110,111]. Other populations at high risk for PCP infection include: patients with acute lymphoblastic leukemia (ALL), patients with prolonged CD4+ T cell counts of <200 cell/μL as the result of immunopressive chemotherapeutics, and patients receiving immunomodulatory therapy such as corticosteroids, calcineurin inhibitors, and anti-tumor necrosis factor [36].

Secondary prophylaxis

HIV-infected patients, who have a history of PCP, should be given chemoprophylaxis for life with TMP-SMX unless immune reconstitution occurs as the result of initiation of effective anti-retroviral therapy (ART). Secondary prophylaxis should be discontinued in adult and adolescent patients whose CD4+ T cell counts have increased to ≥200 cells/μL as the result of ART. If an episode of PCP occurs at a CD4+ T cell count ≥200 cells/μL, it is prudent to continue PCP prophylaxis indefinitely [78].

REFERENCES

1. Chagas C. Tabalho do Instituto de Manguinhos sobre uma nova trypanosomiase humana, pelo dr. Carlos Chagas, assistente do Instituto. *Ann Acad Med Rio de Janiero* 1909;75:188–190.
2. Redhead SA, Cushion ME, Frenkel JK, et al. *Pneumocystis* and *Trypanasoma cruzi*: Nomenclature and typifications. *J Eukaryot Microbiol* 2006;53(1):2–11.
3. Delanoë P, Delanoë M. De la rareté de *Pneumocystis carinii* chez laes cobayes del la region de Paris, absence de kystes chez d'autre animaux (lapin, gernouille, 3 anguilles). *Bull Soc Pathol Exot* 1914;7:271–272.
4. Ammich O. Über die nichtsyphilitische interstitielle Pneumonie des ersten Kidersalters. *Virchows Arch f path Anat* 1938;302:539–554.
5. Benecke E. Eigenartige Bronchiolenerkrangung im ersten Lebersjarh. *Verhandl d deutsch path Gellesch* 1939;31:119–131.
6. Baar HS. Interstitial plasmacellular pneumonia due to *Pneumocystis carinii*. *J Clin Path* 1954;8:19–24.
7. Hamperl H. *Pneumocystis*. Infection and cytomegaly of the lungs in newborn and adult. *Am J Pathol* 1956;32(1):1–11.
8. Vaněk J, Jírovec O. Infection á Pneumocystis chez l'homme et ches les animaux. *Ann Soc belge de méd trop* 1952;22:301–307.
9. Edman JC, Kovacs JA, Masur H, et al. Ribosomal RNA sequence show *Pneumocystis carinii* to be a member of the fungi. *Nature* 1988;334(6182):519–522.
10. Stringer JR, Cushion MT, Wakefield AE. New nomenclature for the genus *Pneumocystis*. *J Eukaryot Microbiol* 2001;48 Suppl:184S–189S.
11. Ma L, Chen Z, Huang DW, et al. Genome analysis of three *Pneumocystis* species reveals adaptation mechanisms to life exclusively in mammalian hosts. *Nat Comm* 2016;7:10740.
12. Cushion, MT. *Pneumocystis*: Unraveling the cloak of obscurity. *Trends Microbiol* 2004;12:243–249.
13. Thomas CF, Jr, Limper AH. Current insights into the biology and pathogenesis of *Pneumocystis* pneumonia. *Nat Rev Microbiol* 2007;5:298–308.
14. Cushion MT, Linke MJ, Ashbaugh A, et al. Echinocandin treatment of *Pneumocystis* pneumonia in rodent models depletes cysts leaving trophic burdens that cannot transmit the infection. *PLoS One* 2010;5: e8524.
15. Stringer JR, Cushion MT. The genome of *Pneumocystis carinii*. *FEMS Immunol Med Microbiol* 1998;22(1–2):15–26.
16. De Stefano JA, Myers JD, Du Pont D, et al. Cell wall antigens of *Pneumocystis carinii* trophozoites and cysts: Purification and carbohydrate analysis of these glycoproteins. *J Eukaryot Microbiol* 1998;45(3):334–343.
17. Kaneshiro ES. The lipids of *Pneumocystis carinii*. *Clin Microbiol Rev* 1998;11(1):27–41.
18. Kaneshiro ES. Biochemical research elucidating metabolic pathways in *Pneumocystis*. *Parasite* 2010;17(4):285–291.
19. Smulian AG, Keely SP, Sunkin SM, et al. Genetic and antigenic variation in *Pneumocystis carinii* organisms: Tools for examining the epidemiology and pathogenesis of infection. *J Lab Clin Med* 1997;130(5):461–468.
20. Linke MF, Sunkin SM, Andrew RP, et al. Expression, structure, and location of epitopes of the major surface glycoprotein of *Pneumocystis carinii* f. sp. Carninii. *Clin Diagn Lab Immunol* 1998;5(1):50–57.
21. Gigliotti F, Hughes TW. Passive immunoprophylaxis with specific monoclonal antibody confers partial protection against *Pneumocystis carinii* pneumonitis in animal models. *J Clin Invest* 1988;81(6):1666–1668.
22. Gigliotti F, Haidras CG, Wright TW, et al. Passive intranasal monoclonal antibody prophylaxis against murine *Pneumocystis carinii* pneumonia. *Infect Immun* 2002;70(3):1069–1074.
23. Theus SA, Smulian AG, Sullivan DW, et al. Cytokine responses to the native and recombinant forms of the major surface glycoprotein of *Pneumocystis carinii*. *Clin Exp Immunol* 1997;109(2):255–260.
24. Theus SA, Andrews RP, Steele P, et al. Adoptive transfer of lymphocytes sensitized to the major surface glycoprotein of *Pneumocystis carinii* confers protection in the rat. *J Clin Invest* 1995;95 (6):2587–2593.
25. Pottratz ST, Paulsrud J, Smith JS, et al. *Pneumocystis carinii* attachment to cultured lung cells by *Pneumocystis* gp120, a fibronectin binding protein. *J Clin Invest* 1991;88(2):403–407.
26. Ezekowitz RA, Williams DJ, Koziel H, et al. Uptake of *Pneumocystis carinii* mediated by the macrophage mannose receptor. *Nature* 1991;351(6322):155–158.
27. Limper AH, Standing JE, Hoffman OA, et al. Vitronectin binds to *Pneumocystis carinii* and mediates organism attachment to cultured lung epithelial cells. *Infect Immun* 1993;61(10):4302–4309.

28. McCormack FX, Festa AL, Andrews RP, et al. The carbohydrate recognition domain of surfactant protein A mediates binding to the major surface glycoprotein of *Pneumocystis carinii*. *Biochemistry* 1997;36(26):8092–8099.

29. O'Riordan DM, Standing JE, Kwon KY, et al. Surfactant protein D interacts with *Pneumocystis carinii* and mediates organism adherence to alveolar macrophages. *J Clin Invest* 1995;95(6):2699–2710.

30. Finkelman MA. *Pneumocystis jirovecii* infection: Cell wall (1→3)-β-D-glucan biology and diagnostic utilities. *Crit Rev Microbiol* 2010;36:271–281.

31. Rahier JF, Ben-Horin S, Chowers Y, et al. European evidence-based consensus on the prevention, diagnosis and management of opportunistic infections in inflammatory bowel disease. *J Crohns Colitis* 2009;3:47–91.

32. Hof F. *Pneumocystis jirovecii*: A peculiar fungus posing particular problems for therapy and prophylaxis. *Mycoses* 2012;55:1–7.

33. Morris A, Lundgren JD, Masur H, et al. Current epidemiology of *Pneumocystis* pneumonia. *Emerg Infect Dis* 2004;10:1713–1720.

34. Hughes WT, Kuhn S, Chaudary S, et al. Successful chemoprophylaxis for *Pneumocystis carinii* pneumonitis. *N Engl J Med* 1977;297:1419–1426.

35. Buchacz K, Lau B, Jing Y, et al. Incidence of AIDS-defining opportunistic infections in a multicohort analysis of HIV-infected persons in the United States and Canada, 2000–2010. *J Infect Dis* 2016;214(6):862–872.

36. Avino LJ, Naylor SM, Roecker AM. *Pneumocystis jirovecii* pneumonia in the non-HIV-infected population. *Ann Pharmacother* 2016;50(8):673–679.

37. Yale SH, Limper AH. *Pneumocystis carinii* pneumonia in patients without acquired immunodeficiency syndrome: Associated illnesses and prior corticosteroid therapy. *Mayo Clin Proc* 1996;71:5.

38. Sepkowitz KA, Brown AE, Telzak EE, et al. *Pneumocystis carinii* pneumonia among patients without AIDS at a cancer hospital. *JAMA* 1992;267:832.

39. Rodriguez M, Fishman JA. Prevention of infection due to *Pneumocystis* spp. in human immunodeficiency virus-negative immunocompromised patients. *Clin Microbiol Rev* 2004;17:770.

40. Sepkowitz KA, Brown AE, Armstrong D. *Pneumocystis carinii* pneumonia without acquired immunodeficiency syndrome. More patients, same risk. *Arch Intern Med* 1995;155:1125.

41. Keely SP, Baughman RP, Smulian AG, et al. Source of *Pneumocystis carinii* in recurrent episodes of pneumonia in AIDS patients. *AIDS* 1996;10(8):881–888.

42. Beard CB, Carter JL, Keely SP, et al. Genetic variation in *Pneumocystis carinii* isolates from different geographic regions: Implications for transmission. *Emerg Infect Dis* 2000;6(3):265–272.

43. Walzer PD, Kim CK, Cushion MT. *Pneumocystis carinii*. In: Walzer PD, Genta RM (Eds.). *Parasitic Infections in the Compromised Host*. New York: Marcel Dekker, 1989:83–178.

44. Benfield TL, Prento P, Junge J, et al. Alveolar damage in AIDS-related *Pneumocystis carinii* pneumonia. *Chest* 1997;111(5):1193–1199.

45. Gent J, Settnes OP. Pathological characteristics for the diagnosis of *Pneumocystis carinii* pneumonia. A retrospective autopsy study. *APMIS* 1990;98(12):1098–1104.

46. Stansell JD, Hopewell PC. *Pneumocystis carinii* pneumonia: Risk factors, clinical presentation and natural history. In: Sattler FR, Walzer PD (Eds.). *Pneumocystis carinii*. London, UK: Bailliére Tindall, 1995:449–459.

47. D'Angelo E, Calderini E, Robatto FM, et al. Lung and chest wall mechanics in patients with acquired immunodeficiency syndrome and severe *Pneumocystis carinii* pneumonia. *Eur Respir J* 1997;10(10):2343–2350.

48. Smulian AG, Ryan M, Staben C, et al. Signal transduction in *Pneumocystis carinii*: Characterization of the genes (pcg1) encoding the alpha subunit of the G protein (PCG1) of *Pneumocystis carinii carinii* and *Pneumocystis carinii* ratti. *Infect Immun* 1996;64(3):691–701.

49. Gustafson MP, Thomas CD Jr, Rusnak F, et al. Differential regulation of growth and checkpoint control mediated by a Cdc25 mitotic phosphatase from *Pneumocystis carinii*. *J Biol Chem* 2001;276(1):835–843.

50. Fox D, Smulian AG. Mitogen-activated protein kinase Mkp1 of *Pneumocystis carinii* complements the slt2Delta defect in the cell integrity pathway of *Saccaromyces cerevisiae*. *Mol Microbiol* 1999;34(3):451–462.

51. Smulian AG, Sesterhenn T, Tanaka R, et al. The ste3 pheromone receptor gene of *Pneumocystis carinii* is surrounded by a cluster of signal transduction genes. *Genetics* 2001;157(3):991–1002.

52. Kottom TJ, Limper AH. Cell wall assembly by *Pneumocystis carinii*. Evidence for a unique gsc-1 subunit mediating beta-1,3-glucan deposition. *J Biol Chem* 2000;275(51):40628–40634.

53. Stansell JD, Osmond DH, Charlebois E, et al. Predictors of *Pneumocystis carinii* pneumonia in HIV-infected persons. Pulmonary Complications of HIV Infection Study Group. *Am J Respir Crit Care Med* 1997;155:60–66.

54. Mansharamani NG, Balachandran D, Vernovsky I, et al. Peripheral blood CD4+ T-lymphocyte counts during *Pneumocystis carinii* pneumonia in immunocompromised patients without HIV infection. *Chest* 2000;118:712–720.

55. Browne MJ, Hubbard SM, Longo DL, et al. Excess prevalence of *Pneumocystis carinii* pneumonia in patients treated for lymphoma with combination chemotherapy. *Ann Intern Med* 1986;104:338–344.

56. Byrd JC, Hargis JB, Kester KE, et al. Opportunistic pulmonary infections with fludarabine in previously treated patients with low-grade lymphoid malignancies: A role for *Pneumocystis carinii* pneumonia prophylaxis. *Am J Hematol* 1995;49:135–142.

57. Hughes WT, Feldman S, Aur RJ, et al. Intensity of immunosuppressive therapy and the incidence of *Pneumocystis carinii* pneumonitis. *Cancer* 1975;36:2004–2009.

58. Peters SG, Prakash UB. *Pneumocystis carinii* pneumonia. Review of 53 cases. *Am J Med* 1987;82:73–78.

59. Sugimoto H, Uchida H, Akiyama N, et al. Improved survival of renal allograft recipients with *Pneumocystis carinii* pneumonia by early diagnosis and treatment. *Transplant Proc* 1992;24:1556–1558.

60. Tuan IZ, Dennison D, Weisdorf DJ. *Pneumocystis carinii* pneumonitis following bone marrow transplantation. *Bone Marrow Transplant* 1992;10:267–272.

61. Smulian AG, Sullivan DW, Theus SA. Immunization with recombinant *Pneumocystis carinii* p55 antigen provides partial protection against infection: Characterization of epitope recognition associated with immunization. *Microbes Infect* 2000;2(2):127–136.

62. Walzer PD, Kim CK, Linke MJ, et al. Outbreaks of *Pneumocystis carinii* pneumonia in colonies of immunodeficient mice. *J Exp Med* 1990;172(3):937–945.

63. Dohn MN, Frame PT. Clinical manifestations in adults. In: Walzer PD (Eds.). *Pneumocystis carinii Pneumonia*. New York: Marcel Dekker, 1994:415–436.

64. Haverkos HW. Assessment of therapy for *Pneumocystis carinii* pneumonia. PCP Therapy Project Group. *Am J Med* 1984;76(3):501–508.

65. Kovacs JA, Hiemenz JW, Macher AM, et al. *Pneumocystis carinii* pneumonia: A comparison between patients with the acquired immunodeficiency syndrome and patients with other immunodeficiencies. *Ann Intern Med* 1984;100(5):663–671.

66. Walzer PD, Smulian AG. *Pneumocystis* species. In: Mandell GL, Bennet JE, Dolin R (Eds.). *Principles and Practice of Infectious Diseases*, 6th ed. Vols. 1 and 2. Philadelphia, PA: Churchill Livingstone, 2005:3080–3090.

67. Fishman JA. Radiological approaches to the diagnosis of *Pneumocystis carinii* pneumonitis. In: Walzer PD (Ed.). *Pneumocystis carinii Pneumonia*. New York: Marcel Dekker, 1994:381–401.

68. Crans CA Jr, Boiselle PM. Imaging features of *Pneumocystis carinii* pneumonia. *Crit Rev Diagn Imaging* 1999;40:251.

69. Hidalgo A, Falcó V, Mauleón S, et al. Accuracy of high-resolution CT in distinguishing between *Pneumocystis carinii* pneumonia and non-*Pneumocystis carinii* pneumonia in AIDS patients. *Eur Radiol* 2003;13:1179.

70. Kennedy CA, Goetz MB. Atypical roentgenographic manifestations of *Pneumocystis carinii* pneumonia. *Arch Intern Med* 1992;152:1390.

71. Edelstein H, McCabe RE. Atypical presentations of *Pneumocystis carinii* pneumonia in patients receiving inhaled pentamidine prophylaxis. *Chest* 1990;98:1366.

72. Uwyyed K, Bar-Ziv J, Kramer MR. Case report: *Pneumocystis carinii* pneumonia presenting as a solitary cavitating lung lesion in non-HIV immunosuppressed patients. *Br J Radiol* 1996;69:472.

73. Pagano L, Fianchi L, Mele L, et al. *Pneumocystis carinii* pneumonia in patients with malignant haematological diseases: 10 years' experience of infection in GIMEMA centres. *Br J Haematol* 2002;117:379.

74. Jacobs JA, Dieleman MM, Cornelissen EI, et al. Bronchoalveolar lavage fluid cytology in patients with *Pneumocystis carinii* pneumonia. *Acta Cytol* 2001;45:317.

75. Thomas CF Jr, Limper AH. Pneumocystis pneumonia: Clinical presentation and diagnosis in patients with and without acquired immune deficiency syndrome. *Semin Respir Infect* 1998;13:289.

76. Shelhamer JH, Gill VJ, Quinn TC, et al. The laboratory evaluation of opportunistic pulmonary infections. *Ann Intern Med* 1996;124:585.

77. Limper AH, Offord KP, Smith TF, Martin WJ 2nd. *Pneumocystis carinii* pneumonia. Differences in lung parasite number and inflammation in patients with and without AIDS. *Am Rev Respir Dis* 1989;140:1204.

78. Panel on Opportunistic Infections in HIV-Infected Adults and Adolescents. Guidelines for the prevention and treatment of opportunistic infections in HIV-infected adults and adolescents: Recommendations from the Centers for Disease Control and Prevention, the National Institutes of Health, and the HIV Medicine Association of the Infectious Diseases Society of America. Available at http://aidsinfo.nih.gov/contentfiles/lvguidelines/adult_oi.pdf (Accessed on December 9, 2016).

79. Alanio A, Hauser PM, Lagrou K, et al. ECIL guidelines for the diagnosis of Pneumocystis jirovecii pneumonia in patients with haematological malignancies and stem cell transplant recipients. *J Antimicrob Chemother* 2016;71:2386.

80. Fischer S, Gill VJ, Kovacs J, et al. The use of oral washes to diagnose *Pneumocystis carinii* pneumonia: A blinded prospective study using a polymerase chain reaction-based detection system. *J Infect Dis* 2001;184:1485.

81. Oz HS, Hughes WT. Search for *Pneumocystis carinii* DNA in upper and lower respiratory tract of humans. *Diagn Microbiol Infect Dis* 2000;37:161.

82. Hughes W, Leoung G, Kramer F, et al. Comparison of atovaquone (566C80) with trimethoprim-sulfamethoxazole to treat *Pneumocystis carinii* pneumonia in patients with AIDS. *N Engl J Med* 1993 May;328(21):1521–1527.

83. Safrin S, Finkelstein DM, Feinberg J, et al. Comparison of three regimens for treatment of mild to moderate *Pneumocystis carinii* pneumonia in patients with AIDS. A double-blind, randomized, trial of oral trimethoprim-sulfamethoxazole, dapsone-trimethoprim, and clindamycin-primaquine. ACTG 108 Study Group. *Ann Intern Med* 1996 May;124(9):792–802.

84. Limper AH, Knox KS, Sarosi GA, et al. An official American Thoracic Society statement: Treatment of fungal infections in adult pulmonary and critical care patients. *Am J Respir Crit Care Med* 2011;183:96.

85. Nielsen TL, Eeftinck Schattenkerk JK, Jensen BN, et al. Adjunctive corticosteroid therapy for *Pneumocystis carinii* pneumonia in AIDS: A randomized European multicenter open label study. *J Acquir Immune Defic Syndr* 1992;5(7):726–731.

86. Bozzette SA, Sattler FR, Chiu J, et al. A controlled trial of early adjunctive treatment with corticosteroids for *Pneumocystis carinii* pneumonia in the acquired immunodeficiency syndrome. California Collaborative Treatment *Group. N Engl J Med* 1990;323(21):1451–1457.

87. The National Institutes of Health-University of California Expert Panel for Corticosteroids as Adjunctive Therapy for Pneumocystis Pneumonia. Consensus statement on the use of corticosteroids as adjunctive therapy for pneumocystis pneumonia in the acquired immunodeficiency syndrome. *N Engl J Med* 1990;323(21):1500–1504.

88. Montaner JS, Lawson LM, Levitt N, Belzberg A, Schechter MT, Ruedy J. Corticosteroids prevent early deterioration in patients with moderately severe *Pneumocystis carinii* pneumonia and the acquired immunodeficiency syndrome (AIDS). *Ann Intern Med* 1990;113(1):14–20.

89. Gallant JE, Chaisson RE, Moore RD. The effect of adjunctive corticosteroids for the treatment of *Pneumocystis carinii* pneumonia on mortality and subsequent complications. *Chest* 1998;114(5):1258–1263.

90. Briel M, Bucher HC, Boscacci R, Furrer H. Adjunctive corticosteroids for *Pneumocystis jirovecii* pneumonia in patients with HIV-infection. *Cochrane Database Syst Rev* 2006;3:CD006150.

91. Medina I, Mills J, Leoung G, et al. Oral therapy for *Pneumocystis carinii* pneumonia in the acquired immunodeficiency syndrome. A controlled trial of trimethoprim-sulfamethoxazole versus trimethoprim-dapsone. *N Engl J Med* 1990;323(12):776–782.

92. Black JR, Feinberg J, Murphy RL, et al. Clindamycin and primaquine therapy for mild-to-moderate episodes of *Pneumocystis carinii* pneumonia in patients with AIDS: AIDS Clinical Trials Group 044. *Clin Infect Dis* 1994;18(6):905–913.

93. Toma E, Thorne A, Singer J, et al; with the CTN-PCP Study Group. Clindamycin with primaquine vs. Trimethoprim-sulfamethoxazole therapy for mild and moderately severe *Pneumocystis carinii* pneumonia in patients with AIDS: A multicenter, double-blind, randomized trial (CTN 004). *Clin Infect Dis* 1998;27(3):524–530.

94. Smego RA, Jr., Nagar S, Maloba B, Popara M. A meta-analysis of salvage therapy for *Pneumocystis carinii* pneumonia. *Arch Intern Med* 2001;161(12):1529–1533.

95. El-Sadr WM, Murphy RL, Yurik TM, et al; with Community Program for Clinical Research on AIDS and the AIDS Clinical Trials Group. Atovaquone compared with dapsone for the prevention of *Pneumocystis carinii* pneumonia in patients with HIV infection who cannot tolerate trimethoprim, sulfonamides, or both. *N Engl J Med* 1998;339(26):1889–1895.

96. Furrer H, Egger M, Opravil M, et al; Swiss HIV Cohort Study. Discontinuation of primary prophylaxis against *Pneumocystis carinii* pneumonia in HIV-1-infected adults treated with combination antiretroviral therapy. *N Engl J Med* 1999;340(17):1301–1306.

97. Dohn MN, Weinberg WG, Torres RA, et al; with the Atovaquone Study Group. Oral atovaquone compared with intravenous pentamidine for *Pneumocystis carinii* pneumonia in patients with AIDS. *Ann Intern Med* 1994;121(3):174–180.

98. Conte JE, Jr, Chernoff D, Feigal DW, Jr, Joseph P, McDonald C, Golden JA. Intravenous or inhaled pentamidine for treating *Pneumocystis carinii* pneumonia in AIDS. A randomized trial. *Ann Intern Med* 1990;113(3):203–209.

99. Wharton JM, Coleman DL, Wofsy CB, et al. Trimethoprim-sulfamethoxazole or pentamidine for *Pneumocystis carinii* pneumonia in the acquired immunodeficiency syndrome. A prospective randomized trial. *Ann Intern Med* 1986;105(1):37–44.

100. Soo Hoo GW, Mohsenifar Z, Meyer RD. Inhaled or intravenous pentamidine therapy for *Pneumocystis carinii* pneumonia in AIDS. A randomized trial. *Ann Intern Med* 1990;113(3):195–202.

101. Montgomery AB, Feigal DW, Jr, Sattler F, et al. Pentamidine aerosol versus trimethoprim-sulfamethoxazole for *Pneumocystis carinii* in acquired immune deficiency syndrome. *Am J Respir Crit Care Med* 1995;151(4):1068–1074.

102. Centers for Disease Controm and Prevention. Guidelines for prophylaxis against *Pneumocystis carinii* pneumonia for persons infected with human immunodeficiency virus. *MMWR Morb Mortal Wkly Rep* 1989;38(Suppl 5):1–9.

103. Bozzette SA, Finkelstein DM, Spector SA, et al; with the NIAID AIDS Clinical Trials Group. A randomized trial of three anti-pneumocystis agents in patients with advanced human immunodeficiency virus infection. *N Engl J Med* 1995;332(11):693–699.

104. Schneider MM, Hoepelman AI, Eeftinck Schattenkerk JK, et al; with The Dutch AIDS Treatment Group. A controlled trial of aerosolized pentamidine or trimethoprim-sulfamethoxazole as primary prophylaxis against *Pneumocystis carinii* pneumonia in patients with human immunodeficiency virus infection. *N Engl J Med* 1992;327(26):1836–1841.

105. Schneider MM, Nielsen TL, Nelsing S, et al; with Dutch AIDS Treatment Group. Efficacy and toxicity of two doses of trimethoprim-sulfamethoxazole as primary prophylaxis against *Pneumocystis carinii* pneumonia in patients with human immunodeficiency virus. *J Infect Dis* 1995;171(6):1632–1636.

106. Phair J, Munoz A, Detels R, Kaslow R, Rinaldo C, Saah A. The risk of *Pneumocystis carinii* pneumonia among men infected with human immunodeficiency virus type 1. Multicenter AIDS Cohort Study Group. *N Engl J Med* 1990;322(3):161–165.

107. Kaplan JE, Hanson DL, Navin TR, Jones JL. Risk factors for primary *Pneumocystis carinii* pneumonia in human immunodeficiency virus-infected adolescents and adults in the United States: Reassessment of indications for chemoprophylaxis. *J Infect Dis* 1998;178(4):1126–1132.

108. Selwyn PA, Pumerantz AS, Durante A, et al. Clinical predictors of *Pneumocystis carinii* pneumonia, bacterial pneumonia and tuberculosis in HIV-infected patients. *AIDS* 1998;12(8):885–893.

109. Tomblyn M, Chiller T, Einsele H, et al. Guidelines for preventing infectious complications among hematopoietic cell transplant recipients: A global perspective. *Biol Blood Marrow Transpl* 2009;15:1143–1238.

110. Wang EZ, Partovi N, Levy RD, et al. *Pneumocystis* pneumonia in solid organ transplant recipients: Not yet an infection of the past. *Transpl Infect Dis* 2012;14:519–525.

111. Martin SI, Fishman JA. AST Infectious Diseases Community of Practice. *Pneumocystis* pneumonia in solid organ transplantation. *Am J Transplant* 2013;13(suppl 4):272–279.

23

Management of mucormycoses

JOHN R. PERFECT AND AHMAD MOURAD

INTRODUCTION

The management of Mucormycosis has always centered around a triad of strategies to cure this unusual, but not rare infection. These three therapeutic areas are (*i*) the control of the underlying disease, (*ii*) surgery, and (*iii*) antifungal therapy [1–3].

Control of underlying disease

The control of an underlying disease is extremely important to the final outcome of these infections [4]. In the past, mucormycete infections such as rhinocerebral disease were frequently linked to poorly-controlled diabetes and at times, specifically related to or linked to ketoacidosis. Diabetes is still a risk factor but the combination of better diabetic control and the use of statins with their antifungal activity may have combined to make this risk group less common [5]. Despite a possible change in epidemiology, it is still critical to optimize diabetic control for successful management of this infection, and it is clear that diabetic renal dysfunction and the use of polyenes make this risk group very difficult to manage. Even more difficult to manage is the enlarging risk group of mucormycosis associated with hematological malignancies and bone marrow transplant recipients. This risk group provides a series of advantages for the fungus over the host. For example, it is associated with voriconazole exposure, which may suggest that the patient had avoided an aspergillus infection only to survive long enough to contract an invasive mucormycosis with these ubiquitous, environmental molds or even a direct interaction with the mold [6]. Furthermore, this

patient population combines other advantageous conditions for the mold's survival in a weakened host such as neutropenia, graft-versus-host disease, high doses of corticosteroids, malnutrition, and relatively high iron states from multiple transfusions. These patients represent the "perfect storm" for the clinical growth of this mold. It is therefore essential to remember that at times this mould infection is an extreme marker for the end stage of a life-threatening underlying disease and this fact needs to be factored into the treatment strategy and outcome.

Surgery

The second major strategic factor in the management of mucormycosis is the need to consider the value of surgical debridement. The well-known pathophysiology of mucormycosis describes the mold's angioinvasive nature within the mammalian host. It invades blood vessels causing ischemia/infarctions and eventually necrotic devitalized tissue. From rhinosinusitis to pneumonitis, it is important that dead necrotic material is surgically removed. Some of this devitalized tissue would not be effectively improved without debridement since an antifungal agent would not be able to penetrate well to the site of infection. Of course, all sites of infections and clinical conditions are not amenable to surgical debridement, and medical therapy alone will be necessary at times. Ideally, the infection site is surgically removed but on a practical basis it will be necessary to judge at the bedside the extent of the surgical debridement of this infection that is necessary and/or feasible. It can range from complete surgical removal of a cutaneous or subcutaneous infection to the very minimal ability to debride a mucormycete brain abscess. In the middle of these two polar extremes is the surgical debridement in the nasal and sinus areas connecting into the orbit or brain, which may require several surgical procedures to remove devitalized tissue. Therefore, although surgical intervention is a critical factor in the successful management of mucormycosis the precision of its use and the technical outcome are hard to develop into robust guidelines and variable quality assurances, respectively.

Antifungal therapy

The third major management factor of mucormycosis is the use of antifungal therapy. This factor has recently engendered renewed enthusiasm for studies and attempts to optimize therapies. With the in vitro susceptibility testing, animal model efficacy studies, and clinical experiences from over 50 years, the optimal regimens for specific antifungal therapy for mucormycosis remain without support of robust comparative clinical trials. In truth, it is extremely difficult to marshal the members of medical centers needed to study this infection, and further complicating the studies is the variable impact of both surgery and the underlying disease on outcome. Therefore, the precision of optimal antifungal therapy is simply lacking, but the literature does provide some insights and guidance.

Polyenes

Historically, amphotericin B deoxycholate (AmBd) was the only active systemic antifungal agent for treatment of mucormycote infections. In 2008, a retrospective review of 70 consecutive hematology patients with mucormycosis found that there was a two-fold higher mortality with delayed AmBd administration [7], and a review of the literature from 1960 to 2016 showed that AmBd is still an effective treatment with a preferred dose of AmBd 1–1.5 mg/kg/day [8]. It is well known that the use of AmBd is accompanied by severe infusional reactions and renal toxicity. This is particularly common in patients who frequently already have compromised renal function and high doses are used. Therefore, the lipid formulations of amphotericin B—liposomal amphotericin B (LAmB), amphotericin B lipid complex (ABLC), and amphotericin B colloidal dispersion—became very attractive therapeutic agents for treatment of mucormycosis. LAmB is usually given in the 5 mg/kg/day range. However, with less toxicity and better tolerability than AmBd, LAmB can be given in higher doses. In a diabetic ketoacidosis murine model, it was found that LAmB at 15 mg/kg/day was superior for treatment compared to a lower dose of 7.5 mg/kg/day or AmBd 1 mg/kg/day [9]. Therefore, there is some suggestion that higher doses may be necessary for treatment success. In humans, a recent study suggested that high doses of LAmB (10 mg/kg/day) were not more effective than lower doses (7.5 mg/kg/day) but were associated with greater rates of renal injury [10]. More data is required to make definitive conclusions about

dosing in humans. Furthermore, although amphotericin B colloidal dispersion has been less frequently used secondary to early reports of increased infusional-related toxicity, the other formulations have been used and particularly ABLC has been reported in open trials to effectively treat zygomycosis [11,12]. Although treatment success in humans has been reported with all three lipid products of amphotericin B there have been no prospective trials directly comparing the agents and/or their dosing to each other. There are retrospective studies with small numbers of patients in which the lipid products generally have some detectable clinical success in over half the patients [8,11–17]. Some animal models have been used to compare LAmB and ABLC. In a disseminated R. oryzae mouse model, there was generally better survival with the use of the LAmB preparation in both the diabetic ketoacidosis and neutropenia models [18]. When examining the CNS burden of infection, the liposomal product appeared to be more potent although ABLC at high doses showed a positive impact on CNS infection [18].

Despite the lack of conclusive evidence about either the best preparation or the proper dose, the compilation of experience supports the continued use of the lipid formulations of amphotericin B as primary induction therapy for disseminated mucormycosis; the dose and duration, however, will need to be carefully adjusted for each case. A reasonable starting point may be LAmB or ABLC at 5 mg/kg/d for an induction period of 4–6 weeks.

Azoles

In vitro activity against the mucormycetes is always the initial platform to base therapy. Although not as effective as amphotericin B, posaconazole and isavuconazole are the two triazoles that have been shown to have reasonable *in vitro* activity against some species in the Mucorales [8].

POSACONAZOLE

Posaconazole has animal model experience in mucormycosis and the results have been mixed and not as consistent as the polyene data. In one study of disseminated R. oryzae infection in both diabetic ketoacidosis and neutropenic models, posaconazole monotherapy had no benefit and there was also no benefit when combined with liposomal amphotericin B [19]. These results were confirmed with another mouse model [20]. However, a third study in a neutropenic model of disseminated R. oryzae using two strains did show that posaconazole monotherapy had antifungal activity but was not as potent as amphotericin B, but the combination did have a positive interaction including impact on CNS fungal burden [21]. Thus, the limited animal models studied would suggest that the use of posaconazole for primary therapy has less assurance of activity compared to the polyene. As is the case with all antifungals and the mucormycosis, the lack of robust prospective therapeutic studies with posaconazole in humans limits the certainty of the conclusions that can be made about optimal therapy. In a retrospective study assessing 91 patients and a difficult-to-treat population, approximately 60%–70% of cases had a favorable treatment outcome with posaconazole salvage therapy [22]. Oral suspension of posaconazole was used at a divided dose of 800 mg/day. Current recommendation for use of oral suspension of posaconazole for salvage therapy is 200 mg four times daily [12]. However, the oral suspension form, which has been used until the recent development of the extended-release tablet and intravenous formulation, did not always result in predictable drug concentrations and had many interactions with coadministered drugs [23]. With the extended- release tablet, more predictable and higher drug concentrations can be achieved compared to the oral suspension form [24]. 300 mg p.o. bid on day 1 followed by 300 mg p.o. once daily is the current recommendation for the extended-release tablet. The intravenous formulation has also shown promise and has utility [25]. It can be given peripherally and used as an alternative in patients who cannot tolerate oral intake. With these new developments it is likely that posaconazole will continue to have a role in the treatment of mucormycosis, with attention being given to drug exposure by drug level monitoring.

ISAVUCONAZOLE

Isavuconazole has shown variable in vitro activity against the Mucorales and several reports have been made of isavuconazole being used for salvage therapy in patients who have failed on or were not able to tolerate other antifungals agents [8,26]. However, there is a promise of isavuconazole being used as primary therapy, with less toxicity and better tolerability compared to amphotericin B. A single arm open label trial revealed that weighted-all-cause mortality at day 42 of therapy was similar in patients that were given isavuconazole as primary treatment compared to a registry cohort of patients receiving a polyene (33% vs. 41% respectively). Overall complete and partial response for primary treatment of mucormycosis with isavuconazole was 32% (36% for salvage therapy) [26]. These figures tend to underestimate the success of the regimens since many patients will be classified as stable and thus not success. In this disease process, stabilization of disease is a positive goal. However, these results allowed isavuconazole to obtain FDA approval for mucormycosis treatment. Isavuconazole is given in the form of the prodrug, isavuconazonium sulfate, and is dosed at a 200 mg equivalent of isavuconazole (oral or intravenous) tid for 6 doses for loading followed by 200 mg daily. Furthermore, the long-term tolerability of isavuconazole was evident with the median time of therapy being over 3 months as compared to amphotericin B being under 3 weeks. Adverse events were a rare cause for discontinuation of therapy with isavuconazole. Although there have been no head to head comparisons between isavuconazole and posaconazole, and it is likely that they are similar in efficacy. However, it appears that isavuconazole will be the azole of choice for primary therapy for patients with mucormycosis or in refractory patients or those intolerant to other antifungal agents.

Echinocandins and combination therapy

ECHINOCANDINS

Interestingly, although the echinocandins have poor antifungal activity against the growth of mucormycetes directly in vitro, there has been demonstrated an immunomodulatory activity of echinocandins against several molds such as *Rhizopus oryzae*. For example, the addition of caspofungin increased mold cell wall beta-glucan exposure and this impact allowed human neutrophil attacks against this remodeled cell wall [27].

Since there are some conflicting results regarding echinocandins in vitro in which there is poor direct antifungal activity against mucormycete growth [28,29], it may alter fungus to allow host cells to attack it and it was necessary to study this antifungal class in animal models of mucormycete infections. The echinocandins as monotherapy appear to have limited antifungal activity in disseminated mucormycete infections in mice [30]. The combination of poor in vitro activity and a very meager response in animal models alone make it unlikely that the echinocandins will have much use as monotherapy in mucormyceate infections.

COMBINATION THERAPY

Some reports of echinocandin-polyene synergy have been published for mouse survival [31,32]. This positive interaction with lipid products of amphotericin B and all the commercially available echinocandins supports the continued investigation of combination therapy in difficult-to-manage cases of mucormycosis, and the echinocandins can be placed into combination consideration for this difficult-to-treat infection.

In regards to the use of adding an echinocandin to amphotericin B, there is one retrospective review of 34 patients with rhino-orbital-cerebral mucormycosis [33]. These patients were primarily diabetics and treatment with the polyene–echinocandin combination was successful in all six evaluable patients compared to approximately 40% success in the amphotericin B monotherapy group. There are great risks in interpreting these small, unrandomized, retrospective studies but with present information, there are no data that the combination causes harm and thus we will need a more robust study before formal recommendations can be made.

Combining amphotericin B with posaconazole has also been studied with 30 different mucormycete strains that found the drug combination often demonstrates a synergistic effect on hyphae more commonly than conidia [20]. In a subset of very difficult patients to treat, the use of a combination of amphotericin B plus posaconazole had a favorable response in approximately half the patients [33]. A common treatment strategy is to induce with a lipid formulation of amphotericin B and then add a triazole (isavuconazole or posaconazole) during later stages of induction and then continue as monotherapy. Unfortunately, the length of antifungal therapy for mucormycosis is not precise but generally continues for months.

Adjunctive therapy

As with all infections with potentially poor outcomes and immunocompromised host, there have been studies to consider adjunctive therapies to provide an advantage for the host. Mucormycete infections are one of those mycoses with a rich history of adjunctive therapies. From cytokine therapies such as GM–CSF and interferon-gamma [34–36] to granulocyte transfusions [37], there have been attempts to bolster the host's immunity. In these few reports it is difficult to evaluate whether there was a positive clinical impact and these immune modulating strategies are generally used when heroic measures are needed and until better studies are performed. There are two other creative measures, which have been used in mucormycosis that are based around changing the local host environment to put the fungus at a disadvantage. First, it has been reported that hyperbaric oxygen was used to improve the oxygenation of devitalized tissue environment and directly kill or inhibit the fungus [38]. It has appeared to cause no harm but on the other hand, there are no convincing data that it provides for a better outcome. It remains in the arena of "should we or can we do it" for specific refractory cases and there is no solid support that it is routinely necessary [12]. Another adjunctive therapy has recently been considered and studied. Iron chelation with deferoxamine has been known as a risk factor for disseminated mucormycosis by its use as a siderophore to enhance iron uptake by the mucormycete and promote its growth [39]. Newer iron-chelating agents, such as deferasirox, have the opposite effect and can steal iron from the mold. Deferasirox has shown antimucormycete activity in vitro and in murine models [39,40]. These results were a platform to try it in human case reports with both success and failure [41,42]. Subsequently, a randomized, double-blinded, placebo-controlled trial revealed that patients with mucormycosis treated with deferasirox had higher mortality [43]. Although, it is difficult to make conclusions due to the limited power of the study and a possible bias against the chelation agent in the randomization process, it is not generally recommended for the management of mucormycosis in hematological patients [12] and should probably be primarily considered in known iron overload states with mucormycosis.

In summary, mucormycosis is generally treated with a three-part strategy: (*i*) surgical debridement, (*ii*) lipid formulation of amphotericin B as primary antifungal agent for serious disease but with isavuconazole or posaconazole as second-line or salvage therapy, and (*iii*) control of the underlying disease. Despite its reputation as a difficult mold infection to treat and significant difficulties to precisely study it for robust recommendations, a careful plan of management can frequently be successful in mucormycosis if there is control of the underlying disease.

REFERENCES

1. Chayakulkeeree M, Ghannoum MA, Perfect JR. Zygomycosis: The re-emerging fungal infection. *Eur J Clin Microbiol Infect Dis* 2006;25(4):215–229.
2. Rogers TR. Treatment of zygomycosis: Current and new options. *J Antimicrob Chemother* 2008;61(Suppl 1):i35–i40.
3. Kauffman CA, Malani AN. Zygomycosis: An emerging fungal infection with new options for management. *Curr Infect Dis Rep* 2007;9(6):435–440.
4. Roden MM, Zaoutis TE, Buchanan WL, Knudsen TA, Sarkisova TA, Schaufele RL, et al. Epidemiology and outcome of zygomycosis: A review of 929 reported cases. *Clin Infect Dis* 2005;41(5):634–653.
5. Bellanger AP, Tatara AM, Shirazi F, Gebremariam T, Albert ND, Lewis RE, et al. Statin concentrations below the minimum inhibitory concentration attenuate the virulence of *Rhizopus oryzae*. *J Infect Dis* 2016;214(1):114–121.
6. Bellanger AP, Albert ND, Lewis RE, Walsh TJ, Kontoyiannis DP. Effect of preexposure to triazoles on susceptibility and virulence of *Rhizopus oryzae*. *Antimicrob Agents Chemother* 2015;59(12):7830–7832.
7. Chamilos G, Lewis RE, Kontoyiannis DP. Delaying amphotericin B-based frontline therapy significantly increases mortality among patients with hematologic malignancy who have zygomycosis. *Clin Infect Dis* 2008;47(4):503–509.
8. Riley TT, Muzny CA, Swiatlo E, Legendre DP. Breaking the mold: A review of mucormycosis and current pharmacological treatment options. *Ann Pharmacother* 2016;50(9):747–757.
9. Ibrahim AS, Avanessian V, Spellberg B, Edwards JE, Jr. Liposomal amphotericin B, and not amphotericin B deoxycholate, improves survival of diabetic mice infected with *Rhizopus oryzae*. *Antimicrob Agents Chemother* 2003;47(10):3343–3344.
10. Lanternier F, Poiree S, Elie C, Garcia-Hermoso D, Bakouboula P, Sitbon K, et al. Prospective pilot study of high-dose (10 mg/kg/day) liposomal amphotericin B (L-AMB) for the initial treatment of mucormycosis. *J Antimicrob Chemother* 2015;70(11):3116–3123.
11. Larkin J, Montero, J.A. Efficacy and safety of amphotericin B lipid complex for zygomycosis. *Infect Med* 2003;20:210–216.
12. Cornely OA, Arikan-Akdagli S, Dannaoui E, Groll AH, Lagrou K, Chakrabarti A, et al. ESCMID and ECMM joint clinical guidelines for the diagnosis and management of mucormycosis 2013. *Clin Microbiol Infect* 2014;20 Suppl 3:5–26.

13. Herbrecht R, Letscher-Bru V, Bowden RA, Kusne S, Anaissie EJ, Graybill JR, et al. Treatment of 21 cases of invasive mucormycosis with amphotericin B colloidal dispersion. *Eur J Clin Microbiol Infect Dis* 2001;20(7):460–466.

14. Strasser MD, Kennedy RJ, Adam RD. Rhinocerebral mucormycosis. Therapy with amphotericin B lipid complex. *Arch Intern Med* 1996;156(3):337–339.

15. Walsh TJ, Hiemenz JW, Seibel NL, Perfect JR, Horwith G, Lee L, et al. Amphotericin B lipid complex for invasive fungal infections: Analysis of safety and efficacy in 556 cases. *Clin Infect Dis* 1998;26(6):1383–1396.

16. Perfect JR. Treatment of non-*Aspergillus* moulds in immunocompromised patients, with amphotericin B lipid complex. *Clin Infect Dis* 2005;40(Suppl 6):S401–S408.

17. Walsh TJ, Goodman JL, Pappas P, Bekersky I, Buell DN, Roden M, et al. Safety, tolerance, and pharmacokinetics of high-dose liposomal amphotericin B (AmBisome) in patients infected with *Aspergillus* species and other filamentous fungi: Maximum tolerated dose study. *Antimicrob Agents Chemother* 2001;45(12):3487–3496.

18. Ibrahim AS, Gebremariam T, Husseiny MI, Stevens DA, Fu Y, Edwards JE, Jr., et al. Comparison of lipid amphotericin B preparations in treating murine zygomycosis. *Antimicrob Agents Chemother* 2008;52(4):1573–1576.

19. Ibrahim AS, Gebremariam T, Schwartz JA, Edwards JE, Jr., Spellberg B. Posaconazole mono- or combination therapy for treatment of murine zygomycosis. *Antimicrob Agents Chemother* 2009;53(2):772–775.

20. Dannaoui E, Meis JF, Loebenberg D, Verweij PE. Activity of posaconazole in treatment of experimental disseminated zygomycosis. *Antimicrob Agents Chemother* 2003;47(11):3647–3650.

21. Rodriguez MM, Serena C, Marine M, Pastor FJ, Guarro J. Posaconazole combined with amphotericin B, an effective therapy for a murine disseminated infection caused by *Rhizopus oryzae*. *Antimicrob Agents Chemother* 2008;52(10):3786–3788.

22. van Burik JA, Hare RS, Solomon HF, Corrado ML, Kontoyiannis DP. Posaconazole is effective as salvage therapy in zygomycosis: A retrospective summary of 91 cases. *Clin Infect Dis* 2006;42(7):e61–e65.

23. Dolton MJ, Bruggemann RJ, Burger DM, McLachlan AJ. Understanding variability in posaconazole exposure using an integrated population pharmacokinetic analysis. *Antimicrob Agents Chemother* 2014;58(11):6879–6885.

24. Durani U, Tosh PK, Barreto JN, Estes LL, Jannetto PJ, Tande AJ. Retrospective comparison of posaconazole levels in patients taking the delayed-release tablet versus the oral suspension. *Antimicrob Agents Chemother* 2015;59(8):4914–4918.

25. Kersemaekers WM, van Iersel T, Nassander U, O'Mara E, Waskin H, Caceres M, et al. Pharmacokinetics and safety study of posaconazole intravenous solution administered peripherally to healthy subjects. *Antimicrob Agents Chemother* 2015;59(2):1246–1251.

26. Marty FM, Ostrosky-Zeichner L, Cornely OA, Mullane KM, Perfect JR, Thompson GR, 3rd., et al. Isavuconazole treatment for mucormycosis: A single-arm open-label trial and case-control analysis. *Lancet Infect Dis* 2016;16(7):828–837.

27. Lamaris GA, Lewis RE, Chamilos G, May GS, Safdar A, Walsh TJ, et al. Caspofungin-mediated beta-glucan unmasking and enhancement of human polymorphonuclear neutrophil activity against *Aspergillus* and non-*Aspergillus* hyphae. *J Infect Dis* 2008;198(2):186–192.

28. Del Poeta M, Schell WA, Perfect JR. In vitro antifungal activity of pneumocandin L-743,872 against a variety of clinically important molds. *Antimicrob Agents Chemother* 1997;41(8):1835–1836.

29. Guembe M, Guinea J, Pelaez T, Torres-Narbona M, Bouza E. Synergistic effect of posaconazole and caspofungin against clinical zygomycetes. *Antimicrob Agents Chemother* 2007;51(9):3457–3458.

30. Ibrahim AS, Bowman JC, Avanessian V, Brown K, Spellberg B, Edwards JE, Jr., et al. Caspofungin inhibits *Rhizopus oryzae* 1,3-beta-D-glucan synthase, lowers burden in brain measured by quantitative PCR, and improves survival at a low but not a high dose during murine disseminated zygomycosis. *Antimicrob Agents Chemother* 2005;49(2):721–727.

31. Ibrahim AS, Gebremariam T, Fu Y, Edwards JE, Jr., Spellberg B. Combination echinocandin-polyene treatment of murine mucormycosis. *Antimicrob Agents Chemother* 2008;52(4):1556–1558.

32. Spellberg B, Fu Y, Edwards JE, Jr., Ibrahim AS. Combination therapy with amphotericin B lipid complex and caspofungin acetate of disseminated zygomycosis in diabetic ketoacidotic mice. *Antimicrob Agents Chemother* 2005;49(2):830–832.

33. Reed C, Bryant R, Ibrahim AS, Edwards J, Jr., Filler SG, Goldberg R, et al. Combination polyene-caspofungin treatment of rhino-orbital-cerebral mucormycosis. *Clin Infect Dis* 2008;47(3):364–371.

34. Gil-Lamaignere C, Simitsopoulou M, Roilides E, Maloukou A, Winn RM, Walsh TJ. Interferon- gamma and granulocyte-macrophage colony-stimulating factor augment the activity of polymorphonuclear leukocytes against medically important zygomycetes. *J Infect Dis* 2005;191(7):1180–1187.

35. Sahin B, Paydas S, Cosar E, Bicakci K, Hazar B. Role of granulocyte colony-stimulating factor in the treatment of mucormycosis. *Eur J Clin Microbiol Infect Dis* 1996;15(11):866–869.

36. Garcia-Diaz JB, Palau L, Pankey GA. Resolution of rhinocerebral zygomycosis associated with adjuvant administration of granulocyte-macrophage colony-stimulating factor. *Clin Infect Dis* 2001;32(12):e145–e150.

37. Safdar A. Difficulties with fungal infections in acute myelogenous leukemia patients: Immune enhancement strategies. *Oncologist* 2007;12(Suppl 2):2–6.

38. Ferguson BJ, Mitchell TG, Moon R, Camporesi EM, Farmer J. Adjunctive hyperbaric oxygen for treatment of rhinocerebral mucormycosis. *Rev Infect Dis* 1988;10(3):551–559.

39. Spellberg B, Edwards J, Jr., Ibrahim A. Novel perspectives on mucormycosis: Pathophysiology, presentation, and management. *Clin Microbiol Rev* 2005;18(3):556–569.

40. Ibrahim AS, Gebermariam T, Fu Y, Lin L, Husseiny MI, French SW, et al. The iron chelator deferasirox protects mice from mucormycosis through iron starvation. *J Clin Invest* 2007;117(9):2649–2657.

41. Reed C, Ibrahim A, Edwards JE, Jr., Walot I, Spellberg B. Deferasirox, an iron-chelating agent, as salvage therapy for rhinocerebral mucormycosis. *Antimicrob Agents Chemother* 2006;50(11):3968–3969.

42. Soummer A, Mathonnet A, Scatton O, Massault PP, Paugam A, Lemiale V, et al. Failure of deferasirox, an iron chelator agent, combined with antifungals in a case of severe zygomycosis. *Antimicrob Agents Chemother* 2008;52(4):1585–1586.

43. Spellberg B, Ibrahim AS, Chin-Hong PV, Kontoyiannis DP, Morris MI, Perfect JR, et al. The Deferasirox-AmBisome Therapy for Mucormycosis (DEFEAT Mucor) study: A randomized, double-blinded, placebo-controlled trial. *J Antimicrob Chemother* 2012;67(3):715–722.

24

Antifungal management in risk groups: Solid organ transplant recipients

JASMINE CHUNG, SYLVIA F. COSTA, AND BARBARA D. ALEXANDER

INTRODUCTION

Over the past decade, the epidemiology of invasive fungal infections (IFIs) in solid organ transplant (SOT) patients has evolved. The use of new antifungal drugs and modifications in transplant practices, including changes in surgical techniques, conditioning regimens, and new immunosuppressive agents, has contributed to the shift in the numbers and types of IFIs encountered. To say the least, treatment of fungal disease in a complex transplant patient is challenging, and optimal outcome requires prompt diagnosis and consideration of several important factors, including coinfection with immunomodulatory viruses, comorbid conditions, and drug interactions. The management of invasive mycoses within the complex milieu of the SOT recipient is discussed in this chapter.

TYPES AND TIMING OF INFECTIONS

For SOT recipients, the timeline for infections following transplantation has traditionally been divided into three phases: the first month, months 2 through 6, and more than 6 months after the transplant procedure (Figure 24.1). The risk for developing an invasive mycosis during each of these periods is linked to the patient's overall net state of immunosuppression, use of prophylactic therapies, and their exposure to fungal pathogens. During the first posttransplant month, technical and anatomical factors including those related to the surgical procedure and its aftermath, such as the presence of foreign bodies, ischemia

with resulting devitalized tissue, remnant fluid collections, and prolonged intensive care support, contribute to the risk. *Candida* is the most common fungal pathogen encountered during this period. During the second through sixth posttransplant months, the SOT recipient has typically left the hospital, but the maximum impact of the induction immunosuppressive regimen begins to manifest in terms of infectious risks. In addition, patients are now routinely exposed to a broad array of fungal pathogens including *Aspergillus* and other molds, *Cryptococcus*, and *Pneumocystis jirovecii*. Latent infections from past exposures to the geographically restricted endemic fungi may also reactivate [1–3]. Beyond the sixth month following transplantation, the risk for IFIs for the majority of SOT recipients begins to decline, as most patients will have been placed on minimal maintenance immunosuppressive therapy. Infections after 6 months tend to occur either in the setting of continued chronic infection [e.g., cytomegalovirus (CMV)] or due to increased immunosuppression such as is required with recurrent or chronic rejection [1–4].

Rates of specific IFIs vary not only by time after transplant, but also by the type of solid organ transplanted. For example, invasive aspergillosis (IA) is rarely encountered in the pancreas transplant recipient, while lung transplant recipients are considered to be at relatively high risk for this infection. The incidence of IA during the first 12 months following lung transplant is 2.4%, compared with 0.8%, 0.3%, and 0.1% after heart, liver, and kidney transplant, respectively [5]. Risk factors unique to each organ transplanted are likely to blame for these differences.

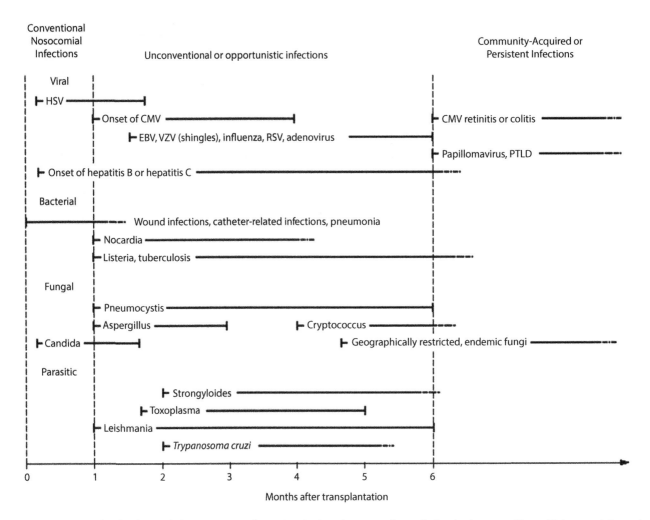

Figure 24.1 Periods of risk in solid organ transplantation in the absence of prophylactic therapy. (From Fishman, J.A. and Rubin, R.H., *N Engl. J. Med.*, 338, 1741–1751, 1998. Copyright © 1998 Massachusetts Medical Society. Reprinted with permission from Massachusetts Medical Society.)

In lung transplant recipients, factors contributing to the risk of IA include a vulnerable anastomotic site, continuous environmental exposure, *Aspergillus* colonization of the airways, CMV pneumonitis, acute rejection, and obliterative bronchiolitis [6]. For liver transplant recipients, retransplantation, large volume intraoperative transfusion, pretransplant fulminant hepatic or renal failure, heavy *Candida* colonization peritransplant, choledochojejunostomy, and bleeding complications requiring reoperation have been identified as major factors for invasive candidiasis (IC) [7–10]. New risk factors for IFIs are being continually identified and most recently, renal failure, thrombocytopenia, human herpes virus-6, extracorporeal membrane oxygenation, delayed sternal closure, and ventricular assist devices have been implicated.

The largest epidemiologic data for IFIs in transplant recipients comes from the CDC-sponsored Transplant Associated Infection Surveillance Network (TRANSNET), which prospectively monitored nearly 17,000 SOT recipients for IFIs between 2001 and 2006. Based on these data, for the SOT population combined as a group, *Candida* remains the most common fungal pathogen, causing 53% of

IFIs, followed by *Aspergillus* (19%), *Cryptococcus* (8%), other molds (6%), endemic molds (5%), *Mucorales* (2%), other yeasts (2%), and *Pneumocystis* (1%). For the two most common pathogens, *Candida* and *Aspergillus*, the median time to diagnosis is 81 and 186 days, respectively [11,12]. Although IC is the most common IFI in the SOT recipients, invasive mold infection (IMI) is, by far, more common in the lung transplant recipients, accounting for 70% of all IFI in this transplant population per overall TRANSNET analysis, with *Aspergillus* (72.7%) being the most common mold infection. In contrast, IMI accounted for 35%, 21% and 18% of all IFIs in the heart, kidney and liver SOT populations, respectively [13].

Endemic mycoses are uncommon with an incidence of ≤5% in SOT recipients. According to the TRANSNET data, endemic mycosis infections follow a bimodal distribution, with 40% of infections occurring in the first 6 months and 34% occurring between 2 and 11 years post transplantation. Although uncommon, it is important to recognize the risk of donor-derived endemic mycoses in SOT patients, especially those who have obtained their organs from foreign sources through commercial and sometimes illegal measures [11,14].

Apart from reactivation of latent infections, endemic mycoses can sometimes be acquired through travel and present as late onset IFIs in the SOT recipient who has been travelling through endemic regions [15,16].

Antifungal prophylaxis strategies are increasingly adopted by the transplant community, although a standardized approach to prophylaxis in SOT populations across institutions is not in place. The use of antifungal prophylaxis is likely to modify the type and timing of IFIs in SOT. Breakthrough IFIs in SOT patients on antifungal prophylaxis are not uncommon. They are either due to pharmacologic failure (often with subtherapeutic antifungal drug levels), lack of source control (e.g., infected prosthetic devices left *in situ* or presence of undrained infected collections) or infection with resistant or rare and emerging fungi (which pose diagnostic and therapeutic challenges). In lung transplant recipients requiring prophylaxis, colonization / infection with pathogens with reduced susceptibility to the drug employed is an emerging phenomenon. Depending on the SOT performed and choice of systemic antifungal prophylaxis agent used, breakthrough infections with fluconazole-resistant *Candida* spp., echinocandin-resistant *C. glabrata* with *FKS1/FKS2* mutations, voriconazole-resistant aspergillus (e.g., *A. fumigatus* with *cyp51A* mutation), *Scedosporium*, *Mucorales* and *Fusarium* are not unexpected. Specifically for echinocandin prophylaxis, breakthrough *Trichosporon* infection is a concern [17–24].

PREVENTION

Preventing fungal infections in the transplant recipient is a worthy goal owing to high associated morbidity and mortality. In order to prevent fungal infections, attention must be given to the mode of transmission of the pathogen, the burden of the epidemiologic exposure, as well as the patient's overall net state of immunosuppression at different points in time. Preventive measures are often multifaceted and may include reducing environmental exposures and/or antifungal drugs, and will vary during unique periods of intense immunosuppression. For example, the majority of invasive mold infections are acquired by inhaling aerosolized fungal spores. Hence, as a first line of defense, heavily contaminated air, such as would occur at construction sites, bird coops, bat caves, and during activities such as soil tilling or mowing grass, should be avoided at all times following any type of transplantation. Patients should wear a mask and avoid areas of renovation or construction in the hospital. Damp mopping should be employed as standard housekeeping practice in order to avoid aerosolization of spores. Some authors also advocate avoiding water aerosols, such as those created while bathing (showering), in addition to using water purification at the general or individual level, in order to protect from a waterborne source of molds. Finally, for *Candida*, potential acquisition from the hands of health care workers exists, so hand washing is strongly recommended [25–27].

Antifungal agents may be employed to prevent invasive disease. Such therapy is typically carefully targeted in SOT recipients, with timing and duration of antifungal therapy variable depending on the type of transplant and window of risk. In this section, we will focus our discussion on the caveats pertaining to antifungal prophylaxis in lung and liver transplant recipients. For more detailed discussion on antifungal prophylaxis, please review the chapter "Antifungal Prophylaxis: An Ounce of Prevention is Worth A Pound of Cure."

In lung transplant recipients, no well-controlled, randomized, multicenter study has been performed to establish a standard prophylactic approach; however, the majority of experts agree that the risk for invasive fungal disease is substantially high enough during the immediate posttransplant period to warrant antifungal prophylaxis. Thus, the majority of all lung transplant programs use some type of antifungal preventive therapy during the immediate post- transplant window, with the duration of prophylaxis varying 1–3 months posttransplant (most are ≤6 months). Aerosolized amphotericin B-based regimens alone or in combination with a systemic azole, such as fluconazole, or systemic therapy alone with a mold active azole, such as itraconazole or voriconazole, are the regimens most often used. Small studies evaluating inhaled aerosolized amphotericin B deoxycholate (AmBd) and amphotericin B lipid complex (ABLC) have demonstrated these drugs to be safe in the lung transplant population. While aerosolized ABLC tends to be better tolerated than aerosolized AmBd, studies have documented minimal systemic absorption for both, and thus few systemic toxicities when amphotericin B-based drugs are administered via aerosolization. This, coupled with the ease of once weekly treatments amenable to long term and outpatient administration, are two of the attractive features of this particular approach to antifungal prophylaxis [28–30].

Centers have different approaches to preventive therapy once the lung transplant recipient has completed the initial prophylactic regimen. For example, if a surveillance bronchoscopy culture grows *Aspergillus*, approximately half of the centers have a protocol to initiate antifungal therapy in order to prevent progression to invasive disease. Duration of therapy in this setting varies by center from <1 month to >6 months [31,32]. Prophylaxis regimens are also not clearly defined when patients are undergoing treatment for rejection. Some centers will use mold active antifungal prophylaxis during treatment for rejection, particularly when alemtuzumab is used. Multicenter studies designed to assess the efficacy of antifungal prophylaxis regimens in the lung transplant population are needed.

Antifungal drugs that have been studied in randomized controlled trials as prophylaxis in the liver transplant population include fluconazole, itraconazole, anidulafungin, micafungin, and amphotericin B [33–40]. Fluconazole is easily absorbed and has adequate tissue penetration while certain formulations of itraconazole have been associated with gastrointestinal intolerance and low serum concentrations. Anidulafungin and micafungin are both well tolerated, have few drug–drug interactions and are non-inferior to fluconazole prophylaxis, and they may potentially reduce the risk of IA in high risk patients. Amphotericin B was administered intravenously in this group, and despite having broad spectrum of activity, infusion-related adverse events or nephrotoxicity were problematic. One suggested and reasonable approach to prophylaxis in the liver transplant population, as well as pancreas and small bowel graft recipients, is to assess the risk for infection in each individual patient and initiate prophylaxis for patients with two or more high risk characteristics (See Tables 24.1 and 24.2).

The newer azoles with mold activity (posaconazole and isavuconazole) have also received attention regarding their potential for use as long-term prophylaxis in higher risk SOT population, but this has not been formally studied in clinical trials.

Alternative strategies to the long-term use of antifungal agents as prophylaxis are needed. One such approach is to use new, minimally invasive diagnostic tests in a preemptive approach to preventing clinically symptomatic fungal disease. In such a strategy, patients would have the diagnostic test performed twice weekly during periods of highest risk for fungal disease. Antifungal therapy would be instituted only if the test is positive. This strategy would be effective only if the test is able to detect the infection very early in the course of disease. Two such tests that are currently FDA approved for the diagnosis of fungal disease, the galactomannan and glucan assays, have been shown to turn positive prior to the development of clinical symptoms

Table 24.1 Risk factors for invasive candidiasis in solid organ transplantation

Organ	Risk factor
Small bowel	Anastomotic disruption
	Graft dysfunction
	Acute rejection
	Enhanced immunosuppression
	Multivisceral transplant
Pancreas	Enteric drainage
	Postperfusion pancreatitis
	Vascular graft thrombosis
	Wound infection with *Candida*
	Older donor age
	Pancreatic after renal or simultaneous pancreatic renal transplant
Liver	Posttransplant dialysis requirement
	Peritransplant colonization with *Candida*
	Antibiotic prophylaxis for spontaneous bacterial peritonitis
	Retransplantation
	Intraabdominal bleeding
	High intratransplant transfusion requirement
	Hyperglycemia requiring insulin and exposure to more than three antibiotics

Source: Husain, S. et al., *Transplantation*, 75, 2023–2029, 2003; Odabasi, Z. et al., *Clin. Infect. Dis.*, 39, 199–205, 2004; Nieto-Rodriguez, J.A. et al., *Ann. Surg.*, 223, 70–76, 1996; Guaraldi, G. et al., *Transplantation*, 80, 1742–1748, 2005; Tzakis, A.G. et al., *Transplantation*, 75, 1512–1517, 2003; Benedetti, E. et al., *J. Am. Coll. Surg.*, 183, 307–316, 1996; Everett, J.E. et al., *Arch. Surg.*, 129, 1310–1316, discussion 6–7, 1994; Nath, D.S. et al., *Transplant Proc.*, 37, 934–936, 2005; Patel, R. et al., *Transplantation*, 62, 926–934, 1996; Hadley, S. et al., *Transplantation*, 59, 851–859, 1995; Collins, L.A. et al., *J. Infect. Dis.*, 170, 644–652, 1994; Castaldo, P. et al., Arch. Surg., 126, 149–156, 1991.

Table 24.2 Risk factors for invasive aspergillosis in solid organ transplantation

Organ	Risk factor
Lung	Unhealed anastomotic site
	Airway ischemia
	Reperfusion injury
	Delayed sternal closure
	Decreased cough and delayed mucociliary clearance
	Receipt of single lung
	Presence of bronchial stents
	CMV pneumonitis
	Acute rejection
	Obliterative bronchiolitis
	Augmented immunosuppression for refractory rejection
	Aspergillus colonization of airways
Liver	Pretransplant fulminant hepatic or renal failure
	Primary allograft failure
	Retransplantation
	Large-volume intraoperative transfusions
	Bleeding requiring reoperation
	Choledochojejunostomy anastomosis
	Requirement of renal replacement therapy
Heart	Reoperation
	Cytomegalovirus disease
	Posttransplant dialysis
	Augmented immunosuppression for cardiac allograft vasculopathy
	Episode of IA in heart transplant program 2 months before or after transplantation date

Source: Singh, N. and Husain, S., *J. Heart Lung Transplant.*, 22, 258–266, 2003; Pappas, P.G. et al., *Am. J. Transplant.*, 6, 386–391, 2006; Singh, N. et al., *Liver Transpl.*, 12, 1205–1209, 2006; Hadley, S. et al., *Transplantation*, 59, 851–859, 1995; Collins, L.A., et al., *J. Infect. Dis.*, 170, 644–652, 1994; Castaldo, P. et al., *Arch. Surg.*, 126, 149–156, 1991; Singh, N. et al., *Med. Mycol.* 44, 445–449, 2006; Briegel, J. et al., *Eur. J. Clin. Microbiol. Infect. Dis.*, 14, 375–382, 1995; Munoz, P. et al., *Am. J. Transplant.*, 4, 636–643, 2004; Husni, R.N. et al., *Clin. Infect. Dis.*, 26, 753–755, 1998; Paradowski, L.J., *J. Heart Lung Transplant.*, 16, 524–531, 1997; Scott, J.P. et al., *J. Heart Lung Transplant.*, 10, 626–636, 1991; discussion 36–37; Paterson, D. L. and Singh, N., Medicine (Baltimore), 78, 123–138, 1999.

Table 24.3 Recommended prophylaxis for *Pneumocystis* pneumonia

Prophylactic agents	
First line	Trimethoprim–sulfamethoxazole
Second line	Dapsone
	Dapsone-pyrimethamine
	Pentamidine
	Atovaquone

Type of transplant	Duration of prophylaxis
Solid Organ Transplant	
Lung Heart/Lung	Prophylaxis for 12 months
When the incidence in institution or region is >5% prophylaxis.	
If patient has history of PCP or frequent opportunistic infections.	
If patient is receiving therapy for acute rejection or Has neutropenia.	
If patient is being treated for CMV or is considered at high risk for CMV infection.	Consider lifelong prophylaxis
Heart, Liver, Kidney, Pancreas, Small Bowel	Prophylaxis for 6–12 months
In patients with multiple rejection episodes and treatment for rejection.	
In patients with graft dysfunction.	
In patients with persistent viral infections such as CMV.	

Source: Rodriguez, M. and Fishman, J.A., *Clin. Microbiol. Rev.*, 17, 770–782, 2004; Cardenal, R. et al., *Eur. J. Cardiothorac. Surg.*, 20, 799–802, 2001; Olsen, S.L. et al., *Transplantation*, 56, 359–362, 1993; Fishman, J.A., *Clin. Infect. Dis.*, 33, 1397–1405, 2001; Branten, A.J. et al., *Nephrol. Dial. Transplant.*, 10, 1194–1197, 1995; Radisic, M. et al., *Transpl. Infect. Dis.*, 5, 84–93, 2003; Elinder, C.G. et al., *Transpl. Int.*, 5, 81–84, 1992; Gordon, S.M. et al., *Clin. Infect. Dis.*, 28, 240–246, 1999.

and radiographic changes. The clinical utility of serial monitoring with each test has been studied in hematologic malignancy/HSCT populations for preemptive treatment strategies, and the results are promising enough to warrant larger multicenter trials in these populations [58,59]. Unfortunately, the few studies of these tests performed to date in SOT populations have been disappointing [60–62].

Prophylaxis for PCP is generally recommended for transplant patients. In fact, prophylaxis has led to a substantial decrease in the rate of PCP infection in the SOT population, with the diagnosis decreasing from 33% (1992–1996) to 8% (1997–2003) in one center [63]. The duration of PCP prophylaxis, as with other fungal pathogens, is variable depending on the type of transplant and prevalence of PCP in the area (See Table 24.3).

ISSUES IN MANAGEMENT

Coinfections

The herpes viruses, cytomegalovirus (CMV), human herpes virus 6 (HHV-6), and human herpes virus 7 (HHV-7), have been described as having immunomodulatory properties that may facilitate infection with other opportunistic pathogens, including fungi [72–77]. Perhaps most compelling are data supporting CMV disease as a risk for opportunistic fungal infections. In one center, 36% of liver transplant recipients with CMV disease developed an IFI over a one-year period compared to 8% without CMV disease [73]. Preceding CMV disease, CMV pneumonitis, and CMV viremia were all associated with the development of an IFI, and being a CMV

seronegative recipient of a CMV seropositive donor organ (CMV R–/D+) increased the risk by 19-fold. The use of prophylactic ganciclovir in heart transplant recipients reduces not only the rate of CMV disease but also of IFIs, with only 7% of IFIs reported in patients on ganciclovir prophylaxis compared to 27% who were not (p = 0.007) [78].

General recommendations have been suggested for the management of CMV in the different transplant groups, and universal or preemptive therapy may be used [72]. Universal prophylaxis is generally given to high-risk SOT patients (CMV R–/D+), with preemptive therapy reserved for SOT recipients considered to be at intermediate risk for CMV disease and for allogeneic HSCT recipients. For preemptive therapy, frequent monitoring for the development of CMV reactivation is required so that therapy can be given when viremia is first detectable, but the patient is still asymptomatic. It appears that both approaches decrease CMV disease compared to no prophylaxis or placebo [79,80]. Whether universal and preemptive regimens are equally effective at also reducing associated fungal infections is still under investigation. In one study of SOT recipients, both regimens reduced the rate of acute allograft rejection; however, only universal prophylaxis significantly decreased bacterial and fungal infections in the population under study [80]. On the other hand, studies in liver transplant recipients receiving preemptive prophylaxis compared with those never requiring prophylaxis and high-risk patients receiving universal prophylaxis showed no difference in the rate of fungal infections, suggesting that CMV preemptive therapy is beneficial [79,81]. The addition of CMV immune globulin alone or when added to ganciclovir appears to confer no additional protection against IFIs [82–84].

HHV-6 has also been implicated as facilitating infection with fungi [74,75,77]. In liver transplant recipients, HHV-6 viremia has been associated with higher rates of IFI; IFI occurred in 32% of patients with HHV-6 viremia compared to 4% of those without viremia (p = 0.009). Further, HHV-6 was present either preceding the IFI or within 1 week of IFI in 80% of those who had both infections. HHV-6 was noted to be a strong predictor of IFI (OR 8.3, 95% CI = 1.2–58; p = 0.0336), thus corroborating previous studies, which showed a potential higher risk for IFI in patients with HHV-6 infection [77].

It is known that HHV-6 facilitates infection with CMV, and in turn, CMV is associated with IFI [75]. Similarly, in a cohort of renal transplant recipients, patients with HHV-7 and coinfected with CMV had a significant increase in CMV disease [76,85]. Thus, both HHV-6 and HHV-7 may indirectly increase the risk for IFI through their effect on CMV. The use of ganciclovir has been shown to reduce the viral load of HHV-6, HHV-7, and CMV, and the incidence of CMV disease [86]. Prophylactic ganciclovir has also been associated with reduced rates of IFI [78]. It is, therefore, postulated that by treating this group of herpes viruses, one may manipulate their immunomodulatory effect and thereby reverse their permissive effect on susceptibility to IFIs.

Epstein–Barr virus (EBV), another herpes virus, may also be independently associated with IFI. In one series of pediatric liver transplant recipients, the rate of IFIs was reported to be 40% during the first year posttransplant. Of the posttransplant variables assessed, only bacterial infection, EBV infection, and tacrolimus administration were independently associated with development of IFI [87].

Comorbid conditions

Comorbid conditions present in the SOT population that have been associated with IFIs include rejection, hypogammaglobulinemia, renal replacement therapy, and diabetes. An immune reconstitution syndrome has also recently been associated with the treatment of cryptococcosis in SOT recipients. It is important to recognize these comorbid conditions in order to ensure the optimal management for transplant recipients during periods of heightened risk for IFI and in order to promote a successful outcome for those patients who develop concomitant IFIs.

REJECTION

Rejection may occur at any time in the posttransplant period in the SOT population. Among the newer immunosuppressive agents, monoclonal antibodies, such as alemtuzumab, are being increasingly used to treat steroid-resistant rejection episodes. With the resulting intense and long-lasting immunosuppression secondary to lymphocyte depletion and other alterations of cellular immunity caused by alemtuzumab, patients are at risk for IFI. In a large study of 547 SOT recipients receiving alemtuzumab for either induction or rejection and followed for 12 months after the first alemtuzumab dose, opportunistic infections occurred in 10% of patients [88]. The risk of developing an opportunistic infection was approximately five times higher when alemtuzumab was given for rejection versus induction (21.5% vs. 4.5%, respectively). Of the opportunistic infections, 32% were IFIs (18/62), 83% (15/18) of which occurred in patients who received alemtuzumab for rejection. The median time to infection was 58 days after alemtuzumab therapy and 245 days after transplant.

Importantly, lymphocyte depletion persisted even after 12 months following alemtuzumab administration. Median CD4 counts at baseline were 626 cells/mm^3, and at 1, 3, 6, 9, and 12 months, median counts were 6, 15, 52, 92, and 127 cells/mm^3, respectively. Patients who experienced rejection and received alemtuzumab had usually received other immunosuppressive agents (methylprednisolone, another lymphocyte-depleting antibody such as rabbit antithymocyte globulin, or monoclonal CD3 antibody) and, thus, had a higher net state of immunosuppression, which increased the risk of IFI. Patients who received alemtuzumab for rejection had also experienced more transplant graft failure than those who received alemtuzumab for induction, and tended to be further out in their posttransplant period. As such, they had longer environmental exposure and generally were on different antimicrobial prophylaxis than those earlier in their posttransplant phase. In some centers, mold active triazoles and/or aerosolized amphotericin B-based prophylaxis are used when alemtuzumab is administered for steroid refractory rejection in lung transplant recipients (personal communication, B.D. Alexander).

IMMUNE RECONSTITUTION SYNDROME

An immune reconstitution syndrome (IRS) has been reported in SOT patients infected with *C. neoformans* [89]. In a review of 22 centers, 83 SOT patients with cryptococcosis were identified. An IRS-like syndrome was diagnosed in four patients based on worsening of a previously responding lesion not explained by failure of therapy or another infection. The four patients received standard treatment with a formulation of amphotericin B +/− flucytosine and were subsequently transitioned to fluconazole. However, the patients developed signs suggestive of worsening infection including increased inflammatory cells in CSF and enhancing CNS lesions. Cytology or histopathology revealed budding yeast cells consistent with *Cryptococcus* and even granuloma; however, all cultures remained negative. It was postulated that antifungal therapy elicited a vigorous proinflammatory Th-1 response in the host, leading to exacerbation of clinical signs and symptoms. The authors emphasized the importance of keeping this phenomenon in mind when faced with a seemingly worsening clinical picture following the initiation of treatment for cryptococcosis and to not merely ascribe it to failure of therapy [89]. Whether or not the use of steroids would be beneficial in SOT patients with IRS requires study.

HYPOGAMMAGLOBULINEMIA

Hypogammaglobulinemia in the posttransplant period has been associated with increased risk of infection in some studies [90–92]. Increased rates of CMV infection as well as a trend in IFIs have been noted in SOT with hypogammaglobulinemia. Several of these patients developed hypogammaglobulinemia after receiving increased immunosuppression to treat rejection or bronchiolitis obliterans syndrome, and some had concomitant neutropenia. In a group of lung transplant recipients with severe hypogammaglobulinemia, IA accounted for 44% of infections [93]. The authors suggest measures to manage these severely hypogammaglobulinemic patients including the reduction of immunosuppression when feasible, increasing prophylaxis for infection, and immunoglobulin replacement therapy. Though one study in liver transplant recipients did not find an increased risk of CMV disease, bacterial infection, or fungal infection with hypogammaglobulinemia in the posttransplant period, hypogammaglobulinemia was associated with increased mortality at 1 and 5 years posttransplant [94].

METABOLIC CONDITIONS

Other comorbid conditions have been associated with an increased risk of IFIs following trans-plantation. Liver transplant recipients have been considered at high risk for invasive mold infection if they required renal replacement therapy on the day of transplant or if hospital discharge was delayed beyond 7 days posttransplant secondary to renal or hepatic insufficiency. Increased risk of IFI may be conferred by transplant for fulminant hepatic failure or retransplant. Both of these groups may warrant antifungal prophylaxis [95]. Posttransplantation dialysis is also a significant predictor of IC following liver transplant [8]. Uremia and renal replacement therapy have been associated with impaired neutrophil function and increased neutrophil apoptosis [96,97].

Diabetes mellitus is frequently encountered following transplantation, often the consequence of steroid use. Poorly controlled diabetes is a well-described risk factor for the development of zygomycosis in the SOT population, and hyperglycemia requiring insulin therapy has been associated with candidemia in liver transplant recipients [41,98,99]. Aggressive control of blood sugars is mandatory for these patients.

Antifungal drug interactions and monitoring

The advent of newer azoles with activity against *Aspergillus* and other molds (voriconazole, posaconazole, isavuconazole) as well as a new class of antifungals, the echinocandins (caspofungin, micafungin, anidulafungin) has increased the armamentarium of drugs available against IFIs [100]. The FDA approved indications for treatment of specific mycoses is presented in Table 24.4. Drug interactions between antifungal agents and immunosuppressive medications exist and require dose modification, monitoring of serum levels, or occasionally, a change in medication regimen.

Itraconazole is the first mold-active triazole available clinically. While it has relatively broad activity, it has a black box warning for cardiac toxicity and is also a potent inhibitor of the cytochrome P450 CYP3A4 enzyme (See Table 24.5). When itraconazole is administered with cyclosporine or tacrolimus, increased plasma concentrations of these immunosuppressants result. The dose of cyclosporine should be decreased by at least 50%, if not more, after an intravenous itraconazole loading dose, and serum levels monitored. Concomitant administration of itraconazole and sirolimus also increase plasma concentrations of sirolimus, requiring dose adjustment or even discontinuation of the latter. Levels of all these immunosuppressants should be monitored frequently, and the dosages adjusted accordingly to achieve the desired serum concentrations and immunosuppressive effect. Certain formulations of itraconazole, such as the capsules, are not reliably absorbed from the gastrointestinal tract, and levels of itraconazole should be monitored or itraconazole changed to a different formulation (oral solution, iv formulation) to achieve therapeutic levels. A loading regimen may be used prior to standard or maintenance dosing to achieve the desired trough levels. Trough levels of itraconazole >0.5 μg/mL have been suggested to achieve higher efficacy [101–103,114,115].

Voriconazole, a derivative of fluconazole, has a broad spectrum of activity. It is metabolized by the human hepatic cytochrome P450 enzymes, with highest affinity for *Cyp*2C19. Inhibition of *Cyp*3A4 by voriconazole is less than that of other azoles, such as ketoconazole and itraconazole (See Table 24.5). Voriconazole has significant drug interaction with calcineurin inhibitors, and caution should be used when these agents are coadministered. Recommendations on dosage adjustment when starting voriconazole in patients already on cyclosporine or tacrolimus include reducing cyclosporine dose by 50% and tacrolimus by 66%. Calcineurin inhibitor levels should subsequently be monitored closely. Dosage adjustments also need to be made once voriconazole is discontinued so that therapeutic concentrations of these immunosuppressive drugs can be maintained. Coadministration of voriconazole and sirolimus is contraindicated by the manufacturer, but a few cases of patients treated with these agents concomitantly have been published. Doses of sirolimus were significantly reduced and serum levels tightly monitored to maintain concentrations in the therapeutic range [119].

In adults receiving voriconazole, variability exists between doses administered and trough levels, and low serum voriconazole levels have been associated with failure of therapy. If a patient is failing treatment with voriconazole, one should check a voriconazole level to ensure absorption. A steady-state trough of at least 0.5 μg/mL suggests adequate absorption. Other data suggest a higher success rate in patients with plasma voriconazole levels >0.5 μg/mL. In addition, an increase in the number of favorable responses was noted in transplant recipients with IA treated with

Table 24.4 Antifungal agents and their FDA approved indications for the treatment of specific mycoses

Drug	FDA approved indication								
	Candidiasis		Aspergillus	Mucormycosis	Fusarium Scedosporium	Endemic mycoses	Febrile Neutropenia	Prophylaxis	Cryptococcosis
	Esopharyn-geal	Invasive							
Amphotericin deoxycholate	✓	✓	✓	✓	✓	Blastomycosis Histoplasmosis Coccidioidomycosis	✓		✓
Lipid formulation of amphotericin	✓	(salvage) ABLC LAMB	(salvage) ABLC LAMB	(salvage) ABLC	(salvage) Fusarium ABLC		✓ LAMB		✓ LAMB ABLC (salvage)
Fluconazole	✓	✓						✓ (Candida)	
Itraconazole	✓		✓ (salvage)			Blastomycosis Histoplasmosis	✓		
Voriconazole	✓	✓ (Non-neutropenic)	✓		✓ (salvage)				
Posaconazole	✓		✓	✓				✓ (IA & Candida)	
Isavuconazole	✓		✓	✓					
Anidulafungin	✓	✓							
Micafungin	✓	✓						✓ (Candida)	
Caspofungin	✓	✓	✓ (salvage)				✓		

Source: Sporanox (Itraconazole) Injection—Package Insert, Ortho Biotech Products LP, Lake Forest, IL, 2001; Sporanox (Itraconazole) Oral Solution—Package Insert, Janssen Pharmaceutica NV, Beerse, Belgium, 2003; Sporanox (Itraconazole) Capsules—Package Insert, Janssen Pharmaceuticals, Ireland, 2001; Vfend (Voriconazole) Tablets, Oral Suspension and Injection—Package Insert, Pfizer, New York, pp. 1–43, 2006; Noxafil (Posaconazole) Tablets, Oral Suspension and Injection—Package Insert, Merck & Co, Whitehouse Station, NJ, 2014; Cresemba (Isavuconazole) Capsules and Injection—Package Insert, Astellas Pharma US, Inc, Northbrook, IL, 2015; Cancidas (Caspofungin Acetate) for Injection—Package Insert, MERCK and Co., Whitehouse Station, NJ, 2005; Mycamine (Micafungin) Package Insert, Astella Pharma, Tokyo, Japan, 2006; Eraxis (Anidulafungin) for Injection—Package Insert, Roerig (Division of Pfizer, Inc.), New York, 2007; Amphotericin B for Injection—Package Insert, X-Gen Pharmaceuticals, Big Flats, NY, 2009; AmBisome (Amphotericin B Liposome) for Injection—Package Insert, Astella Pharmas US, Deerfield, IL, 2012; ABELCET (Amphotericin B Lipid Complex Injection)—Package Insert, Sigma-Tau PharmaSource, Indianapolis, IN, 2013; Diflucan (Fluconazole) Tablets, Oral Suspection and Injection—Package Insert, Roerig (Division of Pfizer, Inc.), New York, 2011.

Table 24.5 Relative inhibition of cytochrome P450 isoenzymes by triazoles

Cytochrome P450 enzyme	Fluconazole	Itraconazole	Voriconazole	Posaconazole	Isavuconazole
2C19	+	-	+++[a]	-	-
2C8/9	++	+	++[a]	-	-
3A4	++	+++[a]	++[a]	+++[a]	+/++[a]

Source: *Sporanox (Itraconazole) Injection—Package Insert*, Ortho Biotech Products LP, Lake Forest, IL, 2001; *Sporanox (Itraconazole) Oral Solution—Package Insert*, Janssen Pharmaceutica NV, Beerse, Belgium, 2003; *Sporanox (Itraconazole) Capsules—Package Insert*, Janssen Pharmaceuticals, Ireland, 2001; *Vfend (Voriconazole) Tablets, Oral Suspension and Injection—Package Insert*, Pfizer, New York, pp. 1–43, 2006; *Noxafil (Posaconazole) Tablets, Oral Suspension and Injection—Package Insert*, Merck & Co, Whitehouse Station, NJ, 2014; *Cresemba (Isavuconazole) Capsules and Injection—Package Insert*, Astellas Pharma US, Inc, Northbrook, IL, 2015; *Diflucan (Fluconazole) Tablets, Oral Suspection and Injection—Package Insert*, Roerig (Division of Pfizer, Inc.), New York, 2011; Dodds-Ashley, E., *Pharmacotherapy*, 30, 842–854, 2010; Theuretzbacher, U. et al., *Clin. Pharmacokinet.*, 45, 649–663, 2006; Bruggemann, R.J. et al., *Clin. Infect. Dis.*, 48, 1441–1458, 2009; Niwa, T. et al., *Biol. Pharm. Bull.*, 28, 1805–1808, 2005; Courtesy of R. Drew, Duke University Hospital.

+ Minimal inhibition.

++ Moderate inhibition.

+++ Strong inhibition.

[a] Antifungal is also a substrate for cytochrome P450 enzyme.

voriconazole when random serum concentrations were above 2 µg/mL [104,119–133].

Although voriconazole is a broad spectrum antifungal agent with good bioavailability, proven efficacy in the treatment of IA, and is also frequently used as prophylaxis in the SOT population, its prolonged use has been associated with photosensitivity reactions and an increased risk of squamous cell carcinoma (SCC), especially in the lung transplant recipients. In one retrospective study, SCC developed in as many as 39.5% of patients receiving voriconazole for prophylaxis or treatment of IFIs. Risk factors for the development of SCC in the lung transplant population include older age at time of transplant, skin cancer pretransplant, prior history of voriconazole exposure, longer voriconazole therapy, and living in geographic locations with high levels of sun exposure. The decision for prolonged voriconazole therapy in at-risk population groups needs to reviewed; skin cancer education, photoprotection, scheduled skin cancer screening and the use of alternative pharmacologic options with no SCC risk needs to be considered [134–138].

Another phenomenon that the transplant physician should be aware of with prolonged voriconazole therapy is voriconazole-induced periostitis. It is associated with bone pain, elevated alkaline phosphate levels, elevated serum fluoride levels, and radiological findings of periostitis (usually involving the ribs, clavicles, scapula, and pelvis) with subsequent resolution of symptoms after drug withdrawal. This phenomenon has been described in a heterogeneous group of patients, including SOT recipients [139–144].

Posaconazole is closely related to itraconazole, though with superior activity and better tolerability. In addition, it has activity against the *Mucorales*. It was first approved by the FDA as an oral suspension in 2006. The bioavailability of the oral suspension is dependent on high fat food intake, gut motility and gastric acidity. In the transplant populations, swallow impairment or severe oral mucositis may limit its use. Posaconazole suspension also has saturable absorption requiring dosing multiple times each day despite a long

half-life. A delayed-release (DR) tablet and intravenous formulations of posaconazole were later approved by the FDA in 2013 and 2014, with the unique features of once daily dosing, improved bioavailability and more reliable blood concentrations. In a single center retrospective cohort study conducted in adult hematological cancer patients, the delayed-release tablets were more likely to achieve levels ≥0.7 µg/mL compared to oral suspension, and tablet levels were not affected by acid suppression, GvHD of gut, mucositis or diarrhea. In another single center retrospective study conducted at Mayo Clinic, which included both SOT and HSCT patients, 90% of patients receiving the DR tablets achieved steady-state levels ≥0.7 µg/mL compared to 58% of patients receiving the oral suspension [105,115,145–151].

When posaconazole therapy is initiated or discontinued, dose adjustment and more frequent clinical monitoring of cyclosporine and tacrolimus levels should be performed. The cyclosporine dose should be reduced to approximately three-fourths of the original dose, and the tacrolimus dose reduced to approximately one-third of the original dose when starting posaconazole [114,152].

Posaconazole is FDA approved for the treatment of oropharyngeal candidiasis and for antifungal prophylaxis in patients with hematologic malignancy and prolonged neutropenia in HSCT recipients. Having said this, in the setting of life-threatening fungal infections, posaconazole is increasingly used as a form of salvage therapy for IA and mucormycosis, with response rates ranging from 42% to 79%. Given that minimal inhibitory concentration (MIC) for fungal pathogens differs by species, we recommend obtaining fungal MICs and optimizing drug exposure to ensure clinical success. Clinical studies have suggested trough levels of >0.7 µg/mL for prophylaxis and trough levels of >1.0–1.25 µg/mL for the treatment of IFI. However, higher trough levels may be needed for some pathogens, and based on Monte Carlo simulations, achieving pharmacodynamics parameters compatible with optimal clinical outcomes

(AUC/MIC $\geq$ 100) may not be possible for some (e.g., MIC > 0.5 µg/mL for *Aspergillus* spp. and the *Mucorales*) [146,153–161].

Isavuconazole is a second-generation broad spectrum triazole with activity against yeasts and molds, including the *Mucorales*. The advantages of this new agent include its broad spectrum of activity, the availability of water-soluble intravenous formulation (without the need for cyclodextrin carrier), making it a favorable alternative in patients with underlying renal impairment. It also has excellent bioavailability, predictable pharmacokinetics, improved tolerability with fewer side effects, and relatively fewer drug interactions compared with the other triazoles. It is metabolized by the human hepatic cytochrome P450 enzymes, with affinity to *Cyp*3A4 but minimal effect on *Cyp*2C19 or *Cyp*2C8/9 (see Table 24.5). Although serum concentrations of sirolimus, tacrolimus and cyclosporine are expected to increase with concurrent isavuconazole use, no formal dose reduction of the immunusuppressants have yet been made. Very close monitoring of immunosuppressant levels is warranted. In a recent case report, the authors have recommended a 50% reduction in tacrolimus dose at the initiation of isavuconazole therapy based on their clinical experience [100,106,162–166].

Unlike voriconazole, posaconazole, and itraconazole, serum concentration monitoring is not currently recommended for isavuconazole. However, isavuconazole is a substrate of *Cyp*3A4 and levels may fluctuate dependent on concurrent administration of inhibitors or inducers of this isoenzyme. In addition, CYP polymorphisms do exist and there may be racial variations in isavuconazole metabolism. More studies to establish the correlation between plasma levels and adverse effects and efficacy are required [115,165–167].

The polyene antifungals, amphotericin B deoxycholate, amphotericin B lipid complex, and liposomal amphotericin, are also used to manage IFIs in the transplant population. Infusion- related side effects (fever, chills, and rigors) and nephrotoxicity (elevated serum creatinine, hypokalemia) are the main adverse events with amphotericin B deoxycholate and, to a lesser degree, the lipid formulations. One should proceed with caution when administering these agents with calcineurin inhibitors and other nephrotoxic agents as altered kidney function may rapidly develop. In transplant recipients, the lipid products of amphotericin B are favored over amphotericin B deoxycholate. Aerosolized amphotericin B, amphotericin B lipid complex, and liposomal amphotericin have been used mainly for prophylaxis in the SOT and HSCT population. They may precipitate bronchospasm and have been associated with nausea, vomiting, and taste disturbance, but were generally well tolerated and not systemically absorbed to a significant degree [29,120,168–176].

Of the echinocandins, caspofungin and anidulafungin are not metabolized by the human cytochrome P450 system.

Micafungin demonstrates weak *Cyp*3A4 inhibition. In general, these drugs are well tolerated and have few adverse effects. Transient elevation of liver transaminases has been reported in healthy volunteers and in SOT patients concomitantly administered caspofungin and calcineurin inhibitors. The coadministration of caspofungin with cyclosporine led to an increase in the AUC of caspofungin by about 35% without increase in maximum concentration (Cmax). The levels of cyclosporine were not increased. The manufacturer recommends caution when coadministering these agents, and they stress the importance of evaluating the risk–benefit ratio prior to use. Monitoring of liver enzymes during concomitant therapy with these agents is recommended. The administration of caspofungin with tacrolimus does not affect caspofungin pharmacokinetics but may reduce tacrolimus concentration by 25%. Careful monitoring of tacrolimus dosages and levels is required to maintain therapeutic concentrations.

Micafungin is well tolerated, and though nausea, vomiting, diarrhea, and hyperbilirubinemia were noted in HSCT recipients on micafungin prophylaxis, this was no different from those on fluconazole prophylaxis. No interactions were noted between micafungin and cyclosporine, tacrolimus, mycophenolate mofetil, fluconazole, or prednisolone. Micafungin has been administered to SOT patients who were receiving calcineurin inhibitors, found to be well tolerated, and no dose modification of either medication was required. When micafungin is coadministered with sirolimus, trough levels of sirolimus may be increased and the AUC increased by 21%. Thus, sirolimus levels should be monitored and dosages adjusted to maintain concentrations in the therapeutic range.

Anidulafungin is also well tolerated though hypokalemia, nausea, and diarrhea were the most common adverse events in one noninferiority study. Coadministration with cyclosporine caused elevation of the steady-state AUC of anidulafungin by 22% without affecting the Cmax, but the manufacturer does not recommend dose adjustment of either drug. Coadministration with tacrolimus did not result in alteration of either Cmax or AUC of either drug, and no dose adjustments are recommended. Coadministration with voriconazole also does not affect these parameters nor is dosage modification recommended [107–109,120,177–185].

Common clinical questions

1. Two years posttransplant, a 49-year-old male orthotopic liver transplant recipient presented with a 2-week history of non-productive cough. Chest radiograph showed a 1.5 cm left pulmonary nodule. His sputum cultures were negative and his serum cryptococcal antigen was 1:32. Blood cultures were negative. His cerebrospinal fluid cryptococcal antigen and fungal cultures were negative. His immunosuppressants

include tacrolimus and mycophenolate. What would you recommend for therapy?

a. Amphotericin B deoxycholate plus flucytosine
b. Liposomal amphotericin plus flucytosine
c. Fluconazole 400 mg daily
d. Fluconazole 200 mg daily
e. Micafungin

Correct Answer: Fluconazole 400 mg daily,
Cryptococcosis has been documented in organ transplant recipients often as a late onset infection. The patient has likely mild-moderate cryptococcosis in a solid organ transplant recipient without evidence of cryptococcemia or central nervous system infection. Treatment of choice is fluconazole 400 mg daily for a duration of 6–12 months. Therapeutic drug monitoring for fluconazole is not required. Drug interactions between fluconazole and tacrolimus exist, and a 40% dose reduction of fluconazole is recommended. In the setting of disseminated infection, severe pulmonary disease or central nervous system infection, induction therapy with liposomal amphotericin and flucytosine followed by consolidation and maintenance therapy with fluconazole is recommended. Echinocandins have no activity against *Cryptococcus spp.* [11,114,115,186,187].

2. A 58 year old with a history of hepatitis B liver cirrhosis complicated by hepatocellular carcinoma had undergone an orthotopic liver transplant (with Roux-en-Y biliary anastomosis) 2 years ago. He is now admitted for cholangitis (associated with extended-spectrum beta-lactamase (ESBL) *E. coli* bacteremia) and progressive liver failure associated with hepatorenal syndrome, requiring hemodialysis support. He has been listed for re-transplant and the surgeons are asking about peri-operative antibiotic cover. He is currently on cyclosporine and prednisone. What would you recommend?

a. He has completed his course of antibiotics for cholangitis and is infection free. We can stop antibiotics.
b. Continue on IV meropenem and add fluconazole for antifungal prophylaxis.
c. Continue on IV meropenem and add IV liposomal amphotericin for antifungal prophylaxis.
d. Continue on IV meropenem and add IV vancomycin for enterococcal cover.
e. Continue on IV meropenem and add IV micafungin for antifungal prophylaxis.

Correct Answer: Continue on IV meropenem and add IV micafungin for antifungal prophylaxis, He is a patient undergoing liver retransplant with potentially increased technical complexity of surgery. He has both hepatic dysfunction and renal dysfunction requiring dialysis support. He is also on broad spectrum antibiotics. This is a fragile immunocompromised patient with >2 risk factors for IFIs. Common IFIs associated with liver transplant include IC and IA, with IC being more common. Leaving him without antibiotic cover would not be prudent. In addition to antibacterial cover, antifungal prophylaxis would be recommended. IV micafungin has both candida and aspergillus coverage and is relatively well tolerated, with less drug-related adverse effects, including hepatotoxicity, and does not require dose adjustments in the setting of renal failure. In the TENPIN study, it has been shown to be non-inferior to fluconazole for antifungal prophylaxis in high risk liver transplant recipients. Although liposomal amphotericin has both Candida and Aspergillus cover, it is associated with nephrotoxicity and the use of this drug in a patient who is on cyclosporin and hemodialysis may not be ideal [4,8,9,11,12,40].

3. An orthotopic lung transplant recipient developed steroid-resistant rejection 6 months posttransplant and was given rabbit antithymocyte globulin (RATG). 8 months posttransplant, he also received alemtuzumab. He was given voriconazole for antifungal prophylaxis. He now presents with shortness of breath, fever, acute renal insufficiency and a left cavitary mass lesion was seen on chest CT. KOH stain of his transbronchial lung biopsy showed aseptate hyphae with irregular branching. What drug should be started now?

a. Continue on voriconazole.
b. Stop voriconazole. Switch to posaconazole.
c. Continue voriconazole and add terbinafine.
d. Stop voriconazole. Switch to liposomal amphotericin.
e. Stop voriconazole. Use high dose Bactrim.

Correct Answer: Stop voriconazole. Switch to liposomal amphotericin, This patient with significant rejection has received intense and long-lasting immunosuppression with lymphocyte depleting agents and cellular immune modulating agents and is at very high risk of IFI. Although IA is the most common IFI in the lung transplant recipient, he has been on voriconazole prophylaxis. Given the clinical picture, radiographic and KOH stain findings, he has breakthrough infection on voriconazole therapy. He has developed pulmonary mucormycosis and the drug of choice is liposomal amphotericin. Other breakthrough infections on voriconazole include voriconazole-resistant *Aspergillus* associated with *cyp51A* mutation, *Fusarium,* and *Scedosporium. Aspergillus, Scedosporium,* and *Fusarium* have septate filamentous hyphae. Although posaconazole has broad spectrum of activity, including mold activity, and has been used in the treatment of *Mucorales* in the salvage setting, it is not FDA approved for this indication and IV liposomal amphotericin is still the drug of choice. Isavuconazole, another new broad spectrum triazole (studied in the VITAL study), has shown activity against mucormycosis and is FDA approved. It is also well tolerated and could potentially be used in this patient, especially in the setting of renal failure. Combination therapy of voriconazole and terbinafine is used for the treatment of *Scedosporium*. The clinical picture is not suggestive of *Pneumocystis jiroveci* [4,105,106,111,164].

4. A bilateral orthotopic lung transplant recipient was recently diagnosed with IA and was started on voriconazole. He is on tacrolimus, azathioprine and prednisone for immunosuppression. Two weeks after starting voriconazole therapy, he presents to the hospital with altered mental status. His wife has commented that in the last week, he was tremulous and was complaining of weakness. What is the most appropriate next course of action?
   a. Check serum voriconazole levels.
   b. Check serum tacrolimus levels.
   c. Perform lumbar puncture to rule out opportunistic infections of the CNS in this immunocompromised host.
   d. Request for an urgent MRI to look for HSV encephalitis / progressive multifocal leukoencephalopathy.
   e. Check both serum voriconazole and tacrolimus levels.

Correct Answer: Check both serum voriconazole and tacrolimus, Voriconazole has significant drug–drug interactions with the calcineurin inhibitors. At the initiation of voriconazole therapy, dose reduction of tacrolimus by 66% is recommended. Tremors and weakness are common side effects associated with tacrolimus toxicity and confusion is associated with both tacrolimus and voriconazole toxicity. Voriconazole exhibits non-linear kinetics and therapeutic drug monitoring is recommended. For the treatment of invasive aspergillosis, a target trough level of >2 µg/mL is recommended [100,115]. Opportunistic infections of the CNS are a possibility; however, the priority would be to rule out both tacrolimus and voriconazole drug toxicity.

REFERENCES

1. Fishman JA, Rubin RH. Infection in organ-transplant recipients. *N Engl J Med* 1998;338(24):1741–1751.
2. Fishman JA. Overview: Fungal infections in the transplant patient. *Transpl Infect Dis* 2002;4 Suppl 3:3–11.
3. Rubin RH. Overview: Pathogenesis of fungal infections in the organ transplant recipient. *Transpl Infect Dis* 2002;4 Suppl 3:12–17.
4. Anesi JA, Baddley JW. Approach to the solid organ transplant patient with suspected fungal infection. *Infect Dis Clin North Am* 2016;30(1):277–2796.
5. Morgan J, Wannemuehler KA, Marr KA, Hadley S, Kontoyiannis DP, Walsh TJ, et al. Incidence of invasive aspergillosis following hematopoietic stem cell and solid organ transplantation: Interim results of a prospective multicenter surveillance program. *Med Mycol* 2005;43 Suppl 1:S49–S58.
6. Singh N, Husain S. Aspergillus infections after lung transplantation: Clinical differences in type of transplant and implications for management. *J Heart Lung Transplant* 2003;22(3):258–266.
7. Pappas PG, Andes D, Schuster M, Hadley S, Rabkin J, Merion RM, et al. Invasive fungal infections in low-risk liver transplant recipients: A multi-center prospective observational study. *Am J Transplant* 2006;6(2):386–391.
8. Husain S, Tollemar J, Dominguez EA, Baumgarten K, Humar A, Paterson DL, et al. Changes in the spectrum and risk factors for invasive candidiasis in liver transplant recipients: Prospective, multicenter, case–controlled study. *Transplantation* 2003;75(12):2023–2029.
9. Singh N, Pruett TL, Houston S, Munoz P, Cacciarelli TV, Wagener MM, et al. Invasive aspergillosis in the recipients of liver retransplantation. *Liver Transpl* 2006;12(8):1205–1209.
10. Singh N, Wagener MM, Marino IR, Gayowski T. Trends in invasive fungal infections in liver transplant recipients: Correlation with evolution in transplantation practices. *Transplantation* 2002;73(1):63–67.
11. Pappas PG, Alexander BD, Andes DR, Hadley S, Kauffman CA, Freifeld A, et al. Invasive fungal infections among organ transplant recipients: Results of the Transplant-Associated Infection Surveillance Network (TRANSNET). *Clin Infect Dis* 2010;50(8):1101–1111.
12. Andes DR, Safdar N, Baddley JW, Alexander B, Brumble L, Freifeld A, et al. The epidemiology and outcomes of invasive Candida infections among organ transplant recipients in the United States: Results of the Transplant-Associated Infection Surveillance Network (TRANSNET). *Transpl Infect Dis* 2016;18(6):921–931.
13. Doligalski CT, Benedict K, Cleveland AA, Park B, Derado G, Pappas PG, et al. Epidemiology of invasive mold infections in lung transplant recipients. *Am J Transplant* 2014;14(6):1328–1333.
14. Kauffman CA, Freifeld AG, Andes DR, Baddley JW, Herwaldt L, Walker RC, et al. Endemic fungal infections in solid organ and hematopoietic cell transplant recipients enrolled in the Transplant-Associated Infection Surveillance Network (TRANSNET). *Transpl Infect Dis* 2014;16(2):213–224.

15. Kotton CN, Hibberd PL, Practice ASTIDCo. Travel medicine and transplant tourism in solid organ transplantation. *Am J Transplant* 2013;13 Suppl 4:337–347.

16. Hart J, Dyer JR, Clark BM, McLellan DG, Perera S, Ferrari P. Travel-related disseminated *Penicillium marneffei* infection in a renal transplant patient. *Transpl Infect Dis* 2012;14(4):434–439.

17. Alexander BD. Prophylaxis of invasive mycoses in solid organ transplantation. *Curr Opin Infect Dis* 2002;15(6):583–589.

18. Peghin M, Monforte V, Martin-Gomez MT, Ruiz-Camps I, Berastegui C, Saez B, et al. Epidemiology of invasive respiratory disease caused by emerging non-*Aspergillus* molds in lung transplant recipients. *Transpl Infect Dis* 2016;18(1):70–78.

19. Peghin M, Monforte V, Martin-Gomez MT, Ruiz-Camps I, Berastegui C, Saez B, et al. 10 years of prophylaxis with nebulized liposomal amphotericin B and the changing epidemiology of *Aspergillus* spp. infection in lung transplantation. *Transpl Int* 2016;29(1):51–62.

20. Vazquez JA, Manavathu EK. Molecular characterization of a voriconazole-resistant, posaconazole-susceptible *Aspergillus fumigatus* isolate in a lung transplant recipient in the United States. *Antimicrob Agents Chemother* 2016;60(2):1129–1133.

21. Alexander BD, Johnson MD, Pfeiffer CD, Jimenez-Ortigosa C, Catania J, Booker R, et al. Increasing echinocandin resistance in *Candida glabrata*: Clinical failure correlates with presence of FKS mutations and elevated minimum inhibitory concentrations. *Clin Infect Dis* 2013;56(12):1724–1732.

22. Ramos A, Cuervas-Mons V, Noblejas A, Banos I, Duran P, Marcos R, et al. Breakthrough rhinocerebral mucormycosis in a liver transplant patient receiving caspofungin. *Transplant Proc* 2009;41(5):1972–1975.

23. Tascini C, Urbani L, Doria R, Catalano G, Leonildi A, Filipponi F, et al. Breakthrough *Fusarium* spp fungemia during caspofungin therapy in an ABO-incompatible orthotopic liver transplant patient. *J Chemother* 2009;21(2):236–238.

24. Almeida Junior JN, Song AT, Campos SV, Strabelli TM, Del Negro GM, Figueiredo DS, et al. Invasive *Trichosporon* infection in solid organ transplant patients: A report of two cases identified using IGS1 ribosomal DNA sequencing and a review of the literature. *Transpl Infect Dis* 2014;16(1):135–140.

25. Warris A, Verweij PE. Clinical implications of environmental sources for *Aspergillus*. *Med Mycol* 2005;43 Suppl 1:S59–S65.

26. Sehulster L, Chinn RY, CDC, HICPAC. Guidelines for environmental infection control in health-care facilities. Recommendations of CDC and the Healthcare Infection Control Practices Advisory Committee (HICPAC). *MMWR Recomm Rep* 2003;52(RR-10):1–42.

27. Avery RK, Michaels MG, Practice ASTIDCo. Strategies for safe living after solid organ transplantation. *Am J Transplant* 2013;13 Suppl 4:304–310.

28. Palmer SM, Perfect JR, Howell DN, Lawrence CM, Miralles AP, Davis RD, et al. Candidal anastomotic infection in lung transplant recipients: Successful treatment with a combination of systemic and inhaled antifungal agents. *J Heart Lung Transplant* 1998;17(10):1029–1033.

29. Drew RH, Dodds Ashley E, Benjamin DK, Jr., Duane Davis R, Palmer SM, Perfect JR. Comparative safety of amphotericin B lipid complex and amphotericin B deoxycholate as aerosolized antifungal prophylaxis in lung-transplant recipients. *Transplantation* 2004;77(2):232–237.

30. Husain S, Sole A, Alexander BD, Aslam S, Avery R, Benden C, et al. The 2015 International Society for Heart and Lung Transplantation guidelines for the management of fungal infections in mechanical circulatory support and cardiothoracic organ transplant recipients: Executive summary. *J Heart Lung Transplant* 2016;35(3):261–282.

31. Husain S, Zaldonis D, Kusne S, Kwak EJ, Paterson DL, McCurry KR. Variation in antifungal prophylaxis strategies in lung transplantation. *Transpl Infect Dis* 2006;8(4):213–218.

32. Dummer JS, Lazariashvilli N, Barnes J, Ninan M, Milstone AP. A survey of anti-fungal management in lung transplantation. *J Heart Lung Transplant* 2004;23(12):1376–1381.

33. Winston DJ, Busuttil RW. Randomized controlled trial of oral itraconazole solution versus intravenous/oral fluconazole for prevention of fungal infections in liver transplant recipients. *Transplantation* 2002;74(5):688–695.

34. Winston DJ, Pakrasi A, Busuttil RW. Prophylactic fluconazole in liver transplant recipients. A randomized, double-blind, placebo-controlled trial. *Ann Intern Med* 1999;131(10):729–737.

35. Sharpe MD, Ghent C, Grant D, Horbay GL, McDougal J, David Colby W. Efficacy and safety of itraconazole prophylaxis for fungal infections after orthotopic liver transplantation: A prospective, randomized, double-blind study. *Transplantation* 2003;76(6):977–983.

36. Shah T, Lai WK, Gow P, Leeming J, Mutimer D. Low-dose amphotericin for prevention of serious fungal infection following liver transplantation. *Transpl Infect Dis* 2005;7(3–4):126–132.

37. Tollemar J, Hockerstedt K, Ericzon BG, Jalanko H, Ringden O. Liposomal amphotericin B prevents invasive fungal infections in liver transplant recipients. A randomized, placebo-controlled study. *Transplantation* 1995;59(1):45–50.

38. Cruciani M, Mengoli C, Malena M, Bosco O, Serpelloni G, Grossi P. Antifungal prophylaxis in liver transplant patients: A systematic review and meta-analysis. *Liver Transpl* 2006;12(5):850–858.

39. Winston DJ, Limaye AP, Pelletier S, Safdar N, Morris MI, Meneses K, et al. Randomized, double-blind trial of anidulafungin versus fluconazole for prophylaxis of invasive fungal infections in high-risk liver transplant recipients. *Am J Transplant* 2014;14(12):2758–2764.

40. Saliba F, Pascher A, Cointault O, Laterre PF, Cervera C, De Waele JJ, et al. Randomized trial of micafungin for the prevention of invasive fungal infection in high-risk liver transplant recipients. *Clin Infect Dis* 2015;60(7):997–1006.

41. Nieto-Rodriguez JA, Kusne S, Manez R, Irish W, Linden P, Magnone M, et al. Factors associated with the development of candidemia and candidemia-related death among liver transplant recipients. *Ann Surg* 1996;223(1):70–76.

42. Guaraldi G, Cocchi S, Codeluppi M, Di Benedetto F, De Ruvo N, Masetti M, et al. Outcome, incidence, and timing of infectious complications in small bowel and multivisceral organ transplantation patients. *Transplantation* 2005;80(12):1742–1748.

43. Tzakis AG, Kato T, Nishida S, Levi DM, Tryphonopoulos P, Madariaga JR, et al. Alemtuzumab (Campath-1H) combined with tacrolimus in intestinal and multivisceral transplantation. *Transplantation* 2003;75(9):1512–1517.

44. Benedetti E, Gruessner AC, Troppmann C, Papalois BE, Sutherland DE, Dunn DL, et al. Intra-abdominal fungal infections after pancreatic transplantation: Incidence, treatment, and outcome. *J Am Coll Surg* 1996;183(4):307–316.

45. Everett JE, Wahoff DC, Statz C, Gillingham KJ, Gruessner A, Gruessner RW, et al. Characterization and impact of wound infection after pancreas transplantation. *Arch Surg* 1994;129(12):1310–1316; discussion 6–7.

46. Nath DS, Kandaswamy R, Gruessner R, Sutherland DE, Dunn DL, Humar A. Fungal infections in transplant recipients receiving alemtuzumab. *Transplant Proc* 2005;37(2):934–936.

47. Patel R, Portela D, Badley AD, Harmsen WS, Larson-Keller JJ, Ilstrup DM, et al. Risk factors of invasive *Candida* and non-Candida fungal infections after liver transplantation. *Transplantation* 1996;62(7):926–934.

48. Hadley S, Samore MH, Lewis WD, Jenkins RL, Karchmer AW, Hammer SM. Major infectious complications after orthotopic liver transplantation and comparison of outcomes in patients receiving cyclosporine or FK506 as primary immunosuppression. *Transplantation* 1995;59(6):851–859.

49. Collins LA, Samore MH, Roberts MS, Luzzati R, Jenkins RL, Lewis WD, et al. Risk factors for invasive fungal infections complicating orthotopic liver transplantation. *J Infect Dis* 1994;170(3):644–652.

50. Castaldo P, Stratta RJ, Wood RP, Markin RS, Patil KD, Shaefer MS, et al. Clinical spectrum of fungal infections after orthotopic liver transplantation. *Arch Surg* 1991;126(2):149–156.

51. Singh N, Limaye AP, Forrest G, Safdar N, Munoz P, Pursell K, et al. Late-onset invasive aspergillosis in organ transplant recipients in the current era. *Med Mycol* 2006;44(5):445–449.

52. Briegel J, Forst H, Spill B, Haas A, Grabein B, Haller M, et al. Risk factors for systemic fungal infections in liver transplant recipients. *Eur J Clin Microbiol Infect Dis* 1995;14(5):375–382.

53. Munoz P, Rodriguez C, Bouza E, Palomo J, Yanez JF, Dominguez MJ, et al. Risk factors of invasive aspergillosis after heart transplantation: Protective role of oral itraconazole prophylaxis. *Am J Transplant* 2004;4(4):636–643.

54. Husni RN, Gordon SM, Longworth DL, Arroliga A, Stillwell PC, Avery RK, et al. Cytomegalovirus infection is a risk factor for invasive aspergillosis in lung transplant recipients. *Clin Infect Dis* 1998;26(3):753–755.

55. Paradowski LJ. Saprophytic fungal infections and lung transplantation—Revisited. *J Heart Lung Transplant* 1997;16(5):524–531.

56. Scott JP, Fradet G, Smyth RL, Mullins P, Pratt A, Clelland CA, et al. Prospective study of transbronchial biopsies in the management of heart-lung and single lung transplant patients. *J Heart Lung Transplant* 1991;10(5 Pt 1):626–636; discussion 36–37.

57. Paterson DL, Singh N. Invasive aspergillosis in transplant recipients. *Medicine (Baltimore)* 1999;78(2):123–138.

58. Odabasi Z, Mattiuzzi G, Estey E, Kantarjian H, Saeki F, Ridge RJ, et al. Beta-D-glucan as a diagnostic adjunct for invasive fungal infections: Validation, cutoff development, and performance in patients with acute myelogenous leukemia and myelodysplastic syndrome. *Clin Infect Dis* 2004;39(2):199–205.

59. *Platelia Aspergillus EIA (Package Insert)*. Redmond, WA: Bio-Rad, 2006. [Ref Type: Generic]

60. Pfeiffer CD, Fine JP, Safdar N. Diagnosis of invasive aspergillosis using a galactomannan assay: A meta-analysis. *Clin Infect Dis* 2006;42(10):1417–1427.

61. Husain S, Kwak EJ, Obman A, Wagener MM, Kusne S, Stout JE, et al. Prospective assessment of Platelia *Aspergillus* galactomannan antigen for the diagnosis of invasive aspergillosis in lung transplant recipients. *Am J Transplant* 2004;4(5):796–802.

62. Kwak EJ, Husain S, Obman A, Meinke L, Stout J, Kusne S, et al. Efficacy of galactomannan antigen in the Platelia *Aspergillus* enzyme immunoassay for diagnosis of invasive aspergillosis in liver transplant recipients. *J Clin Microbiol* 2004;42(1):435–438.

63. Joos L, Chhajed PN, Wallner J, Battegay M, Steiger J, Gratwohl A, et al. Pulmonary infections diagnosed by BAL: A 12-year experience in 1066 immunocompromised patients. *Respir Med* 2007;101(1):93–97.

64. Rodriguez M, Fishman JA. Prevention of infection due to *Pneumocystis* spp. in human immunodeficiency virus-negative immunocompromised patients. *Clin Microbiol Rev* 2004;17(4):770–782.

65. Cardenal R, Medrano FJ, Varela JM, Ordonez A, Regordan C, Rincon M, et al. *Pneumocystis carinii* pneumonia in heart transplant recipients. *Eur J Cardiothorac Surg* 2001;20(4):799–802.

66. Olsen SL, Renlund DG, O'Connell JB, Taylor DO, Lassetter JE, Eastburn TE, et al. Prevention of *Pneumocystis carinii* pneumonia in cardiac transplant recipients by trimethoprim sulfamethoxazole. *Transplantation* 1993;56(2):359–362.

67. Fishman JA. Prevention of infection caused by *Pneumocystis carinii* in transplant recipients. *Clin Infect Dis* 2001;33(8):1397–1405.

68. Branten AJ, Beckers PJ, Tiggeler RG, Hoitsma AJ. *Pneumocystis carinii* pneumonia in renal transplant recipients. *Nephrol Dial Transplant* 1995;10(7):1194–1197.

69. Radisic M, Lattes R, Chapman JF, del Carmen Rial M, Guardia O, Seu F, et al. Risk factors for *Pneumocystis carinii* pneumonia in kidney transplant recipients: A case–control study. *Transpl Infect Dis* 2003;5(2):84–93.

70. Elinder CG, Andersson J, Bolinder G, Tyden G. Effectiveness of low-dose cotrimoxazole prophylaxis against *Pneumocystis carinii* pneumonia after renal and/or pancreas transplantation. *Transpl Int* 1992;5(2):81–84.

71. Gordon SM, LaRosa SP, Kalmadi S, Arroliga AC, Avery RK, Truesdell-LaRosa L, et al. Should prophylaxis for *Pneumocystis carinii* pneumonia in solid organ transplant recipients ever be discontinued? *Clin Infect Dis* 1999;28(2):240–246.

72. Cytomegalovirus. *Am J Transplant* 2004;4 Suppl 10:51–58.

73. George MJ, Snydman DR, Werner BG, Griffith J, Falagas ME, Dougherty NN, et al. The independent role of cytomegalovirus as a risk factor for invasive fungal disease in orthotopic liver transplant recipients. Boston Center for Liver Transplantation CMVIG-Study Group. Cytogam, MedImmune, Inc. Gaithersburg, Maryland. *Am J Med* 1997;103(2):106–113.

74. Dockrell DH, Mendez JC, Jones M, Harmsen WS, Ilstrup DM, Smith TF, et al. Human herpesvirus 6 seronegativity before transplantation predicts the occurrence of fungal infection in liver transplant recipients. *Transplantation* 1999;67(3):399–403.

75. Dockrell DH, Prada J, Jones MF, Patel R, Badley AD, Harmsen WS, et al. Seroconversion to human herpesvirus 6 following liver transplantation is a marker of cytomegalovirus disease. *J Infect Dis* 1997;176(5):1135–1140.

76. Kidd IM, Clark DA, Sabin CA, Andrew D, Hassan-Walker AF, Sweny P, et al. Prospective study of human betaherpesviruses after renal transplantation: Association of human herpesvirus 7 and cytomegalovirus co-infection with cytomegalovirus disease and increased rejection. *Transplantation* 2000;69(11):2400–2404.

77. Rogers J, Rohal S, Carrigan DR, Kusne S, Knox KK, Gayowski T, et al. Human herpesvirus-6 in liver transplant recipients: Role in pathogenesis of fungal infections, neurologic complications, and outcome. *Transplantation* 2000;69(12):2566–2573.

78. Wagner JA, Ross H, Hunt S, Gamberg P, Valantine H, Merigan TC, et al. Prophylactic ganciclovir treatment reduces fungal as well as cytomegalovirus infections after heart transplantation. *Transplantation* 1995;60(12):1473–1477.

79. Hellinger WC, Bonatti H, Machicao VI, Yao JD, Brumble LM, Alvarez S, et al. Effect of antiviral chemoprophylaxis on adverse clinical outcomes associated with cytomegalovirus after liver transplantation. *Mayo Clin Proc* 2006;81(8):1029–1033.

80. Kalil AC, Levitsky J, Lyden E, Stoner J, Freifeld AG. Meta-analysis: The efficacy of strategies to prevent organ disease by cytomegalovirus in solid organ transplant recipients. *Ann Intern Med* 2005;143(12):870–880.

81. Singh N, Wannstedt C, Keyes L, Wagener MM, Gayowski T, Cacciarelli TV. Indirect outcomes associated with cytomegalovirus (opportunistic infections, hepatitis C virus sequelae, and mortality) in liver-transplant recipients with the use of pre-emptive therapy for 13 years. *Transplantation* 2005;79(10):1428–1434.

82. Valantine HA, Luikart H, Doyle R, Theodore J, Hunt S, Oyer P, et al. Impact of cytomegalovirus hyperimmune globulin on outcome after cardiothoracic transplantation: A comparative study of combined prophylaxis with CMV hyperimmune globulin plus ganciclovir versus ganciclovir alone. *Transplantation* 2001;72(10):1647–1652.

83. Kruger RM, Paranjothi S, Storch GA, Lynch JP, Trulock EP. Impact of prophylaxis with cytogam alone on the incidence of CMV viremia in CMV-seropositive lung transplant recipients. *J Heart Lung Transplant* 2003;22(7):754–763.

84. Rea F, Potena L, Yonan N, Wagner F, Calabrese F. Cytomegalovirus hyper immunoglobulin for CMV prophylaxis in thoracic transplantation. *Transplantation* 2016;100 Suppl 3:S19–S26.

85. Osman HK, Peiris JS, Taylor CE, Warwicker P, Jarrett RF, Madeley CR. "Cytomegalovirus disease" in renal allograft recipients: Is human herpesvirus 7 a co-factor for disease progression? *J Med Virol* 1996;48(4):295–301.

86. Mendez JC, Dockrell DH, Espy MJ, Smith TF, Wilson JA, Harmsen WS, et al. Human beta-herpesvirus interactions in solid organ transplant recipients. *J Infect Dis* 2001;183(2):179–184.

87. Verma A, Wade JJ, Cheeseman P, Samaroo B, Rela M, Heaton ND, et al. Risk factors for fungal infection in paediatric liver transplant recipients. *Pediatr Transplant* 2005;9(2):220–225.

88. Peleg AY, Husain S, Kwak EJ, Silveira FP, Ndirangu M, Tran J, et al. Opportunistic infections in 547 organ transplant recipients receiving alemtuzumab, a humanized monoclonal CD-52 antibody. *Clin Infect Dis* 2007;44(2):204–212.

89. Singh N, Lortholary O, Alexander BD, Gupta KL, John GT, Pursell K, et al. An immune reconstitution syndrome-like illness associated with *Cryptococcus neoformans* infection in organ transplant recipients. *Clin Infect Dis* 2005;40(12):1756–1761.

90. Corales R, Chua J, Mawhorter S, Young JB, Starling R, Tomford JW, et al. Significant post-transplant hypogammaglobulinemia in six heart transplant recipients: An emerging clinical phenomenon? *Transpl Infect Dis* 2000;2(3):133–139.

91. Kawut SM, Shah L, Wilt JS, Dwyer E, Maani PA, Daly TM, et al. Risk factors and outcomes of hypogammaglobulinemia after lung transplantation. *Transplantation* 2005;79(12):1723–1726.

92. Yamani MH, Avery RK, Mawhorter SD, Young JB, Ratliff NB, Hobbs RE, et al. Hypogammaglobulinemia following cardiac transplantation: A link between rejection and infection. *J Heart Lung Transplant* 2001;20(4):425–430.

93. Goldfarb NS, Avery RK, Goormastic M, Mehta AC, Schilz R, Smedira N, et al. Hypogammaglobulinemia in lung transplant recipients. *Transplantation* 2001;71(2):242–246.

94. Doron S, Ruthazer R, Werner BG, Rabson A, Snydman DR. Hypogammaglobulinemia in liver transplant recipients: Incidence, timing, risk factors, and outcomes. *Transplantation* 2006;81(5):697–703.

95. Hellinger WC, Bonatti H, Yao JD, Alvarez S, Brumble LM, Keating MR, et al. Risk stratification and targeted antifungal prophylaxis for prevention of aspergillosis and other invasive mold infections after liver transplantation. *Liver Transpl* 2005;11(6):656–662.

96. Anding K, Gross P, Rost JM, Allgaier D, Jacobs E. The influence of uraemia and haemodialysis on neutrophil phagocytosis and antimicrobial killing. *Nephrol Dial Transplant* 2003;18(10):2067–2073.

97. Majewska E, Baj Z, Sulowska Z, Rysz J, Luciak M. Effects of uraemia and haemodialysis on neutrophil apoptosis and expression of apoptosis-related proteins. *Nephrol Dial Transplant* 2003;18(12):2582–2588.

98. Kontoyiannis DP, Lionakis MS, Lewis RE, Chamilos G, Healy M, Perego C, et al. Zygomycosis in a tertiary-care cancer center in the era of *Aspergillus*-active antifungal therapy: A case–control observational study of 27 recent cases. *J Infect Dis* 2005;191(8):1350–1360.

99. Forrest GN, Mankes K. Outcomes of invasive zygomycosis infections in renal transplant recipients. *Transpl Infect Dis* 2007;9(2):161–164.

100. Nett JE, Andes DR. Antifungal agents: Spectrum of activity, pharmacology, and clinical indications. *Infect Dis Clin North Am* 2016;30(1):51–83.

101. *Sporanox (Itraconazole) Injection—Package Insert*. Lake Forest, IL: Ortho Biotech Products, L.P., 2001. [Ref Type: Generic].

102. *Sporanox (Itraconazole) Oral Solution—Package Insert*. Beerse, Belgium: Janssen Pharmaceutica N.V., 2003. [Ref Type: Generic].

103. *Sporanox (Itraconazole) Capsules—Package Insert*. Titusville, NJ: © Janssen Pharmaceuticals, Inc, 2001. [Ref Type: Generic].

104. *Vfend (Voriconazole) Tablets, Oral Suspension and Injection—Package Insert*. New York, NY: Pfizer, Inc., 2006:1–43. [Ref Type: Generic].

105. *Noxafil (Posaconazole) Tablets, Oral Suspension and Injection—Package Insert*. Whitehouse Station, NJ: Merck & Co. Inc, 2014. [Ref Type: Generic].

106. *Cresemba (Isavuconazole) Capsules and Injection—Package Insert*. Northbrook, IL: Astellas Pharma US, Inc, 2015. [Ref Type: Generic].

107. *Cancidas (Caspofungin Acetate) for Injection—Package Insert*. Whitehouse Station, NJ: MERCK and CO., Inc., 2005. [Ref Type: Generic].

108. *Mycamine (Micafungin) Package Insert*. Tokyo, Japan: Astella Pharma, Inc., 2006. [Ref Type: Generic].

109. *Eraxis (Anidulafungin) for Injection—Package Insert*. New York, NY: Roerig (Division of Pfizer, Inc.), 2007. [Ref Type: Generic].

110. *Amphotericin B for Injection—Package Insert*. Big Flats, NY: X-Gen Pharmaceuticals, Inc, 2009. [Ref Type: Generic].

111. *AmBisome (Amphotericin B Liposome) for Injection—Package Insert*. Deerfield, IL: Astella Pharmas US, Inc., 2012. [Ref Type: Generic].

112. *ABELCET (Amphotericin B Lipid Complex Injection)—Package Insert*. Indianapolis, IN: Sigma-Tau PharmaSource, Inc, 2013. [Ref Type: Generic].

113. *Diflucan (Fluconazole) Tablets, Oral Suspension and Injection—Package Insert*. New York, NY: Roerig (Division of Pfizer, Inc.), 2011. [Ref Type: Generic].

114. Dodds-Ashley E. Management of drug and food interactions with azole antifungal agents in transplant recipients. *Pharmacotherapy* 2010;30(8):842–854.

115. Goodwin ML, Drew RH. Antifungal serum concentration monitoring: An update. *J Antimicrob Chemother* 2008;61(1):17–25.

116. Theuretzbacher U, Ihle F, Derendorf H. Pharmacokinetic/pharmacodynamic profile of voriconazole. *Clin Pharmacokinet* 2006;45(7):649–663.

117. Bruggemann RJ, Alffenaar JW, Blijlevens NM, Billaud EM, Kosterink JG, Verweij PE, et al. Clinical relevance of the pharmacokinetic interactions of azole antifungal drugs with other coadministered agents. *Clin Infect Dis* 2009;48(10):1441–1458.

118. Niwa T, Shiraga T, Takagi A. Effect of antifungal drugs on cytochrome P450 (CYP) 2C9, CYP2C19, and CYP3A4 activities in human liver microsomes. *Biol Pharm Bull* 2005;28(9):1805–1808.

119. Marty FM, Lowry CM, Cutler CS, Campbell BJ, Fiumara K, Baden LR, et al. Voriconazole and sirolimus coadministration after allogeneic hematopoietic stem cell transplantation. *Biol Blood Marrow Transplant* 2006;12(5):552–559.

120. Steinbach WJ, Stevens DA. Review of newer antifungal and immunomodulatory strategies for invasive aspergillosis. *Clin Infect Dis* 2003;37(Suppl 3):S157–S187.

121. Sadaba B, Campanero MA, Quetglas EG, Azanza JR. Clinical relevance of sirolimus drug interactions in transplant patients. *Transplant Proc* 2004;36(10):3226–3228.

122. Venkataramanan R, Zang S, Gayowski T, Singh N. Voriconazole inhibition of the metabolism of tacrolimus in a liver transplant recipient and in human liver microsomes. *Antimicrob Agents Chemother* 2002;46(9):3091–3093.

123. Romero AJ, Le Pogamp P, Nilsson LG, Wood N. Effect of voriconazole on the pharmacokinetics of cyclosporine in renal transplant patients. *Clin Pharmacol Ther* 2002;71(4):226–234.

124. Mathis AS, Shah NK, Friedman GS. Combined use of sirolimus and voriconazole in renal transplantation: A report of two cases. *Transplant Proc* 2004;36(9):2708–2709.

125. Husain S, Paterson DL, Studer S, Pilewski J, Crespo M, Zaldonis D, et al. Voriconazole prophylaxis in lung transplant recipients. *Am J Transplant* 2006;6(12):3008–3016.

126. Alkan Y, Haefeli WE, Burhenne J, Stein J, Yaniv I, Shalit I. Voriconazole-induced QT interval prolongation and ventricular tachycardia: A non-concentration-dependent adverse effect. *Clin Infect Dis* 2004;39(6):e49–e52.

127. Trifilio S, Singhal S, Williams S, Frankfurt O, Gordon L, Evens A, et al. Breakthrough fungal infections after allogeneic hematopoietic stem cell transplantation in patients on prophylactic voriconazole. *Bone Marrow Transplant* 2007;40(5):451–456.

128. Trifilio S, Pennick G, Pi J, Zook J, Golf M, Kaniecki K, et al. Monitoring plasma voriconazole levels may be necessary to avoid subtherapeutic levels in hematopoietic stem cell transplant recipients. *Cancer* 2007;109(8):1532–1535.

129. Herbrecht R, Denning DW, Patterson TF, Bennett JE, Greene RE, Oestmann JW, et al. Voriconazole versus amphotericin B for primary therapy of invasive aspergillosis. *N Engl J Med* 2002;347(6):408–415.

130. Smith J, Safdar N, Knasinski V, Simmons W, Bhavnani SM, Ambrose PG, et al. Voriconazole therapeutic drug monitoring. *Antimicrob Agents Chemother* 2006;50(4):1570–1572.

131. Denning DW, Ribaud P, Milpied N, Caillot D, Herbrecht R, Thiel E, et al. Efficacy and safety of voriconazole in the treatment of acute invasive aspergillosis. *Clin Infect Dis* 2002;34(5):563–571.

132. www.fda.gov/ohrms/dockets/ac/01/briefing/3792b2_02_FDA-voriconazole.htm Accessed November 10, 2007; page search term `Voriconazole Efficacy Response Assessment', 2007 [Ref Type: Generic].

133. Johnson HJ, Han K, Capitano B, Blisard D, Husain S, Linden PK, et al. Voriconazole pharmacokinetics in liver transplant recipients. *Antimicrob Agents Chemother* 2010;54(2):852–859.

134. Feist A, Lee R, Osborne S, Lane J, Yung G. Increased incidence of cutaneous squamous cell carcinoma in lung transplant recipients taking long-term voriconazole. *J Heart Lung Transplant* 2012;31(11):1177–1181.

135. Mansh M, Binstock M, Williams K, Hafeez F, Kim J, Glidden D, et al. Voriconazole exposure and risk of cutaneous squamous cell carcinoma, *Aspergillus* colonization, invasive aspergillosis and death in lung transplant recipients. *Am J Transplant* 2016;16(1):262–270.

136. Williams K, Mansh M, Chin-Hong P, Singer J, Arron ST. Voriconazole-associated cutaneous malignancy: A literature review on photocarcinogenesis in organ transplant recipients. *Clin Infect Dis* 2014;58(7):997–1002.

137. Vadnerkar A, Nguyen MH, Mitsani D, Crespo M, Pilewski J, Toyoda Y, et al. Voriconazole exposure and geographic location are independent risk factors for squamous cell carcinoma of the skin among lung transplant recipients. *J Heart Lung Transplant* 2010;29(11):1240–1244.

138. Zwald FO, Spratt M, Lemos BD, Veledar E, Lawrence C, Marshall Lyon G, et al. Duration of voriconazole exposure: An independent risk factor for skin cancer after lung transplantation. *Dermatol Surg* 2012;38(8):1369–1374.

139. Adwan MH. Voriconazole-induced periostitis: A new rheumatic disorder. *Clin Rheumatol* 2017;36(3):609–615

140. Moon WJ, Scheller EL, Suneja A, Livermore JA, Malani AN, Moudgal V, et al. Plasma fluoride level as a predictor of voriconazole-induced periostitis in patients with skeletal pain. *Clin Infect Dis* 2014;59(9):1237–1245.

141. Tarlock K, Johnson D, Cornell C, Parnell S, Meshinchi S, Baker KS, et al. Elevated fluoride levels and periostitis in pediatric hematopoietic stem cell transplant recipients receiving long-term voriconazole. *Pediatr Blood Cancer* 2015;62(5):918–920.

142. Wermers RA, Cooper K, Razonable RR, Deziel PJ, Whitford GM, Kremers WK, et al. Fluoride excess and periostitis in transplant patients receiving long-term voriconazole therapy. *Clin Infect Dis* 2011;52(5):604–611.

143. Chen L, Mulligan ME. Medication-induced periostitis in lung transplant patients: Periostitis deformans revisited. *Skeletal Radiol* 2011;40(2):143–148.

144. Wang TF, Wang T, Altman R, Eshaghian P, Lynch JP, 3rd, Ross DJ, et al. Periostitis secondary to prolonged voriconazole therapy in lung transplant recipients. *Am J Transplant* 2009;9(12):2845–2850.

145. Dolton MJ, Bruggemann RJ, Burger DM, McLachlan AJ. Understanding variability in posaconazole exposure using an integrated population pharmacokinetic analysis. *Antimicrob Agents Chemother* 2014;58(11):6879–6885.

146. Dekkers BG, Bakker M, van der Elst KC, Sturkenboom MG, Veringa A, Span LF, et al. Therapeutic drug monitoring of posaconazole: An update. *Curr Fungal Infect Rep* 2016;10:51–61.

147. Ullmann AJ, Cornely OA, Burchardt A, Hachem R, Kontoyiannis DP, Topelt K, et al. Pharmacokinetics, safety, and efficacy of posaconazole in patients with persistent febrile neutropenia or refractory invasive fungal infection. *Antimicrob Agents Chemother* 2006;50(2):658–666.

148. Krishna G, Ma L, Martinho M, O'Mara E. Single-dose phase I study to evaluate the pharmacokinetics of posaconazole in new tablet and capsule formulations relative to oral suspension. *Antimicrob Agents Chemother* 2012;56(8):4196–4201.

149. Kersemaekers WM, Dogterom P, Xu J, Marcantonio EE, de Greef R, Waskin H, et al. Effect of a high-fat meal on the pharmacokinetics of 300-milligram posaconazole in a solid oral tablet formulation. *Antimicrob Agents Chemother* 2015;59(6):3385–3389.

150. McKeage K. Posaconazole: A review of the gastro-resistant tablet and intravenous solution in invasive fungal infections. *Drugs* 2015;75(4):397–406.

151. Durani U, Tosh PK, Barreto JN, Estes LL, Jannetto PJ, Tande AJ. Retrospective comparison of posaconazole levels in patients taking the delayed-release tablet versus the oral suspension. *Antimicrob Agents Chemother* 2015;59(8):4914–4918.

152. Raad, II, Graybill JR, Bustamante AB, Cornely OA, Gaona-Flores V, Afif C, et al. Safety of long-term oral posaconazole use in the treatment of refractory invasive fungal infections. *Clin Infect Dis* 2006;42(12):1726–1734.

153. Dolton MJ, Ray JE, Marriott D, McLachlan AJ. Posaconazole exposure-response relationship: Evaluating the utility of therapeutic drug monitoring. *Antimicrob Agents Chemother* 2012;56(6):2806–2813.

154. Seyedmousavi S, Mouton JW, Verweij PE, Bruggemann RJ. Therapeutic drug monitoring of voriconazole and posaconazole for invasive aspergillosis. *Expert Rev Anti Infect Ther* 2013;11(9):931–941.

155. Jang SH, Colangelo PM, Gobburu JV. Exposure-response of posaconazole used for prophylaxis against invasive fungal infections: Evaluating the need to adjust doses based on drug concentrations in plasma. *Clin Pharmacol Ther* 2010;88(1):115–119.

156. Walsh TJ, Raad I, Patterson TF, Chandrasekar P, Donowitz GR, Graybill R, et al. Treatment of invasive aspergillosis with posaconazole in patients who are refractory to or intolerant of conventional therapy: An externally controlled trial. *Clin Infect Dis* 2007;44(1):2–12.

157. Alexander BD, Perfect JR, Daly JS, Restrepo A, Tobon AM, Patino H, et al. Posaconazole as salvage therapy in patients with invasive fungal infections after solid organ transplant. *Transplantation* 2008;86(6):791–796.

158. van Burik JA, Hare RS, Solomon HF, Corrado ML, Kontoyiannis DP. Posaconazole is effective as salvage therapy in zygomycosis: A retrospective summary of 91 cases. *Clin Infect Dis* 2006;42(7):e61–e65.

159. Greenberg RN, Mullane K, van Burik JA, Raad I, Abzug MJ, Anstead G, et al. Posaconazole as salvage therapy for zygomycosis. *Antimicrob Agents Chemother* 2006;50(1):126–133.

160. Lewis RE, Albert ND, Kontoyiannis DP. Comparative pharmacodynamics of posaconazole in neutropenic murine models of invasive pulmonary aspergillosis and mucormycosis. *Antimicrob Agents Chemother* 2014;58(11):6767–6772.

161. Seyedmousavi S, Mouton JW, Melchers WJ, Bruggemann RJ, Verweij PE. The role of azoles in the management of azole-resistant aspergillosis: From the bench to the bedside. *Drug Resist Updat* 2014;17(3):37–50.

162. Miceli MH, Kauffman CA. Isavuconazole: A new broad-spectrum triazole antifungal agent. *Clin Infect Dis* 2015;61(10):1558–1565.

163. Maertens JA, Raad, II, Marr KA, Patterson TF, Kontoyiannis DP, Cornely OA, et al. Isavuconazole versus voriconazole for primary treatment of invasive mould disease caused by *Aspergillus* and other filamentous fungi (SECURE): A phase 3, randomised-controlled, non-inferiority trial. *Lancet* 2016;387(10020):760–769.

164. Marty FM, Ostrosky-Zeichner L, Cornely OA, Mullane KM, Perfect JR, Thompson GR, 3rd, et al. Isavuconazole treatment for mucormycosis: A single-arm open-label trial and case–control analysis. *Lancet Infect Dis* 2016;16(7):828–837.

165. Groll AH, Desai A, Han D, Howieson C, Kato K, Akhtar S, et al. Pharmacokinetic assessment of drug–drug interactions of isavuconazole with the immunosuppressants cyclosporine, mycophenolic acid, prednisolone, sirolimus, and tacrolimus in healthy adults. *Clin Pharmacol Drug Dev* 2017;6(1):76–85.

166. Kim T, Jancel T, Kumar P, Freeman AF. Drug–drug interaction between isavuconazole and tacrolimus: A case report indicating the need for tacrolimus drug-level monitoring. *J Clin Pharm Ther* 2015;40(5):609–611.

167. Pettit NN, Carver PL. Isavuconazole: A new option for the management of invasive fungal infections. *Ann Pharmacother* 2015;49(7):825–842.

168. Alexander BD, Dodds Ashley ES, Addison RM, Alspaugh JA, Chao NJ, Perfect JR. Non-comparative evaluation of the safety of aerosolized amphotericin B lipid complex in patients undergoing allogeneic hematopoietic stem cell transplantation. *Transpl Infect Dis* 2006;8(1):13–20.

169. Gubbins PO, Penzak SR, Polston S, McConnell SA, Anaissie E. Characterizing and predicting amphotericin B-associated nephrotoxicity in bone marrow or peripheral blood stem cell transplant recipients. *Pharmacotherapy* 2002;22(8):961–971.

170. Walsh TJ, Goodman JL, Pappas P, Bekersky I, Buell DN, Roden M, et al. Safety, tolerance, and pharmacokinetics of high-dose liposomal amphotericin B (AmBisome) in patients infected with *Aspergillus* species and other filamentous fungi: Maximum tolerated dose study. *Antimicrob Agents Chemother* 2001;45(12):3487–3496.

171. Walsh TJ, Hiemenz JW, Seibel NL, Perfect JR, Horwith G, Lee L, et al. Amphotericin B lipid complex for invasive fungal infections: Analysis of safety and efficacy in 556 cases. *Clin Infect Dis* 1998;26(6):1383–1396.

172. Wingard JR, White MH, Anaissie E, Raffalli J, Goodman J, Arrieta A, et al. A randomized, double-blind comparative trial evaluating the safety of liposomal amphotericin B versus amphotericin B lipid complex in the empirical treatment of febrile neutropenia. L Amph/ABLC Collaborative Study Group. *Clin Infect Dis* 2000;31(5):1155–1163.

173. Taylor AL, Watson CJ, Bradley JA. Immunosuppressive agents in solid organ transplantation: Mechanisms of action and therapeutic efficacy. *Crit Rev Oncol Hematol* 2005;56(1):23–46.

174. Dubois J, Bartter T, Gryn J, Pratter MR. The physiologic effects of inhaled amphotericin B. *Chest* 1995;108(3):750–753.

175. Lowry CM, Marty FM, Vargas SO, Lee JT, Fiumara K, Deykin A, et al. Safety of aerosolized liposomal versus deoxycholate amphotericin B formulations for prevention of invasive fungal infections following lung transplantation: A retrospective study. *Transpl Infect Dis* 2007;9(2):121–125.

176. Palmer SM, Drew RH, Whitehouse JD, Tapson VF, Davis RD, McConnell RR, et al. Safety of aerosolized amphotericin B lipid complex in lung transplant recipients. *Transplantation* 2001;72(3):545–548.

177. Sable CA, Nguyen BY, Chodakewitz JA, DiNubile MJ. Safety and tolerability of caspofungin acetate in the treatment of fungal infections. *Transpl Infect Dis* 2002;4(1):25–30.

178. Marr KA, Hachem R, Papanicolaou G, Somani J, Arduino JM, Lipka CJ, et al. Retrospective study of the hepatic safety profile of patients concomitantly treated with caspofungin and cyclosporin A. *Transpl Infect Dis* 2004;6(3):110–116.

179. Forrest GN, Rasetto F, Akpek G, Philosophe B. Safety and efficacy of micafungin in transplantation recipients. *Transplantation* 2006;82(11):1549.

180. Kuse ER, Chetchotisakd P, da Cunha CA, Ruhnke M, Barrios C, Raghunadharao D, et al. Micafungin versus liposomal amphotericin B for candidaemia and invasive candidosis: A phase III randomised double-blind trial. *Lancet* 2007;369(9572):1519–1527.

181. Reboli AC, Rotstein C, Pappas PG, Chapman SW, Kett DH, Kumar D, et al. Anidulafungin versus fluconazole for invasive candidiasis. *N Engl J Med* 2007;356(24):2472–2482.

182. Dowell JA, Stogniew M, Krause D, Henkel T, Damle B. Lack of pharmacokinetic interaction between anidulafungin and tacrolimus. *J Clin Pharmacol* 2007;47(3):305–314.

183. Dowell JA, Schranz J, Baruch A, Foster G. Safety and pharmacokinetics of coadministered voriconazole and anidulafungin. *J Clin Pharmacol* 2005;45(12):1373–1382.

184. Dowell JA, Stogniew M, Krause D, Henkel T, Weston IE. Assessment of the safety and pharmacokinetics of anidulafungin when administered with cyclosporine. *J Clin Pharmacol* 2005;45(2):227–233.

185. van Burik JA, Ratanatharathorn V, Stepan DE, Miller CB, Lipton JH, Vesole DH, et al. Micafungin versus fluconazole for prophylaxis against invasive fungal infections during neutropenia in patients undergoing hematopoietic stem cell transplantation. *Clin Infect Dis* 2004;39(10):1407–1416.

186. Perfect JR, Dismukes WE, Dromer F, Goldman DL, Graybill JR, Hamill RJ, et al. Clinical practice guidelines for the management of cryptococcal disease: 2010 update by the Infectious Diseases Society of America. *Clin Infect Dis* 2010;50(3):291–322.

187. Sun HY, Wagener MM, Singh N. Cryptococcosis in solid-organ, hematopoietic stem cell, and tissue transplant recipients: Evidence-based evolving trends. *Clin Infect Dis* 2009;48(11):1566–1576.

Prophylaxis and treatment of invasive fungal infections in neutropenic cancer and hematopoietic cell transplant patients

DANIEL R. RICHARDSON, MARCIE L. RICHES, AND HILLARD M. LAZARUS

INTRODUCTION

Invasive fungal infections (IFIs) are a major cause of morbidity and mortality among patients affected with hematologic malignancies, particularly those undergoing hematopoietic cell transplant (HCT) and those affected by acute leukemia. Significant advances in the treatment and prevention of IFIs over the last several decades have contributed to improving HCT and leukemia outcomes. With the number of patients undergoing HCT increasing yearly and the utilization of an increased number of mismatched and unrelated donors, the management of IFIs remains an important clinical opportunity to improve overall patient outcomes.

Pathogens

Previously, *Candida* spp. were the major cause of IFIs among HCT patients; however, with routine fluconazole prophylaxis, there has been a substantial reduction in the rate of IFIs caused by fluconazole-sensitive fungi. Instead, the increasing and extensive use of IFI prophylaxis prompted the emergence not only of resistant *Candida* spp. (i.e., *C. glabrata, C. guillermondii, C. krusei, C. parapsilosis*) [1,2] but also invasive aspergillosis (IA) and more serious IFIs caused by less commonly encountered fungi that frequently exhibit intrinsic resistance to many antifungal agents. With the introduction of mold-active triazole prophylaxis (i.e., voriconazole, posaconazole), the IA incidence has fallen. However, less common but resistant infections, such as fusariosis and mucormycosis, remain a serious concern [3–5]. A retrospective analysis confirmed that non-*Aspergillus* mold infections are associated with high mortality, but the frequency of these infections has not increased in the current antifungal era [6].

In contrast to *Candida* sp. infections, *Aspergillus* sp. IFI predominates in the post-engraftment neutropenic period. The most commonly affected groups include HCT recipients receiving immunosuppressive therapy for graft-versus-host disease (GvHD) as well as those subjects given T-cell depleted grafts [7,8]. The incidence of such infection ranges from 5% to 10% in allogeneic HCT recipients, whereas less than 2% of autologous HCT recipients develop *Aspergillus sp.* IFI [9]. Among acute leukemia patients, those with acute myeloid leukemia (AML) have the highest rates of IFI, roughly 10%–25% [10]. One large multicenter surveillance program reported that infections occurring after HCT included *A. fumigatus* (56%), *A. flavus* (19%), *A. terreus* (16%), *A. niger* (8%), and *A. versicolor* (1.3%) [11]. Other less common but highly virulent mold IFIs include *Fusarium sp.*, *Scedosporium,* and *Zygomycetes* and are associated with mortality rates as high as 87% [11,12]. *Scedosporium* infections usually begin early in the first month after HCT, while zygomycoses may develop as long as 3 months after HCT, usually in association with GvHD and its treatment [11].

Diagnosis

Although data are accumulating regarding the benefits of using molecular-based testing, analysis of tissue and fluid specimens remain the gold-standard for the diagnosis of IFI. The optimal rationale for diagnosis likely is a combined approach guided by clinical, radiographic, and interval screening with several biomarkers. Unfortunately, there remain no agreed upon approaches for the type, frequency or indications for molecular testing.

Diagnostic classification of fungal infection was revised in a consensus statement from the European Organization for Research and Treatment of Cancer/Invasive Fungal Infections Cooperative Group and the National Institute of Allergy and Infectious Diseases Mycoses Study Group (EORTC/MSG) published in 2008 [13]. These guidelines that cover both molds and yeasts, remain the accepted standard for classifying IFIs. IFIs are classified as "possible," "probable," or "proven." Proven IFIs encompass those diagnosed with direct demonstration of fungal elements in diseased tissue. Probable IFIs must include a host factor, clinical features consistent with IFI, and some mycological element to be present (e.g., galactomannan, β-glucan, or fungal elements discovered in sputum, bronchoalveolar lavage (BAL), or sinus aspirate). Possible IFIs are diagnosed when appropriate host and clinical factors are present, but there is no mycological support (Table 25.1).

Because obtaining direct fungal culture can often be invasive and potentially result in a substantial delay from culture to diagnosis, there has been an interest in developing rapid detection tests that can be obtained from serum or other more accessible body fluids. Although insufficient for a diagnosis of proven IFI, these indirect methods contribute to a diagnosis of probable IFI. Galactomannan (GM) is a component of the cell wall released during the replication of *Aspergillosis* and can be detected in patients with IA infection. Recently published guidelines of the Infectious Disease Society of America (IDSA) recommend serum and BAL galactomannan as an accurate marker for the diagnosis of IA in high-risk patients [14]. The sensitivity and specificity of serum GM for IA among immunocompromised patients is 78% and 81%, respectively, though varies based on optical density cut-off [15]. However, for patients actively receiving mold prophylaxis, serum GM is often falsely positive, although BAL specimens are not thought to be effected

Table 25.1 Diagnostic criteria for proven, probable, and possible IFI [13]

Proven IFI	Probable IFI	Possible IFI
Requires one of the following:	Requires all of the following:	Cases meeting appropriate host and clinical criteria of probable IFI but without appropriate mycological criteria
Histopathologic, cytopathologic or direct microscopic examination of specimen from a normally sterile site obtained by biopsy or needle aspiration with characteristic mold or yeast pathology	Host factor (Neutropenia, receipt of HCT, prolonged use of steroids, treatment with T-cell immunosuppressant, or severe immunodeficiency)	
Recovery of either mold or yeast by culture obtained from a normally sterile site	Clinical criteria (Evidence of fungal infection involving lower respiratory tract, tracheobronchitis, sinonasal cavities, CNS)	
Blood culture that yields either a mold or yeast in the context of a compatible clinical picture	Mycological criteria (direct evidence of mold in sputum, BAL, or sinus aspirate; or indirect testing [detection of antigen or cell-wall constituents])	

Abbreviations: IFI, invasive fungal infection; HCT, hematopoietic cell transplantation; CNS, central nervous system; BAL, bronchoalveolar lavage.

by prophylaxis. As the false negative rate of serum GM is high, a single negative test is often not clinically useful. Meta-analysis suggests that BAL is safe and effective and may be useful to guide antifungal therapy in asymptomatic or febrile high-risk patients and can reduce unnecessary antifungal therapy [16].

Other serum assays include those that detect $(1 \rightarrow 3)$-β-D-glucan, a polysaccharide found in the cell wall of many pathogenic fungi. While these approaches are recommended for diagnosing IA in high-risk patients (sensitivity 47%–64% in patients with hematologic malignancy or HCT), such monitoring is not specific for *Aspergillus* infections as $(1 \rightarrow 3)$-β-D-glucan is present on many fungi [17]. Aguado et al. reported the results of a randomized controlled, trial using serum GM versus a combination of GM and polymerase chain reaction (PCR)-based *Aspergillus* DNA detection for IA in high-risk patients [18]. A combined monitoring strategy was associated with an earlier diagnosis (13 vs. 20 days; p = 0.022) and a lower incidence of IA (4.2% vs. 13.1%; odds ratio, 0.29 [95% confidence interval, 0.09–0.91]). Arvanitis and colleagues reported a positive-predictive value of 88% and a negative predictive value of nearly 100% for a combined GM and PCR approach [19]. There are limited data to suggest intermittently screening asymptomatic patients though it may be considered for those who are at high risk for invasive disease. Again, given the rather low sensitivity of the test, a single negative result is not useful. A non-contrast CT scan should be performed in those with suspicion for IA and attempts at biopsy should be made to direct therapy when possible [14].

Blood or tissue cultures remain the gold-standard for the diagnosis of candidemia and invasive candidiasis, respectively. Sensitivity of blood cultures for candidiasis is only 50% [20], though the limit of detection of blood cultures is ≤1 colony-forming unit/mL, below that of PCR [21]. Sensitivities of cultures of tissue and other bodily fluid also is poor at <50% [21]. The role of *Candida* sp. antigen and antibody testing is thought to be limited. All patients diagnosed as having candidemia should have a dilated ophthalmologic examination, preferably performed by an ophthalmologist looking for exudates in the retina and other areas.

Incidence and risk factors

The incidence of IFIs varies by type of HCT, with much higher rates seen among patients undergoing allogeneic HCT. In a prospective, surveillance study of over 1,800 patients undergoing allogeneic HCT, the Italian group GITMO (Gruppo Italiano Trapianto Midollo Osseo) reported an overall incidence at one-year post-HCT of new or recurrent proven or probable IFI of 8.8% with roughly 95% of patients receiving primary or secondary fungal prophylaxis [22]. IA was the most common infection, representing 81% of cases, with candidiasis (11%), zygomycosis (3.7%), fusariosis (1.8%), and others with one case each of *Scedosporium* sp., *Scopulariopsis* sp., *Cryptococcus neoformans*, and *Geotrichum capitatum* [22]. Prospective,

observational data collected in the US and China from allogeneic HCT recipients receiving azole prophylaxis report similar rates of IFIs of 11% and 7.7%, respectively [9,23]. Retrospective data from HCT procedures in Spain, where patients were given triazole prophylaxis, are also similar with a one-year IFIs incidence of roughly 11% [5]. Patients receiving reduced-intensity conditioning regimens appear to have an incidence of IFIs similar to those undergoing myeloablative conditioning regimens [24,25].

Incidence rates of IFIs among patients undergoing autologous HCT appear lower, with published rates of 0%–8% [10,11,23,26]. The significant variation in incidence of IFI may reflect the type of conditioning, duration of neutropenia, and variable patient-related risk factors [10]. Pagano et al. recommend that despite the lower incidence of IFIs among autologous HCT recipients, those patients with any IFI risk factors should be considered intermediate risk for IFI and in most cases receive prophylaxis [10].

The incidence of IFIs among patients affected by acute leukemia and other myelo- and lympho-proliferative disorders vary by type of hematologic disorder. Of 881 Italian AML patients receiving intensive chemotherapy, 77 developed proven or probable IFI (8.7%): 54 (6.1%) were due to invasive mold infections and 23 (2.6%) were yeast infections [27]. In a retrospective review of 969 acute lymphocytic leukemia patients, 65 (6.7%) developed an IFI during induction chemotherapy: 26 (3.3%) IA, 33 (3.4%) invasive candidiasis and six other IFIs [28]. Among 773 Australian patients receiving antimold prophylaxis and undergoing treatment for lymphoproliferative disorders, 29 (3.8%) were diagnosed as having an IFI [29]. Patients with precursor lymphoid neoplasms had the highest IFI rates (29.4%) followed by patients with mature B-cell neoplasms, including small cell lymphocytic lymphoma/chronic lymphocytic leukemia (SLL/CLL) (7.8%), and diffuse large B-cell lymphoma (4.3%) [29].

While the duration and extent of neutropenia clearly correlates with the risk of IFI, large studies have elucidated multiple other significant risk factors (Table 25.2). It remains unclear how much each individual hazard may further compound IFI possibility. Knowledge of risk factors remains critical to identify the most vulnerable patients and to guide empiric and prophylactic strategies. Age over 65 years, the presence of chronic GvHD, CMV reactivation, receiving an unrelated donor allograft, and previous IFI consistently are identified as significant elements contributing to worse patient outcomes [5,10,22]. The Italian group SEIFEM (Sorveglianza Epidemiologica Infezioni Fungine Nelle Emopatie Maligne) provided recommendations to risk-stratify patients for likelihood of developing an IFI [10]. A scoring system and algorithm for risk stratifying patients was proposed although it has not been integrated into current guidelines. Allogeneic HCT recipients receiving unrelated allografts and those AML patients with baseline neutropenia, previous IFI, low complete remission probability, age >65 years, and pulmonary dysfunction as well as persons undergoing induction chemotherapy, and AML/MDS patients receiving salvage regimens were among

Table 25.2 Risk factors for the development of IFI

All patients	Graft-related factors	Post-HCT factors
Patient age >40 yrs. (or >65 yrs.)	Receipt of allogeneic HCT	Severe mucositis
Thrombocytopenia	Graft manipulation (e.g., CD34+ selection)	Development of ≥ grade 2 acute GvHD
Prior history of: Splenectomy; fungal infection; environmental exposure to fungus	Infused CD34+ hematopoietic cell dose ≤2 × 10⁶/kg	Development of chronic GvHD
Prolonged (>10 days) neutropenia (ANC < 500 cells/µL)	HLA-mismatched related donor	Lack of laminar air-flow in transplant room
Presence of viral disease (e.g., CMV)	Matched unrelated donor	
Mucosal fungal colonization	Use of UCB cells	
Use of systemic corticosteroids	Donor lymphocyte infusion	
Disrupted skin integrity	Multiple HCT	
Presence of a central venous catheter device	Transplantation using *in vivo* T-cell depletion (e.g., ATG-, alemtuzumab-containing regimens)	
Pulmonary dysfunction		
High-risk leukemia		
Baseline neutropenia		

Abbreviations: IFI, invasive fungal infection; HCT, hematopoietic stem cell transplantation; ANC, absolute neutrophil count; CMV, cytomegalovirus; HLA, human leukocyte antigen; UCB, umbilical cord blood; ATG, antithymocyte globulin; GvHD, graft-versus-host disease.

the highest risk groups. Although these patients were identified as having higher risk for IFIs, specific prophylactic or treatment recommendations still need to be refined.

Mortality rates

The IFI-attributable mortality has decreased progressively over the last decade for all patients, decreasing from 60%–70% for all IFIs to current rates of about 20%–30% [22]. Case-fatality rates for IA are roughly 48.5% for allogeneic HCT recipients, which has decreased from earlier rates of 70%–90% [22]. Mortality rates due to *Candida* sp. infections are lower among these patients, varying from 20% to 40% [30,31]. Disappointingly, one-year survival from infection by invasive non-*Aspergillus* mold infections is dismal, only reaching 15% with mucormycosis and 21% with fusariosis [6]. Use of non-myeloablative conditioning regimens, unfortunately, exhibit outcomes similar to ablative conditioning regimens [24]. Typically survival is significantly higher among patients receiving autologous HCT [10].

Time intervals for risk of IFIs

A tri-modal distribution for time to IFI occurrence has been noted with infections classified as early (during neutropenia), late (following engraftment) or very late (after 100 days post-HCT) [22]. *Candida* IFIs usually peak early, while IA typically begins prior to engraftment and continues into the second and third months after HCT, overlapping with treatment of GvHD if it develops. Over the past decade, very late infections are of increasing concern. The overall outcome of patients developing late or very late IFIs are poor, significantly higher than early IFIs, with a non-relapse mortality of 40% at 1-year [5].

T-cell depleted grafts are associated with delayed immune reconstitution and increased incidence of viral and fungal infections. A study by Mihu et al. in patients who underwent T-cell depleted HCT showed that beyond 40 days post-HCT, IA developed a median of 164 (range, 68–667) days after HCT [7]. The incidence of late onset IA among unmodified, T-cell depleted, or reduced-intensity conditioning HCT was 2.2%, 4%, and 6.8%, respectively.

IFIs caused by *Candida* and other yeasts are thought to be associated either with the transmigration of *Candida* sp. organisms across damaged mucosal surfaces, or via direct inoculation through use of indwelling venous catheters. By day 100 after HCT, most patients have recovered from barrier damage, have improving immunity and are able to control *Candida* infections. Conversely, invasive mold infections likely result from environmental exposure to *Aspergillosis* sp., *Fusarium* sp., and *Mucormycosis* sp. Effective preventive measures include high-efficiency particulate air (HEPA) filters and laminar airflow systems. Additionally, hospital water distribution systems have been implicated as reservoirs of opportunistic molds [32,33]. Post-HCT, minimization of potential exposures are needed including following hospital discharge [34].

MANAGEMENT OF IFIs

Treatment strategies for IFIs are outlined in Table 25.3. In addition to the use of an antifungal agent, treatment may include surgery (e.g., drainage, debridement) and attempts at immune enhancement through decreasing immune suppression or consideration of granulocyte transfusions [35]. Several of these tools will be discussed later in this chapter. Current antifungal agents are detailed in Table 25.4. The development and FDA approval of the new azole

Table 25.3 Treatment strategies for invasive fungal infections (IFIs)

Treatment strategy	Definitions	Goal
Prophylaxis (primary or secondary)	Administration of antifungal agent for prevention of IFI during the time period of high risk	Prevention
Treatment in empiric fashion	Administration of antifungal agent in patients with persistent fever despite broad-spectrum antibiotic therapy but no signs and symptoms of infection	Treatment
Preemptive therapy	Administration of antifungal agent in patients strongly suspected of having IFI due to fungal colonization, pulmonary/sinus symptoms, sepsis or radiologic findings compatible with IFIs, but no tissue documentation of IFI	Treatment
Definitive treatment of established IFI	Administration of antifungal agent when an IFI has been diagnosed	Treatment

Table 25.4 Class and properties of current antifungal agents

Antifungal agent and class	Spectrum	Formulations	Major toxicity/side effects
Polyenes			
Amphotericin B deoxylate	*Histoplasma, Coccidioides, Candida, Aspergillus, Blastomyces, Rhodotorula, Cryptococcus, Sporothrix schenckil, Mucor* species	IV	Nephrotoxicity, hypotension, tachypnea, nausea, diarrhea, headache, hepatotoxicity
Amphotericin B lipid complex	*Aspergillus, Zygomycetes, Fusarium, Cryptococcus,* and many hard-to-treat *Candida* species	IV	Nephrotoxicity (less than amphotericin B deoxylate)
Liposomal amphotericin B	*Aspergillus, Candida, Cryptococcus* species	IV	Nephrotoxicity (less than amphotericin B deoxylate)
Amphotericin B colloidal dispersion	*Aspergillus, Candida, Mucor, Cryptococcus* species	IV	Nephrotoxicity (less than amphotericin B deoxylate)
Azoles			
Fluconazole	*Candida, Cryptococcus* species	Oral suspension, tablet, IV	Hepatotoxicity, leukopenia, hypokalemia, dose reduction required in renal impairment
Itraconazole	*Blastomyces, Histoplasma, Aspergillus* species	Capsule	Gastrointestinal (nausea, vomiting, diarrhea), rash
Second generation azoles			
Voriconazole	*Aspergillus, Candida* species, *Scedosporium apiospermum, Fusarium* species	Oral suspension, tablet, IV	Abnormal vision, hepatotoxicity, fever, rash, drug–drug interactions
Posaconazole	*Aspergillus, Candida* species, rare mold infections	Oral suspension	Fever, headache, anemia, neutropenia, thrombocytopenia, diarrhea, nausea, vomiting, hypokalemia
Isavuconazole	*Aspergillus, Candida* species, *Scedosporium apiospermum, Fusarium* species, Mucorales	Capsule, IV	Hepatotoxicity, abnormal vision, fever, rash, fewer drug–drug interactions
Echinocandins			
Caspofungin	*Candida, Aspergillus* species	IV	Diarrhea, nausea, pyrexia, hepatotoxicity, rash
Micafungin	*Candida* species	IV	Nausea, vomiting, hypokalemia,
Anidulafungin	*Candida* species	IV	Rare (gastrointestinal)

Table 25.5 Recommendations for antifungal prophylaxis in high-risk hematologic malignancy patients or HCT recipients

Clinical condition	Recommendations
AML: Less-intensive induction or consolidation chemotherapy	Fluconazole 200 mg/day, from admission to resolution of neutropenia
AML: Intensive induction or consolidation or high-dose chemotherapy	Posaconazole 200 mg TID or itraconazole 200 mg BID, from first day of chemotherapy until resolution of neutropenia
Autologous HCT	Fluconazole 200–400 mg/day, from admission to resolution of neutropenia
Allogeneic HCT: Matched-related donor	Fluconazole 400 mg/day, from admission until day 75 after HCT
Allogeneic HCT: Mismatched, haploidentical or unrelated donor or umbilical cord blood cell graft	Posaconazole 200 mg TID or itraconazole 200 mg BID or fluconazole 400 mg/day, from the last day of conditioning to at least day 75 after HCT
Allogeneic HCT: Acute GvHD grade ≥2, or extensive chronic GvHD	Posaconazole 200 mg TID until resolution of GvHD with monitoring of cyclosporine or tacrolimus levels

Abbreviation: HCT, hematopoietic cell transplant.

isavuconazole represents important progress in the treatment of IFIs. It is well tolerated, has activity against yeasts, molds, and dimorphic fungi and has significantly fewer drug–drug interactions than other azoles. This property is especially important given the extensive drug–drug interactions seen among other azoles often used in patients receiving treatment for acute leukemia and for GvHD prophylaxis. Published studies for isavuconazole are encouraging, showing efficacy similar to voriconazole for invasive mold disease as well as demonstrating activity against mucormycosis [36–38]. Though not recommended as first-line therapy currently, it remains a reasonable option in patients who are intolerant to voriconazole or posaconazole and a potential option for resistant organisms.

Primary chemoprophylaxis of IFIs

As mortality rates with IFIs are high, patients considered at increased risk of IFI should receive antifungal prophylaxis as this approach demonstrates a clear decrease in mortality compared to placebo [39]. Nearly all post-transplant HCT patients receive some type of antifungal prophylaxis. Consideration of patient risk factors and the timing for the development of common pathogens guides prophylaxis employed. The risk of invasive candidiasis is significantly higher in the pre-engraftment period whereas invasive mold infection during pre-engraftment is rare in patients without previous infections. Most invasive mold infections occur later in the post-transplant period, usually in the context of significant GvHD [5,10,40,41]. In patients receiving reduced-intensity conditioning (RIC), the duration of neutropenia generally is shorter conferring lower risk as compared to myeloablative (MA) regimens, though

studies have not shown a difference in IFI incidence (14.8% vs. 13.7%, p = 0.89) [5,24]. Acute leukemia patients or those undergoing myeloablative HCT conditioning regimens are at considerable risk for developing prolonged neutropenia and subsequent IFI.

Recommendations for antifungal prophylaxis in hematologic malignancy patients or HCT recipients are detailed in Table 25.5. Available antifungal agents and recommended prophylaxis doses are detailed in Table 25.6. Recent antifungal randomized studies in those patients are shown in Table 25.7 [42–51].

PROPHYLAXIS IN THE PRE-ENGRAFTMENT PERIOD AND NEUTROPENIA FOR PATIENTS WITHOUT A PREVIOUS HISTORY OF IFIs

Azoles

Fluconazole remains the primary agent for prophylaxis for lower risk patients. It is reasonably well-tolerated, has 90% oral bioavailability, and primarily covers most Candida sp. Notably, C. glabrata has variable sensitivity, and C. krusei is resistant. Recommendations from the CDC, Infectious Diseases Society of America (IDSA), and the American Society for Blood and Marrow Transplantation (ASBMT) support its use in this setting. Their recommendations are supported by multiple, older randomized clinical trials (RCTs) comparing fluconazole to placebo that illustrated an overall survival benefit [34]. Duration of treatment is not defined, though treatment should continue at least through resolution of neutropenia; many clinicians advocate for continuing treatment through day 75 in allogeneic HCT patients based on a survival benefit seen in a post-hoc analysis of an RCT [52,53].

Table 25.6 Available antifungal agents and recommended prophylaxis doses

Antifungal agent	Trade name	Recommended prophylactic dose	Recommended treatment dose	Drug level monitoring
Polyenes				
Amphotericin B deoxylate	Fungizone®	0.3 mg/kg/day IV	0.3–1 mg/kg IV	No
Amphotericin B lipid complex	Abelcet®	1 mg/kg/day IV	5 mg/kg IV	No
Liposomal amphotericin B	AmBisome®	1 mg/kg/day IV	3 mg/kg IV	No
Amphotericin B colloidal dispersion	Amphotec™	1 mg/kg/day IV	3–4 mg/kg IV	No
Azoles				
Fluconazole	Diflucan®	100–400 mg/day IV/po	400 mg/day IV	No
Itraconazole	Sporanox®	200 mg/day IV	200 mg/day IV q12 hours	Yes
Second generation azoles				
Voriconazole	Vfend®	4 mg/kg IV q12 hours	6 mg/kg IV q12 hours for 24 hours, then 4 mg/kg IV q12 hours	Yes
Posaconazole	Noxafil®	200 mg po q8 hours	400 mg po q12 hours	Yes
		300 mg IV q12 for 24 hours then 300 mg/day	300 mg IV q12 for 24 hours then 300 mg/day	Yes
Posaconazole delayed-release capsule		300 mg po q12 for 24 hours then 300 mg/day	300 mg po q12 for 24 hours followed by 300 mg/day	Yes
Isavuconazole	Crescemba®	NA	200 mg po/IV q8 hours for 48 hours, then 200 mg/day	No
Echinocandins				
Caspofungin	Cancidas®	50 mg/day IV	70 mg/day IV loading dose, then 50 mg/day IV	No
Micafungin	Mycamine®	50 mg/day IV	100–150 mg/day	No
Anidulafungin	Eraxis®	NA	100–200 mg/day IV, then 50–100 mg/day IV	No

With the introduction of extended-spectrum azoles (itraconazole, voriconazole, posaconazole, and isavuconazole), there has been considerable interest in fluconazole comparative trials in the prophylactic setting. A multicenter, open-label RCT illustrated that itraconazole, when compared to fluconazole for primary prophylaxis until day 100 in HCT patients, significantly decreased proven IFI though no survival benefit was seen [43]. Another open-label, RCT suggested that itraconazole provided better mold coverage, but similar Candida sp. coverage, without a survival benefit [44]. Despite somewhat better efficacy, itraconazole prophylaxis is less attractive due to high rates of GI side effects resulting in poor tolerability.

A large, double-blind RCT compared voriconazole to fluconazole as primary prophylaxis in standard-risk patients and suggested a trend towards fewer IFIs in the voriconazole group though overall survival and fungal-free survival (FFS) were similar [45]. A post-hoc analysis of the study showed that AML patients undergoing allogeneic HCT had significantly fewer IFIs and improved FFS [45]. Compared to itraconazole in another trial, voriconazole had similar efficacy and was better tolerated [54]. These studies suggest that voriconazole is at least as effective fluconazole for yeast while also providing mold coverage. Reported breakthrough Zygomycetes IFIs during voriconazole prophylaxis represent a major concern for using this agent; notably, these infections were not identified in the large double-blind RCT of fluconazole versus voriconazole prophylaxis [45,55–58].

Posaconazole demonstrates superior efficacy compared to standard azole agents as prophylaxis in patients at high risk for IFIs [46,47]. In a randomized study of 602 neutropenic patients with AML or myelodysplastic syndrome (MDS), persons receiving posaconazole prophylaxis had a lower incidence of IFIs compared to those receiving either fluconazole or itraconazole (2% vs. 8%, p < 0.001 and 1% vs. 7%, p < 0.001) [47]. This benefit was seen throughout the entire

Table 25.7 Recent randomized studies involving antifungal prophylaxis in HCT recipients and neutropenic patients with hematologic malignancies

Reference	No. and type of patients	Comparison of antifungal agents	Efficacy	Statistical significance
[42]	837 Neutropenic (155 allo and 261 auto HSCT)	VOR 6 mg/kg IV q12 hours, then 3 mg/kg IV q12 hours vs. Lipo	VOR>Lipo	p = 0.02
[43]	144 Allo HCT	ITRA 200 mg IV q12 hours×2 d, then 200 mg IV q24 hours or 200 mg po q12 hours vs. FLU 400 mg/day IV/po	ITRA>FLU	p = 0.01
[44]	494 Auto HCT	ITRA 2.5 mg/kg bid po vs. FLU	ITRA>FLU	p = 0.03
[45]	600 Allo HCT	VOR 200 mg bid po vs. FLU 400 mg/day po	NS	
[46]	600 Allo HCT	POS 200 mg tid po vs. FLU 400 mg/day po	POS>FLU	1.0% vs. 5.9% IA, p = 0.001
[47]	660 Neutropenic	POS 200 mg tid po vs. either FLU 400 mg/day po or ITRA 200 mg bid po	POS>FLU or ITRA	1% vs. 7% IA, p < 0.001
[48]	882 (405 Auto and allo HCT)	MICA 50 mg/day IV vs. FLU 400 mg/day IV	MICA>FLU	p = 0.03
[49]	106 Allo HCT	MICA 150 mg/day IV vs. FLU 400 mg/day	NS	
[50]	283 Neutropenic HCT (56 Auto and 227Allo HCT)	MICA 50 mg/day IV vs. ITRA 5 mg/kg/day po	NS	
[51]	257 (110 Auto HCT and 140 Allo HCT)	MICA 50 mg/day IV vs. FLU 400 mg/day IV	NS	

Abbreviations: Auto, autologous; Allo, allogeneic; Lipo, liposomal amphotericin B; VOR, voriconazole; MICA, micafungin; FLU, fluconazole; POSA, posaconazole; IA, invasive aspergillosis; NS, not significant.

study period (5% vs. 11%, p = 0.003) and was associated with lower overall (p = 0.048) and IFI-related (p = 0.01) mortality. Other studies in neutropenic HCT patients and in HCT patients receiving treatment for GvHD have illustrated that posaconazole was more effective than fluconazole at preventing IA, IFI-related mortality, and breakthrough IFIs [46,59]. These data have led several groups to recommend posaconazole as prophylaxis in higher risk patients, especially those with or at high risk for GvHD [60]. Although posaconazole has considerable GI side effects and absorption issues, the relatively recently approved IV formulation and delayed release tablets may mitigate these concerns.

The newest triazole, isavuconazole, has not been extensively studied in the prophylactic setting though, due to its favorable side effect profile and pharmacodynamics, likely studies will be forthcoming. The lack of comparative studies and high cost significantly limit its use currently in the prophylactic setting.

Echinocandins

The echinocandins have demonstrated efficacy for primary prophylaxis of IFIs. In a double-blind RCT comparing micafungin to fluconazole in HCT patients in the pre-engraftment setting, micafungin was superior during the neutropenic phase with a lower likelihood of being switched to empiric antifungal therapy and fewer episodes of breakthrough aspergillosis (1.6% vs. 2.4%) [48]. In an

open-label RCT of 287 neutropenic HCT patients, compared to itraconazole, micafungin was shown to be non-inferior and better tolerated [50]. More patients treated with micafungin than itraconazole completed the RCT (82.9% versus 67.3%, respectively); fewer subjects in the micafungin group withdrew due to an adverse event (4.4% versus 21.1%) or drug-related adverse events (8% versus 26.5%) (p < 0.001) [50]. Limited studies have assessed the efficacy of caspofungin although retrospective and phase 2 data show that this agent has efficacy in both primary and secondary prophylaxis [61–63]. Mattiuzzi et al. compared caspofungin to itraconazole in 192 hematologic malignancy patients undergoing induction chemotherapy [64]. Caspofungin prophylaxis was comparable in efficacy to itraconazole without significant differences in IFIs, adverse events or mortality rates. Anidulafungin, another echinocandin, was found to be effective and safe in the prophylaxis of neutropenic children at high risk for IFIs [65]. Although as a group the echinocandins are attractive in the prophylactic setting due to their limited drug–drug interactions and favorable side effect profile, first-line use is limited by cost and only IV formulation.

Conclusions

A systematic review and meta-analysis of 5 trials, with a total of 2,147 patients, concluded that all second generation azoles (viz. posaconazole, voriconazole, and itraconazole) were superior to fluconazole at preventing proven/probable IFI. Posaconazole and voriconazole were superior to itraconazole for preventing IA. All-cause mortality was similar in all patients receiving mold-active prophylaxis [39]. In another recently published network meta-analysis of primary prophylaxis surveying 25 different double-blind trials from 1978 until 2010, posaconazole was shown to be the best overall prophylactic agent although voriconazole was superior to posaconazole at preventing *Candida* sp. infections [66]. Another meta-analysis confirmed the utility of posaconazole suggesting it has the highest probability of being most effective in the prophylactic setting [67].

Although newer-generation azoles and echinocandins have superior efficacy in some measures when compared to fluconazole for primary prophylaxis of IFIs, for patients at very low risk of IFIs, the increased cost and the lack of a clear mortality benefit continue to support the use of fluconazole. Though posaconazole has compelling data supporting its use for higher risk patients, likely long-term tolerability, drug costs, local IFI epidemiology, and route of administration will discriminate between mold-active agents. With the notable exception of isavuconazole, the more recent additions to the IFI armamentarium continue to have significant drug–drug interactions, especially with cyclophosphamide-based conditioning regimens and calcineurin inhibitors [68]. Table 25.8 details some important drug–drug interactions of common antifungal agents.

ANTIFUNGAL PROPHYLAXIS IN THE PRE-ENGRAFTMENT PERIOD FOR PATIENTS WITH A PREVIOUS HISTORY OF IFI

Mold-active agents are recommended as prophylaxis in patients with a prior history of an IFI [69–73]. No published RCTs examine secondary prophylaxis in patients with such a history. A recently published observational database study of 825 patients with a past history of IFI as compared to 10,247 control patients who underwent allogeneic HCT concluded that although pre-HCT IFI was associated with lower progression-free survival (PFS) (RR of relapse or death 1.24, 95% CI [1.11–1.38], p < 0.0001) and overall survival (OS) (RR 1.33, 95% CI [1.19–1.48], p < 0.0001), pre-HCT IFI does not appear to be a contraindication to allogeneic HCT due to significant survivorship [71]. Roughly 30% (95% CI 26%–34%) of patients with a prior history of IFI were alive 5 years following HCT and likely experienced a significant benefit from HCT. Eighty-seven percent of cases received antifungal prophylaxis with a higher proportion receiving mold-active agents. The authors noted that unfortunately information on prophylaxis versus changes in therapy could not be examined in this registry dataset. In the subset analysis, patients who received an HCT prior to 2001 had inferior OS and PFS compared to later cases, perhaps suggesting an improvement in outcomes among patients receiving newer antifungal agents [71]. Similar results were reported among patients with acute leukemia [72].

Table 25.8 Drug–drug interactions of antifungal agents and precaution measures

Antifungal agent	Requires monitoring of antifungal drug blood concentrations	Requires switching to alternative drug when used with	Contraindicated
Fluconazole	Cyclosporine, tacrolimus, phenytoin, warfarin, rifampin	Simvastatin, lovastatin	
Itraconazole	Cyclosporine, tacrolimus, digoxin, warfarin, carbamazepine, rifabutin, ritonavir, amprenavir, indinavir	Simvastatin, lovastatin, alprazolam, diazepam, triazolam, midazolam	Cyclophosphamide, vinca alkaloids, quinidine, ergot alkaloids, cisapride
Voriconazole	Cyclosporine, omeprazole, tacrolimus, warfarin, sulfonylureas, simvastatin, lovastatin, vinca alkaloids, calcium channel blockers, benzodiazepines, phenytoin		Cyclophosphamide, cisapride, ergot alkaloids, quinidine, sirolimus, terfenadine, carbamazepine, barbiturates, rifampin, rifabutin
Posaconazole	Cyclosporine, tacrolimus, venetoclax, calcium channel blockers, benzodiazepines, phenytoin, vincristine	Atorvastatin, lovastatin, simvastatin	Ergot alkaloids, sirolimus, terfenadine, carbamazepine, barbiturates, rifampin, rifabutin
Isavuconazole	Cyclosporine, tacrolimus, benzodiazepines, venetoclax, oxycodone, ibrutinib, metformin, fentanyl, digoxin, tocilizumab		Ketoconazole, carbamazepine, barbiturates, rifampin
Caspofungin	Rifampin, carbamazepine, dexamethasone, phenitoin, tacrolimus, cyclosporine		
Micafungin	Sirolimus, nifedipine		

ANTIFUNGAL PROPHYLAXIS IN THE POST-ENGRAFTMENT PERIOD

Similar to treatment decisions during pre-engraftment, decisions on antifungal prophylaxis in the post-engraftment period are driven by risk stratification and IFI epidemiology. As mentioned above, the duration for prophylaxis remains undefined. Older studies showed an overall improvement at 3 months after HCT when fluconazole prophylaxis continued through day 75 compared to placebo [53]. Protection against *Candida* sp. infection-related death persisted at 8 years post-HCT [52]. Breakthrough infections by fluconazole-resistant organisms, such as *Aspergillus* sp., *C. glabrata,* and *C. krusei,* remain a significant concern [74,75].

Two similar studies comparing itraconazole and fluconazole to prophylaxis through 180 days after HCT found no difference in OS; however, fewer IFIs occurred in the itraconazole group than in the fluconazole cohort (7% vs. 15% and 9% vs. 25%, respectively, p < 0.05 for both) [43,44]. Notably, patients receiving itraconazole experienced significantly more hepatotoxicity and nephrotoxicity that necessitated drug discontinuation (36% vs. 16%, p < 0.01) [44]. Patients receiving cyclophosphamide as part of a conditioning regimen or concomitant vincristine are especially vulnerable to complications with itraconazole [68,76].

In an international, randomized, double-blind study involving 600 hematologic disease patients, Ullmann et al. prospectively compared posaconazole versus fluconazole for infection prophylaxis at the onset of GvHD [46]. At the end of the fixed, 112-day treatment period, posaconazole was as effective as fluconazole in preventing all IFIs (5.3% vs. 9%, p = 0.07) but was superior to fluconazole in preventing proven or probable IA (2.3% vs. 7%, p = 0.006). Fewer overall breakthrough IFIs (2.4% vs. 7.6%, p = 0.004) were noted. In particular, IA occurred at a reduced incidence (1% vs. 5.9%, p = 0.001) in the posaconazole-treated cohort. Overall mortality was similar, but IFI-attributable deaths were marginally significantly reduced in the posaconazole group (1% vs. 4%, p = 0.046). Therefore, posaconazole prophylaxis has been recommended in the post-engraftment period for patients who are at risk for or develop GvHD [60]. For patients intolerant of triazoles, the echinocandins represent potential effective alternatives for prophylaxis in the post-engraftment period. Prophylactic therapy using low-dose amphotericin B deoxycholate is limited due to infusion-related side effects and drug-related toxicity [77].

ANTIFUNGAL PROPHYLAXIS FOR NEUTROPENIA IN HIGH-RISK HEMATOLOGIC MALIGNANCY

Antifungal prophylaxis recommendations for patients with neutropenia and high-risk hematologic malignancy are similar to allogeneic HCT recipients. Most data are derived from AML or MDS patients who are undergoing induction chemotherapy. In a multicenter, randomized study of 304 AML and MDS patients, posaconazole was compared to fluconazole or itraconazole [47]. Patients received prophylaxis with each cycle of chemotherapy for up to 12 weeks,

until recovery from neutropenia or development of IFI. Proven or probable IFIs were less frequent in posaconazole-treated patients (2% vs. 8%, p < 0.001). In addition, fewer IA infections were observed (1% vs. 7%, p < 0.001) and OS was significantly prolonged (p = 0.04) in the posaconazole-treated group. Serious adverse events (predominantly affecting the gastrointestinal tract) were higher in the posaconazole group (6% vs. 2%, p = 0.01). This study has led to the adoption of mold-active azoles as prophylaxis in many high-risk leukemia patients such as those who experienced a prior IFI, were receiving salvage chemotherapy, were age >65 years, had baseline neutropenia, significant pulmonary dysfunction, or had a low probability of obtaining complete remission during induction [78]. Despite a lack of comparative evidence, IV voriconazole or caspofungin may be considered as alternatives to posaconazole.

Duration of antifungal prophylaxis

Most studies demonstrate that for AML or for other hematologic malignancy patients undergoing chemotherapy or autologous HCT, prophylaxis should continue until the neutrophil count has recovered (>500–1,000/μL). For allogeneic HCT recipients, typically patients receive prophylaxis at least through day 75 post-HCT based on post-hoc data from a RCT utilizing fluconazole therapy [53]. Additionally, patients receiving daily corticosteroid doses equivalent to or greater than prednisolone 1 mg/kg for 0–13 days, or 0.25 to 1 mg/kg for 14–27 days are at increased risk of IA and should continue to receive antifungal prophylaxis [40]. The duration of posaconazole prophylaxis during GvHD treatment should reflect the grade of GvHD and the extent of immunosuppressive therapy required though optimal length of therapy is undefined [34].

Secondary prophylaxis after IFI

For patients with a prior IFI, secondary prophylaxis should be administered in the course of further cycles of chemotherapy or for HCT. Recurrent IFI rates are high among patients not given preventative therapy. For example, for patients with a history of IA undergoing HCT, a 62% progression rate was reported in those who did not receive antifungal therapy compared to 16% in treated patients [79]. Unfortunately, there are no large published studies that have been performed in this setting to guide therapeutic choices. In order to minimize the chance of recurrent IFI, clinicians should consider timing of the transplant, duration of prior antifungal therapy, hematopoietic cell source, feasibility of surgical resection of affected tissue, and possibility for use of donor granulocyte transfusions during the period of profound neutropenia. Data from the CIBMTR demonstrated inferior survival but insufficient evidence to preclude consideration of allogeneic HCT in patients with prior IFI [71]. This analysis documented a 24% one-year incidence of IFI in patients with prior IFI, compared to only 17% in patients without prior IFI (p < 0.001); however, details regarding treatment of the IFI and the secondary prophylaxis were limited. The optimal agent for secondary prophylaxis is unknown but clinicians must consider the type of prior IFI and additional risk factors.

Empiric therapy

Neutropenic fever is common among patients at risk for IFIs and often persists despite appropriate empiric antibacterial medication(s). Antifungal therapy administered in empiric fashion often is employed in the setting of persistent neutropenic fever (lasting more than 3–5 days) [80]. Updated IDSA guidelines suggest utilizing empiric antifungal therapy with either lipid formulation AmB or an echinocandin [21]. This recommendation is based, in part, on a multi-national, prospective randomized trial showing equal efficacy of caspofungin to liposomal AmB [81]. Rates of overall response, breakthrough IFI, and resolution of fever during neutropenia were similar between the treatment groups. In contrast, successful resolution of baseline infection and survival through 7 days of follow-up significantly favored the caspofungin group. This result primarily was due to treatment discontinuation as

a result of infusion-related events and nephrotoxicity in the liposomal AmB arm. A comparison of voriconazole and liposomal AmB found fewer breakthrough IFIs with voriconazole (p = 0.003) [42]. A recently published prospective, randomized trial comparing micafungin to itraconazole in the empiric treatment of neutropenic fever suggested non-inferiority of micafungin to itraconazole along with other favorable outcomes in the micafungin-treated group [51]. Posaconazole also was found to be an effective antifungal therapy when given in empiric fashion to 66 neutropenic, febrile patients, but comparative trials are lacking [82]. Empiric therapy should be continued for at least 14 days or until engraftment if patients have a protracted episode of neutropenia [21].

Treatment of IFIs

Table 25.9 details current evidence-based data on prophylactic and empiric use of antifungal agents. Many agents possess significant clinical antifungal activity for the treatment of IFIs. The type of IFI as well as factors such as patient tolerance, drug acquisition cost, and drug–drug interactions inform therapeutic choices.

Table 25.9 Current data on prophylactic and empiric antifungal therapy for neutropenic patients

Antifungal agent	Prophylactic therapy	Empiric therapy	Definitive therapy
Amphotericin B	Effective, but limited due to toxicity	1st line with Echinocandins, though concern for toxicity with long-term use	1st line in Zygomycosis
Fluconazole	1st line in lower risk patients; no mold activity	Strong evidence-based activity during pre-engraftment. Resistant species and pathogens limit use in post-engraftment period	Very limited due to resistant species and pathogens, may be appropriate as step-down therapy or in very low-risk patients
Itraconazole	Effective antifungal but limited due to drug–drug interactions, side effects	Effective antifungal, but limited due to drug–drug interactions, side effects	Strong evidence in Candidiasis, moderate evidence in salvage IA
Voriconazole	Moderate evidence-based efficacy, though limited in practice due to drug–drug interactions	Good evidence-based efficacy	1st line in IA, Strong evidence in Candidiasis
Posaconazole	1st line in higher risk patients	Effective, but comparative trials limited	Strong evidence in candidiasis, moderate evidence in salvage IA
Isavuconazole	Insufficient evidence	Insufficient evidence	Strong evidence for IA and mucormycosis
Micafungin	Good evidence-based efficacy, though limited by cost, IV formulation	1st line	Echinocandins 1st line for Candidiasis
Caspofungin	Good evidence-based efficacy, though limited by cost, IV formulation	1st line	Echinocandins 1st line for Candidiasis, Caspofungin less attractive in IA

Abbreviation: IA, invasive aspergillosis.

CANDIDIASIS

Updated guidelines from the European Conference on Infections in Leukemia (ECIL) and IDSA suggest the use of an enchinocandin for first-line treatment of invasive candidiasis in all hematologic malignancy patients [21,83]. This recommendation is supported by a quantitative review of 7 randomized trials involving more than 1,900 patients in which echinocandin use for treatment of invasive candidiasis was associated with a decreased mortality (Odds ratio 0.65, p = 0.02) when compared to other treatments [84]. Fluconazole is a reasonable alternative in very low risk patients. The transition, from an echinocandin to an azole (typically within 5–7 days), is reasonable if there is no evidence of ongoing candidemia, the isolates are demonstrated to be susceptible to the azole, and the patient is clinically stable. For patients with *C. glabrata*, the data suggest a transition to using high dose fluconazole (800 mg daily) or voriconazole as options. If *C. krusei* is the infecting species, then voriconazole is recommended for step-down therapy. Additionally, if patients warrant coverage against mold, IDSA guidelines support the use of voriconazole [21].

ASPERGILLOSIS

Updated IDSA guidelines continue to recommend voriconazole as first-line treatment [14]. Amphotericin and isavuconazole are recommended alternative treatments. Posaconazole and the echinocandins may have a role in salvage therapy. Notably, Maertens et al. recently published the results of the SECURE trial, a randomized, prospective phase-3 study comparing isavuconazole to voriconazole [36]. A total of 527 patients composed predominantly of hematologic malignancy or allogeneic HCT recipients were randomized. The population included those subjects with possible (36%), probable (39%), or proven (12%) invasive mold infection. The trial demonstrated non-inferiority of isavuconazole as compared to voriconazole. Furthermore, isavuconazole had significantly fewer drug–drug interactions as well as lower rates of hepatobiliary, eye, and skin adverse events. These data led the FDA to recommend approval of the agent for IA and prompted the ECIL guidelines to recommend either isavuconazole or voriconazole in the first-line setting [83]. Ongoing debate continues regarding the utility of combination antifungal therapy with voriconazole and an echinocandin for patients who have invasive pulmonary aspergillosis (IPA). Several small studies demonstrate the success of combining two antifungal therapy regimens, which incorporate new generation antifungals. However, IDSA guidelines recommend against combination therapy due to uncertain benefits, increased costs, and adverse effects [14,85,86]. Certainly further studies are needed. Single agent therapy with an echinocandin for IPA is discouraged unless all other agents are contraindicated. Patients with IPA require prolonged therapy, typically extending 6–12 weeks [14].

TREATMENT OF IFIs CAUSED BY RESISTANT FUNGI IN PATIENTS RECEIVING ANTIFUNGAL PROPHYLAXIS

Prolonged antifungal prophylaxis may be associated with the emergence of multiple resistant fungal species, such as *Zygomycetes*, *C. kruzei*, *Cunninghamella*, *Rhizopus*, disseminated *Aspergillus ustus*, and breakthrough *Candida glabrata* fungemia [87–91]. The emergence of resistant organism simply may be related to selection pressure, though some suggest sub-therapeutic antifungal serum concentrations are contributory. Trifilio et al. noted a weak correlation between lower plasma voriconazole levels and the emergence of resistant IFIs [92]. These and other similar observations have led to considerable discussion about the importance of monitoring voriconazole blood concentrations. A recent randomized, controlled trial investigating the effect of therapeutic drug monitoring showed a benefit, with a complete or partial response seen in 81% of monitored patients as compared to 57% response in non-monitored patients [93]. This result also is supported by observational studies correlating better drug levels with improved responses [94]. The optimal trough concentration remains controversial though most investigators support trough levels >1.0 µg/mL [94].

Treatment of resistant fungal infections is challenging as the efficacy of salvage therapy is disappointing. For example, as second-line antifungal therapy for IA, caspofungin [95], and posaconazole [96] demonstrate 40% to 50% CR or PR rates. Therapy should be individualized with consideration given to previous antifungal exposure, debridement, and options for decreasing immunosuppression [14]. Zygomycosis IFI remains a significant challenge due to the high morbidity and mortality. Recent ECIL recommendations support treatment with amphotericin B (with or without surgery) [83]. Alternative agents include posaconazole and isavuconazole [97]. A single-arm, open label trial suggested that isavuconazole has similar efficacy to amphotericin B and is well-tolerated [37]. *In vitro* studies confirm these findings [38]. A recently published retrospective review illustrated no difference in mortality in patients treated with monotherapy as compared to combination treatment [98].

Immune enhancement strategies

Restoration of immune function is critical for the effective treatment of IFIs though the utility of agents to enhance immune response remains unclear. Table 25.10 details several such treatment options [99–106]. Recombinant hematopoietic growth factors (e.g., granulocyte-macrophage colony-stimulating factor [GM-CSF] and G-CSF) shorten the duration of neutropenia after HCT and are commonly used in neutropenic patients undergoing chemotherapy. Disappointingly, data from a meta-analysis showed no improvement in the outcomes related to fungal disease in patients receiving these agents in prophylactic fashion [107].

Table 25.10 Immune enhancement strategies in hematologic malignancy patients and HSCT recipients with IFIs

Strategy	References	Study groups	Response rate (%)	Survival rate (%)
Clinical				
Donor granulocyte transfusions	[104]	HCT recipients	35	NS
	[101]	HCT recipients	NR	NS
	[102]	HCT recipients	57	28
	[103]	HCT recipients	43	NS
Recombinant				
IFN--y -1	[105]	HCT recipients	45	55
rh-M-CSF	[106]	HCT recipients	NR	27
Adoptive T cells	[108]	HCT recipients	90	NR
Preclinical model				
G-CSF	[99]	Murine		
GM-CSF	[100]	Murine		
Pentraxin	[109]	Murine		
DC vaccine	[110]	Murine		

Abbreviations: IFN, interferon; NS, not significant; NR, not reported; DC, dendritic cell; rh-M-CSF, recombinant macrophage-colony stimulating factor, G-CSF, granulocyte-colony stimulating factor; GM-CSF, granulocyte-macrophage-colony stimulating factor.

Though there is only weak evidence supporting their use in other settings, IDSA guidelines suggest that GM-CSF and G-CSF may be considered in patients with IA or in patients with persistent candidemia expected to have prolonged neutropenia [14]. The IDSA also notes that granulocyte infusions could be considered in this setting. Although accrual was low, data from a recently published randomized controlled trial illustrates no significant clinical benefit between patients receiving granulocyte transfusions and control groups [103]. Post-hoc analysis shows a trend toward better outcomes in patients receiving higher doses of granulocytes per kilogram.

CONCLUSIONS

Even with an expanding arsenal of better-tolerated and more effective agents administered in a prophylaxis setting, IFIs remain a highly feared complication of prolonged neutropenia and immunosuppression in patients who suffer from hematologic malignancy or who undergo HCT. Mortality rates of invasive infections remain unacceptably high, especially among patients who develop less common types of infections. Given multiple effective agents for prophylaxis, a further refined risk stratification strategy incorporating patient-, disease-, and treatment-related factors, local fungal epidemiology, drug toxicity, and drug–drug interactions is essential. Although the development of novel diagnostic tools is promising, a significant challenge remains at defining best practices for fungal surveillance as well as early and definitive diagnosis. The introduction of isavuconazole with a much better drug interaction profile and broadened spectrum of activity is welcomed. This experience highlights both the marginal gains that are being made in IFI treatment and the significant financial costs associated with utilizing newer agents. Although theoretically promising, use of immune enhancement strategies have been clinically disappointing. Perhaps larger gains in the treatment and prevention of IFIs will be made with improvement of immune function during HCT and leukemia treatments in the future.

REFERENCES

1. Pagano L, Caira M, Nosari A, Van Lint MT, Candoni A, Offidani M, et al. Fungal infections in recipients of hematopoietic stem cell transplants: Results of the SEIFEM B-2004 study—Sorveglianza epidemiologica infezioni fungine nelle emopatie maligne. *Clin Infect Dis* 2007;45(9):1161–1170.
2. Conen A, Weisser M, Jorg CO, Battegay M, Trampuz A, Frei R, et al. *Candida krusei*—A serious complication in patients with hematological malignancies: Successful treatment with caspofungin. *Transpl Infect Dis* 2008;10(1):66–70.
3. Winston DJ, Bartoni K, Territo MC, Schiller GJ. Efficacy, safety, and breakthrough infections sssociated with standard long-term posaconazole antifungal prophylaxis in allogeneic stem cell transplantation recipients. *Biol Blood Marrow Transplant* 2011;17(4):507–515.
4. Garnica M, da Cunha MO, Portugal R, Maiolino A, Colombo AL, Nucci M. Risk factors for invasive fusariosis in patients with acute myeloid leukemia and in hematopoietic cell transplant recipients. *Clin Infect Dis* 2015;60(6):875–880.

5. Montesinos P, Rodriguez-Veiga R, Boluda B, Martinez-Cuadron D, Cano I, Lancharro A, et al. Incidence and risk factors of post-engraftment invasive fungal disease in adult allogeneic hematopoietic stem cell transplant recipients receiving oral azoles prophylaxis. *Bone Marrow Transplant* 2015;50(11):1465–1472.

6. Riches ML, Trifilio S, Chen M, Ahn KW, Langston A, Lazarus HM, et al. Risk factors and impact of non-*Aspergillus* mold infections following allogeneic HCT: A CIBMTR infection and immune reconstitution analysis. *Bone Marrow Transplant* 2016;51(2):277–282.

7. Mihu CN, King E, Yossepovitch O, Taur Y, Jakubowski A, Pamer E, et al. Risk factors and attributable mortality of late aspergillosis after T-cell depleted hematopoietic stem cell transplantation. *Transpl Infect Dis* 2008;10(3):162–167.

8. Baddley JW, Stroud TP, Salzman D, Pappas PG. Invasive mold infections in allogeneic bone marrow transplant recipients. *Clin Infect Dis* 2001;32(9):1319–1324.

9. Schuster MG, Cleveland AA, Dubberke ER, Kauffman CA, Avery RK, Husain S, et al. Infections in hematopoietic cell transplant recipients: Results from the organ transplant infection project, a multicenter, prospective, cohort study. *Open Forum Infect Dis* 2017;4(2).

10. Pagano L, Busca A, Candoni A, Cattaneo C, Cesaro S, Fanci R, et al. Risk stratification for invasive fungal infections in patients with hematological malignancies: SEIFEM recommendations. *Blood Rev* 2017;31(2):17–29.

11. Marr KA, Carter RA, Crippa F, Wald A, Corey L. Epidemiology and outcome of mould infections in hematopoietic stem cell transplant recipients. *Clin Infect Dis* 2002;34(7):909–917.

12. Nucci M, Marr KA, Queiroz-Telles F, Martins CA, Trabasso P, Costa S, et al. Fusarium infection in hematopoietic stem cell transplant recipients. *Clin Infect Dis* 2004;38(9):1237–1242.

13. De Pauw B, Walsh TJ, Donnelly JP, Stevens DA, Edwards JE, Calandra T, et al. Revised definitions of invasive fungal disease from the European Organization for Research and Treatment of Cancer/Invasive Fungal Infections Cooperative Group and the National Institute of Allergy and Infectious Diseases Mycoses Study Group (EORTC/MSG) Consensus Group. *Clin Infect Dis* 2008;46(12):1813–1821.

14. Patterson TF, Thompson GR, Denning DW, Fishman JA, Hadley S, Herbrecht R, et al. Practice guidelines for the diagnosis and management of aspergillosis: 2016 Update by the Infectious Diseases Society of America. *Clin Infect Dis* 2016;63(4):E1–E60.

15. Leeflang MM, Debets-Ossenkopp YJ, Visser CE, Scholten R, Hooft L, Bijlmer HA, et al. Galactomannan detection for invasive aspergillosis in immunocompromized patients. *Cochrane Database Syst Rev* 2008(4): CD007394. DOI:10.1002/14651858.CD007394.

16. Chellapandian D, Lehrnbecher T, Phillips B, Fisher BT, Zaoutis TE, Steinbach WJ, et al. Bronchoalveolar lavage and lung biopsy in patients with cancer and hematopoietic stem-cell transplantation recipients: A systematic review and meta-analysis. *J Clin Oncol* 2015;33(5):501–509.

17. Hachem RY, Kontoyiannis DP, Chemaly RF, Jiang Y, Reitzel R, Raad I. Utility of galactomannan enzyme immunoassay and (1,3) beta-D-glucan in diagnosis of invasive fungal infections: Low sensitivity for *Aspergillus fumigatus* infection in hematologic malignancy patients. *J Clin Microbiol* 2009;47(1):129–133.

18. Aguado JM, Vazquez L, Fernandez-Ruiz M, Villaescusa T, Ruiz-Camps I, Barba P, et al. Serum galactomannan versus a combination of galactomannan and polymerase chain reaction-based *Aspergillus* DNA detection for early therapy of invasive aspergillosis in high-risk hematological patients: A randomized controlled trial. *Clin Infect Dis* 2015;60(3):405–414.

19. Arvanitis M, Anagnostou T, Mylonakis E. Galactomannan and polymerase chain reaction-based screening for invasive aspergillosis among high-risk hematology patients: A diagnostic meta-analysis. *Clin Infect Dis* 2015;61(8):1263–1272.

20. Clancy CJ, Nguyen MH. Finding the "missing 50%" of invasive candidiasis: How nonculture diagnostics will improve understanding of disease spectrum and transform patient care. *Clin Infect Dis* 2013;56(9):1284–1292.

21. Pappas PG, Kauffman CA, Andes DR, Clancy CJ, Marr KA, Ostrosky-Zeichner L, et al. Clinical practice guideline for the management of candidiasis: 2016 Update by the Infectious Diseases Society of America. *Clin Infect Dis* 2016;62(4):E1–E50.

22. Girmenia C, Raiola AM, Piciocchi A, Algarotti A, Stanzani M, Cudillo L, et al. Incidence and outcome of invasive fungal diseases after allogeneic stem cell transplantation: A prospective study of the Gruppo Italian Trapianto Midollo Osseo (GITMO). *Biol Blood Marrow Transplant* 2014;20(6):872–880.

23. Sun YQ, Meng FY, Han MZ, Zhang X, Yu L, Huang H, et al. Epidemiology, management, and outcome of invasive fungal disease in patients undergoing hematopoietic stem cell transplantation in china: A multicenter prospective observational study. *Biol Blood Marrow Transplant* 2015;21(6):1117–1126.

24. Hagen EA, Stern H, Porter D, Duffy K, Foley K, Luger S, et al. High rate of invasive fungal infections following nonmyeloablative allogeneic transplantation. *Clin Infect Dis* 2003;36(1):9–15.

25. Fukuda T, Boeckh M, Carter RA, Sandmaier BM, Maris MB, Maloney DG, et al. Risks and outcomes of invasive fungal infections in recipients of allogeneic hematopoietic stem cell transplants after nonmyeloablative conditioning. *Blood* 2003;102(3):827–833.

26. Morgan J, Wannemuehler KA, Marr KA, Hadley S, Kontoyiannis DP, Walsh TJ, et al. Incidence of invasive aspergillosis following hematopoietic stem cell and solid organ transplantation: Interim results of a prospective multicenter surveillance program. *Med Mycol.* 2005;43:S49–S58.

27. Caira M, Candoni A, Verga L, Busca A, Delia M, Nosari A, et al. Pre-chemotherapy risk factors for invasive fungal diseases: Prospective analysis of 1,192 patients with newly diagnosed acute myeloid leukemia (SEIFEM 2010-a multicenter study). *Haematologica* 2015;100(2):284–292.

28. Mariette C, Tavernier E, Hocquet D, Huynh A, Isnard F, Legrand F, et al. Epidemiology of invasive fungal infections during induction therapy in adults with acute lymphoblastic leukemia: A GRAALL-2005 study. *Leuk Lymphoma* 2017;58(3):586–593.

29. Teng JC, Slavin MA, Teh BW, Lingaratnam SM, Ananda-Rajah MR, Worth LJ, et al. Epidemiology of invasive fungal disease in lymphoproliferative disorders. *Haematologica* 2015;100(11):E462–E466.

30. Marr KA, Seidel K, White TC, Bowden RA. Candidemia in allogeneic blood and marrow transplant recipients: Evolution of risk factors after the adoption of prophylactic fluconazole. *Scand J Infect Dis* 2000;181(1):309–316.

31. Girmenia C, Barosi G, Piciocchi A, Arcese W, Aversa F, Bacigalupo A, et al. Primary prophylaxis of invasive fungal diseases in allogeneic stem cell transplantation: Revised recommendations from a consensus process by Gruppo Italiano Trapianto Midollo Osseo (GITMO). *Biol Blood Marrow Transplant* 2014;20(8):1080–1088.

32. Anaissie EJ, Kuchar RT, Rex JH, Francesconi A, Kasai M, Muller FMC, et al. Fusariosis associated with pathogenic *Fusarium* species colonization of a hospital water system: A new paradigm for the epidemiology of opportunistic mold infections. *Clin Infect Dis* 2001;33(11):1871–1878.

33. Anaissie EJ, Stratton SL, Dignani MC, Summerbell RC, Rex JH, Monson TP, et al. Pathogenic *Aspergillus* species recovered from a hospital water system: A 3-year prospective study. *Clin Infect Dis* 2002;34(6):780–789.

34. Tomblyn M, Chiller T, Einsele H, Gress R, Sepkowitz K, Storek J, et al. Guidelines for preventing infectious complications among hematopoietic cell transplantation recipients: A global perspective. *Biol Blood Marrow Transplant* 2009;15(10):1143–1238.

35. Pappas PG. Immunotherapy for invasive fungal infections: From bench to bedside. *Drug Resist Updat* 2004;7(1):3–10.

36. Maertens JA, Raad, II, Marr KA, Patterson TF, Kontoyiannis DP, Cornely OA, et al. Isavuconazole versus voriconazole for primary treatment of invasive mould disease caused by *Aspergillus* and other filamentous fungi (SECURE): A phase 3, randomised-controlled, non-inferiority trial. *Lancet* 2016;387(10020):760–769.

37. Marty FM, Ostrosky-Zeichner L, Cornely OA, Mullane KM, Perfect JR, Thompson GR, et al. Isavuconazole treatment for mucormycosis: A single-arm open-label trial and case–control analysis. *Lancet Infect Dis* 2016;16(7):828–837.

38. Verweij PE, Gonzalez GM, Wiederhold NP, Lass-Florl C, Warn P, Heep M, et al. *In vitro* antifungal activity of isavuconazole against 345 mucorales isolates collected at study centers in eight countries. *J Chemother* 2009;21(3):272–281.

39. Bow EJ, Vanness DJ, Slavin M, Cordonnier C, Cornely OA, Marks DI, et al. Systematic review and mixed treatment comparison meta-analysis of randomized clinical trials of primary oral antifungal prophylaxis in allogeneic hematopoietic cell transplant recipients. *BMC Infect Dis* 2015;15:128.

40. Thursky K, Byrnes G, Grigg A, Szer J, Slavin M. Risk factors for post-engraftment invasive aspergillosis in allogeneic stem cell transplantation. *Bone Marrow Transplant* 2004;34(2):115–121.

41. Grow WB, Moreb JS, Roque D, Manion K, Leather H, Reddy V, et al. Late onset of invasive *Aspergillus* infection in bone marrow transplant patients at a university hospital. *Bone Marrow Transplant* 2002;29(1):15–19.

42. Walsh TJ, Pappas P, Winston DJ, Lazarus HM, Petersen F, Raffalli J, et al. Voriconazole compared with liposomal amphotericin B for empirical antifungal therapy in patients with neutropenia and persistent fever. *N Engl J Med* 2002;346(4):225–234.

43. Winston DJ, Maziarz RT, Chandrasekar PH, Lazarus HM, Goldman M, Blumer JL, et al. Intravenous and oral itraconazole versus intravenous and oral fluconazole for long-term antifungal prophylaxis in allogeneic hematopoietic stem-cell transplant recipients—A multicenter, randomized trial. *Ann Intern Med* 2003;138(9):705–713.

44. Marr KA, Crippa F, Leisenring W, Hoyle M, Boeckh M, Balajee SA, et al. Itraconazole versus fluconazole for prevention of fungal infections in patients receiving allogeneic stem cell transplants. *Blood* 2004;103(4):1527–1533.

45. Wingard JR, Carter SL, Walsh TJ, Kurtzberg J, Small TN, Baden LR, et al. Randomized, double-blind trial of fluconazole versus voriconazole

for prevention of invasive fungal infection after allogeneic hematopoietic cell transplantation. *Blood* 2010;116(24):5111–5118.

46. Ullmann AJ, Lipton JH, Vesole DH, Chandrasekar P, Langston A, Tarantolo SR, et al. Posaconazole or fluconazole for prophylaxis in severe graft-versus-host disease. *N Engl J Med* 2007;356(4):335–347.

47. Cornely OA, Maertens J, Winston DJ, Perfect J, Ullmann AJ, Walsh TJ, et al. Posaconazole vs. fluconazole or itraconazole prophylaxis in patients with neutropenia. *N Engl J Med* 2007;356(4):348–359.

48. van Burik JAH, Ratanatharathorn V, Stepan DE, Miller CB, Lipton JH, Vesole DH, et al. Micafungin versus fluconazole for prophylaxis against invasive fungal infections during neutropenia in patients undergoing hematopoietic stem cell transplantation. *Clin Infect Dis* 2004;39(10):1407–1416.

49. Hiramatsu Y, Maeda Y, Fujii N, Saito T, Nawa Y, Hara M, et al. Use of micafungin versus fluconazole for antifungal prophylaxis in neutropenic patients receiving hematopoietic stem cell transplantation. *Int J Hematol* 2008;88(5):588–595.

50. Huang XJ, Chen H, Han MZ, Zou P, Wu DP, Lai YR, et al. Multicenter, randomized, open-label study comparing the efficacy and safety of micafungin versus itraconazole for prophylaxis of invasive fungal infections in patients undergoing hematopoietic stem cell transplant. *Biol Blood Marrow Transplant* 2012;18(10):1509–1516.

51. Jeong SH, Kim DY, Jang JH, Mun YC, Choi CW, Kim SH, et al. Efficacy and safety of micafungin versus intravenous itraconazole as empirical antifungal therapy for febrile neutropenic patients with hematological malignancies: A randomized, controlled, prospective, multicenter study. *Ann Hematol* 2016;95(2):337–344.

52. Marr KA, Seidel K, Slavin MA, Bowden RA, Schoch HG, Flowers MED, et al. Prolonged fluconazole prophylaxis is associated with persistent protection against candidiasis-related death in allogeneic marrow transplant recipients: Long-term follow-up of a randomized, placebo-controlled trial. *Blood* 2000;96(6):2055–2061.

53. Slavin MA, Osborne B, Adams R, Levenstein MJ, Schoch HG, Feldman AR, et al. Efficacy and safety of fluconazole prophylaxis for fungal-infections after marrow transplantation—A prospective, randomized, double-blind-study. *J Infect Dis* 1995;171(6):1545–1552.

54. Marks DI, Pagliuca A, Kibbler CC, Glasmacher A, Heussel CP, Kantecki M, et al. Voriconazole versus itraconazole for antifungal prophylaxis following allogeneic haematopoietic stem-cell transplantation. *Br J Haematol* 2011;155(3):318–327.

55. Siwek GT, Dodgson KJ, de Magalhaes-Silverman M, Bartelt LA, Kilborn SB, Hoth PL, et al. Invasive zygomycosis in hematopoietic stem cell transplant recipients receiving voriconazole prophylaxis. *Clin Infect Dis* 2004;39(4):584–587.

56. Imhof A, Balajee SA, Fredricks DN, Englund JA, Marr KA. Breakthrough fungal infections in stem cell transplant recipients receiving voriconazole. *Clin Infect Dis* 2004;39(5):743–746.

57. Marty FM, Cosimi LA, Baden LR. Breakthrough zygomycosis after voriconazole treatment in recipients of hematopoietic stem-cell transplants. *N Engl J Med* 2004;350(9):950–952.

58. Vigouroux S, Morin O, Moreau P, Mechinaud F, Morineau N, Mahe B, et al. Zygomycosis after prolonged use of voriconazole in immunocompromised patients with hematologic disease: Attention required. *Clin Infect Dis* 2005;40(4):E35–E37.

59. Sanchez-Ortega I, Patino B, Arnan M, Peralta T, Parody R, Gudiol C, et al. Clinical efficacy and safety of primary antifungal prophylaxis with posaconazole vs itraconazole in allogeneic blood and marrow transplantation. *Bone Marrow Transplant* 2011;46(5):733–739.

60. Hahn J, Stifel F, Reichle A, Holler E, Andreesen R. Clinical experience with posaconazole prophylaxis—A retrospective analysis in a haematological unit. *Mycoses* 2011;54:12–16.

61. Vehreschild JJ, Sieniawski M, Reuter S, Arenz D, Reichert D, Maertens J, et al. Efficacy of caspofungin and itraconazole as secondary antifungal prophylaxis: Analysis of data from a multinational case registry. *Int J Antimicrob Agents* 2009;34(5):446–450.

62. Chou LS, Lewis RE, Ippoliti C, Champlin RE, Kontoyiannis DP. Caspofungin as primary antifungal prophylaxis in stem cell transplant recipients. *Pharmacotherapy* 2007;27(12):1644–1650.

63. de Fabritiis P, Spagnoli A, Di Bartolomeo P, Locasciulli A, Cudillo L, Milone G, et al. Efficacy of caspofungin as secondary prophylaxis in patients undergoing allogeneic stem cell transplantation with prior pulmonary and/or systemic fungal infection. *Bone Marrow Transplant.* 2007;40(3):245–249.

64. Mattiuzzi GN, Alvarado G, Giles FJ, Ostrosky-Zeichner L, Cortes J, O'Brien S, et al. Open-label, randomized comparison of itraconazole versus caspofungin for prophylaxis in patients with hematologic malignancies. *Antimicrob Agents Chemother* 2006;50(1):143–147.

65. Benjamin DK, Driscoll T, Seibel NL, Gonzalez CE, Roden MM, Kilaru R, et al. Safety and pharmacokinetics of intravenous anidulafungin in children with neutropenia at high risk for invasive fungal infections. *Antimicrob Agents Chemother* 2006;50(2):632–638.

66. Leonart LP. A network meta-analysis of primary prophylaxis for invasive fungal infection in haematological patients. *J Clin Pharm Ther* 2017; 42(5):530–538.

67. Pechlivanoglou P, Le HH, Daenen S, Snowden JA, Postma MJ. Mixed treatment comparison of prophylaxis against invasive fungal infections in neutropenic patients receiving therapy for haematological malignancies: A systematic review. *J Antimicrob Chemother* 2014;69(1):1–11.

68. Marr KA, Leisenring W, Crippa F, Slattery JT, Corey L, Boeckh M, et al. Cyclophosphamide metabolism is affected by azole antifungals. *Blood* 2004;103(4):1557–1559.

69. Abernethy AP, Zafar SY, Uronis H, Wheeler JL, Coan A, Rowe K, et al. Validation of the Patient Care Monitor (Version 2.0): A review of system assessment instrument for cancer patients. *J Pain Symptom Manage* 2010;40(4):545–558.

70. Hill BT, Kondapalli L, Artz A, Smith S, Rich E, Godley L, et al. Successful allogeneic transplantation of patients with suspected prior invasive mold infection. *Leuk Lymphoma* 2007;48(9):1799–1805.

71. Maziarz RT, Brazauskas R, Chen M, McLeod AA, Martino R, Wingard JR, et al. Pre-existing invasive fungal infection is not a contraindication for allogeneic HSCT for patients with hematologic malignancies: A CIBMTR study. *Bone Marrow Transplant* 2017;52(2):270–278.

72. Penack O, Tridello G, Hoek J, Socie G, Blaise D, Passweg J, et al. Influence of pre-existing invasive aspergillosis on allo-HSCT outcome: A retrospective EBMT analysis by the Infectious Diseases and Acute Leukemia Working Parties. *Bone Marrow Transplant* 2016;51(3):418–423.

73. Kruger WH, Russmann B, de Wit M, Kroger N, Renges H, Sobottka I, et al. Haemopoietic cell transplantation of patients with a history of deep or invasive fungal infection during prophylaxis with liposomal amphotericin B. *Acta Haematol* 2005;113(2):104–108.

74. Marr KA, White TC, vanBurik JAH, Bowden RA. Development of fluconazole resistance in *Candida albicans* causing disseminated infection in a patient undergoing marrow transplantation. *Clin Infect Dis* 1997;25(4):908–910.

75. Wingard JR, Merz WG, Rinaldi MG, Miller CB, Karp JE, Saral R. Association of *Torulopsis glabrata* infections with fluconazole prophylaxis in neutropenic bone marrow transplant patients. *Antimicrob Agents Chemother* 1993;37(9):1847–1849.

76. Gillies J, Hung KA, Fitzsimons E, Soutar R. Severe vincristine toxicity in combination with itraconazole. *Clin Lab Haematol* 1998;20(2):123–124.

77. Barrett JP, Vardulaki KA, Conlon C, Cooke J, Daza-Ramirez P, Evans EGV, et al. A systematic review of the antifungal effectiveness and tolerability of amphotericin B formulations. *Clin Ther* 2003;25(5):1295–1320.

78. Nucci M, Anaissie E. How we treat invasive fungal diseases in patients with acute leukemia: The importance of an individualized approach. *Blood* 2014;124(26):3858–3869.

79. Sipsas NV, Kontoyiannis DP. Clinical issues regarding relapsing aspergillosis and the efficacy of secondary antifungal prophylaxis in patients with hematological malignancies. *Clin Infect Dis* 2006;42(11):1584–1591.

80. Wingard JR. Empirical antifungal therapy in treating febrile neutropenic patients. *Clin Infect Dis* 2004;39:S38–S43.

81. Walsh TJ, Teppler H, Donowitz GR, Maertens JA, Baden LR, Dmoszynska A, et al. Caspofungin versus liposomal amphotericin B for empirical antifungal therapy in patients with persistent fever and neutropenia. *N Engl J Med* 2004;351(14):1391–1402.

82. Ullmann AJ, Cornely OA, Burchardt A, Hachem R, Kontoyiannis DP, Topelt K, et al. Pharmacokinetics, safety, and efficacy of posaconazole in patients with persistent febrile neutropenia or refractory invasive fungal infection. *Antimicrob Agents Chemother* 2006;50(2):658–666.

83. Tissot F, Agrawal S, Pagano L, Petrikkos G, Groll AH, Skiada A, et al. ECIL-6 guidelines for the treatment of invasive candidiasis, aspergillosis and mucormycosis in leukemia and hematopoietic stem cell transplant patients. *Haematologica* 2017;102(3):433–444.

84. Andes DR, Safdar N, Baddley JW, Playford G, Reboli AC, Rex JH, et al. Impact of treatment strategy on outcomes in patients with candidemia and other forms of invasive candidiasis: A patient-level quantitative review of randomized trials. *Clin Infect Dis* 2012;54(8):1110–1122.

85. Safdar A, Rodriguez G, Rolston KVI, O'Brien S, Khouri IF, Shpall EJ, et al. High-dose caspofungin combination antifungal therapy in patients with hematologic malignancies and hematopoietic stem cell transplantation. *Bone Marrow Transplant* 2007;39(3):157–164.

86. Gahn B, Schub N, Repp R, Gramatzki M. Triple antifungal therapy for severe systemic candidiasis allowed performance of allogeneic stem cell transplantation. *Eur J Med Res* 2007;12(8):337–340.

87. Girmenia C, Moleti ML, Micozzi A, Iori AP, Barberi W, Foa R, et al. Breakthrough *Candida krusei* fungemia during fluconazole prophylaxis followed by breakthrough zygomycosis during caspofungin therapy in a patient with severe aplastic anemia who underwent stem cell transplantation. *J Clin Microbiol* 2005;43(10):5395–5396.

88. Kontoyiannis DP, Marr KA, Park BJ, Alexander BD, Anaissie EJ, Walsh TJ, et al. Prospective surveillance for invasive fungal infections in hematopoietic stem cell transplant recipients, 2001–2006: Overview of

the Transplant-Associated Infection Surveillance Network (TRANSNET) database. *Clin Infect Dis* 2010;50(8):1091–1100.

89. Alexander BD, Schell WA, Miller JL, Long GD, Perfect JR. *Candida glabrata* fungemia in transplant patients receiving voriconazole after fluconazol. *Transplantation* 2005;80(6):868–871.

90. Trifilio S, Singhal S, Williams S, Frankfurt O, Gordon L, Evens A, et al. Breakthrough fungal infections after allogeneic hematopoietic stem cell transplantation in patients on prophylactic voriconazole. *Bone Marrow Transplant* 2007;40(5):451–456.

91. Pavie J, Lacroix C, Hermoso DG, Robin M, Ferry C, Bergeron A, et al. Breakthrough disseminated *Aspergillus ustus* infection in allogeneic hematopoietic stem cell transplant recipients receiving voriconazole or caspofungin prophylaxis. *J Clin Microbiol* 2005;43(9):4902–4904.

92. Trifilio S, Pennick G, Pi J, Zook J, Golf M, Kaniecki K, et al. Monitoring plasma voriconazole levels may be necessary to avoid subtherapeutic levels in hematopoietic stem cell transplant recipients. *Cancer* 2007;109(8):1532–1535.

93. Park WB, Kim NH, Kim KH, Lee SH, Nam WS, Yoon SH, et al. The effect of therapeutic drug monitoring on safety and efficacy of voriconazole in invasive fungal infections: A randomized controlled trial. *Clin Infect Dis* 2012;55(8):1080–1087.

94. Troke PF, Hockey HP, Hope WW. Observational study of the clinical efficacy of voriconazole and its relationship to plasma concentrations in patients. *Antimicrob Agents Chemother* 2011;55(10):4782–4788.

95. Maertens J, Raad I, Petrikkos G, Boogaerts M, Selleslag D, Petersen FB, et al. Efficacy and safety of caspofungin for treatment of invasive aspergillosis in patients refractory to or intolerant of conventional antifungal therapy. *Clin Infect Dis* 2004;39(11):1563–1571.

96. Walsh TJ, Raad I, Patterson TF, Chandrasekar P, Donowitz GR, Graybill R, et al. Treatment of invasive aspergillosis with posaconazole in patients who are refractory to or intolerant of conventional therapy: An externally controlled trial. *Clin Infect Dis* 2007;44(1):2–12.

97. van Burik JAH, Hare RS, Solomon HF, Corrado ML, Kontoyiannis DP. Posaconazole is effective as salvage therapy in zygomycosis: A retrospective summary of 91 cases. *Clin Infect Dis* 2006;42(7):E61–E65.

98. Kyvernitakis A, Torres HA, Jiang Y, Chamilos G, Lewis RE, Kontoyiannis DP. Initial use of combination treatment does not impact survival of 106 patients with haematologic malignancies and mucormycosis: A propensity score analysis. *Clin Microbiol Infect* 2016;22(9):811.e1.

99. Sionov E, Mendlovic S, Segal E. Experimental systemic murine aspergillosis: Treatment with polyene and caspofungin combination and G-CSF. *J Antimicrob Chemother* 2005;56(3):594–597.

100. Brummer E, Maqbool A, Stevens DA. *In vivo* GM-CSF prevents dexamethasone suppression of killing of *Aspergillus fumigatus* conidia by bronchoalveolar macrophages. *J Leukoc Biol* 2001;70(6):868–872.

101. Hubel K, Carter RA, Liles WC, Dale DC, Price TH, Bowden RA, et al. Granulocyte transfusion therapy for infections in candidates and recipients of HPC transplantation: A comparative analysis of feasibility and outcome for community donors versus related donors. *Transfusion* 2002;42(11):1414–1421.

102. Price TH, Bowden RA, Boeckh M, Bux J, Nelson K, Liles WC, et al. Phase I/II trial of neutrophil transfusions from donors stimulated with G-CSF and dexamethasone for treatment of patients with infections in hematopoietic stem cell transplantation. *Blood* 2000;95(11):3302–3309.

103. Price TH, Boeckh M, Harrison RW, McCullough J, Ness PM, Strauss RG, et al. Efficacy of transfusion with granulocytes from G-CSF/dexamethasone-treated donors in neutropenic patients with infection. *Blood* 2015;126(18):2153–2161.

104. Safdar A, Hanna HA, Boktour M, Kontoyiannis DP, Hachem R, Lichtiger B, et al. Impact of high-dose granulocyte transfusions in patients with cancer with candidemia—Retrospective case–control analysis of 491 episodes of *Candida* species bloodstream infections. *Cancer* 2004;101(12):2859–2865.

105. Safdar A, Rodriguez GH, Lichtiger B, Dickey BF, Kontoyiannis DP, Freireich EJ, et al. Recombinant interferon gamma 1b immune enhancement in 20 patients with hematologic malignancies and systemic opportunistic infections treated with donor granulocyte transfusions. *Cancer* 2006;106(12):2664–2671.

106. Nemunaitis J, Shannondorcy K, Appelbaum FR, Meyers J, Owens A, Day R, et al. Long-term follow-up of patients with invasive fungal disease who received adjunctive therapy with recombinant human macrophage-colony-stimulating factor. *Blood* 1993;82(5):1422–1427.

107. Sung L, Nathan PC, Alibhai SMH, Tomlinson GA, Beyene J. Meta-analysis: Effect of prophylactic hematopoietic colony-stimulating factors on mortality and outcomes of infection. *Ann Intern Med* 2007;147(6):400–411.

108. Perruccio K, Tosti A, Burchielli E, Topini F, Ruggeri L, Carotti A, et al. Transferring functional immune responses to pathogens after haploidentical hematopoietic transplantation. *Blood* 2005;106(13):4397–4406.

109. Gaziano R, Bozza S, Bellocchio S, Perruccio K, Montagnoli C, Pitzurra L, et al. Anti-*Aspergillus fumigatus* efficacy of pentraxin 3 alone and in combination with antifungals. *Antimicrob Agents Chemother* 2004;48(11):4414–4421.

110. Bozza S, Perruccio K, Montagnoli C, Gaziano R, Bellocchio S, Burchielli E, et al. A dendritic cell vaccine against invasive aspergillosis in allogeneic hematopoietic transplantation. *Blood* 2003;102(10):3807–3814.

26

Antifungal use in transplant recipients: Selection, administration, and monitoring

RICHARD H. DREW, MARY L. TOWNSEND, MELANIE W. POUND, AND STEVEN W. JOHNSON

INTRODUCTION

Invasive fungal infections (IFIs) cause significant morbidity and mortality in both hematologic stem cell transplant (HSCT) and solid organ transplant (SOT) recipients. For example, the 12-month incidence of first IFIs among HSCT recipients was 7.7 cases per 100 transplants for matched unrelated allogeneic, 8.1 cases per 100 transplants for mismatched-related allogeneic, 5.8 cases per 100 transplants for matched-related allogeneic, and 1.2 cases per 100 transplants for autologous HSCT. Invasive aspergillosis (43%), invasive candidiasis (28%), and zygomycosis (now known as mucormycosis) (8%) were the most common IFIs in these patients [1]. In SOT recipients, invasive candidiasis (53%), invasive aspergillosis (19%), cryptococcosis (8%), non-*Aspergillus* molds (8%), endemic fungi (5%), and mucormycosis (2%) were the most common IFIs, occurring at a cumulative incidence between 1.3%–11.6% (depending upon transplant type) [2].

HSCT and SOT recipients at highest risk of IFIs should receive antifungals as prophylaxis [3,4]. Selection of the optimal antifungal should be based on patient- and drug-specific factors, including (but not limited to) degree and duration of immunosuppression, transplant type, comorbidities

(notably cytomegalovirus (CMV) infections and graft-vs-host disease), organ function, safety and efficacy of the antifungal selected, and likely fungal pathogens. However, based on such criteria, none of the agents currently available would be considered "ideal." Appropriate selection, dosing and timely administration of antifungals is also essential to transplant recipients with IFIs, especially those with severe, invasive forms of the disease [5,6]. However, several challenges exist in optimizing IFI therapy for HSCT and SOT transplant recipients. Diagnostic uncertainty often leads to delays in therapy, given the nonspecific nature of many presenting signs and symptoms of IFIs in these patients. Prior exposure to antifungals (either as prevention or previous treatment) can increase the risk of drug resistance to select agents (notably echinocandins and azoles) [7] and decrease the sensitivity of some of the diagnostic techniques, such as the galactomannan assay [8]. Selection and administration of antifungals may also be significantly influenced by the limited ability to take oral therapy, organ dysfunction, treatment-limiting drug toxicities, and drug interactions seen with select antifungals [9]. As a result of these complexities, significant variation can be observed in both the prevention [10–12] and treatment [10,12] of IFIs in both HSCT and SOT recipients.

This chapter provides an overview of agents for systemic fungal infections. Our objective is to provide sufficient information to guide clinicians as to the selection, dosing, and administration of these agents for the prevention and treatment of IFIs in HSCT and SOT recipients. Readers are referred to other chapters in this text regarding disease-specific treatment recommendations.

ANTIFUNGALS FOR PREVENTION AND TREATMENT OF INVASIVE FUNGAL INFECTIONS

Polyenes

Among the polyenes (amphotericin B and nystatin), only amphotericin B (formulated as amphotericin B deoxycholate [AmBd], liposomal amphotericin B [L-AmB], amphotericin B lipid complex [ABLC], and amphotericin B cholesteryl sulfate complex [ABCD]) is utilized for prevention and treatment of IFIs. Despite its broad-spectrum and fungicidal activity against many yeasts and molds, use has been limited due to the recent introduction of newer and safer alternatives (namely the echinocandins and broad-spectrum triazoles for both IFI prevention and treatment). Amphotericin B binds to ergosterol (a cholesterol-like derivative) in the fungal cell membrane, resulting in escape of intracellular ions and constituents [13,14]. While the binding affinity of amphotericin B greatly favors ergosterol over cholesterol (found in mammalian cells), the nonselective nature of the binding is thought to explain some of the drug's toxicity [15]. Resistance to amphotericin B is most often linked to target site alterations (notably a decrease in cell wall ergosterol mediated through alterations in enzymes responsible for ergosterol) [7]. Concentration-dependent fungicidal activity has been demonstrated *in vitro* and *in vivo* at higher concentrations against susceptible pathogens [16]. Peak serum to minimum inhibitory concentration (MIC) ratio (Cmax: MIC) is the pharmacodynamic endpoint, which best correlates with efficacy [17,18]. A post-antifungal effect ranging from 3 to 14 hours (depending on the species) has been reported with amphotericin B [16,19].

Despite the introduction of newer antifungals, amphotericin B continues to be the broadest-spectrum antifungal agent currently available [9,20]. Resistance to amphotericin B is rare among *Candida* spp., but higher MICs have been reported with *C. krusei* and *C. glabrata* and intrinsic resistance has been reported with *C. lusitaniae* [21–23]. Amphotericin B also displays activity against most *Aspergillus* spp. (with the exception of *A. terreus*) [9,20]. Among endemic mycoses, amphotericin has demonstrated *in vitro* activity against *Histoplasma capsulatum*, *Coccidioides immitis*, and *Blastomyces dermatitidis* [20,24]. Amphotericin is also active *in vitro* against *Rhodotorula* spp., *Cryptococcus neoformans*, *Sporothrix schenkii*, *Saccharomyces cerevisiae*, *Fusarium* spp., *Cladosporium* spp., *Scytalidium* spp., *Scedosporium* spp., and Mucorales [20,24].

Amphotericin B is only available in an intravenous (IV) formulation due to its limited oral bioavailability (5%–9%) [9,20,25]. Following IV administration, amphotericin B distributes widely into tissues, such as the liver, spleen, lung, kidney, and to a lesser extent, the cerebrospinal fluid (<2.5% of simultaneous serum concentrations) [15,26]. Differences in tissue distribution between amphotericin B deoxycholate and lipid-based formulations of amphotericin B have been reported [9,27,28]. For example, liver and spleen concentrations have been noted to be higher following administration of lipid-based formulations when compared to amphotericin B deoxycholate [27]. ABLC distributes rapidly in lung tissue and poorly into kidneys, while ABCD distributes poorly into the kidneys, lungs, and brain. Protein binding of amphotericin B is approximately 90% [26]. The major metabolic pathway of amphotericin B is largely undetermined. Trivial amounts can be detected in bile, while active drug excreted in urine accounts for only 2.5%–5% of a dose [9]. The elimination half-life of amphotericin B may (on average) be as much as 15 days [9,29].

Adverse events associated with amphotericin B are frequent and sometimes treatment-limiting. Infusion-related reactions (such as pain at the injection site, chills, rigors, fever, phlebitis, headache, bronchospasm, hypotension, nausea, and vomiting) occur in 70%–90% of patients and may diminish despite continued therapy [9,20,30,31]. Amphotericin B-induced nephrotoxicity is also common. Azotemia, hypokalemia, hypomagnesemia, hyperchloremia, renal tubular acidosis, or nephrocalcinosis have all been reported as manifestations of such toxicity [9]. Depending on the manifestation, patient risk factors and formulation of amphotericin B, such reactions occur in 24%–80% of patients [30,32].

Historically, amphotericin B has been used as a prophylactic strategy in a variety of high-risk patient populations, including HSCT and SOT recipients [9,20]. However, many of the populations whose IFIs were due primarily to yeast (i.e., autologous HSCT, liver transplant, etc.) were transitioned to fluconazole prophylaxis as a primary strategy. While amphotericin B is still considered an option for the prophylaxis of select patient populations at increased risk of mold infections, such use of amphotericin B has largely been replaced by the extended-spectrum triazoles (i.e., voriconazole and posaconazole) or echinocandins [3,4,33–35]. Published reports of empiric use of amphotericin B in patients at risk of IFIs have generally involved cancer patients with neutropenia (secondary to chemotherapy) and fever [33,36,37]. More recently, such comparisons have involved the use of a lipid-based formulation (i.e., LAmB) in comparison to caspofungin [36]. Survival rates were 92.6% versus 89.2% for caspofungin and amphotericin B, respectively, (p = 0.05). Caspofungin was better tolerated than amphotericin B, with a decreased incidence of nephrotoxicity (2.6% vs. 11.5%, respectively, p < 0.001). Alternatively, amphotericin B may be used first-line for empirical or preemptive therapy in select high-risk patients (i.e., prolonged neutropenic patients) with a suspected invasive aspergillosis infection [38].

The efficacy of amphotericin B has been reported in a variety of documented IFIs, most notably for candidiasis [3], aspergillosis [38], cryptococcal infections [39], and central nervous system infections due to endemic mycoses [40,41]. Controlled clinical trials for the treatment of invasive candidal infections [42–44], along with a more recent meta-analysis [45], have observed the lack of significant differences in mortality rates between AmBd and the comparative agent. In contrast, both echinocandins and fluconazole demonstrate significant reductions in overall adverse effects, specifically nephrotoxicity [45]. Although not included in the meta-analysis, voriconazole was subsequently found to be non-inferior to amphotericin B for treatment of candidemia [46]. Therefore, while amphotericin B is identified in current consensus treatment guidelines for the treatment of invasive candidiasis [3], its role is likely to be largely as an alternative to triazoles and echinocandins for refractory infection, endophthalmitis, endocarditis, and CNS infections [3]. For treatment of invasive aspergillosis, amphotericin B is currently recommended as an alternative to voriconazole therapy [38]. This recommendation is based largely on a randomized study, which compared voriconazole and amphotericin B deoxycholate (1–1.5 mg/kg/day) [47]. Twelve-week response rates (52.8% vs. 31.6%, absolute difference 21.2%; 95% CI, 10.4–32.9) and survival (70.8% vs. 57.9%, HR 0.59; 95% CI, 0.40–0.88) both favored voriconazole over amphotericin B, respectively.

In contrast to its role as alternate therapy in most patients with candidiasis and aspergillosis, amphotericin B (in combination with flucytosine) is still recommended as a "first-line" agent for induction treatment of severe cryptococcal disease, notably meningitis, severe pulmonary infections, and cryptococcemia [39]. Amphotericin B also continues to play a role in the treatment of severe, invasive histoplasmosis and blastomycosis [40,48–50]. In patients with AIDS-associated histoplamosis, clinical response rates with conventional amphotericin B (0.7 mg/kg) or liposomal amphotericin (3.0 mg/kg) for 2 weeks, followed by itraconazole consolidation for 10 weeks were 64% and 88%, respectively, (p = 0.014) [48]. Amphotericin B is generally restricted to initial treatment of severe pulmonary infections or in cases of severe, disseminated disease, or CNS histoplasmosis [50]. For moderate to severe cases of blastomycosis, amphotericin B is also considered first-line treatment based on clinical cure rates ranging from 70% to 91% [40,49]. Use in infections due to *Coccidiodes* spp. is generally restricted to treatment of serious, invasive infections such as pneumonia and meningitis (the later as an intrathecal administration) [51].

Flucytosine

Flucytosine (5-FC) is a fluorinated pyrimidine analog that must be metabolized into its active form in order to exert its antifungal properties [52,53]. Flucytosine is deaminated by cytosine deaminase to produce 5-fluorouracil, then converted to metabolites, which inhibit protein and DNA synthesis [52,53]. While flucytosine monotherapy is fungistatic against most isolates, combinations with amphotericin B results in fungicidal activity against most species [54]. Intrinsic or acquired resistance can occur through a variety of mechanisms, including decreases in transport into the cell via cytosine permease, alterations of metabolic enzymes (cytosine deaminase and uridine monophosphate pyrophosphorylate [uPRTase]), and increases in production of competitive pyrimidines [7,55–57]. Combinations with other agents reduce the rate of resistance development against flucytosine [58–62]. Time above the minimum inhibitory concentration (T > MIC) best characterizes it's pharmacodynamics properties [63]. A post-antifungal effect (up to 7.4 or 5.4 hours) can be observed for *Candida* spp. and *C. neoformans*, respectively [64].

Flucytosine exhibits activity *in vitro* against most *Candida* spp. Overall susceptibility of 1,448 *Candida* spp. against flucytosine in isolates obtained from 2006 to 2007 was 95.9%. Of note, however, only 3.4% of *C. krusei* were considered susceptible [65]. Against 1,811 isolates of *Cryptococcus neoformans* obtained between 1990–2004, flucytosine resistance varied widely based on geographic location, ranging from 35% in the United States (US) to 68% in Latin America [66]. Other *in vitro* activity has been documented against *Rhodotorula* spp., *Saccharomyces cerevisiae*, and certain causative pathogens of chromoblastomycosis (i.e., *Fonsecaea* spp., *Phialophora* spp., *Cladosporium* spp.) [67].

Flucytosine is available in the United States only in an oral formulation. Bioavailability is high (78%–89%), and maximum serum concentrations occur approximately 2 hours after an oral dose [68,69]. Protein binding is minimal (2.9%–4%) [68,69]. While tissue concentrations comparable to serum concentrations have been reported in a variety of tissues (spleen, heart, liver, kidney, and lung), they are generally lower in cerebrospinal fluid (80%) [67]. Approximately 90% of a dose is excreted renally as active drug [68,69]. Its half-life (2.4–4.8 hours) is significantly prolonged (range 29.9–250 hours) in patients with renal insufficiency [68–70].

Gastrointestinal side effects (nausea, vomiting, diarrhea, and abdominal discomfort) occurred in approximately 6% of patients receiving flucytosine therapy [69,71]. Hepatotoxicity associated with flucytosine use (reported with a range of 0%–41%) most commonly manifests as reversible elevations in transaminases and/or alkaline phosphatase [69,71–73]. Reversible myelosupression (in up to 27% of patients) most commonly manifests after 2–4 weeks of therapy as either leukopenia or thrombocytopenia [71,73,74].

Flucytosine is rarely used for IFIs prevention or empiric therapy of suspected IFIs, largely due to the rapid development of resistance when used as monotherapy, availability only in an oral formulation, and its toxicity profile [9,20]. More commonly, flucytosine is used in combination with other antifungals (notably amphotericin B) to treat cryptococcal infections [39,62], select infections caused by *Candida* spp. [3] and chromoblastomycosis [62,75]. For the initial treatment of invasive cryptococcal infections, flucytosine is used in combination with amphotericin B due to poor clinical response rates with either fluconazole or amphotericin B monotherapy [58,72,76–78]. Sterilization of the cerebral spinal fluid (CSF) occurs at a more rapid rate with combination flucytosine plus amphotericin B when compared to AmB-d monotherapy [39,58]. Furthermore, clinical rates have been shown to improve with combination therapy [39,58]. Cryptococcal eradication from the CSF was considerably more rapid with AmB-d plus flucytosine than with AmB-d alone (p = 0.0006) [58]. Amphotericin B in combination with flucytosine improves survival compared to amphotericin B monotherapy or in combination with fluconazole. Significantly fewer deaths occurred in patients receiving amphotericin B with flucytosine than those receiving amphotericin B monotherapy (HR, 0.61; 95% CI, 0.39 to 0.97; unadjusted p = 0.04). Combination therapy with fluconazole had no significant effect on survival, as compared with monotherapy (HR, 0.71; 95% CI, 0.45 to 1.11; p = 0.13) [79]. Current Infectious Diseases Society of America treatment guidelines recommend amphotericin B plus flucytosine as first-line treatment for the initial management of invasive cryptococcal infections [39]. Less frequently, flucytosine in combination with amphotericin B has been used for select candidal infections (such as endocarditis, meningitis, and endophthalmitis) [3]. Controlled clinical data to support such a combination is lacking. Given the availability of newer treatment options for these infections (i.e., echinocandins and triazoles), such a combination is rarely encountered in current clinical practice. Finally, although flucytosine has also been used in the treatment of chromoblastomycosis, efficacy data is limited to case reports [75].

Triazoles

The triazole class of antifungals consists of fluconazole, itraconazole, voriconazole, posaconazole and most recently, isavuconazole. These agents share many characteristics; however, they vary greatly in regards to pharmacokinetics, clinical use, and toxicity [80–83]. Triazoles work within the fungal cell membrane and prevent the conversion of lanosterol to ergosterol by inhibiting the cytochrome P450 dependent 14-α-demethylase. As a result of this inhibition, there is an accumulation of methylsterols, which causes cellular disruption and inhibition of growth and cellular replication [9,20].

Resistance to triazoles may occur due to mechanisms such as mutations in the azole binding pocket of 14α-demethylase, over-expression of MDR1 efflux pumps impacting fluconazole, and CDR1 and CDR2 efflux pumps, which affect all triazoles [7]. Intrinsic fluconazole resistance in *C. krusei* is due to impaired binding to 14α-demethylase and is not seen with newer triazoles due to enhanced enzyme binding [7]. Increases in fluconazole MICs can be

predictive of a decrease in susceptibility to other triazoles for *Candida* spp. [7,84]. Cross-resistance between triazoles among *Candida* spp. isolates can occur due to multi-drug efflux pumps (i.e., CDR pumps), which has been especially noted among *C. glabrata* [85]. While data are limited with isavuconazole, cross resistance between other triazoles is expected to affect isavuconazole as well. The clinical outcome is yet to be characterized; consequently, patients failing prior triazole therapy may require an alternative antifungal class [80,82,83].

In vitro and *in vivo* data have demonstrated that triazoles have a concentration-independent fungistatic activity against *Candida* spp., and mold-active triazoles have a slow concentration-dependent fungicidal activity against *Aspergillus* spp. [18,86–89]. The pharmacokinetic/pharmacodynamic parameter that best correlates efficacy outcomes with triazoles is the area under the curve to MIC ratio (AUC:MIC) [80,90–94]. For fluconazole, treatment success has been correlated with an AUC:MIC ratio of greater than 25 for mucosal and invasive candidiasis [90,91,95]. A post-antifungal effect with mold-active triazoles against *Aspergillus* spp. has been demonstrated (0.5 hours) but is lacking against *Candida* spp. [89].

As a class, the triazoles demonstrate favorable activity *in vitro* against most *Candida* spp. commonly encountered clinically (i.e., *C. albicans*, *C. lusitaniae*, *C. parapsilosis*, and *C. tropicalis*) [20,96,97]. However, fluconazole often exhibits dose-dependent activity against *C. glabrata*, while *C. krusei* is inherently resistant [96]. Voriconazole, posaconazole, and isavuconazole demonstrate increased activity *in vitro* (relative to fluconazole) against both *C. glabrata* and *C. krusei* [9,20,98]. Triazoles also demonstrate activity *in vitro* against most endemic mycoses, such as *Coccidioides* spp., *Blastomyces*, and *Histoplasma* spp. [9,20,96,97,99]. Furthermore, triazoles demonstrate activity *in vitro* against *Cryptococcus neoformans* [9,20,96,97,99]. In contrast to the other triazoles, fluconazole lacks activity against *Aspergillus* spp. [9,20,96,97]. Additionally, itraconazole, voriconazole, posaconazole, and isavuconazole exhibit activity against *Fusarium* spp., and *Scedosporium apiospermum* [9,20,99]. Finally, posaconazole and isavuconazole demonstrate activity *in vitro* against Mucorales [96,99].

Historically, among the triazoles, fluconazole exhibits the most favorable pharmacokinetic profile; however, recently this is being challenged with the addition of isavuconazole and new dosage formulations of posaconazole. Available in both intravenous and oral (tablets and suspension) dosage formulations, fluconazole exhibits linear pharmacokinetics [9,20,96]. Bioavailability following oral administration is high (>90%) and independent of gastric pH or the presence of food for absorption [20,96,100,101]. In contrast, the oral bioavailability of itraconazole is highly variable and pH dependent based on the formulation utilized [20,96]. Itraconazole oral solution is best absorbed under fasting conditions and has a bioavailability of 50% [20,96,102]. Overall, the capsule formulation has a decrease in bioavailability in comparison to the solution [96]. The oral capsule formulation has optimal absorption when given with food or in the presence of low gastric pH [102]. Voriconazole is available as both intravenous and oral (tablets and suspension) formulations [103]. Oral bioavailability is approximately 96%, but may be reduced by about 20% and delayed by an hour when administered with food [20,103–105]. High-fat meals have also been shown to reduce both the peak serum concentration (Cmax) and area under the time-concentration curve (AUC) [103,104]. Therefore, oral voriconazole is recommended to be administered either 1 hour before or 1 hour after meals [103,104]. Posaconazole was previously only available as an oral suspension [97,106]. Absorption of posaconazole suspension is slow (time to Cmax ~ 3–6 hours), saturable, highly variable, and dependent on dosing regimen and food administration [106–109]. Single doses of posaconazole suspension exceeding 800 mg are not fully absorbed, and dividing the total daily dose into two to four doses appears to increase the bioavailability [108,109]. Optimal posaconazole suspension absorption also occurs when administered with a high-fat meal or carbonated acidic beverage (i.e., ginger ale) [106,107,110]. Despite efforts to improve the absorption of posaconazole suspension, such measures may still result in suboptimal serum concentrations among many high-risk patients. Recently, a new delayed-release and intravenous formulation of posaconazole has been developed. These dosage forms produce higher and more predictable serum posaconazole concentrations compared to the suspension formulation. Furthermore, the tablet formulation is not affected by stomach pH given the delayed release into the small intestine to maximize absorption. Consequently, dosing is different from that of the oral suspension [111,112]. Isavuconazole is administered as a prodrug (isavuconazonium), making it unique compared to the other triazoles. Available as both intravenous and oral (capsule) formulations, isavuconazole does not require cyclodextrin for solubilization; therefore, both formulations are cyclodextrin-free. Bioavailability following oral administration is high (98%) and independent of gastric pH or the presence of food for absorption [113,114].

In general, triazoles undergo wide distribution into body fluids and tissues. Fluconazole is hydrophilic and undergoes extensive distribution, with a volume of distribution (Vd) of 0.56–0.82 L/kg [20,100,115,116]. It obtains good CSF (>60%), vitreal (28%–75%) and urine penetration (90%) [20,100,115,116]. Protein binding with fluconazole is 11%–12%, but increases with chronic renal failure (23%) [100,117]. Itraconazole is lipophilic (with a Vd of 11 L/kg), highly protein bound (>99%), and penetrates well into tissues (with the exception of the CSF [<10%]) [20,96]. Voriconazole is also lipophilic (estimated Vd of 4.6 L/kg) and distributes well into tissues, including the CSF (42%–67%) and vitreous fluid (38%) [20,103]. The plasma protein binding of the drug is ~58% [103]. Posaconazole and isavuconazole are both highly protein bound (>98% and >99%, respectively) and have

extensive volume of distributions (226–295 L and 450 L, respectively) [110,113,114,118].

Most triazoles undergo extensive hepatic metabolism and renal elimination. In contrast to the other triazoles, fluconazole is minimally metabolized (10%) and elimination primarily occurs renally as unchanged drug in the urine (80%) [9,20]. Itraconazole is extensively metabolized through the liver by cytochrome P450 (Cyp3A4) with a half-life of 29–35 hours [20,96,102]. The major metabolite, hydroxyitraconazole, also possesses antifungal properties [102]. Excretion occurs mostly as inactive metabolites into the urine (~40%) and feces (3%–18%) [102]. Likewise, voriconazole is also metabolized hepatically, with the isoenzyme Cyp2C19 as the major metabolic pathway and (to a lesser extent) Cyp3A4 and Cyp2C9 [105]. Plasma concentrations may vary between patients due to Cyp2C19 genetic polymorphism. Cyp2C19 "poor metabolizers" (seen in 15%–20% of Asians and 3%–5% of Caucasians and African Americans) can exhibit up to a 4-fold increase in voriconazole concentrations [103,105,119,120]. Saturation of the metabolic clearance of voriconazole can lead to disproportional increases in the Cmax and AUC with increasing doses [105]. The major metabolite of voriconazole (N-oxide) is inactive and primarily eliminated through the urine, with a half-life of 6–12 hours [103,105]. Posaconazole is metabolized by UDP-glucuronosyltransferase to an inactive metabolite. The half-life ranges between 20 and 66 hours (depending on formulation) and is eliminated primarily as unchanged drug (66%) in the feces (71%) and urine (13%) [106,113,114,118,121,122]. The prodrug isavuconazonium sulfate is rapidly hydrolyzed in blood to isavuconazole by esterases. Isavuconazole is cleared through hepatic metabolism with renal elimination accounting for <1% of the administered dose. The half-life ranges between 56–77 hours for oral and 76–104 hours for the intravenous formulation [113,114].

Adverse effects most commonly associated or clinically significant with triazoles include gastrointestinal (nausea, vomiting, hepatic enzyme elevations) and cardiovascular (i.e., QTc prolongation [shortening for isavuconazole]) effects [9,20,113,114,123]. Therefore, patients with underlying risk factors for hepatic insufficiency and/or QTc prolongation should use all triazoles cautiously. Fluconazole is generally well-tolerated [100,124]. Elevations in transaminases resulting in hepatic failure are infrequent and not dose-dependent or related to duration of exposure to fluconazole [124,125]. Administration of itraconazole solution has been associated with gastrointestinal side effects (nausea, vomiting, diarrhea, and abdominal pain) in up to one-third of patients, and is likely due primarily to the cyclodextrin vehicle [102]. Hypokalemia, rash, edema, headache, fever, hepatotoxicity, and dizziness have also been reported with itraconazole [102]. Furthermore, heart failure in patients receiving itraconazole can occur; thus itraconazole is contraindicated in patients with or a history of ventricular dysfunction, patients receiving other negative inotropic drugs, or erythromycin [126]. The mechanism of this adverse effect is thought to be related to itraconazole's negative inotropic effect [102]. Gastrointestinal disturbances (including mild to moderate elevations in serum transaminases [12%]) can occur in patients taking voriconazole [103]. Typically, dose-dependent transaminase elevations occur after several weeks of voriconazole therapy and may resolve with continued use [103]. In addition, voriconazole administration has been associated with visual disturbances (14%–44%) and CNS effects (such as mental confusion) [103,127]. Visual disturbances associated with the administration of voriconazole are often transient in nature and may include photophobia, color vision changes, and hallucinations. These changes often dissipate within the first week of therapy [103,127]. Mild photosensitivity, Stevens-Johnson syndrome, QT prolongation, arrhythmias, and sudden cardiac deaths have also been reported with voriconazole therapy in post-marketing surveillance and clinical studies [103,127,128]. In contrast to voriconazole, posaconazole seems to be well-tolerated. The most common adverse effects associated with oral posaconazole use include gastrointestinal (diarrhea, nausea, vomiting), fever, and headache [106]. Intravenous posaconazole is associated with similar adverse effects to those of oral; however, thrombophlebitis was seen if the drug was administered through a peripheral line. Therefore, intravenous posaconazole should be administered through a central line [111,112]. Additionally, reversible mild to moderate elevations in transaminases and QTc prolongation have also been noted in clinical studies [129]. Isavuconazole has a similar tolerability profile to that of fluconazole [80]. In phase I and II studies, no serious adverse effects occurred. The most common adverse effects reported were gastrointestinal side effects (mild upper abdominal pain, diarrhea, nausea, elevation in transaminases). Unlike voriconzole, no visual disturbances were reported. Furthermore, adverse events caused by isavuconazole were statistically fewer relative to voriconazole, including hepatobiliary (9% vs. 16%) and skin (34% vs. 43%). In addition, isavuconazole showed statistically fewer study drug-related adverse events relative to voriconazole (42% vs. 60%). Lastly, since isuvaconazole is not formulated with cyclodextrin, unlike intravenous posaconazole and voriconzole, nephrotoxicity due to cyclodextrin is not a concern [80,113,114].

Fluconazole has been employed as prophylaxis against invasive candidiasis in transplant populations (such as liver or pancreatic transplant patients, autologous and low-risk allogeneic HSCT patients with neutropenia) [3,4,34]. Fluconazole may also be used to prevent donor-derived candidiasis in kidney transplant recipients [130]. Furthermore, posaconazole and voriconazole may be used for prophylaxis in patients with increased risk factors for aspergillosis infections, such as lung transplant patients and allogeneic HSCT with graft versus host disease (GvHD) [4,34,38,130]. The utility of isavuconazole for prophylaxis against IFIs is yet to be determined, however, given its favorable profile (spectrum of activity similar to posaconazole, oral formulation with excellent bioavailability, possibly fewer drug interactions than voriconazole and itraconazole and adverse effect profile similar to fluconazole), isavuconazole is an attractive possibility [131–133]. Currently, limited data exists for the use of isavuconazole for prophylaxis against IFIs.

The use of triazoles for empiric treatment of IFIs or for documented infections varies among members of the class, largely due to differences in pharmacokinetic profiles, available dosage forms, in vitro activity, drug interactions, and published clinical experience. This is summarized in more detail elsewhere (see Chapters 48–54). In brief, fluconazole may be used empirically for suspected candidiasis in patients without risk factors for non-albicans infections, while voriconazole (or other antifungals) is preferred in higher-risk patients [3]. Itraconazole or voriconazole can be used empirically for treatment of aspergillosis, with voriconazole preferred in most cases [38]. Posaconazole's role in the treatment of invasive aspergillosis is less well-established, and is generally reserved for patients refractory or intolerant to alternate therapies [134]. For endemic mycoses, both fluconazole and intraconazole may be used in select cases of IFIs due to Blastomyces dermatitidis and Coccidioides spp. infections [40,41]. Fluconazole therapy is generally the preferred triazole for the management of select cryptococcal infections [39], while fluconazole, posaconazole, and voriconazole are considered alternatives to itraconazole in the treatment of histoplasmosis [50]. Itraconazole can be used as step down therapy in Sporothrix schenckii infections [135], while posaconazole is emerging as a treatment of select IFIs due to Mucorales [136]. In regards to the new triazole isavuconazole, the treatment of IFIs will be better defined as clinical experience increases. Isavuconazole is currently indicated for the treatment of invasive aspergillosis and mucormycosis. In a phase 3 study evaluating the safety and efficacy of once-daily isavuconazole versus twice-daily voriconazole in the primary treatment of invasive fungal disease caused by Aspergillus species or other filamentous fungi, isavuconazole was noninferior to voriconazole [137]. Isavuconazole is currently considered an alternative to voriconazole in aspergillosis management [38]. Furthermore, in an open-label trial that studied primary as well as salvage therapy of invasive mucormycosis, isavuconazole showed efficacy that was similar to that reported for amphotericin B and posaconazole [138]. Isavuconazole's use in candidemia and other invasive infections by Candida is currently being evaluated.

Echinocandins

The echinocandin class consists of caspofungin, micafungin, and anidulafungin. Echinocandins inhibit fungal cell wall synthesis. The resulting concentration-dependent activity is fungicidal against many of the Candida spp. and generally fungistatic against Aspergillus spp. [139–141]. A post-antifungal effect has been observed with all the echinocandins ranging from 0.9 hours to ≥20.1 hours depending upon the Candida spp. and the specific echinocandin and concentration studied [142]. The primary mechanism of resistance of the echinocandin class appears to be related to mutations in the gene that encodes for FKS 1 (one of the main building blocks for the fungal cell wall). Cross-resistance among agents is common in the presence of such a mutation [143].

Echinocandins possess comparable spectrums of antifungal activity, including *Candida spp.* and *Aspergillus spp.* [144–146]. Specifically, the echinocandins are active *in vitro* against *C. albicans, C. glabrata, C. krusei, C. lusitaniae,* and *C. tropicalis* with variable activity against *C. parapsilosis* [20]. Despite this uncertain *in vitro* activity against *C. parapsilosis*, it does not appear to be clinically significant as demonstrated in clinical trials, although close monitoring for fungemic patients may be necessary [147–149]. They also display activity *in vitro* against *A. flavus, A. fumigatus, A. niger,* and *A. terreus* [20]. A study evaluating *Aspergillus* spp. isolates (including *A. fumigatus, A. flavus, A. niger,* and *A. terreus*) in transplant patients revealed minimum effective concentrations at or below the epidemiological cut-off values ($\leq$0.06 mcg/mL) for caspofungin, micafungin, and anidulafungin [150].

All echinocandins require intravenous administration due to poor oral bioavailability [144–146]. Caspofungin, micafungin, and anidulafungin are highly protein bound to albumin (>~97%) [144–146]. Caspofungin displays extensive tissue distribution with animal reports demonstrating concentrations at 16-, 3-, and 2-fold plasma concentration in the liver, kidneys, and large intestines, respectively. Other organs such as the small intestines, lungs, and spleen show comparable caspofungin plasma concentrations, while the brain and heart have considerably lower concentrations [9,20]. In addition, high concentrations of caspofungin have been reported in the alveolar cells (ACs) of a lung transplant patient as noted in a case report [151]. The pharmacokinetics of micafungin was studied among lung transplant patients specifically evaluating micafungin concentrations in the plasma, epithelial lining fluid (ELF), and ACs [152]. Peak concentrations in the ACs were 3.5-fold higher than the plasma concentrations and 12.6-fold higher than the ELF. Caspofungin is primarily metabolized by hydrolysis and N-acetylation and is unaffected by the CYP-enzyme pathway and does not inhibit P-glycoprotein [144]. Anidulafungin does not undergo hepatic metabolism, but rather the medication is slowly degraded via a chemical breakdown at the body's physiologic temperature and pH [146]. Caspofungin's elimination half-life of 13 ± 1.9 hours was reported in patients with esophageal candidiasis [144], and is comparable to a study with micafungin in patients with invasive candidiasis [145] and among patients undergoing bone marrow or peripheral stem cell transplants [153]. In contrast, a healthy volunteer study reported a half-life of 52 hours for anidulafungin [146]. Peak, trough, and AUCs for caspofungin do not appear to be significantly altered when coadministered with liposomal amphotericin B in allogeneic HSCT recipients [154]. Micafungin is metabolized in the liver by catechol-O-methyltransferase, as well

as by hydroxylation. In addition, it appears to be affected *in vitro* by the *CyP*3A system, although it does not appear to be clinically relevant nor does it appear to be affected by the P-glycoprotein system [145].

The echinocandins are generally well-tolerated although patients should be monitored for the development of adverse reactions throughout therapy. Such reactions include infusion-related reactions, hypersensitivity reactions, and hepatic effects. In particular, patients receiving any of the echinocandins should be monitored for liver function test (LFT) elevations during therapy; if abnormal, the risk-to-benefit ratio should be considered if the echinocandin is to be continued. In addition, BUN and serum creatinine concentrations should be monitored in patients receiving micafungin [144–146].

Echinocandin antifungals have been investigated for their safety and efficacy in the prevention of IFIs in transplant recipients [33,34,155,156]. The majority of published guidelines focus on their use in prevention of IFIs in HSCT recipients [4,34,155]. Specifically, micafungin is considered an alternative (to posaconazole or voriconazole) in the prophylaxis of invasive aspergillosis for neutropenic patients undergoing HSCT [38]. Caspofungin can also be considered as antifungal prophylaxis for candidiasis among high-risk allogeneic HSCT patients or acute leukemia patients undergoing induction chemotherapy [33]. More recently, caspofungin has been compared to fluconazole for prophylaxis in high-risk liver transplant recipients [156]. Among SOT recipients, guidelines recommend the use of echinocandins as alternative (to fluconazole) prophylaxis or treatment for kidney, liver or pancreas transplant patients in which *Candida* spp. isolates are detected in the preservation fluid or if the surgeries to retrieve the organ may have intestinal leakage [130]. Of note, an alternative approach is prophylactic use of echinocandins in high-risk patients in the ICU. Recently, a pivotal study evaluated the use of echinocandin prophylaxis for invasive candidiasis in the ICU. This randomized, double-blind, placebo-controlled trial of caspofungin prophylaxis followed by preemptive therapy for invasive candidiasis did not have sufficient power to demonstrate a significant reduction in the incidence of invasive candidiasis with echinocandin prophylaxis [35]. Therefore, prophylaxis among nonneutropenic patients should be restricted to patient populations with proven benefit (e.g., liver, pancreas, or small-bowel transplant) [3].

The echinocandin class can be considered for empiric therapy in high-risk cancer patients with unexplained fever and neutropenia. Specifically, the echinocandins, as well as voriconazole or an amphotericin B preparation, can be considered for mold coverage in these high-risk patients who have received prophylactic fluconazole with fever beyond a 4-day duration [33]. For treatment of documented infections, echinocandins are considered as first-line treatment for candidemia or suspected candidiasis in both neutropenic and non-neutropenic patients [3]. In addition, they are also considered first-line options for suppurative thrombophlebitis, infected pacemakers, implantable cardiac defibrillators

(ICDs) and esophageal candidiasis [3]. Although variable *in vitro* activity against *C. parapsilosis*, if patients with documented infection are responding to an echinocandin, it is reasonable to continue echinocandin therapy to completion according to current Candidiasis guidelines [3]. The echinocandins (caspofungin and micafungin) are considered alternative (salvage) treatment options for invasive pulmonary aspergillosis and other *Aspergillus spp.* infections [38].

Administration and monitoring of antifungals in transplant recipients

Expert guidelines have been published to aid in the selection, dosing, and administration of antifungals for both prevention and treatment of IFIs, including HSCT and SOT patient populations. These include specific patient populations such as critical care patients with pulmonary IFIs [157], febrile neutropenic cancer patients [4,33], and organism-specific recommendations for the treatment of aspergillosis [38], blastomycoses [40], coccidioidomycosis [51], cryptococcosis [39], candidiasis [3], histoplasmosis [50], and sporotrichosis [135].

POLYENES

Selection. Published efficacy data for many IFIs utilize AmBd. For select indications (notably cryptococcal infections), both liposomal amphotericin B (LAmB) and amphotericin B lipid complex (ABLC) show comparable efficacy to amphotericin B deoxycholate [39,158–161]. Lipid formulations were superior to amphotericin B deoxycholate in one study involving SOT patients with CNS cryptococcal infections [162] and have been recommended over amphotericin B deoxycholate for the treatment of cryptococcal meningoencephalitis in transplant recipients. For empiric therapy of fever in neutropenic cancer patients, lipid formulations demonstrate reductions in toxicity, but superior efficacy has not been demonstrated [163]. Since lipid-based formulations exhibit reductions in the incidence of nephrotoxicity when compared to amphotericin B deoxycholate [164–168], their use is preferred in patients at increased risk of amphotericin B-induced toxicity, including those receiving concomitant nephrotoxins, higher doses (daily or cumulative), and in the presence of underlying renal insufficiency. Therefore, lipid formulation may be also preferred to amphotericin B deoxycholate for mucormycosis in SOT and HSCT recipients [169–171].

While lipid-based formulations demonstrate reduced nephrotoxicity relative to amphotericin B deoxycholate, the optimal choice among these formulations is less clear [9,20,28,103,172]. Although combining AmBd with lipid emulsions had demonstrated reductions in nephrotoxicity (relative to amphotericin B deoxycholate) [168,172], pharmacokinetic and efficacy data are presently lacking and such preparations cannot be routinely recommended. As previously discussed in this chapter, significant pharmacokinetic differences exist among lipid-based formulations currently FDA-approved (LAmB, ABLC, and ABCD)

[28]. Potential implications of such differences would be preference of one preparation over another based on infection site. However, clinical data from adequately controlled trials are lacking to detect significant differences in clinical efficacy between ABLC and LAmB [20,103,172]. Relative to safety, LAmB demonstrated less infusion-related reactions than ABLC after administration of the first dose in patients not receiving premedications for infusion-related reactions [173]. Therefore, in patients experiencing infusion-related reactions, liposomal amphotericin B may be preferred to amphotericin B deoxycholate [173]. While this study also indicated a reduction in nephrotoxicity with LAmB (relative to ABLC), this has not been consistently supported from other trial data. In contrast, ABCD has been associated with significant infusion-related reactions [174]. Combined with the limited published efficacy data, this has significantly limited use of ABCD relative to other lipid-based formulations. Finally, all lipid-based formulations have significant increases in acquisition costs relative to AmBd. Pharmacoeconomic comparisons evaluating cost-effectiveness differences between ABLC and LAmB have generally demonstrated a high dependency on drug acquisition cost to demonstrate significant differences between preparations [175].

Dosing and adminstration. Doses of amphotericin B are dependent upon pathogen, site of infection, and preparation. Intravenous doses of amphotericin B deoxycholate for IFIs range from 0.6–1.5 mg/kg administered once daily. The highest doses are generally reserved for refractory IFIs (such as mucormycosis). For lipid-based formulations, usual daily doses range 3–5 mg/kg administered once daily (see Table 26.1).

Because of its concentration-dependent activity, dose intensification of amphotericin B has been investigated in attempts to increase its efficacy. LAmB has been investigated in doses of up to 10 mg/kg/day [180]. Neutropenic, allogeneic HSCT patients with IFIs due to molds were randomized to receive either 3 or 10 mg/kg/day for 14 days, followed by 3 mg/kg/day thereafter [180]. No difference was observed in clinical efficacy within 14 days despite increased rates of nephrotoxicity and hypokalemia in the 10 mg/kg group. Therefore, dose intensification (i.e., >5 mg/kg/d of a lipid formulation) is generally reserved for LAmB as salvage therapy in cases of severe, refractory mucormycosis [181]. A clinical trial evaluating liposomal amphotericin B 10 mg/kg/d in this patient population is underway [182].

Although not eliminated renally, alternate day administration (without reduction of the total weekly dose) was often recommended for patients with renal dysfunction requiring continued administration of amphotericin B. Given the availability of lipid-based formulations of amphotericin B and their relative safety in patients with renal insufficiency requiring amphotericin B administration, there is little need for alternate day administration of AmBd. The pharmacokinetic profile of LAmB administered 7.5 mg/kg once weekly or 15 mg/kg single dose as prophylaxis in HSCT patients

Table 26.1 Usual adult doses of systemic antifungals

Drug class	Agent	Indication	Standard dosing	Renal impairment dosing	Hepatic impairment dosing	References
Triazoles	Fluconazole	Candidemia/candidiasis	50–800 mg/day	Crcl ≤50 mL/minute decrease standard dose by 50% Hemodialysis-standard dose after each dialysis session	None	[3,4,33,38,40,41,62,100,135]
			800 mg (12 mg/kg) loading dose, then 400 mg/day (6 mg/kg/day)			
		Cryptococcosis—pulmonary disease	400 mg/day			
		Cryptococcal meningitis/disseminated disease	400–800 mg/day			
		Consolidation	200 mg/day			
		Maintenance				
		Histoplasmosis	800 mg/day			
		Coccidioidomycosis	200–400 mg/day			
		Prophylaxis	400–800 mg/day			
		Non-life threatening /meningitis				
		Stem cell transplant (neutropenic) prophylaxis	400 mg/day (6 mg/kg/day)			
		Solid organ transplant prophylaxis	200–400 mg/day (3–6 mg/kg/day)			
	Itraconazole	Candida infections oropharyngeal/esophageal	200 mg/day	NR-use caution	NR-use caution	[3,38,40,41,50,62,102,135]
		Histoplasmosis/blastomycosis	200 mg three times daily X 3 days, then 200 mg twice daily			
		Aspergillosis prophylaxis treatment	200 mg two to four times daily (capsule) or 2.5 mg/kg twice daily (solution)			
			200 mg three times daily X 3 days then 200 mg twice daily			
		Sporotrichosis	100 mg–200 mg/day			
		Paracoccidioidomycosis	100 mg/day			
		Chromomycosis	100–200 mg/day			
		Coccidioidomycosis	200 mg twice to three times daily			

(Continued)

Table 26.1 (Continued) Usual adult doses of systemic antifungals

Drug class	Agent	Indication	Standard dosing	Renal impairment dosing	Hepatic impairment dosing	References
	Posaconazole	Prophylaxis of invasive fungal infection	200 mg three times daily (suspension) 300 mg twice daily on day 1, then 300 mg daily (IV/delayed-release tablet)	CrCl <50 mL/minute - after IV loading dose switch to PO	None	[38,41,50, 110,177]
		Aspergillosis	200 mg four times daily until stable, then 400 mg twice daily (suspension)			
		Oropharyngeal candidiasis	100 mg twice daily on day 1, then 100 mg once daily (suspension)			
		Oropharyngeal candidiasis refractory to itraconazole and/or fluconazole	400 mg twice daily (suspension)			
		Histoplasmosis/coccidioidomycosis	400 mg twice daily (suspension)			
		Mucormycosis	200 mg four times daily or 400 mg twice daily (suspension)	None	None	
	Voriconazole	Candida infections; aspergillosis, scedosporiosis, histoplasmosis, coccidioidomycosis, fusariosis	IV: 6 mg/kg twice daily– day 1 then 4 mg/kg twice daily PO: 400 mg twice daily—day 1 then 200 mg twice daily[a,b]	CrCl <50 mL/minute - after IV loading dose switch to PO	Mild-to-moderate dysfunction (Child-Pugh A or B)—Following standard loading dose, reduce maintenance by 50% Severe dysfunction – NR—use caution	[3,38,40,41, 50,62,103]
	Isavuconazole	Aspergillosis; mucormycosis	IV/PO: 200 mg (372 mg prodrug) three times daily for 6 doses (48 hours) then 200 mg once daily (372 mg prodrug)	None	Severe dysfunction—NR—use caution	[176]
Echinocandins	Anidulafungin	Candidemia, Candida intraabdominal infections, including abscess and peritonitis	200 mg IV load on day 1, then 100 mg/day IV	None	None	[146]
		Esophageal candidiasis	200 mg/day			

(Continued)

Table 26.1 (*Continued*) Usual adult doses of systemic antifungals

Drug class	Agent	Indication	Standard dosing	Renal impairment dosing	Hepatic impairment dosing	References
	Caspofungin	Febrile neutropenia-empiric treatment, candidemia, *Candida* intraabdominal infections, including abscess and peritonitis, *Candida* infections of the pleural space, invasive aspergillosis, esophageal candidiasis	70 mg IV load on day 1, then 50 mg/day IV	None	Child-Pugh score 7–9: 70 mg IV load on day 1, then 35 mg/day IV	[3,38,144]
		Invasive pulmonary aspergillosis prophylaxis	50 mg/day			
		Invasive pulmonary aspergillosis-(alternative therapy) or empiric aspergillosis treatment	70 mg/day load on day 1, then 50 mg/day IV			
	Micafungin	Candidemia, disseminated candidiasis-acute, *Candida* intraabdominal infections, including abscess and peritonitis	100 mg/day IV	None	Child-Pugh score 7–9: 70 mg IV load on day 1, then 35 mg/day IV	[3,38,145]
		Esophageal candidiasis	150 mg/day IV		None	
		HSCT prophylaxis of *Candida* infections	50 mg/day IV			
		Invasive aspergillosis (salvage treatment)	100–150 mg/day IV (dose not established)			
		Invasive aspergillosis prophylaxis	50–100 mg/day			

(*Continued*)

Table 26.1 (*Continued*) Usual adult doses of systemic antifungals

Drug class	Agent	Indication	Standard dosing	Renal impairment dosing	Hepatic impairment dosing	References
flucytosine		Candidiasis, cryptococcosis	25 mg/kg PO every 6 hours + amphotericin B (or lipid formulations of amphotericin)	CrCl 20–40 mL/minute: reduce dose by 50%; CrCl <20 mL/minute: reduce dose by 75%	NR	[3,29,39, 68,69,178]
		Cryptococcal meningitis-HIV infection, pulmonary Crytococcus-HIV infection	25 mg/kg PO every 6 hours + amphotericin B (or lipid formulations of amphotericin) for induction phase ++			
Polyenes	Amphotericin B deoxycholate	Candidemia or suspected candidiasis (non-neutropenic patients), osteomyelitis, septic arthritis, esophageal candidiasis	0.5–1 mg/kg/d IV (0.5–0.7 mg/kg/d IV for esophageal candidiasis)[c]	No specific adjustment recommended, but monitor renal function	NR	[3,15,38,40, 41,50,62]
		Invasive *Aspergillus* spp. infections	0.25–1 mg/kg/d IV			
		Acute pulmonary histoplasmosis or progressive disseminated histoplasmosis-moderate to severe	0.7–1 mg/kg/d IV			
		Cryptococcal meningitis (transplant patients)	0.7 mg/kg/d IV			
		Sporotrichosis	0.7–1 mg/kg/d IV			
		Blastomycosis	0.7–1 mg/kg/d IV			
		Mucormycosis	1–1.5 mg/kg/d IV			

(*Continued*)

Table 26.1 (Continued) Usual adult doses of systemic antifungals

Drug class	Agent	Indication	Standard dosing	Renal impairment dosing	Hepatic impairment dosing	References
	Amphotericin B lipid complex	Candida spp. infections, sporotrichosis and blastomycosis	3–5 mg/kg/d IV	No specific adjustment recommended, but monitor renal function	NR	[3,38,40, 41,50,62]
			Aspergillus spp. infections	5 mg/kg/d IV		
			Histoplasmosis	5 mg/kg/d IV		
			Cryptococcal meningitis (transplant patients)	5 mg/kg/d IV (with 5-FC)		
	Liposomal amphotericin B	Candida spp. infections, Aspergillus spp. infections, sporotrichosis, and blastomycosis	3–5 mg/kg/d IV	No specific adjustment recommended, but monitor renal function	NR	[3,38,40,41,50,62,179]
			Histoplasmosis	3–5 mg/kg/d IV		
			Cryptococcal meningitis (transplant patients)	3–4 mg/kg/d IV (with 5-FC)		
			Mucormycosis	5 mg/kg/d IV		
	Amphotericin B cholesteryl sulfate	Candidiasis	3.9–6 mg/kg/d IV	No specific adjustment recommended, but monitor renal function	NR	[3,38,40,135]
		Aspergillosis	3–4 mg/kg/d IV			
		Blastomycosis	Sporotrichosis			
		3–5 mg/kg/d IV	3–5 mg/kg/d IV			

Abbreviation: NR = No recommendations.

a For patients >40 kg; maintenance dose can be increased to 300 mg twice daily if poor response.

b For patients <40 kg; loading dose 200 mg twice a day on day 1 followed by 100 mg twice daily; if poor response maintenance dose can be increased to 150 mg twice daily.

c Other Candida spp. infections can be treated with AmBd ranging from 0.3 to 1 mg/kg/day depending on type of infection.

has been investigated [183]. While amphotericin B concentrations in these patients at the end of the week were thought to be sufficient against most *Candida* and *Aspergillus* strains for prophylaxis, they experienced nephrotoxicity significantly faster than the patients in a comparator (daily dosing) cohort. Such a strategy is not currently recommended in prophylaxis guidelines. Finally, intermittent administration of liposomal amphotericin B (i.e., 5 mg/kg 2–3 times per week following 3–4 weeks of daily therapy) has been identified as a potential option for select patients requiring long-term amphotericin B therapy (as part of combination therapy) for the treatment of mucormycosis [181].

Medications to prevent or treat infusion-related reactions may include corticosteroids to prevent phlebitis, antihistamines to diminish allergic response, and analgesics (acetaminophen or ibuprofen) to prevent fever and chills [30,184]. A 1 mg test dose prior to the initial dose has been recommended to screen for patients at risk of acute hypersensitivity reaction [15,31]. This is best accomplished by calculating the aliquot from the first dose necessary to deliver the test dose, and monitoring the patient for 15–30 minutes for reaction. While extending the infusion time (from the standard of 4–6 hours to 24 hours) has been reported to decrease some of the infusion-related reactions [185–187], clinical response data in patients receiving such therapy for documented IFIs is sparse. Finally, while not evaluated in controlled clinical trials, administration of 500–1000 mL of normal saline prior to the administration of amphotericin B may decrease the incidence of nephrotoxicity [188,189]. Coadministration of amphotericin B with leukocytes should be avoided whenever possible due to the potential for acute pulmonary toxicity [190].

While not FDA-approved for aerosol administration, numerous case reports and limited clinical trials have been published evaluating the use of various formulations of amphotericin B given via aerosol in select transplant populations, including HSCT and lung transplant recipients [191–193]. Much of the focus for such administration has been on the prevention and/or adjunctive treatment of invasive aspergillosis in high-risk patients, with the goal of providing high antifungal concentrations at the site of initial infection (i.e., lung) while minimizing systemic side effects [191,194]. Reports in the transplant patient population for prevention of IFIs include both bone marrow transplant recipients [195,196] and SOT recipients (most commonly lung transplant recipients) [197–200]. Doses of AmBd range from 5–20 mg once daily to three times daily delivered from a variety of nebulizers and durations of drug exposure. Use of added systemic prophylaxis also varies between reports. Lipid-based formulations of amphotericin B, notably ABLC and LAmB, have also been reported as a prophylactic strategy (alone or in combination with systemic agents) in transplant patients [200–203]. Human data regarding the role of aerosolized formulations of amphotericin B for IFI treatment are restricted to the use of case reports or case series in patients receiving concomitant systemic therapy [204–211]. Adverse events associated with the administration of aerosolized amphotericin B include nausea, bad taste, cough, dizziness, chest tightness, mild bronchospasm, and sputum production [195–199,203,211–214]. The optimal preparation, dose, delivery system, need for concomitant systemic antifungals, timing, and duration of therapy for aerosolized amphotericin B formulations require further study [215,216].

Monitoring. Amphotericin B concentrations are not routinely monitored. Drug interactions are limited primarily to other agents, which undergo primary renal elimination, since amphotericin-induced renal dysfunction may decrease clearance of such agents. Routine monitoring should include renal function studies (BUN, creatinine), LFTs, serum electrolytes (Mg and K), and complete blood counts [9,15,20,189].

Drug interactions. Most clinically-relevant drug interactions with amphotericin B are due to its potential to cause nephrotoxicity and significant electrolyte abnormalities (such as hypokalemia). Therefore, reduced clearance of renally eliminated agents may occur as a consequence of amphotericin B-induced nephrotoxicity [217]. Amphotericin B-induced hypokalemia may potentiate the toxicity of select agents (such as cardiac glycosides) or cause additive hypokalemia from these other agents (i.e., loop or thiazide diuretics) [217]. See Table 26.2.

FLUCYTOSINE

Selection. Flucytosine is available in the United States only as an oral formulation.

Dosing/Administration. Flucytosine is administered orally as 75–100 mg/kg/day in three or four divided doses. The daily dose should be adjusted depending on the degree of renal function. A 50% dose reduction has been recommended for patients with a creatinine clearance of 20–40 mL/minute, and a 75% reduction for a creatinine clearance of <20 mL/minute [29,68,178]. Flucytosine is highly removed during hemodialysis; therefore administration after dialysis sessions is recommended (see Table 26.1).

Monitoring. Risks of flucytosine-induced myelosupression and hepatotoxicity can be reduced through monitoring peak serum concentrations, serum creatinine, liver function tests, and complete blood counts at regularly scheduled intervals during therapy. Steady-state peak concentrations are reached after 3–5 days of therapy and should be measured 2 hours post-dose with a target concentration of 30 to 80 µg/mL [67]. Flucytosine concentrations greater than 100 µg/mL have been associated with increased risk of toxicity and should be avoided [226]. Additionally, flucytosine spot serum concentrations should be maintained below 100 µg/mL [67]. However, the lack of local laboratory availability of flucytosine concentration measurements makes such monitoring impractical in some clinical settings.

Drug Interactions. Pharmacokinetic drug interactions with flucytosine are minimal (see Table 26.2). Because of its potential to cause hematologic toxicity, flucytosine should be used with caution in combination with other agents

Table 26.2 Significant drug-drug interactions among the antifungal agents[a]

Antifungal class	Specific medication	Drug interactions	Clinical significance	References
Azoles	Fluconazole	Cyclosporine[c], tacrolimus[c], sirolimus[c], alfentanil, amitriptyline, nortriptyline, statins (atorvastatin, simvastatin, lovastatin, fluvastatin), sulfonylureas (glimepride, glipizide, glyburide), benzodiazepines (triazolam, midazolam, alprazolam), omeprazole, phenytoin, cyclophosphamide, fentanyl, ibuprofen, warfarin, calcium channel blockers (i.e., nifedipine, isradipine, amlodipine, felodipine), theophylline, prednisone, celecoxib, carbamazepine, methadone, dofetilide, erthryomycin Rifampin, clopidogrel **Contraindicated:** cisapride, astemizole, pimozide, quinidine, terfinadine, conivaptan, tolvaptan, ranolazine	• Fluconazole increases drug concentrations of all drugs listed • Monitor for adverse effects related to supratherapeutic concentrations of each drug • Methadone, dofetilide, and erythromycin also have increased risk of QT prolongation and torsades de pointes • Rifampin decreases fluconazole concentrations • Fluconazole decreases concentrations of active metabolites of clopidogrel • Fluconazole increases cisapride, astemizole, pimozide, quinidine, and terfinadine serum concentrations; increased risk of QT prolongation and torsades de pointes. • Fluconazole increases conivaptan, tolvaptan, and ranolazine serum concentrations	[100,218,219,220,221]

(Continued)

Table 26.2 (Continued) Significant drug-drug interactions among the antifungal agents[a]

Antifungal class	Specific medication	Drug interactions	Clinical significance	References
	Itraconazole	Cyclosporine[d], tacrolimus[d], sirolimus, carbamazepine, terfenadine, vinca alkaloids, docetaxel, busulfan, statins (simvastatin, lovastatin, atorvastatin), digoxin, disopyramide, calcium channel blockers (i.e., dihydropyridines, verapamil), benzodiazepines (diazepam, alprazolam), nevirapine, cyclophosphamide, steroids (fluticasone, budesonide, dexamethasone, methylprednisolone), haloperidol, loperamide, Repaglinide, risperidone, rifabutin, fentanyl, warfarin, protease inhibitors (indinavir, ritonavir, saquinavir)	• Itraconazole increases drug concentrations of all drugs listed • Monitor for adverse effects related to supratherapeutic concentrations of each drug	[102,218,219,221]
		Rifampin, rifabutin, isoniazid, phenytoin, carbamazepine, phenobarbital, omeprazole[b], antacids[b], H2 blockers[b], nevirapine	• Itraconazole concentrations decrease • Monitor for breakthrough fungal infections or suboptimal clinical efficacy	
		Clarithromycin, erythromycin, indinavir, lopinavir/ritonavir, ritonavir	• Itraconazole concentrations increase • Monitor for adverse effects of itraconazole	
		Contraindicated: cisapride, pimozide, quinidine, dofetilide, dronedarone, levacetylmethadol, methadone, midazolam, triazolam, eplerenone, nisoldipine, ergot alkaloids, eletriptan, aliskiren, apixaban, conivaptan, tolvaptan, ranolazine	• Itraconazole increases cisapride, pimozide, quinidine, dofetilide, dronedarone, methadone, and levacetylmethadol serum concentrations; increased risk of QT prolongation and torsades de pointes • Itraconazole increases serum concentrations of other drugs listed resulting in serious life-threatening adverse effects related to supratherapeutic concentrations of the other drugs (i.e., prolonged sedative effects with midazolam/triazolam)	

(Continued)

Table 26.2 (Continued) Significant drug-drug interactions among the antifungal agents[a]

Antifungal class	Specific medication	Drug interactions	Clinical significance	References
	Posaconazole	Cyclosporine[e], tacrolimus[e], statins, calcium channel blockers (i.e., nifedipine, felodipine, diltiazem, verapamil), vinca alkaloids, benzodiazepines (midazolam, triazolam, alprazolam), phenytoin, protease inhibitors (ritonavir, atazanavir), digoxin, steroids (i.e., salmeterol, fluticasone) Rifampin, rifabutin, phenytoin, omeprazole, cimetidine, metoclopramide (suspension only), efavirenz **Contraindicated:** Ergot alkaloids, pimozide, dofetilide, dronedarone, cisapride, quinidine, sirolimus, simvastatin, eplerenone apixaban, conivaptan, tolvaptan, methadone, ranolazine	• Posaconazole increases drug concentrations of all drugs listed • Monitor for adverse effects related to supratherapeutic concentrations of each drug • Posaconazole concentrations decrease • Monitor for breakthrough fungal infections or suboptimal clinical efficacy • Posaconazole increases cisapride, pimozide, quinidine, dofetilide, dronedarone, and methadone serum concentrations; increased risk of QT prolongation and torsades de pointes • Posaconazole increases serum concentrations of other drugs listed resulting in serious life-threatening adverse effects related to supratherapeutic concentrations of the other drug	[110,218,219,221,222]

(Continued)

Table 26.2 (*Continued*) Significant drug-drug interactions among the antifungal agents[a]

Antifungal class	Specific medication	Drug interactions	Clinical significance	References
	Voriconazole	Cyclosporine[f], tacrolimus[f], phenytoin, sulfonylureas (i.e., glipizide, glyburide), statins (i.e., simvastatin, lovastatin), vinca alkaloids, calcium channel blockers (i.e., felodipine), benzodiazepines (i.e., midazolam, alprazolam, triazolam), prednisolone, oral contraceptives, cimetidine, fentanyl, oxycodone, methadone, ibuprofen, warfarin Clopidogrel, omeprazole Phenytoin, efavirenz **Contraindicated:** rifampin, ritonavir, carbamazepine, phenobarbital rifabutin, sirolimus, quinidine, pimozide, dofetilide, dronedarone, terfenadine ergot alkaloids, cisapride, apixaban, conivaptan, tolvaptan, eplerenone, fluticasone, salmeterol, ranolazine	• Voriconazole increases drug concentrations of all drugs listed • Monitor for adverse effects related to supratherapeutic concentrations of each drug • Methadone also has increased risk of QT prolongation and torsades de pointes • Voriconazole decreases serum concentrations of active metabolites of clopidogrel • Voriconazole concentrations increase with omeprazole; omeprazole concentrations increase with voriconazole • Voriconazole concentrations decrease with all of these drugs • Efavirenz concentrations also increase with voriconazole • Voriconazole concentrations decrease with rifampin, ritonavir, carbamezepine, phenobarbital, and rifabutin • Rifabutin concentrations increase with voriconazole • Voriconazole increases cisapride, pimozide, quinidine, dofetilide, and dronedarone serum concentrations; increased risk of QT prolongation and torsades de pointes • Voriconazole increases serum concentrations of other drugs listed resulting in serious life-threatening adverse effects related to supratherapeutic concentrations of the other drug	[103,105,127,218, 219,221,222]

(Continued)

Table 26.2 (*Continued*) Significant drug–drug interactions among the antifungal agents[a]

Antifungal class	Specific medication	Drug interactions	Clinical significance	References
	Isavuconazole	Rifampin	• Isavuconazole concentrations decrease with coadministration with rifampin. • Use with caution	[113,114,132,176]
		Lopinavir/ritonavir	• Isavuconazole concentrations increase with coadministration with lopinavir/ritonavir • Use with caution	
		Bupropion	• Isavuconazole increases drug concentrations of bupropion • Dose increase of bupropion may be necessary when coadministered with isavuconazole	
		Atorvastatin, cyclosporine, sirolimus, tacrolimus, midazolam, mycophenolate mofetil, digoxin	• Isavuconazole increases drug concentrations of all drugs listed • Therapeutic drug monitoring should be performed with sirolimus, tacrolimus, cyclosporine and digoxin	
Echinocandins	Anidulafungin	None	NA	[146]
	Caspofungin	Cyclosporine	• Cyclosporin may increase capsofungin concentrations and may increase hepatotoxic risk	[144,223,224,225]
		Tacrolimus	• Caspofungin may decrease tacrolimus concentrations; close monitoring of tacrolimus recommended	
		Rifampin	• Rifampin reduces caspofungin concentrations by 30%	
		Efavirenz, nevirapine, phenytoin, dexamethasone and carbamazepine	• These drugs induce metabolism of caspofungin; increasing the daily dose of caspofungin to 70 mg/day is recommended with concomitant use	
	Micafungin	None	NA	[145]

(*Continued*)

Table 26.2 (*Continued*) Significant drug–drug interactions among the antifungal agents[a]

Antifungal class	Specific medication	Drug interactions	Clinical significance	References
Flucytosine (5-FC)		Amphotericin B formulations, zidovudine	• Increased risk for hematologic toxicity with zidovudine; amphotericin products can increase concentrations of 5-FC	[69,217]
Polyenes	Amphotericin B deoxycholate Liposomal amphotericin B Amphotericin B lipid complex Amphotericin B colloidal dispersion	Cyclosporine, tacrolimus, digoxin, aminoglycosides, cisplatin, foscarnet, NSAIDs, corticosteroids, thiazide and loop diuretics, flucytosine	• Increased risk for nephrotoxicity and electrolyte disturbances; reduced clearance of 5-FC from nephrotoxicity may result in increased 5-FC toxicities	[217]

Abbreviations: NA = not applicable.

[a] Not intended to be a complete list.

[b] Capsule formulation.

[c] When administered with fluconazole ≥200 mg/day—cyclosporine dose decreases by 21%–50%; tacrolimus dose decreases by 40%; sirolimus dose decrease by 50%–70%.

[d] With itraconazole—cyclosporine dose decreases by 50%–60%; tacrolimus dose decreases by 50–60%.

[e] With posaconazole—cyclosporine dose—three-fourths of original dose; tacrolimus dose—one-third of original dose.

[f] With voriconazole—cyclosporine dose—one-half of the original dose; tacrolimus dose—one-third of original dose.

with similar toxicity. While potential exists for cytarabine to antagonize the antifungal activity of flucytosine, the clinical significance of such an interaction in humans is unknown [69].

TRIAZOLES

Selection. Unlike other classes of antifungals, significant differences exist amongst the triazoles in pharmacokinetic profiles, available dosage forms, *in vitro* activity, drug interactions, and published clinical experience. Fluconazole, the first triazole on the market, is typically a preferred agent for susceptible fungi, such as *Candida* spp., *Coccidioides*, and *Cryptococcus* spp. due to its excellent bioavailabilty, availability in both parenteral and oral formulations, favorable pharmacokinetics, and lower cost in comparison to the other triazoles [3,41,62,96]. However, fluconazole's use can be limited due to its lack of activity against *C. krusei*, molds, and some *C. glabrata* isolates [96]. While itraconazole's spectrum of activity includes *Aspergillus* spp., it is only available orally, has erratic absorption, and more adverse effects compared to fluconazole [9,96]. Itraconazole is often used for the treatment of endemic fungal infections, such as histoplasmosis, blastomycosis, sporotrichosis, and coccidiomycosis [40,41,50,135]. Voriconazole, posaconazole and isavuconazole exhibit activity against *Aspergillus spp.* and have enhanced activity (relative to fluconazole) against *Candida spp.,* such as *C. krusei* and *C. glabrata,* including those with an elevated MIC to fluconazole and itraconazole [9,96,98,227]. However, activity against *C. glabrata* can be variable with the newer triazoles and cross-resistance within the triazole class has occurred. For example, while voriconazole has demonstrated activity against fluconazole-resistant *Candida* spp., only 30% of the pathogens were susceptibile to voriconazole in an *in vitro* study [228]. In addition to being a drug-of-choice for invasive aspergillosis, voriconazole has been used to treat infections caused by *Fusarium spp.* and *Scedosporium apiospermum* [38,229,230]. Posaconazole can be used as step-down therapy for invasive mucormycosis and is considered an alternative agent in the treatment of aspergillosis [38,134,169,177,231,232]. Isavuconazole is a promising alternative for the prophylaxis and treatment of *Candida* infections. This assumption is based on *in vitro* activity and animal model data [98,227,233,234]. However, clinical data is lacking. On the other hand, recent clinical data supports the use of isavuconazole for the treatment of invasive aspergillosis and mucormycosis [137]. Isavuconazole has the potential to become first-line treatment for invasive aspergillosis and mucormycosis; however, there is a need for more clinical data and experience with its use [80].

Pharmacokinetic differences exist between the agents in terms of penetration into the CNS and urine, with fluconazole and voriconazole having the highest penetration into the CNS (isavuconazole has low CNS penetration but high penetration in brain) and only fluconazole achieves reliable concentrations in the urine [9,20,80,96,113,114].

The patient's inability to take oral therapy should be considered, as itraconazole is unavailable in parenteral dosage form in the United States. Renal function (i.e., fluconazole requires dose reduction and intravenous voriconazole and posaconazole are not recommended in renal impairment), and hepatic impairment (i.e., voriconazole requires a maintenance dose reduction) also should be considered when determining which triazole is utilized [9,20,96,112]. Despite its broader spectrum of activity against yeasts and molds, voriconazole has a higher incidence of adverse reactions, more drug–drug interactions, and a wide intra- and inter-patient variability in serum concentrations in comparison to fluconazole [9,96,133]. Therapeutic drug monitoring (TDM) in serious life-threatening fungal infections is warranted when using itraconazole, posaconazole, and voriconazole to ensure adequate concentrations to achieve optimal efficacy [235].

In addition to patient-, drug-, and disease-specific factors to consider when selecting a triazole for IFI treatment as previously summarized, risk of breakthrough IFIs and promotion/selection of resistance are additional considerations when selecting triazoles as IFI prophylaxis. IFI prophylaxis studies with triazoles have been conducted in a variety of transplantation settings such as HSCT patients and lung transplant recipients. Most of these studies evaluate the efficacy of fluconazole. For example, fungal-free survival at 180 days was evaluated in allogeneic HSCT patients ($n = 600$) receiving either fluconazole or voriconazole for the prevention of IFIs (in the setting of a structured fungal screening program utilizing serum galactomannan testing) [236]. No difference in survival between the drugs (75% for voriconazole vs. 78% for fluconazole; p = 0.49) was detected. Additionally, prophylactic posaconazole has been shown to be superior to fluconazole in allogeneic HSCT patients ($n = 600$) with GvHD in preventing aspergillosis (2.3% vs. 7.0%; odds ratio 0.31; 95% CI 0.13 to 0.75; p = 0.006) and decreasing the incidence of IFI-related death (1% vs. 4%; p = 0.046); however, both agents were effective in preventing all IFIs and adverse events were similar between both groups (36% in posaconazole vs. 38% in fluconazole) [237]. Fluconazole-resistant *C. glabrata* as well as breakthrough *C. krusei* infections have been reported in patients receiving prophylactic fluconazole therapy [238–240]. Therefore, while prevention of candidiasis can be routinely accomplished with the use of fluconazole in many transplant patient populations, those at higher risk for non-*albicans Candida* spp. infections and/or invasive aspergillosis should be considered for alternate prophylaxis. Itraconazole can also be used, but does not have any advantage over fluconazole in the prevention of IFIs with *Candida* spp. [3,4]. Newer trizoles (such as voriconazole and posaconazole) are often being used instead of itraconazole in patients at an increased risk for mold infections (such a lung transplant receipients) due to itraconazole's erratic absorption, drug–drug interactions, and high incidence of gastrointestinal intolerance [38,96,133]. In allogeneic HSCT patients ($n = 489$), voriconazole was found to be superior to itraconazole in the composite endpoints of success of prophylaxis (48.7% vs. 33.2%, p < 0.01), ability to tolerate study drug for ≥100 days (53.6% vs. 39.0%, p < 0.01), and survival to day 180 without IFIs (81.9% for voriconazole and 80.9% for itraconazole, p = NS) [241]. A general concern in patients receiving voriconazole for prophylaxis has been the increased incidence of elevated LFTs [241,242]. As previously mentioned, isavuconazole may be an attractive option for prophylaxis, but clinical data and experiences are limited [80].

Dosing/Administration. Fluconazole dosing is dependent on indication, pathogen susceptibility, and the patient's renal function (see Table 26.1). Loading doses (800 mg/day or 12 mg/kg/day) of fluconazole are recommended for candidemia or suspected invasive candidiasis [3]. Doses of intravenous and oral fluconazole are identical. Dosing adjustment is required in patients with renal dysfunction, including those requiring hemodialysis. Limited data exists regarding pharmacokinetic parameters of fluconazole in transplant patients. Small studies conducted in HSCT patients receiving oral fluconazole suggest comparable AUC and Cmax to healthy volunteers despite the fact that time to peak serum concentration (Tmax) was prolonged and plasma steady state was not reached within 14 days in these patients [243,244].

While AUC/MIC ratios provide useful information for optimal dose selection with fluconazole, individual patient AUC determinations are impractical. As a result, other parameters such as the dose:MIC ratio have also been evaluated for fluconazole. Studies evaluating the dose:MIC ratio in candidemia and mucosal candidiasis have found that a ratio greater than 50 had a better response rate to treatment in comparison to those with lower ratios [95,245]. Utilizing this data, patients infected with *Candida* spp. whose MIC to fluconazole was 32 mcg/mL would require higher doses of fluconazole (>400 mg/day). Based on proposed *in vitro* interpretive breakpoints, *C. albicans*, *C. tropicalis*, and *C. parapsilosis* isolates with MICs >4 mcg/mL would not be able to a reach target dose:MIC ratio with fluconazole doses of 400 mg/day [228]. Similarly with *C. glabrata*, MICs of ≤32 mcg/mL would be considered susceptible using a higher target dose of fluconazole 800 mg/day [228].

Itraconazole dosing recommendations are also summarized in Table 26.1. Loading doses (200 mg TID X 3 days) have been recommended in the treatment of aspergillosis [38]. While itraconazole is available as a capsule and a solution, the solution is more extensively and reliably absorbed. Studies of itraconazole capsules conducted in HSCT patients have reported reductions in itraconazole serum concentrations (in comparison to healthy adults) and high inter-individual variability (likely secondary to patients' concurrent medications, comorbidities, and food consumption) [246,247]. Similar results of reduced and variable absorption were noted in a small study evaluating itraconazole serum concentrations in lung transplant patients [248]. Itraconazole oral solution is best absorbed under fasting conditions and has a bioavailability of 50%

[20,96,102]. The solution should be taken on an empty stomach and the capsules with food or an acidic beverage (i.e., cola) to enhance absorption [96,102]. Based on current (limited) data, no dosing adjustments are recommended for patients with renal impairment or those requiring either hemo- or peritoneal dialysis. While recommendations regarding dosing adjustments in patients with hepatic impairment are lacking, it is known that the half-life of the drug is prolonged in these patients [9,20].

Voriconazole is available as both intravenous and oral (tablets and suspension) formulations (see Table 26.1). The recommended dose for intravenous therapy is weight-based, while oral therapy is a standard fixed dose. Oral bioavailability is approximately 96%, but may be reduced by about 20% and delayed by an hour when administered with food [20,103,104]. High-fat meals have been shown to reduce both the peak serum concentration (Cmax) and AUC, therefore oral voriconazole is recommended to be administered either 1 hour before or 1 hour after meals [103,104]. Administration of a loading dose can achieve target concentrations more rapidly (within 24 hours) [103,105]. A study evaluating the conversion of weight-based IV to fixed standard oral doses of voriconazole suggests that one may not be able to achieve similar serum concentrations in patients of extreme weights [249]. Following a standard loading dose, the maintenance dose should be reduced by 50% in patients with mild-to-moderate hepatic impairment (Child-Pugh class A or B) [103,250]. Currently, no pharmacokinetic studies or recommendations are available for patients with more severe hepatic impairment (Child-Pugh class C) [103]. While no dosing adjustments are recommended in patients with mild to severe renal impairment, the intravenous formulation of voriconazole is solubilized in sulfobutylether-B-cyclodextrin (SBECD) and accumulation of SBECD can occur in patients with a creatinine clearance of <50 mL/minute [103,251]. Therefore, these patients should avoid receiving the intravenous formulation of voriconazole for maintenance dosing unless the benefits outweigh the risks of SBECD accumulation [103,251]. A recent study evaluating the safety and treatment outcomes in acutely ill patients with candidemia and renal insufficiency compared patients receiving intravenous voriconazole with SBECD to amphotericin B deoxycholate followed by fluconazole [252]. Patients with moderate (CrCl 30–50 mL/minute) to severe (CrCl <30 mL/minute) renal failure receiving voriconazole (median of 7 days IV therapy) had less acute renal failure or worsening renal insufficiency (39% vs. 53%) in comparison to amphotericin B.

Studies in allogeneic HSCT, liver, and lung transplant recipients have documented poor absorption with high inter- and intra-patient variability in voriconazole concentrations [253–257]. In one report in HSCT recipients, 15% had undetectable trough concentrations [254]. The pharmacokinetics and bioavailability of voriconazole were evaluated in adult lung transplant patients (n = 13) during the early postoperative period [256]. Bioavailability in cystic fibrosis (CF) patients was significantly lower compared to non-CF patients, suggesting that they would require higher doses. Bioavailabilty improved with postoperative time. Liver transplant patients receiving voriconazole immediately following transplant also demonstrated highly variable voriconazole serum concentrations [62]. While genetic polymorphisms of *Cyp2C19* can also significantly impact voriconazole metabolism and (subsequently) serum concentrations, *Cyp2C19* genotyping in patients prior to starting voriconazole therapy has not been routinely performed. Finally, pediatric patients metabolize voriconazole at a faster rate than adults and therefore may require higher doses in order to achieve comparable concentrations achieved in adults [250].

Posaconazole is available as an oral suspension, intravenous solution, and oral tablet (delayed-release). Typical doses of posaconazole suspension range between 600 and 800 mg/day in divided doses. With the tablet and intravenous formulations, a loading dose of 300 mg (three 100 mg tablets) is taken twice daily on the first day, followed by a 300 mg daily maintenance dose on the second day and thereafter (see Table 26.1). Host factors (such as chemotherapy-induced mucositis, gastrointestinal impairment secondary to GvHD, diarrhea, and a decrease in dietary intake) can lead to poor posaconazole suspension absorption [258,259]. Patients who exhibit poor absorption of posaconazole suspension may not benefit solely from increasing doses [260]. Dividing the total daily dose into two or four doses (i.e., 200 mg QID) is recommended and appears to increase the bioavailability [108,109]. Optimal posaconazole suspension absorption also occurs when administered with a high-fat meal, a liquid nutritional supplement or carbonated acidic beverage (i.e., ginger ale) [107,110]. Furthermore, coadministration of posaconazole suspension with H2 blockers or proton pump inhibitors should be avoided as a high gastric pH can decrease posaconazole concentrations [110]. Regardless of such attempts to improve posaconazole suspension absorption, these measures may still result in inadequate blood concentrations. Therefore, posaconazole tablet formulation will likely replace the older suspension. A study evaluating the tablet formulation in IFIs among subjects considered high risk with neutropenia found average steady-state serum concentrations significantly higher than those achieved with the highest absorbable dose of posaconazole suspension (1.1 mcg/mL vs. 0.52 mcg/mL). Of note, the average serum concentration with the delayed-release tablet is higher than the proposed target concentrations for prophylaxis and treatment of IFIs [109,261]. Given its delayed-release design, posaconazole tablets cannot be crushed or chewed. Its absorption is independent of stomach pH; however, the tablets should be administered with food [262]. A phase 3 study evaluated the pharmacokinetics of intravenous and suspension formulations of posaconazole in high-risk patients for IFIs. The study found that the intravenous formulation was well tolerated and resulted in adequate steady-state serum concentrations. Furthermore, individuals who remained on the intravenous formulation compared to those who switched to the suspension formulation had a higher mean steady-state serum concentration [112]. The delayed release tablet and intravenous formulation are capable of predictably achieving higher serum posaconazole concentrations [112,261].

Pharmacokinetic studies with oral posaconazole performed in patients with mild-to-moderate renal impairment indicated no dosage adjustments are necessary for this patient population [110,262,263]. However, individuals with hemodialysis-dependent renal failure did demonstrate variable posaconazole AUC values [263]. Therefore, it is recommended to monitor these patients closely for clinical response [110,263]. In contrast, intravenous posaconazole, like intravenous voriconazole, is solubilized in cyclodextrin and accumulation of cyclodextrin can occur in patients with a creatinine clearance of <50 mL/minute [264]. In a study evaluating a single dose of posaconazole in patients with varying degrees of hepatic impairment ($n = 19$), pooled Cmax values indicated that there was a 36% increase in the AUC in patients with hepatic impairment (relative to healthy controls), as well as a prolonged elimination half-life [265]. While the authors concluded that dosing adjustments were probably unnecessary in patients with hepatic impairment receiving posaconazole, larger studies need to be conducted and monitoring of posaconazole serum concentrations is likely needed.

Similar to that observed for voriconazole, pharmacokinetic studies conducted in HSCT patients have demonstrated high posaconazole (suspension formulation) inter- and intra-patient variability [258,259,266,267]. As much as a 50% decrease in drug exposure has been reported with conditions such as mucositis, diarrhea, and GvHD [258,259,266,267]. Posaconazole serum concentrations in cardiothoracic transplant patients ($n = 17$) also found decreases in drug exposure (47% of patients had concentrations ≤ 0.5 µg/mL), but was thought to be related to concurrent proton pump inhibitor use [268]. Furthermore, pharmacokinetic parameters in lung transplant patients ($n = 20$) receiving posaconazole 400 mg twice a day with high-fat meals for 14 days was also evaluated, but found to be dissimilar to HSCT and cardiothoracic transplant patients. Posaconazole plasma concentrations, pulmonary ELF, and AC concentrations in these patients were measured and were above the MIC_{90} for *Aspergillus* spp., thus indicating that this dose could be used in this patient population for prevention and treatment of infection [269].

Isavuconazole is administered as a water-soluble prodrug. It is available as an intravenous solution and oral capsule. Dosing is the same for both invasive mucormycosis and aspergillosis. A loading dose is required for the first 48 hours, then a maintenance dose follows 12–24 hours after the last loading dose (see Table 26.1). Bioequivalence between the intravenous and oral formulations has been demonstrated; therefore, dosing is the same and switching between formulations doesn't require an additional loading dose. Dosing is not affected by renal impairment (including end-stage renal disease), hepatic impairment (mild or moderate), gastric pH, or age. Oral isavuconazole may be administered with or without food [113,114,176,270].

Monitoring. Serum concentration monitoring of fluconazole is generally not required due to its favorable pharmacokinetic profile and wide therapeutic range in comparison to other triazoles [96,235]. Similarly, serum concentration monitoring of isavuconazole is not currently recommended; however, since the correlation between serum concentrations, adverse effects, and efficacy have not been fully assessed at this time and the utility of TDM remains uncertain [132]. In contrast, itraconazole, voriconazole, and posaconazole demonstrate significant intra- and inter-patient variability in serum concentrations secondary to alterations in absorption, metabolism, elimination, and drug–drug interactions [235]. Therapeutic serum drug concentration monitoring can be beneficial in select, high-risk patients receiving these triazoles in order to ensure adequate target concentrations. Drug and indication-specific recommended target concentrations for the triazoles are summarized in Table 26.3. Samples for analysis are obtained once steady state has been achieved (usually 5–7 days after initiation of therapy) [271]. Although the trough concentration (obtained just prior to the dose) does not provide verification of optimal triazole absorption and AUC, such information can aid in determining if a patient has subtherapeutic drug exposure [271]. Limited data are available with select triazoles to correlate trough concentrations with successful prevention or treatment of IFIs as well as toxicity [134,272–278]. Recently, a cohort study in patients with hematological malignancies, compared posaconazole trough concentrations and concentrations obtained at 4 and 8 hours post dose [279]. A majority of the trough concentrations and 4 hour post-dose concentrations differed by <20%. Therefore, although troughs are likely preferred, this study suggested posaconazole concentrations taken several hours prior to the trough may still be helpful. Monitoring of concentrations should be performed monthly in patients receiving prolonged courses of triazoles (and in some cases twice a month) depending on changes in concurrent interacting medications, disease progression, toxicity, or changes in the host (i.e., development of mucositis, diarrhea, or vomiting) [271].

Itraconazole serum concentrations of <0.5 μg/mL (by high performance liquid chromatography—[HPLC]) for IFI prophylaxis have been associated with an increased risk of breakthrough fungal infections [273,281]. For treatment of various IFIs due to *Candida, Aspergillus, Cryptococcus,* and *Coccidioides* spp., a higher likelihood of treatment success occurred when itraconazole serum concentrations exceed 1–2 μg/mL (by HPLC) or 6 μg/mL (by bioassay) [271,272,282]. In terms of toxicity, itraconazole serum trough concentrations greater than 5 μg/mL (by HPLC) or 17 μg/mL (by bioassay) were associated with an increased risk of peripheral edema and GI adverse effects [277].

Multiple studies evaluating voriconazole concentrations and their correlation to prophylaxis and treatment outcomes have been evaluated. Prophylactic use of voriconazole has also been evaluated in allo-HSCT patients [275,276]. Voriconazole trough concentrations of <0.5 μg/mL were more likely to develop breakthrough fungal infections versus those with trough concentrations >2 μg/mL. For treatment, patients in several studies with mean plasma concentrations of less than 0.5 μg/mL had a lower treatment response in comparison to those with concentrations between 0.5 μg/mL and 5 μg/mL (not statistically significant) [103]. In another study of patients (60% with hematological malignancy) with IFIs ($n = 52$), where half the patients were being treated for aspergillosis infections, 46% of patients with voriconazole trough concentrations of ≤1 μg/mL failed therapy in comparison to 12% of patients with concentrations >1 μg/mL [274]. Logistic regression modeling of data indicated that successful treatment had a probability of 70% if a trough of 1 μg/mL was obtained. For treatment of aspergillosis, random concentrations of <2.05 μg/mL were associated with poor outcomes [283].

Several studies have evaluated the correlation between voriconazole serum concentrations and toxicity [254,274,278]. Conclusions regarding relationships between voriconazole serum concentrations and LFT abnormalities are conflicting. In HSCT patients, a correlation was made between voriconazole serum concentrations with AST ($r = 0.5$, $p = 0.0009$) and alkaline phosphatase (ALP) ($r = 0.34$, $p = 0.03$) [254]. However, there was no correlation with ALT or bilirubin. The high incidence of liver dysfunction after HSCT and confounding factors made the establishment of a cause-and-effect relationship difficult. Other studies have reported non-statistically significant increased incidence of liver abnormalities in patients with voriconazole concentrations >5.5 mg/L in comparison to patients with lower concentrations (19% vs. 8%) [274]. No correlations were found between voriconazole troughs and ALP or γ-glutamyl transpeptidase. In a retrospective analysis

Table 26.3 Relative inhibition of cytochrome P450 isoenzymes by triazoles [100,102,103,105,110,133,176,218,220,280]

Cytochrome P450 Enzyme	Fluconazole	Itraconazole	Voriconazole	Posaconazole	Isavuconazole
2C19	+	–	+++^	–	–
2C8/9	++	+	++^	–	–
3A4	++	+++^	++^	+++^	+/++^

+   Minimal inhibition.
++ Moderate inhibition.
+++ Strong inhibition.
^   Antifungal is also a substrate for cytochrome P450 enzyme.

of ten phase 2 and 3 safety and pharmacokinetic studies, a weak but statistically significant correlation between voriconazole serum concentrations and risk of AST (OR, 1.13; 95% CI 1.06 to 1.20), ALP (OR, 1.16; 95% CI 1.08 to 1.25), or bilirubin (OR, 1.17; 95% CI 1.08 to 1.27) abnormalities were noted [278]. Additionally, utilizing the receiver operator curve analysis, no single voriconazole concentration was predictive of subsequent AST, ALT, ALP, or bilirubin abnormalities. Elevated voriconazole serum concentrations were thought likely the result of hepatic impairment and not the etiology. Data regarding CNS toxicity and voriconazole serum concentrations have been more consistent, with serum concentrations >5 mg/L being associated with an increased risk [274,284]. For example, in one study of patients with IFIs (n = 52), the incidence of neurotoxicity was 31% in patients with trough concentrations >5.5 mg/L [274].

Several studies have evaluated correlations between posaconazole serum concentrations administered prophylactically and breakthrough fungal infections. In patients with GvHD following HSCT and AML/MDS patients with chemotherapy-induced neutropenia, breakthrough IFIs were more likely to occur in patients with random plasma concentrations of <0.719 µg/mL [237,285,286]. In another study conducted in cardiothoracic transplant recipients receiving either posaconazole for prophylaxis or treatment, trough concentrations that were >500 ng/mL were more likely to predict success in both preventing and treating IFIs [268]. For treatment as salvage therapy for invasive aspergillosis, clinical response was higher in patients whose mean plasma concentrations were between 0.719 and 1.250 µg/mL [134]. Patients with concentrations in the highest quartile (1.25 µg/mL) had a clinical response rate of 70%. To date, studies have not been able to establish a clear relationship between posaconazole serum concentrations and adverse effects [285,287]. Given this lack of correlation, target posaconazole trough concentrations for IFI prophylaxis of >0.7 µg/mL have been proposed [285]. Target posaconazole trough concentrations for treatment have been recommended to be >0.7 µg/mL with an upwards titration to >1.25 µg/mL if needed [134]. See Table 26.3.

Other tests. All of the triazoles have been associated with elevations in transaminases and bilirubin that are typically transient in nature. It is recommended that baseline and subsequent serial monitoring of liver function tests, including total bilirubin, be performed in patients considered to be at an increased risk of developing transaminitis (i.e., patients with underlying hepatic dysfunction, patients receiving progressive dose escalation of voriconazole) [100, 102,103,110,113,114,127]. Minimal data exist regarding hepatotoxicity and triazole cross-reactivity. Case reports have suggested that patients who have experienced elevations in liver function tests while receiving fluconazole, itraconazole, or posaconazole can be switched to voriconazole safely [288,289]. Patients taking concurrent drugs that can prolong the QT interval should also use triazoles with caution as this class of agents has been associated with QT

prolongation and torsades, with the exception of isavuconazole. In clinical trials, isavuconazole was noted to cause dose- and concentration-related QTc interval shortening. QTc shortening occurred with an incidence of 0.4%. The clinical significance of isavuconazole-induced QTc shortening is unknown at this time [113,176]. Additionally, patients receiving voriconazole should be monitored for visual disturbances during therapy (transient and resolve with continued drug use), skin reactions, such as rash or phototoxicity (reversible once discontinued and not preventable with sunscreen), as well as neurotoxicity. Patients with renal impairment should be monitored closely for declining renal function if receiving intravenous voriconazole or posaconazole, as patients with an estimated CrCl of <50 mL/minute should not receive intravenous voriconazole or posaconazole unless the benefit outweighs the risk of cyclodextrin toxicity [103].

Drug Interactions. The triazoles have a significant number of drug–drug interactions, including medications commonly used in the transplant patient population [133,218]. They are mediated primarily through their variable inhibition of the cytochrome P450 system (most notably *Cyp*3A4) [218]. See Table 26.4. Among the triazoles, voriconazole exhibits the most drug–drug interactions secondary to its inhibitory properties of *Cyp*3A4, 2C8/9, and 2C19 as well as being a substrate for all three isoenzymes [218]. Genetic polymorphisms of individual patients with *Cyp*450, 2C19, and 2C9 isoenzymes can also play a factor in determining the extent of the drug interactions [120,219]. Fluconazole is considered to be a moderate inhibitor of the isoenzymes 3A4, 2C8/9, and to a lesser extent 2C19 [96,218,219]. Itraconazole is also a potent inhibitor of *Cyp*3A4 isoenzyme, and to a lesser degree *Cyp*2C8/9 [218]. Although posaconazole is not metabolized via the CYP450 system, drug–drug interactions do occur through this system due to posaconazole's ability to inhibit *Cyp*3A4 [220]. Isavuconazole appears to be a mild to moderate inhibitor of *Cyp*3A4. The drug's interaction profile most closely resembles fluconazole and itraconazole [113,114,132,176]. All of the triazoles are substrates for P-glycoprotein with the exception of voriconazole and isavuconazole [176,218]. Additionally, itraconazole, posaconazole, and isavuconazole are inhibitors of P-glycoprotein [176,218,290]. Furthermore, the uridine 5′-diphosphate (UDP)-glucuronosyltransferases (UGT) enzyme system, a part of phase II metabolism, is responsible for glucuronidation of some drugs, particularly posaconazole [121,218]. Drug interactions occur with fluconazole as a result of its ability to inhibit glucuronidation of some drugs metabolized through uridine diphosphate glucuronosyltransferases (UDP-UGTs) [96].

Inhibition of *Cyp*3A4 (which may occur immediately following the first dose of the triazole) may result in increases in serum concentrations of immunosuppressive agents, such as cyclosporine, tacrolimus, and sirolimus [218,219]. These immunosupressives are also substrates and inhibitors of P-glycoprotein [218]. Therefore, inhibition of P-glycoprotein by itraconazole, posaconazole, and

Table 26.4 Therapeutic drug monitoring for select antifungal agents [39,102,103,134,235,271–278,285,287,291–296]

Drug	Timing of sample	Target concentration(s)	Recommendations for subtherapeutic concentrations
Amphotericin B	NA	Not established	• NA
Flucytosine	Days 3–5—Peak (2 hours post dose)	Treatment: (cryptococcal meningitis) 30–80 µg/mL[#] (candidal meningitis) 40–60 µg/mL Toxicity: >100 µg/mL	• Increase dose
Itraconazole	> Day 7—Trough[a]	Prophylaxis: ≥0.5 µg/mL Treatment: 1–2 µg/mL Toxicity: >5 µg/mL[b]	• Switch from capsule to solution formulation • Avoid acid suppressing agents • Increase dose up to 200 mg three times daily
Posaconazole	Day 5–7—Trough[a]	Prophylaxis: >0.7 µg/mL Treatment: >1.0 µg/mL Toxicity: not established	• Switch from suspension to DR tablets • Take with fatty meal and carbonated acidic beverage (suspension) • Avoid acid suppressing agents (suspension) • Change dosing regimen to 200 mg four times daily (produces higher concentrations than 400 mg twice daily) (suspension)
Voriconazole	Day 5–7—Trough[a]	Prophylaxis: ≥0.5 µg/mL Treatment: >1 µg/mL Toxicity associated with Trough: >5 µg/mL	• Avoid taking with meals • Increase daily dose by 100 mg and recheck concentration in 1 week
Isavuconazole	(not established)	(not established)	
Anidulafungin Caspofungin Micafungin	NA	Not established	• NA

Abbreviations: NA = not applicable.
[#] By HPLC (high-performance liquid chromatography)
[a] Trough concentration taken prior to next dose
[b] HPLC value estimated from microbiologic assay. Microbiologic assay is twofold to threefold higher in value than HPLC because it also measures active metabolite of hydroxyitraconazole. [235,277]

isavuconazole can also contribute to additional increased concentrations of these agents [176,218,219]. Dose reductions of these immunosupressives (ranging from 30% to 90% depending on triazole) followed by immunosuppressive serum concentration and close adverse event monitoring are recommended when transplant patients are initiating a triazole [100,102,103,110,218,219]. Once the triazole therapy is discontinued, immunosuppressants should be closely monitored and doses adjusted as appropriate. Serum concentrations of immunosuppressants commonly return to baseline after 7–10 days of triazole discontinuation [219]. See Table 26.2.

Corticosteroids, chemotherapeutic agents, proton pump inhibitors, H2 antagonists, cardiovascular drugs, benzodiazepines, and rifamycins may also interact with triazoles (see Table 26.2). Triazoles may increase corticosteroid concentrations, leading to adrenal insufficiency [218]. Triazoles

that are pH-dependent for absorption (i.e., itraconazole capsules, posaconazole suspension) may exhibit decreased absorption if concomitantly administered with H2 antagonists or proton pump inhibitors [218]. This decrease has been reported to be as much as 32% change in healthy volunteers [110]. Benzodiazepines metabolized by $Cyp3A4$ (i.e., midazolam, triazolam, and alprazolam) may exhibit increased concentrations secondary to triazole-induced inhibition [102,110,218,220].

Several different classes of cardiovascular medications interact with triazoles. Triazole-induced inhibition of $Cyp3A4$ can lead to increased concentrations of some statins (such as atorvastatin, simvastatin, lovastatin) and calcium channel blockers (such as diltiazem, verapamil) [218,220]. Itraconazole and isavuconazole may increase digoxin serum concentrations through P-glycoprotein inhibition and warfarin prothrombin time can be prolonged with fluconazole and voriconazole in some instances due to inhibition of *Cyp*3A4 and 2C9 [100,102,103,176,218,220,221]. Pharmacodynamic interactions may also occur between cardiovascular medications and triazoles due to possible potentiation of QT prolongation (such as dofetilide) and, therefore, are contraindicated with some triazoles. An extensive review of azoles and transplant drug interactions can be found elsewhere [218,219].

ECHINOCANDINS

Selection. Although FDA-approved indications differ between the echinocandins, agents within the echinocandin class are generally considered comparable based on pharmacokinetic profiles, *in vitro* activity and existing clinical data regarding efficacy and safety. All are approved for the treatment of candidemia, esophageal candidiasis and other suspected *Candida* spp. infections. In addition, caspofungin is FDA-approved for the treatment of invasive aspergillosis for those patients who have failed or cannot tolerate other therapies [144–146]. Relative to other echinocandins, the utility of caspofungin in transplant patients may be limited due to a significant drug interaction with cyclosporine and also the need for dosage adjustments with hepatic dysfunction [144].

Published experience with echinocandins in pediatric patients is somewhat limited. Reports describe caspofungin use for invasive candidiasis and as salvage therapy (alone or in combination for other types of infection) for aspergillosis [297]. Micafungin pharmacokinetics have recently been reported in pediatric patients [298,299], and it has been studied among pediatric patients for invasive candidiasis [300]. These studies demonstrate comparable efficacy to other agents with fewer adverse effects. While anidulafungin previously was not recommended for use in the pediatric population (due to its reconstitution requirement with ethanol), reformulation has now permitted reconstitution with sterile water for injection [146,297]. Although there are currently no pediatric efficacy data for anidulafungin, one study demonstrated it was safe in the infant and neonate population with similar concentrations to older children at comparable doses [301].

Dosing/Administration. The echinocandins require once-daily, intravenous infusions. Depending upon indication, both anidulafungin and caspofungin may require a loading dose on day 1 (see Table 26.1). Alternate-day dosing of micafungin 3 mg/kg IV every other day as prophylaxis has also been investigated in pediatric HSCT recipients ($n = 15$) [302]. While plasma concentrations measured at 48 hours were higher than the MIC of "highly susceptible fungal pathogens" (mean, 0.8 mg/L, range of 0.3–2.0 mg/L), clinical data to support such dosing is presently lacking.

Similar to amphotericin B, dose escalation has been investigated with the echinocandin class due to their concentration-dependent pharmacodynamic profile. In one study, patients with invasive candidiasis were randomized to receive either the usual dose caspofungin (70 mg loading dose followed by 50 mg/day) or high-dose caspofungin (150 mg/day) [303]. While no differences in the secondary outcome of treatment response could be detected (likely due to an inadequate sample size), similar rates of adverse effects were observed in both groups. Micafungin has also been studied in a dose-escalation study [153]. Overall, there were no toxicities that were directly related to the dosing of micafungin. Further attempts of dose escalation of the echinocandins may be hindered by the echinocandin-specific, organism-specific paradoxic attenuation of *in vitro* activity at higher concentrations [142]. The clinical relevance of such an effect is unknown.

The effects of organ dysfunction on echinocandin dosing requirements vary between members of the class. Although micafungin is affected by hepatic dysfunction, the degree to which it is affected generally does not require dosage adjustments for patients with liver disease [145]. The exception may be liver dysfunction (as reflected by total bilirubin) in liver transplant recipients [304]. Micafungin concentrations relative to dose was significantly higher in patients with total bilirubin concentrations >5 mg/dL (p < 0.0001) [304]. Therefore, while more studies are needed, a reduction in micafungin dose should be considered among patients with elevated total bilirubin levels. In patients with moderate hepatic impairment (Child-Pugh score 7–9), the dose of caspofungin should be adjusted from 50 mg/day to the adjusted daily dose to 35 mg/day (both following the initial 70 mg dose load on day 1) [144]. Infusion-related reactions (such as fever, peripheral edema, rash, and other histamine-related reactions) may occur with echinocandin administration [144–146]. Infusions over at least 1 hour are recommended.

Dose adjustments of the echinocandin (specifically caspofungin) may be needed when certain medications are co-administered. For example, when caspofungin is used in combination with medications that induce metabolism (i.e., carbamazepine, dexamethasone, efavirenz, nevirapine, and phenytoin), the daily caspofungin dose should be increased to 70 mg/day [144,305]. Studies of caspofungin in combination with rifampin in healthy subjects revealed a 30% reduction in caspofungin concentrations [144,305]. Neither anidulafungin nor micafungin requires dosage adjustments when given concomitantly with other medications.

Monitoring. Echinocandin serum concentration monitoring is not routinely performed. Liquid chromatography-tandem mass spectrometry methods are under investigation currently [306–308]. Patients should be monitored for the development of adverse reactions of the medications throughout therapy; such reactions include hypersensitivity, infusion-related reactions, and hepatic adverse effects. In particular, patients receiving any of the echinocandins should be monitored for LFT elevations during therapy; if abnormal, the risk-to-benefit ratio should be considered if the echinocandin is to be continued. In addition, BUN and serum creatinine concentrations should be monitored in patients receiving micafungin [144–146].

Drug Interactions. Clinically-significant drug interactions for the echinocandin class are summarized in Table 26.2. Despite the lack of pharmacokinetic interactions due to CYP-450, echinocandins increase the incidence or severity of side effects from immunosuppressive therapies [144,309]. In one report, seven of the ten caspofungin-treated HSCT patients experienced a potential worsening of cyclosporine (CyA)-induced hepatotoxicity [144,223,309,310]. In another retrospective evaluation of twenty HSCT patients administered CyA and caspofungin, ALT and aspartate aminotransferase (AST) concentrations peaked at 104- and 203-fold times the upper limit of normal (respectively) during the 15 days of co-administration [223]. Alkaline phosphatase and total bilirubin concentrations also increased during treatment. All elevations decreased after caspofungin was discontinued [223]. Despite these findings, other reports have been published showing a negligible effect on hepatic function for this combination [224,225]. Increased liver enzymes (thought likely due to bacterial sepsis) was observed in only one of seven liver transplant recipients co-administered caspofungin and CyA [225]. Based on pharmacokinetic data in healthy adults demonstrating reductions in tacrolimus AUC_{0-12} and Cmax by 20% and 16%, respectively; close monitoring of tacrolimus concentrations are recommended in patients receiving caspofungin [144]. No significant interactions were observed when micafungin was studied in combination with tacrolimus in six HSCT patients as well as healthy volunteers [311,312]. Although a micafungin-CyA interaction has been reported among healthy volunteers ($n = 28$), no significant interactions between these agents were noted in the package insert [145].

Micafungin co-administration may increase serum concentrations of sirolimus, nifedipine and itraconazole. Thus, careful monitoring for toxicity and possible dosage reductions of these agents may be required when used concomitantly with micafungin [145]. Since anidulafungin does not undergo hepatic metabolism, it lacks CYP enzyme pathway and P-glycoprotein-mediated interactions [146]. Specifically, CyA, voriconazole, tacrolimus, liposomal amphotericin B and rifampin have all been studied with anidulafungin with no significant interactions noted [146,313].

Combination antifungal therapy

A comprehensive discussion of the application of combination therapy is beyond the scope of this chapter, and the reader is referred elsewhere for such discussions [62]. With rare exception, most of the data supporting such approaches are from animal models, *in vitro* studies and uncontrolled clinical observations [62]. Results of such studies may be conflicting, depending upon the model, definitions, dosing and sequencing of the antifungals [62].

With little exception, combination antifungal therapy is often restricted to patients with severe, life-threatening, treatment-refractory IFIs (invasive candidiasis, invasive aspergillosis, and rare mold infections). Combination therapy for invasive candidiasis is poorly studied and not routinely recommended [3]. The exception would be in cases of *Candida* CNS infections, endocarditis or opthalmitis where combinations of amphotericin B/flucytosine have been recommended [3]. Echinocandin combinations (with azoles, flucytosine or amphotericin B) may also be considered for *Candida* endocarditis [3]. For invasive aspergillosis, the role of combination therapy is for salvage therapy [38]. However, while combinations of caspofungin plus voriconazole are mentioned for CNS infections, little clinical data is available to support such recommendations. Recently, a pivotal randomized study evaluating monotherapy voriconazole versus combination therapy with voriconazole plus anidulafungin for the primary treatment of invasive aspergillosis was conducted. The primary endpoint of all-cause mortality did not show combination therapy was superior based on predefined criteria of a 10% difference. Mortality rates at 6 weeks were 19.3% (26 of 135) for combination therapy and 27.5% (39 of 142) for monotherapy (8.2% difference [95% CI, 19.0 to 1.5]; p = 0.087). However, in a post-hoc analysis of individuals with galactomannan-diagnosed infection, the difference in mortality was 11.5% (15.7% [17 of 108] for combination therapy vs. 27.3% [30 of 110] for monotherapy: 11.5% difference [CI, 22.7 to 0.4]; p = 0.037). Therefore, clinicians must consider whether an 8.2%–11.5% improvement in survival is clinically significant, despite not showing statistical significance in this study [314].

Perhaps the indication best-studied for combination antifungals in humans is the treatment of cryptococcal meningitis, where amphotericin B plus flucytosine combinations are recommended as initial (induction) therapy for patients with HIV in developed nations [39]. Other combinations considered alternatives to this first-line therapy for such patients include amphotericin B plus fluconazole or fluconazole plus flucytosine [39]. Likewise, controlled human data are lacking regarding combination therapy for endemic mycoses. Combinations of amphotericin B plus either fluconazole or itraconazole may be considered for severe coccidioidomycosis [41].

Due largely to the high mortality rates in patients with invasive mucormycosis, there has been a growing interest in the use of newer antifungal treatment strategies in this patient population, including (but not limited to) combinations of antifungal agents [169,181,232]. Such combinations may include the use of an amphotericin B (most commonly a lipid-based formulation such as LAmB) in combination with either posaconazole or an echinocandin [169,171,181,232]. The utility of isavuconazole in combination with another antifungal for the treatment of mucormycosis is unknown. Regardless of the agents used, prompt recognition and rapid institution of antifungal therapy are keys to successful treatment of this infection.

CONCLUSION

Optimizing the choice, dose and administration of antifungals for prevention and treatment in HSCT and SOT recipients can significantly impact IFI-related morbidity and mortality. Systemic administration of the broad-spectrum antifungal amphotericin B (in its various formulations) is often limited by its toxicities (primarily nephrotoxicity and electrolyte wasting) and (in many situations) has been replaced by newer antifungals. For prophylaxis in select transplant patients, the use of aerosolized amphotericin B formulations is also being used. Flucytosine administration is limited primarily to oral administration (as part of a combination regimen) for the treatment of cryptococcal infections because of concerns over toxicity (primarily hematologic) and the rapid development of resistance when given as monotherapy. The triazoles (fluconazole, itraconazole, voriconazole, posaconazole, and isavuconazole) differ in their pharmacokinetic characteristics. Fluconazole possesses an optimal pharmacokinetic profile and can be administered orally and intravenously for the treatment of invasive candidiasis in select patients with susceptible *Candida* spp. However, its potency against non-*albicans Candida* (relative to voriconazole, posaconazole, and isavuconazole) is limited. In addition, these newer triazoles offer the potential to treat a variety of mold infections, notably invasive aspergillosis. However, triazoles possess significant (but varying) interactions with a variety of immunosuppressive agents used in the transplant population. In addition, the administration of itraconazole, voriconazole, or posaconazole in patients with documented IFIs should be guided by serum drug concentration monitoring. Echinocandins are parenteral antifungals, which possess potent activity against a broad spectrum of *Candida* spp. and have been used as part of salvage therapy in the treatment of invasive aspergillosis. Advantages to this class include minimal drug interactions and a favorable safety profile. Finally, little data are available to support the routine administration of combinations of antifungals outside the use of flucytosine-containing combinations for the treatment of cryptococcal infections.

REFERENCES

1. Kontoyiannis DP, Marr KA, Park BJ, et al. Prospective surveillance for invasive fungal infections in hematopoietic stem cell transplant recipients, 2001–2006: Overview of the Transplant-Associated Infection Surveillance Network (TRANSNET) Database. *Clin Infect Dis* 2010;50:1091–1100.
2. Pappas PG, Alexander BD, Andes DR, et al. Invasive fungal infections among organ transplant recipients: Results of the Transplant-Associated Infection Surveillance Network (TRANSNET). *Clin Infect Dis* 2010;50:1101–1111.
3. Pappas PG, Kauffman CA, Andes DR, et al. Executive summary: Clinical practice guideline for the management of candidiasis: 2016 Update by the Infectious Diseases Society of America. *Clin Infect Dis* 2016;62:409–417.
4. National Comprehensive Cancer Network. Prevention and Treatment of Cancer-related Infections. NCCN Guidelines Version 1.2018. https://www.nccn.org/professionals/physician_gls/pdf/infections.pdf. Accessed 9 Oct 2018.
5. Patel GP, Simon D, Scheetz M, Crank CW, Lodise T, Patel N. The effect of time to antifungal therapy on mortality in candidemia associated septic shock. *Am J Ther* 2009;16:508–511.
6. Zilberberg MD, Kollef MH, Arnold H, et al. Inappropriate empiric antifungal therapy for candidemia in the ICU and hospital resource utilization: A retrospective cohort study. *BMC Infect Dis* 2010;10:150.
7. Drew R, Townsend M. Antifungal drug resistance: Clinical relevance and impact of antifungal drug use. *Curr Fung Infect Rep* 2010;4:129–136.
8. Marr KA, Laverdiere M, Gugel A, Leisenring W. Antifungal therapy decreases sensitivity of the *Aspergillus* galactomannan enzyme immunoassay. *Clin Infect Dis* 2005;40:1762–1769.
9. Pound MW, Townsend ML, Dimondi V, Wilson D, Drew RH. Overview of treatment options for invasive fungal infections. *Med Mycol* 2011;49:561–580.
10. Munoz P, Rojas L, Cervera C, et al. Poor compliance with antifungal drug use guidelines by transplant physicians: A framework for educational guidelines and an international consensus on patient safety. *Clin Transplant* 2012;26:87–96.
11. Neoh CF, Snell GI, Kotsimbos T, et al. Antifungal prophylaxis in lung transplantation—A world-wide survey. *Am J Transplant* 2011;11:361–366.
12. Singh N, Wagener MM, Cacciarelli TV, Levitsky J. Antifungal management practices in liver transplant recipients. *Am J Transplant* 2008;8:426–431.
13. Brajtburg J, Bolard J. Carrier effects on biological activity of amphotericin B. *Clin Microbiol Rev* 1996;9:512–531.
14. Vertut-Croquin A, Bolard J, Gary-Bobo CM. Transfer of amphotericin B from gel state vesicles to mycoplasma cells: Biphasic action on potassium transport and permeability. *Antimicrob Agents Chemother* 1985;28:167–171.
15. *Amphotericin B deoxycholate Package Insert*. X-Gen Pharmaceuticals, Horseheads, NY, April 2010. (Available at http://www.x-gen.us/wp-content/uploads/sites/21/2014/03/XGSS_TSM_AM.0118.pdf). Accessed 9 Oct 2018).
16. DiBonaventura G, Spedicato I, Picciani C, D'Antonio D, Piccolomini R. *In vitro* pharmacodynamic characteristics of amphotericin B, caspofungin, fluconazole, and voriconazole against bloodstream

isolates of infrequent *Candida* species from patients with hematologic malignancies. *Antimicrob Agents Chemother* 2004;48:4453–4456.

17. Andes D, Stamsted T, Conklin R. Pharmacodynamics of amphotericin B in a neutropenic-mouse disseminated-candidiasis model. *Antimicrob Agents Chemother* 2001;45:922–926.

18. Klepser ME, Wolfe EJ, Jones RN, Nightingale CH, Pfaller MA. Antifungal pharmacodynamic characteristics of fluconazole and amphotericin B tested against *Candida albicans*. *Antimicrob Agents Chemother* 1997;41:1392–1395.

19. Vitale RG, Meis JF, Mouton JW, et al. Evaluation of the post-antifungal effect (PAFE) of amphotericin B and nystatin against 30 zygomycetes using two different media. *J Antimicrob Chemother* 2003;52:65–70.

20. Dodds-Ashley E, Lewis R, Lewis J, Martin C, Andes D. Pharmacology of systemic antifungal agents. *Clin Infect Dis* 2006;43:S28–S39.

21. Young LY, Hull CM, Heitman J. Disruption of ergosterol biosynthesis confers resistance to amphotericin B in *Candida lusitaniae*. *Antimicrob Agents Chemother* 2003;47:2717–2724.

22. Pfaller MA, Messer SA, Boyken L, Tendolkar S, Hollis RJ, Diekema DJ. Geographic variation in the susceptibilities of invasive isolates of *Candida glabrata* to seven systemically active antifungal agents: A global assessment from the ARTEMIS antifungal surveillance program conducted in 2001 and 2002. *J Clin Microbiol* 2004;42:3142–146.

23. Pfaller MA, Messer SA, Hollis RJ. Strain delineation and antifungal susceptibilities of epidemiologically related and unrelated isolates of *Candida lusitaniae*. *Diagn Microbiol Infect Dis* 1994;20:127–133.

24. Drew RH. Polyenes for the prevention and treatment of invasive fungal infections. In: Ghannoum MA, Perfect J (Eds.). *Antifungal Therapy*. New York: Informa Healthcare; 2010:163–183.

25. Robbie G, Wu TC, Chiou WL. Poor and unusually prolonged oral absorption of amphotericin B in rats. *Pharm Res* 1999;16:455–458.

26. Christiansen KJ, Bernard EM, Gold JW, Armstrong D. Distribution and activity of amphotericin B in humans. *J Infect Dis* 1985;152:1037–1043.

27. Wong-Beringer A, Jacobs RA, Guglielmo BJ. Lipid formulations of amphotericin B: Clinical efficacy and toxicities. *Clin Infect Dis* 1998;27:603–618.

28. Frothingham R. Lipid formulations of amphotericin B for empirical treatment of fever and neutropenia. *Clin Infect Dis* 2002;35:896–897.

29. Daneshmend TK, Warnock DW. Clinical pharmacokinetics of systemic antifungal drugs. *Clin Pharmacokinet* 1983;8:17–42.

30. Goodwin SD, Cleary JD, Walawander CA, Taylor JW, Grasela TH, Jr. Pretreatment regimens for adverse events related to infusion of amphotericin B. *Clin Infect Dis* 1995;20:755–761.

31. Gallis HA, Drew RH, Pickard WW. Amphotericin B: 30 years of clinical experience. *Rev Infect Dis* 1990;12:308–329.

32. Nicholl TA, Nimmo CR, Shepherd JD, Phillips P, Jewesson PJ. Amphotericin B infusion-related toxicity: Comparison of two- and four-hour infusions. *Ann Pharmacother* 1995;29:1081–1087.

33. Freifeld AG, Bow EJ, Sepkowitz KA, et al. Clinical practice guideline for the use of antimicrobial agents in neutropenic patients with cancer: 2010 Update by the Infectious Diseases Society of America. *Clin Infect Dis* 2011;52:427–431.

34. Marr KA, Bow E, Chiller T, et al. Fungal infection prevention after hematopoietic cell transplantation. *Bone Marrow Transplant* 2009;44:483–487.

35. Ostrosky-Zeichner L, Shoham S, Vazquez J, et al. MSG-01: A randomized, double-blind, placebo-controlled trial of caspofungin prophylaxis followed by preemptive therapy for invasive candidiasis in high-risk adults in the critical care setting. *Clin Infect Dis* 2014;58:1219–1226.

36. Walsh TJ, Teppler H, Donowitz GR, et al. Caspofungin versus liposomal amphotericin B for empirical antifungal therapy in patients with persistent fever and neutropenia. *N Engl J Med* 2004;351:1391–1402.

37. Ellis M, Bernsen R, li-Zadeh H, et al. A safety and feasibility study comparing an intermittent high dose with a daily standard dose of liposomal amphotericin B for persistent neutropenic fever. *J Med Microbiol* 2009;58:1474–1485.

38. Patterson TF, Thompson GR, 3rd, Denning DW, et al. Practice guidelines for the diagnosis and management of aspergillosis: 2016 Update by the Infectious Diseases Society of America. *Clin Infect Dis* 2016;63:e1–e60.

39. Perfect JR, Dismukes WE, Dromer F, et al. Clinical practice guidelines for the management of cryptococcal disease: 2010 Update by the Infectious Diseases Society of America. *Clin Infect Dis* 2010;50:291–322.

40. Chapman SW, Dismukes WE, Proia LA, et al. Clinical practice guidelines for the management of blastomycosis: 2008 Update by the Infectious Diseases Society of America. *Clin Infect Dis* 2008;46:1801–1812.

41. Galgiani JN, Ampel NM, Blair JE, et al. Coccidioidomycosis. *Clin Infect Dis* 2005;41:1217–1223.

42. Anaissie EJ, Darouiche RO, bi-Said D, et al. Management of invasive candidal infections: Results of a prospective, randomized, multicenter study of fluconazole versus amphotericin B and review of the literature. *Clin Infect Dis* 1996;23:964–972.

43. Phillips P, Shafran S, Garber G, et al. Multicenter randomized trial of fluconazole versus amphotericin B for treatment of candidemia in non-neutropenic patients. Canadian Candidemia Study Group. *Eur J Clin Microbiol Infect Dis* 1997;16:337–345.

44. Rex JH, Bennett JE, Sugar AM, et al. A randomized trial comparing fluconazole with amphotericin B for the treatment of candidemia in patients without neutropenia. Candidemia Study Group and the National Institute of Health. *N Engl J Med* 1994;331:1325–1330.

45. Gafter-Gvili A, Vidal L, Goldberg E, Leibovici L, Paul M. Treatment of invasive candidal infections: Systematic review and meta-analysis. *Mayo Clin Proc* 2008;83:1011–1121.

46. Kullberg BJ, Sobel JD, Ruhnke M, et al. Voriconazole versus a regimen of amphotericin B followed by fluconazole for candidaemia in non-neutropenic patients: A randomised non-inferiority trial. *Lancet* 2005;366:1435–1442.

47. Herbrecht R, Denning DW, Patterson TF, et al. Voriconazole versus amphotericin B for primary therapy of invasive aspergillosis. *N Engl J Med* 2002;347:408–415.

48. Johnson PC, Wheat LJ, Cloud GA, et al. Safety and efficacy of liposomal amphotericin B compared with conventional amphotericin B for induction therapy of histoplasmosis in patients with AIDS. *Ann Intern Med* 2002;137:105–109.

49. Bradsher RW. Histoplasmosis and blastomycosis. *Clin Infect Dis* 1996;22 Suppl 2:S102–S111.

50. Wheat LJ, Freifeld AG, Kleiman MB, et al. Clinical practice guidelines for the management of patients with histoplasmosis: 2007 Update by the Infectious Diseases Society of America. *Clin Infect Dis* 2007;45:807–825.

51. Galgiani JN, Ampel NM, Blair JE, et al. Executive summary: 2016 Infectious Diseases Society of America (IDSA) Clinical Practice Guideline for the Treatment of Coccidioidomycosis. *Clin Infect Dis* 2016;63:717–722.

52. Polak A, Scholer HJ. Mode of action of 5-fluorocytosine and mechanisms of resistance. *Chemotherapy* 1975;21:113–130.

53. Waldorf AR, Polak A. Mechanisms of action of 5-fluorocytosine. *Antimicrob Agents Chemother* 1983;23:79–85.

54. Polak A. Mode of action of 5-fluorocytosine and 5-fluorouracil in dematiaceous fungi. *Sabouraudia* 1983;21:15–25.

55. Polak A. 5-Fluorocytosine—Current status with special references to mode of action and drug resistance. *Contrib Microbiol Immunol* 1977;4:158–167.

56. Hope WW, Tabernero L, Denning DW, Anderson MJ. Molecular mechanisms of primary resistance to flucytosine in *Candida albicans*. *Antimicrob Agents Chemother* 2004;48:4377–4386.

57. Fasoli M, Kerridge D. Isolation and characterization of fluoropyrimidine-resistant mutants in two *Candida* species. *Ann N Y Acad Sci* 1988;544:260–263.

58. Brouwer AE, Rajanuwong A, Chierakul W, et al. Combination antifungal therapies for HIV-associated cryptococcal meningitis: A randomised trial. *Lancet* 2004;363:1764–1767.

59. Cuenca-Estrella M. Combinations of antifungal agents in therapy—what value are they? *J Antimicrob Chemother* 2004;54:854–869.

60. Lewis RE, Diekema DJ, Messer SA, Pfaller MA, Klepser ME. Comparison of Etest, chequerboard dilution and time-kill studies for the detection of synergy or antagonism between antifungal agents tested against *Candida* species. *J Antimicrob Chemother* 2002;49:345–351.

61. Martin E, Maier F, Bhakdi S. Antagonistic effects of fluconazole and 5-fluorocytosine on candidacidal action of amphotericin B in human serum. *Antimicrob Agents Chemother* 1994;38:1331–1338.

62. Johnson MD, Perfect JR. Use of antifungal combination therapy: Agents, order, and timing. *Curr Fungal Infect Rep* 2010;4:87–95.

63. Andes D, vanOgtrop M. *In vivo* characterization of the pharmacodynamics of flucytosine in a neutropenic murine disseminated candidiasis model. *Antimicrob Agents Chemother* 2000;44:938–942.

64. Turnidge JD, Gudmundsson S, Vogelman B, Craig WA. The postantibiotic effect of antifungal agents against common pathogenic yeasts. *J Antimicrob Chemother* 1994;34:83–92.

65. Messer SA, Moet GJ, Kirby JT, Jones RN. Activity of contemporary antifungal agents, including the novel echinocandin anidulafungin, tested against *Candida* spp., *Cryptococcus* spp., and *Aspergillus* spp.: Report from the SENTRY Antimicrobial Surveillance Program (2006 to 2007). *J Clin Microbiol* 2009;47:1942–1946.

66. Pfaller MA, Messer SA, Boyken L, et al. Global trends in the antifungal susceptibility of *Cryptococcus neoformans* (1990 to 2004). *J Clin Microbiol* 2005;43:2163–2167.

67. Drew RH. Flucytosine. In: Ghannoum MA, Perfect J (Eds.). *Antifungal Therapy*. New York: Informa; 2010:184–198.

68. Cutler RE, Blair AD, Kelly MR. Flucytosine kinetics in subjects with normal and impaired renal function. *Clin Pharmacol Ther* 1978;24:333–342.

69. *Flucytosine Package Insert*. Valeant Pharmaceuticals International, Quebec, Canada. November 2013. Available at https://dailymed.nlm.nih.gov/dailymed/archives/fdaDrugInfo.cfm?archiveid=2352.

70. Schonebeck J, Polak A, Fernex M, Scholer HJ. Pharmacokinetic studies on the oral antimycotic agent 5-fluorocytosine in individuals with normal and impaired kidney function. *Chemotherapy* 1973;18:321–336.

71. Vermes A, van Der SH, Guchelaar HJ. Flucytosine: Correlation between toxicity and pharmacokinetic parameters. *Chemotherapy* 2000;46:86–94.

72. Bennett JE, Dismukes WE, Duma RJ, et al. A comparison of amphotericin B alone and combined with flucytosine in the treatment of cryptoccal meningitis. *N Engl J Med* 1979;301:126–131.

73. Stamm AM, Diasio RB, Dismukes WE, et al. Toxicity of amphotericin B plus flucytosine in 194 patients with cryptococcal meningitis. *Am J Med* 1987;83:236–242.

74. Hiddemann W, Essink ME, Fegeler W, Zuhlsdorf M, Sauerland C, Buchner T. Antifungal treatment by amphotericin B and 5-fluorocytosine delays the recovery of normal hematopoietic cells after intensive cytostatic therapy for acute myeloid leukemia. *Cancer* 1991;68:9–14.

75. Mauceri AA, Cullen SI, Vandevelde AG, Johnson JE, III. Flucytosine. An effective oral treatment for chromomycosis. *Arch Dermatol* 1974;109:873–876.

76. Bicanic T, Wood R, Meintjes G, et al. High-dose amphotericin B with flucytosine for the treatment of cryptococcal meningitis in HIV-infected patients: A randomized trial. *Clin Infect Dis* 2008;47:123–130.

77. van der Horst CM, Saag MS, Cloud GA, et al. Treatment of cryptococcal meningitis associated with the acquired immunodeficiency syndrome. National Institute of Allergy and Infectious Diseases Mycoses Study Group and AIDS Clinical Trials Group. *N Engl J Med* 1997;337:15–21.

78. Saag MS, Powderly WG, Cloud GA, et al. Comparison of amphotericin B with fluconazole in the treatment of acute AIDS-associated cryptococcal meningitis. The NIAID Mycoses Study Group and the AIDS Clinical Trials Group. *N Engl J Med* 1992;326:83–89.

79. Day JN, Chau TT, Lalloo DG. Combination antifungal therapy for cryptococcal meningitis. *N Engl J Med* 2013;368:2522–2523.

80. Falci DR, Pasqualotto AC. Profile of isavuconazole and its potential in the treatment of severe invasive fungal infections. *Infect Drug Resist* 2013;6:163–174.

81. Girmenia C. New generation azole antifungals in clinical investigation. *Expert Opin Investig Drugs* 2009;18:1279–1295.

82. Livermore J, Hope W. Evaluation of the pharmacokinetics and clinical utility of isavuconazole for treatment of invasive fungal infections. *Expert Opin Drug Metab Toxicol* 2012;8:759–765.

83. Pasqualotto AC, Denning DW. New and emerging treatments for fungal infections. *J Antimicrob Chemother* 2008;61 Suppl 1:i19–i30.

84. Sanglard D, Coste AT. Activity of isavuconazole and other azoles against *Candida* slinical isolates and yeast model systems with known azole resistance mechanisms. *Antimicrob Agents Chemother* 2015;60:229–238.

85. Pfaller MA, Messer SA, Hollis RJ, et al. Variation in susceptibility of bloodstream isolates of *Candida glabrata* to fluconazole according to patient age and geographic location in the United States in 2001 to 2007. *J Clin Microbiol* 2009;47:3185–3190.

86. Klepser ME, Malone D, Lewis RE, Ernst EJ, Pfaller MA. Evaluation of voriconazole pharmacodynamics using time-kill methodology. *Antimicrob Agents Chemother* 2000;44(7):1917–1920.

87. Lewis RE, Wiederhold NP, Klepser ME. *In vitro* pharmacodynamics of amphotericin B, itraconazole, and voriconazole against *Aspergillus*, *Fusarium*, and *Scedosporium* spp. *Antimicrob Agents Chemother* 2005;49(3):945–951.

88. Oakley KL, Morrissey G, Denning DW. Efficacy of SCH-56592 in a temporarily neutropenic murine model of invasive aspergillosis with an itraconazole-susceptible and an itraconazole-resistant isolate of *Aspergillus fumigatus*. *Antimicrob Agents Chemother* 1997;41:1504–1507.

89. Manavathu EK, Ramesh MS, Baskaran I, Ganesan LT, Chandrasekar PH. A comparative study of the post-antifungal effect (PAFE) of amphotericin B, triazoles and echinocandins on *Aspergillus fumigatus* and *Candida albicans*. *J Antimicrob Chemother* 2004;53:386–389.

90. Andes D. Pharmacokinetics and pharmacodynamics of antifungals. *Infect Dis Clin North Am* 2006;20:679–697.

91. Baddley JW, Patel M, Bhavnani SM, Moser SA, Andes DR. Association of fluconazole pharmacodynamics with mortality in patients with candidemia. *Antimicrob Agents Chemother* 2008;52:3022–3028.

92. Mavridou E, Bruggemann RJ, Melchers WJ, Verweij PE, Mouton JW. Impact of *cyp51A* mutations on the pharmacokinetic and pharmacodynamic properties of voriconazole in a murine model of disseminated aspergillosis. *Antimicrob Agents Chemother* 2010;54:4758–4764.

93. Andes D, Marchillo K, Lowther J, Bryskier A, Stamstad T, Conklin R. *In vivo* pharmacodynamics of HMR 3270, a glucan synthase inhibitor, in a murine candidiasis model. *Antimicrob Agents Chemother* 2003;47:1187–1192.

94. Andes D, Marchillo K, Conklin R, et al. Pharmacodynamics of a new triazole, posaconazole, in a murine model of disseminated candidiasis. *Antimicrob Agents Chemother* 2004;48:137–142.

95. Pai MP, Turpin RS, Garey KW. Association of fluconazole area under the concentration-time curve/MIC and dose/MIC ratios with mortality in nonneutropenic patients with candidemia. *Antimicrob Agents Chemother* 2007;51:35–39.

96. Lass-Florl C. Triazole antifungal agents in invasive fungal infections: A comparative review. *Drugs* 2011;71:2405–2419.

97. Thompson GR, III, Cadena J, Patterson TF. Overview of antifungal agents. *Clin Chest Med* 2009;30:203–215, v.

98. Seifert H, Aurbach U, Stefanik D, Cornely O. In vitro activities of isavuconazole and other antifungal agents against *Candida* bloodstream isolates. *Antimicrob Agents Chemother* 2007;51:1818–1821.

99. Thompson GR, 3rd, Wiederhold NP. Isavuconazole: A comprehensive review of spectrum of activity of a new triazole. *Mycopathologia* 2010;170:291–313.

100. *Diflucan (fluconazole) Package Insert*. Pfizer, Inc, New York, NY. March 2018. (Available at http://www.pfizer.com/files/productsuspi_diflucan.pdf).

101. Zimmermann T, Yeates RA, Laufen H, Pfaff G, Wildfeuer A. Influence of concomitant food intake on the oral absorption of two triazole antifungal agents, itraconazole and fluconazole. *Eur J Clin Pharmacol* 1994;46:147–150.

102. *Sporanox (itraconazole oral solution) Package Insert*. Janssen Pharmaceuticals, Inc. Titusville, NJ, March 2017. (Available at http://www.janssen.com/us/sites/www_janssen_com_usa/files/products-documents/pi-sporanoxcapsules.pdf). Accessed 9 Oct 2018.

103. Vfend (voriconazole) Package Insert. Pfizer, Inc, New York, NY, February 2015. (Available at http://labeling.pfizer.com/ShowLabeling.aspx?id=618).

104. Purkins L, Wood N, Kleinermans D, Greenhalgh K, Nichols D. Effect of food on the pharmacokinetics of multiple-dose oral voriconazole. *Br J Clin Pharmacol* 2003;56 Suppl 1:17–23.

105. Theuretzbacher U, Ihle F, Derendorf H. Pharmacokinetic/pharmacodynamic profile of voriconazole. *Clin Pharmacokinet* 2006;45:649–663.

106. *Noxafil (posaconazole) Package Insert*. Merck and Co, Inc. White Plains, NJ, August 2016. Available at https://www.merck.com/product/usa/pi_circulars/n/noxafil/noxafil_pi.pdf.

107. Courtney R, Wexler D, Radwanski E, Lim J, Laughlin M. Effect of food on the relative bioavailability of two oral formulations of posaconazole in healthy adults. *Br J Clin Pharmacol* 2004;57:218–222.

108. Courtney R, Pai S, Laughlin M, Lim J, Batra V. Pharmacokinetics, safety, and tolerability of oral posaconazole administered in single and multiple doses in healthy adults. *Antimicrob Agents Chemother* 2003;47:2788–2795.

109. Ezzet F, Wexler D, Courtney R, Krishna G, Lim J, Laughlin M. Oral bioavailability of posaconazole in fasted healthy subjects: Comparison between three regimens and basis for clinical dosage recommendations. *Clin Pharmacokinet* 2005;44:211–220.

110. Krishna G, Moton A, Ma L, Medlock MM, McLeod J. Pharmacokinetics and absorption of posaconazole oral suspension under various gastric conditions in healthy volunteers. *Antimicrob Agents Chemother* 2009;53:958–966.

111. Dekkers BG, Bakker M, van der Elst KC, et al. Therapeutic drug monitoring of posaconazole: An update. *Curr Fungal Infect Rep* 2016;10:51–61.

112. Maertens J, Cornely OA, Ullmann AJ, et al. Phase 1B study of the pharmacokinetics and safety of posaconazole intravenous solution in patients at risk for invasive fungal disease. *Antimicrob Agents Chemother* 2014;58:3610–3617.

113. Schmitt-Hoffmann A, Roos B, Heep M, et al. Single-ascending-dose pharmacokinetics and safety of the novel broad-spectrum antifungal triazole BAL4815 after intravenous infusions (50, 100, and 200 milligrams) and oral administrations (100, 200, and 400 milligrams) of its prodrug, BAL8557, in healthy volunteers. *Antimicrob Agents Chemother* 2006;50:279–285.

114. Schmitt-Hoffmann A, Roos B, Maares J, et al. Multiple-dose pharmacokinetics and safety of the new antifungal triazole BAL4815 after intravenous infusion and oral administration of its prodrug, BAL8557, in healthy volunteers. *Antimicrob Agents Chemother* 2006;50:286–293.

115. Lewis RE. Pharmacokinetic Considerations for the use of newer antifungal agents. *Curr Fungal Infect Rep* 2008;2:5–11.

116. Foulds G, Brennan DR, Wajszczuk C, et al. Fluconazole penetration into cerebrospinal fluid in humans. *J Clin Pharmacol* 1988;28:363–366.

117. Buijk SL, Gyssens IC, Mouton JW, Verbrugh HA, Touw DJ, Bruining HA. Pharmacokinetics of sequential intravenous and enteral fluconazole in critically ill surgical patients with invasive mycoses and compromised gastro-intestinal function. *Intensive Care Med* 2001;27:115–121.

118. Li Y, Theuretzbacher U, Clancy CJ, Nguyen MH, Derendorf H. Pharmacokinetic/pharmacodynamic profile of posaconazole. *Clin Pharmacokinet* 2010;49:379–396.

119. Ikeda Y, Umemura K, Kondo K, Sekiguchi K, Miyoshi S, Nakashima M. Pharmacokinetics of voriconazole and cytochrome P450 2C19 genetic status. *Clin Pharmacol Ther* 2004;75:587–588.

120. Desta Z, Zhao X, Shin JG, Flockhart DA. Clinical significance of the cytochrome P450 2C19 genetic polymorphism. *Clin Pharmacokinet* 2002;41:913–958.

121. Ghosal A, Hapangama N, Yuan Y, et al. Identification of human UDP-glucuronosyltransferase enzyme(s) responsible for the glucuronidation of posaconazole (Noxafil). *Drug Metab Dispos* 2004;32:267–271.

122. Krieter P, Flannery B, Musick T, Gohdes M, Martinho M, Courtney R. Disposition of posaconazole following single-dose oral administration in healthy subjects. *Antimicrob Agents Chemother* 2004;48:3543–3551.

123. Pham CP, de Feiter PW, van der Kuy PH, van Mook WN. Long QTc interval and torsade de pointes caused by fluconazole. *Ann Pharmacother* 2006;40:1456–1461.

124. Stevens DA, Diaz M, Negroni R, et al. Safety evaluation of chronic fluconazole therapy. Fluconazole Pan-American Study Group. *Chemotherapy* 1997;43:371–377.

125. Gearhart MO. Worsening of liver function with fluconazole and review of azole antifungal hepatotoxicity. *Ann Pharmacother* 1994;28:1177–1781.

126. Ahmad SR, Singer SJ, Leissa BG. Congestive heart failure associated with itraconazole. *Lancet* 2001;357:1766–1767.

127. Johnson LB, Kauffman CA. Voriconazole: A new triazole antifungal agent. *Clin Infect Dis* 2003;36:630–637.

128. Philips J, Marty F, Stone R, Koplan B, Katz J, Baden L. Torsades de pointes associated with voriconazole use. *Transpl Infect Dis* 2007;9:33–36.

129. Raad II, Graybill JR, Bustamante AB, et al. Safety of long-term oral posaconazole use in the treatment of refractory invasive fungal infections. *Clin Infect Dis* 2006;42:1726–1734.

130. Singh N, Huprikar S, Burdette SD, Morris MI, Blair JE, Wheat LJ. Donor-derived fungal infections in organ transplant recipients: Guidelines of the American Society of Transplantation, Infectious Diseases Community of Practice. *Am J Transplant* 2012;12:2414–2428.

131. Miceli MH, Kauffman CA. Isavuconazole: A new broad-spectrum triazole antifungal agent. *Clin Infect Dis* 2015;61:1558–1565.

132. Pettit NN, Carver PL. Isavuconazole: A new option for the management of invasive fungal infections. *Ann Pharm* 2015;49:825–842.

133. Girmenia C, Iori AP. An update on the safety and interactions of antifungal drugs in stem cell transplant recipients. *Expert Opin Drug Saf* 2017;16:329–339.

134. Walsh TJ, Raad I, Patterson TF, et al. Treatment of invasive aspergillosis with posaconazole in patients who are refractory to or intolerant of conventional therapy: An externally controlled trial. *Clin Infect Dis* 2007;44:2–12.

135. Kauffman CA, Bustamante B, Chapman SW, Pappas PG. Clinical practice guidelines for the management of sporotrichosis: 2007 update by the Infectious Diseases Society of America. *Clin Infect Dis* 2007;45:1255–1265.

136. Enoch DA, Aliyu SH, Sule O, Lewis SJ, Karas JA. Posaconazole for the treatment of mucormycosis. *Int J Antimicrob Agents* 2011;38:465–473.

137. Maertens JA, Raad, II, Marr KA, et al. Isavuconazole versus voriconazole for primary treatment of invasive mould disease caused by *Aspergillus* and other filamentous fungi (SECURE): A phase 3, randomised-controlled, non-inferiority trial. *Lancet* 2016;387:760–769.

138. Marty FM, Ostrosky-Zeichner L, Cornely OA, et al. Isavuconazole treatment for mucormycosis: A single-arm open-label trial and case-control analysis. *Lancet Infect Dis* 2016;16:828–837.

139. Antachopoulos C, Meletiadis J, Sein T, Roilides E, Walsh TJ. Concentration-dependent effects of caspofungin on the metabolic activity of *Aspergillus* species. *Antimicrob Agents Chemother* 2007;51:881–887.

140. Kurtz MB, Heath IB, Marrinan J, Dreikorn S, Onishi J, Douglas C. Morphological effects of lipopeptides against *Aspergillus fumigatus* correlate with activities against (1,3)-beta-D-glucan synthase. *Antimicrob Agents Chemother* 1994;38:1480–1489.

141. Nakai T, Uno J, Ikeda F, Tawara S, Nishimura K, Miyaji M. *In vitro* antifungal activity of micafungin (FK463) against dimorphic fungi: Comparison of yeast-like and mycelial forms. *Antimicrob Agents Chemother* 2003;47:1376–1381.

142. Pound MW, Townsend ML, Drew RH. Echinocandin pharmacodynamics: Review and clinical implications. *J Antimicrob Chemother* 2010;65:1108–1118.

143. Perlin DS. Resistance to echinocandin-class antifungal drugs. *Drug Resist Updat* 2007;10:121–130.

144. Cancidas (caspofungin) Package Insert [Internet]. Merck and Co, Inc., White Plains, NJ, April 2016. Available at https://www.merck.com/product/usa/pi_circulars/c/cancidas/cancidas_pi.pdf.

145. Mycamine [package insert]. Astellas Pharma US, Inc. Deerfield, IL, USA; June 2011. (Available at: http://www.mycamine.com/docs/mycamine.pdf). Accessed March 23, 2012. Package Insert. 2012.

146. Eraxis [package insert]. Pfizer Inc., NY, NY, USA. November 2010. (Available at: http://labeling.pfizer.com/ShowLabeling.aspx?id=566). Accessed March 23, 2012. Package Insert. 2012.

147. Bennett JE. Echinocandins for candidemia in adults without neutropenia. *N Engl J Med* 2006;355:1154–1159.

148. Mora-Duarte J, Betts R, Rotstein C, et al. Comparison of caspofungin and amphotericin B for invasive candidiasis. *N Engl J Med* 2002;347:2020–2029.

149. Walsh TJ. Echinocandins—An advance in the primary treatment of invasive candidiasis. *N Engl J Med* 2002;347:2070–2072.

150. Lockhart SR, Zimbeck AJ, Baddley JW, et al. *In vitro* echinocandin susceptibility of *Aspergillus* isolates from patients enrolled in the Transplant-Associated Infection Surveillance Network. *Antimicrob Agents Chemother* 2011;55:3944–3946.

151. Burkhardt O, Ellis S, Burhenne H, et al. High caspofungin levels in alveolar cells of a lung transplant patient with suspected pulmonary aspergillosis. *Int J Antimicrob Agents* 2009;34:491–492.

152. Walsh TJ, Goutelle S, Jelliffe RW, et al. Intrapulmonary pharmacokinetics and pharmacodynamics of micafungin in adult lung transplant patients. *Antimicrob Agents Chemother* 2010;54:3451–3459.

153. Hiemenz J, Cagnoni P, Simpson D, et al. Pharmacokinetic and maximum tolerated dose study of micafungin in combination with fluconazole versus fluconazole alone for prophylaxis of fungal infections in adult patients undergoing a bone marrow or peripheral stem cell transplant. *Antimicrob Agents Chemother* 2005;49:1331–1336.

154. Groll AH, Silling G, Young C, et al. Randomized comparison of safety and pharmacokinetics of caspofungin, liposomal amphotericin B, and the combination of both in allogeneic hematopoietic stem cell recipients. *Antimicrob Agents Chemother* 2010;54:4143–4149.

155. Maertens J, Marchetti O, Herbrecht R, et al. European guidelines for antifungal management in leukemia and hematopoietic stem cell transplant recipients: Summary of the ECIL 3—2009 update. *Bone Marrow Transplant* 2011;46:709–718.

156. Fortun J, Muriel A, Martin-Davila P, et al. Caspofungin versus fluconazole as prophylaxis of invasive fungal infection in high-risk liver transplantation recipients: A propensity score analysis. *Liver Transplant* 2016;22:427–435.

157. Limper AH, Knox KS, Sarosi GA, et al. An official American Thoracic Society statement: Treatment of fungal infections in adult pulmonary and critical care patients. *Am J Respir Crit Care Med* 2011;183:96–128.

158. Sharkey PK, Graybill JR, Johnson ES, et al. Amphotericin B lipid complex compared with amphotericin B in the treatment of cryptococcal meningitis in patients with AIDS. *Clin Infect Dis* 1996;22:315–321.

159. Baddour LM, Perfect JR, Ostrosky-Zeichner L. Successful use of amphotericin B lipid complex in the treatment of cryptococcosis. *Clin Infect Dis* 2005;40 Suppl 6:S409–S413.

160. Coker RJ, Viviani M, Gazzard BG, et al. Treatment of cryptococcosis with liposomal amphotericin B (AmBisome) in 23 patients with AIDS. *AIDS* 1993;7:829–835.

161. Hamill RJ, Sobel JD, El-Sadr W, et al. Comparison of 2 doses of liposomal amphotericin B and conventional amphotericin B deoxycholate for treatment of AIDS-associated acute cryptococcal meningitis: A randomized, double-blind clinical trial of efficacy and safety. *Clin Infect Dis* 2010;51:225–232.

162. Sun HY, Alexander BD, Lortholary O, et al. Lipid formulations of amphotericin B significantly improve outcome in solid organ transplant recipients with central nervous system cryptococcosis. *Clin Infect Dis* 2009;49:1721–1728.

163. Johansen HK, Gotzsche PC. Amphotericin B lipid soluble formulations vs. amphotericin B in cancer patients with neutropenia. *Cochrane Database Syst Rev* 2000;3:CD000969.

164. Tiphine M, Letscher-Bru V, Herbrecht R. Amphotericin B and its new formulations: Pharmacologic characteristics, clinical efficacy, and tolerability. *Transpl Infect Dis* 1999;1:273–283.

165. Walsh TJ, Finberg RW, Arndt C, et al. Liposomal amphotericin B for empirical therapy in patients with persistent fever and neutropenia. National Institute of Allergy and Infectious Diseases Mycoses Study Group. *N Engl J Med* 1999;340:764–771.

166. Herbrecht R, Letscher V, Andres E, Cavalier A. Safety and efficacy of amphotericin B colloidal dispersion. An overview. *Chemotherapy* 1999;45 Suppl 1:67–76.

167. Gurwith M, Mamelok R, Pietrelli L, Du MC. Renal sparing by amphotericin B colloidal dispersion: Clinical experience in 572 patients. *Chemotherapy* 1999;45 Suppl 1:39–47.

168. Mistro S, Maciel IM, de Menezes RG, Maia ZP, Schooley RT, Badaro R. Does lipid emulsion reduce amphotericin B nephrotoxicity? A systematic review and meta-analysis. *Clin Infect Dis* 2012;54:1774–1777.

169. Lanternier F, Sun HY, Ribaud P, Singh N, Kontoyiannis DP, Lortholary O. Mucormycosis in organ and stem cell transplant recipients. *Clin Infect Dis* 2012;54:1–8.

170. Pagano L, Offidani M, Fianchi L, et al. Mucormycosis in hematologic patients. *Haematologica* 2004;89:207–214.

171. Sun HY, Singh N. Mucormycosis: Its contemporary face and management strategies. *Lancet Infect Dis* 2011;11:301–311.

172. Barrett JP, Vardulaki KA, Conlon C, et al. A systematic review of the antifungal effectiveness and tolerability of amphotericin B formulations. *Clin Ther* 2003;25:1295–1320.

173. Wingard JR, White MH, Anaissie E, Raffalli J, Goodman J, Arrieta A. A randomized, double-blind comparative trial evaluating the safety of liposomal amphotericin B versus amphotericin B lipid complex in the empirical treatment of febrile neutropenia. L Amph/ABLC Collaborative Study Group. *Clin Infect Dis* 2000;31:1155–1163.

174. White MH, Bowden RA, Sandler ES, et al. Randomized, double-blind clinical trial of amphotericin B colloidal dispersion vs. amphotericin B in the empirical treatment of fever and neutropenia. *Clin Infect Dis* 1998;27:296–302.

175. Kuti JL, Kotapati S, Williams P, Capitano B, Nightingale CH, Nicolau DP. Pharmacoeconomic analysis of amphotericin B lipid complex versus liposomal amphotericin B in the treatment of fungal infections. *Pharmacoeconomics* 2004;22:301–310.

176. US AP. Product Information: CRESEMBA(R) oral capsules, intravenous injection, isavuconazonium sulfate oral capsules, intravenous injection. Astellas Pharma US, Northbrook, IL, 2015.

177. Greenberg RN, Mullane K, van Burik JA, et al. Posaconazole as salvage therapy for zygomycosis. *Antimicrob Agents Chemother* 2006;50:126–133.

178. Block ER, Bennett JE, Livoti LG, Klein WJ, Jr., MacGregor RR, Henderson L. Flucytosine and amphotericin B: Hemodialysis effects on the plasma concentration and clearance. Studies in man. *Ann Intern Med* 1974;80:613–617.

179. Ambisome Package Insert. Astellas Pharma US, Northbrook, IL, May 2012. Available at https://www.astellas.us/docs/ambisome.pdf.

180. Cornely OA, Maertens J, Bresnik M, et al. Liposomal amphotericin B as initial therapy for invasive mold infection: A randomized trial comparing a high-loading dose regimen with standard dosing (AmBiLoad trial). *Clin Infect Dis* 2007;44:1289–1297.

181. Kontoyiannis DP, Lewis RE. How I treat mucormycosis. *Blood* 2011;118:1216–1224.

182. Lanternier F, Lortholary O. [AMBIZYGO: Phase II study of high dose liposomal amphotericin B (AmBisome) [10 mg/kg/j] efficacy against zygomycosis]. *Medecine et maladies infectieuses* 2008;38 Suppl 2:S90–S91.

183. Gubbins PO, Amsden JR, McConnell SA, Anaissie EJ. Pharmacokinetics and buccal mucosal concentrations of a 15 milligram per kilogram of body weight total dose of liposomal amphotericin B administered as a single dose (15 mg/kg), weekly dose (7.5 mg/kg), or daily dose (1 mg/kg) in peripheral stem cell transplant patients. *Antimicrob Agents Chemother* 2009;53:3664–3674.

184. Paterson DL, David K, Mrsic M, et al. Pre-medication practices and incidence of infusion-related reactions in patients receiving AMPHOTEC: Data from the Patient Registry of Amphotericin B Cholesteryl Sulfate Complex for Injection Clinical Tolerability (PRoACT) registry. *J Antimicrob Chemother* 2008;62:1392–1400.

185. Eriksson U, Seifert B, Schaffner A, Eriksson U, Seifert B, Schaffner A. Comparison of effects of amphotericin B deoxycholate infused over 4 or 24 hours: Randomised controlled trial. *BMJ* 2001;322:579–582.

186. Falci DR, Lunardi LW, Ramos CG, Bay MB, Aquino VR, Goldani LZ. Continuous infusion of amphotericin B deoxycholate in the treatment of cryptococcal meningoencephalitis: Analysis of safety and fungicidal activity. *Clin Infect Dis* 2010;50:e26–e29.

187. Peleg AY, Woods ML. Continuous and 4 h infusion of amphotericin B: A comparative study involving high-risk haematology patients. *J Antimicrob Chemother* 2004;54:803–808.

188. Moen MD, Lyseng-Williamson KA, Scott LJ. Liposomal amphotericin B: A review of its use as empirical therapy in febrile neutropenia and in the treatment of invasive fungal infections. *Drugs* 2009;69:361–392.

189. Llanos A, Cieza J, Bernardo J, et al. Effect of salt supplementation on amphotericin B nephrotoxicity. *Kidney Int* 1991;40:302–308.

190. Wright DG, Robichaud KJ, Pizzo PA, Deisseroth AB. Lethal pulmonary reactions associated with the combined use of amphotericin B and leukocyte transfusions. *N Engl J Med* 1981;304:1185–1189.

191. Drew R. Potential role of aerosolized amphotericin B formulations in the prevention and adjunctive treatment of invasive fungal infections. *Int J Antimicrob Agents* 2006;27 Suppl 1:36–44.

192. Monforte V, Roman A, Gavalda J, et al. Nebulized amphotericin B concentration and distribution in the respiratory tract of lung-transplanted patients. *Transplantation* 2003;75:1571–1574.

193. Borro JM, Sole A, de la Torre M, et al. Efficiency and safety of inhaled amphotericin B lipid complex (Abelcet) in the prophylaxis of invasive fungal infections following lung transplantation. *Transplant Proc* 2008;40:3090–3093.

194. Klepser M. Amphotericin B in lung transplant recipients. *Ann Pharmacother* 2002;36:167–169.

195. Conneally E, Cafferkey M, Daly P, Keane C, McCann S. Nebulized amphotericin B as prophylaxis against invasive aspergillosis in granulocytopenic patients. *Bone Marrow Transplant* 1990;5:403–406.

196. Hertenstein B, Kern W, Schmeiser T, et al. Low incidence of invasive fungal infections after *bone marrow transplant*ation in patients receiving amphotericin B inhalations during neutropenia. *Ann Hematol* 1994;68:21–26.

197. Reichenspurner H, Gamberg P, Nitschke M, et al. Significant reduction in the number of fungal infections after lung-, heart-lung, and heart transplantation using aerosolized amphotericin B prophylaxis. *Transplant Proc* 1997;29:627–628.

198. Calvo V, Borro J, Morales P, et al. Antifungal prophylaxis during the early postoperative period of lung transplantation. Valencia Lung Transplant Group. *Chest* 1999;115:1301–1304.

199. Monforte V, Roman A, Gavalda J, et al. Nebulized amphotericin B prophylaxis for *Aspergillus* infection in lung transplantation: Study of risk factors. *J Heart Lung Transplant* 2001;20:1274–1281.

200. Drew RH, Ashley ED, Benjamin DK, Davis RD, Palmer SM, Perfect JR. Comparative safety of amphotericin B lipid complex and amphotericin B deoxycholate as aerosolized antifungal prophylaxis in lung-transplant recipients. *Transplantation* 2004;77:232–237.

201. Palmer S, Drew R, Whitehouse J, et al. Safety of aerosolized amphotericin B lipid complex in lung transplant recipients. *Transplantation* 2001;72:545–548.

202. Alexander BD, Dodds Ashley ES, Addison RM, Alspaugh JA, Chao NJ, Perfect JR. Non-comparative evaluation of the safety of aerosolized amphotericin B lipid complex in patients undergoing allogeneic hematopoietic stem cell transplantation. *Transplant Infect Dis* 2006;8:13–20.

203. Rijnders BJ, Cornelissen JJ, Slobbe L, et al. Aerosolized liposomal amphotericin B for the prevention of invasive pulmonary aspergillosis during prolonged neutropenia: A randomized, placebo-controlled trial. *Clin Infect Dis* 2008;46:1401–1408.

204. Dalconte I, Riva G, Obert R, et al. Tracheobronchial aspergillosis in a patient with AIDS treated with aerosolized amphotericin B combined with itraconazole. *Mycoses* 1996;39:371–374.

205. Palmer S, Perfect J, Howell D, et al. Candidal anastomotic infection in lung transplant recipients: Successful treatment with a combination of systemic and inhaled antifungal agents. *J Heart Lung Transplant* 1998;17:1029–1033.

206. Kanj S, Welty-Wolf K, Madden J, et al. Fungal infections in lung and heart-lung transplant recipients. Report of 9 cases and review of the literature. *Medicine (Baltimore)* 1996;75:142–156.

207. Birsan T, Taghavi S, Klepetko W. Treatment of *Aspergillus*-related ulcerative tracheobronchitis in lung transplant recipients. *J Heart Lung Transplant* 1998;17:437–438.

208. Casey P, Garrett J, Eaton T. Allergic bronchopulmonary aspergillosis in a lung transplant patient successfully treated with nebulized amphotericin. *J Heart Lung Transplant* 2002;21:1237–1241.

209. Suzuki K, Iwata S, Iwata H. Allergic bronchopulmonary aspergillosis in a 9-year-old boy. *Eur J Pediatr* 2002;161:408–409.

210. Oehling A, Giron M, Subira M. Aerosol chemotherapy in bronchopulmonary candidiasis. *Respiration* 1975;32:179–184.

211. Kilburn K. The innocuousness and possible therapeutic use of aerosol amphotericin B. *Am Rev Respir Dis* 1959;80:441–442.

212. Behre G, Schwartz S, Lenz K, et al. Aerosol amphotericin B inhalations for prevention of invasive pulmonary aspergillosis in neutropenic cancer patients. *Ann Hematol* 1995;71:287–291.

213. Schwartz S, Behre G, Heinemann V, et al. Aerosolized amphotericin B inhalations as prophylaxis of invasive *Aspergillus* infections during prolonged neutropenia: Results of a prospective randomized multicenter trial. *Blood* 1999;93:3654–3661.

214. De Laurenzi A, Matteocci A, Lanti A, Pescador L, Blandino F, Papetti C. Amphotericin B prophylaxis against invasive fungal infections in neutropenic patients: A single center experience from 1980 to 1995. *Infection* 1996;24:361–366.

215. Perfect JR, Ashley ED, Drew R. Design of aerosolized amphotericin B formulations for prophylaxis trials among lung transplant recipients. *Clin Infect Dis* 2004;39:S207–S210.

216. (anon). Fungal infections. *Am J Transplant* 2004;4:110–134.

217. Gubbins PO, Heldenbrand S. Clinically relevant drug interactions of current antifungal agents. *Mycoses* 2010;53:95–113.

218. Dodds-Ashley E. Management of drug and food interactions with azole antifungal agents in transplant recipients. *Pharmacotherapy* 2010;30:842–854.

219. Saad AH, DePestel DD, Carver PL. Factors influencing the magnitude and clinical significance of drug interactions between azole antifungals and select immunosuppressants. *Pharmacotherapy* 2006;26:1730–1744.

220. Bruggemann RJ, Alffenaar JW, Blijlevens NM, et al. Clinical relevance of the pharmacokinetic interactions of azole antifungal drugs with other coadministered agents. *Clin Infect Dis* 2009;48:1441–1458.

221. Lipp HP. Antifungal agents—Clinical pharmacokinetics and drug interactions. *Mycoses* 2008;51 Suppl 1:7–18.

222. Wilson DT, Drew RH, Perfect JR. Antifungal therapy for invasive fungal diseases in allogeneic stem cell transplant recipients: An update. *Mycopathologia* 2009;168:313–327.

223. Christopeit M, Eikam M, Behre G. Comedication of caspofungin acetate and cyclosporine A after allogeneic haematopoietic stem cell transplantation leads to negligible hepatotoxicity. *Mycoses* 2008;51 Suppl 1:19–24.

224. Anttila VJ, Piilonen A, Valtonen M. Co-administration of caspofungin and cyclosporine to a kidney transplant patient with pulmonary *Aspergillus* infection. *Scand J Infect Dis* 2003;35:893–894.

225. Saner F, Gensicke J, Rath P, et al. Safety profile of concomitant use of caspofungin and cyclosporine or tacrolimus in liver transplant patients. *Infection* 2006;34:328–332.

226. Pasqualotto AC, Howard SJ, Moore CB, Denning DW. Flucytosine therapeutic monitoring: 15 years experience from the UK. *J Antimicrob Chemother* 2007;59:791–793.

227. Guinea J, Pelaez T, Recio S, Torres-Narbona M, Bouza E. In vitro antifungal activities of isavuconazole (BAL4815), voriconazole, and fluconazole against 1,007 isolates of zygomycete, *Candida, Aspergillus, Fusarium,* and *Scedosporium* species. *Antimicrob Agents Chemother* 2008;52:1396–1400.

228. Pfaller MA, Diekema DJ, Gibbs DL, et al. Results from the ARTEMIS DISK Global Antifungal Surveillance Study, 1997 to 2007: A 10.5-year analysis of susceptibilities of *Candida* species to fluconazole and voriconazole as determined by CLSI standardized disk diffusion. *J Clin Microbiol* 2010;48:1366–1377.

229. Lortholary O, Obenga G, Biswas P, et al. International retrospective analysis of 73 cases of invasive fusariosis treated with voriconazole. *Antimicrob Agents Chemother* 2010;54:4446–4450.

230. Munoz P, Marin M, Tornero P, Martin Rabadan P, Rodriguez-Creixems M, Bouza E. Successful outcome of *Scedosporium apiospermum* disseminated infection treated with voriconazole in a patient receiving corticosteroid therapy. *Clin Infect Dis* 2000;31:1499–1501.

231. van Burik JA, Hare RS, Solomon HF, Corrado ML, Kontoyiannis DP. Posaconazole is effective as salvage therapy in zygomycosis: A retrospective summary of 91 cases. *Clin Infect Dis* 2006;42:e61–e65.

232. Song Y, Qiao J, Giovanni G, et al. Mucormycosis in renal transplant recipients: Review of 174 reported cases. *BMC Infect Dis* 2017;17:283.

233. Majithiya J, Sharp A, Parmar A, Denning DW, Warn PA. Efficacy of isavuconazole, voriconazole and fluconazole in temporarily neutropenic murine models of disseminated *Candida tropicalis* and *Candida krusei. J Antimicrob Chemother* 2009;63:161–166.

234. Warn PA, Sharp A, Parmar A, Majithiya J, Denning DW, Hope WW. Pharmacokinetics and pharmacodynamics of a novel triazole, isavuconazole: Mathematical modeling, importance of tissue concentrations, and impact of immune status on antifungal effect. *Antimicrob Agents Chemother* 2009;53:3453–3461.

235. Andes D, Pascual A, Marchetti O. Antifungal therapeutic drug monitoring: Established and emerging indications. *Antimicrob Agents Chemother* 2009;53:24–34.

236. Wingard JR, Carter SL, Walsh TJ, et al. Randomized, double-blind trial of fluconazole versus voriconazole for prevention of invasive fungal infection after allogeneic hematopoietic cell transplantation. *Blood* 2010;116:5111–118.

237. Ullmann AJ, Lipton JH, Vesole DH, et al. Posaconazole or fluconazole for prophylaxis in severe graft-versus-host disease. *N Engl J Med* 2007;356:335–347.

238. Fortun J, Lopez-San RA, Velasco JJ, et al. Selection of *Candida glabrata* strains with reduced susceptibility to azoles in four liver transplant patients with invasive candidiasis. *Eur J Clin Microbiol Infect Dis* 1997;16:314–318.

239. Wingard JR, Merz WG, Rinaldi MG, Johnson TR, Karp JE, Saral R. Increase in *Candida krusei* infection among patients with bone marrow transplantation and neutropenia treated prophylactically with fluconazole. *N Engl J Med* 1991;325:1274–1277.

240. Wingard JR, Merz WG, Rinaldi MG, Miller CB, Karp JE, Saral R. Association of *Torulopsis glabrata* infections with fluconazole prophylaxis in neutropenic bone marrow transplant patients. *Antimicrob Agents Chemother* 1993;37:1847–1849.

241. Marks DI, Pagliuca A, Kibbler CC, et al. Voriconazole versus itraconazole for antifungal prophylaxis following allogeneic haematopoietic stem-cell transplantation. *Br J Haematol* 2011;155:318–327.

242. Cadena J, Levine DJ, Angel LF, et al. Antifungal prophylaxis with voriconazole or itraconazole in lung transplant recipients: Hepatotoxicity and effectiveness. *Am J Transplant* 2009;9:2085–2091.

243. el-Yazigi A, Ellis M, Ernst P, Spence D, Hussain R, Baillie FJ. Pharmacokinetics of oral fluconazole when used for prophylaxis in bone marrow transplant recipients. *Antimicrob Agents Chemother* 1997;41:914–917.

244. el-Yazigi A, Ellis M, Ernst P, Hussein R, Baillie FJ. Effect of repeat dosing on the pharmacokinetics of oral fluconazole in bone marrow transplant patients. *J Clin Pharmacol* 1997;37:1031–1037.

245. Clancy CJ, Yu VL, Morris AJ, Snydman DR, Nguyen MH. Fluconazole MIC and the fluconazole dose/MIC ratio correlate with therapeutic response among patients with candidemia. *Antimicrob Agents Chemother* 2005;49:3171–3177.

246. Persat F, Marzullo C, Guyotat D, Rochet MJ, Piens MA. Plasma itraconazole concentrations in neutropenic patients after repeated high-dose treatment. *Eur J Cancer* 1992;28A:838–841.

247. Prentice AG, Warnock DW, Johnson SA, Phillips MJ, Oliver DA. Multiple dose pharmacokinetics of an oral solution of itraconazole in autologous bone marrow transplant recipients. *J Antimicrob Chemother* 1994;34:247–252.

248. Patterson TF, Peters J, Levine SM, et al. Systemic availability of itraconazole in lung transplantation. *Antimicrob Agents Chemother* 1996;40:2217–2220.

249. Purkins L, Wood N, Ghahramani P, Greenhalgh K, Allen MJ, Kleinermans D. Pharmacokinetics and safety of voriconazole following intravenous- to oral-dose escalation regimens. *Antimicrob Agents Chemother* 2002;46:2546–2553.

250. Jeu L, Piacenti FJ, Lyakhovetskiy AG, Fung HB. Voriconazole. *Clin Ther* 2003;25:1321–1381.

251. Hoffman HL, Rathbun RC. Review of the safety and efficacy of voriconazole. *Expert Opin Investig Drugs* 2002;11:409–429.

252. Oude Lashof AM, Sobel JD, Ruhnke M, et al. Safety and tolerability of voriconazole in patients with baseline renal insufficiency and candidemia. *Antimicrob Agents Chemother* 2012;56:3133–3137.

253. Trifilio S, Pennick G, Pi J, et al. Monitoring plasma voriconazole levels may be necessary to avoid subtherapeutic levels in hematopoietic stem cell transplant recipients. *Cancer* 2007;109:1532–1535.

254. Trifilio S, Ortiz R, Pennick G, et al. Voriconazole therapeutic drug monitoring in allogeneic hematopoietic stem cell transplant recipients. *Bone Marrow Transplant* 2005;35:509–513.

255. Bruggemann RJ, Blijlevens NM, Burger DM, Franke B, Troke PF, Donnelly JP. Pharmacokinetics and safety of 14 days intravenous voriconazole in allogeneic haematopoietic stem cell transplant recipients. *J Antimicrob Chemother* 2010;65:107–113.

256. Han K, Capitano B, Bies R, et al. Bioavailability and population pharmacokinetics of voriconazole in lung transplant recipients. *Antimicrob Agents Chemother* 2010;54:4424–4431.

257. Johnson HJ, Han K, Capitano B, et al. Voriconazole pharmacokinetics in liver transplant recipients. *Antimicrob Agents Chemother* 2010;54:852–859.

258. Ullmann AJ, Cornely OA, Burchardt A, et al. Pharmacokinetics, safety, and efficacy of posaconazole in patients with persistent febrile neutropenia or refractory invasive fungal infection. *Antimicrob Agents Chemother* 2006;50:658–666.

259. Gubbins PO, Krishna G, Sansone-Parsons A, et al. Pharmacokinetics and safety of oral posaconazole in neutropenic stem cell transplant recipients. *Antimicrob Agents Chemother* 2006;50:1993–1999.

260. Cornely OA, Helfgott D, Langston A, et al. Pharmacokinetics of different dosing strategies of oral posaconazole in patients with compromised gastrointestinal function and who are at high risk for invasive fungal infection. *Antimicrob Agents Chemother* 2012;56:2652–2658.

261. Duarte RF, Lopez-Jimenez J, Cornely OA, et al. Phase 1b study of new posaconazole tablet for prevention of invasive fungal infections in high-risk patients with neutropenia. *Antimicrob Agents Chemother* 2014;58:5758–5765.

262. Krishna G, Ma L, Martinho M, Preston RA, O'Mara E. A new solid oral tablet formulation of posaconazole: A randomized clinical trial to investigate rising single- and multiple-dose pharmacokinetics and safety in healthy volunteers. *J Antimicrob Chemother* 2012;67:2725–2730.

263. Courtney R, Sansone A, Smith W, et al. Posaconazole pharmacokinetics, safety, and tolerability in subjects with varying degrees of chronic renal disease. *J Clin Pharmacol* 2005;45:185–192.

264. Noxafil(R) intravenous injection, oral delayed release tablets, oral suspension, posaconazole intravenous injection, oral delayed release tablets, oral suspension. Merck and Co, Inc, Whitehouse Station, NJ, 2014. Available. at http://labeling. pfizer.com/ShowLabeling.aspx?id=618.

265. Moton A, Krishna G, Ma L, et al. Pharmacokinetics of a single dose of the antifungal posaconazole as oral suspension in subjects with hepatic impairment. *Curr Med Res Opin* 2010;26:1–7.

266. Kohl V, Muller C, Cornely OA, et al. Factors influencing pharmacokinetics of prophylactic posaconazole in patients undergoing allogeneic stem cell transplantation. *Antimicrob Agents Chemother* 2010;54:207–212.

267. Krishna G, Martinho M, Chandrasekar P, Ullmann AJ, Patino H. Pharmacokinetics of oral posaconazole in allogeneic hematopoietic stem cell transplant recipients with graft-versus-host disease. *Pharmacotherapy* 2007;27:1627–1636.

268. Shields RK, Clancy CJ, Vadnerkar A, et al. Posaconazole serum concentrations among cardiothoracic transplant recipients: Factors impacting trough levels and correlation with clinical response to therapy. *Antimicrob Agents Chemother* 2011;55:1308–1311.

269. Conte JE, Jr., DeVoe C, Little E, Golden JA. Steady-state intrapulmonary pharmacokinetics and pharmacodynamics of posaconazole in lung transplant recipients. *Antimicrob Agents Chemother* 2010;54:3609–3613.

270. Schmitt-Hoffmann A, Desai A, Kowalski D, Pearlman H, Yamazaki T, Townsend R. Isavuconazole absorption following oral administration in healthy subjects is comparable to intravenous dosing, and is not affected by food, or drugs that alter stomach pH. *Int J Clin Pharm Ther* 2016;54:572–580.

271. Hope WW, Billaud EM, Lestner J, Denning DW. Therapeutic drug monitoring for triazoles. *Curr Opin Infect Dis* 2008;21:580–586.

272. Poirier JM, Cheymol G. Optimisation of itraconazole therapy using target drug concentrations. *Clin Pharmacokinet* 1998;35:461–473.

273. Glasmacher A, Hahn C, Leutner C, et al. Breakthrough invasive fungal infections in neutropenic patients after prophylaxis with itraconazole. *Mycoses* 1999;42:443–451.

274. Pascual A, Calandra T, Bolay S, Buclin T, Bille J, Marchetti O. Voriconazole therapeutic drug monitoring in patients with invasive mycoses improves efficacy and safety outcomes. *Clin Infect Dis* 2008;46:201–211.

275. Trifilio SM, Bennett CL, Yarnold PR, et al. Breakthrough zygomycosis after voriconazole administration among patients with hematologic malignancies who receive hematopoietic stem-cell transplants or intensive chemotherapy. *Bone Marrow Transplant* 2007;39:425–429.

276. Trifilio S, Singhal S, Williams S, et al. Breakthrough fungal infections after allogeneic hematopoietic stem cell transplantation in patients on prophylactic voriconazole. *Bone Marrow Transplant* 2007;40:451–456.

277. Lestner JM, Roberts SA, Moore CB, Howard SJ, Denning DW, Hope WW. Toxicodynamics of itraconazole: Implications for therapeutic drug monitoring. *Clin Infect Dis* 2009;49:928–930.

278. Tan K, Brayshaw N, Tomaszewski K, Troke P, Wood N. Investigation of the potential relationships between plasma voriconazole concentrations and visual adverse events or liver function test abnormalities. *J Clin Pharmacol* 2006;46:235–243.

279. Heinz WJ, Zirkel J, Kuhn A, et al. Relevance of timing for determination of posaconazole plasma concentrations. *Antimicrob Agents Chemother* 2011;55:3621–3623.

280. Niwa T, Shiraga T, Takagi A. Effect of antifungal drugs on cytochrome P450 (CYP) 2C9, *Cyp*2C19, and *Cyp*3A4 activities in human liver microsomes. *Biol Pharm Bull* 2005;28:1805–1808.

281. Glasmacher A, Prentice A, Gorschluter M, et al. Itraconazole prevents invasive fungal infections in neutropenic patients treated for hematologic malignancies: Evidence from a meta-analysis of 3,597 patients. *J Clin Oncol* 2003;21:4615–4626.

282. Cartledge JD, Midgely J, Gazzard BG. Itraconazole solution: Higher serum drug concentrations and better clinical response rates than the capsule formulation in acquired immunodeficiency syndrome patients with candidosis. *J Clin Pathol* 1997;50:477–480.

283. Smith J, Safdar N, Knasinski V, et al. Voriconazole therapeutic drug monitoring. *Antimicrob Agents Chemother* 2006;50:1570–1572.

284. Zonios DI, Gea-Banacloche J, Childs R, Bennett JE. Hallucinations during voriconazole therapy. *Clin Infect Dis* 2008;47:e7–e10.

285. Jang SH, Colangelo PM, Gobburu JV. Exposure-response of posaconazole used for prophylaxis against invasive fungal infections: Evaluating the need to adjust doses based on drug concentrations in plasma. *Clin Pharmacol Ther* 2010;88:115–119.

286. Cornely OA, Maertens J, Winston DJ, et al. Posaconazole vs. fluconazole or itraconazole prophylaxis in patients with neutropenia. *N Engl J Med* 2007;356:348–359.

287. Moton A, Krishna G, Wang Z. Tolerability and safety profile of posaconazole: Evaluation of 18 controlled studies in healthy volunteers. *J Clin Pharm Ther* 2009;34:301–311.

288. Foo H, Gottlieb T. Lack of cross-hepatotoxicity between voriconazole and posaconazole. *Clin Infect Dis* 2007;45:803–805.

289. Spellberg B, Rieg G, Bayer A, Edwards JE, Jr. Lack of cross-hepatotoxicity between fluconazole and voriconazole. *Clin Infect Dis* 2003;36:1091–1093.

290. Wang EJ, Lew K, Casciano CN, Clement RP, Johnson WW. Interaction of common azole antifungals with P glycoprotein. *Antimicrob Agents Chemother* 2002;46:160–165.

291. Goodwin ML, Drew RH. Antifungal serum concentration monitoring: An update. *J Antimicrob Chemother* 2008;61:17–25.

292. Howard SJ, Felton TW, Gomez-Lopez A, Hope WW. Posaconazole: The case for therapeutic drug monitoring. *Ther Drug Monit* 2012;34:72–76.

293. Lewis RE. Antifungal Therapeutic Drug Monitoring. *Curr Fungal Infect Rep* 2010;4:158–167.

294. Dolton MJ, Ray JE, Marriott D, McLachlan AJ. Posaconazole exposure-response relationship: Evaluating the utility of therapeutic drug monitoring. *Antimicrob Agents Chemother* 2012;56:2806–2813.

295. Hussaini T, Ruping MJ, Farowski F, Vehreschild JJ, Cornely OA. Therapeutic drug monitoring of voriconazole and posaconazole. *Pharmacotherapy* 2011;31:214–225.

296. Smith J, Andes D. Therapeutic drug monitoring of antifungals: Pharmacokinetic and pharmacodynamic considerations. *Ther Drug Monit* 2008;30:167–172.

297. Cohen-Wolkowiez M, Moran C, Benjamin DK, Jr., Smith PB. Pediatric antifungal agents. *Curr Opin Infect Dis* 2009;22:553–558.

298. Benjamin DK, Jr., Smith PB, Arrieta A, et al. Safety and pharmacokinetics of repeat-dose micafungin in young infants. *Clin Pharmacol Ther* 2010;87:93–99.

299. Hope WW, Smith PB, Arrieta A, et al. Population pharmacokinetics of micafungin in neonates and young infants. *Antimicrob Agents Chemother* 2010;54:2633–2637.

300. Queiroz-Telles F, Berezin E, Leverger G, et al. Micafungin versus liposomal amphotericin B for pediatric patients with invasive candidiasis: Substudy of a randomized double-blind trial. *Pediatr Infect Dis J* 2008;27:820–826.

301. Cohen-Wolkowiez M, Benjamin DK, Jr., Piper L, et al. Safety and pharmacokinetics of multiple-dose anidulafungin in infants and neonates. *Clin Pharmacol Ther* 2011;89:702–707.

302. Mehta PA, Vinks AA, Filipovich A, et al. Alternate-day micafungin antifungal prophylaxis in pediatric patients undergoing hematopoietic stem cell transplantation: A pharmacokinetic study. *Biol Blood Marrow Transplant* 2010;16:1458–1462.

303. Betts RF, Nucci M, Talwar D, et al. A Multicenter, double-blind trial of a high-dose caspofungin treatment regimen versus a standard caspofungin treatment regimen for adult patients with invasive candidiasis. *Clin Infect Dis* 2009;48:1676–1684.

304. Muraki Y, Iwamoto T, Kagawa Y, et al. The impact of total bilirubin on plasma micafungin levels in living-donor liver transplantation recipients with severe liver dysfunction. *Biol Pharm Bull* 2009;32:750–754.

305. Stone JA, Migoya EM, Hickey L, et al. Potential for interactions between caspofungin and nelfinavir or rifampin. *Antimicrob Agents Chemother* 2004;48:4306–4314.

306. Decosterd LA, Rochat B, Pesse B, et al. Multiplex ultra-performance liquid chromatography-tandem mass spectrometry method for simultaneous quantification in human plasma of fluconazole, itraconazole, hydroxyitraconazole, posaconazole, voriconazole, voriconazole-N-oxide, anidulafungin, and caspofungin. *Antimicrob Agents Chemother* 2010;54:5303–5315.

307. Farowski F, Cornely OA, Vehreschild JJ, et al. Quantitation of azoles and echinocandins in compartments of peripheral blood by liquid chromatography-tandem mass spectrometry. *Antimicrob Agents Chemother* 2010;54:1815–1819.

308. Kirchhoff F, Maier B, Rieger C, Ostermann H, Spohrer U, Vogeser M. An on-line solid phase extraction procedure for the routine quantification of caspofungin by liquid chromatography-tandem mass spectrometry. *Clin Chem Lab Med* 2011;50:521–524.

309. Egger SS, Meier S, Leu C, et al. Drug interactions and adverse events associated with antimycotic drugs used for invasive aspergillosis in hematopoietic SCT. *Bone Marrow Transplant* 2010;45:1197–1203.

310. Morrissey CO, Slavin MA, O'Reilly MA, et al. Caspofungin as salvage monotherapy for invasive aspergillosis in patients with haematological malignancies or following allogeneic stem cell transplantation: Efficacy and concomitant cyclosporin A. *Mycoses* 2007;50 Suppl 1:24–37.

311. Hebert MF, Blough DK, Townsend RW, et al. Concomitant tacrolimus and micafungin pharmacokinetics in healthy volunteers. *J Clin Pharmacol* 2005;45:1018–1024.

312. Fukuoka N, Imataki O, Ohnishi H, et al. Micafungin does not influence the concentration of tacrolimus in patients after allogeneic hematopoietic stem cell transplantation. *Transplant Proc* 2010;42:2725–2730.

313. Dowell JA, Stogniew M, Krause D, Henkel T, Damle B. Lack of pharmacokinetic interaction between anidulafungin and tacrolimus. *J Clin Pharmacol* 2007;47:305–314.

314. Marr KA, Schlamm HT, Herbrecht R, et al. Combination antifungal therapy for invasive aspergillosis: A randomized trial. *Ann Intern Med* 2015;162:81–89.

27

Infants: Yeasts are beasts in early life

RACHEL G. GREENBERG AND DANIEL K. BENJAMIN JR.

EPIDEMIOLOGY

Candida species are the third most common pathogen in nosocomial blood stream infections among premature infants [1–4]. In a large multicenter cohort of ELBW ($\leq$1000 g birth weight) infants admitted to the Neonatal Intensive Care Unit (NICU) between 2004 and 2007, invasive candidiasis occurred in 9.0% (137/1515) [5]. Another large cohort study demonstrated that the incidence of invasive candidiasis in the NICU decreased from 1997 to 2010, possibly due to increased use of antifungal prophylaxis and decreased use of broad-spectrum antibiotics [6]. Mortality from all *Candida* species in premature infants has been consistently reported at 20% [2,3,7–9]. In addition to high mortality, candidiasis in infants is associated with significant morbidities in survivors including: poor neurodevelopmental outcome, periventricular leukomalacia, chronic lung disease, and severe retinopathy of prematurity [9–13].

C. albicans is the most commonly isolated species in infants [5,14–16]. However, the epidemiology of candidiasis is changing, and the percentage of cases caused by *C. albicans* has recently declined from 80% to as low as 29% in some centers [14,17]. In one center, 5% (1/22) of cases of neonatal candidiasis from 1981 to 1990 were due to *C. parapsilosis* [18]. This percentage increased to 60% (53/89) from 1991 to 1995. *C. albicans* continues to be associated with increased rates of end organ damage and higher attributable mortality relative to the other *Candida* species [8,19]. *C. glabrata, C. krusei, C. lusitaniae,* and *C. tropicalis* are less commonly isolated in infants [17,20,21].

RISK FACTORS

Specific risk factors for invasive disease tend to fall in one of two categories—those that increase colonization of mucosal surfaces or those that disrupt or impair immune function.

Increased colonization

Infants are initially colonized vertically at birth or horizontally in the nursery by parents or caregivers [22,23]. On admission to the NICU, 5%–10% of all infants were found to be colonized with *Candida* [24]. By 7 days of life, colonization rates increased to 50% and rose to 64% by one month of age [23,25,26].

Third-generation cephalosporins and other broad-spectrum antibiotics enhance fungal colonization by destroying competing bacterial flora [15]. In a cohort of over 6000 infants, multivariable modeling revealed that third-generation cephalosporin or carbapenem use in the past 7 days was associated with candidiasis [27]. Gastric acidity is considered to be protective against *Candida* infection by suppressing fungal growth in the upper gastrointestinal tract.

The use of H_2 blockers has been linked to an increased risk of candidemia in infants [5,28].

Impaired immune system

Prematurity is the strongest risk factor for candidiasis in infants. The immune system of the preterm infant has defects in chemotaxis, cytokine and antibody production, and phagocytosis [29,30]. Invasive medical devices such as central venous catheters and endotracheal tubes compromise an already underdeveloped layer of skin and place the premature infant at an especially high risk for candidiasis [5]. Administration of intravenous lipids supports the growth of *Candida* and was found to be associated with candidiasis in a study of 1515 ELBW infants from 19 centers [5,31]. The use of steroids such as hydrocortisone and dexamethasone has been associated with increased risk of candidiasis in infants [32–35].

CLINICAL MANIFESTATIONS

Candidemia

Signs and symptoms of candidemia are often non-specific and subtle in infants and may include: temperature instability, lethargy, apnea, hypotension, respiratory distress, abdominal distension, hyperglycemia, and feeding intolerance [36,37]. Although longer periods of candidemia are associated with increased risk of dissemination, dissemination can occur in the setting of only a single positive blood culture [29,36].

Meningoencephalitis

Meningitis complicates approximately 15% of cases of candidemia in infants; a rate that has been falling over the last 30 years but is still much higher than the rate of meningitis observed in candidemic adult patients. This fact has important implications for diagnostic workup and therapeutic approaches, as clinicians cannot assume that the central nervous system (CNS) is not involved in otherwise seemingly straightforward candidemia.

Candidiasis of the CNS often results in granulomas, parenchymal abscesses, and vasculitis, and unremarkable CSF parameters in the presence of CNS infection are common [13,15,38]. Only 25% of infants in one series of infants with *Candida* meningitis had abnormalities noted on CSF examination [10].

Urinary tract infections

Renal disease may present with rising creatinine, hypertension, flank mass, or acute urinary obstruction from fungal mycetoma [39,40]. Patients with candiduria should have a renal ultrasound to detect the two types of renal involvement: non-shadowing echogenic foci and parenchymal infiltration [39]. Often, radiographic findings persist despite proper therapy, negative cultures, and clinical recovery [41].

Optic complications

Optic infections may result in chorioretinal infections or, more rarely, lens abscesses [42,43]. As with meningitis, rates of chorioretinal lesions complicating candidemia are falling [44,45]. A recent review of 123 candidemic VLBW infants found only 1 patient with optic involvement [44]. However, infants with candidemia in the absence of direct optic infections have been shown to be at increased risk for the development of severe retinopathy of prematurity [11–13,42,46].

Other organs

Endocarditis is documented in <5% of candidemic infants. Candidemia may also result in infections of the bones and joints. Assessment of end-organ damage in the presence of neonatal candidemia should include an ultrasound of the head and abdomen, lumbar puncture, ophthalmologic exam, and an echocardiogram.

PROPHYLAXIS

A survey of 219 US neonatologists revealed that 34% used antifungal prophylaxis in their practice, while a survey of 193 NICUs from 28 European countries reported 55% used antifungal prophylaxis [47,48]. Agents used for prophylaxis included fluconazole, oral nystatin, and amphotericin B deoxycholate. Data regarding amphotericin B deoxycholate for *Candida* prophylaxis in premature infants are limited to one small trial of 40 VLBW infants, 20 of whom were randomized to receive liposomal amphotericin B deoxycholate once weekly [49]. While the drug seemed well-tolerated, the trial was not powered to evaluate efficacy.

Non-absorbable agents

Use of non-absorbable oral agents for prevention of candidemia in infants is controversial [50]. Nystatin is the most commonly used non-absorbable agent in infants, and miconazole has also been studied [47,51]. In a placebo-controlled trial of infants <1750 g in a NICU in South Africa, oral miconazole was associated with decreased rectal *Candida* colonization; there was no effect on systemic *Candida* infection [51]. A small randomized controlled trial of infants <1250 g birth weight given nystatin (100,000 units every 8 hours) or placebo demonstrated a significant decrease in both colonization rates and invasive *Candida* infections, 6% (2/33) in the nystatin group versus 32% (11/34) in the placebo group [52]. A recent larger study of nystatin prophylaxis evaluated 3991 infants randomly assigned to nystatin or nystatin only if orally colonized with *Candida* [53]. In this study, the rate of candidiasis for VLBW infants not receiving prophylaxis was 45% (104/232). This rate of candidiasis is an order magnitude higher than rates observed for VLBW infants in other multicenter cohort studies [7,9]. Although nystatin administration decreased the incidence of candidiasis, the significance of this decrease is difficult to interpret in the presence of such a high rate of candidiasis in the control group. Similarly, a randomized study of VLBW infants in Turkey, which compared oral nystatin to placebo, found that nystatin was associated with a decreased rate of colonization and a decreased incidence of invasive *Candida* infections, 4% (4/94) in the nystatin group vs. 16% (15/91) in the placebo group. A Cochrane review of available data for non-absorbable antifungal prophylaxis found a significant reduction in the risk of invasive *Candida* infection [54]. However, the authors suggest the findings should be interpreted with caution given methodological weaknesses of the trials and the high rates of invasive *Candida* infections in the control groups.

There is concern that nystatin may be inactivated prior to reaching the intestines, the target region for the drug [55]. Nystatin is also ineffective in protecting against invasion of other anatomic sites: skin, respiratory tract, and catheter sites.

Fluconazole

Several randomized placebo-controlled trials have been completed evaluating fluconazole prophylaxis in preterm infants (Table 27.1). A study of 103 VLBW infants

demonstrated lower rates of colonization in the fluconazole group but no difference in invasive disease [26]. A second study of 100 ELBW infants found a significant decrease in both *Candida* colonization and the incidence of candidiasis [56]. The placebo arm in this single center study had one of the highest rates (13/50; 26%) of invasive candidiasis reported in ELBW infants. A subsequent study of fluconazole prophylaxis at the same institution evaluated 3 mg/kg twice weekly dosing (12 doses total) versus the previous regimen (26 doses) in ELBW infants [57]. Rates of candidiasis were similar between the twice weekly dosing group 3% (1/40) and the older regimen 5% (2/41), p = 0.68. Twice weekly dosing might decrease drug toxicity and cost versus the more frequent dosing schedule. Several cohort studies have demonstrated decreased incidence of candidiasis using fluconazole prophylaxis [58–61].

A large 8-center study evaluated fluconazole prophylaxis in 322 VLBW infants [62]. The infants were randomized 1:1:1 to receive placebo, fluconazole prophylaxis at 3 mg/kg/dose, or fluconazole prophylaxis at 6 mg/kg/dose. The rate of candidiasis in the 2 prophylaxis groups was 3% (7/127) and the rate in the placebo group was 14% (14/106). The rate of candidiasis in the placebo group ELBW infants, 14% (6/43), was twice of that observed in previous large multicenter studies [7,9]. Rates of candidiasis in the infants 1000–1499 g birth weight were over 10 times as high as previous observational studies, 13% (8/63) versus 1% in the 16 center

Table 27.1 Fluconazole prophylaxis randomized controlled trials

Study	Population	N	Results (systemic fungal infection)
Violaris (1998)	<1500 g	80	Nystatin: 44% (4/9) Fluconazole: 0% (0/8), p < 0.05
Kicklighter (2001)	<1500 g	103	Placebo: 4% (2/50) Fluconazole: 4% (2/53), p = NS
Kaufman (2001)	<1000 g	100	Placebo: 20% (10/50) Fluconazole: 0% (0/50), p < 0.01
Kaufman (2005)	<1000 g	81	Previous dosing: 5% (2/41) Twice weekly: 2% (1/40), p = 0.83
Manzoni (2007)	<1500 g	322	Placebo: 13.2% (14/106) Fluconazole 3 mg: 3.2% (7/216), p = 0.02 Fluconazole 6 mg: 2.7% (3/112), p = 0.05
Parikh (2007)	<1500 g	120	Placebo: 25% (15/60) Fluconazole: 27% (16/60), p = 0.84
Violaris (2010)	<1500 g	80	Nystatin: 14% (16/42) Fluconazole: 5% (2/38); p = NS
Aydemir (2011)	<1500 g	278	Placebo: 16.5% (15/91) Fluconazole: 3.2% (3/93); p < 0.001
Mersal (2013)	<1200 g	59	Nystatin: 0% (0/24) Fluconazole: 0% (0/33); p = NS
Benjamin (2014)	<750 g	361	Placebo: 11% (19/173) Fluconazole: 4% (8/188); p = 0.02
Kirpal (2015)	<1500 g	80	Placebo: 43% (16/37) Fluconazole: 21% (8/38); p = 0.04

Note: RCT, randomized controlled trial.

NICHD Neonatal Research Network. In a subsequent trial of 361 infants <750 g birth weight, infants were randomized to fluconazole prophylaxis at 6 mg/kg/dose twice weekly vs. Placebo [63]. The study's primary endpoint was a composite of death or invasive candidiasis. While invasive candidiasis occurred less frequently in the fluconazole group, 3% (6/188), vs. the placebo group, 9% (16/173), there was no difference in the composite primary outcome of the study. In addition to these trials, a number of smaller randomized trials of fluconazole prophylaxis have been performed [26,57,64–68]. A Cochrane review of all available trials on fluconazole prophylaxis suggested that systemic fluconazole therapy reduces the incidence of invasive *Candida* infection in preterm infants but does not affect mortality [69]. Similarly, a meta-analysis of patient-level data from 4 trials found that fluconazole prophylaxis reduced the odds of invasive candidiasis or death, invasive candidiasis, and *Candida* colonization [70]. Resistance to fluconazole was not observed in during the courses of these randomized trials and side effects of fluconazole were minimal. A recent cost analysis indicated that the use of fluconazole prophylaxis would result in cost savings in NICUs where the rate of invasive candidiasis is >2.8% [71].

EMPIRIC THERAPY

Antifungal therapy initiated the day before or the day of the first positive culture in infected ELBW infants has been associated with improved mortality and morbidity [13,72]. In a study of 136 ELBW infants with invasive candidiasis, infants who received empiric antifungal therapy had a lower incidence of death or NDI, 50% (19/38) compared to infants who did not receive empiric antifungal therapy, 64% (55/86) (odds ratio 0.27, 95% confidence interval 0.08–0.86) [72]. The decision to initiate empiric therapy in adult patients is largely based on a predictive model of risk in the treatment of neutropenic patients with prolonged febrile episodes, but until recently, no such model exists for infants [73]. Several efforts have been made to develop a similar model for infants with candidiasis. A retrospective multicenter cohort study examined risk factors and subsequent candidiasis from blood cultures of 6,172 premature infants and developed a model that was 85% sensitive and 47% specific in predicting candidemia [27]. Building on this work, a prospective cohort study evaluated the ability of a clinical prediction model against clinician judgment to predict invasive *Candida* infection. Significant predictors of *Candida* infection in the clinical prediction model included a *Candida*-like dermatitis, presence of a central catheter, vaginal delivery, lack of enteral feeding, lower gestational age, hypoglycemia, and thrombocytopenia. The clinical prediction model (area under the ROC curve [AUC] = 0.79) was superior to clinical judgement, as determined by administration of empiric antifungal therapy (AUC 0.70; p = 0.0022). The available data suggest that if empirical antifungal therapy is being considered in a premature infant, the decision should be made based on the evaluation of clinical risk factors rather than bedside judgment.

TREATMENT

Removal of the central venous catheter within 24 hours of a positive blood culture is a critical component of treatment [74]. Delayed removal of central venous catheters in candidemic infants has been associated with increased mortality and morbidity, including worse neurodevelopmental outcomes [8,74,75].

Amphotericin B deoxycholate

Amphotericin B deoxycholate is the most often used agent for invasive candidiasis in infants [76]. However, there are limited pharmacokinetic data in infants. Two studies involving a total of 17 infants demonstrated a longer half-life of the drug in infants compared with adults [77,78]. Test doses are not recommended as the drug is much better tolerated in infants than in adults [77,79]. CSF penetration is poor in adult patients but was found to reach 40%–90% of serum levels in preterm infants [77]. Side effects observed in infants include electrolyte abnormalities and nephrotoxicity [80,81]. Amphotericin B deoxycholate is effective against most *Candida* species causing disease in infants except for *C. lusitaniae* [82]. A prospective observational study of 59 infants with invasive candidiasis found that all isolates were sensitive to amphotericin B deoxycholate [16].

There are only 3 published randomized controlled trials for treatment of candidemia in infants (Table 27.2). One of these is a 23-patient study comparing amphotericin B deoxycholate (1 mg/kg/day) versus fluconazole (10 mg/kg loading dose followed by 5 mg/kg/day) [83]. Although the study was not sufficiently powered for non-inferiority, there was no observed difference in survival between the two groups. Five (45%) of the infants in the amphotericin group suffered thrombophlebitis leading to abscess formation compared with only 1/12 (8%) of the infants receiving fluconazole. One infant in the amphotericin B deoxycholate group suffered acute renal toxicity and 2 additional infants demonstrated an increase in liver enzymes. Only 1 infant receiving fluconazole experienced an increase in liver enzymes. The other 2 randomized controlled trials for treatment of candidemia included amphotericin B deoxycholate in the comparison group and will be discussed in the section on echinocandins.

Lipid preparations of amphotericin B

Published experience with lipid preparations of amphotericin B in infants is also limited [79]. Serum levels on day 1 and day 28 of therapy were reported for 17 infants receiving 1 mg/kg/day of liposomal amphotericin B (LAmB) [84]. Levels were lower than in adults and children receiving similar doses. Population pharmacokinetics of amphotericin B lipid complex (ABLC) were evaluated in 28 infants with a median birth weight of 910 grams [85]. Serum level in infants receiving both 2.5 mg/kg/day and 5 mg/kg/day were similar to levels reported in adults. There was no accumulation of

Table 27.2 Prospective trials of antifungals for invasive *Candida* infection

Author	Type of study	Drug	Survival
Fasano (1994)	Prospective cohort	Fluconazole	97% (30/31)
Driessen (1996)	RCT	Amphotericin B	54.5% (6/11)
		Fluconazole	67% (8/12)
Wainer (1997)	Prospective cohort	Fluconazole	70% (14/20)
Huttova (1998)	Prospective cohort	Fluconazole	80% (32/40)
Adler-Shohet (2001)	Prospective cohort	ABLC	82% (9/11)
Scarcella (2003)	Prospective cohort	LAmB	73% (32/44)
Juster-Reicher (2003)	Prospective cohort	LAmB	95% (35/37)
Linder (2003)	Prospective cohort	Amphotericin B	85% (29/34)
		LAmB	83% (5/6)
		ABCD	86% (12/14)
Lopez Sastre (2003)	Prospective cohort	Amphotericin b	100% (4/4)
		LAmB	64% (52/81)
		ABLC	76% (22/29)
Odio (2004)	Prospective cohort	Caspofungin	90% (9/10)
Mohamed (2012)	RCT	Caspofungin	93% (14/15)
		Amphotericin B	82% (14/17)
Benjamin (2015)	RCT	Micafungin	85% (17/20)
		Amphotericin B	90% (9/10)

Note: RCT, randomized controlled trial.

drug noted after multiple doses. Although therapeutic levels of amphotericin B were detected in urine samples, little to no amphotericin B was detected in the CSF.

Amphotericin B colloidal dispersion (ABCD) and LAmB were compared with amphotericin B deoxycholate in 56 candidemic infants [86]. Infants with a serum creatinine <1.2 mg/dL were given 1 mg/kg/day of amphotericin B deoxycholate (*n* = 34) while the remaining infants were given either 5 mg/kg/day of ABCD (*n* = 16) or LAmB (*n* = 6). Potassium supplementation was required in 16 (47%) of the infants receiving amphotericin B deoxycholate and none of the 22 infants receiving the lipid preparations. Renal function improved during the course of treatment of all three groups. In a separate cohort of 44 infants treated with 1–5 mg/kg/day of LAmB, the only side effect noted was hypokalemia occurring in 16 (36%) of the infants [87]. A total of 32 (73%) of the infants responded to therapy, including 5/6 (83%) of the infants with meningitis. Another report observed 118 infants given LAmB (*n* = 81) or ABLC (*n* = 29) [88]. Both antifungals were started at 1 mg/kg/day and increased as tolerated to a maximum dose of 5 mg/kg/day. No difference in mortality was observed between the two groups and efficacy was 94% and 86% with LAmB and ABLC respectively. LAmB was used in a series of 41 infants with candidiasis with a success rate of 95% (39/41) [79]. The authors noted that eradication of infection occurred earlier when the target dose of 5–7 mg/kg/day was reached faster and concluded that clinicians should initiate therapy with this dose. A large cohort study showed increased mortality and treatment failure for infants with *Candida* infection treated with lipid preparations compared with AmB [81].

There is some concern about the ability of the lipid preparations to clear renal and CSF *Candida* infections [85,89]. However, successful treatment of infants with *Candida* meningitis has been reported [87,90].

Flucytosine

Flucytosine is not an option for candidiasis as monotherapy because resistance develops rapidly. Use of 5-FC for candidiasis is further limited by lack of a parenteral formulation in the United States, and it is not approved for use in infants. However, 5-FC is occasionally administered in combination with other antifungals for *Candida* meningoencephalitis [91]. In a cohort of 17 cases of *Candida* meningitis (including 11 infants), improvement was noted in 15 patients on combination therapy of amphotericin B deoxycholate and 5-FC [92]. An analysis of 27 ELBW infants with *Candida* meningitis revealed that time to clear infection was longer in infants given combination flucytosine and amphotericin B than those treated with amphotericin B alone [8]. Bone marrow suppression is the predominant toxicity.

The azoles

Fluconazole is used frequently in the NICU due to the predominance of fungal infections due to *C. albicans* and *C. parapsilosis,* both species that are generally susceptible. Recently, population pharmacokinetics studies in infants have evaluated the appropriate therapeutic dose of fluconazole in infants. Because fluconazole clearance was associated with gestational age, postnatal age, weight, and serum creatinine, loading dose of 25 mg/kg/day and a maintenance dose of at least 12 mg/kg/d in the first 90 days after birth is needed to achieve therapeutic concentrations in ≥90% of infants <30 weeks gestation and 80% of infants 30–40 weeks gestation [93,94].

A group of 19 premature infants with a mean birth weight of 1725 g treated with fluconazole experienced clearance of infection in 18 cases (95%) [95]. The one failure was caused by *C. glabrata*. The infants were given a 10 mg/kg loading dose followed by 5 mg/kg/day. Only one infant, with syphilitic hepatitis, required a dosing change because of elevation in liver function tests. A prospective report of 40 infants given 6 mg/kg/day of fluconazole reported an overall mortality of 20% (8/40) [96]. Elevated liver function tests were observed in 2 (5%) infants.

Voriconazole, a second-generation triazole, has been found to be active *in vitro* against both *C. glabrata* and *C. krusei*, as well as some isolates that have developed resistance to fluconazole. However, voriconazole should be used with caution in instances where fluconazole resistance is likely [97]. To emphasize this point, we have observed an infant at our institution that developed resistance to both azoles while on treatment doses of fluconazole [98]. Voriconazole is not recommended in patients with renal insufficiency as its cyclodextrin carrier is renally cleared [99]. The drug is metabolized by the liver, and good CSF penetration has been observed. Torsades de pointes has rarely been seen during therapy in adult patients. Other side effects include allergic reactions, elevated transaminases, and visual disturbances.

A 10-week-old infant with hemaphagocytic lymphohistiocytosis with a cutaneous *Trichosporon beigelii* infection was given 6 mg/kg every 12 hours of voriconazole [100]. Serum levels obtained were subtherapeutic for invasive fungal infections. The authors recommended a dose of 8 mg/kg every 8 hours based on their findings. Another 18-day-old infant born at 24 weeks gestational age with *Aspergillus fumigatus* was treated successfully with voriconazole after failing multiple other therapies [101]. Therapeutic drug monitoring data from 9 additional children <3 years of age who received voriconazole revealed that weight-based dosing did not reliably predict plasma concentrations, and thus therapeutic drug monitoring is necessary to achieve adequate concentrations and avoid adverse effects [101].

The echinocandins

Caspofungin was not tested in infants prior to market approval, and there remains very little experience with caspofungin in infants. Odio et al reported on a series of 10 infants receiving caspofungin as salvage therapy after initial therapy with amphotericin B deoxycholate [102]. In this report 9/10 (90%) infants survived, and no adverse drug events were observed. The infants were given a dose of 1 mg/kg/day for 2 days before increasing the dose to 2 mg/kg/day for the duration of treatment. Another retrospective study of 13 infants with refractory candidemia after traditional therapy (amphotericin B, fluconazole, or flucytosine) received add-on therapy with caspofungin [103]. Sterilization of blood cultures was achieved in 85% (11/13) of infants. Adverse events included elevation of liver enzymes in 4 infants, hypokalemia in 2 infants, and thrombophlebitis in 1 infant. We have reported hypercalcemia in an infant given a loading dose of 100 mg/m^2 followed by 70 mg/m^2/day [98]. No further electrolyte abnormalities were noted once the dose of caspofungin was decreased to 35 mg/m^2/day. Only one randomized controlled trial of caspofungin has been performed in infants. Thirty-two infants were randomized to receive caspofungin or amphotericin B [104]. Although the numbers were small, infants receiving caspofungin were more likely to show efficacy of treatment and had significantly fewer adverse events.

One pharmacokinetics study of caspofungin has been performed specifically in neonates and young infants [105]. Patients were enrolled to receive either single-dose ($n = 6$) or multiple-dose (b-n = 12) caspofungin at 25 mg/m^2/day. This dose appeared to provide relatively similar plasma exposures to those obtained in adults receiving 50 mg/day. Adverse events were reported in 5/18 (28%) infants who received caspofungin.

Micafungin was evaluated in premature infants in a single dose (0.75–3.0 mg/kg) pharmacokinetic study [106]. The half-life in infants weighing >1000 g was 8 hours and 5.5 hours in infants 500–1000 g. The area under the curve (AUC) in infants >1000 g was approximately 50% less than that observed in older children; and the AUC was approximately 50% less in infants 500–1000 g compared to infants >1000 g. The substantially reduced AUC observed in infants is extremely important because the echinocandins (as a class) have shown a dose-response relationship. We also performed several pharmacokinetics studies of micafungin in infants. We reported the safety and non-compartmental pharmacokinetics of micafungin in infants at 7, 10, and 15 mg/kg [107,108]. When data from these 3 trials were combined, we demonstrated that the population pharmacokinetics are linear in the range of 0.75 to 15 mg/kg. We also demonstrated that the dosage of 10 mg/kg resulted in near-maximal decline in fungal burden within the central nervous system [109].

A 2014 meta-analysis of available micafungin trial data for infants (<2 years of age) showed a reasonable safety profile and efficacy in this age group [110]. A trial was recently performed in infants were randomized 2:1 to micafungin 10 mg/kg/day to amphotericin B 1 mg/kg/day [111]. The trial was terminated early due to insufficient recruitment, with 30 infants enrolled (20 received micafungin, 10 received amphotericin B). The study's primary outcome of fungal-free survival was achieved in 60% (95% confidence interval: 36%–81%) in the micafungin group and 70% (95% confidence interval: 35%–93%) in the amphotericin B group. Serious adverse events were common, with 60% (12/20) in the micafungin group and 70% (7/10) in the amphotericin B group having at least 1 serious adverse event. Because it was underpowered, the study results are difficult to interpret.

The pharmacokinetics of anidulafungin has been recently studied in infants [112]. Intravenous anidulafungin (1.5 mg/kg/day) was administered to 15 infants and neonates over 3–5 days. No drug-related serious adverse events were observed, and the study results indicated that neonates and infants receiving 1.5 mg/kg/day of anidulafungin had similar exposures to older children receiving the same weight-based dosing and adult patients receiving 100 mg/day. However, the safety data of anidulafungin are sufficiently limited that we do not recommend it as first line therapy in the nursery.

CONCLUSION

Candida infections are of increasing importance as physicians care for a growing number of immunocompromised, premature infants. *Candida* speciation patterns continue to change with the introduction of newer antifungals for both prophylaxis and empiric therapy. Treatment options are greater now than ever before, but physicians are hampered by a lack of randomized controlled trials in this special population. Amphotericin B deoxycholate (1 mg/kg/day) and fluconazole (25 mg/kg loading dose, 12 mg/kg/day maintenance) should continue to be used as first line agents for candidiasis. Micafungin (10 mg/kg/day) should be considered as a second line agent. Antifungal prophylaxis with fluconazole (6 mg/kg twice weekly) should be considered for NICUs with a high baseline incidence of fungal infection.

Common clinical questions

1. What are some of the most important factors for invasive *Candida* infection in infants?
2. What factors should be considered when deciding whether antifungal prophylaxis is warranted for a particular infant?
3. If central nervous system infection is suspected in an infant with invasive *Candida* infection, which antifungal medications are most appropriate to be used for empiric therapy?
4. If appropriate therapy is selected to an infant with proven candidemia, can indwelling catheters remain in place so that the therapy can be administered?

ANSWERS TO COMMON CLINICAL QUESTIONS

1. Risk factors generally fall into 2 categories – those that increase colonization and those that disrupt or impair immune function. Risk factors that increase colonization include exposure to broad spectrum antibiotics, poor hand hygiene techniques, and exposure to H$_2$ blocking agents. Risk factors that result in impaired immune function include the presence of foreign devices, systemic corticosteroid use, and prematurity.

2. Important considerations include: the presence of *Candida* risk factors for the particular infant, the rate of invasive *Candida* infection at the unit, and cost and resources available.
3. Reasonable empirical therapy choices for an infant at risk for central nervous system *Candida* infection include amphotericin B, fluconazole, and micafungin. Voriconazole also has good central nervous system penetration but is less preferred due to need for therapeutic drug monitoring. Liposomal forms of amphotericin B do not achieve adequate central nervous system concentrations.
4. No, indwelling catheters and other devices should be removed as soon as possible. Delayed removal of catheters is associated with increased length of time to clear infection and increased morbidity and mortality.

REFERENCES

1. Kaufman D. Strategies for prevention of neonatal invasive candidiasis. *Semin Perinatol* 2003;27:414–424.
2. Stoll BJ, Gordon T, Korones SB, et al. Late-onset sepsis in very low birth weight neonates: A report from the National Institute of Child Health and Human Development Neonatal Research Network. *J Pediatr* 1996;129:63–71.
3. Benjamin DK, DeLong E, Cotten CM, Garges HP, Steinbach WJ, Clark RH. Mortality following blood culture in premature infants: Increased with Gram-negative bacteremia and candidemia, but not Gram-positive bacteremia. *J Perinatol* 2004;24:175–180.
4. Boghossian NS, Page GP, Bell EF, et al. Late-Onset sepsis in very low birth weight infants from singleton and multiple-Gestation Births. *J Pediatr* 2013;162(6):1120–1124.
5. Benjamin DK, Jr., Stoll BJ, Gantz MG, et al. Neonatal candidiasis: Epidemiology, risk factors, and clinical judgment. *Pediatrics* 2010;126:e865–e873.
6. Aliaga S, Clark RH, Laughon M, et al. Changes in the incidence of candidiasis in neonatal intensive care units. *Pediatrics* 2014;133:236–242.
7. Stoll BJ, Hansen N, Fanaroff AA, et al. Late-onset sepsis in very low birth weight neonates: The experience of the NICHD Neonatal Research Network. *Pediatrics* 2002;110:285–291.
8. Benjamin DK, Jr., Stoll BJ, Fanaroff AA, et al. Neonatal candidiasis among infants <1000g birthweight: Risk factors, mortality, and neurodevelopmental outcomes at 18–22 months. *Interscience Conference on Antimicrobial Agents and Chemotherapy*; 2004; Washington, DC.
9. Benjamin DK, Jr., Stoll BJ, Fanaroff AA, et al. Neonatal candidiasis among extremely low birth weight infants: Risk factors, mortality rates, and neurodevelopmental outcomes at 18 to 22 months. *Pediatrics* 2006;117:84–92.

10. Lee BE, Cheung PY, Robinson JL, Evanochko C, Robertson CM. Comparative study of mortality and morbidity in premature infants (birth weight, <1,250 g) with candidemia or candidal meningitis. *Clinical Infectious Diseases: An Official Publication of the Infectious Diseases Society of America* 1998;27:559–565.

11. Kremer I, Naor N, Davidson S, Arbizo M, Nissenkorn I. Systemic candidiasis in babies with retinopathy of prematurity. *Graefes Arch Clin Exp Ophthalmol* 1992;230:592–594.

12. Mittal M, Dhanireddy R, Higgins RD. *Candida* sepsis and association with retinopathy of prematurity. *Pediatrics* 1998;101:654–657.

13. Friedman S, Richardson SE, Jacobs SE, O'Brien K. Systemic *Candida* infection in extremely low birth weight infants: Short term morbidity and long term neurodevelopmental outcome. *Pediatr Infect Dis J* 2000;19:499–504.

14. Makhoul IR, Kassis I, Smolkin T, Tamir A, Sujov P. Review of 49 neonates with acquired fungal sepsis: Further characterization. *Pediatrics* 2001;107:61–66.

15. Kaufman D, Fairchild KD. Clinical microbiology of bacterial and fungal sepsis in very-low-birth-weight infants. *Clin Microbiol Rev* 2004;17:638–680, table of contents.

16. Roilides E, Farmaki E, Evdoridou J, et al. Neonatal candidiasis: Analysis of epidemiology, drug susceptibility, and molecular typing of causative isolates. *Eur J Clin Microbiol Infect Dis* 2004;23:745–750.

17. Mullen CA, Abd El-Baki H, Samir H, Tarrand JJ, Rolston KV. Non-albicans *Candida* is the most common cause of candidemia in pediatric cancer patients. *Support Care Cancer* 2003;11:321–325.

18. Kossoff EH, Buescher ES, Karlowicz MG. Candidemia in a neonatal intensive care unit: Trends during fifteen years and clinical features of 111 cases. *Pediatr Infect Dis J* 1998;17:504–508.

19. Benjamin DK, Jr., Poole C, Steinbach WJ, Rowen JL, Walsh TJ. Neonatal candidemia and end-organ damage: A critical appraisal of the literature using meta-analytic techniques. *Pediatrics* 2003;112:634–640.

20. Manzoni P, Farina D, Leonessa M, et al. Risk factors for progression to invasive fungal infection in preterm neonates with fungal colonization. *Pediatrics* 2006;118:2359–2364.

21. Fridkin SK, Kaufman D, Edwards JR, Shetty S, Horan T. Changing incidence of *Candida* bloodstream infections among NICU patients in the United States: 1995–2004. *Pediatrics* 2006;117:1680–1687.

22. Waggoner-Fountain LA, Walker MW, Hollis RJ, et al. Vertical and horizontal transmission of unique *Candida* species to premature newborns. *Clin Infect Dis* 1996;22:803–808.

23. Bendel CM. Colonization and epithelial adhesion in the pathogenesis of neonatal candidiasis. *Semin Perinatol* 2003;27:357–364.

24. Baley JE, Kliegman RM, Boxerbaum B, Fanaroff AA. Fungal colonization in the very low birth weight infant. *Pediatrics* 1986;78:225–232.

25. Rowen JL, Rench MA, Kozinetz CA, Adams JM, Jr., Baker CJ. Endotracheal colonization with *Candida* enhances risk of systemic candidiasis in very low birth weight neonates. *J Pediatr* 1994;124:789–794.

26. Kicklighter SD, Springer SC, Cox T, Hulsey TC, Turner RB. Fluconazole for prophylaxis against candidal rectal colonization in the very low birth weight infant. *Pediatrics* 2001;107:293–298.

27. Benjamin DK, Jr., DeLong ER, Steinbach WJ, Cotton CM, Walsh TJ, Clark RH. Empirical therapy for neonatal candidemia in very low birth weight infants. *Pediatrics* 2003;112:543–547.

28. Saiman L, Ludington E, Pfaller M, et al. Risk factors for candidemia in neonatal intensive care unit patients. The national epidemiology of mycosis survey study group. *Pediatr Infect Dis J* 2000;19:319–324.

29. Chapman RL, Faix RG. Persistently positive cultures and outcome in invasive neonatal candidiasis. *Pediatr Infect Dis J* 2000;19:822–827.

30. Lewis DB, Wilson CB. *Infectious Diseases of the Fetus and Newborn Infant*. Philadelphia, PA: The W. B. Saunders; 2001.

31. Swindell K, Lattif AA, Chandra J, Mukherjee PK, Ghannoum MA. Parenteral lipid emulsion induces germination of *Candida albicans* and increases biofilm formation on medical catheter surfaces. *J Infect Dis* 2009;200:473–480.

32. Botas CM, Kurlat I, Young SM, Sola A. Disseminated candidal infections and intravenous hydrocortisone in preterm infants. *Pediatrics* 1995;95:883–887.

33. Pera A, Byun A, Gribar S, Schwartz R, Kumar D, Parimi P. Dexamethasone therapy and *candida* sepsis in neonates less than 1250 grams. *J Perinatol* 2002;22:204–208.

34. Hovi L, Saarinen-Pihkala UM, Vettenranta K, Saxen H. Invasive fungal infections in pediatric bone marrow transplant recipients: Single center experience of 10 years. *Bone Marrow Transplant* 2000;26:999–1004.

35. Krupova Y, Sejnova D, Dzatkova J, et al. Prospective study on fungemia in children with cancer: Analysis of 35 cases and comparison with 130 fungemias in adults. *Support Care Cancer* 2000;8:427–430.

36. Benjamin DK, Jr., Ross K, McKinney RE, Jr., Benjamin DK, Auten R, Fisher RG. When to suspect fungal infection in neonates: A clinical comparison of *Candida albicans* and *Candida parapsilosis* fungemia with coagulase-negative *staphylococcal* bacteremia. *Pediatrics* 2000;106:712–718.

37. Fanaroff AA, Korones SB, Wright LL, et al. Incidence, presenting features, risk factors and significance of late onset septicemia in very low birth weight infants. The National Institute of Child Health and Human Development Neonatal Research Network. *Pediatr Infect Dis J* 1998;17:593–598.

38. Cohen-Wolkowiez M, Smith PB, Mangum B, et al. Neonatal *Candida* meningitis: Significance of cerebrospinal fluid parameters and blood cultures. *J Perinatol* 2007;27:97–100.

39. Bryant K, Maxfield C, Rabalais G. Renal candidiasis in neonates with candiduria. *Pediatr Infect Dis J* 1999;18:959–963.

40. Fanaroff A, Martin R. *Neonatal-Perinatal Medicine*. 7th ed. St. Louis, MO: Mosby, 2002.

41. Benjamin DK, Jr., Fisher RG, McKinney RE, Jr., Benjamin DK. Candidal mycetoma in the neonatal kidney. *Pediatrics* 1999;104:1126–1129.

42. Baley JE, Ellis FJ. Neonatal candidiasis: Ophthalmologic infection. *Seminars in Perinatology* 2003;27:401–405.

43. Pickering LK. *Red Book*. 26th ed. Elk Grove Village, IL: American Academy of Pediatrics; 2003.

44. Fisher RG, Gary Karlowicz M, Lall-Trail J. Very low prevalence of endophthalmitis in very low birthweight infants who survive candidemia. *J Perinatol* 2005;25:408–411.

45. Baley JE, Annable WL, Kliegman RM. *Candida* endophthalmitis in the premature infant. *J Pediatr* 1981;98:458–461.

46. Haroon Parupia MF, Dhanireddy R. Association of postnatal dexamethasone use and fungal sepsis in the development of severe retinopathy of prematurity and progression to laser therapy in extremely low-birth-weight infants. *J Perinatol* 2001;21:242–247.

47. Burwell LA, Kaufman D, Blakely J, Stoll BJ, Fridkin SK. Antifungal prophylaxis to prevent neonatal candidiasis: A survey of perinatal physician practices. *Pediatrics* 2006;118:e1019–e1026.

48. Kaguelidou F, Pandolfini C, Manzoni P, Choonara I, Bonati M, Jacqz-Aigrain E. European survey on the use of prophylactic fluconazole in neonatal intensive care units. *Eur J Pediatr* 2012;171:439–445.

49. Arrieta AC, Shea K, Dhar V, et al. Once-weekly liposomal amphotericin B as *Candida* prophylaxis in very low birth weight premature infants: A prospective, randomized, open-label, placebo-controlled pilot study. *Clin Ther* 2010;32:265–271.

50. Weitkamp JH, Poets CF, Sievers R, et al. *Candida* infection in very low birth-weight infants: Outcome and nephrotoxicity of treatment with liposomal amphotericin B (AmBisome). *Infection* 1998;26:11–15.

51. Wainer S, Cooper PA, Funk E, Bental RY, Sandler DA, Patel J. Prophylactic miconazole oral gel for the prevention of neonatal fungal rectal colonization and systemic infection. *Pediatr Infect Dis J* 1992;11:713–716.

52. Sims ME, Yoo Y, You H, Salminen C, Walther FJ. Prophylactic oral nystatin and fungal infections in very-low-birthweight infants. *Am J Perinatol* 1988;5:33–36.

53. Ozturk MA, Gunes T, Koklu E, Cetin N, Koc N. Oral nystatin prophylaxis to prevent invasive candidiasis in neonatal intensive care unit. *Mycoses* 2006;49:484–492.

54. Austin N, Cleminson J, Darlow BA, McGuire W. Prophylactic oral/topical non-absorbed antifungal agents to prevent invasive fungal infection in very low birth weight infants. *Cochrane Database Syst Rev* 2015:Cd003478.

55. Hofstra W, de Vries-Hospers HG, van der Waaij D. Concentrations of nystatin in faeces after oral administration of various doses of nystatin. *Infection* 1979;7:166–170.

56. Kaufman D, Boyle R, Hazen KC, Patrie JT, Robinson M, Donowitz LG. Fluconazole prophylaxis against fungal colonization and infection in preterm infants. *N Engl J Med* 2001;345:1660–1666.

57. Kaufman D, Boyle R, Hazen KC, Patrie JT, Robinson M, Grossman LB. Twice weekly fluconazole prophylaxis for prevention of invasive *Candida* infection in high-risk infants of <1000 grams birth weight. *J Pediatr* 2005;147:172–179.

58. Uko S, Soghier LM, Vega M, et al. Targeted short-term fluconazole prophylaxis among very low birth weight and extremely low birth weight infants. *Pediatrics* 2006;117:1243–1252.

59. Bertini G, Perugi S, Dani C, Filippi L, Pratesi S, Rubaltelli FF. Fluconazole prophylaxis prevents invasive fungal infection in high-risk, very low birth weight infants. *J Pediatr* 2005;147:162–165.

60. Healy CM, Baker CJ, Zaccaria E, Campbell JR. Impact of fluconazole prophylaxis on incidence and outcome of invasive candidiasis in a neonatal intensive care unit. *J Pediatr* 2005;147:166–171.

61. Manzoni P, Arisio R, Mostert M, et al. Prophylactic fluconazole is effective in preventing fungal colonization and fungal systemic infections in preterm neonates: A single-center, 6-year, retrospective cohort study. *Pediatrics* 2006;117:e22–32.

62. Manzoni P, Stolfi I, Pugni L, et al. A multicenter, randomized trial of prophylactic fluconazole in preterm neonates. *N Engl J Med* 2007;356:2483–2495.

63. Benjamin DK, Jr., Hudak ML, Duara S, et al. Effect of fluconazole prophylaxis on candidiasis and mortality in premature infants: A randomized clinical trial. *JAMA* 2014;311:1742–1749.

64. Manzoni P, Stolfi I, Pugni L, et al. A multicenter, randomized trial of prophylactic fluconazole in preterm neonates. *N Engl J Med* 2007;356:2483–2495.

65. Aydemir C, Oguz SS, Dizdar EA, et al. Randomised controlled trial of prophylactic fluconazole versus nystatin for the prevention of fungal colonisation and invasive fungal infection in very low birth weight infants. *Arch Dis Child Fetal Neonatal Ed* 2011;96:F164–F168.

66. Kirpal H, Gathwala G, Chaudhary U, Sharma D. Prophylactic fluconazole in very low birth weight infants admitted to neonatal intensive care unit: Randomized controlled trial. *The Journal of Maternal-fetal & Neonatal Medicine: The Official Journal of the European Association of Perinatal Medicine, the Federation of Asia and Oceania Perinatal Societies, the International Society of Perinatal Obstet* 2016;29:624–628.

67. Violaris K, Carbone T, Bateman D, Olawepo O, Doraiswamy B, LaCorte M. Comparison of fluconazole and nystatin oral suspensions for prophylaxis of systemic fungal infection in very low birthweight infants. *Am J Perinatol* 2010;27:73–78.

68. Mersal A, Alzahrani I, Azzouz M, et al. Oral Nystatin versus intravenous fluconazole as neonatal antifungal prophylaxis: Non-inferiority trial. *J Clin Neonatol* 2013;2:88–92.

69. Cleminson J, Austin N, McGuire W. Prophylactic systemic antifungal agents to prevent mortality and morbidity in very low birth weight infants. *Cochrane Database Syst Rev* 2015:Cd003850.

70. Ericson JE, Kaufman DA, Kicklighter SD, et al. Fluconazole prophylaxis for the prevention of candidiasis in premature infants: A meta-analysis using patient-level data. *Clinical Infectious Diseases: An Official Publication of the Infectious Diseases Society of America* 2016;63:604–610.

71. Swanson JR, Vergales J, Kaufman DA, Sinkin RA. Cost analysis of fluconazole prophylaxis for prevention of neonatal invasive candidiasis. *Pediatr Infect Dis J* 2016;35:519–523.

72. Greenberg RG, Benjamin DK, Gantz MG, et al. Empiric antifungal therapy and outcomes in extremely low birth weight infants with invasive candidiasis. *J Pediatr* 2012;161:264–269.e2.

73. Pizzo PA, Robichaud KJ, Gill FA, Witebsky FG. Empiric antibiotic and antifungal therapy for cancer patients with prolonged fever and granulocytopenia. *Am J Med* 1982;72:101–111.

74. Eppes SC, Troutman JL, Gutman LT. Outcome of treatment of candidemia in children whose central catheters were removed or retained. *Pediatr Infect Dis J* 1989;8:99–104.

75. Karlowicz MG, Rowen JL, Barnes-Eley ML, et al. The role of birth weight and gestational age in distinguishing extremely low birth weight infants at high risk of developing candidemia from infants at low risk: A multicenter study. *Pediatr Res* 2002;51:301A (abstract).

76. Rowen JL, Tate JM. Management of neonatal candidiasis. Neonatal candidiasis study group. *Pediatr Infect Dis J* 1998;17:1007–1011.

77. Baley JE, Meyers C, Kliegman RM, Jacobs MR, Blumer JL. Pharmacokinetics, outcome of treatment, and toxic effects of amphotericin B and 5-fluorocytosine in neonates. *J Pediatr* 1990;116:791–797.

78. Starke JR, Mason EO, Jr., Kramer WG, Kaplan SL. Pharmacokinetics of amphotericin B in infants and children. *J Infect Dis* 1987;155:766–774.

79. Juster-Reicher A, Flidel-Rimon O, Amitay M, Even-Tov S, Shinwell E, Leibovitz E. High-dose liposomal amphotericin B in the therapy of systemic candidiasis in neonates. *Eur J Clin Microbiol Infect Dis* 2003;22:603–607.

80. Baley JE, Kliegman RM, Fanaroff AA. Disseminated fungal infections in very-low-birth-weight infants: Therapeutic toxicity. *Pediatrics* 1984;73:153–157.

81. Le J, Adler-Shohet FC, Nguyen C, Lieberman JM. Nephrotoxicity associated with amphotericin B deoxycholate in neonates. *Pediatr Infect Dis J* 2009;28:1061–1063.

82. Minari A, Hachem R, Raad I. *Candida* lusitaniae: A cause of breakthrough fungemia in cancer patients. *Clinical Infectious Diseases: An Official Publication of the Infectious Diseases Society of America* 2001;32:186–190.

83. Driessen M, Ellis JB, Cooper PA, et al. Fluconazole vs. amphotericin B for the treatment of neonatal fungal septicemia: A prospective randomized trial. *Pediatr Infect Dis J* 1996;15:1107–1112.

84. Kotwani RN, Gokhale PC, Bodhe PV, Kirodian BG, Kshirsagar NA, Pandya SK. A comparative study of plasma concentrations of liposomal amphotericin B (L-AMP-LRC-1) in adults, children and neonates. *Int J Pharm* 2002;238:11–15.

85. Wurthwein G, Groll AH, Hempel G, Adler-Shohet FC, Lieberman JM, Walsh TJ. Population pharmacokinetics of amphotericin B lipid complex in neonates. *Antimicrob Agents Ch* 2005;49:5092–5098.

86. Linder N, Klinger G, Shalit I, et al. Treatment of candidaemia in premature infants: Comparison of three amphotericin B preparations. *J Antimicrob Chemother* 2003;52:663–667.

87. Scarcella A, Pasquariello MB, Giugliano B, Vendemmia M, de Lucia A. Liposomal amphotericin B treatment for neonatal fungal infections. *Pediatr Infect Dis J* 1998;17:146–148.

88. Lopez Sastre JB, Coto Cotallo GD, Fernandez Colomer B. Neonatal invasive candidiasis: A prospective multicenter study of 118 cases. *Am J Perinatol* 2003;20:153–163.

89. Bekersky I, Fielding RM, Dressler DE, Lee JW, Buell DN, Walsh TJ. Pharmacokinetics, excretion, and mass balance of liposomal amphotericin B (AmBisome) and amphotericin B deoxycholate in humans. *Antimicrob Agents Ch* 2002;46:828–833.

90. Jarlov JO, Born P, Bruun B. *Candida albicans* meningitis in a 27 weeks premature infant treated with liposomal amphotericin-B (AmBisome). *Scand J Infect Dis* 1995;27:419–420.

91. Rao HK, Myers GJ. *Candida* meningitis in the newborn. *South Med J* 1979;72:1468–1471.

92. Smego RA, Jr., Perfect JR, Durack DT. Combined therapy with amphotericin B and 5-fluorocytosine for *Candida* meningitis. *Rev Infect Dis* 1984;6:791–801.

93. Wade KC, Benjamin DK, Jr., Kaufman DA, et al. Fluconazole dosing for the prevention or treatment of invasive candidiasis in young infants. *Pediatr Infect Dis J* 2009;28:717–723.

94. Piper L, Smith PB, Hornik CP, et al. Fluconazole loading dose pharmacokinetics and safety in infants. *Pediatr Infect Dis J* 2011;30:375–378.

95. Wainer S, Cooper PA, Gouws H, Akierman A. Prospective study of fluconazole therapy in systemic neonatal fungal infection. *Pediatr Infect Dis J* 1997;16:763–767.

96. Huttova M, Hartmanova I, Kralinsky K, et al. *Candida* fungemia in neonates treated with fluconazole: Report of forty cases, including eight with meningitis. *Pediatr Infect Dis J* 1998;17:1012–1015.

97. Muller FM, Weig M, Peter J, Walsh TJ. Azole cross-resistance to ketoconazole, fluconazole, itraconazole and voriconazole in clinical *Candida albicans* isolates from HIV-infected children with oropharyngeal candidosis. *J Antimicrob Chemother* 2000;46:338–340.

98. Smith PB, Steinbach WJ, Cotten CM, et al. Caspofungin for the treatment of azole resistant candidemia in a premature infant. *J Perinatol* 2007;27:127–129.

99. Sabo JA, Abdel-Rahman SM. Voriconazole: A new triazole antifungal. *Ann Pharmacother* 2000;34:1032–1043.

100. Maples HD, Stowe CD, Saccente SL, Jacobs RF. Voriconazole serum concentrations in an infant treated for Trichosporon beigelii infection. *Pediatr Infect Dis J* 2003;22:1022–1024.

101. Doby EH, Benjamin DK, Jr., Blaschke AJ, et al. Therapeutic monitoring of voriconazole in children less than three years of age: A case report and summary of voriconazole concentrations for ten children. *Pediatr Infect Dis J* 2012;31:632–635.

102. Odio CM, Araya R, Pinto LE, et al. Caspofungin therapy of neonates with invasive candidiasis. *Pediatr Infect Dis J* 2004;23:1093–1097.

103. Natarajan G, Lulic-Botica M, Rongkavilit C, Pappas A, Bedard M. Experience with caspofungin in the treatment of persistent fungemia in neonates. *J Perinatol* 2005;25:770–777.

104. Mohamed WA, Ismail M. A randomized, double-blind, prospective study of caspofungin vs. amphotericin B for the treatment of invasive candidiasis in newborn infants. *J Trop Pediatr* 2012;58:25–30.

105. Saez-Llorens X, Macias M, Maiya P, et al. Pharmacokinetics and safety of caspofungin in neonates and infants less than 3 months of age. *Antimicrob Agents Ch* 2009;53:869–875.

106. Heresi GP, Gerstmann DR, Reed MD, et al. The pharmacokinetics and safety of micafungin, a novel echinocandin, in premature infants. *Pediatr Infect Dis J* 2006;25:1110–1115.

107. Benjamin DK, Jr., Smith PB, Arrieta A, et al. Safety and pharmacokinetics of repeat-dose micafungin in young infants. *Clin Pharmacol Ther* 2010;87:93–99.

108. Smith PB, Walsh TJ, Hope W, et al. Pharmacokinetics of an elevated dosage of micafungin in premature neonates. *Pediatr Infect Dis J* 2009;28:412–415.

109. Hope WW, Smith PB, Arrieta A, et al. Population pharmacokinetics of micafungin in neonates and young infants. *Antimicrob Agents Ch* 2010;54:2633–2637.

110. Manzoni P, Wu C, Tweddle L, Roilides E. Micafungin in premature and non-premature infants: A systematic review of 9 clinical trials. *Pediatr Infect Dis J* 2014;33:e291–e298.

111. Benjamin DK, Hope WW, Kaufman D, et al. Micafungin (MCA) versus Conventional Amphotericin B (CAB) in the Treatment of Invasive Candidiasis (IC) in infants. *Interscience Conference of Antimicrobial Agents and Chemotherapy* (ICAAC); 2015; San Diego, CA.

112. Cohen-Wolkowiez M, Benjamin DK, Jr., Piper L, et al. Safety and pharmacokinetics of multiple-dose anidulafungin in infants and neonates. *Clin Pharmacol Ther* 2011;89:702–707.

28

Newer antifungal agents in pediatrics

WILLIAM J. STEINBACH

INTRODUCTION

The antifungal landscape has been changing rapidly, with several newer agents approved and clinicians striving to determine the optimal niches for each agent in the overall therapeutic armamentarium. Unfortunately, studies with these antifungal agents in pediatric patients are slow and often clinical investigation stops after only initial pharmacokinetic exploration. Even the limited data we have on pediatric antifungals points to interesting differences between both adult and pediatric pharmacokinetics for the same agent, as well as differences among pediatric pharmacokinetics within the individual drug classes. For example, voriconazole displays non-linear pharmacokinetics in adult patients but linear pharmacokinetics in children, demanding higher doses in smaller patients and possibly explaining treatment failures due to under-dosing using the approved adult dosing regimen. Likewise, caspofungin requires higher doses in pediatric compared to adult patients, and dosing is best accomplished by using a body surface area regimen rather than a body weight scheme. Micafungin displays a clear trend towards lower plasma drug levels obtained in neonatal patients, emphasizing the importance of the neonatal period as a separate age group among pediatric patients.

These unique attributes to pediatric dosing underscore the necessity to more fully evaluate antifungals in children and not merely extrapolate data from adult studies to our smallest patients, as well as the overall difficulty for pediatricians managing sick children to effectively utilize antifungals. This chapter provides an overview of the current state of systemic antifungal therapy in pediatric patients, yet focuses exclusively on newer antifungal agents more recently approved and the available date in pediatric and neonatal patients.

TRIAZOLES

The triazole antifungals are heterocyclic synthetic compounds that inhibit the cytochrome P450 dependent 14 α-lanosterol demethylation, a vital step in fungal cell membrane ergosterol synthesis [1,2]. The drugs bind through a nitrogen group in their 5-membered azole ring to the heme group in the target protein and block demethylation of the C14 of lanosterol, leading to substitution of methylated sterols in the membrane and depletion of ergosterol. The result is an accumulation of precursors leading to abnormal fungal membrane permeability, membrane-bound enzyme activity, and coordination of chitin synthesis. The azoles are subdivided into imidazoles and triazoles on the basis of the number of nitrogens in the azole ring, with the structural differences resulting in different binding affinities of the azole pharmacophore for the cytochrome P450 (CYP) enzyme system. Triazoles can be subdivided into first (fluconazole and itraconazole) and second generation (voriconazole, posaconazole, and isavuconazole) agents. Three triazoles (itraconazole, voriconazole, posaconazole) need therapeutic drug monitoring with trough levels within the first 4–7 days (when patient is at pharmacokinetic steady-state); it is unclear at present if isavuconazole will require drug-level monitoring. It is less clear if therapeutic drug monitoring is required during primary azole prophylaxis, although low levels have been associated with a higher probability of breakthrough infection.

VORICONAZOLE

Pediatric pharmacokinetics

Voriconazole (VFend®; Pfizer Inc., New York, NY), a synthetic derivative of fluconazole, was the first available second generation triazole and was approved in 2002 by the US Food and Drug Administration (FDA). It has potent activity against a broad spectrum of clinically relevant fungal pathogens, including *Aspergillus, Candida, Cryptococcus,* and some less common molds [3] (Table 28.1).

Voriconazole is available in IV, oral tablet, and oral suspension formulations. In adults, its oral bioavailability is greater than 90%; however, its oral bioavailability is more modest in children, ranging from 44%–65% [4,5]. Pharmacokinetic modeling suggests that this difference can be accounted for by intestinal first pass metabolism occurring in children but not adults [6]. Voriconazole is extensively distributed to tissues, including the CNS, and has been used successfully to treat CNS fungal infections [7,8]. Voriconazole undergoes extensive hepatic metabolism by the cytochrome P450 system and dose adjustment is recommended in individuals with hepatic impairment. High inter-patient variability has been observed in voriconazole drug concentrations over a range of doses and coincides in part with genetic polymorphisms in the CYP enzymes [9].

As a result of genetic polymorphisms in the gene encoding Cyp2C19, some individuals are poor metabolizers, and some are extensive metabolizers [10]. About 5% of white people and 15%–20% of non-Indian Asians have a slow metabolizer phenotype.

In addition to genetic variation in voriconazole metabolism, there are important age-related differences with implications for pediatric dosing. In contrast to adults and older children, in whom voriconazole metabolism is nonlinear (resulting in marked increases in drug exposure related to relatively small changes in dose), young children have linear metabolism and therefore require much larger proportional doses to achieve adequate drug exposure.

An open, multi-center study investigated the safety, tolerability, and pharmacokinetics of intravenous voriconazole in immunocompromised pediatric patients [11]. This study included a single-dose-study of 11 patients ages 2–11 years (mean age 5.9 years) receiving 3 or 4 mg/kg of body weight and a multiple-dose-study of 24 patients ages 2–11 years (mean age 6.4 years) receiving a loading dose of 6 mg/kg twice daily (BID) on day 1, followed by 3 mg/kg BID on day 2 to day 4 and 4 mg/kg BID on day 4 to day 8. In contrast to the previously established nonlinear elimination of voriconazole in healthy adult volunteers [12] and adult patients [13], this study found linear pharmacokinetics of voriconazole in children over a dosage range of 3 and 4 mg/kg BID. Therefore, children require higher dosages of voriconazole than adults to achieve comparable serum levels and a maintenance dose of 4 mg/kg BID in children approximates only 3 mg/kg BID in adults [11]. Extrapolation of area under the curve (AUC) and maximum serum pharmacokinetic levels in children revealed an estimated 11 mg/kg/dose would be required to achieve adult values obtained with only 4 mg/kg/dose if linear pharmacokinetics were maintained throughout the full dosage interval (Table 28.2).

A subsequent pharmacokinetic study evaluated higher voriconazole doses and studied 9 patients in each of two

Table 28.1 Spectrum of activity of selected antifungal agents

Antifungal	Important clinical uses
Amphotericin B	*Blastomyces dermatitidis, Coccidioides immitis, Cryptococcus neoformans, Histoplasma capsulatum, Paracoccidioides brasiliensis, Sporotrix schenckii,* most *Candida* species, *Aspergillus,* Zygomycetes (NOT: *C. lusitaniae;* LESS EFFECTIVE: *Scedosporium, Fusarium, Trichosporon*)
Fluconazole	Most *Candida, C. neoformans, B. dermatitidis, H. capsulatum, C. immitis, P. brasiliensis* (NOT: *C. krusei, Aspergillus;* LESS EFFECTIVE: *C. glabrata,*)
Itraconazole	*Candida, Aspergillus, B. dermatitidis, H. capsulatum, C. immitis, P. brasiliensis*
Voriconazole	*Candida, Aspergillus, Fusarium, B. dermatitidis, H. capsulatum, C. immitis, Malassezia* species, *Scedosporium,* dematiaceous molds (NOT: Zygomycetes; LESS EFFECTIVE: *C. glabrata*)
Posaconazole	Same as voriconazole, except does have activity against Zygomycetes and *C. glabrata*
Isavuconazole	Same as posaconazolre
Caspofungin Micafungin Anidulafungin	*Candida, Aspergillus* (NOT: *C. neoformans, Fusarium,* Zygomycetes)

Table 28.2 Preferred pediatric dosing of approved systemic antifungal agents

Drug class	Antifungal drug	Preferred adult dosing	Preferred pediatric dosing
Polyene	Amphotericin B deoxycholate	1–1.5 mg/kg/day	1–1.5 mg/kg/day
	Amphotericin B Lipid Complex	5 mg/kg/day	5 mg/kg/day
	Amphotericin B Colloidal Dispersion	5 mg/kg/day	5 mg/kg/day
	Liposomal Amphotericin B	5 mg/kg/day	5 mg/kg/day
Triazole	Fluconazole	100–800 mg/day; 3–6 mg/kg/day	6–12 mg/kg/day
	Voriconazole	Load: 6 mg/kg/dose BID x 1 day Maintenance: 4 mg/kg/dose BID	Load: 9 mg/kg/dose BID x 1 day Maintenance: 8 mg/kg/dose IV BID
	Posaconazole	400 mg BID	Unknown
Echinocandin	Isavuconazole	Load:	Unknown
	Caspofungin	200 mg TID x 2 days Maintenance: 200 mg QD Load: 70 mg QD x 1 day Maintenance: 50 mg QD	Load: 70 mg/m^2 QD x 1 day Maintenance: 50 mg/m^2 QD
	Micafungin	50–100 mg QD	2–10 mg/kg QD
	Anidulafungin	50–100 mg QD	0.75–1.5 mg/kg QD

Abbreviations: QD = once daily; BID = twice daily

age groups (2–6 years, 6–12 years) [14]. Each child received either 4 mg/kg/dose followed by 6 mg/kg/dose or 6 mg/kg/dose followed by 8 mg/kg/dose. Each child also received at least two different doses in escalating order and then was switched to oral voriconazole. The intravenous doses had similar pharmacokinetic parameters within each age cohort, except a greater AUC level in the 8 mg/kg/dose range in the older age cohort. After oral dosing, the older age group had higher AUC and maximum serum levels compared to the younger children. However, even at the 8 mg/kg/dose, the AUC (34,681 ng × h/mL) in children was still less than that seen with adult patients (42,000 ng × h/mL) at the 4 mg/kg/dose level. Interestingly, the bioavailability of oral voriconazole was lower (65%) than seen in adult patients (96%) [14]. This study also demonstrated a high interpatient pharmacokinetic variability, as has been reported for studies concerning voriconazole drug level monitoring, but no significant differences were seen in the 2–6 year vs. 6–12 year age groups except at the 8 mg/kg/dose.

A subsequent population pharmacokinetic study predicted that an IV dose of 7 mg/kg twice daily for children less than 12 years of age provided exposure similar to that of adults [4] The European Medicines Agency (EMEA) approved dosing for voriconazole in children was then to load with 7 mg/kg/dose for 1 day and then continue with the same 7 mg/kg/dose as a maintenance dose. However, this pharmacokinetic study raised several important points that remain inconclusively investigated. The higher dose of 8 mg/kg/dose still yielded an AUC level lower than in adult patients received a standard dosing, suggesting that the optimal voriconazole dose in children is likely even higher.

Studies using therapeutic drug monitoring to guide voriconazole dosing have shown that even higher doses are required in many cases to achieve goal trough concentrations above 1 μ/L, with a median dose of 16mg/kg/day required in children age 2–12 years [5,9] Current recommendations for voriconazole in children are for an IV loading dose of 9 mg/kg/dose BID for 1 day, followed by a maintenance IV dose of 8 mg/kg/dose BID. Transition to oral dosing should increase to 9 mg/kg/dose BID [15] (Table 28.3).

Given the substantial inter-individual variability in voriconazole pharmacokinetics, therapeutic drug monitoring of voriconazole levels is recommended to gauge adequacy of treatment and to avoid potential toxicities; target trough concentrations between 1 and 5 μg/L are recommended [16]. With linear pharmacokinetics in children, clinicians have a wider therapeutic window with which to safely increase the voriconazole dose. These dosing concerns are especially problematic with the known differences in metabolism across patient subpopulations and the concerns of a lack of standard effective voriconazole level goals.

For children, voriconazole is available as an orange-flavored suspension (40 mg/mL). A common practice in pediatrics is to crush tablets and administer them to pediatric patients through a gastric or duodenal tube. A study examined the bioavailability of crushed or whole voriconazole tablets in an open-label, randomized, two-way crossover study in 20 health volunteers [17]. While there was a slightly faster time to maximum serum concentration with the crushed tablets (0.5 hours vs. 1.5 hours), the bioavailability was equivalent in crushed and whole tablets.

Table 28.3 Pharmacokinetic differences in pediatric antifungal dosing

Antifungal drug	Unique pediatric trait
Amphotericin B products	No known dosing differences, but children can generally tolerate higher doses than adults
Fluconazole	Dose higher in children due to shorter half-life
Voriconazole	*Linear* pharmacokinetics in children as compared to non-linear pharmacokinetics in adults
	Optimal pediatric dose still not yet determined, and it is possible to increase dose further if needed
Posaconazole	Pharmacokinetic studies are ongoing
Isavuconazole	Pharmacokinetic studies are ongoing
Caspofungin	Need to use body-surface area dosing scheme and not weigh-based dosing in children due to rapid clearance
Micafungin	Dosing depends on age, with smaller children requiring high doses and neonates requiring even higher doses
Anidulafungin	Appears to be no difference in dosing between children and adults

Voriconazole's main side effects include reversible dose-dependent visual disturbances (increased brightness, blurred vision) [18] in as many as one-third of treated patients; elevated serum hepatic transaminases with higher doses; [19] and occasional skin reactions, likely due to photosensitization [20]. Less common but serious toxicities include neurotoxicity with prominent visual hallucinations [21], which is associated with serum trough levels above 5.5 μg/L and must be distinguished from the more common visual disturbances, and prolongation of the QT interval with associated cardiac arrhythmias. Voriconazole produces some unique transient visual field abnormalities in about 10% of adults and children. There are an increasing number of reports, seen in as high as 20% of patients, of a photosensitive sunburn-like erythema that is not aided by sunscreen (only sun avoidance). In some rare long-term (mean of 3 years of therapy) cases, this voriconazole phototoxicity has developed into cutaneous squamous cell carcinoma [22]. Similar to the other triazoles, drug interactions can be problematic due to inhibition of the CYP enzyme system. Intravenous voriconazole is solubilized in sulfobutyl ether β-cyclodextrin (SBECD) and because elimination of cyclodextrin is dependent on glomerular filtration, the vehicle can accumulate in patients with severely impaired renal function, but the clinical significance of this accumulation has yet to be determined fully.

Clinical experience and pediatric data

A multi-center, randomized, open trial compared the outcome of patients receiving either intravenous voriconazole or amphotericin B deoxycholate for primary therapy of invasive aspergillosis [23]. In the voriconazole arm a total of 144 patients (13–79 years, mean 48.5 years) received a loading dose of 6 mg/kg IV BID on day 1, followed by 4 mg/kg IV BID for at least 7 days and 200 mg BID orally for a total of 12 weeks. In the amphotericin B treatment group, 133 patients (12–75 years, mean 50.5 years) were administered 1.0–1.5 mg/kg IV once daily. The overall response rate at 12 weeks showed statistically significantly more complete and partial responses in patients treated with voriconazole (52.8%) compared to patients treated with amphotericin B (31.6%). Voriconazole-treated patients also had a higher survival rate than Amphotericin B–treated patients (70.8% vs. 57.9%; p = 0.02) and showed significantly fewer drug-related severe adverse side effects. While this study revolutionized the landscape of invasive aspergillosis treatment, the study did not include children younger than 12 years and enrolled very few under 18 years of age. Therefore, no firm conclusions can be made on the superiority of voriconazole over amphotericin B in this age group.

A minority of 52/144 (36%) patients in the voriconazole group and a majority of 107/133 (80%) patients in the amphotericin B group received another licensed antifungal therapy besides their primary study drug, resulting in a smaller final group of patients receiving only voriconazole or only amphotericin B. Patients receiving voriconazole as initial therapy and then switching to another antifungal drug still had a higher rate of complete and partial responses than patients who obtained amphotericin B as initial drug followed by another antifungal agent (48% vs. 38%) [24], suggesting that the initial therapy with the triazole was more effective.

An additional open study confirmed these promising data by administering voriconazole as primary (52%) or salvage therapy (48%) to 116 patients with invasive aspergillosis [25]. Up to 48% of the patients demonstrated a complete or partial response, whereas in 21% the disease was stable and in 31% failed. The results of these clinical studies have led experts to recommend voriconazole as the preferred antifungal against invasive aspergillosis [26].

Voriconazole is also effective in the treatment of *Candida* infections. In a randomized, double-blind multicenter trial including 391 immunocompromised patients with esophageal candidiasis, oral voriconazole (200 mg BID) showed a primary success rate of 98.3% compared to 95.1% in patients treated with oral fluconazole (200 mg once daily) [27]. In another multicenter study of 422 patients with candidemia, voriconazole was as efficacious as amphotericin B followed by fluconazole [28]. Moreover, voriconazole also demonstrates similar success rates and less breakthrough fungal infections compared to liposomal Amphotericin B in patients with neutropenia and persistent fever [29].

The largest pediatric study reported on 58 children (ages 9 months-15 years, mean 8.2 years) with invasive fungal infections refractory to or intolerant of conventional antifungal therapy [30]. Voriconazole was administered as a loading dose of 6 mg/kg IV BID on the first day of therapy, followed by 4 mg/kg IV BID. If feasible, the IV dose was then later switched to an oral dose of 100 or 200 mg BID for children weighing <40 kg or ≥40 kg, respectively. Responses to the therapy with voriconazole were complete or partial in 26 (45%), stable in 4 (7%) and failed in 25 (43%) patients. *Aspergillus* spp. was the most common infecting organism (72%) and 43% of those patients responded to the therapy. In a subsequent case series, voriconazole was utilized as salvage therapy in 7 children (age range 2–13 years, median 5 years) with invasive aspergillosis [31]. Complete and partial response was observed in each of 2 patients, stable response in 1 patient and failure of the voriconazole treatment in 2 patients. These are the largest published reports of voriconazole use in children, and while they demonstrated that voriconazole is generally as effective in children as adults, the incorrect dosages utilized don't answer the fundamental question of true efficacy in children.

At present, there are no studies available in neonates. There are ongoing concerns about the effect of voriconazole on the developing retina in neonates due to the well-documented visual disturbances in pediatric and adult patients.

POSACONAZOLE

Pharmacokinetics

Posaconazole (Noxafil®, Schering-Plough Research Institute, Kenilworth, NJ) is a second-generation extended-spectrum triazole and derivative of itraconazole that was approved by the FDA in 2006. Posaconazole has excellent activity against both yeast and mold infections, specifically including activity against zygomycosis where voriconazole has no antifungal efficacy [32].

Posaconazole was initially available only as an oral suspension, but delayed-release tablets and an IV formulation are now available. Both oral formulations are FDA approved for use in children age 13 and older; the IV formulation is approved for individuals 18 and older. The pharmacokinetics and appropriate dosing differ for each formulation. Absorption of the oral suspension is variable and is greatly

improved when it is given with a high-fat meal or in multiple divided doses [33]. The bioavailability of posaconazole increases significantly when administered in divided doses. One study showed the highest bioavailability of posaconazole in fasting healthy volunteers receiving 800 mg/day divided in 4 doses compared to 800 mg/day divided in either 1 or 2 doses [34]. When administered in the fed state, 800 mg/day divided in two doses gave similar serum levels to dosing four times daily and is more practical for compliance. Another study reported on posaconazole in 98 adult patients with febrile neutropenia or refractory fungal infections [35]. Posaconazole was administered in 3 different regimes: 400 mg BID, 600 mg BID or 800 mg once daily. A daily dose of 800 mg/day given as 400 mg BID provided the greatest posaconazole exposure.

Absorption of the tablet formulation is less variable and is not dependent on food intake; it can also be given once daily with the 300 mg daily adult dose achieving similar drug exposure to the 200 mg oral suspension dose given three times daily [36]. Posaconazole has dose-proportional pharmacokinetics up to 800 mg/day, and has a large apparent volume of distribution with slow elimination, suggesting an extensive distribution into tissues. Posaconazole has lower central nervous system penetration than voriconazole; however, there are well-documented cases of clinical success for treatment of CNS fungal infection. Posaconazole is metabolized by glucuronidation and primarily eliminated via the fecal route. Mild or moderate chronic renal impairment has no appreciable effect on the pharmacokinetics of oral posaconazole, but avoidance of the IV formulation is recommended in the setting of moderate or severe renal impairment due to potential accumulation of the vehicle, SBECD.

Posaconazole is an inhibitor of *Cyp*3A4 metabolism and P-glycoprotein transport and is subject to drug interactions with substrates for these pathways, such as calcineurin inhibitors or benzodiazepines. Posaconazole is overall well tolerated. The most common drug-related adverse events are gastrointestinal (nausea, vomiting, abdominal pain) and hepatic (elevated hepatic enzymes and alanine aminotransferase) [37,38]. Rare, but serious adverse events include hepatotoxicity and QT interval prolongation with associated cardiac arrhythmias. Administration of the IV formulation as a slow infusion via central venous catheter is recommended due to infusion site reactions noted with repeated administration.

There are currently very limited pediatric pharmacokinetic data for posaconazole. Serum samples obtained on 12 pediatric (ages 8–17 years) and 194 adult (ages 18–64 years) patients from a multicenter, phase 3, open-label study of patients with invasive fungal infections refractory to standard antifungal therapies were analyzed as preliminary comparisons of adult versus child pharmacokinetics [39]. All patients received a maintenance dose of 800 mg/day in divided doses except 1 pediatric patient who obtained 400 mg/day as a divided dose on the day of sample collection. The mean plasma concentrations of posaconazole in children and adults were 776 ng/mL (median 579 ng/mL; range 85.3–2,891 ng/mL) and 817 ng/mL (median 626 ng/mL; range 0–3,710 ng/mL), respectively, suggesting similar plasma concentrations in pediatric and adult patients. One limitation with this study is that while the age range of the 12 pediatric patients was 8–17 years, it consisted of a single 8 year-old patient, a single 10-year old patient, and all other patients were ≥12 years old. This skew toward teenagers could explain the results similar to adult dosage findings. Pediatric experience with posaconazole therapy is very limited in general.

Clinical experience and pediatric data

In adult patients with severe graft-versus-host disease posaconazole was as effective as fluconazole as antifungal prophylaxis, but more effectively prevented invasive aspergillosis as well as breakthrough invasive fungal infections and reduced deaths due to invasive fungal infections [40]. Moreover, in adult patients with neutropenia posaconazole was superior to either fluconazole or itraconazole in preventing invasive fungal infections (2% vs. 8%) [41].

Posaconazole has also been evaluated for treatment of oropharyngeal and esophageal candidiasis in HIV-positive patients. It demonstrated comparable efficacy to fluconazole in the treatment of oropharyngeal candidiasis, with significantly lower rates of relapse [42].

Although its current FDA-approved indications are limited to antifungal prophylaxis and oropharyngeal candidiasis, promising data have emerged for posaconazole in treatment of other invasive fungal infections. Posaconazole showed a survival benefit over historic controls in treating invasive aspergillosis as salvage antifungal therapy [43], and demonstrated a success rate of 72% in treating invasive aspergillosis that was refractory to voriconazole [44], but has not been examined as primary therapy. Due to voriconazole's lack of activity against the Mucorales group, there is excitement due to posaconazole's *in vitro* activity as well as clinical efficacy as a salvage therapy against these emerging infections. A review of 96 case reports describing posaconazole as a combination or second-line therapy for mucormycosis found an approximately 70% rate of complete or partial response, but the true success rate is likely lower due to publication bias [45].

Experience with posaconazole in children is limited. A retrospective cohort study of 60 children less than 12 years of age who received posaconazole prophylaxis after allogeneic HSCT demonstrated no breakthrough invasive fungal infections occurring during the prophylaxis period (up to 200 days post-transplantation), and no severe adverse events [46] The oral suspension was given at doses of either 5 mg/kg/dose twice daily or 4mg/kg/dose three times daily, with higher trough levels noted on the three times daily regimen.

Segal and colleagues reported on 7 pediatric (ages 9–18 years) and 1 adult patient (age 36 years) with chronic granulomatous disease and invasive filamentous fungal infections who received posaconazole as salvage therapy [37]. Except

one patient who received posaconazole as a dosage of 200 mg three times daily, the remaining 7 patients received 400 mg BID. Treatment with posaconazole led to a complete response in 7/8 adult including 6/7 pediatric patients. Importantly, in that study, the prior antifungal drug was voriconazole in 7/8 patients and was discontinued due to failure ($n = 6$) or intolerance ($n = 1$). Two open-label, multicenter, compassionate trials investigated the outcome of 24 patients including 3 pediatric patients (ages 7, 17, and 18 years) with active zygomycosis treated with posaconazole oral suspension (200 mg four times daily or 400 mg BID [47]. Overall, 79% of patients had a complete or partial response while all 3 pediatric patients were treated successfully (1 complete response and 2 partial responses).

A subsequent multicenter retrospective survey of 15 children age 3–17 years with invasive fungal infections refractory to first-line therapy demonstrated complete or partial response to therapy in 9 patients and no severe adverse events, though mild adverse events were reported in 11 patients [48]. Posaconazole will have an important role in antifungal management in the future, but devoted pediatric clinical studies, both to define the optimal dosing in children and for comparative efficacy, have yet to be performed.

The pediatric oral suspension dose recommended by some experts for treating invasive disease is 18 mg/kg/day divided 3 times daily, but the true answer is likely higher and serum trough level monitoring is recommended. A study with a new pediatric formulation for suspension, essentially the tablet form that is able to be suspended, is underway. Importantly, the current tablet cannot be broken for use due to its chemical coating. Pediatric dosing with the current IV or extended-release tablet dosing is completely unknown, but adolescents can likely follow the adult dosing schemes. In adult patients, IV posaconazole is loaded at 300 mg twice daily on the first day, and then 300 mg once daily starting on the second day. Similarly, in adult patients, the extended-release tablet is dosed as 300 mg twice daily on the first day, and then 300 mg once daily starting on the second day. In adult patients, the maximum amount of posaconazole oral suspension given is 800 mg per day due to its excretion, and that has been given as 400 mg twice daily or 200 mg 4 times a day in severely ill patients due to findings of a marginal increase in exposure with more frequent dosing. Greater than 800 mg per day is not indicated in any patient. Like voriconazole and itraconazole, trough levels should be monitored, and most experts feel that posaconazole levels for treatment should be at least greater than 700 ng/mL (0.7 µg/mL).

ISAVUCONAZOLE

Pharmacology and toxicities

Isavuconazole, formulated in IV and oral capsule preparations as a prodrug, isavuconazonium sulfate, was approved by the FDA in 2015 for treatment of invasive aspergillosis and mucormycosis in adults. It has a broad spectrum of activity including *Candida, Cryptococcus, Aspergillus,* and the Mucorales. The prodrug, isavuconazonium, is rapidly cleaved by plamsa esterases to isavuconazole. Oral bioavailability is 98% with low intersubject variability and no clinically significant food effect. It is water soluble with high protein binding, a large volume of distribution indicating likely high tissue penetration. It exhibits dose-proportional pharmacokinetics with moderate deviation from linearity. Elimination is primarily though hepatic metabolism; its prolonged half-life allows once daily dosing following initial loading doses [49,50]. Because it is highly water soluble, the IV formulation of isavuconazole does not require the SBECD carrier that is needed for voriconazole and posaconazole IV formulations; thus it can be used in the setting of significant renal impairment without risk of accumulation.

Isavuconazole is both a substrate and an inhibitor of *Cyp*3A4 and is therefore subject to clinically significant drug-drug interactions with *Cyp*3A4 substrates, inhibitors or inducers. The most frequently reported adverse events in clinical trials have been gastrointestinal symptoms, headache, elevated hepatic enzymes, hypokalemia, dyspnea, cough, peripheral edema, and back pain. The overall occurrence rates of adverse events were similar between isavuconazole and voriconazole, but drug-related adverse events were less frequent with isavuconazole, and the frequency of dermatologic and visual adverse events was lower with isavuconazole [51].

Clinical experience and pediatric data

In a phase 2 randomized controlled trial comparing three isavuconazole oral dosing regimens (including a once weekly regimen) to oral fluconazole for treatment of esophageal candidiasis in immunocompromised patients, all three regimens were non-inferior to fluconazole [52]. Rates of endoscopically confirmed cure were 95%–98% for the isavuconazole regimens and 95% for fluconazole. A phase 3 randomized controlled trial compared isavuconazole to voriconazole for treatment of invasive aspergillosis and other invasive mold infections in 516 immunocompromised adults [51]. On the primary endpoint of all-cause mortality at 6 weeks, isavuconazole was non-inferior to voriconazole, with 18.6% mortality vs. 20% mortality for voriconazole. Overall treatment success at the end of treatment was also comparable between groups. An open-label non-comparative trial evaluated isavuconazole for treatment of 37 patients with proven or probable invasive mucormycosis, either as primary or salvage therapy [53]. All-cause mortality at 6 weeks was 38% and overall response at end of therapy was 31%; in light of the severe natural history of invasive mucormycosis, this trial supports clinical efficacy of isavuconazole in treatment of mucormycosis. An additional clinical trial is underway evaluating isavuconazole for treatment of invasive candidiasis. There are currently no reported pediatric clinical studies of isavuconazole.

ECHINOCANDINS

The echinocandins are a class of antifungal agents that noncompetitively inhibit the synthesis of β-(1,3)-D-glucan, which is an essential component of the fungal cell wall that provides structural integrity and is essential for fungal cell growth and division [1,54]. As β-(1,3)-D-glucan is not shared by mammalian cells, these are highly selective for fungi [55]. Of significance, the cell wall of *Cryptococcus neoformans* and *Zygomycetes* lack this glucan or significant amounts of it and therefore the echinocandins are not affective against these fungal pathogens [56]. Because of their large molecular weight, echinocandins are not well absorbed orally and must be administered intravenously [1].

The echinocandins are not metabolized through the CYP system, so fewer drug interactions are problematic, compared with the azoles. There is no need to dose-adjust in renal failure, but one needs a lower dosage in the setting of very severe hepatic dysfunction. As a class, these antifungals generally have poor CSF penetration, although animal studies have shown adequate brain parenchyma levels, and do not penetrate the urine well. While the 3 clinically available echinocandins, each individually have some unique and important dosing and pharmacokinetic parameters, especially in children, efficacy is generally equivalent. Opposite the azole class, the echinocandins are fungicidal against yeasts but fungistatic against molds. The fungicidal activity against yeasts has elevated the echinocandins to the preferred therapy against invasive candidiasis. Echinocandins are thought to be best utilized against invasive aspergillosis only as salvage therapy if a triazole fails or in a patient with suspected triazole resistance, but not as primary monotherapy against invasive aspergillosis or any other mold infection. Improved efficacy with combination therapy with the echinocandins and triazoles against *Aspergillus* infections is unclear, with disparate results in multiple smaller studies and a definitive clinical trial demonstrating minimal benefit over voriconazole monotherapy in only certain patient populations. Some experts have used combination therapy in invasive aspergillosis with a triazole plus echinocandin only during the initial phase of waiting for triazole drug levels to be appropriately high. There are reports of echinocandin resistance in *Candida* spp, as high as 12% in *C. glabrata* in some studies, and the echinocandins as a class are often somewhat less active against *Candida parapsilosis* isolates (approximately 10%–15% respond poorly, but most are still susceptible).

CASPOFUNGIN

Pharmacokinetics

Caspofungin (Cancidas®; Merck Co., Whitehouse, NJ) was the first echinocandin to receive approval from the FDA in 2001 and is a semisynthetic derivate of the natural product pneumocandin B_0 [1,57]. Caspofungin is primarily excreted by the liver and not metabolized by the cytochrome

P450 enzymes [58,59]. Tissue distribution accounts for an initial rapid decline in plasma levels, and subsequently the drug undergoes slow hepatic metabolism via hydrolysis and N-acetylation. The drug also undergoes spontaneous degradation; these processes together account for a terminal half-life of 27 to 50 hours.

Caspofungin shows linear pharmacokinetics after single dosing but modest nonlinearity after multiple dosing [59]. In adults, a loading dose of 70 mg on the first day, followed by a maintenance dose of 50 mg daily is recommended [59]. Dose reduction is not necessary in patients with renal impairment or mild hepatic insufficiency [60,61]. However, in patients with moderate hepatic insufficiency, reduction of the maintenance dose to 35 mg/day after the initial 70 mg loading dose is recommended [61]. A slight reduction of tacrolimus exposure by approximately 20% was seen with coadministration of caspofungin, and therefore close monitoring of tacrolimus concentrations is recommended [62]. Moreover, caspofungin interacts with cyclosporine A resulting in an increased plasma concentration of caspofungin by about 35% without an alteration of the cyclosporine A plasma levels [60].

Walsh and colleagues reported on 39 children (2–11 years) and adolescents (12–17 years) (mean 7.7 years) with a new onset of fever and neutropenia in whom caspofungin was administered either on a basis of weight (1 mg/kg/day) or body surface area (BSA) (50 or 70 mg/m²/day) [63]. Pediatric pharmacokinetic data were compared to those in adult patients receiving caspofungin 50 or 70 mg/day for mucosal candidiasis. The weight-based regimen in 7 children (1 mg/kg/day) yielded a significantly smaller area under the concentration-time curve over 24 hours (AUC_{0-24}) compared to adults (50 mg/day) and was therefore discontinued. However, in children ($n = 10$) and adolescents ($n = 8$) receiving 50 mg/m²/day using the BSA regimen the AUC_{0-24} following multiple doses was similar to that of adult patients receiving the FDA-approved 50-mg daily regimen. Moreover, children ($n = 12$) taking 70 mg/m²/day showed comparable AUC_{0-24} values after multiple doses to adult patients (70 mg/day). The β-phase half-life of caspofungin was approximately one third (37%; p = 0.001) less in children than in adults. Even BSA dosing revealed that adolescent and pediatric concentrations descend more rapidly than in adult patients, with statistically significant decreases in end-of-infusion concentrations of caspofungin with increasing age. Therefore, a BSA dosing regimen is now recommended for caspofungin therapy in pediatric patients. Only 5 patients (12.8%) experienced drug-related clinical adverse events (fever, diarrhea, phlebitis, proteinuria, and skin rash) and 2 patients (5.1%) laboratory adverse events (hypokalemia and increased serum aspartate transaminase).

To investigate efficacy and safety of caspofungin at 50 mg/m²/day also in a younger age group a pharmacokinetic study was conducted in 8 immunosuppressed children ages 3–24 months with fever and neutropenia [64]. In young children clearance ($t_{1/2}$ = 8.04 hours) was reduced ~38%

relative to adults at 50 mg/day ($t_{1/2}$ = 13.0 hours) and no confirmed invasive fungal infection during study course was observed. The authors concluded that caspofungin administered at 50 mg/m²/day in young children 3 to 24 months of age reaches comparable plasma exposure to that of adults receiving 50 mg/day.

Another study investigated retrospectively the safety of caspofungin in 25 pediatric immunocompromised patients (ages 0.3–26.2 years, median 9.8 years) who obtained caspofungin for documented ($n = 13$) or suspected ($n = 8$) fungal infections or for prophylaxis ($n = 4$) [65]. Caspofungin doses ranged from 0.8 to 1.6 mg/kg/day for patients weighing <50 kg and from 50 to 75 mg/day for patients weighing ≥50 kg. Caspofungin was generally well tolerated with side effects occurring only in 3/25 (12%) patients (hypokalemia and elevated total serum bilirubin).

Clinical experience and pediatric data

A multicenter, retrospective, non-comparative survey in Germany reported on 64 immunocompromised pediatric patients ages 0.4–17.9 years (median 11.5 years) who received caspofungin for proven (26.6%), probable (21.8%) and possible (26.6%) invasive fungal infections or empirical treatment (25%) [66]. The mean daily maintenance dose was 1.07 mg/kg (0.40–2.92 mg/kg) or 34.3 mg/m² (16–57 mg/m²) for a median treatment duration of 37.0 days (3–218 days). An overall successful outcome was achieved in 67.7% of patients and the overall survival rate was 75% at the end of treatment. However, the majority of patients (68.7%) received caspofungin in combination with another antifungal treatment regimen, resulting in only one-third of patients receiving caspofungin as monotherapy. Moreover, the BSA regimen (50 mg/m²), which has been shown to result in a more optimal caspofungin exposure to pediatric patients compared to the weight-based regimen, was utilized in only 5/64 patients [63].

Two smaller studies investigated the efficacy of caspofungin in children with invasive fungal infections. One preliminary report from an ongoing prospective, multicenter trial study showed good overall response to caspofungin in 28 children with documented fungal infections (loading dose 70 mg/m² on day one, followed by a maintenance dose of 50 mg/m²) [67]. Success rates were 88% and 50% in patients with invasive candidiasis and invasive aspergillosis, respectively. Another study reported on an overall 50% survival rate and 65% of response rate in 20 pediatric patients with invasive fungal infections who received caspofungin for salvage or first-line therapy [68]. Caspofungin is also effective in the treatment of children with febrile neutropenia. Khayat and colleagues showed in 26 pediatric patients that caspofungin is as least as effective as liposomal amphotericin B and demonstrates better tolerability [69].

A retrospective analysis of compassionate-use caspofungin in 25 immunocompromised children, most of whom also received other antifungal agents, noted that only 3 (12%) had a possible drug-related adverse event, which included hypokalemia and elevated serum bilirubin or hepatic transaminases [70]. Another study of 64 immunocompromised children revealed that caspofungin was not discontinued in any patients due to adverse events, and clinical adverse events were mild to moderate and observed in 34 patients (53%) [66] Mean aspartate aminotransferase and alanine aminotransferase values were slightly higher at end of therapy, but creatinine, bilirubin, and alkaline phosphatase levels were not different from baseline.

To date the use of caspofungin in neonates with invasive candidiasis has been limited. Odio and colleagues reported on the use of caspofungin for salvage therapy in 10 neonates (9 premature and 1 term) with invasive candidiasis refractory to the treatment with amphothericin B deoxycholate [71]. In this patient population, invasive candidiasis was caused by *Candida albicans* ($n = 4$), *Candida parapsilosis* ($n = 3$), *Candida tropicalis* ($n = 2$), and *Candida glabrata* ($n = 1$). Despite initial therapy with amphothericin B deoxycholate, blood cultures remained positive in all patients for 13–49 days. Caspofungin was initiated with a dose of 1 mg/kg/day for 2 days followed by 2 mg/kg/day for 15–21 days in 9 patients or with a dose of 0.5 mg/kg/day for 3 days followed by 1 mg/kg/day for 28 days in 1 patient. Between 3 and 7 days all positive blood cultures cleared. A total of 8/10 neonates resolved on caspofungin therapy, one patient responded after relapsing and a second administration of caspofungin was needed, and one patient died of an overwhelming bacterial septicemia. There were no clinical or laboratory adverse events attributable to caspofungin administration.

In a subsequent study, 6 premature neonates with invasive candidiasis refractory to amphothericin B deoxycholate received caspofungin as monotherapy at an initial dose of 0.5–1 mg/kg/day (days 1–3) and a maintenance dose of 1–3 mg/kg/day [72]. All 6 neonates were successfully treated (complete response) and tolerated caspofungin therapy very well. A linear scaling of the observed pharmacokinetic data was performed and compared to historical pharmacokinetic data in pediatric patients (either children 2–11 years or adolescents 12–17 years) receiving 50 mg/m²/day and adults receiving the standard dose of 50 mg/day. Caspofungin plasma concentrations at doses of 2 mg/kg/day or 25 mg/m²/day in premature neonates corresponded to 50 mg/day given in adults and are therefore this dose has been recommended for further evaluation in neonates.

The largest retrospective neonatal report showed that caspofungin (1 mg/kg IV once daily) added to amphothericin B, fluconazole or flucytosine treatment in 13 neonates (12 premature and 1 term) with persistent candidemia sterilized blood cultures in 11/13 patients within 3 days (range 1–21 days) [73]. Adverse events included elevation of liver enzymes ($n = 4$), hypokalemia ($n = 2$) and severe thrombophlebitis ($n = 1$).

MICAFUNGIN

Pharmacokinetics

Micafungin (Mycamine®, Astellas PharmaUS, Inc., Deerfield, IL) is the second available echinocandin and was approved by the FDA in 2005 for esophageal candidiasis and for prophylaxis in patients undergoing hematopoietic stem cell transplantation [74]. It is a water-soluble lipopeptide synthesized after cleavage of the hexapeptide FR901370, a natural product of the fungus *Coleoptioma empedri* [74]. Micafungin is metabolized in the liver and excreted into bile and urine and there is no metabolism by the cytochrome P450 enzymes. It exhibits a linear dose-dependent relationship in both adult and pediatric patients [75,76] as well as premature infants [77]. In contrast to caspofungin, it has simple linear elimination kinetics. It undergoes limited hepatic metabolism by arylsulfatase, catechol O-methyltransferase, and hydroxylation, with predominantly biliary excretion. Dose reduction is not necessary in patients with moderate hepatic or renal dysfunction [78]. There does not appear to be a drug interaction with micafungin and tacrolimus [79] but a mild inhibition of cyclosporin A metabolism by micafungin [80].

A multicenter, phase I, open-label dose escalation study assessed the pharmacokinetics and safety of micafungin in neutropenic pediatric patients and included 77 children stratified by age (2–12 and 13–17 years) [75]. They received an initial micafungin dose of 0.5 mg/kg/day, which was then escalated to higher dose levels of 1.0, 1.5, 2.0, 3.0 and 4.0 mg/kg/day. Plasma half-life, clearance and volume of distribution did not differ over time or across dosage cohorts and were similar to adult pharmacokinetics as also reported by Townsend et al. [81]. Interestingly, there was an inverse relation between increased clearance and decreased age, suggesting higher doses of micafungin might be needed in younger age groups.

Arrieta and colleagues performed a meta-analysis of the use and safety of micafungin in 244 pediatric patients (<16 years of age) from 5 clinical trials [82]. Pediatric patients were treated with up to 8.6 mg/kg/day for up to 681 days. The safety profile was similar to that of adults and in only 25% of patients ≥1 adverse event possibly related to micafungin occurred. In a subpopulation of 77 neutropenic febrile pediatric patients who received micafungin for prophylaxis at doses between 0.5 to 4 mg/kg/day, there was an inverse relation for age and clearance again noted as described earlier [75,82]. The average clearance in this patient subpopulation was found to be 1.5 to 2 times greater in patients 8 years and younger compared to patients older than 8 years [82]. Another study in Japan involving 19 pediatric patients with deep fungal infections caused by either *Aspergillus* or *Candida* species reported linear pharmacokinetics for micafungin (1 to 6 mg/kg/day) as well as similar dose-proportionality when compared with adult data [76]. In contrast to the two previous studies, no age dependent pharmacokinetic profile was noticed among the 3 different age groups (<2 years, 2 to 5 years and 6 to 15 years) regarding plasma half-life [76]. Furthermore, Hope and colleagues reported a linear relationship of clearance and weight in 72 children [83]. In pediatric patients. drug related adverse events occurred in approximately 12% of patients and included diarrhea, vomiting, and headache [75]. No attributable nephrotoxicity and infusion-related toxicity was noted, but minimal hepatotoxicity was observed.

In addition to the pediatric data there are two pharmacokinetic studies in neonates available. Heresi and colleagues evaluated micafungin in 18 premature infants weighing >1000 g using three dosages (0.75, 1.5, and 3.0 mg/kg/day) and in 5 premature infants weighing 500 to 1000 g using 0.75 mg/kg/day [77]. There was a shorter half-life and a more rapid clearance per body weight in the smaller weight group compared with the >1000 g group. Moreover, clearance for micafungin in neonates weighing <1000 g was 1.7-fold and 2.6-fold greater than the clearance of 2 to 8 years- and 9 to 17 years-old children, respectively, reported previously by Seibel et al. [75]. A shorter plasma half-life and a higher clearance of micafungin was also seen in neonates after a single dosing compared to children ages 2 to 8 years [82]. Overall, micafungin was well tolerated in neonates and no serious drug-related adverse events were reported [77].

A study of safety and pharmacokinetics of micafungin in young infants with suspected *Candida* infection found that micafungin doses of 7 and 10 mg/kg/day were well tolerated and provided exposure shown in animal models to be adequate for treatment of CNS infection [84]. In preterm infants, a dose of 15 mg/kg was shown to approximate drug exposure of a 5 mg/kg adult doses [85]. A population pharmacokinetic study based on these clinical studies showed that desired target attainment was likely at a dose of 10 mg/kg/day for the majority of neonates and young infants [86].

Micafungin doses up to 4.5 mg/kg/day have been shown to be well tolerated in children and adolescents with pharmacokinetics more similar to adults [87]. A population pharmacokinetic study of micafungin in children and adolescents found that a dose of 2 mg/kg/day was appropriate for most children to achieve target exposure for treatment of invasive candidiasis [88]. Doses in children are generally thought to be 2 mg/kg/day, with higher doses likely needed for younger patients, and premature neonates dosed at 10 mg/kg/day. Adult micafungin dosing (100 or 150 mg once daily) is to be used in patients who weigh more than 40 kg. Unlike the other echinocandins, a loading dose is not required for micafungin.

Clinical experience and pediatric data

A pediatric multi-center, randomized, double blind trial compared the efficacy of micafungin versus liposomal amphotericin B (LAmB) as first-line therapy in 98 pediatric patients with proven invasive candidiasis [89]. The study included 19 premature infants, 57 patients younger than 2 years, and 41 patients ages 2 to 15 years. Micafungin and LAmB were administered at a daily dose of 2 mg/kg and 3 mg/kg, respectively, to premature infants ($n = 19$), children younger than 2 years ($n = 57$) and children ages 2–15 years ($n = 41$). Treatment success, as determined by both clinical and microbiologic response, and survival during treatment and the 12-week follow-up were similar in both the micafungin and LAmB treatment group (72.9% vs. 76.0% and 75% vs. 76%, respectively). Notably, micafungin compared to LAmB was more effective in patients with neutropenia (85.3% vs. 76.9%) but less effective in patients 2 to 15 years old (63.6% vs. 73.7%).

Another multicenter, randomized, double blind phase III study compared the efficacy and safety of micafungin with that of fluconazole for prophylaxis against invasive fungal infections during neutropenia [90]. A total of 882 patients were enrolled including 84 pediatric patients (<16 years). Success rate, defined as the absence of suspected, proven or probable fungal infection at the end of treatment and at follow-up after 4 weeks, was better in patients receiving micafungin than in patients receiving fluconazole (80.0% vs. 73.5%, p = 0.03). Micafungin was also superior to fluconazole in pediatric patients with success rates of 69.2% and 53.3%. Despite the improved efficacy over fluconazole in pediatric patients, the treatment success rates in children (69.2%) was lower than adults aged 16–64 years (81.1%) and adults >64 years (97.0%). It is unclear if this lowered success rate in children is due to an ineffectively low pediatric dose of micafungin and this rate could be increased with optimal dosing. This lowered success rate in pediatric patients was also seen in an open-label non-comparative study of candidemia, which enrolled 126 patients including 20 (15.9%) children (<16 years of age) [91]. In patients receiving at least 5 doses of micafungin 84.9% of adult ($n = 106$), but only 75% (15 of 20) of pediatric patients responded to micafungin therapy, possibly because of inadequate dosing in children.

There are several non-comparative studies investigating the efficacy of micafungin in patients with invasive aspergillosis and candidiasis. Denning and colleagues investigated the outcome of 225 patients with proven or probable invasive aspergillosis including 58 children (<16 years of age) [92]. A total of 26/58 (44.8%) pediatric patients responded to micafungin therapy including 12/27 (44.4%) children younger than 10 years compared to a 35.6% overall response rate. However, only 34/225 patients received micafungin as monotherapy with a 50% response rate when administered as primary therapy but only a 40.9% response rate when given as salvage therapy. In a further analysis of those 58 pediatric patients (<16 years) with probable or proven invasive aspergillosis, micafungin was administered in 2 children as monotherapy and in 56 children in combination with other antifungal agents [93]. The overall response rate was 45%, complete and partial responses were seen in 16% and 29%, respectively. In pediatric ($n = 16$) and adult ($n = 69$) bone marrow transplant recipients who had refractory invasive aspergillosis micafungin in combination with their existing antifungal regimen, an overall complete and partial response was revealed in 39% of the adult patients and 38% of the pediatric patients [94].

Another study showed, that micafungin is more effective in *Candida* than in *Aspergillus* infections [82]. Fifty-three children with invasive candidiasis and 58 children with invasive aspergillosis received micafungin at a dose of 1–2 mg/kg/day and showed complete and partial responses in 72% and 49%, respectively [82].

ANIDULAFUNGIN

Pharmacokinetics

Anidulafungin (Eraxis®, Pfizer, New York, NY) was approved by the FDA in February 2006 for esophageal candidiasis, candidemia, peritonitis and intra-abdominal abscesses [95]. Antifungal dosing in adult patients for anidulafungin was studied at 50 and 100 mg/day for esophageal candidiasis and invasive candidiasis, respectively [1]. Anidulafungin has linear pharmacokinetics and the longest β-half-life compared to caspofungin and micafungin. The volume of distribution and clearance is greater in anidulafungin than in micafungin [54].

A multicenter, phase I/II dose escalation study investigated the pharmacokinetic profile and safety of anidulafungin in neutropenic pediatric patients at high risk for invasive fungal infections [96]. A total of 25 patients, 12 patients in the 2- to 11-year old group and 12 patients in the 12- to 17-year old group, received anidulafungin at either 0.75 mg/kg/day (*n* = 13) or 1.5 mg/kg/day (*n* = 12). Plasma drug concentrations and drug exposures were similar for patients between age groups and a weight-adjusted clearance was consistent across age. In children receiving anidulafungin at 0.75 mg/kg/day or 1.5 mg/kg/day, pharmacokinetic data were similar compared to adult patients obtaining doses of 50 or 100 mg/day. This important feature distinguishes anidulafungin from caspofungin where a higher dosing based on body-surface area is recommended. No drug-related serious adverse events occurred. Anidulafungin was well tolerated and its dosing can be based on body weight.

Clinical experience and pediatric data

To date there are no reports available on the efficacy of anidulafungin in pediatric patients and neonates.

CONCLUSION

The recent explosion of newer antifungal agents has greatly augmented the clinical spectrum of drugs available against invasive fungal infections. However, the importance of devoted pediatric data has been largely underestimated. Pharmacokinetics appear more complex in children than in adults, and at times the pharmacokinetics are directly opposite that seen in adults. While limited pharmacokinetic studies have begun active discussions about correct pediatric antifungal dosing, there has been only a small body of work studying the efficacy of antifungal agents in pediatric patients. This situation seems paradoxical, as the known dosing differences would clearly led to efficacy differences when adult doses were studied in children. It will only be through the performance of larger pediatric trials that pediatric dosing and indications will be improved and benefit children.

COMMON CLINICAL QUESTIONS AND ANSWERS

1. What is the dose of voriconazole for children and how does it differ than in adults?

   Answer: Voriconazole is metabolized in a linear fashion in children and dosing is higher. Therefore, for IV administration, load with 9 mg/kg/dose BID on day 1, and then a maintenance dose of 8 mg/kg/dose BID. Oral maintenance is at 9 mg/kg/dose. Dosing at higher doses is especially important in the youngest children.

2. What is the bioavailability of voriconazole in children and how is it different than in adults?

   Answer: Voriconazole has an approximately 96% bioavailability in adults, but only approximately 40–60% in children.

3. How is micafungin dosed in neonates?

   Answer: Micafungin in neonates is given at 10 mg/kg/day, which is significantly higher than in children (2 mg/kg/day) and due to the very rapid clearance of the drug in neonates.

4. How is caspofungin dosed in children and how does that differ than in adults?

   Answer: Caspofungin in children is dosed based on a body-surface area approach, loading with 70 mg/m² on day 1 and then continuing with 50 mg/m² as maintenance dosing. In adult patients, loading is 70 mg on day 1 and then continued with 50 mg per day.

REFERENCES

1. Steinbach WJ. Antifungal agents in children. *Pediatr Clin North Am* 2005;52:895–915, viii.
2. Sanati H, Belanger P, Fratti R, Ghannoum M. A new triazole, voriconazole (UK-109,496), blocks sterol biosynthesis in *Candida albicans* and *Candida krusei*. *Antimicrob Agents Chemother* 1997;41:2492–2496.
3. Perfect JR, Cox GM, Lee JY, et al. The impact of culture isolation of *Aspergillus* species: A hospital-based survey of aspergillosis. *Clin Infect Dis* 2001;33:1824–1833.
4. Karlsson MO, Lutsar I, Milligan PA. Population pharmacokinetic analysis of voriconazole plasma concentration data from pediatric studies. *Antimicrob Agents Chemother* 2009;53:935–944.

5. Walsh TJ, Driscoll T, Milligan PA, et al. Pharmacokinetics, safety, and tolerability of voriconazole in immunocompromised children. *Antimicrob Agents Chemother* 2010;54:4116–4123.

6. Zane NR, Thakker DR. A physiologically based pharmacokinetic model for voriconazole disposition predicts intestinal first-pass metabolism in children. *Clin Pharmacokinet* 2014;53:1171–1182.

7. Schwartz S, Ruhnke M, Ribaud P, et al. Improved outcome in central nervous system aspergillosis, using voriconazole treatment. *Blood* 2005;106:2641–2645.

8. Weiler S, Fiegl D, MacFarland R, et al. Human tissue distribution of voriconazole. *Antimicrob Agents Chemother* 2011;55:925–928.

9. Bartelink IH, Wolfs T, Jonker M, et al. Highly variable plasma concentrations of voriconazole in pediatric hematopoietic stem cell transplantation patients. *Antimicrob Agents Chemother* 2013;57:235–240.

10. Mikus G, Scholz IM, Weiss J. Pharmacogenomics of the triazole antifungal agent voriconazole. *Pharmacogenomics* 2011;12:861–872.

11. Walsh TJ, Karlsson MO, Driscoll T, et al. Pharmacokinetics and safety of intravenous voriconazole in children after single- or multiple-dose administration. *Antimicrob Agents Chemother* 2004;48:2166–2172.

12. Purkins L, Wood N, Ghahramani P, Greenhalgh K, Allen MJ, Kleinermans D. Pharmacokinetics and safety of voriconazole following intravenous- to oral-dose escalation regimens. *Antimicrob Agents Chemother* 2002;46:2546–2553.

13. Lazarus HM, Blumer JL, Yanovich S, Schlamm H, Romero A. Safety and pharmacokinetics of oral voriconazole in patients at risk of fungal infection: A dose escalation study. *J Clin Pharmacol* 2002;42:395–402.

14. Walsh TJ, Driscoll TA, Arietta AC, et al. *Pharmacokinetics, Safety, and Tolerability of Voriconazole in Hospitalized Children*, 2006; San Francisco CA: ICAAC.

15. Friberg LE, Ravva P, Karlsson MO, Liu P. Integrated population pharmacokinetic analysis of voriconazole in children, adolescents, and adults. *Antimicrob Agents Chemother* 2012;56:3032–3042.

16. Andes D, Pascual A, Marchetti O. Antifungal therapeutic drug monitoring: Established and emerging indications. *Antimicrob Agents Chemother* 2009;53:24–34.

17. Dodds Ashley ES, Zaas AK, Fang AF, Damle B, Perfect JR. Comparative pharmacokinetics of voriconazole administered orally as either crushed or whole tablets. *Antimicrob Agents Chemother* 2007;51:877–880.

18. Lazarus HM, Blummer JL, Yanovich S, Schlamm H, Romero A. Safety and pharmacokinetics of oral voriconazole in patients at risk of fungal infection: A dose escalation study. *J Clin Pharmacol* 2002;42:395–402.

19. Tan K, Brayshaw N, Tomaszewski K, Troke P, Wood N. Investigation of the potential relationships between plasma voriconazole concentrations and visual adverse events or liver function test abnormalities. *J Clin Pharmacol* 2006;46:235–243.

20. Denning DW, Griffiths CE. Muco-cutaneous retinoid-effects and facial erythema related to the novel triazole antifungal agent voriconazole. *Clin Exp Dermatol* 2001;26:648–653.

21. Pascual A, Calandra T, Bolay S, Buclin T, Bille J, Marchetti O. Voriconazole therapeutic drug monitoring in patients with invasive mycoses improves efficacy and safety outcomes. *Clin Infect Dis* 2008;46:201–211.

22. Levine MT, Chandrasekar PH. Adverse effects of voriconazole: Over a decade of use. *Clin Transplant* 2016;30:1377–1386.

23. Herbrecht R, Denning DW, Patterson TF, et al. Voriconazole versus amphotericin B for primary therapy of invasive aspergillosis. *N Engl J Med* 2002;347:408–415.

24. Patterson TF, Boucher HW, Herbrecht R, et al. Strategy of following voriconazole versus amphotericin B therapy with other licensed antifungal therapy for primary treatment of invasive aspergillosis: Impact of other therapies on outcome. *Clin Infect Dis* 2005;41:1448–1452.

25. Denning DW, Ribaud P, Milpied N, et al. Efficacy and safety of voriconazole in the treatment of acute invasive aspergillosis. *Clin Infect Dis* 2002;34:563–571.

26. Patterson TF, Thompson III GR, Denning DW, et al. Practice guidelines for the diagnosis and management of aspergillosis: 2016 update by the Infectious Diseases Society of America. *Clin Infect Dis* 2016;6(4):e1–e60.

27. Ally R, Schurmann D, Kreisel W, et al. A randomized, double-blind, double-dummy, multicenter trial of voriconazole and fluconazole in the treatment of esophageal candidiasis in immunocompromised patients. *Clin Infect Dis* 2001;33:1447–1454.

28. Kullberg BJ, Sobel JD, Ruhnke M, et al. Voriconazole versus a regimen of amphotericin B followed by fluconazole for candidaemia in non-neutropenic patients: A randomised non-inferiority trial. *Lancet* 2005;366:1435–1442.

29. Walsh TJ, Pappas P, Winston DJ, et al. Voriconazole compared with liposomal amphotericin B for empirical antifungal therapy in patients with neutropenia and persistent fever. *N Engl J Med* 2002;346:225–234.

30. Walsh TJ, Lutsar I, Driscoll T, et al. Voriconazole in the treatment of aspergillosis, scedosporiosis and other invasive fungal infections in children. *Pediatr Infect Dis J* 2002;21:240–248.

31. Cesaro S, Strugo L, Alaggio R, et al. Voriconazole for invasive aspergillosis in oncohematological patients: A single-center pediatric experience. *Support Care Cancer* 2003;11:722–727.

32. Torres HA, Hachem RY, Chemaly RF, Kontoyiannis DP, Raad, II. Posaconazole: A broad-spectrum triazole antifungal. *Lancet Infect Dis* 2005;5:775–785.

33. Courtney R, Wexler D, Radwanski E, Lim J, Laughlin M. Effect of food on the relative bioavailability of two oral formulations of posaconazole in healthy adults. *Br J Clin Pharmacol* 2004;57:218–222.

34. Ezzet F, Wexler D, Courtney R, Krishna G, Lim J, Laughlin M. Oral bioavailability of posaconazole in fasted healthy subjects: Comparison between three regimens and basis for clinical dosage recommendations. *Clin Pharmacokinet* 2005;44:211–220.

35. Ullmann AJ, Cornely OA, Burchardt A, et al. Pharmacokinetics, safety, and efficacy of posaconazole in patients with persistent febrile neutropenia or refractory invasive fungal infection. *Antimicrob Agents Chemother* 2006;50:658–666.

36. Duarte RF, Lopez-Jimenez J, Cornely OA, et al. Phase 1b study of new posaconazole tablet for prevention of invasive fungal infections in high-risk patients with neutropenia. *Antimicrob Agents Chemother* 2014;58:5758–5765.

37. Segal BH, Barnhart LA, Anderson VL, Walsh TJ, Malech HL, Holland SM. Posaconazole as salvage therapy in patients with chronic granulomatous disease and invasive filamentous fungal infection. *Clin Infect Dis* 2005;40:1684–1688.

38. Walsh TJ, Raad I, Patterson TF, et al. Treatment of invasive aspergillosis with posaconazole in patients who are refractory to or intolerant of conventional therapy: An externally controlled trial. *Clin Infect Dis* 2007;44:2–12.

39. Krishna G, Sansone-Parsons A, Martinho M, Kantesaria B, Pedicone L. Posaconazole plasma concentrations in juvenile patients with invasive fungal infection. *Antimicrob Agents Chemother* 2007;51:812–818.

40. Ullmann AJ, Lipton JH, Vesole DH, et al. Posaconazole or fluconazole for prophylaxis in severe graft-versus-host disease. *N Engl J Med* 2007;356:335–347.

41. Cornely OA, Maertens J, Winston DJ, et al. Posaconazole vs. fluconazole or itraconazole prophylaxis in patients with neutropenia. *N Engl J Med* 2007;356:348–359.

42. Vazquez JA, Skiest DJ, Nieto L, et al. A multicenter randomized trial evaluating posaconazole versus fluconazole for the treatment of oropharyngeal candidiasis in subjects with HIV/AIDS. *Clin Infect Dis* 2006;42:1179–1186.

43. Walsh TJ, Raad I, Patterson TF, et al. Treatment of invasive aspergillosis with posaconazole in patients who are refractory to or intolerant of conventional therapy: An externally controlled trial. *Clin Infect Dis* 2007;44:2–12.

44. Heinz WJ, Egerer G, Lellek H, Boehme A, Greiner J. Posaconazole after previous antifungal therapy with voriconazole for therapy of invasive *aspergillus* disease, a retrospective analysis. *Mycoses* 2013;56:304–310.

45. Vehreschild JJ, Birtel A, Vehreschild MJ, et al. Mucormycosis treated with posaconazole: Review of 96 case reports. *Crit Rev Microbiol* 2013;39:310–324.

46. Doring M, Muller C, Johann PD, et al. Analysis of posaconazole as oral antifungal prophylaxis in pediatric patients under 12 years of age following allogeneic stem cell transplantation. *BMC Infect Dis* 2012;12:263.

47. Greenberg RN, Mullane K, van Burik JA, et al. Posaconazole as salvage therapy for zygomycosis. *Antimicrob Agents Chemother* 2006;50:126–133.

48. Lehrnbecher T, Attarbaschi A, Duerken M, et al. Posaconazole salvage treatment in paediatric patients: A multicentre survey. *Eur J Clin Microbiol Infect Dis* 2010;29:1043–1045.

49. Schmitt-Hoffmann A, Roos B, Heep M, et al. Single-ascending-dose pharmacokinetics and safety of the novel broad-spectrum antifungal triazole BAL4815 after intravenous infusions (50, 100, and 200 milligrams) and oral administrations (100, 200, and 400 milligrams) of its prodrug, BAL8557, in healthy volunteers. *Antimicrob Agents Chemother* 2006;50:279–285.

50. Schmitt-Hoffmann A, Roos B, Maares J, et al. Multiple-dose pharmacokinetics and safety of the new antifungal triazole BAL4815 after intravenous infusion and oral administration of its prodrug, BAL8557, in healthy volunteers. *Antimicrob Agents Chemother* 2006;50:286–293.

51. Maertens JA, Raad, II, Marr KA, et al. Isavuconazole versus voriconazole for primary treatment of invasive mould disease caused by *Aspergillus* and other filamentous fungi (SECURE): A phase 3, randomised-controlled, non-inferiority trial. *Lancet* 2016;387:760–769.

52. Viljoen J, Azie N, Schmitt-Hoffmann AH, Ghannoum M. A phase 2, randomized, double-blind, multicenter trial to evaluate the safety and efficacy of three dosing regimens of isavuconazole compared with fluconazole in patients with uncomplicated esophageal candidiasis. *Antimicrob Agents Chemother* 2015;59:1671–1679.

53. Marty FM, Ostrosky-Zeichner L, Cornely OA, et al. Isavuconazole treatment for mucormycosis: A single-arm open-label trial and case-control analysis. *The Lancet infectious diseases* 2016;16:828–837.

54. Denning DW. Echinocandin antifungal drugs. *Lancet* 2003;362:1142–1151.

55. Maschmeyer G, Glasmacher A. Pharmacological properties and clinical efficacy of a recently licensed systemic antifungal, caspofungin. *Mycoses* 2005;48:227–234.

56. Franzot SP, Casadevall A. Pneumocandin L-743,872 enhances the activities of amphotericin B and fluconazole against Cryptococcus neoformans *in vitro*. *Antimicrob Agents Chemother* 1997;41:331–336.

57. Abruzzo GK, Gill CJ, Flattery AM, et al. Efficacy of the echinocandin caspofungin against disseminated aspergillosis and candidiasis in cyclophosphamide-induced immunosuppressed mice. *Antimicrob Agents Chemother* 2000;44:2310–2318.

58. Hoang A. Caspofungin acetate: An antifungal agent. *Am J Health Syst Pharm* 2001;58:1206–1214; quiz 15–17.

59. Stone JA, Holland SD, Wickersham PJ, et al. Single- and multiple-dose pharmacokinetics of caspofungin in healthy men. *Antimicrob Agents Chemother* 2002;46:739–745.

60. Merck. Cancidas® (caspofungin acetate). *Prescribing Information*. Whitehouse Station, NJ: Merck, 2001.

61. Stone JA, Holland SD, Li SX. Effect of hepatic insufficiency on the pharmacokinetics of caspofungin. *41st Interscience Conference on Antimicrobial Agents and Chemotherapy*; Chicago, IL, 2001 p. 45.

62. Holland SD, Stone JA, Li SX. Drug interactions between caspofungin and tacrolimus. *Program and abstracts of the 41st Interscience Conference on Antimicrobial Agents and Chemotherapy*; Chicago, IL, 2001 p. A-13.

63. Walsh TJ, Adamson PC, Seibel NL, et al. Pharmacokinetics, safety, and tolerability of caspofungin in children and adolescents. *Antimicrob Agents Chemother* 2005;49:4536–4545.

64. Neely MN, Jafri H, Seibel NL, et al. Pharmacokinetics (PK) and safety of caspofungin (CAS) in young children ages 3 to 24 months. *Pediatric Academic Societies' Annual Meeting*; 2007; Toronto, ON, Canada.

65. Franklin JA, McCormick J, Flynn PM. Retrospective study of the safety of caspofungin in immunocompromised pediatric patients. *Pediatr Infect Dis J* 2003;22:747–749.

66. Groll AH, Attarbaschi A, Schuster FR, et al. Treatment with caspofungin in immunocompromised paediatric patients: A multicentre survey. *J Antimicrob Chemother* 2006;57:527–535.

67. Jafri H, Zaoutis T, Keller N, et al. Prospective, Multicenter Study of Caspofungin (CAS) for Treatment (Rx) of Documented Fungal Infections in Pediatric Patients (Ped Pts). *46th Interscience Conference on Antimicrobial Agents and Chemotherapy*; San Francisco CA; 2006.

68. Merlin E, Galambrun C, Ribaud P, et al. Efficacy and safety of caspofungin therapy in children with invasive fungal infections. *Pediatr Infect Dis J* 2006;25:1186–1188.

69. Khayat N, Amsallem D, Nerich V, et al. Caspofungin versus liposomal amphotericin B for empirical therapy in children with persistently febrile neutropenia. *45th Interscience Conference on Antimicrobial Agents and Chemotherapy*; 2005.

70. Franklin JA, McCormick J, Flynn PM. Retrospective study of the safety of caspofungin in immunocompromised pediatric patients. *Pediatr Infect Dis J* 2003;22:747–749.

71. Odio CM, Araya R, Pinto LE, et al. Caspofungin therapy of neonates with invasive candidiasis. *Pediatr Infect Dis J* 2004;23:1093–1097.

72. Odio CM, Pinto LE, Alfaro B, et al. *Pharmacokinetics Of Caspofungin In Six Premature Neonates With Invasive Candidiasis At A Neonatal Intensive Care Unit*. ICAAC; Washington, DC, 2005.

73. Natarajan G, Lulic-Botica M, Rongkavilit C, Pappas A, Bedard M. Experience with caspofungin in the treatment of persistent fungemia in neonates. *J Perinatol* 2005;25:770–777.

74. Chandrasekar PH, Sobel JD. Micafungin: A new echinocandin. *Clin Infect Dis* 2006;42:1171–1178.

75. Seibel NL, Schwartz C, Arrieta A, et al. Safety, tolerability, and pharmacokinetics of Micafungin (FK463) in febrile neutropenic pediatric patients. *Antimicrob Agents Chemother* 2005;49:3317–3324.

76. Tabata K, Katashima M, Kawamura A, Tanigawara Y, Sunagawa K. Linear pharmacokinetics of micafungin and its active metabolites in Japanese pediatric patients with fungal infections. *Biol Pharm Bull* 2006;29:1706–1711.

77. Heresi GP, Gerstmann DR, Reed MD, et al. The pharmacokinetics and safety of micafungin, a novel echinocandin, in premature infants. *Pediatr Infect Dis J* 2006;25:1110–1115.

78. Hebert MF, Smith HE, Marbury TC, et al. Pharmacokinetics of micafungin in healthy volunteers, volunteers with moderate liver disease, and volunteers with renal dysfunction. *J Clin Pharmacol* 2005;45:1145–1152.

79. Hebert MF, Blough DK, Townsend RW, et al. Concomitant tacrolimus and micafungin pharmacokinetics in healthy volunteers. *J Clin Pharmacol* 2005;45:1018–1024.

80. Hebert MF, Townsend RW, Austin S, et al. Concomitant cyclosporine and micafungin pharmacokinetics in healthy volunteers. *J Clin Pharmacol* 2005;45:954–960.

81. Townsend RW, Bekersky I, Buell DN, Buell NS. Pharmacokinetic evaluation of echinocandin FK463 in pediatric and adult patients. *Focus on Fungal Infections* 2001;11.

82. Arrieta A, Seibel NL, Kovanda L, et al. *Safety, Efficacy and Pharmacokinetics (pk) of Micafungin (mica) in Pediatric (ped) Patients (pts)*. San Francisco, CA: ICAAC, 2006.

83. Hope WW, Keirns J, Buell D, et al. *Population Pharmacokinetics (Pk) Of Micafungin In Neonates And Children*. San Francisco, CA: ICAAC, 2006.

84. Benjamin DKJ, Smith PB, Arrieta A, et al. Safety and pharmacokinetics of repeat-dose micafungin in young infants. *Clin Pharmacol Ther* 2010;87:93–99.

85. Smith PB, Walsh TJ, Hope W, et al. Pharmacokinetics of an elevated dosage of micafungin in premature neonates. *Pediatr Infect Dis J* 2009;28:412–415.

86. Hope WW, Smith PB, Arrieta A, et al. Population pharmacokinetics of micafungin in neonates and young infants. *Antimicrob Agents Chemother* 2010;54:2633–2637.

87. Seibel NL, Schwartz C, Arrieta A, et al. Safety, tolerability, and pharmacokinetics of micafungin (FK463) in febrile neutropenic pediatric patients. *Antimicrob Agents Chemother* 2005;49:3317–3324.

88. Hope WW, Kaibara A, Roy M, et al. Population pharmacokinetics of micafungin and its metabolites M1 and M5 in children and adolescents. *Antimicrob Agents Chemother* 2015;59:905–913.

89. Arrieta A, Telles Filho F, Berezin E, Freire A, Diekmann-Berndt H. *A Randomized, Double-blind Trial Comparing Micafungin (MCFG) and Liposomal Amphotericin B (L-AMB) in Pediatric Patients with Invasive Candidiasis*. San Francisco, CA: ICAAC, 2006.

90. van Burik JA, Ratanatharathorn V, Stepan DE, et al. Micafungin versus fluconazole for prophylaxis against invasive fungal infections during neutropenia in patients undergoing hematopoietic stem cell transplantation. *Clin Infect Dis* 2004;39:1407–1416.

91. Ostrosky-Zeichner L, Kontoyiannis D, Raffalli J, et al. International, open-label, noncomparative, clinical trial of micafungin alone and in combination for treatment of newly diagnosed and refractory candidemia. *Eur J Clin Microbiol Infect Dis* 2005;24:654–661.

92. Denning DW, Marr KA, Lau WM, et al. Micafungin (FK463), alone or in combination with other systemic antifungal agents, for the treatment of acute invasive aspergillosis. *J Infect* 2006;53:337–349.

93. Flynn P, Seibel NL, Arrieta A, et al. Treatment of invasive aspergillosis (IA) in pediatric patients (pts) with micafungin (MICA) alone or in combination with other systemic antifungal agents. San Francisco, CA: ICAAC, 2006.

94. Ratanatharathorn V, Flynn P, van Burik JA, McSweeney P, Niederwieser D, Kontoyiannis D. Micafungin in combination with systemic antifungal agents in the treatmentof refractory aspergillosis in bone marrow transplant patients. *American Society of Hematology 44th Annual Meeting*; Philadelphia, Pennsylvania, 2002.

95. Cohen-Wolkowiez M, Benjamin DK, Jr., Steinbach WJ, Smith PB. Anidulafungin: A new echinocandin for the treatment of fungal infections. *Drugs Today (Barc)* 2006;42:533–544.

96. Benjamin DK, Jr., Driscoll T, Seibel NL, et al. Safety and pharmacokinetics of intravenous anidulafungin in children with neutropenia at high risk for invasive fungal infections. *Antimicrob Agents Chemother* 2006;50:632–638.

29

Fungal infections in burn patients

NOUR HASAN

INTRODUCTION

Despite major advances in the care of burn patients, infectious complications remain an important cause of morbidity and mortality from extensive burn injuries [1]. Although the incidence of bacterial wound infections has significantly decreased with the broad acceptance of topical antibiotics, early burn wound excision, and patient isolation practices, the incidence of fungal wound infections remain unchanged [2,3]. Fungal infections remain a common cause of morbidity, mortality, and cost in burn patients [1–4].

EPIDEMIOLOGY

The incidence of fungal contamination and infection in burn patients is reported to be 6.3%–15%, although there are significant differences between individual burn centers ranging from 0.7% up to 24.1% [5,6]. This variation may be the result of different standards in the performance of surveillance cultures and may reflect differences in the frequency, quality, and quantity of diagnostic efforts in suspected cases [5]. In a North American multicenter analysis of 435 burn patients with positive fungal cultures, cultures obtained from burn wounds comprised over one half of all reported fungal cultures. Respiratory cultures were the second most common culture, site followed by urine, blood, and other sources [6]. In a review of the U.S. Army Institute of Surgical Research (USAISR) Burn Center's electronic database [2], the reported rate of fungal wound infection (FWI) over the 12-year study period was 2% of patients admitted with thermal burns (4.5 patients per year), while fungal wound colonization (FWC) was reported in 4.6% of patients. FWI progressed from FWC in 15.4% of patients

with FWC, and these 15.4% represented 40% of patients who ultimately developed a FWI. Progression to FWI was related only to the size of the wound. Fungal wound involvement (FWI or FWC) was detected on median postburn day 16. FWI, but not FWC, was an independent risk factor for mortality, along with age, burn size, and inhalation injury. The presence of FWI increased mortality by an odds ratio of 8.16, which was higher than the impact of inhalation injury on mortality odds and about the same impact as augmenting the total body surface area by 33%. However, the impact of FWI on mortality was only remarkable in patients with a burn size of 30%–60% of total body surface area (mortality rate of 80% in patients with FWI vs. 18% in patients with FWC and no fungus patients pooled). However, whether fungal invasion itself contributed causally to mortality or just represented a marker for other contributors was not definitely assessed in this report [2]. In a more recent 5 year retrospective study from the same institution [7], the incidence of FWI was 0.69 per 1000 hospital days and similarly the overall mortality of patients with FWI was significantly higher than that seen in those with FWC (79% vs. 24% respectively). In addition to wound infections, burn patients are also cited as being among the highest risk groups for invasive fungal infections. Data from the National Nosocomial Infection Surveillance Program demonstrated that burn patients with central venous catheters have the highest risk of candidemia of any hospitalized group [8].

In an attempt to determine the contribution of fungal infections to mortality in burn patients, 97 autopsies over a 12-year period were reviewed [9] and, out of 44% patients with fungal elements on histopathology, mortality was attributed to the fungal infection in 33% (14 out of 42 patients). The most common sites of infections with attributable mortality were wounds (86%) and the pulmonary system (14%), followed by abdomen, kidney, and fungemia, with some patients having multiple sites. *Aspergillus* and *Candida* were the most frequently recovered fungi; however, in cases where fungus was an attributable cause of death, *Aspergillus* was more commonly recovered alone or in association with other fungi. Similarly, among the 175 patients identified in the previously mentioned 12-year retrospective study performed by USAISR (2), *Aspergillus*-like fungi (parallel-walled, branching, septate hyphae) were seen in the greatest fraction of patients on wound pathology (83%), followed by yeast-like structures (budding yeasts or rounded yeast-like structures) in 36% of patients, and *Mucor*-like (wide, ribbon-like, rarely septate hyphae) structures in the smallest fraction (15%). *Aspergillus*-like fungi and *Mucor*-like fungi were more likely to be seen in FWI than in FWC patients, with no difference in frequency for yeast-like fungi. However, correlation between histopathologic and culture identification of fungi is not always consistent [7]. The most commonly encountered opportunistic fungal pathogens in burn patients include *Candida* spp., *Aspergillus* spp. (including *A. fumigatus, A. flavus, A. terreus*), *Zygomycetes, Fusarium* spp., *Trichosporon, Penicillium, Cladosporium, Cryptococcus, Acremonium, Coccidioides*, Curvuleria, and *Bipolaris* [2–9].

RISK FACTORS

The mechanical barrier of the intact skin is destroyed after burn injury, providing a port of entry for fungi and other microorganisms to invade easily. In addition, necrotic or degenerated tissues are favorable culture media for colonization and growth of various microorganisms including fungi. Broad-spectrum antibiotics, commonly administered to patients after severe burn injuries, total parental nutrition, long term invasive monitoring, and deep venous catheters are additional risk factors for fungal infections [10]. Furthermore, serious thermal injuries induce a state of immunosuppression that predisposes burn patients to infectious complications [11]. The mechanisms responsible for this decreased resistance to infection remain poorly understood but several perturbations of both the innate and adaptive immune systems have been documented in animal models and patients [12]. Previous studies demonstrated that burn injuries result in alteration in T-cell function [12]. Following a significant burn injury, it was observed that T-cell response becomes skewed from a Th1 CD4+ cell response toward a Th2 CD4+ cell response [13–15] with increased production of cytokines IL-4 and IL-10, which are significant anti-inflammatory cytokines. Diminished IL-12 (induces differentiation of Naive T to TH1 phenotype) production by mononuclear cells after burn injury has also been documented [16]. Further impairment of T-lymphocyte

activity is reflected by depressed proliferative responses of peripheral blood mononuclear cells and sometimes development of global T-cell anergy [17]. Furthermore, excessive monocyte production of the inhibitory factors PGE2 in burn patients may also play a role in the overall immunosuppressive status [18,19]. Alterations to innate immunity following burn injury have also been reported and include impaired production and release of granulocytes and macrophages from the bone marrow [20], diminished macrophage phagocytic capacity [11] and neutrophil dysfunction [21–23]. Initially, the immunologic response to severe burn injury is pro-inflammatory but later becomes predominately anti-inflammatory in an effort to maintain homeostasis and restore normal physiology [11]. As a result of the secondary anti-inflammatory state and subsequent alterations to the adaptive and innate immune systems, burn patients are more susceptible to bacterial and fungal wound infections and severe sepsis [11,12,15].

CLINICAL MANIFESTATIONS OF FUNGAL BURN WOUND INFECTIONS

Invasive fungal infection after burn injury is characterized by local or systemic inflammation, tissue and cell damage caused by colonization, growth and proliferation of various fungi in wounds, blood stream, internal organs, or tissues of burn patients [10].

Although burn wounds are sterile immediately after the thermal injury, these wounds eventually become colonized with hospital-associated microorganisms, including fungi. As with bacterial wound infections, fungal burn wound infections tend to have a late onset, generally occurring after the second week of thermal injury [2], and are usually diagnosed after a period of burn wound colonization with the yeast or molds that are normally seen in the patient's surrounding environment [2]. The main concern regarding colonized and infected wounds is not only the fact that they have a propensity to heal much slower, but that they are also a significant source of systemic infection and can rapidly lead to the development of invasive fungal infections. Furthermore, fungal colonization and wound infection will also prevent adequate wound healing and skin grafting [10].

Although there are no classic or typical manifestations associated with an invasive burn wound infection, it is not uncommon for the edges of the wound to darken initially in the periphery and subsequently throughout the entire wound area, with an appearance similar to ecthyma gangrenosum. Occasionally, burn wounds may also become infected with different genera of zygomycetes, especially with *Rhizopus* or *Mucor* spp. Although infections due to these molds are not very common, they are important to diagnose early because of their ability to spread rapidly across different facial tissue planes. Additionally, they have

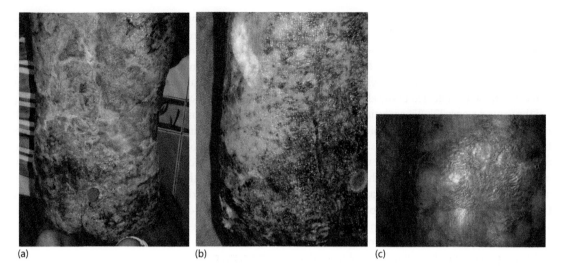

(a) (b) (c)

Figure 29.1 **(a)** Wounds of a child with 50% scalds deteriorating despite higher antibiotic therapy showing early separation of eschar at subcutaneous level due to fat necrosis in fungal wound invasion. Wound biopsy confirmed FWI by C. krusei. **(b)** 10 days after starting antifungal treatment the wound condition improved remarkably. **(c)** Same patient grafted after wound biopsy was negative. (Reprinted from *Burns*, 28, Sarabahi, S. et al. Changing pattern of fungal infection in burn patients, 520–528, Copyright 2012, with permission from Elsevier.)

the ability to invade the local vasculature, producing diffuse small vessel thrombosis resulting in local progressive tissue necrosis and occasional systemic dissemination of the infection. Inflammation around wounds infected with fungi is obvious. Granulation tissue looks gray or bright red but is fragile and bleeds easily. Mucoidal exudate frequently covers the wound. Skin graft appears patent initially but is unable to grow or expand. Hematogenous spread of *Aspergillus* and *Mucor* leads to extensive skin hemorrhage or necrosis. Hemorrhagic spots and disseminated erythematous nodules may be found on normal skin [3]. Other local signs of fungal wound infection may include separation of eschar layer, conversion of partial thickness injury into full thickness necrosis, green pigment of the subcutaneous fat, and subcutaneous edema with central wound necrosis [3] (See Figure 29.1). Fungal infection should also be suspected in patients with fever, despite the intake of broad-spectrum antibiotics for >7–15 days, and deteriorating condition [24].

Due to burn-wound-related permanent inflammation and consequent physiological reactions, common definitions of sepsis are not applicable to burn patients [25,26]. Standardized definitions for sepsis and infection that are specifically applicable to the burn patient were developed in 2007 [27]. These definitions distinguish the change in patient status as a result of an infection from changes that occur secondary to the hypermetabolic response of the burn itself (Table 29.1). Furthermore, laboratory tests may have limited impact. The efficacy of biochemical markers of inflammation, such as C-reactive protein, procalcitonin, and interleukin-6 to diagnose sepsis in burn patients, has

Table 29.1 American Burn Association criteria for burn wound sepsis

At least three of the following parameters:
- Temperature >39°C or <36.5°C
- Progressive tachycardia (adults >110 beats per minute; children >2 standard deviations above age-specific normal values)
- Progressive tachypnea (adults >25 breathes per minute; children >2 SD above age-specific normal values)
- Thrombocytopenia (applies three days after resuscitation) (adults <100,000 platelets per microliter; children <2 SD below age-specific normal values)
- Hyperglycemia or insulin resistance
- Inability to tolerate enteral feedings for more than 24 hours secondary to abdominal distension, feeding intolerance or uncontrollable diarrhea.

Plus one of the following criteria:
- Infection is confirmed on a culture
- Pathologic tissue source identified (e.g., microbial or fungal invasion into an unburned tissue)
- Clinical improvement in response to antimicrobial administration

not been proven. These markers are not routinely measured, and their interpretation remains unclear [27]. However, a recent systematic review suggests that procalcitonin may be a useful biomarker for early diagnosis of sepsis in burn patients [28].

DIAGNOSIS OF FUNGAL BURN WOUND INFECTIONS

The diagnosis of burn wound infections when suspected clinically or on routine surveillance can only reliably be made by histological examination of affected tissue along with fungal cultures of the wound biopsy [7]. It is essential to recognize the difference between the significance of a positive superficial wound culture and "true" infection. In most situations, fungal pathogens recovered from an open wound will be considered colonizers unless there is evidence that these pathogens have become invasive, or there are local signs or symptoms of infection. The differentiation is made by pathology, in which fungal wound infection is defined as invasion of fungal elements into viable tissue; in contrast, fungal wound colonization is defined as fungal elements in eschar (nonviable burned skin) or "neo-eschar" (a previously excised, now necrotic wound surface), but not viable tissue [2].

TREATMENT

Patients with FWC should be treated by aggressive surgical debridement and, in the case of FWI, an intravenous antifungal drug, most commonly liposomal amphotericin B or an echinocandin, should additionally be initiated. Therapy should subsequently be tailored based on the fungal speciation and antifungal susceptibility [24].

Once invasive fungal infection through burnt tissue is identified, especially with *Aspergillus* or *Mucor* infection that preserves angioinvasive potential, immediate and extensive wound debridement and early closure of wound defect are the surgical approaches to the treatment. The coverage of a burn area by skin grafts or flaps should be performed only when wound infection is controlled (negative swab cultures and biopsies) and there is no clinical evidence of fungal sepsis [24]. Where infected tissue may not be removed, an exposure or semi-exposure method of wound closure is recommended, with the treated wound kept clean and dry [10].

The topical treatment of burn wounds with nystatin powder at a concentration of 6 million U/g has been proven effective in small numbers of patients for treatment of burn wound infections caused by *Candida* spp., *Aspergillus,* or *Fusarium* spp., as it was shown to be effective in eradicating invasive clusters of fungi in deep wound tissues [29].

PROPHYLAXIS

Early surgical intervention and early wound closure are key functions in limiting the risk of fungal infection in burn patients [24]. Adequate infection control practices and minimizing modifiable predisposing factors are important prevention strategies. The use of indwelling catheters should be minimized as far as practicable. Broad-spectrum antibiotics should be avoided for long periods and focused to culture results as soon as possible [10]. When potent topical antimicrobial agents are applied continuously, nystatin powder may be combined with silver sulfadiazine and mafenide acetate to prevent overgrowth of fungi at the wound site [26]. Silver-based topical antimicrobials, such as silver sulfadiazine, possess potent bactericidal and fungicidal properties related to their effect on respiratory enzymes in cells of microorganisms [30]. However, these topical agents have the potential for direct toxicity and have been shown to retard wound healing [29]. Silver impregnated dressings provide controlled and more prolonged silver ion release and sustained concentrations to the burn wounds; additionally, they reduce the risk of nosocomial infection, given limited number of dressing changes [31]. However, a conclusive evidence on the effect of silver-containing dressings or agents to prevent wound infection is lacking [32].

REFERENCES

1. Atiyeh BS, Gunn SW, Hayak SN. State of the art in burn treatment. *World J Surg* 2005; 29(2):131–148.
2. Horvath EE, Murray CK, Vaughan GM, et al. Fungal wound infection (not colonization) is independently associated with mortality in burn patients. *Ann Surg* 2007;245(6):978–985.
3. Becker WK, Cioffi WG Jr, McManus AT, et al. Fungal burn wound infection. A 10-year experience. *Arch Surg* 1991;126:44–48.
4. Cochran A, Morris SE, Edelman LS, Saffle JR. Systemic *Candida* infection in burn patients: A case-control study of management patterns and outcomes. *Surg Infect* (Larchmt) 2002;3:367–374.
5. Struck MF, Gille J. Fungal infections in burns: A comprehensive review. *Ann Burns Fire Disasters* 2013;26(3):147–153.
6. Ballard J, Edelman L, Saffle J, et al. Positive fungal cultures in burn patients: A multicenter review. *J Burn Care Res* 2008;29:213–221.
7. Schofield CM, Murray CK, Horvath EE, Cancio LC, Kim SH, Wolf SE, Hospenthal DR. Correlation of culture with histopathology in fungal burn wound colonization and infection. *Burns* 2007;33(3):341–346.
8. Jarvis WR. Epidemiology of nosocomial fungal infections, with emphasis on *Candida* species. *Clin Infect Dis* 1995;20:1526–1530.
9. Murray CK, Loo FL, Hospenthal DR, Cancio LC, Jones JA, Kim SH, Holcomb JB, Wade CE, Wolf SE. Incidence of systemic fungal infection and related mortality following severe burns. *Burns* 2008;34(8):1108–1112.
10. Gaoxing Luo, Jianglin Tan, Yizhi Peng, et al. Guideline for diagnosis, prophylaxis and treatment of invasive fungal infection post burn injury in China 2013. *Burns Trauma* 2014; 2(2): 45–52.
11. Church D, Elsayed S, Reid O, et al. Burn wound infections. *Clin Microbiol Rev* 2006;19:403–434.
12. Cioffi WG. What's new in burns and metabolism. *J Am Coll Surg* 2001;192:241–254.

13. DiPiro JT, Howdieshell TR, Goddard JK, Callaway DB, Hamilton RG, Mansberger, Jr. AR 1995. Association of interleukin-4 plasma levels with traumatic injury and clinical course. *Arch Surg* 1995;130(11):1159–1163.

14. Yeh FL, Lin WL, Shen HD, et al. Changes in circulating levels of an anti-inflammatory cytokine interleukin 10 in burned patients. *Burns* 2000;26:454–459.

15. Gosain A, Gamelli RL 2005. A primer in cytokines. *J Burn Care Rehabil* 26:7–12.

16. Goebel A, Kavanagh E, Lyons A, Saporoschetz IB, Soberg C, Lederer JA, Mannick JA, Rodrick ML. Injury induces deficient interleukin-12 production, but interleukin-12 therapy after injury restores resistance to infection. *Ann Surg* 2000;231:253–261.

17. De AD, Kodys KM, Pellegrini J, et al. Induction of global anergy rather than inhibitory Th2 lymphokines mediates posttrauma T-cell immunodepression. *Clin Immunol* 2000;96:52–66.

18. Gamelli RL, He LK, Liu LH. Macrophage mediated suppression of granulocyte and macrophage growth after burn wound infection reversal by means of anti-PGE2. *J Burn Care Rehabil* 2000;21:64–69.

19. Santangelo S, Shoup M, Gamelli RL, Shankar R. Prostaglandin E2 receptor antagonist (SC-19220) treatment restores the balance to bone marrow myelopoiesis after burn sepsis. *J Trauma Inj Infect Crit Care* 2000;48:826–831.

20. Gamelli RL, He LK, H Liu. Marrow granulocyte-macrophage progenitor cell response to burn injury as modified by endotoxin and indomethacin. *J Trauma* 1994;37:339–346.

21. Grogan JB. Altered neutrophil phagocytic function in burn patients. *J. Trauma* 1976; 16:734–738.

22. Grogan JB, Miller RC. Impaired function of polymorphonuclear leukocytes in patients with burns and other trauma. *Surg Gynecol Obstet* 1973;137:784–788.

23. McManus AT, Kim SH, McManus WF, et al. Comparison of quantitative microbiology and histopathology in divided burn-wound biopsy specimens. *Arch Surg* 1987;122:74–76.

24. Capoor MR, Sarabahi S, Tiwari VK, Narayanan RP. Fungal infections in burns: Diagnosis and management. *Indian J Plast Surg* 2010;43(Suppl): S37–S42.

25. Jeschke MG, Chinkes DL, Finnerty CC, Kulp G, Suman OE, Norbury WB, Branski LK, Gauglitz GG, Mlcak RP, Herndon DN. Pathophysiologic response to severe burn injury. *Ann Surg* 2008;248(3):387–401.

26. Jeschke MG, Gauglitz GG, Kulp GA, Finnerty CC, Williams FN, Kraft R, Suman OE, Mlcak RP, Herndon DN. Long-term persistance of the pathophysiologic response to severe burn injury. *PLoS One* 2011;6(7):e21245.

27. Greenhalgh DG, Saffle JR, Holmes JH IV, Gamelli RL, Palmieri TL, Horton JW, Tompkins RG, et al. American Burn Association consensus conference to define sepsis and infection in burns. *J Burn Care Res* 2007;28(6):776–790.

28. Ren H, Li Y, Han C, Hu H. Serum procalcitonin as a diagnostic biomarker for sepsis in burned patients: A meta-analysis. *Burns* 2015;41(3):502.

29. Gallagher JJ, Branski LK, Williams-Bouyer N, Villarreal C, Herndon DN Treatment of infections in burns. Chapter 12, In: Herndon DN (Ed.), *Total burn care*, 4th ed. Amsterdam, the Netherlands: Elsevier Science Health Science division, 2012:137–156.

30. Wright JB, Lam K, Hansen D, et al. Efficacy of topical silver against fungal burn wound pathogens. *Am J Infect Control* 1999;27(4):344–350.

31. Elliott C. The effects of silver dressings on chronic and burns wound healing. *Br J Nurs* 2010;19(15):S32–S36.

32. Storm-Versloot MN, Vos CG, Ubbink DT, Vermeulen H. Topical silver for preventing wound infection. *Cochrane Database Syst Rev* 2010;(3):CD006478.

33. Sarabahi S, Tiwari VK, Arora S, Capoor MR, Pandey A. Changing pattern of fungal infection in burn patients. *Burns* 2012;28(4):520–528.

30

Allergic bronchopulmonary aspergillosis

NOUR HASAN

INTRODUCTION

Allergic bronchopulmonary aspergillosis (ABPA) is a lung disease caused by an immunologic response to the mold *Aspergillus fumigatus*. The disease is mostly described in genetically susceptible asthmatics and cystic fibrosis (CF) patients. An exaggerated host immune response involving Th2 CD4+T cells is central to the pathogenesis of ABPA. The diagnosis of ABPA requires the combination of clinical, radiographic, and laboratory criteria.

This chapter reviews the major pathologic manifestations of ABPA, clinical, radiographic, and laboratory features of the disease and current knowledge about its pathogenesis and treatment.

EPIDEMIOLOGY OF ALLERGIC BRONCHOPULMONARY ASPERGILLOSIS

Sensitization to *A. fumigatus* (AS), defined as immediate cutaneous reactivity to *A. fumigatus* antigens or the presence of specific immunoglobulin E (IgE) antibodies to this species, is proposed to be the first step in the development of ABPA [1]. The National Health and Nutrition Examination Survey 2005–2006, which provides the largest and most recent nationally representative data on IgE-mediated sensitization in the US population, reported a prevalence of *Aspergillus* sensitization of 6.5% [2]. Despite being diagnosed with increasing frequency, the true prevalence of ABPA remains unclear due to the lack of large population-based surveillance studies and the variation in the criteria used in the diagnosis [1]. The prevalence of ABPA in patients with

asthma ranges from 1% to 32% in reported studies [3]. While globally, the burden of ABPA was estimated by Denning et al. [4] to exceed 4.8 million patients (range 1.4–6.8 millions) in an estimated global adult asthma prevalence of 193 million people. The prevalence of ABPA in patients with CF also ranges from 3% to 25% where different diagnostic criteria used in these reports [5]. The Epidemiologic Study of Cystic Fibrosis (ESCF) in North America reported a prevalence rate of only 2.2% [6]. While, the European Epidemiologic Registry of Cystic Fibrosis (ERCF) reported an overall prevalence of 7.8%. ABPA has also been described in patients with hyper-IgE syndrome, chronic granulomatous disease [7,8], and in lung transplant recipient [9].

GENETIC PREDISPOSITION

It is hypothesized that ABPA develops in asthmatic and CF patients due to a combination of genetic susceptibility factors. Genetic studies suggest that HLA-DR2 and DR5 (possibly DR4, DR7) restriction is associated with increased susceptibility to ABPA [10,11]. Furthermore, within HLA-DR2 and HLA-DR5, there are restricted genotypes. In particular, HLA-DRB1*1501, -DRB1*1503, -DRB1*1104, -DRB1*1101, -DRB1*04 and -DRB1*0701 were reported to provide high relative risk. Whereas HLA-DQ2 molecules (especially -DQB1*0201) are associated with resistance [12]. Single nucleotide polymorphisms (SNP) of the IL-4 receptor alpha chain (IL-4Ra) was also reported as a likely susceptibility factor that leads to an increased sensitivity to IL-4 stimulation [13], which, in turn, increases expression of other receptors, including CD23 and CD86 on B cells, and IgE isotype switching and IgE synthesis

[14]. IL-10 polymorphisms were shown to be associated with *Aspergillus* colonization and the development of ABPA in patients with CF [15]. Single nucleotide polymorphisms (SNP) of the IL-13 previously reported to be associated with atopy and asthma may also be important with the development of ABPA [16]. Also, single nucleotide polymorphisms (SNPs) in the collagen region of surfactant proteins A1 (SP-A2) and mannose binding lectin (MBL) may contribute to differential susceptibility of the host to ABPA [17–19]. Susceptibility to allergic bronchopulmonary aspergillosis was also associated with polymorphism of Toll-like receptor 9 [20]. Another possible association of ABPA with duplication of the CHIT1 gene has been reported [21]. CHIT1 gene encodes chitotriosidase, an enzyme that catalyzes the cleavage of chitin present in fungal cell walls, and duplication in the gene is associated with decreased levels and enzymatic activity of chitotriosidase. Interestingly, there is a possible pathogenetic link between CFTR mutations and ABPA [22].

PATHOGENESIS OF ALLERGIC BRONCHOPULMONARY ASPERGILLOSIS

In the proposed model of the immunopathogenesis (see Figure 30.1) of ABPA, *A. fumigatus* spores, 3–5 μm in

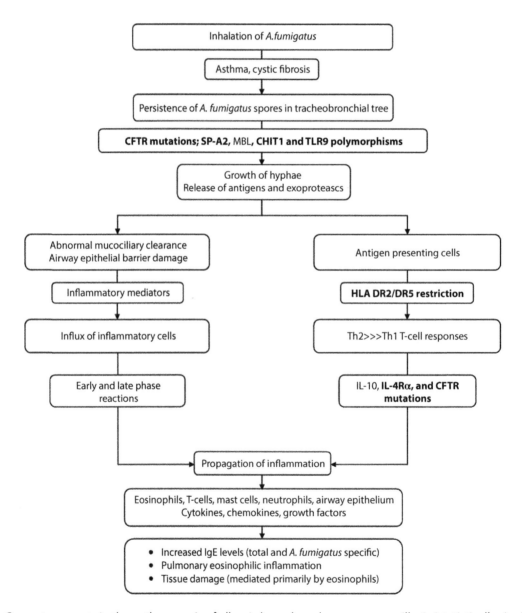

Figure 30.1 Current concepts in the pathogenesis of allergic bronchopulmonary aspergillosis (statistically significant genetic associations have been indicated in bold font). CFTR, CF transmembrane conductance regulator; HLA, human leucocyte antigen; IL, interleukin; SP, surfactant protein; TLR, toll-like receptor. (From Agarwal, R. et al.: ABPA complicating asthma ISHAM working group. Allergic bronchopulmonary aspergillosis: Review of literature and proposal of new diagnostic and classification criteria. *Clin. Exp. Allergy*, 2013, 43, 859. Copyright 2013 by John Wiley & Sons. Reprinted with permission.)

size, are inhaled into the bronchial airway. Fungal conidia are immunologically inert due to the presence of surface hydrophobin that prevents immune recognition of airborne fungal spores [23]. In asthma and cystic fibrosis patients and secondary to defective airway clearance, spores are trapped by the luminal mucus and subsequently germinate, and form mycelia [24]. Normally the hyphal forms are killed by lung macrophages and neutrophils, which are the first line of defense [25,26]. In ABPA, genetic polymorphism defects in the innate immunity can lead to either persistence of *A. fumigatus* in the airways or modify the subsequent immune responses in genetically susceptible asthma and CF patients [27]. *A. fumigatus* releases a variety of proteins, organic acids and fatty acids, such as superoxide dismutases, catalases, proteases, ribotoxin, phospholipases, hemolysin, gliotoxin, phthioic acid, and other toxins [28–35]. In the development of ABPA, it is proposed that *Aspergillus* proteins have a direct effect on the pulmonary epithelia and macrophage inflammation, as it was demonstrated that *Aspergillus* proteases induced epithelial cell detachment [36,37] and induced bronchial cells to produce pro-inflammatory chemokines and cytokines, such as IL-8, IL-6, and monocyte chemoattractant protein (MCP)-1. This protease activity allows for enhanced allergen exposure to the bronchoalveolar lymphoid tissue (BALT) immune system [38]. Hyphae can also be identified within the interstitia of the pulmonary parenchyma in ABPA further allowing for *A. fumigatus* allergens to be exposed to the respiratory epithelium and immune system at high concentrations. Allergens produced by *Aspergillus* mycelia are processed by antigen-presenting cells bearing HLA-DR2 or -DR5 and presented to T-cells within the BALT [38] and on the background of genetic susceptibility [27] in AS and ABPA (The allergic inflammatory response in patients with ABPA appears to be quantitatively greater than that in *Aspergillus* sensitive atopic asthma patients and patients with CF), the T-cell response to *Aspergillus* allergens becomes skewed from a Th1 CD4+ cell response toward a Th2 CD4+ cell response, with synthesis and secretion of IL-4, IL-5, and IL-13 cytokines [38]. This leads to a profound inflammatory reaction including total and *A. fumigatus* specific IgE synthesis, mast cell degranulation and promotion of a strong eosinophilic response. In addition, formation of IgG and IgA antibodies to antigens of *A. fumigatus* also occurs.

The consequences of this response are intense airway inflammation, airway damage, and remodeling with the development of bronchiectasis and fibrosis.

CLINICAL FEATURES AND STAGING OF ABPA

The clinical and diagnostic manifestations of ABPA arise from an allergic response to multiple antigens expressed by *A. fumigatus*, colonizing the bronchial mucus. Patients usually manifest with uncontrolled asthma, wheezing and productive cough. Systemic symptoms of fever, weight loss, malaise and fatigue may also occur. Expectoration of

brownish mucus plugs and hemoptysis can also be seen. Some asthmatic patients may be diagnosed during the screening process [39].

The International Society for Human and Animal Mycology (ISHAM) working group for ABPA proposed a new clinical staging of ABPA in asthma [1] (see Table 30.1).

DIAGNOSIS

The diagnosis of ABPA is currently made on a combination of clinical, radiological and immunological findings. The classic case usually fulfills the following criteria (Patterson criteria) [40–42]: (1) Asthma, (2) current or past chest infiltrates, (3) immediate cutaneous reactivity to *Aspergillus* species, (4) elevated total serum IgE (>417 IU/mL or >1000 ng/mL), (5) serum precipitating antibodies to *A. fumigatus*, (6) central bronchiectasis on chest CT, (7) peripheral blood eosinophilia, (8) elevated serum IgE and/or IgG to *A. fumigatus*. The minimal essential criteria for diagnosis of ABPA include (14): (1) asthma, (2) immediate cutaneous reactivity to *Aspergillus* species, (3) elevated total serum IgE concentration (>417 IU/mL or >1000 ng/mL), (4) elevated serum IgE and IgG to *A. fumigatus*, and (5) central bronchiectasis.

However, the above criteria seem to be too rigid [24]. Although considered a diagnostic feature of ABPA, precipitating antibodies (*A. fumigatus* specific IgG) are present in 69%–90% in patients with ABPA and patients with CF and asthma without ABPA [1,43]. Also, the presence of distal airway obstruction has a low specificity as high percentage of patients with CF have this symptom because of their primary disease [44]. In addition, use of steroids can reduce the total serum IgE concentration to <1000 ng/mL in some patients with ABPA. Furthermore, although peripheral eosinophilia is considered an important criterion for ABPA diagnosis, peripheral eosinophil counts have been found to be of limited value, as only 40% of patients with ABPA presented with an eosinophil count >1000 cells/μL at diagnosis in one of the recent studies [45]. In ABPA, the pulmonary eosinophilia is far greater than peripheral blood with little correlation between the two; thus, a low eosinophil count does not exclude ABPA [46]. Moreover, bronchiectasis often seem to occur too late in the progression of the disease to be valuable in making the diagnosis [47], and, specifically in patients with CF, these findings are often present because of the nature of the disease.

Given that the diagnosis of ABPA in CF is difficult, and may often be delayed, because many of the diagnostic criteria overlap with common manifestations of CF, the Cystic Fibrosis Foundation Consensus proposed the following **minimum criteria** for the diagnosis of ABPA in CF patients [24]:

1. Acute or subacute clinical deterioration not attributable to another etiology.
2. Total serum IgE concentration of >500 IU/mL (1200 ng/mL). If the total IgE level is 200–500 IU/mL, but ABPA is still considered, repeat testing is

Table 30.1 Newly proposed clinical staging of ABPA in asthma

Stage	Definition	Features
0	Asymptomatic	• GINA definition of controlled asthma • On investigation fulfils the diagnostic criteria of ABPA • Has not been previously diagnosed to have ABPA
1	Acute	• Patient has uncontrolled asthma/constitutional symptoms • Fulfils diagnostic criteria for ABPA • Not previously diagnosed to have ABPA
1a	With mucoid impaction	Meets all the criteria and there is documented mucoid impaction on chest radiograph, CT chest or bronchoscopy
1b	Without mucoid impaction	Meets all the criteria and there is no documented mucoid impaction on CT chest or bronchoscopy
2	Response	• Clinical improvement (resolution of constitutional symptoms, improvement in asthma control) • Major radiological improvement[a] • IgE decline by ≥25% of baseline at 8 weeks
3	Exacerbation	Clinical and/or radiological deterioration associated with an increase in IgE by ≥50%
4	Remission	Sustained clinicoradiological improvement with IgE levels remaining at or below baseline (or increase by <50%) for ≥6 months on or off therapy other than systemic glucocorticoids
5a	Treatment-dependent ABPA	If patient has relapse on two or more consecutive occasions within 6 months of stopping treatment or has worsening of clinical, radiological or immunological parameters on tapering oral steroids/azoles
5b	Glucocorticoid-dependent asthma	If the patient requires oral or parenteral glucocorticoids for control of asthma while the activity of ABPA is controlled as reflected by IgE levels and chest radiograph
6	Advanced ABPA	Presence of type II respiratory failure and/or cor pulmonale with radiological evidence of fibrotic findings consistent with ABPA on HRCT of the chest after excluding reversible causes of acute respiratory failure

Source: Agarwal, R. et al.: ABPA complicating asthma ISHAM working group. Allergic bronchopulmonary aspergillosis: Review of literature and proposal of new diagnostic and classification criteria. Clin. Exp. Allergy, 2013, 43, 850–873. Copyright 2013 by John Wiley & Sons. With permission.
Note: Permanent changes like cystic opacities/fibrosis should not be considered in radiological remission.
[a] CT, computed tomography; HRCT, high-resolution CT; GINA, global initiative for asthma.

recommended in 1–3 months or after steroids are discontinued.

3. Positive Aspergillus skin test or presence of serum A. fumigatus specific IgE antibody
4. One of the following:
   a. Precipitins or serum IgG antibodies to A. fumigatus
   b. New or recent abnormalities on chest radiography (infiltrates or mucus plugging) or chest CT (central bronchiectasis) that have not cleared with standard therapy.

While the **classic case** of ABPA is defined by meeting all the previous criteria with a total IgE concentration of >1000 IU/mL (2400 ng/mL), unless patient is receiving systemic corticosteroids in such case, testing should be repeated after steroid treatment is discontinued.

More recent studies evaluated IgE cutoffs to differentiate ABPA from Aspergillus-sensitized asthma or CF patients [1,48].

In a series of 146 CF patients [48], serologic ABPA and Aspergillus-sensitized CF patients were separated from each other using total IgE levels. Applying consensus criteria in ROC-curve analysis, showed that a value of >500 IU/mL (minimum diagnostic criteria for ABPA) separates ABPA from all other patient groups with a sensitivity of 70% and a specificity of 99%, whereas a level of >1000 IU/mL (classic ABPA) gives a sensitivity of 39% and a specificity of 100%. ROC-curve analysis shows that the optimum level is >185 IU/mL, giving 91% sensitivity and 90% specificity (AUC 0.97). On the other hand, in another series [1] of 372 asthmatic patients, ABPA (56 patients) was separated from asthma using the best cut-off values of total IgE of 2346.5 IU/mL (sensitivity 87.5%, specificity 66.9%, AUC 87.7%). So a cut-off of 500 IU/mL may lead to over-diagnosis of ABPA as these levels are often encountered in AS.

In 2013, The International Society for Human and Animal Mycology (ISHAM) working group for ABPA formulated new diagnostic criteria with an aim to improve the diagnosis and care of patients with ABPA and limit the weaknesses of the previous criteria. According to the new proposed criteria, the diagnosis of allergic bronchopulmonary aspergillosis requires the following [1]:

Predisposing conditions (one must be present):
- Bronchial asthma
- Cystic fibrosis

Obligatory criteria (both should be present):
- Positive *Aspergillus* skin test or elevated IgE levels against *A. fumigatus* (cut-off >0.35kUA/L)
- Elevated total IgE levels (>1000 IU/mL) and if the patient meets all other criteria, an IgE value <1000 IU/mL may be acceptable

Other criteria (at least two of three):
- IgG antibodies against *A. fumigatus* in serum
- Radiographic pulmonary opacities consistent with ABPA
- Total eosinophil count >500 cells/μL in steroid naive patients (may be historical)

RADIOLOGICAL FEATURES AND CLASSIFICATION

Chest radiographic findings [75–77] include consolidations, nodules, tram-track opacities (dilated bronchus visualized in a coronal plane), ring shadows (dilated bronchi seen in an en face orientation), finger-in-glove opacities (mucoid impaction

in the large airways), and fleeting opacities. High resolution CT scan is more sensitive than chest X-ray for the detection of abnormalities and is considered the radiologic modality of choice. Findings on CT chest include bronchiectasis (central bronchiectasis is believed to be one of the hallmarks of ABPA, but it can also extend into the periphery), mucus impaction, atelectasis, and nodules. Cavities and pleuropulmonary fibrosis are usually suggestive of the development of chronic pulmonary aspergillosis (see Table 30.2) for the newly proposed radiological classification of APBA by the International Society for Human and Animal Mycology (ISHAM) working group for ABPA in asthma [1].

SCREENING FOR ABPA

In order to investigate ABPA in patients with asthma [1], it is recommended to perform cutaneous testing for *Aspergillus* or *A. fumigatus* specific IgE levels with the latter being more sensitive [49] (see Figure 30.2). If either is positive, total serum IgE level should be obtained and if it is above 1000 IU/mL further serologic and radiologic testing should follow to determine whether minimum diagnostic criteria are met. The Cystic Fibrosis Foundation Consensus recommendations for screening for ABPA in CF [24] advocate to maintain a high level of suspicion for ABPA in patients >6 years of age and to measure total serum IgE annually. Two scenarios are described: if total serum IgE is >500 IU/mL, immediate cutaneous reactivity to *A. fumigatus* should be done and the diagnosis of ABPA should be considered based on the minimal criteria described above. If total serum IgE level is between 200 and 500 IU/mL, it is recommended to repeat IgE level measurement and perform further diagnostic tests if suspicion is high.

Table 30.2 Newly proposed radiological classification of ABPA based on computed tomographic (CT) chest findings

Classification	Features
ABPA-S (Serological ABPA)	All the diagnostic features of ABPA but no abnormality resulting from ABPA on HRCT chest[a]
ABPA-B (ABPA with bronchiectasis)	All the diagnostic features of ABPA including bronchiectasis on HRCT chest
ABPA-HAM (ABPA with high-attenuation mucus)	All the diagnostic features of ABPA including presence of high-attenuation mucus
ABPA-CPF (ABPA with chronic pleuropulmonary fibrosis)	ABPA with at least two to three other radiological features such as pulmonary fibrosis, parenchymal scarring, fibro-cavitary lesions, aspergilloma and pleural thickening without presence of mucoid impaction, or high-attenuation mucus

Source: Agarwal, R. et al.: ABPA complicating asthma ISHAM working group. Allergic bronchopulmonary aspergillosis: Review of literature and proposal of new diagnostic and classification criteria. *Clin. Exp. Allergy*, 2013, 43, 850–873. Copyright 2013 by John Wiley & Sons. With permission.

Abbreviations: HRCT, high-resolution CT; ABPA, allergic bronchopulmonary aspergillosis.

[a] Findings resulting from co-existent disease, bullae from asthma, tracheomalacia, etc. should not be considered while labelling the patients as ABPA-S.

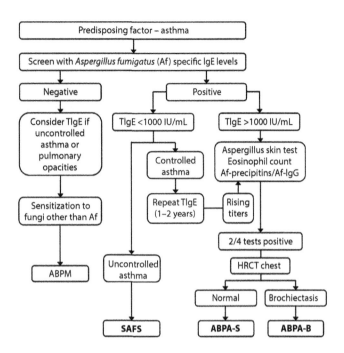

Figure 30.2 Protocol for investigating allergic bronchopulmonary aspergillosis (ABPA) in patients with asthma. (From Agarwal, R. et al.: ABPA complicating asthma ISHAM working group. Allergic bronchopulmonary aspergillosis: Review of literature and proposal of new diagnostic and classification criteria. *Clin, Exp. Allergy*, 2013, 43, 859. Copyright 2013 by John Wiley & Sons. Reprinted with permission.)

TREATMENT

Therapy for ABPA consists of prevention and treatment of acute exacerbations, to prevent development of bronchiectasis and end-stage fibrotic disease [50]. There are two strategies for treatment of ABPA [50]. The first is the attenuation of the inflammation and immunologic response, for which corticosteroids are the mainstay of therapy. The second is the attenuation of the antigen burden arising from fungal colonization of the bronchial tree. Oral corticosteroids are the mainstay of treatment of ABPA. Two regimens of oral corticosteroids are used in clinical practice [39,51]. One regimen [51] uses an initial dose of 0.5 mg/kg daily of prednisone for two weeks, followed by alternate days for 6–8 weeks, this is followed by further tapering by 5–10 mg every two weeks and discontinuation at 3 months. The other regimen [39] uses an initial dose of 0.75 mg/kg for 6 weeks, followed by 0.5 mg/kg for 6 weeks, then taper by 5 mg every 6 weeks to continue for a total duration of at least 6–12 months. The efficacy and safety of the two steroids regimens for the treatment of treatment-naive ABPA patients complicating asthma was compared in a recent randomized controlled trial [52]. There was no difference

in the numbers of subjects with exacerbation after 1 year and glucocorticoid-dependent ABPA after 2 years between the two groups. Furthermore, improvement in lung function and time to first exacerbation were similar in the two groups. However, cumulative glucocorticoid dose and side-effects were significantly higher in the high-dose group suggesting that medium-dose oral glucocorticoids are as effective and safer than high-dose in treatment of ABPA.

Reducing the fungal burden in the respiratory tract by using an antifungal might decrease antigenic stimulation, reduce inflammatory response, ameliorate symptoms, and possibly reduce the long-term risk of disease progression. In this regard, two double blinded randomized control studies have evaluated itraconazole in ABPA. One trial [53] randomized patients with stable ABPA to receive itraconazole (200 mg twice daily orally for 16 weeks) or placebo. Treatment with itraconazole reduced eosinophilic airway inflammation, serum IgE levels and exacerbations requiring oral corticosteroids therapy compared to the control group. The second study [54] randomized patient with corticosteroid-dependent ABPA to receive itraconazole or placebo. Treatment group was reported to have more response defined as a reduction of at least 50% in the corticosteroid dose, a decrease of at least 25% in the serum IgE concentration and improvement of at least 25% in exercise tolerance or pulmonary-function tests or resolution or absence of pulmonary infiltrates. A randomized controlled [1] trial to study the efficacy of itraconazole monotherapy vs. prednisolone in ABPA (MIPA study; clinical trials.gov; NCT01321827) is underway. Newer antifungal agents, including voriconazole and posaconazole, seem to be effective [55] but were not compared to itraconazole in controlled studies. Inhaled amphotericin B has been reported to be effective in case reports and case series [56] as an adjunctive treatment in ABPA. Two randomized controlled trails are underway comparing nebulized amphotericin B combined with an inhaled GCS to inhaled GCS monotherapy or placebo in the maintenance of ABPA remission (NCT01857479 and NCT02273661 respectively).

High dose pulse- IV- steroids therapy seems to be effective in patients with CF and refractory ABPA in uncontrolled studies [57,58]. Omalizumab, a humanized monoclonal antibody against IgE was effective in the treatment of ABPA in the setting of poorly-controlled asthma [59] in a randomized, double-blind, placebo-controlled in adult asthmatics with ABPA using a cross-over design and dose of 750 mg monthly. Exacerbations occurred less frequently during the active treatment phase compared to placebo periods. Proof of efficacy in the treatment of ABPA in patients with cystic fibrosis (CF) awaits validation in clinical trials. Several case reports and small series described the clinical benefit of using inhaled steroid (ICS) in the treatment of ABPA in asthmatic patients [60–63]. However, the only double-blind, placebo-controlled trial of inhaled steroids using beclomethasone at a dose of 400 μg daily for ABPA conducted by the British Thoracic Society failed to show a statistically significant benefit [64]. Furthermore, there are now numerous reports of toxicity associated with using budesonide in combination with itraconazole resulting in adrenal suppression in both asthma and CF patients with ABPA [65–69] owing to itraconazole inhibition of the hepatic cytochrome P4503A4, which is responsible for metabolic detoxification of budesonide. The lack of clearly established benefit coupled with concerns for toxicity lead to great caution when considering use of inhaled steroids especially budesonide in combination with itraconazole to treat ABPA. Thus, high dose of ICS alone has no role in the management of ABPA and can be used for the control of asthma once oral prednisone dose is reduced to below 10 mg/day [1].

1. **Choice of therapy:**
    The Cystic Fibrosis Foundation Consensus recommends treating all exacerbations of ABPA in CF with systemic steroids unless there is a contradiction to their use [24].

    While combination therapy with itraconazole is recommended if slow or poor response to corticosteroids, relapse, corticosteroid-dependent, or corticosteroid toxicity.

    The International Society for Human and Animal Mycology (ISHAM) working group for ABPA in asthma [1] recommends treatment with oral steroids in ABPA with mucoid impaction or ABPA with significant deterioration of lung function attributed to worsening asthma or ABPA (and not intercurrent infection). Azoles were recommended (with or without concomitant steroids) for the treatment of ABPA with recurrent exacerbations (to prevent exacerbations after controlling the exacerbation with glucocorticoids) and in glucocorticoid-dependent ABPA. In addition, the Infectious Disease Society of America [50] suggests treatment with oral itraconazole therapy with therapeutic drug monitoring (TDM) in asthmatic patients with bronchiectasis or mucoid impaction who remain symptomatic despite oral or inhaled corticosteroid therapy.

2. **Follow up and monitoring:**
    Patients on treatment should initially be followed every 6–8 weeks with serum IgE levels, chest radiograph, and lung function test [1]. Effectiveness of therapy is reflected by decrease in the patient's total serum IgE levels (by 25%–50%) along with symptomatic and radiological improvements.

COMPLICATIONS

Complications [1] of ABPA include recurrent exacerbations, atelectasis due to mucus impaction, bronchiectasis, aspergilloma [70], chronic pulmonary aspergillosis [71], and pulmonary hypertension, if not treated appropriately [72].

OTHER PULMONARY ALLERGIC CONDITIONS

1. **Allergic bronchopulmonary mycosis:**
    Allergic bronchopulmonary mycosis is an ABPA-like syndrome caused by fungi other than *A. fumigatus* with similar diagnostic criteria except sensitization to other fungi needs to be documented [72].
2. **Severe asthma with fungal sensitization:**
    Severe asthma with fungal sensitization (SAFS) is characterized by persistent severe asthma (despite standard treatment) and evidence of fungal sensitization, as defined by positive prick test, or fungal antigen-specific blood IgE testing, that do not meet the criteria for ABPA (total IgE <1000 IU/mL) (Figure 30.2) [73,74].

CHAPTER QUESTIONS

Q: Is demonstration of central bronchiectasis on chest imaging is required for diagnosis of ABPA?

A: No, central bronchiectasis should be considered a complication of ABPA and not a major diagnostic criteria. Patients who meet diagnostic criteria but has no abnormalities resulting from ABPA on high-resolution CT scan of the chest (including bronchiectasis) are considered to have serological ABPA. Ideally, these individuals should be identified early in the course of the disease to mitigate or even prevent the progressive bronchial injury that may lead to central bronchiectasis.

Q: What is the first step for the diagnosis of ABPA?

A: ABPA is an advanced stage of *Aspergillus* sensitization (AS) with AS being the first pathogenetic step in development of ABPA. Thus, the first step in diagnosis is documenting sensitivity to *Aspergillus* with either immediate cutaneous hypersensitivity or elevated IgE levels against *A. fumigatus*.

Q: What is the diagnostic value of total IgE level during workup of ABPA?

A: Total IgE level is a useful test in diagnosis of ABPA. A normal total IgE level in the absence of systemic steroid therapy generally excludes active ABPA as the cause of patient's current symptoms.

Q: What is the role of total IgE level in follow up of ABPA?

A: Total IgE level is used to follow up response to treatment in ABPA patients. Response to treatment is associated with 25%–50% decline (but not normalization) of total IgE levels along with clinical and radiologic improvement. An exacerbation of ABPA is associated with an increase in IgE level by 50% of baseline along with clinical and radiologic worsening.

REFERENCES

1. Agarwal R, Chakrabarti A, Shah A, Gupta D, Meis JF, Guleria R, Moss R, Denning DW; ABPA complicating asthma ISHAM working group. Allergic broncho-pulmonary aspergillosis: Review of literature and proposal of new diagnostic and classification criteria. *Clin Exp Allergy* 2013;43:850–873.

2. Gergen PJ, Arbes SJ Jr, Calatroni A, Mitchell HE, Zeldin DC. Total IgE levels and asthma prevalence in the US population: Results from the National Health and Nutrition Examination Survey 2005–2006. *J Allergy Clin Immunol* 2009;124:447–453.

3. Agarwal R, Aggarwal AN, Gupta D, Jindal SK. *Aspergillus* hypersensitivity and allergic broncho-pulmonary aspergillosis in patients with bronchial asthma: Systematic review and meta-analysis. *Int J Tuberc Lung Dis* 2009;13(8):936–944.

4. Denning DW, Pleuvry A, Cole DC. Global burden of allergic bronchopulmonary aspergillosis with asthma and its complication chronic pulmonary aspergillosis in adults. *Med Mycol* 2013;51(4):361–370.

5. Maturu VN, Agarwal R. Prevalence of *Aspergillus* sensitization and allergic bronchopulmo-nary aspergillosis in cystic fibrosis: Systematic review and meta-analysis. *Clin Exp Allergy* 2015;45(12):1765–1778.

6. Mastella G, Rainisio M, Harms HK, et al. Allergic bronchopulmonary aspergillosis in cystic fibrosis. A European epidemiological study. Epidemiologic registry of cystic fibrosis. *Eur Respir J* 2000;16 (3):464–471.

7. Geller DE, Kaplowitz H, Light MJ, et al. Allergic bronchopulmonary aspergillosis in cystic fibro-sis: Reported prevalence, regional distribution, and patient characteristics. Scientific Advisory Group, Investigators, and Coordinators of the Epidemiologic Study of Cystic Fibrosis. *Chest* 1999;116(3):639–646.

8. Eppinger TM, Greenberger PA, White DA, et al. Sensitization to Aspergillus species in the congenital neutrophil disorders chronic granulomatous disease and hyper-IgE syndrome. *J Allergy Clin Immunol* 1999;104(6):1265–1272.

9. Cerceo E, Kotloff RM, Hadjiliadis D, et al. Central airways obstruction due to *Aspergillus fumigatus* after lung transplantation. *J Heart Lung Transplant.* 2009;28(5):515–519.

10. Aron Y, Bienvenu T, Hubert D, Dusser D, Dall'Ava J, Polla BS. HLA-DR polymorphism in allergic bron-chopulmonary aspergillosis. *J Allergy Clin Immunol* 1999;104:891–892.

11. Chauhan B, Santiago L, Hutcheson PS, et al. Evidence for the involvement of two different MHC class II regions in susceptibility or protection in aller-gic bronchopulmonary aspergillosis. *J Allergy Clin Immunol* 2000;106:723–729.

12. Muro M, Mondejar-Lopez P, Moya-Quiles MR, et al. HLA-DRB1 and HLADQB1 genes on susceptibility to and protection from allergic bronchopulmo-nary aspergillosis in patients with cystic fibrosis. *Microbiol Immunol* 2013;57:193–197.

13. Knutsen AP, Kariuki B, Consolino JD, Warrier MR. IL-4 alpha chain receptor (IL-4Ralpha) polymorphisms in allergic bronchopulmonary sspergillosis. *Clin Mol Allergy* 2006;4:3.

14. Khan SP, McClellan JS, Knutsen AP. Increased sensitivity to IL-4 in patients with allergic bronchopulmonary aspergillosis and atopy. *Int Arch Allergy Immunol* 2000;123:319–326.

15. Brouard J, Knauer N, Boelle PY, et al. Influence of interleukin-10 on *Aspergillus fumigatus* infec-tion in patients with cystic fibrosis. *J Infect Dis* 2005;191:1988–1989.

16. Knutsen A. Genetic and respiratory tract risk fac-tors for aspergillosis: ABPA and asthma with fungal sensitization. *Med Mycol* 2006;44:S61–S70.

17. Vaid M, Kaur S, Sambatakou H, Madan T, Denning DW, Sarma PU. Distinct alleles of mannose-binding lectin (MBL) and surfactant proteins A (SP-A) in patients with chronic cavitary pulmonary aspergil-losis and allergic bronchopulmonary aspergillosis. *Clin Chem Lab Med* 2007;45:183–186.

18. Kaur S, Gupta VK, Shah A, Thiel S, Sarma PU, Madan T. Elevated levels of mannan-binding lectin (MBL) and eosinophilia in patients of bronchial asthma with allergic rhinitis and allergic bronchopulmonary aspergillosis associate with a novel intronic polymor-phism in MBL. *Clin Exp Immunol* 2006;143:414–419.

19. Harrison E, Singh A, Morris J, et al. Mannose-binding lectin genotype and serum levels in patients with chronic and allergic pulmonary aspergillosis. *Int J Immunogenet* 2012;39:224–232.

20. Carvalho A, Pasqualotto AC, Pitzurra L, Romani L, Denning DW, Rodrigues F. Polymorphisms in toll-like receptor genes and susceptibility to pulmonary aspergillosis. *J Infect Dis* 2008;197:618–621.

21. Vicencio AG, Chupp GL, Tsirilakis K, et al. CHIT1 mutations: Genetic risk factor for severe asthma with fungal sensitization? *Pediatrics* 2010;126:e982–e985.

22. Agarwal R, Khan A, Aggarwal AN, Gupta D. Link between CFTR mutations and ABPA: A systematic review and meta-analysis. *Mycoses* 2012;55:357–365.

23. Aimanianda V, Bayry J, Bozza S, et al. Surface hydro-phobin prevents immune recognition of airborne fungal spores. *Nature.* 2009;460(7259):1117.

24. Stevens DA, Moss RB, Kurup VP, et al. Allergic bron-chopulmonary aspergillosis in cystic fibrosis—State of the art: Cystic Fibrosis Foundation Consensus Conference. *Clin Infect Dis* 2003;37(Suppl 3):S225–S264.

25. Schaffner A, Douglas H, Braude A. Selective protec-tion against conidia by mononuclear and mycelia by polymorphonuclear phagocytes in resistance

to *Aspergillus*: Observations on these two lines of defense in vivo and in vitro with human and mouse phagocytes. *J Clin Invest* 1982;69: 617–631.

26. Roilides E, Uhlig K, Venzon D, Pizzo PA, Walsh TJ. Prevention of corticosteroid-induced suppression of human polymorphonuclear leukocyte-induced damage of *Aspergillus fumigatus* hyphae by granulocyte colony-stimulating factor and gamma interferon. *Infect Immun* 1993;61: 4870–4877.

27. Agarwal R. Allergic bronchopulmonary aspergillosis: Lessons learnt from genetics. *Indian J Chest Dis Allied Sci* 2011;53:137–140.

28. Markaryan A, Morozova I, Yu H, et al. Purification and characterization of an elastinolytic metalloprotease from *Aspergillus fumigatus* and immunoelectron microscopic evidence of secretion of this enzyme by the fungus invading the murine lung. *Infect Immun* 1994;62(6):2149–2157.

29. Reichard U, Monod M, Odds F, et al. Virulence of an aspergillopepsin-deficient mutant of *Aspergillus fumigatus* and evidence for another aspartic proteinase linked to the fungal cell wall. *J Med Vet Mycol* 1997;35(3):189–196.

30. Latge JP, Moutaouakil M, Debeaupuis JP, et al. The 18-kilodalton antigen secreted by *Aspergillus fumigatus*. *Infect Immun* 1991;59(8):2586–2594.

31. Arruda LK, Mann BJ, Chapman MD. Selective expression of a major allergen and cytotoxin, Asp f I, in *Aspergillus* fumigatus. Implications for the immunopathogenesis of *Aspergillus*-related diseases. *J Immunol* 1992;149(10):3354–3359.

32. Birch M, Robson G, Law D, et al. Evidence of multiple extracellular phospholipase activities of *Aspergillus fumigatus*. *Infect Immun* 1996;64(3):751–755.

33. Ebina K, Sakagami H, Yokota K, et al. Cloning and nucleotide sequence of cDNA encoding Asp- hemolysin from *Aspergillus* fumigatus. *Biochim Biophys Acta* 1994;1219(1):148–150.

34. Sutton P, Waring P, Mullbacher A. Exacerbation of invasive aspergillosis by the immunosuppressive fungal metabolite, gliotoxin. *Immunol Cell Biol* 1996;74(4):318–322.

35. Birch M, Drucker DB, Boote V, et al. Prevalence of phthioic acid in *Aspergillus* species. *J Med Vet Mycol* 1997;35(2):143–145.

36. Robinson BW, Venaille TJ, Mendis AH, McAleer R. Allergens as proteases: An *Aspergillus fumigatus* proteinase directly induces human epithelial cell detachment. *J Allergy Clin Immunol.* 1990;86:726–731.

37. Tomee JFC, Wierenga ATJ, Hiemstra PS, Kauffman HF. Proteases from *Aspergillus fumigatus* induce release of proinflammatory cytokines and cell detachment in airway epithelial cell lines. *J Infect Dis* 1997;176: 300–303.

38. Knutsen AP, Bellone C, Kauffman H. Immunopathogenesis of allergic bronchopulmonary aspergillosis in cystic fibrosis. *J Cyst Fibros* 2002;1(2):76–89.

39. Agarwal R, Gupta D, Aggarwal AN, Behera D, Jindal SK. Allergic bronchopulmonary aspergillosis: Lessons from 126 patients attending a chest clinic in north India. *Chest* 2006;130:442–448.

40. Rosenberg M, Patterson R, Mintzer R, Cooper BJ, Roberts M, Harris KE. Clinical and immunologic criteria for the diagnosis of allergic bronchopulmonary aspergillosis. *Ann Intern Med* 1977;86:405–414.

41. Greenberger PA, Patterson R. Diagnosis and management of allergic bronchopulmonary aspergillosis. *Ann Allergy* 1986;56:444–452.

42. Patterson R, Greenberger PA, Halwig JM, Liotta JL, Roberts M. Allergic bronchopulmonary aspergillosis. Natural history and classification of early disease by serologic and roentgenographic studies. *Arch Intern Med* 1986;146:916–918.

43. Hutcheson PS, Knutsen AP, Rejent AJ, Slavin RG. A 12-year longitudinal study of *Aspergillus* sensitivity in cystic fibrosis patients. *Chest* 1996;110:363–366.

44. Hodson ME. Respiratory system—adults. In: Hodson ME, Geddes D, editors. *Cystic Fibrosis*. London UK: Chapman & Hall, 1995:pp. 37–57.

45. Agarwal R, Khan A, Aggarwal AN, et al. Clinical relevance of peripheral blood eosinophil count in allergic bronchopulmonary aspergillosis. *J Infect Public Health* 2011;4:235–243.

46. Wark PA, Saltos N, Simpson J, Slater S, Hensley MJ, Gibson PG. Induced sputum eosinophils and neutrophils and bronchiectasis severity in allergic bronchopulmonary aspergillosis. *Eur Respir J* 2000;16:1095–1101.

47. Laufer P, Fink JN, Burns WT, et al. Allergic bronchopulmonary aspergillosis in cystic fibrosis. *J Allergy Clin Immunol* 1984;73:44–48.

48. Baxter CG, Dunn G, Jones AM, Webb K, Gore R, Richardson MD, Denning DW. Novel immunologic classification of aspergillosis in adult cystic fibrosis. *J Allergy Clin Immunol* 2013;132:560–566.e10.

49. Agarwal R, Maskey D, Aggarwal AN, et al. Diagnostic performance of various tests and criteria employed in allergic bronchopulmonary aspergillosis: A latent class analysis. *PLoS One* 2013;8:e61105.

50. Patterson TF, Thompson GR 3rd, Denning DW, Fishman JA, Hadley S, Herbrecht R, Kontoyiannis DP, Marr KA, Morrison VA, Nguyen MH, Segal BH, Steinbach WJ, Stevens DA, Walsh TJ, Wingard JR, Young JH, Bennett JE. Practice guidelines for the diagnosis and management of Aspergillosis: 2016 Update by the Infectious Diseases Society of America. *Clin Infect Dis* 2016;pii: ciw326.

51. Vlahakis NE, Aksamit TR. Diagnosis and treatment of allergic bronchopulmonary aspergillosis. *Mayo Clin Proc* 2001;76:930–938.

52. Agarwal R, Aggarwal AN, Dhooria S, Singh Sehgal I, Garg M, Saikia B, Behera D, Chakrabarti A. A randomised trial of glucocorticoids in acute-stage allergic bronchopulmonary aspergillosis complicating asthma. *Eur Respir J* 2016;47:490–498.

53. Wark PA, Hensley MJ, Saltos N, et al. Anti-inflammatory effect of itraconazole in stable allergic bronchopulmonary aspergillosis: A randomized controlled trial. *J Allergy Clin Immunol* 2003;111(5):952–957.

54. Stevens DA, Schwartz HJ, Lee JY, et al. A randomized trial of itraconazole in allergic bronchopulmonary aspergillosis. *N Engl J Med* 2000;342(11):756–762.

55. Chishimba L, Niven RM, Cooley J, Denning DW. Voriconazole and posaconazole improve asthma severity in allergic bronchopulmonary aspergillosis and severe asthma with fungal sensitization. *J Asthma* 2012;49:423–433.

56. Sehgal IS, Agarwal R. Role of inhaled amphotericin in allergic bronchopulmonary aspergillosis. *J Postgrad Med* 2014;60:41–45.

57. Skov M, Pressler T. High-dose IV-pulse methylprednisolone (HDIVPM) successful treatment of allergic bronchopulmonary aspergillosis (ABPA). *Pediatr Pulmonol* 2010;45:365.

58. Thomas MF. Life-threatening allergic bronchopulomnary aspergillosis treated with methylprednisolone and anti-IgE monoclonal antibody. *J R Soc Med* 2009;102: 49–53.

59. Voskamp AL, Gillman A, Symons K, Sandrini A, Rolland JM, O'Hehir RE, Douglass JA. Clinical efficacy and immunologic effects of omalizumab in allergic bronchopulmonary aspergillosis. *J Allergy Clin Immunol Pract* 2015;3(2):192–199. Epub 2015 Jan 29.

60. Balter MS, Rebuck AS. Treatment of allergic bronchopulmonary aspergillosis with inhaled corticosteroids. *Respir Med* 1992;86(5):441–442.

61. Seaton A, Seaton RA, Wightman AJ. Management of allergic bronchopulmonary aspergillosis without maintenance oral corticosteroids: A fifteen-year follow-up. *QJM* 1994;87(9):529–537.

62. Imbeault B, Cormier Y. Usefulness of inhaled high-dose corticosteroids in allergic bronchopulmonary aspergillosis. *Chest* 1993;103(5):1614–1617.

63. Heinig JH, Weeke ER, Groth S, et al. High-dose local steroid treatment in bronchopulmonary aspergillosis. A pilot study. *Allergy* 1988;43(1):24–31.

64. Inhaled beclomethasone dipropionate in allergic bronchopulmonary aspergillosis. Report to the Research Committee of the British Thoracic Association. *Br J Dis Chest* 1979;73(4):349–356.

65. Parmar JS, Howell T, Kelly J, et al. Profound adrenal suppression secondary to treatment with low dose inhaled steroids and itraconazole in allergic bronchopulmonary aspergillosis in cystic fibrosis. *Thorax* 2002;57(8):749–750.

66. Bolland MJ, Bagg W, Thomas MG, et al. Cushing's syndrome due to interaction between inhaled corticosteroids and itraconazole. *Ann Pharmacother* 2004;38(1):46–49.

67. De Wachter E, Malfroot A, De Schutter I, et al. Inhaled budesonide induced Cushing's syndrome in cystic fibrosis patients, due to drug inhibition of cytochrome P450. *J Cyst Fibros* 2003;2(2):72–75.

68. De Wachter E, Vanbesien J, De Schutter I, et al. Rapidly developing Cushing syndrome in a 4-year-old patient during combined treatment with itraconazole and inhaled budesonide. *Eur J Pediatr* 2003;162(7–8):488–489.

69. Skov M, Main KM, Sillesen IB, et al. Iatrogenic adrenal insufficiency as a side-effect of combined treatment of itraconazole and budesonide. *Eur Respir J* 2002;20(1):127–133.

70. Shah A, Panjabi C. Contemporaneous occurrence of allergic bronchopulmonary aspergillosis, allergic Aspergillus sinusitis, and aspergilloma. *Ann Allergy Asthma Immunol* 2006;96(6):874–878.

71. Lowes D, Chishimba L, Greaves M, Denning DW. Development of chronic pulmonary aspergillosis in adult asthmatics with ABPA. *Respir Med* 2015;109(12):1509.

72. Chowdhary A, Agarwal K, Kathuria S, Gaur SN, Randhawa HS, Meis JF. Allergic bronchopulmonary mycosis due to fungi other than *Aspergillus*: A global overview. *Crit Rev Microbiol* 2014;40(1):30–48.

73. Pasqualotto AC, Powell G, Niven R, Denning DW. The effects of antifungal therapy on severe asthma with fungal sensitization and allergic bronchopulmonary aspergillosis. *Respirology* 2009;14:1121–1127.

74. Denning DW, O'Driscoll BR, Hogaboam CM, Bowyer P, Niven R. The link between fungi and asthma—a summary of the evidence. *Eur Respir J* 2006;27: 615–626.

75. Greenberger PA. Allergic bronchopulmonary aspergillosis. *J Allergy Clin Immunol* 2002;110(5):685–692.

76. Agarwal R, Khan A, Garg M, Aggarwal AN, Gupta D. Chest radiographic and computed tomographic manifestations in allergic bronchopulmonary aspergillosis. *World J Radiol* 2012;4:141–150.

77. Shah A. Allergic bronchopulmonary and sinus aspergillosis: The roentgenologic spectrum. *Front Biosci* 2003;8:e138–e146.

31

Fungal infections of the genitourinary tract

RAYMOND R. RACKLEY AND JESSICA C. LLOYD

INTRODUCTION

Fungal infections of the urinary tract encompass a broad variety of fungi including the endemic mycoses, *Cryptococcus* species, and opportunistic pathogens such as *Aspergillus* species [1–3]. However, the overwhelming majority of fungal infections of the urinary tract are caused by *Candida* spp. The escalating use of broad-spectrum antimicrobial agents, corticosteroids, and immunosuppressive and cytotoxic drugs with the frequent use of indwelling urinary catheters have been implicated as risk factors for *Candida* urinary tract infections (UTIs) [4]. The Presence of candiduria may signal diverse pathological states including invasive renal parenchymal disease, fungal bezoars in obstructed ureters, superficial lower urinary tract infection, and lower urinary tract candidal colonization associated with urinary catheterization. Accordingly, the spectrum of clinical disease embraces asymptomatic candiduria, cystitis, pyelonephritis and renal candidiasis. *Candida* spp. have the propensity to cause renal disease by either the hematogenous or the ascending route which is the most common route of *Candida* UTI generally occurring in the setting of bladder instrumentation. Candiduria has always posed a diagnostic and therapeutic challenge as its presence does not always mean infection and may not require treatment. Unfortunately, there are no established diagnostic tests that reliably distinguish infection from colonization. Guidelines for the treatment of candiduria based almost entirely on anecdotal reports and experts' opinion rather than on controlled clinical trials have been suggested by

the Infectious Diseases Society of America (IDSA) and the Mycoses Study Group [5].

The urinary tract is also susceptible to infection by another group of fungi, namely the endemic fungi including *Histoplasma*, *Blastomyces*, and *Coccidioides* spp. However, these pathogens are rarely responsible for the common clinical syndromes of urethritis, cystitis, and pyelonephritis. Instead, they occasionally cause prostatitis, epididymitis, chronic bladder inflammation or ulceration, ureteric obstruction and chronic renal disease [1].

This chapter focuses on the pathogenesis and the spectrum of clinical manifestations of fungal UTIs with a special emphasis placed on various therapeutic approaches.

GENITOURINARY CANDIDIASIS

Epidemiology

Candida is a frequent saprophytic inhabitant of the oral cavity, intestinal tract, external genitalia, urethra, mouth and gastrointestinal tract where 30%–50% of normal individuals are colonized with *Candida* spp. Point prevalence studies indicate that 20%–25% of healthy women have positive vaginal cultures for *Candida albicans* [6]. However, isolation of *Candida* from urine cultures of healthy individuals is rather infrequent. In one study, funguria was found in only 1% of patients; half of them had diabetes mellitus and were receiving antibiotics [7]. In contrast, candiduria is a common problem in hospitalized patients with indwelling urinary catheters occurring in up to 83% of patients with urinary tract drainage devices [4]. *Candida* spp. is responsible for 10%–15% of nosocomial UTIs and up to 26.5% of UTIs in catheterized patients [8–11]. *C. albicans* is the most common pathogen implicated in UTIs in patients admitted to the intensive care unit (ICU) and it ranks second after *Escherichia coli* in non-ICU patients [12,13].

Microbiology

C. albicans is the most common fungal pathogen in UTIs accounting for more than half of the cases of fungal UTIs [4,14]. *C. glabrata* accounts for 25%–35% of infections whereas other *Candida* spp., including *C. tropicalis*, *C. krusei*, and *C. parapsilosis*, account for 8%–28% of cases [1]. *C. parapsilosis* is found more often in urine from neonates and is usually associated with systemic infection in this population [15]. In about 10% of cases, more than one species of *Candida* can be isolated and candiduria cancoexist with or follow bacteriuria [14]. Since many hospital laboratories do not speciate fungus when recovered from urinary culture unless requested to do so, changes in species trends cannot be easily tracked.

Pathogenesis and risk factors

Ascending infection is the most common route for infection of the urinary tract. Women have a shorter urethra and are more prone to develop UTIs by the ascending route secondary to vulvovestibular colonization by *Candida* spp. The presence of urinary devices facilitates the introduction of the organism into the bladder. The pathogenesis of ascending infection with *Candida* spp. is not well known since no animal models exist to study this condition. Ascending infection might lead to upper urinary tract infection in the setting of vesicoureteral reflux or obstruction of the urinary flow resulting in pyelonephritis but rarely leading to disseminated infection such as candidemia. A fungus bezoar consisting of yeast cells, hyphal elements, epithelial and inflammatory cells can form in dilated areas of the urinary tract resulting in a complicated UTI [1,16].

Renal candidiasis is the result of hematogenous seeding of the renal parenchyma. The pathogenesis of hematogenous seeding of *Candida* spp. to the kidney is well established [16–19]. Multiple microabscesses will develop over the cortex secondary to candidemia. *Candida* cells thereafter penetrate through the glomeruli into the proximal tubules to be shed in the urine [19,20]. The presence of yeast in the urine might imply widespread dissemination to many organs. It is believed that *Candida* spp. express special tropism to the kidney. In an autopsy study, renal involvement was noted in 90% of patients dying from disseminated candidiasis. Multiple abscesses in the renal interstitium, the glomeruli, and peritubular vessels associated with papillary necrosis were seen in these autopsies [20,21].

Risk factors for *Candida* UTIs are well described in the literature and include diabetes mellitus, previous use of broad-spectrum antibiotics, corticosteroids and cytotoxic agents, indwelling urinary catheters, old age, malignancy, prior surgical procedures, recent hospitalization, as well as structural and functional abnormalities of the urinary tract [22,23]. Candiduria is a common finding in renal transplant recipients with an incidence rate reaching 11% in one study [24]. Risk factors for *Candida* UTIs in renal transplant recipients are similar to those in hospitalized patients who have not received a transplant. However, in these patients, non-*albicans* spp. are more frequently isolated from the urine. In one study, *C. glabrata* accounted for more than one half (53%) of *Candida* UTIs, followed by *C. albicans* (35%) and *C. parapsilosis* (4%) [23]. This increase in the incidence of *C. glabrata* could be attributed to the overuse of fluconazole prescribed for antifungal prophylaxis which selects for the emergence of *C. glabrata* [24].

Diabetes mellitus is the single most common underlying disease noted in most studies about funguria [4,14]. In one retrospective study, 30% of patients with fungal UTI were diabetic, and in a prospective multicenter surveillance study in the United States, up to 40% of patients with funguria had diabetes [4,22]. This association is related in part to insulin deficiency, which affects the intracellular killing system including the myeloperoxidase, hydrogen peroxide, and the superoxide anion system of polymorphonuclear leukocytes leading to impairment of the phagocytic and fungicidal activity of neutrophils against *Candida* spp. Furthermore, the growth of *Candida* in urine is more enhanced when urinary levels of glucose exceed 150 mg/dl. In addition, female diabetic patients have a higher rate of *Candida* colonization of their perineum putting them at higher risks for *Candida* UTIs. The most important predisposing factor for *Candida* UTIs in the diabetic population is the presence of diabetic autonomic neuropathy leading to a neurogenic bladder that sets up a favorable milieu for fungal UTIs due to stasis of the urine, and in some cases, to the frequent need for instrumentation and use of drainage devices.

Additional risk factors for the development of candiduria include the frequent use of broad-spectrum antibiotics. Antibiotics suppress the normal flora of the perineum and allows the overgrowth of opportunistic fungi with subsequent ingress over the urethra and colonization or infection of the bladder. In one study, *Candida* was found in the urine of 93% of patients who had recently received antibiotics [14]. No antibiotic is exempt from this complication. However, carbapenems and third-generation cephalosporin, such as ceftazidime, were found to be associated with the highest rates of *Candida* colonization [25]. Several mechanisms have been incriminated for the association between antibiotic use and candiduria. Sulfonamides, for example, reduce the neutrophil intracellular killing mechanism of *Candida*. Whereas, tetracycline, doxycycline and aminoglycosides have been shown to suppress neutrophil phagocytosis [26–29]. Besides antibacterial agents, antifungal agents, such as fluconazole, have been shown to favor colonization with *C. glabrata* over *C. albicans* [22]. The time between the onset of candiduria and the use of antibiotics is not well defined. Candiduria might occur during or immediately following antibiotic therapy [1]. Indwelling urinary drainage devices play a major role in predisposition to candiduria. These devices include indwelling urethral catheters, suprapubic catheters, ureteral stents, and nephrostomy tubes. These devices inevitably become colonized with time and serve as a portal of entry for microorganisms into the urinary system. As foreign bodies, they mechanically damage the urinary epithelium and glycosaminoglycan layer and disrupt adequate antibacterial neutrophil function allowing yeast overgrowth. In one study, urinary tract drainage devices were present at the time or within 30 days prior to funguria in 83% of patients [4]. The underlying cause of catheter associated UTIs is related to the formation of a pathogenic biofilm on the surface of the indwelling urinary catheter. A biofilm is a collection of microbial cells on a surface that is surrounded by an extracellular matrix made up of primarily polysaccharide. Formation of biofilm by *Candida* spp. has been demonstrated on a number of devices including central venous catheters, joint devices, dialysis access devices, cardiovascular devices, urinary catheters, penile implants, voice prostheses, dentures, and ocular implants [30,31]. Fluorescence and confocal scanning laser microscopy (CSLM) utilizing carbohydrate specific dyes (e.g., calcofluor and concanavalin A, Con-A) indicated that the *C. albicans* biofilms are encased within a polysaccharide-rich extracellular matrix. *C. albicans* biofilm formation proceeds in an organized fashion through the early, intermediate, and maturation phases of development. Similar stages of development and the presence of extracellular polysaccharide matrix have also been reported for bacterial biofilms [32–34]. In a scanning electron microscopy study of 50 urethral catheters that had been indwelling for a mean of 35 days, 44 catheters had evidence of biofilm formation. Biofilm ranged from 3–490 µm in depth and had visible fungus [35]. Like their bacterial counterparts, biofilm-grown *C. albicans* cells are highly resistant to antimicrobials which explains the high relapse rate of candiduria in the setting of urinary device. Multifactorial mechanisms of resistance in fungal biofilms have been proposed including the physiological state of fungal cells, the steric hindrance or barrier function of the extracellular matrix, the overexpression of drug efflux pumps, the variations in fungal membrane sterol composition, and different developmental phases. Such a broad spectrum of defense is effective against many types of antifungal agents and would explain the difficulty in eradicating candiduria in the presence of urinary catheters [36–38].

It is important to note that all the aforementioned risk factors for candiduria also pre-dispose a patient to bacteriuria. In fact, candiduria per se is almost invariably preceded by bacteriuria. Specific factors that predispose a patient to candiduria but not bacteriuria other than duration of hospitalization have not been identified. More studies are needed to elucidate such factors.

Clinical manifestations

ASYMPTOMATIC CANDIDURIA

Asymptomatic candiduria is the hallmark of hospitalized, debilitated elderly patients with indwelling urinary catheters [16]. Most patients with candiduria have no urinary symptoms. Asymptomatic candiduria is usually a benign condition that rarely leads to candidemia except in the setting of urinary tract obstruction [39]. Conversely, asymptomatic candiduria might be an early predictor or a sign of hematogenous dissemination in critically and chronically ill patients associated with high mortality rates if left untreated [40]. Ultimately, there are only a few widely agreed upon situations in which asymptomatic patients should be treated for candiduria including those with neutropenia or a pending urologic procedure. Additionally, very low birth weight neonates should also be treated as there is a high likelihood that candiduria represents candidemia [41,42].

Finding *Candida* spp. in the urine of an asymptomatic patient is often challenging for clinicians. Such a finding may represent contamination, colonization or a true infection. Contamination can usually be differentiated from urinary tract colonization or UTI by repeating urine cultures to see if yeasts persist. In older women, to eliminate potential contamination by perineal flora, it is often necessary to obtain other samples of urine by sterile bladder catheterization. If the second specimen yields no growth of yeast, contamination by the perineal flora is the likely cause of candiduria and no further action should be undertaken [16]. Diagnostic criteria differentiating between colonization and infection in patients with asymptomatic candiduria are lacking. Pyuria and quantitative cultures of urine have proved to be of little value in separating infection from colonization. Infection occurs at any colony count ranging between 10 and 106 colony forming units (CFU/mL). Kozinn et al. showed that in patients without indwelling urinary catheters, colony counts of more than 10,000 CFU/mL of urine were associated with infection rather than colonization [43]. However, quantitative urine colony counts are of much less value in the catheterized patients. Furthermore, the presence of pyuria in catheterized patients has not been shown to be helpful in differentiating infection from colonization, as an indwelling catheter may in itself lead to pyuria from mechanical irritation of the bladder mucosa. On the other hand, it has been suggested, but never proven, that the presence of pseudohyphae could distinguish fungi causing infection from those colonizing the bladder [16]. In fact, some *Candida* spp. such as *C. glabrata* cannot make pseudohyphae, and *C. albicans* can be induced to form pseudohyphae merely by varying the pH and nutrients in the urine. In the 1970s, it was thought that antibody-coated fungi in the urine could be used as a marker for infection [44–46]. However, this was shown to be a nonspecific finding present in most urine samples tested including those who had no evidence on autopsy of invasive *Candida* spp. in their urinary tract [44].

This diagnostic dilemma of colonization versus infection directly affects the clinician's decision to treat or not to treat when *Candida* spp. are found in the urine of an asymptomatic patient. This dilemma may also influences the interpretation of the results following treatment. Given the benign nature of asymptomatic candiduria and the infrequency of secondary candidemia, there is evidence now to suggest that the most effective treatment modality in patients with asymptomatic candiduria is risk factors modification [10,39]. This approach includes control of diabetes, removal of indwelling catheters, and discontinuation of antibiotics whenever possible. In a prospective, multicenter, placebo-controlled study comparing the efficacy of fluconazole versus placebo in the eradication of candiduria in asymptomatic patients, Sobel et al. found that asymptomatic candiduria resolved with catheter removal in 41% of hospitalized, catheterized patients [15]. After a new catheter was inserted, untreated candiduria resolved in 20% of patients. Although, high short-term rates of eradication of candiduria occurred in patients who received fluconazole therapy, the rate of candiduria 2 weeks after stopping treatment were similar in the fluconazole and placebo arms [15]. In another study, funguria cleared in 75% of untreated patients compared to 35% of patients who underwent catheter removal and 50% of patients who received antifungal therapy [4]. Moreover, there is no evidence that study groups of patients (as opposed to individuals) benefit from therapy and relapse is frequent. Several open randomized trials comparing amphotericin B bladder irrigation and oral fluconazole in the treatment of candiduria have shown similar rates of candiduria recurrence 1 month after therapy [47–49]. However, not all experts agree that persistent asymptomatic candiduria in noncatheterized subjects can simply be observed. They believe that persistent candiduria in non-catheterized subjects should be investigated, since the likelihood of obstruction with stasis is high. The IDSA has issued guidelines for the treatment of candiduria [5]. Because of the increased risk of disseminated disease, they recommend to have the following groups of patients with candiduria treated with antifungal agents: all symptomatic patients, infants with very low birth weights, patients undergoing genitourinary procedures, patients with neutropenia and renal transplant recipients. These recommendations are based on moderate evidence [clinical experience, opinions of respected authorities, descriptive studies, or reports of expert committees (grade III B)].

CYSTITIS

Patients usually present with signs and symptoms of bladder irritation including dysuria, hematuria, frequency, urgency, and suprapubic pain. Cystoscopy typically reveals soft, white, elevated patches with friable mucosa as seen in Figure 31.1 [1]. *Candida* cystitis can lead to the formation of fungus bezoars in the bladder and emphysematous cystitis. Symptomatic cystitis is rare in catheterized and non-catheterized patients as the bladder is usually resistant to *Candida* invasion. In symptomatic patients,

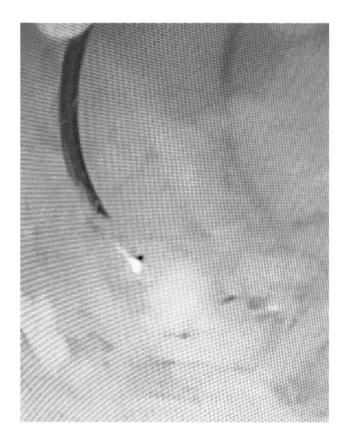

Figure 31.1 Cystoscopic appearance of Candida cystitis reveals the pink and white bladder mucosa with capillaries behind the resection loop and soft, white elevated patches of fungus in the foreground.

candiduria represents true infection; therefore, treatment is recommended. However, many patients with *Candida* cystitis have concomitant bacterial UTI making it difficult to determine whether the symptoms are attributable to *Candida*. Despite these uncertainties, patients with signs and symptoms of cystitis and with only fungus found in culture should be considered as candidates for treatment [5]. Several antifungal agents have been used for the treatment of *Candida* cystitis mainly fluconazole, amphotericin B bladder irrigation and flucytosine [50,51].

Fluconazole, administered orally, remains the first-line treatment regimen for patients with *Candida* UTI because of its favorable pharmacokinetic and safety profiles. Fluconazole is a water-soluble triazole that has an oral bioavailability of more than 90% and is excreted unchanged in the urine to a large degree (80%), with urinary concentration reaching 10 times that of blood [52]. Published experience with other azoles, such as itraconazole and voriconazole, are limited since these agents undergo a high degree of hepatic metabolism and achieve limited concentrations in the urinary tract [52]. The IDSA recommends the use of oral fluconazole in the treatment of *Candida* cystitis at 200 mg daily for 7–14 days [5] Based on the results of a multicenter, randomized, controlled clinical trial, the IDSA recommends 400 mg as the initial dose, followed by 200 mg daily for 14 days [41,53]. Lower doses and shorter courses are discouraged, as *Candida* cystitis should be treated as a complicated urinary tract infection requiring higher dose and longer duration therapy [54].

Continuous bladder irrigation with amphotericin B through an indwelling urinary catheter is an old modality of treatment of *Candida* cystitis first described in 1960 [55]. The eradication rate of candiduria using this therapeutic approach varied from 43% to 100% depending on the study [56,57]. The optimal dose and/or concentration of amphotericin B in bladder irrigation have not been defined yet. Concentrations in most reports ranged from 5 to 50 mg/L [57]. Two randomized trials have compared different concentrations of amphotericin B in bladder irrigation used for the treatment of funguria [48,58–60]. The first one compared concentrations of 5, 100, and 200 mg/L, each administered three times daily for 3 days [48].

Although, on day 1, the efficacy rates for elimination of funguria (~80%–85% for all treatment groups) were significantly better for amphotericin B bladder irrigations than for placebo, by day 10, clearance rates for the three concentrations fell to 42.9%, 68.4%, and 68.2%, respectively. Another randomized study comparing concentrations of 10 mg/L and 50 mg/L administered by continuous irrigation for 72 hours to 26 patients reported efficacy rates of 67% and 100%, respectively [58]. Descriptions of drug administration range from intermittent instillation (up to three times daily with medication dwell times of 2–3 hours) to continuous irrigation (usually via a 3-way Foley catheter) [57]. In spite of all these studies, the optimal method of delivery for amphotericin B bladder irrigation has not been established. A randomized, prospective study compared the efficacy on day 1 of treatment delivered as continuous irrigation of 50 mg/L for 48 hours with that of intermittent instillation of 10 mg/100 mL three times daily [59]. Eight out of ten patients in the continuous infusion group had clearance of fungus from the urine at 72 hours, compared with three of the ten patients in the intermittent treatment group. By day 7, relapse was seen in two patients in the continuous treatment group.

Moreover, the optimal duration of therapy of amphotericin B bladder irrigation is unknown. A single dose has shown limited success for patients without apparent upper tract disease [60] and may not be significantly different from drug delivery for 7 days [47]. A 2-day regimen has also been evaluated with efficacy rates of 75% reported in one study [61]. Despite the lack of solid evidence for the use of amphotericin B bladder irrigation for the treatment of *Candida* cystitis, such treatment strategy is still recommended by some authorities in clinical practice [62]. Adverse effects associated with amphotericin B bladder irrigation have not been frequent and include hematuria, lower abdominal cramping, bladder discomfort, dysuria, and burning during irrigation [58,59].

A single dose of amphotericin B deoxycholate in dosages of 0.3 to 1 mg/kg/day for 1–7 days given intravenously has also been proposed for treatment of funguria but requires parenteral administration and has increased adverse effects compared to fluconazole [63]. Finally, flucytosine has been successfully used in the treatment of urinary candidiasis with response rates of over 90% [64]. It has excellent activity against non-*albicans Candida* spp., especially *C. glabrata*. Flucytosine achieves a high concentration in the urine of patients who do not have advanced renal failure. Its limitation includes bone marrow, hepatic and gastrointestinal toxicity, de novo resistance (25%) observed in *C. albicans* strains, and a rapid tendency to acquired resistance when used as monotherapy. Its use should only be restricted to cases of azole-resistant strains at a dose of 25 mg/kg four times daily given orally for 7–14 days [5].

PYELONEPHRITIS

Patients with infection of the upper urinary tract or pyelonephritis present with fever, leukocytosis, abdominal pain and costovertebral angle tenderness. *Candida* pyelonephritis occurs almost invariably in the setting of urinary obstruction, particularly in patients with diabetes and nephrolithiasis. Candidemia is a rare complication reported only in 3%–10% of cases [39,40]. Fungal bezoar formation is the most serious complication of *Candida* pyelonephritis. While rare, they are typically found in the pelvis or upper ureters, and their presence is suggested by signs of ureteral obstruction associated with candiduria. Upper tract imaging should be strongly considered in patients with fungal pyelonephritis to investigate urinary obstruction; if this is discovered, decompression with a stent or nephrostomy tube is required. Renal colic may occur with the passage of fungal stones, which are portions of fungus bezoars. Excretory urography or retrograde pyelography shows a filling defect in the collecting system. Other complications of *Candida* pyelonephritis include papillary necrosis and local suppurative diseases resulting in pyonephrosis and perinephric or intrarenal abscess formation.

Upper urinary tract infections usually require systemic antifungal therapy, as well as immediate investigation and imaging of the urinary system to exclude obstruction, papillary necrosis, and fungus-ball formation. Amphotericin B bladder irrigation has no role in the treatment of patients with pyelonephritis. Systemic antifungal therapy with either parenteral amphotericin B deoxycholate at >0.6 mg/kg/day, or fluconazole at 6 mg/kg/day is recommended [5]. Flucytosine is occasionally combined with amphotericin B to cover for resistant *Candida* spp. [64]. Efficacy data on the use of the lipid formulation of amphotericin B is lacking. Their use in the treatment of pyelonephritis is not advisable because their structure, which protects the kidney from the toxic effect of amphotericin B, may impair their urinary excretion [65].

Adequate drainage of the urinary tract system by placement of a stent or nephrostomy tube, as well as surgical removal of fungus balls is always essential. Irrigation of nephrostomy tube with either amphotericin B or fluconazole is advisable in some cases to achieve high concentrations of the antifungal agent at the site of infection. Long-term drainage is often needed after clearance of candiduria.

Published experience with the echinocandin caspofungin in the treatment of ascending fungal UTI is limited [66]. One of the major pharmacokinetic disadvantages of echinocandins is the poor glomerular filtration or tubular secretion resulting in subtherapeutic antifungal concentration in the urine. Accordingly, despite their favorable *in-vitro* activity, echinocandins are not considered among the preferred agents for the treatment of candiduria. However, the echinocandins achieve a high tissue concentration independent of glomerular filtration making them a suitable alternative for the treatment of renal candidiasis caused by resistant non-*albicans* strain in the absence of urinary tract obstruction [67,68].

RENAL CANDIDIASIS

Renal candidiasis develops almost exclusively secondary to hematogenous seeding of the kidney during an episode of candidemia. Patients present with high-grade fever, hemodynamic instability and renal insufficiency. Candiduria along with a subtle decline in urinary function is often the only diagnostic clue of disseminated candidiasis. Other clinical features include skin rash and endophthalmitis. Candidemia is detected in 50% of cases making the diagnosis difficult to establish. Moreover, finding of candidal casts in the urine is a specific diagnostic marker for detection of renal candidiasis; however, this marker is a very insensitive tool [20]. The diagnosis of renal candidiasis relies on clinical presentation mostly. Hematogenous renal candidiasis should be treated with high dose systemic amphotericin B or fluconazole. Lipid formulations of amphotericin B, although less nephrotoxic than the standard deoxycholate form, have not been shown to be superior to the latter and are not currently regarded as first-line therapy for disseminated candidiasis [5].

EPIDIDYMITIS, ORCHITIS, AND PROSTATITIS

Epididymo-orchitis and prostatitis caused by *Candida* spp. are an uncommon manifestation of *Candida* urinary tract disease [69–80]. They are mostly described in diabetic and HIV-positive patients or following bladder instrumentation. Epididymo-orchitis usually results from retrograde spread of UTI via the ejaculatory duct and vas deferens. Epididymal infections are rarely caused by hematogenous dissemination of systemic fungal infection [71]. Both *C. albicans* and *C. glabrata* were reported in the setting of epididymo-orchitis. Patients present with scrotal swelling and pain typical of epididymo-orchitis, which is bilateral and complicated in most cases [75]. Failure to isolate a causative bacterium in association with the presence of candiduria and risk factors for candidal infection is highly suggestive of a diagnosis of *Candida* epididymo-orchitis. Percutaneous or open drainage should be considered in complicated cases to obtain specimens for diagnostic microbiology and histology [80]. Treatment requires the combination of orchiectomy or surgical drainage and systemic antifungal therapy according to the species susceptibility pattern. Oral fluconazole is the preferred regimen; however, in case of fluconazole-resistant *Candida* spp., amphotericin B with or without flucytosine would be an appropriate choice [80].

Isolated *Candida* prostatitis is extremely rare [78,79,81]. It occurs usually secondary to systemic infections in immunosuppressed patients and is complicated by prostatic abscess formation. Patients present with irritative voiding symptoms, perineal pain, fever, and acute urinary retention. Surgical drainage in case of abscess formation along with systemic antifungal therapy is recommended.

GENITOURINARY TRACT ASPERGILLOSIS

Aspergillosis of the genitourinary tract is an uncommon infection. It has been mainly reported in patients with malignancies, diabetes, intravenous drug use, chronic alcoholism and in renal transplant recipients [82–86]. Three disease patterns of genitourinary aspergillosis have been described in the literature. The first and most common pattern results from hematogenous spread of disseminated *Aspergillus* infection and is associated with multiorgan involvement including kidney and prostate. The primary site of infection in such cases is either the lungs or the skin [2]. The second pattern is the result of a panurothelial ascending infection, involving the urethra, bladder, ureters, prostate, and kidneys and is secondary to iatrogenic bladder instrumentation [87,88]. The third pattern consists of a localized parenchymal necrosis with an obstructing fungal bezoar formation that can be seen in any part of the urinary tract. This pattern is mostly reported in patients with diabetes, HIV infection, and renal transplant recipients where corticosteroid therapy is a major risk factor [84,87].

Patients with genitourinary tract aspergillosis usually present with fever and microscopic hematuria. Localizing symptoms such as flank pain and dysuria are uncommon. Urine culture is invariably negative making the diagnosis of urinary tract aspergillosis difficult in the absence of clinical suspicion. Repeated large volume urine culture on Sabouraud dextrose medium or brain–heart enriched infusion broth has been suggested. However, the yield is poor because *Aspergillus* organisms have a propensity for tissue attachment and invasion. Tissue culture or pathological examination showing the fungal hyphae in renal tissue remains the standard diagnostic modality [89,90].

Management of urinary tract aspergillosis requires the combination of medical and surgical interventions [91–96]. Systemic amphotericin B alone or combined with flucytosine is the first line treatment [88]. Irrigation with amphotericin B or a liposomal preparation of amphotericin B through a urinary catheter or percutaneous nephrostomy tube has been tried successfully [91]. Open surgical operative drainage via stent or nephrostomy tube is indicated for obstructing fungal bezoars [85]. Infection limited to the prostate could be surgically treated without additional antifungal therapy [96]. Earlier *in vitro* data suggesting that rifampin potentiates the activity of amphotericin B against

Aspergillus spp. has not been proven in clinical studies [97]. Data supporting the use of itraconazole in the treatment of genitourinary aspergillosis is weak since the drug is poorly excreted in the urine. The new azoles, such as voriconazole and posaconazole, and the echinocandins have excellent *in vitro* and *in vivo* activity against a variety of *Aspergillus* infections. However, their use in the treatment of genitourinary aspergillosis has not been validated. Voriconazole undergoes extensive liver metabolism and less than 2% of its active metabolite is excreted in the urine, making it a less suitable antifungal agent for the treatment of urinary tract aspergillosis [98]. The pharmacokinetic properties of posaconazole and caspofungin preclude their use in the treatment of genitourinary aspergillosis. Posaconazole is primarily degraded in the liver to inactive metabolites and excreted in the feces, and caspofungin undergoes primarily liver metabolism as stated previously [99]. Clinical evidence for their success in the treatment of such infections is still awaited.

CRYPTOCOCCUS INFECTIONS OF THE GENITOURINARY TRACT

Cryptococcosis is an infection caused by *Cryptococcus neoformans*, a fungus commonly found in the soil, mostly in pigeon excreta. The disease is acquired by inhalation of the organism which may then disseminate to the meninges, lymph nodes, skin and the genitourinary tract. Therefore, infection of the urinary tract is almost always equivalent to systemic infection. Individuals at risk include patients with AIDS and patients with other immunocompromising conditions, such as hematological malignancies, collagen vascular diseases, diabetes mellitus, renal transplantation, and corticosteroids therapy [100–105]. Cryptococcal infection of the urinary tract can present as pyelonephritis, prostatitis or as occult cryptococcal UTI without a rise in serum cryptococcal antigen. Prostatic cryptococcosis is usually asymptomatic. The prostate gland is considered a site for yeast sequestration after an occult or treated disseminated cryptococcal infection. It has been recognized as a potential clinical site for sanctuary of *C. neoformans* from antifungal treatment. It is an important reservoir for relapse of cryptococcosis in patients who have a high burden of yeasts [105]. A latent *C. neoformans* infection of the prostate has even been found to spread into the blood during prostatic surgery [106]. Diagnosis of prostatic cryptococcosis can be achieved by using ultrasound-guided prostatic biopsy with fungal culture or histopathology of prostatic tissue. High levels of prostate-specific antigen (PSA), which may have represented prostatic inflammation, were recognized in prostatic cryptococcosis in a patient who underwent renal transplantation [107]. After initial induction antifungal treatment of cryptococcal meningoencephalitis in patients who have AIDS, urine or seminal fluid cultures may still be positive for yeasts [108]. Therefore, the prostate might be an important site for relapsed infections if therapy is discontinued early and immune reconstitution has not occurred.

The treatment of genitourinary cryptococcal infection necessitates systemic antifungal therapy with amphotericin B or fluconazole. It has been suggested that antifungal therapy should continue for 6 weeks if the patient is immunocompetent. However, in AIDS patients a lifetime suppressive therapy with fluconazole is recommended. The use of flucytosine in combination with amphotericin B has been proposed based on the response rates of patients with cryptococcal meningitis treated with this combination regimen [109].

HISTOPLASMOSIS OF THE GENITOURINARY TRACT

Histoplasma capsulatum infection is usually a benign self-limited respiratory disease that is most commonly seen in areas of endemicity in the upper Mississippi River and Ohio River valleys. Most of these infections are clinically silent and resolve without consequences [110]. Disseminated disease is uncommon but well-recognized sequelae of histoplasmosis that occurs primarily in patients with impaired cellular defenses or after introduction of a large inoculum [111]. Genitourinary and prostatic involvement with disseminated histoplasmosis rarely occurs. Most cases were only identified at autopsy [112,113]. Of note, many large series reported no evidence of *Histoplasma* prostatitis including a large review of 102 cases of disseminated histoplasmosis [110]. Most patients with prostatic histoplasmosis described in the literature had no identifiable immunodeficiency; however, the disease is currently being reported with higher frequency in patients with HIV infection or AIDS where all cases were detected at the stage of prostatic abscess formation [114–116]. Well-characterized relapses of cryptococcal disease from prostatic reservoirs raise questions about this form of histoplasmosis functioning in the same manner. Treatment data regarding disseminated histoplasmosis involving the prostate are limited. In the genitourinary tract, surgery may not be an option because of the possibility of further dissemination with surgical intervention [117]. Treatment is indicated for all patients with progressive disseminated histoplasmosis. In immunocompetent hosts and immunocompromised hosts without AIDS, Amphotericin B is recommended for patients who are sufficiently ill to require hospitalization [118]. Experience using the lipid formulations of amphotericin B for treating histoplasmosis has not been reported. Most patients respond quickly to amphotericin B and can then be switched to itraconazole to continue the therapeutic course. Itraconazole is the treatment of choice for patients with mild or only moderately severe symptoms who do not require hospitalization and continuation of therapy in those whose condition has improved in response to amphotericin B. Fluconazole should be used only in patients who cannot take itraconazole [119]. *H. capsulatum* may develop resistance to fluconazole during therapy leading to relapse, thus necessitating careful follow-up assessment, including measurement of

H. capsulatum antigen concentration in blood and urine [120]. In patients with AIDS, treatment is divided into an initial 12-week intensive phase to induce a remission in the clinical illness followed by a chronic maintenance phase to prevent relapse. A similar approach may be appropriate in other patients without AIDS who have relapsed after appropriate courses of therapy.

BLASTOMYCOSIS OF THE GENITOURINARY TRACT

Blastomyces dermatitidis is a dimorphic fungus existing in the mycelial form in soil and in the yeast form in tissue. All systemic blastomycosis infections arise from inhalation of spores aerosolized from soil. The skin, bone, genitourinary, and central nervous systems are the most commonly involved extrapulmonary sites. Genitourinary involvement by *B. dermatitidis* occurs secondary to hematogenous dissemination where the lung is usually the primary site of infection. Blastomycosis is a relatively uncommon source of genitourinary disease; however, it remains an important diagnostic consideration particularly in endemic areas including the Mississippi, Missouri, Ohio River valleys, and the Great Lakes region [121]. Genitourinary involvement has been noted in 45% of cases [122]. The prostate and epididymis are most frequently affected, but renal, testicular and preputial disease has also been reported. Genitourinary symptoms may be the primary complaint in 2% of systemic cases [123]. Definitive diagnosis is made by culture or histological identification of the characteristic budding yeast form. Because they lack both sensitivity and specificity, serological tests are generally not helpful for diagnosing blastomycosis. A negative serological test should never be used to rule out disease, nor should a positive titer be an indication to start treatment.

Patients with life-threatening disseminated disease should be treated with amphotericin B. Therapy for some patients may be switched to itraconazole after clinical stabilization with amphotericin B. Patients with mild-to-moderate disseminated blastomycosis should be treated with itraconazole for at least 6 months. Ketoconazole and fluconazole are alternatives to itraconazole [124]. Although voriconazole has been successfully used in the treatment of cerebral blastomycosis, data about its efficacy in the treatment of genitourinary tract blastomycosis is lacking [125,126]. One study showed that high dose posaconazole is effective in curing pulmonary blastomycosis in a murine model; however, this antifungal has not been studied in humans with *B. dermatitis* infection [127].

COCCIDIOIDOMYCOSIS OF THE GENITOURINARY TRACT

Coccidioidomycosis is a fungal infection endemic to the southwestern United States [128]. Humans acquire infection by inhalation of airborne fungal spores of *Coccidioides immitis*. Clinical manifestations are typically a flu-like illness or self-limited pneumonia. Immunocompromised patients are at increased risk for disseminated disease, which most commonly involves the meninges, bones, joints or skin. The genitourinary tract is infrequently affected. An autopsy series of 214 patients with disseminated Coccidioidomycosis showed kidney involvement in 57 (27%), prostatic infection in 4 (1.8%), and epididymal involvement in 2 (0.9%) patients [129–131]. Kidneys are the sixth most common site of dissemination. Patients with coccidioidal prostatitis may be asymptomatic or may present with obstructive symptoms. Most patients with epididymal infection present with scrotal swelling, epididymal induration and tenderness. Urinalysis is often abnormal showing pyuria and hematuria. Urine culture is helpful for establishing the diagnosis of genitourinary coccidioidomycosis. *C. immitis* grows well on most commonly used media. The yield of urine culture can be increased by prostatic massage. Definitive diagnosis requires pathologic tissue examination in which characteristic endospore containing spherules are seen. The IDSA has published guidelines for the management of coccidioidomycosis. Extrapulmonary and nonmeningeal infections are generally treated medically but surgical debridement is an adjunctive measure in some cases. The treatment of isolated genital tract diseases has not been well defined. Surgical resection alone of the involved genital organ with no antifungal therapy in immunocompetent patients would probably be sufficient [132].

Special acknowledgement is made to Rana Traboulsi and Souha Kanj for the help they made to the authors of this book chapter.

COMMON CLINICAL QUESTIONS AND ANSWERS

1. The overwhelming majority of urinary tract infections are caused by:
   a. *Cryptococcus* spp
   b. *Histoplasmosis* spp
   c. *Aspergillus* spp
   d. *Candida* spp

Answer: d, Fungal infections of the urinary tract encompass a broad variety of fungi including the endemic mycosis, *Cryptococcus* species, and opportunistic pathogens such as *Aspergillus* species. However, the overwhelming majority of fungal infections of the urinary tract are caused by *Candida* spp. The escalating use of broad-spectrum antimicrobial agents, corticosteroids, and immunosuppressive and cytotoxic drugs with the frequent use of indwelling urinary catheters have been implicated as risk factors for *Candida* urinary tract infections (UTI). The presence of candiduria may signal diverse pathological states, including invasive renal parenchymal disease, fungal balls in obstructed ureters, superficial lower urinary tract infection, and lower urinary tract candidal colonization associated with urinary catheterization. Accordingly, the spectrums of clinical disease embrace asymptomatic candiduria, cystitis, pyelonephritis, and renal candidiasis

2. Indwelling urinary catheters present a risk factor for *candida* UTI. TRUE OR FALSE

Answer: True, Risk factors for *Candida* UTI are well described in the literature and include poorly controlled diabetes mellitus, previous use of broad-spectrum antibiotics, corticosteroids and cytotoxic agents, indwelling urinary catheters, old age, malignancy, prior surgical procedures, history of renal transplantation, recent hospitalization, and structural or functional abnormalities of the urinary tract.

3. Relative to adult patients, *Candida* _____ is the more likely to be isolated from the urine of hospitalized neonates and usually is associated with systemic infection in this population.
   a. *C. parapsilosis*
   b. *C. albicans*
   c. *C. glabrate*
   d. *C. krusei*

Answer: a, *C. parapsilosis* is found more often in urine from neonates and is usually associated with systemic infection in this population. In adult patients, *C. albicans* is the most common fungal pathogen in UTIs accounting for more than half of the cases of fungal UTIs. *C. glabrata* accounts for 25%–35% of infections whereas other *Candida* spp., including *C. tropicalis*, *C. krusei*, and *C. parapsilosis*, account for 8%–28% of cases in adults. In about 10% of cases, more than one species of *Candida* can be isolated and candiduria can coexist with or follow bacteriuria. Speciation of yeasts when recovered from urinary culture is encouraged.

4. A key principle for management of upper tract candida urinary tract infection is:
   a. Antegrade instillation of antifungal agents
   b. Decompress any sites of urinary tract obstruction
   c. Urinary catheterization
   d. Long term oral antifungal therapy

Answer: b, Patients with infection of the upper urinary tract or pyelonephritis present with fever, leukocytosis, abdominal pain, and costovertebral angle tenderness. *Candida* pyelonephritis occurs almost invariably in the setting of urinary obstruction, particularly in patients with diabetes and nephrolithiasis. Upper tract imaging should be strongly considered in patients with fungal pyelonephritis to investigate urinary obstruction; if this is discovered, decompression with a stent or nephrostomy tube is required.

5. Urinary tract Cryptococcus infections can usually be effectively treated with 7 to 14 days of antibiotic therapy. TRUE OR FALSE.

Answer: False, Cryptococcosis is an infection caused by *Cryptococcus neoformans*, a fungus commonly found in the soil, mostly in pigeon excreta. The disease is acquired by inhalation of the organism, which may then disseminate to the meninges, lymph nodes, skin, and the genitourinary tract. Therefore, infection of the urinary tract is almost always equivalent to systemic infection. Individuals at risk include patients with AIDS or other immunocompromising conditions, such as hematological malignancies, collagen vascular diseases, diabetes mellitus, renal transplantation, and corticosteroids therapy. Cryptococcal infection of the urinary tract can present as pyelonephritis, prostatitis, or as occult cryptococcal UTI without a rise in serum cryptococcal antigen.

The treatment of genitourinary cryptococcal infection necessitates systemic antifungal therapy with amphotericin B or fluconazole. It has been suggested that antifungal therapy should continue for six weeks if the patient is immunocompetent. However, in AIDS patients a lifetime suppressive therapy with fluconazole is recommended.

REFERENCES

1. Sobel JD, Vazquez JA. Fungal infections of the urinary tract. *World J Urol* 1999;17(6):410–414.
2. Flechner SM, McAninch JW. Aspergillosis of the urinary tract: Ascending route of infection and evolving patterns of disease. *J Urol* 1981;125(4):598–601.
3. Bibler MR, Gianis JT. Acute ureteral colic from an obstructing renal aspergilloma. *Rev Infect Dis* 1987;9(4):790–794.
4. Kauffman CA, Vazquez JA, Sobel JD, et al. Prospective multicenter surveillance study of funguria in hospitalized patients. The National Institute for Allergy and Infectious Diseases (NIAID) Mycoses Study Group. *Clin Infect Dis* 2000;30(1):14–18.
5. Pappas PG, Rex JH, Sobel JD, et al. Guidelines for treatment of candidiasis. *Clin Infect Dis* 2004;38(2):161–189.
6. Sobel JD. Pathogenesis and epidemiology of vulvovaginal candidiasis. *Ann N Y Acad Sci* 1988;544:547–557.
7. Michigan S. Genitourinary fungal infections. *J Urol* 1976;116(4):390–397.
8. Phillips JR, Karlowicz MG. Prevalence of *Candida* species in hospital-acquired urinary tract infections in a neonatal intensive care unit. *Pediatr Infect Dis J* 1997;16(2):190–194.
9. Febre N, Silva V, Medeiros EA, et al. Microbiological characteristics of yeasts isolated from urinary tracts of intensive care unit patients undergoing urinary catheterization. *J Clin Microbiol* 1999;37(5):1584–1586.
10. Rivett AG, Perry JA, Cohen J. Urinary candidiasis: A prospective study in hospital patients. *Urol Res* 1986;14(4):183–186.

11. Johansen TE, Cek M, Naber KG, et al. Hospital acquired urinary tract infections in urology departments: Pathogens, susceptibility and use of antibiotics. Data from the PEP and PEAP-studies. *Int J Antimicrob Agents* 2006;28(Suppl 1):S91–S107.

12. Platt R, Polk BF, Murdock B, et al. Risk factors for nosocomial urinary tract infection. *Am J Epidemiol* 1986;124(6):977–985.

13. National Nosocomial Infections Surveillance (NNIS). System Report, data summary from January 1992 through June 2003, issued August 2003. *Am J Infect Control* 2003;31(8):481–498.

14. Richards MJ, Edwards JR, Culver DH, et al. Nosocomial infections in medical intensive care units in the United States. National nosocomial infections surveillance system. *Crit Care Med* 1999;27(5):887–892.

15. Sobel JD, Kauffman CA, McKinsey D, et al. Candiduria: A randomized, double-blind study of treatment with fluconazole and placebo. The National Institute of Allergy and Infectious Diseases (NIAID) Mycoses Study Group. *Clin Infect Dis* 2000;30(1):19–24.

16. Kauffman CA. Candiduria. *Clin Infect Dis* 2005;41(Suppl 6):S371–S376.

17. Goldstein E, Grieco MH, Finkel G, et al. Studies on the pathogenesis of experimental *Candida parapsilosis* and *Candida guilliermondii* infections in mice. *J Infect Dis* 1965;115:293–302.

18. Louria DB, Buse M, Brayton RG, et al. The pathogenesis of *Candida tropicalis* infections in mice. *Sabouraudia* 1966;5(1):14–25.

19. Baghian A, Lee KW. Elimination of *Candida albicans* from kidneys of mice during short-term systemic infections. *Kidney Int* 1991;40(3):400–405.

20. Navarro EE, Almario JS, King C, et al. Detection of *Candida* casts in experimental renal candidiasis: Implications for the diagnosis and pathogenesis of upper urinary tract infection. *J Med Vet Mycol* 1994;32(6):415–426.

21. Lehner T. Systemic candidiasis and renal involvement. *Lancet* 1964;1(7348):1414–1416.

22. Harris AD, Castro J, Sheppard DC, et al. Risk factors for nosocomial candiduria due to *Candida glabrata* and *Candida albicans*. *Clin Infect Dis* 1999;29(4):926–928.

23. Ayeni O, Riederer KM, Wilson FM, et al. Clinicians' reaction to positive urine culture for *Candida* organisms. *Mycoses* 1999;42(4):285–289.

24. Safdar N, Slattery WR, Knasinski V, et al. Predictors and outcomes of candiduria in renal transplant recipients. *Clin Infect Dis* 2005;40(10):1413–1421.

25. Wainstein MA, Graham RC Jr, Resnick MI. Predisposing factors of systemic fungal infections of the genitourinary tract. *J Urol* 1995;154(1):160–163.

26. Weinberger M, Sweet S, Leibovici L, et al. Correlation between candiduria and departmental antibiotic use. *J Hosp Infect* 2003;53(3):183–186.

27. Lehrer RI. Inhibition by sulfonamides of the candidacidal activity of human neutrophils. *J Clin Invest* 1971;50(12):2498–2505.

28. Forsgren A, Schmeling D, Quie PG. Effect of tetracycline on the phagocytic function of human leukocytes. *J Infect Dis* 1974;130(4):412–415.

29. Ferrari FA, Pagani A, Marconi M, et al. Inhibition of candidacidal activity of human neutrophil leukocytes by aminoglycoside antibiotics. *Antimicrob Agents Chemother* 1980;17(1):87–88.

30. Kojic EM, Darouiche RO. *Candida* infections of medical devices. *Clin Microbiol Rev* 2004;17(2):255–267.

31. Jain N, Kohli R, Cook E, et al. Biofilm formation by and antifungal susceptibility of *Candida* isolates from urine. *Appl Environ Microbiol* 2007;73(6):1697–1703.

32. Lane RK, Matthay MA. Central line infections. *Curr Opin Crit Care* 2002;8(5):441–448.

33. Chandra J, Kuhn DM, Mukherjee PK, et al. Biofilm formation by the fungal pathogen *Candida albicans*: Development, architecture, and drug resistance. *J Bacteriol* 2001;183(18):5385–5394.

34. Davey ME, O'Toole GA. Microbial biofilms: From ecology to molecular genetics. *Microbiol Mol Biol Rev* 2000;64(4):847–867.

35. Ganderton L, Chawla J, Winters C, et al. Scanning electron microscopy of bacterial biofilms on indwelling bladder catheters. *Eur J Clin Microbiol Infect Dis* 1992;11(9):789–796.

36. Sauer K, Camper AK, Ehrlich GD, et al. Pseudomonas aeruginosa displays multiple phenotypes during development as a biofilm. *J Bacteriol* 2002;184(4):1140–1154.

37. O'Toole G, Kaplan HB, Kolter R. Biofilm formation as microbial development. *Annu Rev Microbiol* 2000;54:49–79.

38. Chandra J, Mukherjee PK, Leidich SD, et al. Antifungal resistance of candidal biofilms formed on denture acrylic *in vitro*. *J Dent Res* 2001;80(3):903–908.

39. Ang BS, Telenti A, King B, et al. Candidemia from a urinary tract source: Microbiological aspects and clinical significance. *Clin Infect Dis* 1993;17(4):662–666.

40. Nassoura Z, Ivatury RR, Simon RJ, et al. Candiduria as an early marker of disseminated infection in critically ill surgical patients: The role of fluconazole therapy. *J Trauma* 1993;35(2):290–294, discussion 294–295.

41. Pappas PG, Kauffman CA, Andes DR, et al. Clinical practice guideline for the management of candidiasis: 2016 update by the ISDA. *Clin Infect Dis* 2016;62(4):e1–50.

42. Fisher JF, Sobel JD, Kauffman CA, Newman CA. *Candida* urinary tract infections—treatment. *Clin Infect Dis* 2011;52 Suppl 6:S457–S466.

43. Kozinn PJ, Goldberg PK, Gambino SR. Bacteriuria: Colonization or infection. *JAMA* 1985;253(13):1878–1879.

44. Everett ED, Eickhoff TC, Ehret JM. Immunofluorescence of yeast in urine. *J Clin Microbiol* 1976;2(2):142–143.

45. Harding SA, Merz WG. Evaluation of antibody coating of yeasts in urine as an indicator of the site of urinary tract infection. *J Clin Microbiol* 1975;2(3):222–225.

46. Hall WJ. Study of antibody-coated fungi in patients with funguria and suspected disseminated fungal infections or primary fungal pyelonephritis. *J R Soc Med* 1980;73(8):567–569.

47. Fan-Havard P, O'Donovan C, Smith SM, et al. Oral fluconazole versus amphotericin B bladder irrigation for treatment of candidal funguria. *Clin Infect Dis* 1995;21(4):960–965.

48. Leu HS, Huang CT. Clearance of funguria with short-course antifungal regimens: A prospective, randomized, controlled study. *Clin Infect Dis* 1995;20(5):1152–1157.

49. Jacobs LG, Skidmore EA, Freeman K, et al. Oral fluconazole compared with bladder irrigation with amphotericin B for treatment of fungal urinary tract infections in elderly patients. *Clin Infect Dis* 1996;22(1):30–35.

50. Tacker JR. Successful use of fluconazole for treatment of urinary tract fungal infections. *J Urol* 1992;148(6):1917–1978.

51. Graybill JR, Galgiani JN, Jorgensen JH, et al. Ketoconazole therapy for fungal urinary tract infections. *J Urol* 1983;129(1):68–70.

52. Boucher HW, Groll AH, Chiou CC, et al. Newer systemic antifungal agents: Pharmacokinetics, safety and efficacy. *Drugs* 2004;64(18):1997–2020.

53. Sobel JD, Kauffman CA, McKinsey D, et al. Candiduria: A randomized, double-blind study of treatment with fluconazole and placebo. the national institute of allergy and infectious diseases (NIAID) mycoses study group. *Clin Infect Dis* 2000;30(1):19–24.

54. Kauffman CA. Diagnosis and management of fungal urinary tract infection. *Infect Dis Clin North Am* 2014;28(1):61–74.

55. Goldman HJ, Littman ML, Oppenheimer GD, et al. Monilial cystitis-effective treatment with instillations of amphotericin B. *JAMA* 1960;174:359–362

56. Drew RH, Arthur RR, Perfect JR. Is it time to abandon the use of amphotericin B bladder irrigation? *Clin Infect Dis* 2005;40(10):1465–1470.

57. Arthur RR, Drew RH, Perfect JR. Novel modes of antifungal drug administration. *Expert Opin Investig Drugs* 2004;13(8):903–932.

58. Nesbit SA, Katz LE, McClain BW, et al. Comparison of two concentrations of amphotericin B bladder irrigation in the treatment of funguria in patients with indwelling urinary catheters. *Am J Health Syst Pharm* 1999;56(9), 872–875.

59. Trinh T, Simonian J, Vigil S, et al. Continuous versus intermittent bladder irrigation of amphotericin B for the treatment of candiduria. *J Urol* 1995;154(6):2032–2034.

60. Fong IW. The value of a single amphotericin B bladder washout in candiduria. *J Antimicrob Chemother* 1995;36(6):1067–1071.

61. Hsu CC, Ukleja B. Clearance of *Candida* colonizing the urinary bladder by a two-day amphotericin B irrigation. *Infection* 1990;18(5):280–202.

62. Wise GJ. Do not abandon amphotericin B as an antifungal bladder irrigant. *Clin Infect Dis* 2005;41(7):1073–1074.

63. Fisher JF, Hicks BC, Dipiro JT, et al. Efficacy of a single intravenous dose of amphotericin B in urinary tract infections caused by *Candida*. *J Infect Dis* 1987;156(4):685–687.

64. Wise GJ, Kozinn PJ, Goldberg P. Flucytosine in the management of genitourinary candidiasis: 5 years of experience. *J Urol* 1980;124(1):70–72.

65. Agustin J, Lacson S, Raffalli J, et al. Failure of a lipid amphotericin B preparation to eradicate candiduria: Preliminary findings based on three cases. *Clin Infect Dis* 1999;29(3):686–687.

66. Sobel JD, Bradshaw SK, Lipka CJ, et al. Caspofungin in the treatment of symptomatic candiduria. *Clin Infect Dis* 2007;44(5):e46–e49.

67. Abruzzo GK, Gill CJ, Flattery AM, et al. Efficacy of the echinocandin caspofungin against disseminated aspergillosis and candidiasis in cyclophosphamide-induced immunosuppressed mice. *Antimicrob Agents Chemother* 2000;44(9):2310–2318.

68. McCormack PL, Perry CM. Caspofungin: A review of its use in the treatment of fungal infections. *Drugs* 2005;65(14):2049–2068.

69. Swartz DA, Harrington P, Wilcox R. Candidal epididymitis treated with ketoconazole. *N Engl J Med* 1988;319(22):1485.

70. Gordon DL, Maddern J. Treatment of *candida* epididymo-orchitis with oral fluconazole. *Med J* 1992;156(10):744.

71. Docimo SG, Rukstalis DB, Rukstalis MR, et al. *Candida* epididymitis: Newly recognized opportunistic epididymal infection. *Urology* 1993;41(3):280–282.

72. Sheaff M, Ahsan Z, Badenoch D, et al. A rare cause of epididymo-orchitis. *Br J Urol* 1995;75(2):250–251.

73. Jenks P, Brown J, Warnock D, et al. *Candida glabrata* epididymo-orchitis: An unusual infection rapidly cured with surgical and antifungal treatment. *J Infect* 1995;31(1):71–72.

74. Lyne JC, Flood HD. Bilateral fungal epididymo-orchitis with abscess. *Urology* 1995;46(3):412–414.

75. Jenkin GA, Choo M, Hosking P, et al. Candidal epididymo-orchitis: Case report and review. *Clin Infect Dis* 1998;26(4):942–945.

76. Giannopoulos A, Giamarellos-Bourboulis EJ, Adamakis I, et al. Epididymitis caused by *Candida glabrata*: A novel infection in diabetic patients? *Diabetes Care* 2001;24(11):2003–2004.

77. Bartkowski DP, Lanesky JR. Emphysematous prostatitis and cystitis secondary to *Candida albicans*. *J Urol* 1988;139(5):1063–1065.

78. Indudhara R, Singh SK, Vaidyanathan S, et al. Isolated invasive candidal prostatitis. *Urol Int* 1992;48(3):362–364.

79. Collado A, Ponce de Leon J, Salinas D, et al. Prostatic abscess due to *Candida* with no systemic manifestations. *Urol Int* 2001;67(2):186–188.

80. Parr NJ, Prasad BR, Hayhurst V, et al. Suppurative epididymo-orchitis in young 'high risk' patients—A new problem? *Br J Urol* 1993;72(6):949–951.

81. Haas CA, Bodner DR, Hampel N, et al. Systemic candidiasis presenting with prostatic abscess. *Br J Urol* 1998;82(3):450–451.

82. Weiland D, Ferguson RM, Peterson PK, et al. Aspergillosis in 25 renal transplant patients. Epidemiology, clinical presentation, diagnosis, and management. *Ann Surg* 1983;198(5):622–629.

83. Denning DW, Stevens DA. Antifungal and surgical treatment of invasive aspergillosis: Review of 2,121 published cases. *Rev Infect Dis* 1990;12(6):1147–1201.

84. Singer AJ, Kubak B, Anders KH. Aspergillosis of the testis in a renal transplant recipient. *Urology* 1998;51(1):119–121.

85. Hadaya K, Akposso K, Costa de Beauregard MA, et al. Isolated urinary aspergillosis in a renal transplant recipient. *Nephrol Dial Transplant* 1998;13(9):2382–2384.

86. Raghavan R, Date A, Bhaktaviziam A. Fungal and nocardial infections of the kidney. *Histopathology* 1987;11(1):9–20.

87. Irby PB, Stoller ML, McAninch JW. Fungal bezoars of the upper urinary tract. *J Urol* 1990;143(3):447–451.

88. Halpern M, Szabo S, Hochberg E, et al. Renal aspergilloma: An unusual cause of infection in a patient with the acquired immunodeficiency syndrome. *Am J Med* 1992;92(4):437–440.

89. Khan ZU, Gopalakrishnan G, al-Awadi K, et al. Renal aspergilloma due to *Aspergillus flavus*. *Clin Infect Dis* 1995;21(1):210–212.

90. Abbas F, Kamal MK, Talati J. Prostatic aspergillosis. *J Urol* 1995;153(3 Pt 1):748–750.

91. Khawand N, Jones G, Edson M. Aspergillosis of prostate. *Urology* 1989;34(2):100–101.

92. Campbell TB, Kaufman L, Cook JL. Aspergillosis of the prostate associated with an indwelling bladder catheter: Case report and review. *Clin Infect Dis* 1992;14(4):942–944.

93. Ludwig M, Schneider H, Lohmeyer J, et al. Systemic aspergillosis with predominant genitourinary manifestations in an immunocompetent man: What we can learn from a disastrous follow-up. *Infection* 2005;33(2):90–92.

94. Guleria S, Seth A, Dinda AK, et al. Ureteric aspergilloma as the cause of ureteric obstruction in a renal transplant recipient. *Nephrol Dial Transplant* 1998;13(3):792–793.

95. Maranes A, Portoles J, Blanco J, et al. Aspergillus infection of a renal allograft without evidence of a site of origin. *Nephrol Dial Transplant* 1996;11(8):1639–1642.

96. Shirwany A, Sargent SJ, Dmochowski RR, et al. Urinary tract aspergillosis in a renal transplant recipient. *Clin Infect Dis* 1998;27(5):1336.

97. Hughes CE, Harris C, Peterson LR, et al. Enhancement of the *in vitro* activity of amphotericin B against *Aspergillus* spp. by tetracycline analogs. *Antimicrob Agents Chemother* 1984;26(6):837–840.

98. Leveque D, Nivoix Y, Jehl F, et al. Clinical pharmacokinetics of voriconazole. *Int J Antimicrob Agents* 2006;27(4):274–284.

99. Dodds Ashley ES, Alexander BD. Posaconazole. *Drugs Today* (Barc) 2005;41(6):393–400.

100. Lief M, Sarfarazi F. Prostatic cryptococcosis in acquired immune deficiency syndrome. *Urology* 1986;28(4):318–319.

101. Adams JR Jr, Mata JA, Culkin DJ, et al. Acquired immunodeficiency syndrome manifesting as prostate nodule secondary to cryptococcal infection. *Urology* 1992;39(3):289–291.

102. Hinchey WW, Someren A. Cryptococcal prostatitis. *Am J Clin Pathol* 1981;75(2):257–260.

103. Milchgrub S, Visconti E, Avellini J. Granulomatous prostatitis induced by capsule-deficient cryptococcal infection. *J Urol* 1990;143(2):365–366.

104. Salyer WR, Salyer DC. Involvement of the kidney and prostate in cryptococcosis. *J Urol* 1973;109(4):695–698.

105. Larsen RA, Bozzette S, McCutchan JA, et al. Persistent Cryptococcus neoformans infection of the prostate after successful treatment of meningitis. California Collaborative Treatment Group. *Ann Intern Med* 1989;111(2):125–128.

106. Allen R, Barter CE, Chachoua LL, et al. Disseminated cryptococcosis after transurethral resection of the prostate. *Aust N Z J Med* 1982;12(4):296–299.

107. Siddiqui TJ, Zamani T, Parada JP. Primary cryptococcal prostatitis and correlation with serum prostate specific antigen in a renal transplant recipient. *J Infect* 2005;51(3):e153–e157.

108. Staib F, Seibold M, L'Age M. Persistence of *Cryptococcus neoformans* in seminal fluid and urine under itraconazole treatment. The urogenital tract (prostate) as a niche for *Cryptococcus neoformansMycoses* 1990;33(7–8):369–373.

109. Bennett JE, Dismukes WE, Duma RJ, et al. A comparison of amphotericin B alone and combined with flucytosine in the treatment of cryptoccal meningitis. *N Engl J Med* 1979;301(3):126–131.

110. Goodwin RA Jr, Shapiro JL, Thurman GH, et al. Disseminated histoplasmosis: Clinical and pathologic correlations. *Medicine* (Baltimore) 1980;59(1):1–33.

111. Wheat J. Histoplasmosis. Experience during outbreaks in Indianapolis and review of the literature. *Medicine* (Baltimore) 1997;76(5):339–354.

112. Reddy PA, Sutaria M, Brasher CA, et al. Disseminated histoplasmosis: Cutaneous (subcutaneous abscess), vesical and prostatic histoplasmosis. *South Med J* 1970;63(7):819–821.

113. Orr WA, Mulholland SG, Walzak MP Jr. Genitourinary tract involvement with systemic mycosis. *J Urol* 1972;107(6):1047–1050.

114. Marans HY, Mandell W, Kislak JW, et al. Prostatic abscess due to histoplasma capsulatum in the acquired immunodeficiency syndrome. *J Urol* 1991;145(6):1275–1276.

115. Zighelboim J, Goldfarb RA, Mody D, et al. Prostatic abscess due to Histoplasma capsulatum in a patient with the acquired immunodeficiency syndrome. *J Urol* 1992;147(1):166–168.

116. Shah RD, Nardi PM, Han CC. Histoplasma prostatic abscess: Rare cause in an immunocompromised patient. *AJR Am J Roentgenol* 1996;166(2):471.

117. Mawhorter SD, Curley GV, Kursh ED, et al. Prostatic and central nervous system histoplasmosis in an immunocompetent host: Case report and review of the prostatic histoplasmosis literature. *Clin Infect Dis* 2000;30(3):595–598.

118. Wheat J, Sarosi G, McKinsey D, et al. Practice guidelines for the management of patients with histoplasmosis. Infectious Diseases Society of America. *Clin Infect Dis* 2000;30(4):688–695.

119. McKinsey DS, Kauffman CA, Pappas PG, et al. Fluconazole therapy for histoplasmosis. The National Institute of Allergy and Infectious Diseases Mycoses Study Group. *Clin Infect Dis* 1996;23(5):996–1001.

120. Wheat J, Marichal P, Vanden Bossche H, et al. Hypothesis on the mechanism of resistance to fluconazole in Histoplasma capsulatum. *Antimicrob Agents Chemother* 1997;41(2):410–414.

121. Klein BS, Vergeront JM, Davis JP. Epidemiologic aspects of blastomycosis, the enigmatic systemic mycosis. *Semin Respir Infect* 1986;1(1):29–39.

122. Bergner DM, Kraus SD, Duck GB, et al. Systemic blastomycosis presenting with acute prostatic abscess. *J Urol* 1981;126(1):132–133.

123. Seo R, Oyasu R, Schaeffer A. Blastomycosis of the epididymis and prostate. *Urology* 1997;50(6):980–982.

124. Chapman SW, Bradsher RW Jr, Campbell GD Jr, et al. Practice guidelines for the management of patients with blastomycosis. Infectious Diseases Society of America. *Clin Infect Dis* 2000;30(4):679–683.

125. Bakleh M, Aksamit AJ, Tleyjeh IM, et al. Successful treatment of cerebral blastomycosis with voriconazole. *Clin Infect Dis* 2005;40(9):e69–e71.

126. Borgia SM, Fuller JD, Sarabia A, et al. Cerebral blastomycosis: A case series incorporating voriconazole in the treatment regimen. *Med Mycol* 2006;44(7):659–664.

127. Sugar AM, Liu XP. *In vitro* and *in vivo* activities of SCH 56592 against Blastomyces dermatitidis. *Antimicrob Agents Chemother* 1996;40(5):1314–1316.

128. Galgiani JN. Coccidioidomycosis: A regional disease of national importance. Rethinking approaches for control. *Ann Intern Med* 1999;130(4 Pt 1):293–300.

129. Rohn JG, Davila JC, Gibson TE. Urogenital aspects of coccidioidomycosis: Review of the literature and report of two cases. *J Urol* 1951;65(4):660–667.

130. Sohail MR, Andrews PE, Blair JE. Coccidioidomycosis of the male genital tract. *J Urol* 2005;173(6):1978–1982.

131. Truett AA, Crum NF. Coccidioidomycosis of the prostate gland: Two cases and a review of the literature. *South Med J* 2004;97(4):419–422.

132. Galgiani JN, Ampel NM, Blair JE, et al. Coccidioidomycosis. *Clin Infect Dis* 2005;41(9):1217–1223.

32

Mycobiome in health and disease

NAJLA EL-JURDI, JYOTSNA CHANDRA, AND PRANAB K. MUKHERJEE

INTRODUCTION

The importance of commensal microorganisms inhabiting the human body is now undeniable. Research describing the microbiota living in close association with the host in *symbiosis*, or health, opened new doors for investigating the changes that happen in case of *dysbiosis*, or imbalance. Microbiome refers to microorganisms and their genomes co-existing with their hosts. These microbiotas include millions of bacterial, fungal, viral, protozoa, and parasites. In recognition of the central role that the microbiome plays, some researchers coined the term *second genome* to emphasize the importance of their collective genetic repertoire.

The term *bacteriome* refers to the bacterial component of the microbiome that has been the focus of microbiome research until scientists recently started recognizing the role of the *mycobiome,* or fungal component, as well. The importance of characterizing the human and microbial genome, referred to as metagenome, was further supported by the National Institutes of Health (NIH) and the European Commission to create the Human Microbiome Project (HMP) [1]. While the *in utero* environment is considered sterile, commensal microorganisms, primarily bacterial, start developing since childbirth. Research indicates that the first three years of life are crucial for the establishment of the host microbiome and for the development of the immune system [2]. The development of this microbiome repertoire that is unique to each host, much like a fingerprint, is a result of complex multi-directional interactions and exposures including childbirth, breast feeding, environmental exposures and host genetic factors [3]. A fine balance, or symbiosis, is crucial to maintain healthy host physiologic, metabolic and immunologic processes; while imbalance, or dysbiosis, is associated with disease states.

The human microbiota are now believed to be required for normal human development, physiology, immunity, and nutrition [4–6]. Thus, alterations in the microbiome make-up, away from what is considered to be healthy, may have serious consequences. In this regard, recent research has implicated that microbiome imbalances may be associated with disorders as diverse as cancer, obesity, inflammatory bowel disease, psoriasis, asthma, and even autism [7].

Thriving biomedical and clinical research is providing more evidence that the microbiome is associated with disease states including allergy, atopic dermatitis, wounds, metabolic disorders, obesity, diabetes mellitus, cystic fibrosis, chronic obstructive lung disease, chronic kidney disease, rheumatoid arthritis, Alzheimer's disease, Parkinson's, autism, HIV, liver cirrhosis, liver transplant outcomes, inflammatory bowel disease, *clostridium difficile* colitis, colorectal cancer, esophageal cancer, graft-vs-host disease, and others [8–21]. Although much more work is needed to understand the mechanism of interaction between the human host and the microbiome, we now know that the association between the two is undeniable and has various implications on health and disease states.

In this chapter, we aim to describe the bacteriome and more specifically the mycobiome in health and to describe and explore the role of the microbiome in various diseases and/or restoration of health.

DESCRIPTION OF THE BACTERIOME AND MYCOBIOME IN HEALTH

Characterization of the human bacteriome

Collaborative national and international effort to describe the microbiome resulted in major advancement towards characterizing and understanding the microbial constituent. When exploring the literature, it is important to keep in mind that there are significant variations in the experimental design and methodology among the different studies. It is therefore crucial to examine the details involving sample collection and storage, DNA extraction, target amplification, PCR, and sequencing techniques, as well as database and bioinformatics before interpreting and generalizing the findings of the published studies. The National Institute of Standards and Technology (NIST) recently held a workshop to standardize the methodologies in human microbiome research and unify international effort in this field.

More than two decades of research have resulted in profiling the different bacterial organisms that inhabit different body sites, including the skin, oral cavity, gastrointestinal tract, and recently the genitourinary tract and urine microbiome [22]. By far, the larger number of investigations have historically focused on studying the gut bacteriome due to its intimate association with the human host and impact on the immune system since birth. It is no surprise that much research was dedicated to studying the gut bacteriome since the genome of the collective commensal bacteria in the gastrointestinal tract is thought to outnumber the human genome by more than 100 times [23].

Traditional bacterial 16S ribosomal RNA gene sequence-based techniques, revealed that Bacteroidetes and Firmicutes account for the majority of phyla inhabiting the distal gastrointestinal tract (over 90%) [24], with diversity between healthy individuals [24]. Novel metagenomic sequencing techniques are now providing more detailed description of bacterial and fungal genomes comprising the gastrointestinal microbiota [25]. Beyond profiling these microbiota, research is now focusing on the mechanism by which their metabolic products (metabolome), cytokines, and neurohormones maintain homeostasis or contribute to disease states [26].

Characterization of the human mycobiome

It was not until relatively recently that the scientific community and microbiologists recognized the importance of the fungal component of the microbiome and dedicated more research to characterize the fungal profile in different locations. The mission of accurately defining the human mycobiome was possible with the advent of high-throughput, next generation sequencing (NGS) approaches that provide large amounts of sequence data rapidly and at a low cost and the use of internal transcribed spacer (ITS) primers, which are pan fungal primers that have broad fungal specificity.

The basal oral mycobiome of 20 non-smoking healthy volunteers was described by Ghannoum et al. [27], where investigators used a novel multitag pyrosequencing approach (MTPS) to identify oral fungal taxa using ITS primers. This approach revealed the presence of 11 nonculturable and 74 culturable genera, with a total of 101 species. The core oral mycobiome (COM), which was defined to be present in at least 20% of the study participants, included *Candida* species (75%), *Cladosporium* species (60%), *Aureobasidium* species (50%), Saccharomycetales (50%), *Aspergillus* species (35%), *Fusarium* species (30%), and *Cryptococcus* species (20%). Using the Principal Coordinate (PCO) method to group and analyze the MTPS results, the investigators found that the White and Asian male study participants cluster differently from each other, whereas Asian and White females cluster together. This study highlights a few important messages: (1) the establishment of human mycobiome is the result of a complex interplay between genetic and environmental factors; (2) one-third of the detected oral fungi are not culturable; that is, not recovered on a culture medium, and therefore would not be identified without the use of next generation sequencing approaches [27].

The different components of the skin mycobiome in healthy individuals was described by Findley et al. [28], where investigators sampled 14 skin sites in 10 healthy adults. The genus *Malassezia* prevailed in 11/14 body and arm sites, and the plantar heel had the highest fungal diversity with *Malassezia*, *Aspergillus*, *Cryptococcus*, *Rhodotorula*, *Epicoccum* detected among others [28]. Jo et al. [29] compared the skin mycobiome of healthy children and adults, and showed that the lipophilic fungi *Malassezia* predominated on the trunk, head, and arm skin of adults (age 18–39), while children (age < 14) had more diverse fungal communities (including Eurotiomycetes, which comprises common dermatophytes). Since children have less sebaceous skin before puberty, these investigators suggested that changes in the fungal communities during puberty may be due to alterations in sebaceous gland activation and sebum composition. In a recent study, Leung et al. [30] characterized the skin mycobiome and its correlation with bacterial community in healthy Chinese individuals in Hong Kong and reported that effects of gender and age on diversity analyses were test- and site-specific. These investigators showed that the major fungal skin colonizers were common among the studied Chinese and Western populations, and cohabitation (living in the same house) did not appear to play a major role in shaping mycobiome differences between individuals. In summary, it is important to keep in mind that the skin mycobiome can vary according to body site, tissue structure, and skin topography, local outdoor environments, as well as lifestyles.

Recent research [18,31–34] has also shown that there is a substantial difference in the mycobiome between healthy control and disease states (as summarized in the following sections and Table 32.1).

Table 32.1 The human mycobiome: Diverse fungal species living in association with the human host

Body site	Nonpathogenic genera	Potentially pathogenic genera
Oral cavity	*Alternaria*	*Aspergillus*
	Aureobasidium	*Candida*
	Cladosporium	*Cryptococcus*
	Gibberella	*Fusarium*
	Glomus	
	Pichia	
	Saccharomyces	
	Teratosphaeria	
Lungs	*Cladosporium*	*Aspergillus*
	Penicillium	*Candida*
		Cryptococcus
Gastrointestinal Tract	*Cladosporium*	*Aspergillus*
	Penicillium	*Candida*
	Mucor	*Cryptococcus*
	Saccharomyces	*Fusarium*
		Pneumocystis
Skin	*Chrysosporium*	*Aspergillus*
	Debaryomyces	*Candida*
	Epicoccum	*Cryptococcus*
	Epidermophyton	
	Leptosphaerulina	
	Penicillium	
	Phoma	
	Rhodotorula	
	Saccharomyces	
	Ustilago	

ROLE OF MYCOBIOME IN DERMATOLOGICAL CONDITIONS

Studies exploring the skin mycobiome are important since fungi, particularly dermatophytes, and yeast (*Malassezia* and *Candida*) are known fungal skin pathogens. Investigations into the skin microbiome have recently been initiated, with a major focus on bacteriome, although early investigations have also been reported with mycobiome [28,35,36]. In addition, changes in skin mycobiome composition have been associated with non-infectious skin diseases including dandruff, diffuse systemic sclerosis, eczema, and psoriasis [37–39]. Dandruff is a chronic non-inflammatory scaling of the scalp, and often grouped with seborrheic dermatitis and psoriasis (both of which are inflammatory in nature) [40,41].

Dandruff

Dandruff etiology is both non-microbial and microbial in nature [42,43], with the microbial etiology involving the lipophilic yeast *Malassezia*. Park et al. [44] characterized the fungal mycobiome associated with dandruff compared to healthy human scalp (5 healthy subjects and 2 subjects with dandruff) using PCR-amplification of the fungal 26S rRNA gene and showed a decrease in fungal diversity in dandruff-afflicted cases (24 versus 37 fungal species, respectively).

Diffuse systemic sclerosis, allergic rhinitis, and mucormycosis

Separate studies have explored the association of changes in the skin mycobiome with diffuse systemic sclerosis, allergic rhinitis, and mucormycosis. Arron et al. [45] profiled the skin transcriptome of patients with diffuse systemic sclerosis ($n = 4$), and showed that levels of *Rhodotorula* sequences were elevated compared to normal controls ($n = 4$), while bacterial microbiome and viral read counts were similar. Interestingly, there was a significant difference between the read counts for the fungus *R. glutinis*, suggesting that this fungus may be involved in inflammatory response in this disease. Jung et al. [46] analyzed the nasal vestibule mycobiome in patients with allergic rhinitis by culture-independent pyrosequencing methods and identified *Malassezia* as the predominant fungal genus in the nasal vestibule, compared to healthy controls, with *M. restricta* being the most abundant *Malassezia* species. Shelburne et al. [47] published a case report characterizing the infecting pathogen, host, micro-, and mycobiomes in a leukemia patient who developed invasive mucormycosis. These investigators discovered that the patient was infected with a strain of the recently described *Mucor velutinosus* species, which was hypervirulent in a *Drosophila* challenge model and had a predisposition for skin dissemination. In addition, infection was associated with microbial dysbiosis, dominated by staphylococci. Whole exome sequencing revealed multiple non-synonymous polymorphisms in genes critical to control of fungal proliferation (e.g., *NOD2*, *TLR6*, and *PTX3*), as well as maintenance of microbiome diversity (*FUT2*).

Atopic dermatitis and psoriasis

Our group presented findings from microbiome analyses of lesional and non-lesional skin in atopic dermatitis and psoriasis patients [48,49]. Atopic dermatitis (AD) is an itchy, inflammatory skin condition that flares periodically and is associated with changes in skin microbes, barrier defects, and immune dysregulation. We used Ion-Torrent sequencing to identify AD-associated changes in the skin bacteriome and mycobiome, compared to allergic contact dermatitis (ACD) [49]. Skin swabs were obtained from affected and unaffected skin in post-pubertal patients ($n = 13$) with AD or ACD. Both bacteriome and mycobiome clustered closely in affected skin samples of AD but were variable in unaffected samples. Richness of bacteriome and mycobiome in AD was higher in unaffected sites (324 and 65, respectively) compared to affected sites (294 and 42, respectively). Similar patterns were noted for ACD patients. Unlike in ACD, diversity of both bacteriome and mycobiome in AD was reduced in affected skin samples (2.37 and 2.26, respectively) compared to unaffected (2.73 and 2.63, respectively) skin. *Sphingobacetrium* was unique to affected sites and 7 genera were unique to unaffected sites. Twelve fungal genera were unique to affected sites, 35 were unique to unaffected sites, and 30 were differentially present. Levels of *Alternaria alternata* and *Staphylococcus aureus* were increased and positively correlated with each other in affected samples. These results demonstrated that AD was associated with specific changes in diversity and abundance of bacteriome and mycobiome. Further investigations revealed that *A. alternata* and *S. aureus* interact with each other in mixed-species biofilm environment [50]. Similarly, analysis of bacteriome and mycobiome in skin swabs of psoriasis patients revealed changes in the abundance fungi and bacteria in lesional areas [48]. In summary, these results showed that lesional skin in atopic dermatitis and psoriasis are associated with changes in abundance of bacterial and fungal microbiota, and that significant correlations exist between these two microbial kingdoms in the setting of dermatological disease. Moreover, these microbes closely interact with each other in the biofilm milieu, which may provide protection from the host immune system and other antimicrobial defenses.

These studies revealed that the skin mycobiome is complex and influenced by multiple variables, including the environment and host immune response. A major caveat of these studies is the small sample size. The mechanisms by which members of the skin mycobiome affect these diseases have not been elucidated and need to be explored using robust clinical and preclinical studies.

ROLE OF MYCOBIOME IN GASTROINTESTINAL DISEASES

Recent studies have linked fungi with a number of gastrointestinal diseases, including IBD (including Crohn's disease [CD] and ulcerative colitis [UC]) [51], peptic ulcers [52], IBS [53], antibiotic-associated diarrhea [54], and chemotherapy-induced gastrointestinal mucositis [55]. IBD is associated with an inappropriate inflammatory response to intestinal microbial dysbiosis in a genetically susceptible host. Ott et al. [51] profiled the variable regions of the 18S rDNA and showed that mycobiome of fecal samples was different from that of the mucosal samples (dominated by Ascomycota [92.3%] and Basidiomycota [7.7%]). Trojanowska et al. [56] reported a shift in the profile of non-*albicans Candida* species in the gastrointestinal tract of IBD patients with the same *C. albicans* strains isolated from the oral cavity and the gastrointestinal tract. Separate studies have also associated CD with changes in levels of *Candida* species in patients [57], murine colitis [58], and increase in antibodies directed against *C. albicans* and *S. cerevisiae* antigens (such as ASCA). Iliev et al. [59] used a murine model of DSS-induced colitis to demonstrate that severity of CD was higher in Dectin-1 deficient mice (*Clec7a$^{-/-}$*) compared to wild-type mice, and that the proportion of pathogenic fungi (*Candida* and *Trichosporon*) increased with a concomitant increase in inflammation. Notably, levels of the nonpathogenic *Saccharomyces* decreased in the knockout mice. These results hinted at a critical role of mycobiome in IBD-associated inflammation, especially in a Dectin-1 deficient background. These investigators showed that *C. tropicalis* exacerbates the disease by exploiting the lack of Dectin-1 in these mice.

Recently, we used Ion-Torrent sequencing to characterize the gut bacteriome and mycobiome of patients with CD and their non-diseased first-degree relatives (NCDR) in 9 familial clusters living in Northern France/Belgium and in healthy individuals from 4 families living in the same area (non-CD unrelated, NCDU) [60]. CD and NCDR groups clustered together in the mycobiome but not in bacteriome profile. Microbiota of familial (CD, NCDR) samples were distinct from that of non-familial (NCDU) samples. Abundance of *Serratia marcescens* and *Escherichia coli* were high in CD patients, while that of beneficial bacteria was decreased. Abundance of *C. tropicalis* was significantly higher in CD compared to NCDR (p = 003) and positively correlated with *S. marcescens* and *E. coli* (Figure 32.1), with levels of ASCA. The biomass and thickness of triple species biofilms were significantly higher than single and double species biofilm (Figure 32.2a and b). *C. tropicalis* biofilms comprised of blastospores, while double and triple species biofilms were enriched in hyphae and exhibited close

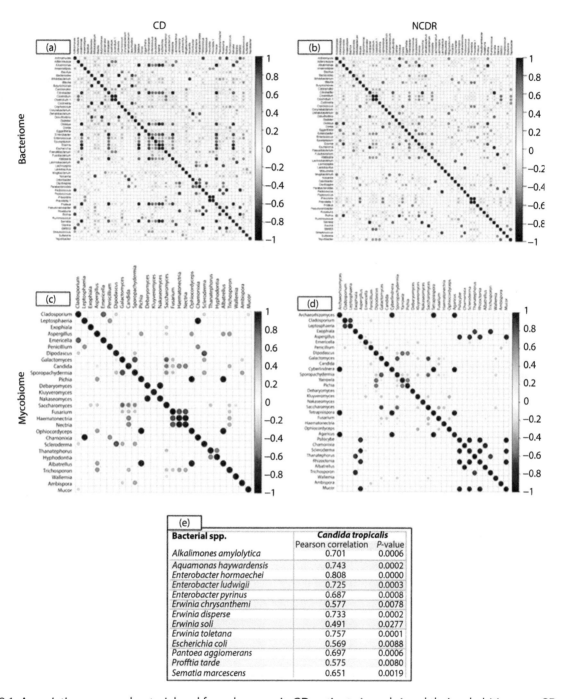

(e)		
Bacterial spp.	Candida tropicalis	
	Pearson correlation	P-value
Alkalimones amylolytica	0.701	0.0006
Aquamonas haywardensis	0.743	0.0002
Enterobacter hormaechei	0.808	0.0000
Enterobacter ludwigii	0.725	0.0003
Enterobacter pyrinus	0.687	0.0008
Erwinia chrysanthemi	0.577	0.0078
Erwinia disperse	0.733	0.0002
Erwinia soli	0.491	0.0277
Erwinia toletana	0.757	0.0001
Escherichia coli	0.569	0.0088
Pantoea agglomerans	0.697	0.0006
Profftia tarde	0.575	0.0080
Sematia marcescens	0.651	0.0019

Figure 32.1 Associations among bacterial and fungal genera in CD patients (a and c) and their cohabiting non-CD relatives (b and d). (a and b) Bacteriome. (c and d) Mycobiome. Red circles indicate negative associations, while blue circles indicate positive associations. Diameters of circles indicate the magnitude of the correlation (−1 through +1) for each fungal pair. Only significant associations (p < 0.05) are shown. (e) Table showing interactions of C. tropicalis with bacteria. (From Hoarau, G. et al., MBio, 7, 2016.)

interactions, as shown by transmission electron microscopy (Figure 32.2c–e). These findings are also supported by other studies showing that members of a family share genetics, environment, diet, and bacterial microbiota, and that family members are more similar to each other than they are to unrelated individuals [61,62]. Since C. tropicalis is also known to interact with specific immune pathways

[63], it is possible that microbial dysbiosis may exacerbate the disease in CD patients by modulating metabolic and host immune response pathways.

These studies provide insight into the roles of bacteria and fungi in CD and suggest that this disease is a manifestation of the complex interplay between host genetic factors and endogenous microbial communities (Figure 32.3).

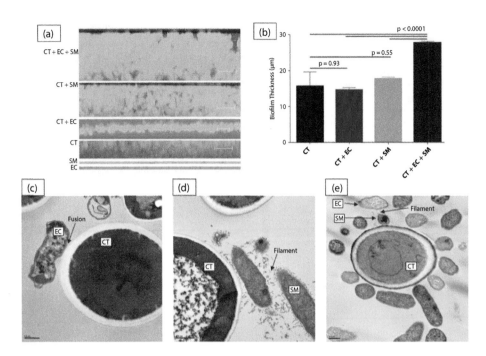

Figure 32.2 Confocal analysis of biofilms formed by *C. tropicalis* (CT) alone or in combination with *E. coli* (EC) and/or *S. marcescens* (SM). **(a)** Side view of biofilms formed by *C. tropicalis* plus *E. coli* plus *S. marcescens*, *C. tropicalis* plus *S. marcescens*, *C. tropicalis* plus *E. coli*, *C. tropicalis* alone, *S. marcescens* alone, or *E. coli* alone. **(b)** Mean thickness of biofilms. Transmission electron microscopy analyses of biofilms formed by *C. tropicalis* (CT) in combination with **(c)** *E. coli* (EC; bar, 0.5° μm), **(d)** *S. marcescens* (SM; bar, 500 nm), or **(e)** *E. coli* and *S. marcescens* (bar, 0.5° μm). SM cells interact with EC and CT through fimbriae (filaments). (From Saunders, C.W. et al., *PLoS Pathog.*, 8, e1002701, 2012.)

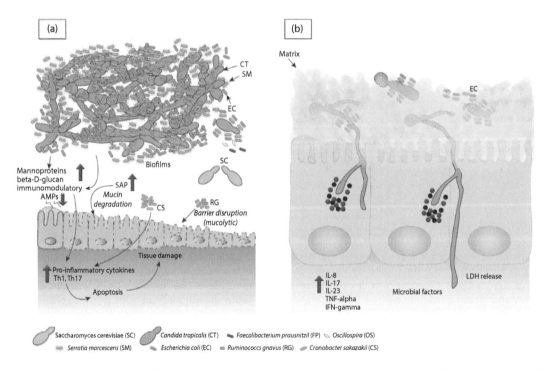

Figure 32.3 Schema showing potential interactions between bacteria, fungi and the host in the gut in Crohn's disease (CD). Inter- and intra-kingdom interactions impact the host immune system in the setting of CD, resulting in increased levels of pro-inflammatory cytokines (e.g., Th17 cytokines) under the influence of enteric pathogens and immunomodulatory components of biofilms (e.g., fungal β-glucans, bacterial lipopolysaccharides), causing increased oxidative damage and apoptotic cell death. Additionally, microbial-induced production of mucolytic enzymes may lead to barrier dysfunction, resulting in tissue damage and lesion formation. **(a)** Interactions between fungi, bacteria and the host in the hut of CD patients - showing increase in the levels of *C. tropicalis*, *E. coli*, and *S. marcescens*; **(b)** Biofilm formation by gut microbiota can influence host response to microbial dysbiosis.

THE MYCOBIOME AND HEPATITIS

The correlation between infection due to the Hepatitis B virus (HBV) and the composition and diversity of the gastrointestinal mycobiome was investigated by Chen et al. [64] in 161 participants including: (1) hepatitis B cirrhosis patients ($n = 38$), (2) chronic hepatitis B patients ($n = 35$), (3) HBV carriers ($n = 33$), and (4) healthy volunteers ($n = 55$). Both culture-dependent and independent (18S rRNA sequencing) methods were used. As expected, the culture-dependent approach detected Candida species (C. albicans, C. glabrata, C. krusei and C. tropicalis) and S. cerevisiae. The culture-independent method identified 37 operational taxonomic units (OTUs, clusters of nearly-identical sequence tags or phylotypes, commonly used to define microbial taxa) [65] representing different fungi, including: Saccharomyces spp., Penicillium spp., Galactomyces spp., and Cryptococcus spp., results that are in agreement with other studies investigating the gastrointestinal mycobiome [51]. The number of fungi detected was positively correlated with disease progression. Abundance of Candida and Saccharomyces spp. were higher in volunteers with increasing severity of HBV infection. Moreover, patients with HBV-related cirrhosis or chronic HBV infection had greater fungal diversity than HBV carriers and healthy controls. These results confirmed earlier findings regarding the relationship between increasing fungal burden and disease severity in HBV infection [66,67]. A potential link between increase in fungal abundance and HBV infection could be an underlying deficiency in the host immune response. For example, Thomas et al. [68] reported an association between mutation in the mannose binding protein (MBP) and persistent HBV infection in Caucasian patients. This protein is a pattern recognition receptor (PRR) that binds to mannan on fungal cell walls, triggering a host immune response, and, thus, plays a key role in defense against fungal pathogens. It is possible that lack or dysfunction of MBP during HBV infection leads to attenuated defense against fungi, and, thus, results in increased colonization by these pathogens. Further research is required to confirm the underlying mechanisms.

ROLE OF MYCOBIOME IN HUMAN IMMUNOCOMPROMISED VIRUS (HIV) INFECTION

Changes in bacteriome and mycobiome have also been explored in the setting of HIV infection. Aas et al. [69] analyzed sub-gingival plaque of HIV-infected patients and reported the presence of two fungal species (Saccharomyces cerevisiae and C. albicans in 4 and 2 patients, respectively). Our group analyzed the oral bacteriome and mycobiome of HIV-infected patients and matched uninfected controls ($n = 12$ for both groups) [70], and showed 8–14 bacterial and 1–9 fungal genera were present in uninfected and HIV-infected participants. The core oral mycobiome (COM), but not the core oral bacteriome (COB) differed between HIV-infected and uninfected individuals, with Candida being the predominant fungus in both groups. C. albicans was the most common Candida species (58% in uninfected and 83% in HIV-infected participants). Moreover, increase in Candida colonization was negatively associated with Pichia, and spent medium from Pichia cultures inhibited growth (including biofilms) of Candida, Aspergillus and Fusarium. The mechanism of PSM-mediated inhibition involved nutrient limitation, modulation of growth, and virulence factors. These results were validated in an experimental murine model of oral candidiasis, where mice treated with PSM exhibited significantly lower infection score (p = 011), fungal burden (p = 04), and tissue invasion compared to untreated mice. These findings provide the first evidence of interaction among members of the oral mycobiota.

In a subsequent study, we implemented a Systems Biology approach using Correlation Difference Network (CDN) analysis to provide insights into the statistically significant functional differences between HIV-infected patients and uninfected individuals [31]. We correlated bacteriome, mycobiome, and metabolome data to model the underlying biological processes. CDN indicated that Rothia, Candida, and the metabolites phenylacetate (PAA), sorbitol, and histamine have a significant correlation differences between the uninfected group and the HIV-infected group. We also identified other interactions between components of the oral microbiome, such as Pasteurella with Clostridia, and Neisseria with Capnocytophaga. These results supported the role of cyclic mono- and dipeptides in quorum sensing between oral bacterial and fungal genera in both uninfected individual controls and the HIV-infected patients. Further studies into the role of microbiome and its functional implications in HIV are warranted.

FUNGAL–BACTERIAL INTERACTIONS

Interactions between bacteria and fungi are of central importance to numerous biological questions in medicine, as they impact pathogenicity, nutritional influence (cooperativity or competition), and biochemical modulations [20]. Such interactions, mediated by different molecular mechanisms, and have been noted since the mid-1990s, especially related to use of antibiotics [71–77]. Recent microbiome analyses have also demonstrated significant correlations between the abundance of fungi and bacteria in the oral cavity, a major port of entry for microorganisms into the human body. Kraneveld et al. [78] combined 16S rRNA gene profiling with real time qPCR measurements to explore the relationship between Candida load, bacterial load, and the bacterial microbiome composition of saliva in elderly subjects. After comparison of the 16S rRNA to Candida ITS qPCR ratios, it was seen that in most subjects bacteria outnumbered Candida. However, in one subject, Candida appeared at much higher levels than bacteria. Interestingly, the authors found that in samples with high Candida load, there was an increase in relative abundance of saccharolytic species from the genera Streptococcus, Lactobacillus, and Scardovia, among others, suggesting a relationship between an acidogenic flora and Candida.

In a separate study, Mukherjee et al. [70] characterized the oral bacteriome and mycobiome in oral wash samples collected from study participants with or without HIV infection and reported that the abundance of bacteria and fungi were negatively correlated (increasing abundance of bacteria was associated with the deceasing abundance of fungi). In samples from uninfected patients, a negative correlation was found between *Rothia* and *Cladosporium*, and between *Granulicatella* and *Cryptococcus*. A similar correlation was identified between *Campylobacter* and *Candida* in patients infected with HIV. Such interactions were also reported by Navazesh et al. [79] and Cruz et al. [80] who reported negative interactions between *Campylobacter* and *Candida*, and *Enterococcus faecalis* and *C. albicans*, respectively. In a separate study, Workman et al. [81] reported that secretory proteins produced by *Campylobacter* inhibit the growth of *C. albicans*. Faust et al. [82] identified a global network of 3005 significant co-occurrence and co-exclusion relationships between 197 clades (genetically similar organisms with a common ancestor) occurring throughout the human microbiome and dependent on the body site. More recently, Sokol et al. [83] showed inter-kingdom microbial associations in CD where several fungal genera (including *Saccharomyces* and *Malassezia*) were positively correlated with bacterial taxa. However, these investigators did not observe correlations between *Candida* and bacteria (in contrast with our study), which could be because they used samples from unrelated controls as comparators, while we used non-diseased relatives to identify disease-associated changes and interactions. These differences between different studies also bring our attention to the need for development of standardized methods for microbiome analyses.

Several studies have reported Mitis group streptococci (MGS) interact with *C. albicans* in oral candidiasis [84–86]. To begin to study interactions between *C. albicans* and MGS members in models relevant to oral disease, Diaz et al. [87–89] developed an *in vitro* organotypic mucosal model that incorporates salivary flow and an oral polymicrobial infection mouse model. Using these models, these investigators showed that when *C. albicans* is co-inoculated with *S. oralis* on mucosal surfaces, streptococcal mucosal biofilm formation is enhanced. Evidence was also provided using the mouse model of oral infection for the role of MGS as accessory pathogens in oral candidiasis [88], where two MGS species were tested (*S. oralis* and *S. gordonii*) and neither showed virulence on their own, even when animals were immunocompromised and inoculated with a high number of organisms. However, when co-inoculated with *C. albicans*, *S. oralis* (but not *S. gordonii*) triggered increased frequency and severity of oral lesions, and greater weight loss. Oral co-inoculation with both organisms also triggered an exaggerated mucosal inflammatory response [89]. Similar interactions have been reported for cystic fibrosis and pulmonary infections [90–92].

Our group recently used Ion-Torrent sequencing to explore atopic dermatitis (AD) and psoriasis-associated changes in bacteriome and mycobiome [48,49]. Levels of *Alternaria alternata* and *Staphylococcus aureus* were increased and positively correlated with each other in affected (AD) samples. We also reported that *Aspergillus nidulans* and *Staphylococcus aureus* were elevated in psoriasis patients. Further investigations revealed that *A. alternata/S. aureus* and *Aspergillus nidulans/S. aureus* interact with each other in mixed-species biofilm environment and that significant correlations exist between these microbial kingdoms in the setting of dermatological disease [48–50].

Dollive et al. [93] investigated the effect of antibiotic treatment on the gut mycobiome in a mouse model using quantitative PCR and pyrosequencing, and reported that antibiotic treatment reduced bacterial abundance with a concomitant increase in fungal abundance. However, the microbial profile reported was affected by the cages in which the animals were housed. Therefore, it is suggested that studies on microbiota should address husbandry practices (e.g., caging, feed) that might affect experimental results.

Taken together, these studies suggest the existence of interkingdom relationships within the microbiota, which are likely mediated by multiple mechanisms, including secretory products, cooperativity, and nutrient competition.

FUNGAL–FUNGAL INTERACTIONS

Our groups described fungal–fungal interactions in the oral human mycobiome in healthy individuals [27] and in HIV-infected patients [70]. In the study involving HIV-infected patients [70], several bacterial and fungal genera were common to both uninfected controls and HIV-infected patients, and 23 statistically significant correlations among different fungi were identified in uninfected individuals, while 6 such correlations were observed in patients. The interactions observed in patients infected with HIV included: *Candida-Epicoccum*, *Candida-Trichosporon*, *Penicillium-Corynespora*, *Penicillium-Fusarium*, *Epicoccum-Trichosporon*, and *Alternaria-Serpula*. An increase in the abundance of *Candida* was associated with a concomitant decrease in the abundance of *Pichia*, suggesting antagonism between these two fungi, which was subsequently confirmed using *in vitro* assays. The *in vitro* results were validated in an experimental mouse model of oral candidiasis showing that *Pichia* was efficacious in the treatment of oral candidiasis. Other examples of the advantages of fungal–fungal interactions include the use of *S. cerevisiae* strains (e.g., *S. boulardii*) as potential probiotics against *C. albicans* infections [94–97]. Further investigations of fungal–fungal interactions are warranted since they could prompt the discovery of novel drugs.

CONCLUSION AND FUTURE DIRECTIONS

This chapter provided ample evidence of an undeniable fact: the host microbiota, both bacteria and fungi, with their collective genome (metagenome) and metabolites (metabolome) play a key role in health and disease states. As we highlighted in this chapter, much remains to be elucidated regarding the mechanisms by which these organisms interact with each other and with their host. In this regard, the microbiota is believed to interact at several levels with the host, including nutritional status and behavioral responses, and can affect local and distant organ systems. Elucidating the functional role of these microbiota in health and disease will be advanced greatly by studies, such as metabolomics, glycomics, and other systems biology analyses. Finally, the evidence regarding these functional roles will need to be corroborated using relevant cell culture and animal models.

QUESTIONS

Are these statements True or False:

Question 1: Culture-based techniques and next generation sequencing are equivalent in the ability to accurately characterize the oral mycobiome of healthy individuals.

Answer: False

Explanation: Investigations of the oral mycobiome in healthy individuals and patients showed that one-third of identified fungal genera were non-culturable.

Question 2: Each individual has a unique skin mycobiome that is similar among different body sites and different than other individuals.

Answer: False

Explanation: The skin mycobiome is highly variable among body sites, and skin topography as well as tissue structure are key determinants of the microbiome composition.

Question 3. The core oral bacteriome and mycobiome differs significantly between HIV-positive and HIV-negative individuals.

Answer: False

Explanation: The core oral bacteriome (COB) is similar between the two groups, whereas the core oral mycobiome (COM) was different and *Candida* was the most common fungus in both groups.

Question 4. Fungal diversity increases with the severity of Hepatitis B virus infection and is higher than that of healthy controls.

Answer: True

Explanation: Investigators identified a higher abundance of *Candida* and *Saccharomyces* with increased severity of HBV infection, and patients with HBV-cirrhosis or chronic HBV infection had greater fungal diversity than HBV carriers and healthy controls.

Question 5. The bacteriome and mycobiome of families with Crohn's disease (CD) and their non-diseased first-degree relatives (NCDR) are similar to each but significantly different as compared to and healthy non-CD unrelated (NCDU) volunteers from the same geographic area.

Answer: False

Explanation: The microbiome diversity and abundance analysis revealed that the CD and NCDR groups clustered together and had similar mycobiome but not bacteriome profile.

REFERENCES

1. Manzo VE, Bhatt AS. The human microbiome in hematopoiesis and hematologic disorders. *Blood* 2015;126(3):311–318.
2. Hooper LV, Littman DR, Macpherson AJ. Interactions between the microbiota and the immune system. *Science* 2012;336(6086):1268–1273.
3. Vieira AT, Fukumori C, Ferreira CM. New insights into therapeutic strategies for gut microbiota modulation in inflammatory diseases. *Clinical & translational immunology* 2016;5(6):e87.
4. IOM (Institute of Medicine). *The Human Microbiome, Diet, and Health: Workshop Summary.* Washington, DC: Food Forum, Food and Nutrition Board, Institute of Medicine, The National Academies Press; 2012.
5. Turnbaugh PJ, Hamady M, Yatsunenko T, Cantarel BL, Duncan A, Ley RE, Sogin ML, Jones WJ, Roe BA, Affourtit JP et al. A core gut microbiome in obese and lean twins. *Nature* 2009;457(7228):480–484.
6. Turnbaugh PJ, Ley RE, Mahowald MA, Magrini V, Mardis ER, Gordon JI. An obesity-associated gut microbiome with increased capacity for energy harvest. *Nature* 2006;444(7122):1027–1031.
7. Balter M. Taking stock of the human microbiome and disease. *Science* 2012;336(6086):1246–1247.
8. Arthur JC, Jobin C. The struggle within: Microbial influences on colorectal cancer. *Inflamm Bowel Dis* 2011;17(1):396–409.
9. Breban M. Gut microbiota and inflammatory joint diseases. *Joint, bone, spine: Revue du rhumatisme* 2016;83(6):645–649.
10. Doycheva I, Leise MD, Watt KD. The intestinal microbiome and the liver transplant recipient: What we know and what we need to know. *Transplantation* 2016;100(1):61–68.
11. Hsiao EY, McBride SW, Hsien S, Sharon G, Hyde ER, McCue T, Codelli JA et al. Microbiota modulate behavioral and physiological abnormalities associated with neurodevelopmental disorders. *Cell* 2013;155(7):1451–1463.

12. Jangi S, Gandhi R, Cox LM, Li N, von Glehn F, Yan R, Patel B, Mazzola MA, Liu S, Glanz BL et al. Alterations of the human gut microbiome in multiple sclerosis. *Nat Commun* 2016;7:12015.

13. Nallu A, Sharma S, Ramezani A, Muralidharan J, Raj D. Gut microbiome in chronic kidney disease: Challenges and opportunities. *Transl Res* 2017;179:24–37.

14. Qin J, Li Y, Cai Z, Li S, Zhu J, Zhang F, Liang S, Zhang W, Guan Y, Shen D et al. A metagenome-wide association study of gut microbiota in type 2 diabetes. *Nature* 2012;490(7418):55–60.

15. Qin N, Yang F, Li A, Prifti E, Chen Y, Shao L, Guo J, Le Chatelier E, Yao J, Wu L et al. Alterations of the human gut microbiome in liver cirrhosis. *Nature* 2014;513(7516):59–64.

16. Serrano-Villar S, Rojo D, Martinez-Martinez M, Deusch S, Vazquez-Castellanos JF, Sainz T, Vera M, Moreno S, Estrada V, Gosalbes MJ et al. HIV infection results in metabolic alterations in the gut microbiota different from those induced by other diseases. *Sci Rep* 2016;6:26192.

17. Stefka AT, Feehley T, Tripathi P, Qiu J, McCoy K, Mazmanian SK, Tjota MY, Seo GY, Cao S, Theriault BR et al. Commensal bacteria protect against food allergen sensitization. *Proc Natl Acad Sci USA* 2014;111(36):13145–13150.

18. Suhr MJ, Banjara N, Hallen-Adams HE. Sequence-based methods for detecting and evaluating the human gut mycobiome. *Lett Appl Microbiol* 2016;62(3):209–215.

19. Zilberman-Schapira G, Zmora N, Itav S, Bashiardes S, Elinav H, Elinav E. The gut microbiome in human immunodeficiency virus infection. *BMC Med* 2016;14(1):83.

20. Ghannoum M. Cooperative evolutionary strategy between the bacteriome and mycobiome. *MBio* 2016;7(6):e01951.

21. Huang YJ, Erb-Downward JR, Dickson RP, Curtis JL, Huffnagle GB, Han MK. Understanding the role of the microbiome in chronic obstructive pulmonary disease: Principles, challenges, and future directions. *Transl Res* 2017;179:71–83.

22. Schneeweiss J, Koch M, Umek W. The human urinary microbiome and how it relates to urogynecology. *International Urogynecology Journal* 2016;27(9):1307–1312.

23. Bull MJ, Plummer NT. Part 1. The human gut microbiome in health and disease. *Integrative Medicine (Encinitas, Calif)* 2014;13(6):17–22.

24. Eckburg PB, Bik EM, Bernstein CN, Purdom E, Dethlefsen L, Sargent M, Gill SR, Nelson KE, Relman DA. Diversity of the human intestinal microbial flora. *Science* 2005;308(5728):1635–1638.

25. Qin J, Li R, Raes J, Arumugam M, Burgdorf KS, Manichanh C, Nielsen T, Pons N, Levenez F, Yamada T et al. A human gut microbial gene catalogue established by metagenomic sequencing. *Nature* 2010;464(7285):59–65.

26. Levy M, Blacher E, Elinav E. Microbiome, metabolites and host immunity. *Curr Opin Microbiol* 2016;35:8–15.

27. Ghannoum MA, Jurevic RJ, Mukherjee PK, Cui F, Sikaroodi M, Naqvi A, Gillevet PM. Characterization of the oral fungal microbiome (Mycobiome) in healthy individuals. *PLoS Pathogens* 2010;6(1):e1000713.

28. Findley K, Oh J, Yang J, Conlan S, Deming C, Meyer JA, Schoenfeld D, Nomicos E, Park M, Kong HH et al. Topographic diversity of fungal and bacterial communities in human skin. *Nature* 2013;498(7454):367–370.

29. Jo JH, Deming C, Kennedy EA, Conlan S, Polley EC, Ng WL, Segre JA, Kong HH. Diverse human skin fungal communities in children converge in adulthood. *J Invest Dermatol* 2016;136(12):2356–2363.

30. Leung MH, Chan KC, Lee PK. Skin fungal community and its correlation with bacterial community of urban Chinese individuals. *Microbiome* 2016;4(1):46.

31. Brown RE, Ghannoum MA, Mukherjee PK, Gillevet PM, Sikaroodi M. Quorum-Sensing dysbiotic shifts in the HIV-Infected Oral Metabiome. *PLoS One* 2015;10(4):e0123880.

32. Ostaff MJ, Stange EF, Wehkamp J. Antimicrobial peptides and gut microbiota in homeostasis and pathology. *EMBO Mol Med* 2013;5(10):1465–1483.

33. Singh B, Qin N, Reid G. Microbiome regulation of autoimmune, gut and liver associated diseases. *Inflammation & Allergy Drug Targets* 2015;14(2):84–93.

34. Suhr MJ, Hallen-Adams HE. The human gut mycobiome: Pitfalls and potentials—A mycologist's perspective. *Mycologia* 2015;107(6):1057–1073.

35. Grice EA, Segre JA. The skin microbiome. *Nat Rev Microbiol* 2011;9(4):244–253.

36. Kong HH. Skin microbiome: Genomics-based insights into the diversity and role of skin microbes. *Trends Mol Med* 2011;17(6):320–328.

37. Gioti A, Nystedt B, Li W, Xu J, Andersson A, Averette AF, Munch K, Wang X, Kappauf C, Kingsbury JM et al. Genomic insights into the atopic eczema-associated skin commensal yeast Malassezia sympodialis. *MBio* 2013;4(1):e00572–00512.

38. Saunders CW, Scheynius A, Heitman J. Malassezia fungi are specialized to live on skin and associated with dandruff, eczema, and other skin diseases. *PLoS Pathog* 2012;8(6):e1002701.

39. Sanfilippo AM, Barrio V, Kulp-Shorten C, Callen JP. Common pediatric and adolescent skin conditions. *J Pediatr Adolesc Gynecol* 2003;16(5):269–283.

40. Guttman-Yassky E, Nograles KE, Krueger JG. Contrasting pathogenesis of atopic dermatitis and psoriasis—part I: Clinical and pathologic concepts. *J Allergy Clin Immunol* 2011;127(5):1110–1118.

41. Johnson MA, Armstrong AW. Clinical and histologic diagnostic guidelines for psoriasis: A critical review. *Clin Rev Allergy Immunol* 2013;44(2):166–172.

42. Pierard-Franchimont C, Xhauflaire-Uhoda E, Pierard GE. Revisiting dandruff. *Int J Cosmet Sci* 2006;28(5):311–318.

43. Jo JH, Jang HS, Ko HC, Kim MB, Oh CK, Kwon YW, Kwon KS. Pustular psoriasis and the Kobner phenomenon caused by allergic contact dermatitis from zinc pyrithione-containing shampoo. *Contact Dermatitis* 2005;52(3):142–144.

44. Park HK, Ha MH, Park SG, Kim MN, Kim BJ, Kim W. Characterization of the fungal microbiota (mycobiome) in healthy and dandruff-afflicted human scalps. *PLoS One* 2012;7(2):e32847.

45. Arron ST, Dimon MT, Li Z, Johnson ME, T AW, Feeney L, J GA, Lafyatis R, Whitfield ML. High Rhodotorula sequences in skin transcriptome of patients with diffuse systemic sclerosis. *J Invest Dermatol* 2014;134(8):2138–2145.

46. Jung WH, Croll D, Cho JH, Kim YR, Lee YW. Analysis of the nasal vestibule mycobiome in patients with allergic rhinitis. *Mycoses* 2015;58(3):167–172.

47. Shelburne SA, Ajami NJ, Chibucos MC, Beird HC, Tarrand J, Galloway-Pena J, Albert N, Chemaly RF, Ghantoji SS, Marsh L et al. Implementation of a pan-Genomic approach to investigate holobiont-Infecting microbe interaction: A case report of a leukemic patient with invasive mucormycosis. *PLoS One* 2015;10(11):e0139851.

48. Mukherjee PK, Chandra J, Retuerto M, Consolo M, Baron E, Nedorost ST, Cooper KD, Ghannoum MA, McCormick TS. Changes in skin bacteriome and mycobiome correlated with disease in psoriasis patients: A pilot study. In: *National Psoriasis Foundation National Volunteer Conference: July 24–26 2015*; San Francisco, CA: National Psoriasis Foundation; 2015.

49. Mukherjee PK, Chandra J, Hammond M, Retuerto M, Ghannoum MA, Nedorost ST. Disease–Specific changes in skin bacteriome and mycobiome in Atopic Dermatitis (AD) patients. In: *2015 Annual Meeting: May 6–9 2015*; Atlanta, GA: Society for Investigative Dermatology; 2015.

50. Hammond M, Chandra J, Retuerto M, Sherif RA, Ghannoum MA, Nedorost S, Mukherjee PK. Skin Microbiome in Atopic Dermatitis (AD): Interactions Between Bacteria (Staphyloccocus) and Fungi (Alternaria). In: *Society for Investigative Dermatology Meeting: 2016*; Phoenix, AZ; 2016.

51. Ott SJ, Kuhbacher T, Musfeldt M, Rosenstiel P, Hellmig S, Rehman A, Drews O, Weichert W, Timmis KN, Schreiber S. Fungi and inflammatory bowel diseases: Alterations of composition and diversity. *Scand J Gastroenterol* 2008, 43(7):831–841.

52. Ramaswamy K, Correa M, Koshy A. Non-healing gastric ulcer associated with *Candida* infection. *Indian J Med Microbiol* 2007;25(1):57–58.

53. Santelmann H, Howard JM. Yeast metabolic products, yeast antigens and yeasts as possible triggers for irritable bowel syndrome. *Eur J Gastroenterol Hepatol* 2005;17(1):21–26.

54. Krause R, Reisinger EC. *Candida* and antibiotic-associated diarrhoea. *Clin Microbiol Infect* 2005;11(1):1–2.

55. Stringer AM, Gibson RJ, Logan RM, Bowen JM, Yeoh AS, Hamilton J, Keefe DM: Gastrointestinal microflora and mucins may play a critical role in the development of 5-Fluorouracil-induced gastrointestinal mucositis. *Exp Biol Med (Maywood)* 2009;234(4):430–441.

56. Trojanowska D, Zwolinska-Wcislo M, Tokarczyk M, Kosowski K, Mach T, Budak A. The role of *Candida* in inflammatory bowel disease. Estimation of transmission of *C. albicans* fungi in gastrointestinal tract based on genetic affinity between strains. *Med Sci Monit* 2010;16(10):CR451–CR457.

57. Standaert-Vitse A, Sendid B, Joossens M, Francois N, Vandewalle-El Khoury P, Branche J et al. *Candida* albicans colonization and ASCA in familial Crohn's disease. *Am J Gastroenterol* 2009;104(7):1745–1753.

58. Jawhara S, Thuru X, Standaert-Vitse A, Jouault T, Mordon S, Sendid B, Desreumaux P, Poulain D. Colonization of mice by *Candida albicans* is promoted by chemically induced colitis and augments inflammatory responses through galectin-3. *J Infect Dis* 2008;197(7):972–980.

59. Iliev ID, Funari VA, Taylor KD, Nguyen Q, Reyes CN, Strom SP, Brown J, Becker CA, Fleshner PR, Dubinsky M et al. Interactions between commensal fungi and the C-Type lectin receptor dectin-1 influence colitis. *Science* 2012;336(6086):1314–1317.

60. Hoarau G, Mukherjee PK, Gower-Rousseau C, Hager C, Chandra J, Retuerto MA, Neut C, Vermeire S, Clemente J, Colombel JF et al. Bacteriome and mycobiome interactions underscore microbial dysbiosis in familial crohn's disease. *MBio* 2016;7(5).

61. Joossens M, Huys G, Cnockaert M, De Preter V, Verbeke K, Rutgeerts P, Vandamme P, Vermeire S. Dysbiosis of the faecal microbiota in patients with Crohn's disease and their unaffected relatives. *Gut* 2011;60(5):631–637.

62. Schloss PD, Iverson KD, Petrosino JF, Schloss SJ. The dynamics of a family's gut microbiota reveal variations on a theme. *Microbiome* 2014;2:25.

63. Whibley N, Jaycox JR, Reid D, Garg AV, Taylor JA, Clancy CJ, Nguyen MH, Biswas PS, McGeachy MJ, Brown GD et al. Delinking CARD9 and IL-17: CARD9 Protects against *Candida tropicalis* Infection through a TNF-alpha-dependent, IL-17-Independent mechanism. *J Immunol* 2015, 195(8):3781–3792.

64. Chen Y, Chen Z, Guo R, Chen N, Lu H, Huang S, Wang J, Li L. Correlation between gastrointestinal fungi and varying degrees of chronic hepatitis B virus infection. *Diagn Microbiol Infect Dis* 2011;70(4):492–498.

65. Morgan XC, Huttenhower C. Chapter 12: Human microbiome analysis. *PLoS Comput Biol* 2012;8(12):e1002808.

66. Brown KS, Ryder SD, Irving WL, Sim RB, Hickling TP. Mannan binding lectin and viral hepatitis. *Immunol Lett* 2007;108(1):34–44.

67. Knoke M. [Gastrointestinal microecology of humans and *Candida*]. *Mycoses* 1999;42 Suppl 1:30–34.

68. Thomas HC, Foster GR, Sumiya M, McIntosh D, Jack DL, Turner MW, Summerfiled JA. Mutation of gene of mannose-binding protein associated with chronic hepatitis B viral infection. *Lancet* 1996;348(9039):1417–1419.

69. Aas JA, Barbuto SM, Alpagot T, Olsen I, Dewhirst FE, Paster BJ. Subgingival plaque microbiota in HIV positive patients. *Journal of Clinical Periodontology* 2007;34(3):189–195.

70. Mukherjee PK, Chandra J, Retuerto M, Sikaroodi M, Brown RE, Jurevic R, Salata RA, Lederman MM, Gillevet PM, Ghannoum MA. Oral mycobiome analysis of HIV-infected patients: Identification of Pichia as an antagonist of opportunistic fungi. *PLoS Pathog* 2014;10(3):e1003996.

71. Gencosmanoglu R, Kurtkaya-Yapicier O, Tiftikci A, Avsar E, Tozun N, Oran ES. Mid-esophageal ulceration and candidiasis-associated distal esophagitis as two distinct clinical patterns of tetracycline or doxycycline-induced esophageal injury. *J Clin Gastroenterol* 2004;38(6):484–489.

72. Sano T, Ozaki K, Kodama Y, Matsuura T, Narama I. Antimicrobial agent, tetracycline, enhanced upper alimentary tract *Candida albicans* infection and its related mucosal proliferation in alloxan-induced diabetic rats. *Toxicol Pathol* 2012;40(7):1014–1019.

73. Wiesner SM, Jechorek RP, Garni RM, Bendel CM, Wells CL. Gastrointestinal colonization by *Candida albicans* mutant strains in antibiotic-treated mice. *Clin Diagn Lab Immunol* 2001;8(1):192–195.

74. Mellado E, Cuenca-Estrella M, Regadera J, Gonzalez M, Diaz-Guerra TM, Rodriguez-Tudela JL. Sustained gastrointestinal colonization and systemic dissemination by *Candida albicans*, *Candida tropicalis* and *Candida parapsilosis* in adult mice. *Diagn Microbiol Infect Dis* 2000;38(1):21–28.

75. DeMaria A, Buckley H, von Lichtenberg F. Gastrointestinal candidiasis in rats treated with antibiotics, cortisone, and azathioprine. *Infect Immun* 1976;13(6):1761–1770.

76. Helstrom PB, Balish E. Effect of oral tetracycline, the microbial flora, and the athymic state on gastrointestinal colonization and infection of BALB/c mice with *Candida albicans*. *Infect Immun* 1979;23(3):764–774.

77. Clark JD. Influence of antibiotics or certain intestinal bacteria on orally administered *Candida albicans* in germ-free and conventional mice. *Infect Immun* 1971;4(6):731–737.

78. Kraneveld EA, Buijs MJ, Bonder MJ, Visser M, Keijser BJ, Crielaard W, Zaura E. The relation between oral *Candida* load and bacterial microbiome profiles in Dutch older adults. *PLoS One* 2012, 7(8):e42770.

79. Navazesh M, Mulligan R, Pogoda J, Greenspan D, Alves M, Phelan J, Greenspan J, Slots J. The effect of HAART on salivary microbiota in the Women's Interagency HIV Study (WIHS). *Oral Surg Oral Med Oral Pathol Oral Radiol Endod* 2005;100(6):701–708.

80. Cruz MR, Graham CE, Gagliano BC, Lorenz MC, Garsin DA. Enterococcus faecalis *inhibits hyphal morphogenesis and virulence of Candida albicans*. *Infect Immun* 2012.

81. Workman SN, Been FE, Crawford SR, Lavoie MC. Bacteriocin-like inhibitory substances from *Campylobacter* spp. *Antonie Van Leeuwenhoek* 2008;93(4):435–436.

82. Faust K, Sathirapongsasuti JF, Izard J, Segata N, Gevers D, Raes J, Huttenhower C. Microbial co-occurrence relationships in the human microbiome. *PLoS Comput Biol* 2012;8(7):e1002606.

83. Sokol H, Leducq V, Aschard H, Pham HP, Jegou S, Landman C, Cohen D, Liguori G, Bourrier A, Nion-Larmurier I et al. Fungal microbiota dysbiosis in IBD. *Gut* 2017;66(6):1039–1048.

84. Frandsen EV, Pedrazzoli V, Kilian M. Ecology of viridans streptococci in the oral cavity and pharynx. *Oral Microbiol Immunol* 1991;6(3):129–133.

85. Diaz PI, Dupuy AK, Abusleme L, Reese B, Obergfell C, Choquette L, Dongari-Bagtzoglou A, Peterson DE, Terzi E, Strausbaugh LD.

Using high throughput sequencing to explore the biodiversity in oral bacterial communities. *Mol Oral Microbiol* 2012;27(3):182–201.

86. Lalla RV, Patton LL, Dongari-Bagtzoglou A. Oral candidiasis: Pathogenesis, clinical presentation, diagnosis and treatment strategies. *J Calif Dent Assoc* 2013;41(4):263–268.

87. Diaz PI, Xie Z, Sobue T, Thompson A, Biyikoglu B, Ricker A, Ikonomou L, Dongari-Bagtzoglou A: Synergistic interaction between Candida albicans and commensal oral streptococci in a novel in vitro mucosal model. *Infect Immun* 2012;80(2):620–632.

88. Xu H, Sobue T, Thompson A, Xie Z, Poon K, Ricker A, Cervantes J, Diaz PI, Dongari-Bagtzoglou A: Streptococcal co-infection augments Candida pathogenicity by amplifying the mucosal inflammatory response. *Cell Microbiol* 2014;16(2):214–231.

89. Diaz PI, Strausbaugh LD, Dongari-Bagtzoglou A: Fungal-bacterial interactions and their relevance to oral health: Linking the clinic and the bench. *Front Cell Infect Microbiol* 2014;4:101.

90. Johnston C, Hinds J, Smith A, van der Linden M, Van Eldere J, Mitchell TJ. Detection of large numbers of pneumococcal virulence genes in streptococci of the mitis group. *J Clin Microbiol* 2010;48(8):2762–2769.

91. Yokoyama T, Sasaki J, Matsumoto K, Koga C, Ito Y, Kaku Y, Tajiri M, Natori H, Hirokawa M. A necrotic lung ball caused by co-infection with Candida and Streptococcus pneumoniae. *Infec Drug Resist* 2011;4:221–224.

92. Denapaite D, Bruckner R, Hakenbeck R, Vollmer W. Biosynthesis of teichoic acids in Streptococcus pneumoniae and closely related species. lessons from genomes. *Microb Drug Resist* 2012;18(3):344–358.

93. Dollive S, Chen YY, Grunberg S, Bittinger K, Hoffmann C, Vandivier L, Cuff C, Lewis JD, Wu GD, Bushman FD. Fungi of the murine gut: Episodic variation and proliferation during antibiotic treatment. *PLoS One* 2013;8(8):e71806.

94. Jawhara S, Habib K, Maggiotto F, Pignede G, Vandekerckove P, Maes E, Dubuquoy L, Fontaine T, Guerardel Y, Poulain D. Modulation of intestinal inflammation by yeasts and cell wall extracts: Strain dependence and unexpected anti-inflammatory role of glucan fractions. *PLoS One* 2012;7(7):e40648.

95. Jawhara S, Poulain D. *Saccharomyces boulardii* decreases inflammation and intestinal colonization by *Candida albicans* in a mouse model of chemically-induced colitis. *Med Mycol* 2007;45(8):691–700.

96. Samonis G, Falagas ME, Lionakis S, Ntaoukakis M, Kofteridis DP, Ntalas I, Maraki S. *Saccharomyces boulardii* and *Candida albicans* experimental colonization of the murine gut. *Med Mycol* 2011;49(4):395–399.

97. Demirel G, Celik IH, Erdeve O, Saygan S, Dilmen U, Canpolat FE. Prophylactic *Saccharomyces boulardii* versus nystatin for the prevention of fungal colonization and invasive fungal infection in premature infants. *Eur J Pediatr* 2013;172(10):1321–1326.

Index

Note: Page numbers in italic and bold refer to figures and tables respectively.

Printed and bound by CPI Group (UK) Ltd, Croydon, CR0 4YY

24/10/2024

01778298-0017